FIFTH EDITION

Human Anatomy

COLOR ATLAS AND TEXTBOOK

J.A. GOSLING, MD, MB CHB, FRCS
Professor of Anatomy
Stanford University
USA

P.F. HARRIS MD, MB CHB, MSC
Emeritus Professor of Anatomy
University of Manchester
UK

J.R. HUMPHERSON MB CHB
Formerly Senior Lecturer in Anatomy
Faculty of Life Sciences
University of Manchester
UK

I. WHITMORE MD, MB BS, LRCP MRCS
Professor of Anatomy
Stanford University
USA

P.L.T. WILLAN MB CHB, FRCS
Formerly Professor of Anatomy
University of UAE
Al-Ain
United Arab Emirates

Photography by:
A.L. BENTLEY ABIPP, AIMBI, MBKS
Medical Photographer
Faculty of Life Sciences
University of Manchester
UK

Embalming and section cutting by:
J.T. DAVIES LIAS
Formerly Senior Anatomical Technician
Faculty of Life Sciences
University of Manchester
UK

Contributors to previous editions:
J.L. HARGREAVES BA(HONS)
Medical Photographer

MOSBY

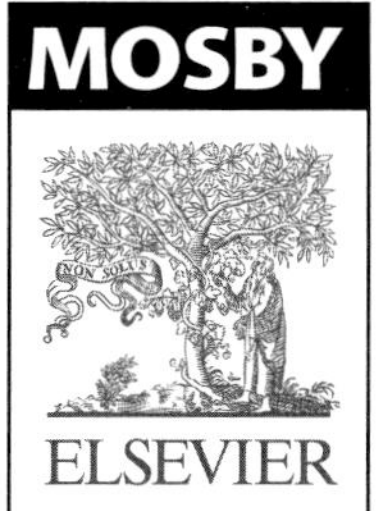

MOSBY
ELSEVIER
An imprint of Elsevier Limited

First edition 1985
Second edition 1990
Third edition 1996
Fourth edition 2002

ISBN: 978-0-7234-3451-1

British Library Cataloguing in Publication Data
A catalogue record for this book is available from the British Library

Library of Congress Cataloging in Publication Data
A catalog record for this book is available from the Library of Congress

Notice
Medical knowledge is constantly changing. Standard safety precautions must be followed, but as new research and clinical experience broaden our knowledge, changes in treatment and drug therapy may become necessary or appropriate. Readers are advised to check the most current product information provided by the manufacturer of each drug to be administered to verify the recommended dose, the method and duration of administration, and contraindications. It is the responsibility of the practitioner, relying on experience and knowledge of the patient, to determine dosages and the best treatment for each individual patient. Neither the Publisher nor the author assume any liability for any injury and/or damage to persons or property arising from this publication.

The Publisher

Printed in Spain
Last digit is the print number: 9 8 7 6 5 4 3 2 1

Preface to fifth edition

This edition maintains the unique combination of concise yet comprehensive text with images of dissections, each undertaken to illustrate features described in the text. Typically the illustrations and text are grouped together on the left and right sides of self-contained spreads, making for easy cross-reference.

In this fifth edition we have been driven by a desire to improve the contents and enhance their relevance as new courses evolve. The text has been refined by remedying omissions and removing ambiguities. In addition, all the diagrams accompanying the dissections have been checked and, where necessary, amended to improve clarity and accuracy. Several free-standing diagrams, including those illustrating dermatomes, have been redrawn. The introductory pages for the chapters on the abdomen and back have been expanded and improved.

In many institutions changing educational approaches have resulted in the phasing out of traditional topographical anatomy courses that included dissection. In their place have appeared integrated courses which incorporate imaging and clinical anatomical relevance. We have responded to this trend by enhancing the radiographic content; for example, in the observation skills pages for the upper and lower limbs scans are accompanied by corresponding cadaver sections. New chest radiographs appear in the thorax chapter and several radiographs have been replaced by higher quality images. New material describing clinical correlations has been integrated throughout the text and none of the anatomical content of the fourth edition has been deleted.

The terminology conforms to the internationally agreed *Terminologia Anatomica*. In addition this edition possesses a list of "alternative terms", including eponyms, which have been selected because they are used frequently. The larger font size for text introduced in the fourth edition has been retained and the font for figure labels changed.

J.A.G., P.F.H., J.R.H., I.W., P.L.T.W.,
2008

Acknowledgements for all editions
The authors are indebted to Dr Waqar Bhatti, Professors R.S. Harris and A.R. Moody and to the Department of Radiology at Manchester University for the provision of radiographs, CT and MR scans.

Our families deserve a special mention, as without their untiring support and patience these editions would certainly not have come to publication.

We thank them all.

Preface to first edition

Despite the many anatomical atlases and textbooks currently available, there appeared to be a need for a book which combined the advantages of each of these forms of presentation. This book was conceived with the intention of filling that need. With a unique combination of photographs of dissections, accompanying diagrams and concise text, this volume aims to provide the student with a better understanding of human anatomy.

The basis of this work is the cadaver as seen in the dissecting room; therefore, reference to surface and radiological anatomy is minimal. Likewise, comments on the clinical and functional significance of selected anatomical structures are brief. However, comparison is made where appropriate between the anatomy of the living and that of the cadaver.

Each dissection was specially prepared and photographed to display only a few important features. However, since photographs of dissections are inherently difficult to interpret, each is accompanied by a guide in the form of a drawing. Each drawing is coloured and labelled to highlight the salient features of the dissection and is accompanied by axes to indicate the orientation of the specimen. Adjacent photographs often depict different stages of the same dissection to help the student construct a three-dimensional image.

The first chapter introduces anatomical terminology, provides general information about the basic tissues of the body, and includes overall views of selected systems. Because the six subsequent chapters describe anatomy primarily through dissection, a regional approach has been employed. Features of bones are described only when considering their related structures, especially muscles and joints; osteology is not considered in its own right. The internal structure of the ear and eye are beyond the scope of this book since the study of these topics requires microscopy; the anatomy of the brain and spinal cord are also excluded as they are usually taught in special courses.

The level of detail contained in this book is appropriate for current courses in topographical anatomy for medical and dental undergraduates. In addition, it will be of value to postgraduates and to students entering those professions allied to medicine in which anatomy is part of the curriculum.

The terminology employed is that which is most frequently used in clinical practice. Where appropriate, alternatives (such as those recommended in *Nomina Anatomica*) are appended in brackets.

Preparation of the dissections and the text has occupied the authors for nearly five years. Our objective was to create a high quality and visually attractive anatomical work and we hope that the time and effort spent in its preparation is reflected in the finished product.

J.A.G., P.F.H., J.R.H., I.W., P.L.T.W.
Manchester, 1985

Contents

Human Anatomy User Guide

Organization

This book begins with a chapter on basic anatomical concepts. Then there are seven chapters, each with its own introduction, on the different regions of the body. Information is usually presented in dissection order, progressing from the surface to deeper structures. The limbs are described from proximal to distal with the joints considered last.

Texts and Photographs

Where possible the text and photographs are arranged on self-contained two-page spreads, so that the reader can locate relevant illustrations without turning a page. In these cases, the references in brackets appear as "(Fig.x.xx)". Additional cross-references to illustrations or text are given as "(see Fig. y.yy)" or "(see page z)" which direct the reader to a different spread.

Accompanying Diagrams

Adjacent to each photograph is a line diagram in which colour is used to focus attention on particular structures in the dissection. The colours conform to the following code:

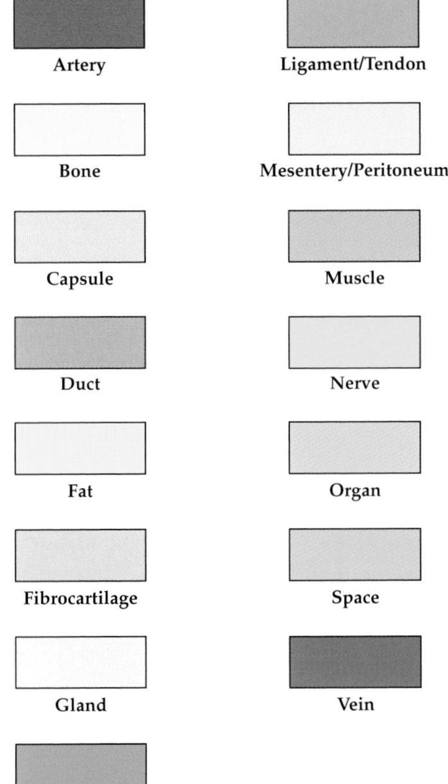

In diagrams showing muscle attachments on bone, the areas are shown using the muscle colour enclosed by different coloured lines. Similarly, in other diagrams coloured lines indicate the extent of a compartment or space.

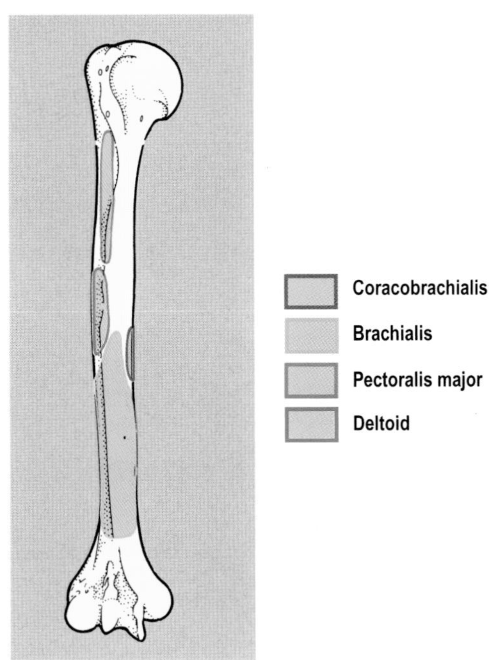

Labels and Leader Lines

The structures of particular interest in each diagram are labelled. A single structure is named in a label either with a single leader line or by a leader line which branches to show different parts of the same structure. However, if two or more structures are named, the first has the main leader line terminating on it while the subsequent structures are indicated by side branches given off at progressively shorter distances from the label. A leader line ending in an arrow indicates a space or cavity.

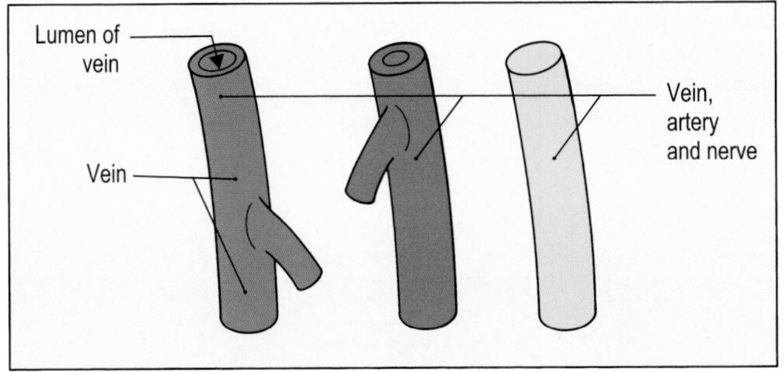

Orientation Guides

Next to the diagrams are orientation guides in which the following abbreviations are used:

L left	**P** posterior	**pr** proximal
R right	**A** anterior	**d** distal
S superior	**la** lateral	
I inferior	**m** medial	

Orientation guides in oblique views employ large and small arrow heads and long and short arrow shafts. Here are four examples:

from in front;

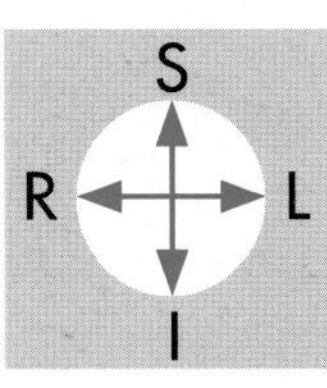

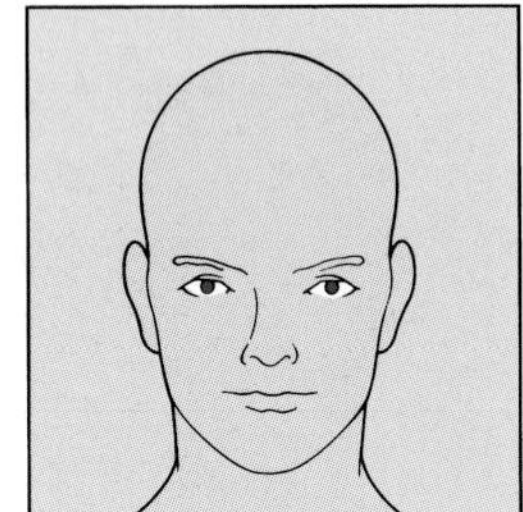

from behind;

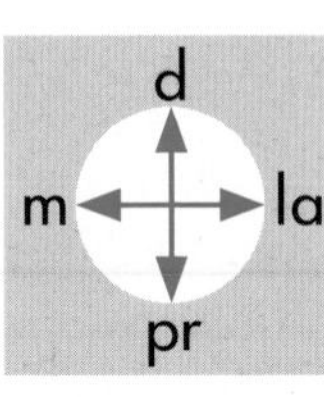

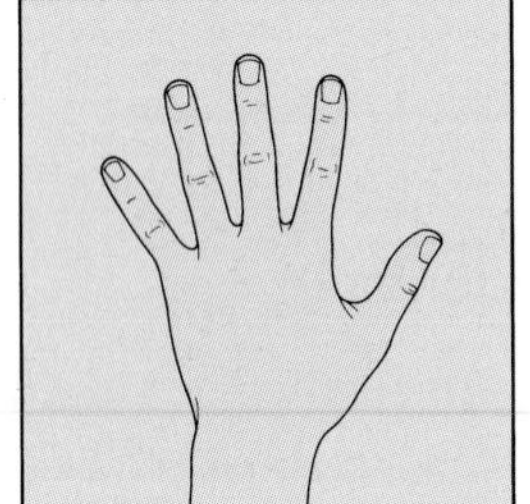

from the left side and slightly in front;

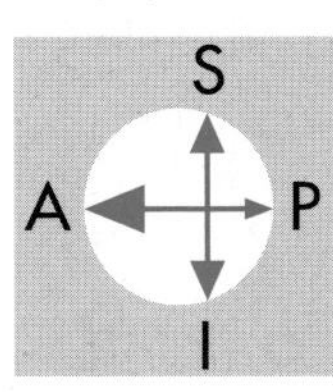

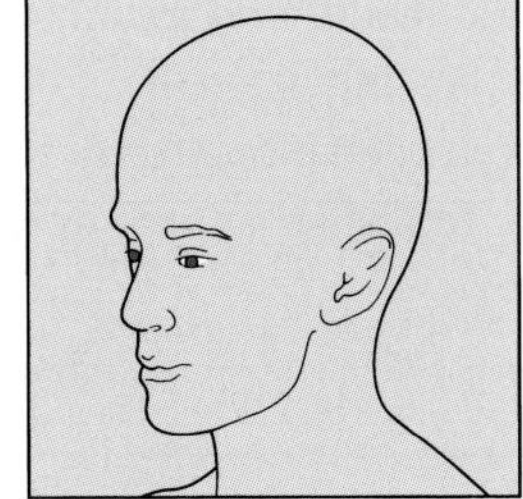

from the left side, slightly above and in front.

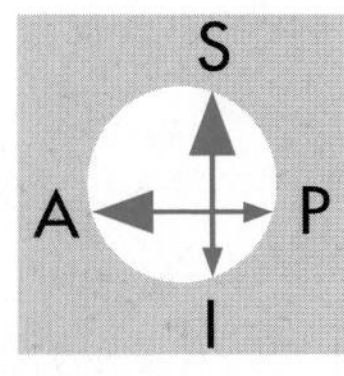

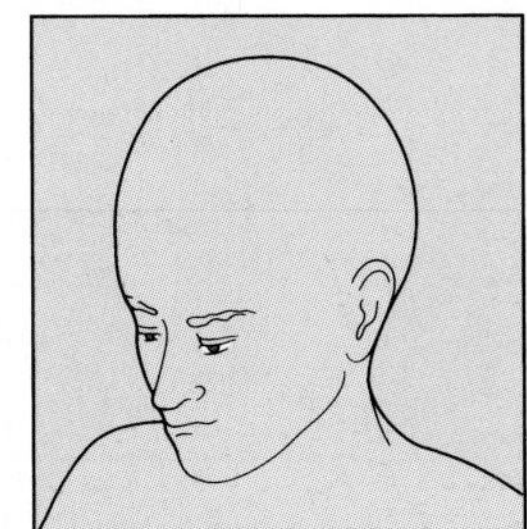

Terminology

The book conforms to *Terminologia Anatomica,* using the English terms. The list of alternative terms relates older non-official terms to their modern equivalent.

Self-assessment

The photographs in the main body of each chapter are unfettered by labels, leader lines or other superimposed markings; thus, readers can readily test their knowledge by either masking the whole of the accompanying diagram and studying the photograph alone, or covering only the labels.

Exams Skills, Clinical Skills & Observations Skills are provided after each chapter to allow readers to further self test themselves. Answers to Exam Skills and Clinical Skills are at the end of the book; those for Observation Skills are at the bottom of the same page as the picture.

Basic anatomical concepts

CHAPTER 1

Terms of Position and Movement

To avoid ambiguity and confusion, anatomical terms of position and movement are defined according to an internationally accepted convention. This convention defines the 'anatomical position' as one in which the human body stands erect with the feet together and the face, eyes and palms of the hands directed forwards (Fig. 1.1).

With the subject in the anatomical position, three sets of planes, mutually at right angles, can be defined.

Vertical (or longitudinal) planes are termed either coronal or sagittal. Coronal (or frontal) planes (Fig. 1.2) pass from one side to the other while sagittal planes (Fig. 1.3) pass from front to back.

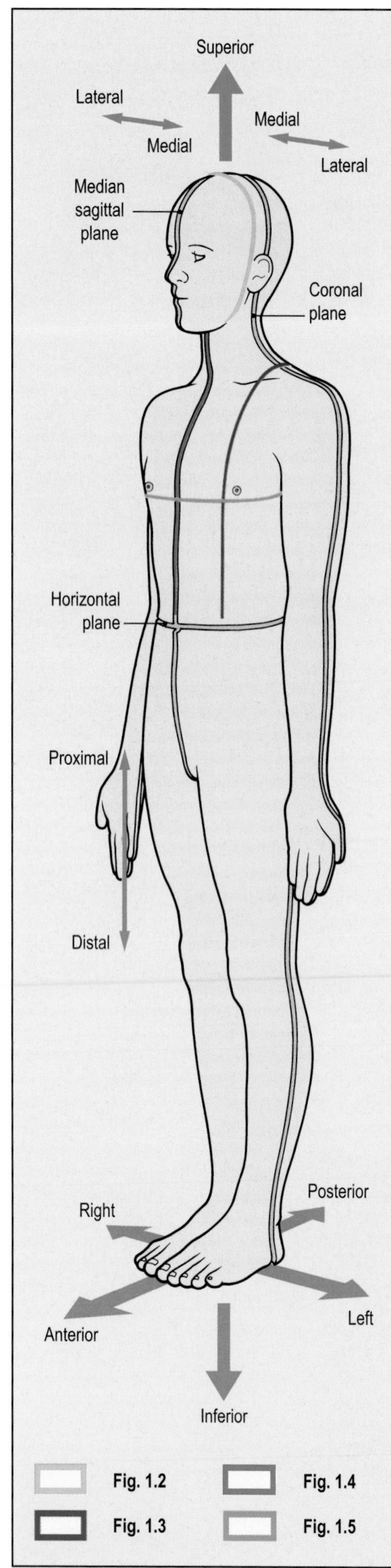

Fig. 1.1 Anatomical position and the terms used in anatomical description.

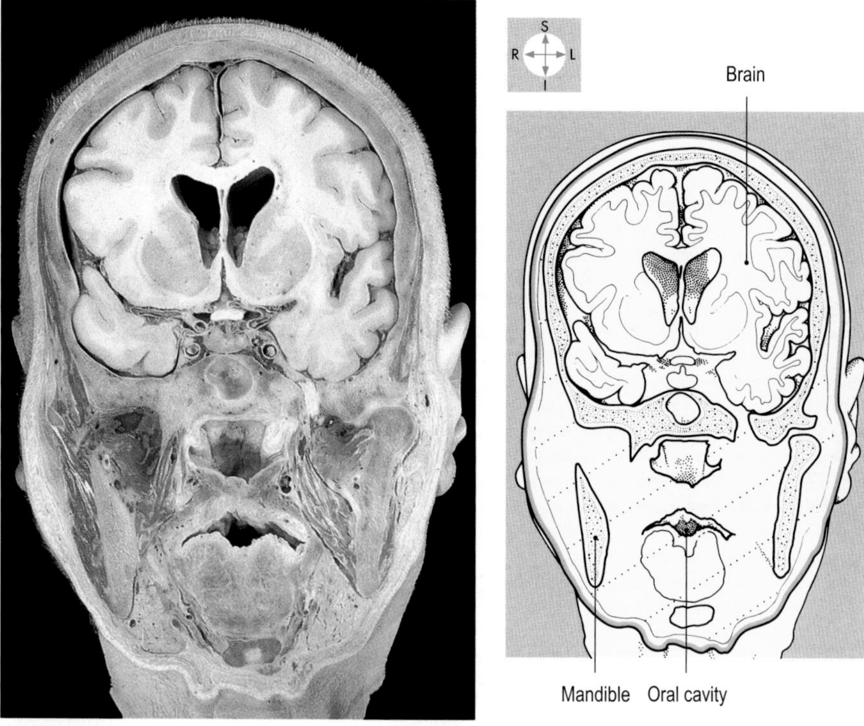

Fig. 1.2 Coronal section through the head.

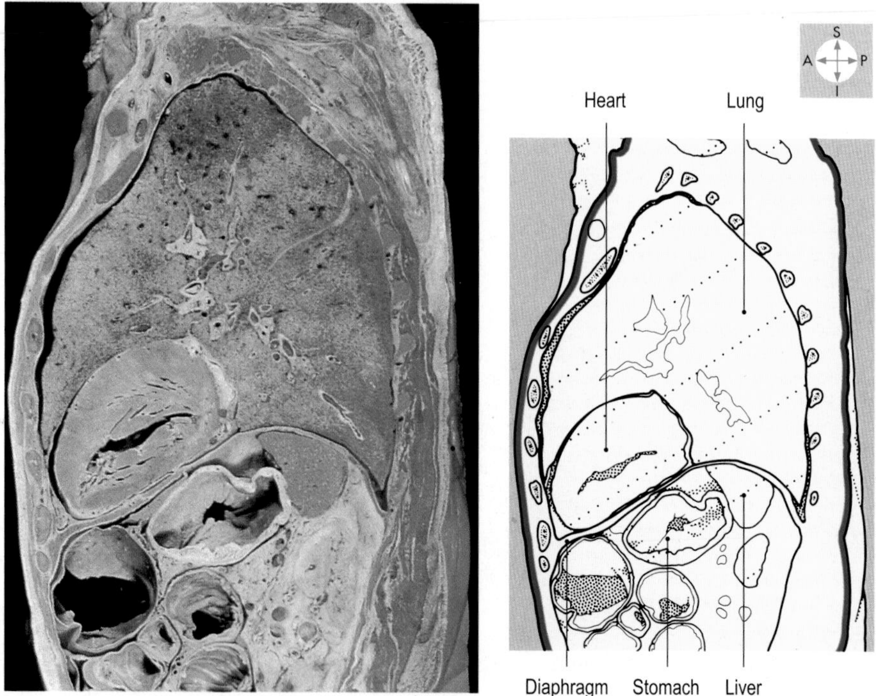

Fig. 1.3 Sagittal section through the trunk. This section lies to the left of the median sagittal plane.

One particular sagittal plane, the median sagittal plane, lies in the midline and divides the body into right and left halves (Fig. 1.4).

Horizontal (or transverse) planes (Fig. 1.5) transect the body from side to side and front to back.

Sections cut at right angles to the long axis of an organ or part of the body are also known as transverse. Similarly, longitudinal sections are cut parallel to the long axis.

The terms medial and lateral are used to indicate the position of structures relative to the median sagittal plane. For example, the ring finger lies lateral to the little finger but medial to the thumb. The front and back of the body are usually termed the anterior (or ventral) and posterior (or dorsal) surfaces respectively (Fig. 1.1). Thus one structure is described as anterior to another because it is placed further forwards.

Superior and inferior are terms used to indicate the relative head/foot positions of structures (Fig. 1.1). Those lying towards the head (or cranial) end of the body are described as superior to others which are inferior (or caudal). Thus the heart lies superior to the diaphragm; the diaphragm is inferior to the heart. In the limbs, the terms proximal and distal have comparable meanings. For example, the elbow joint is proximal to the wrist but distal to the shoulder.

The terms superficial and deep indicate the location of structures in relation to the body surface. Thus the ribs lie superficial to the lungs but deep to the skin of the chest wall (Fig. 1.5).

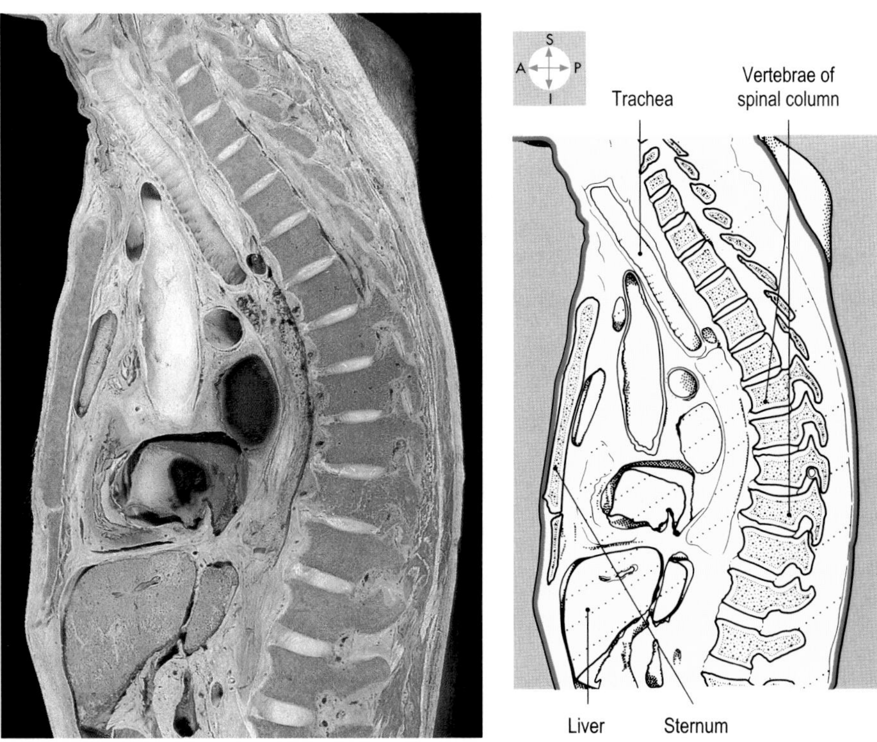

Fig. 1.4 Median sagittal section through the trunk.

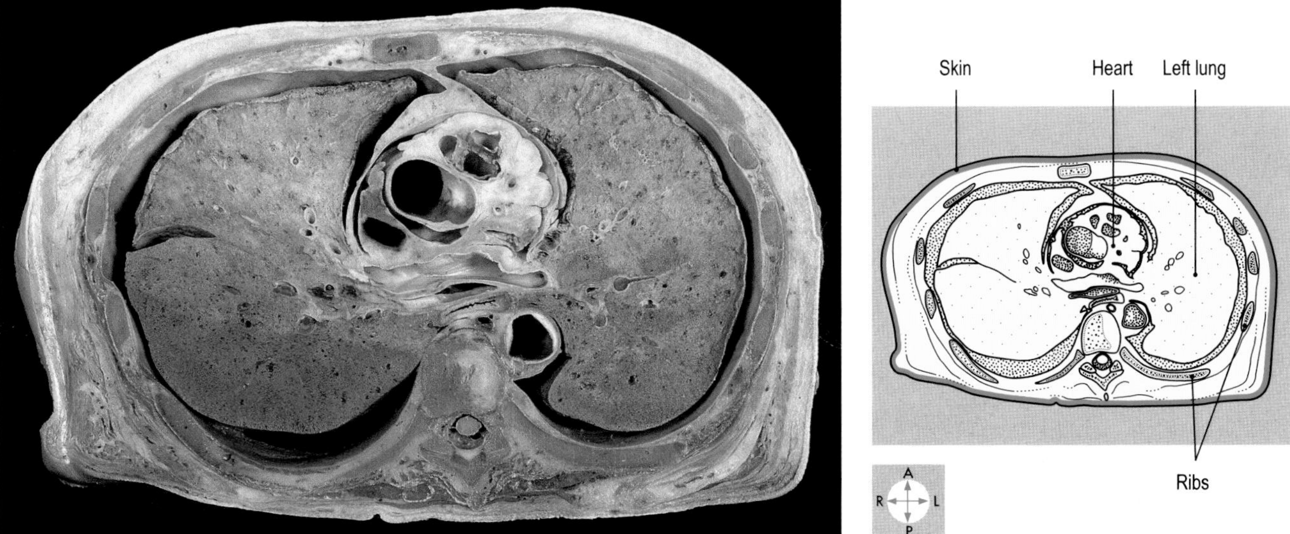

Fig. 1.5 Transverse section through the thorax at the level of the intervertebral disc between the sixth and seventh thoracic vertebrae. Inferior aspect. Compare Fig. 2.69.

Movements at joints are also described by specific terms. From the anatomical position, forward movement of one part in relation to the rest of the body is called flexion. Extension carries the same part posteriorly (Fig. 1.6). However, because in the fetus the developing upper and lower limbs rotate in different directions, the movements of flexion and extension in all joints from the knee downwards occur in opposite directions to the equivalent joints in the upper limb. In abduction, the structure moves away from the median sagittal plane in a lateral direction, whereas adduction moves it towards the midline (Fig. 1.7). For the fingers and toes, the terms abduction and adduction are used in reference to a longitudinal plane passing along the middle finger or the second toe respectively. Movement around the longitudinal axis of part of the body is called rotation. In medial (or internal) rotation the anterior surface of a limb rotates medially, whilst lateral (or external) rotation turns the anterior surface laterally (Fig. 1.8). Movements that combine flexion, extension, abduction, adduction and medial and lateral rotation (for instance, the 'windmilling' action seen at the shoulder joint) are known as circumduction.

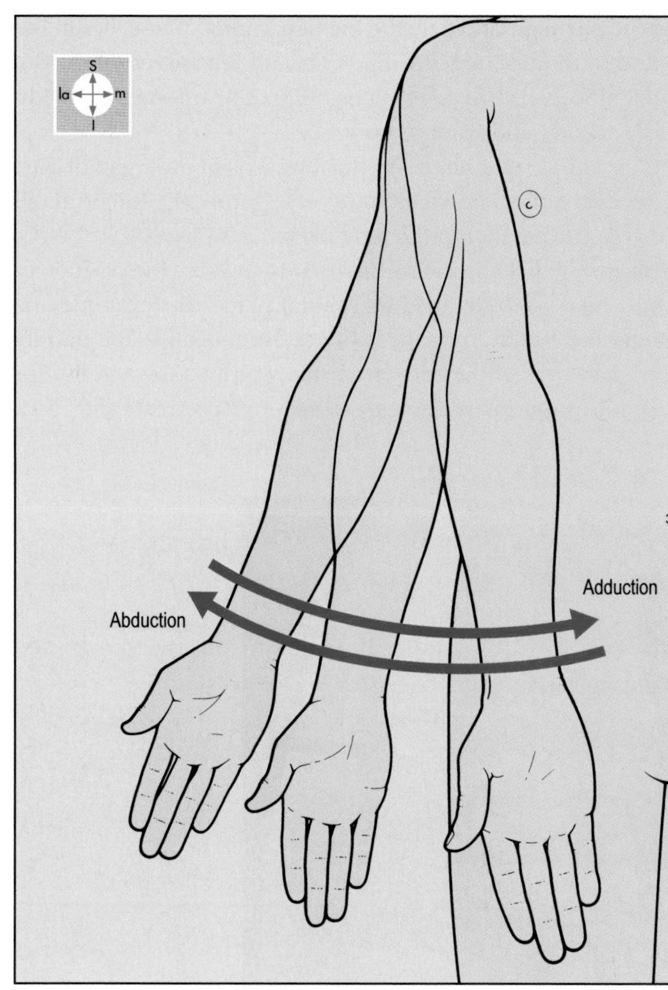

Fig. 1.7 Movements of abduction and adduction. In adduction, flexion of the shoulder joint allows the limb to be carried anterior to the trunk.

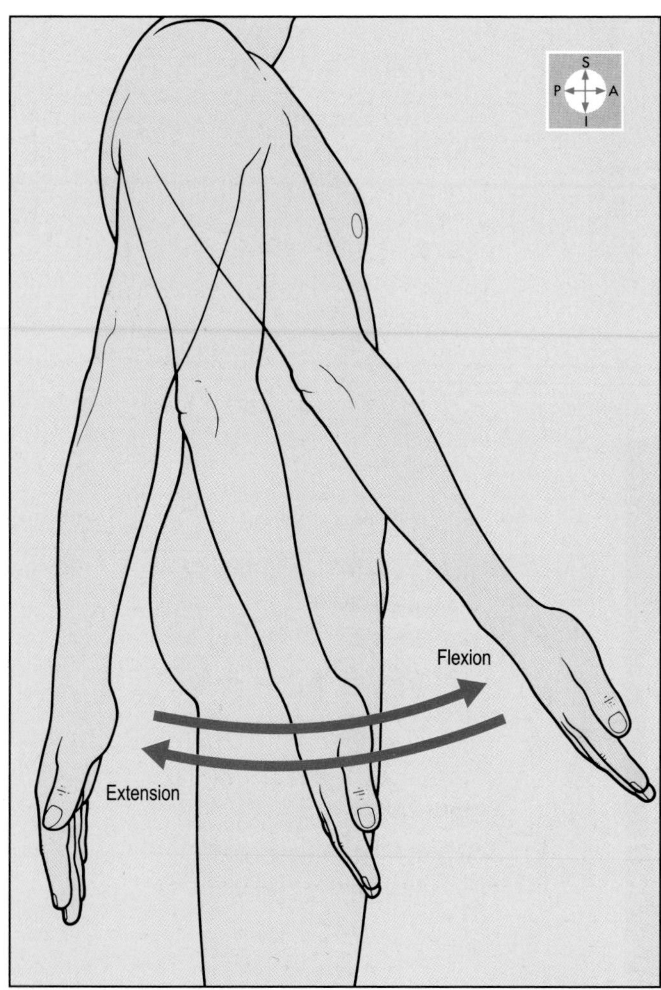

Fig. 1.6 Movements of flexion and extension of the shoulder joint.

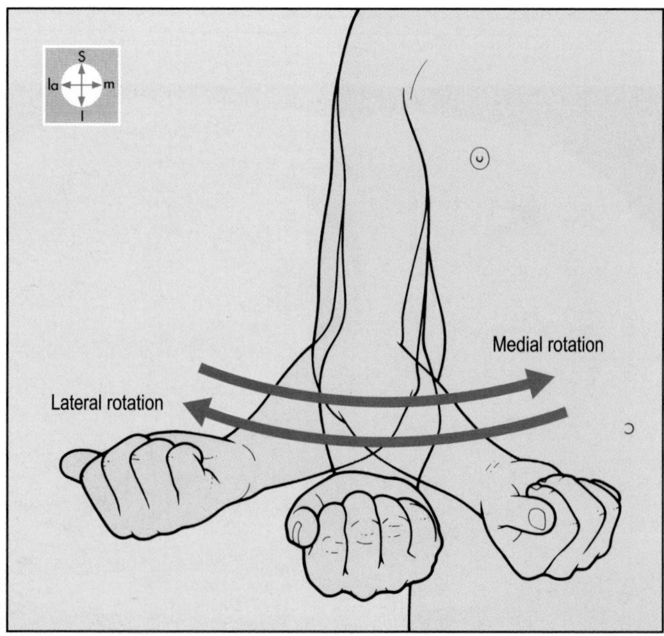

Fig. 1.8 Movement of the forearm indicates medial and lateral rotation at the shoulder joint. The elbow is flexed.

Basic Tissues and Structures

Skin

Skin (Fig. 1.9) is a protective covering for the surface of the body and comprises a superficial layer, called the epidermis, and a deeper layer, the dermis. The epidermis is an epithelium consisting of a surface layer of dead cells which are continually shed and replaced by cells from its deeper germinal layer. The dermis is a layer of connective tissue containing blood vessels, lymphatics and nerves. In most areas of the body the skin is thin and mobile over the underlying structures. Specializations of the skin include fingernails and toenails, hair follicles and sweat glands. On the palms of the hands and soles of the feet (and corresponding surfaces of the digits), hair follicles are absent and the epidermis is relatively thick. The skin in these regions is also firmly anchored to the underlying structures, reducing its mobility during gripping and standing. Lines of tension (Langer's lines) occur within skin and are of importance to surgeons. Scars following surgical incisions made along these lines tend to be narrower than those made across the lines of tension.

Skin is usually well vascularized and receives blood from numerous subcutaneous vessels. Knowledge of this vascular supply is important when operations that involve the use of skin flaps are undertaken. Skin has a rich nerve supply, responding to touch, pressure, heat, cold, vibration and pain. In certain areas, such as the fingertips, the skin is especially sensitive to touch and pressure. Skin is innervated by superficial (cutaneous) branches of spinal or cranial nerves. The area of skin supplied by each cranial or spinal nerve is known as a dermatome (see Figs 1.37 & 1.38).

Subcutaneous tissue (superficial fascia)

Immediately deep to the skin is a layer of loose connective tissue, the subcutaneous tissue (Fig. 1.9), which contains networks of superficial veins and lymphatics and is traversed by cutaneous nerves and arteries. It also contains fat, which varies considerably in thickness from region to region and between individuals. For example, over the buttock the fat is particularly thick whilst on the back of the hand it is relatively thin. Over the lower abdomen this tissue is subdivided into two layers, a superficial fatty layer and a deeper membranous layer.

Deep fascia

The deep fascia (Fig. 1.9) consists of a layer of dense connective tissue immediately beneath the subcutaneous tissue. Although thin over the thorax and abdomen, it forms a substantial layer in the limbs (for example, fascia lata; see p. 260) and neck (for example, investing fascia; see p. 322). Near the wrist and ankle joints the deep fascia is thickened to form retinacula, which maintain the tendons in position as they cross the joints. Deep fascia also provides attachment for muscles and gives anchorage to intermuscular septa, which separate the muscles into compartments. Bleeding and swelling within muscle compartments due to crushing injuries or fractures may raise the pressure so much that it compresses blood vessels and reduces blood flow. The resulting ischaemia may be followed by scarring and deformity with contracture of muscles.

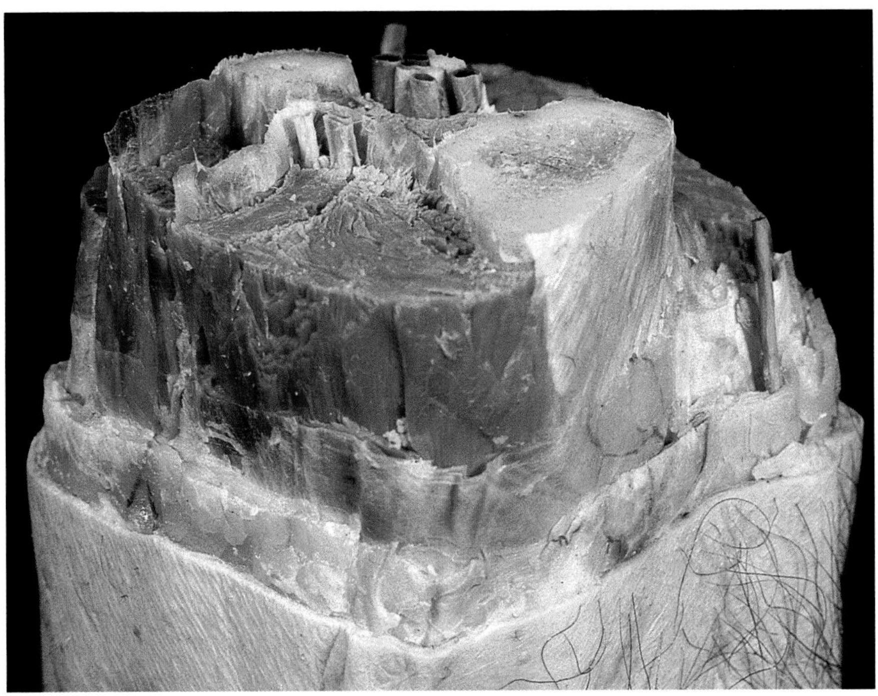

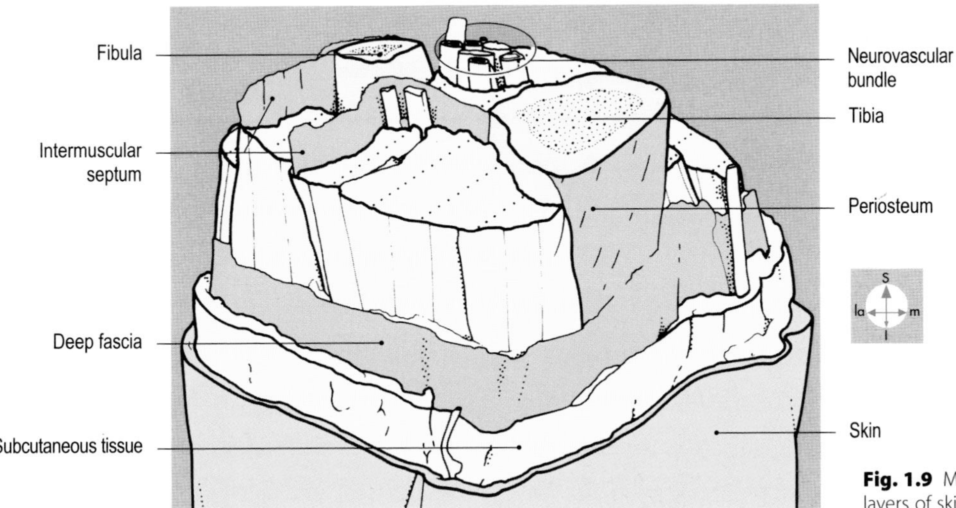

Fig. 1.9 Multilevel 'step' dissection through the right midcalf to show layers of skin, fascia and intermuscular septa.

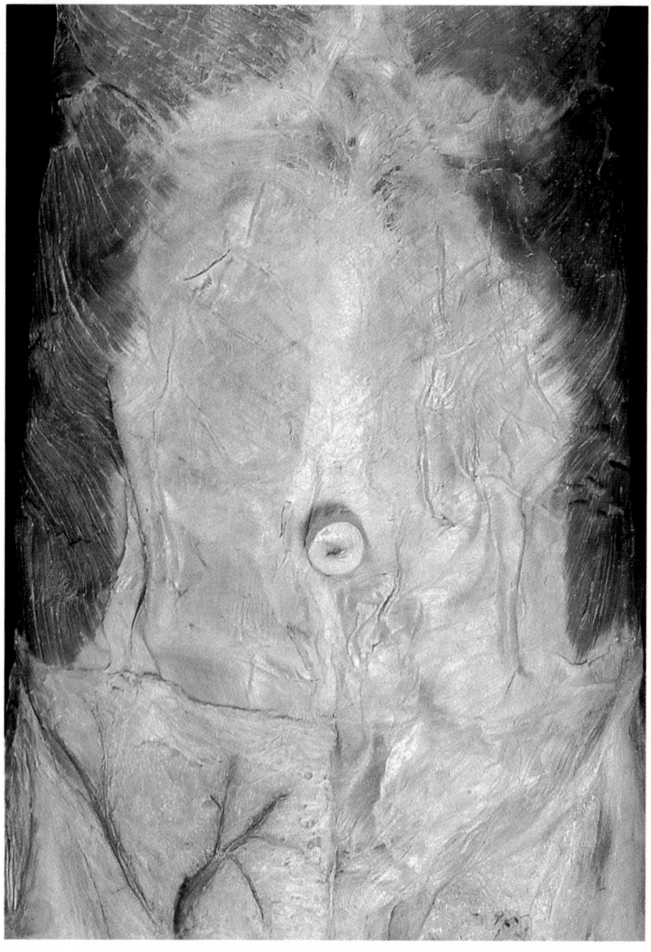

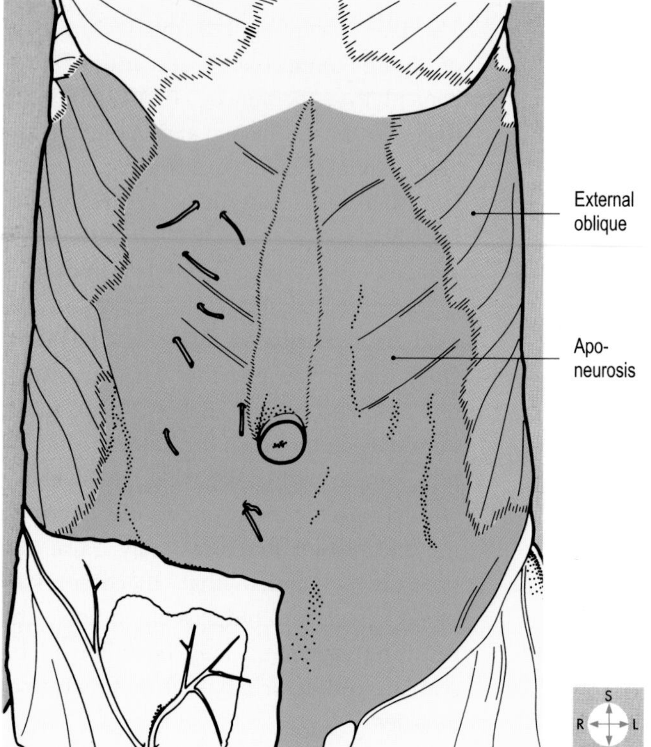

Fig. 1.10 External oblique is a flat muscle with an extensive aponeurosis.

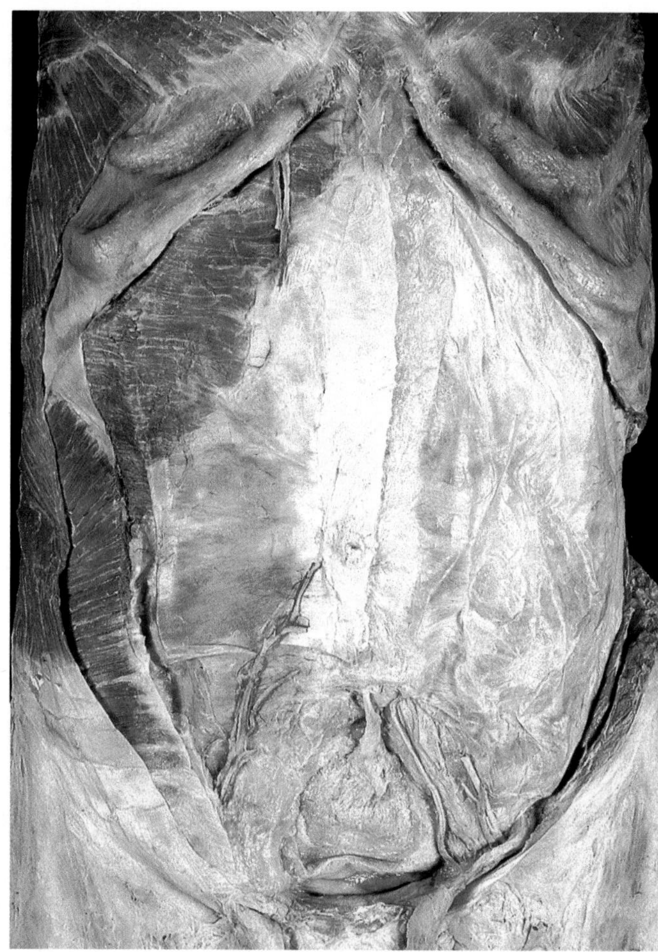

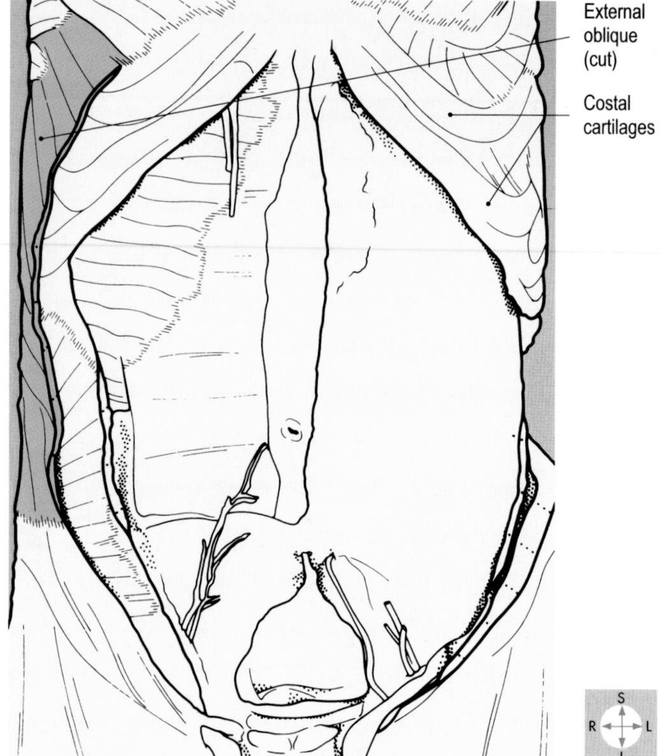

Fig. 1.11 External oblique cut to show its thickness.

Muscle

Muscle is a tissue in which active contraction either shortens its component cells or generates tension along their length. There are three basic types: smooth muscle; cardiac striated muscle; voluntary striated muscle. 'Striated' and 'smooth' describe the microscopic appearance of the muscle.

Smooth muscle is present in the organs of the alimentary, genitourinary and respiratory systems and in the walls of blood vessels. Capable of slow, sustained contraction, smooth muscle is usually controlled by the autonomic nervous system (see p. 22), and, in some organs, by endocrine secretions (hormones).

Cardiac striated muscle (myocardium) is confined to the wall of the heart and is able to contract spontaneously and rhythmically. Its cyclical activity is coordinated by the specialized conducting tissue of the heart and can be modified by the autonomic nervous system.

Skeletal muscle (voluntary striated muscle) is the basic component of those muscles that produce movements at joints. These actions are controlled by the somatic nervous system (see p. 20) and may be voluntary or reflex. Each muscle cell (fibre) has its own motor nerve ending, which initiates contraction of the fibre. Muscles may be attached to the periosteum of bones either directly or by fibrous connective tissue in the form of deep fascia, intermuscular septa or tendons. Direct fleshy attachment can be extensive but tendons are usually attached to small areas of bone. Muscles with similar actions tend to be grouped together, and in limbs these groups occur in compartments (for instance, extensor compartment of forearm).

Usually, each end of a muscle has an attachment to bone. The attachment that remains relatively fixed when the muscle performs its prime action is known as the origin whereas the insertion is the more mobile attachment. However, in some movements the origin moves more than the insertion; therefore, these terms are of only limited significance.

The muscle fibres within voluntary muscle are arranged in differing patterns which reflect the function of the muscle. Sometimes they are found as thin flat sheets (as in external oblique, Figs 1.10 & 1.11). Strap muscles (such as sartorius, Fig. 1.12) have long fibres that reach without interruption from one end of the muscle to the other.

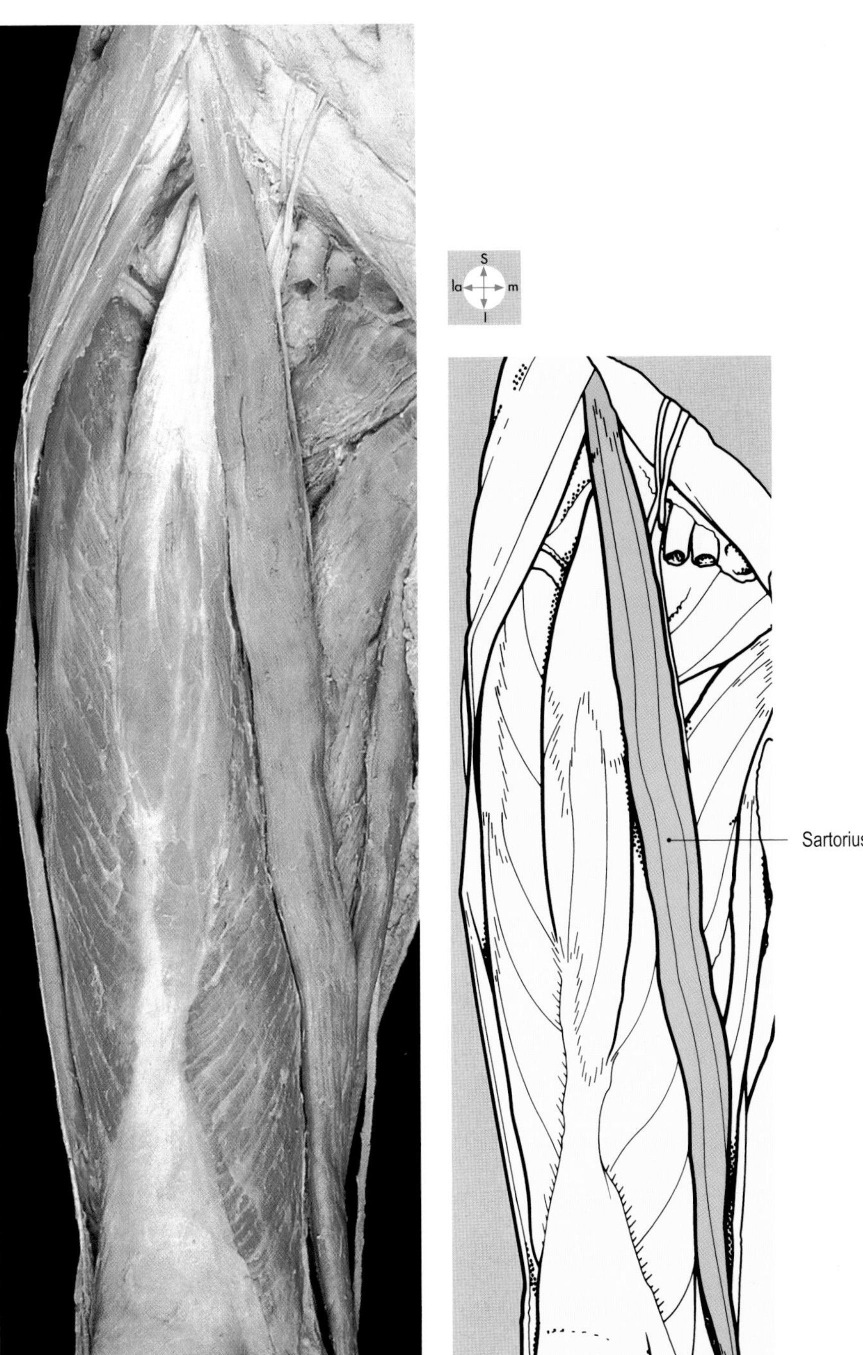

Fig. 1.12 Sartorius is a strap muscle.

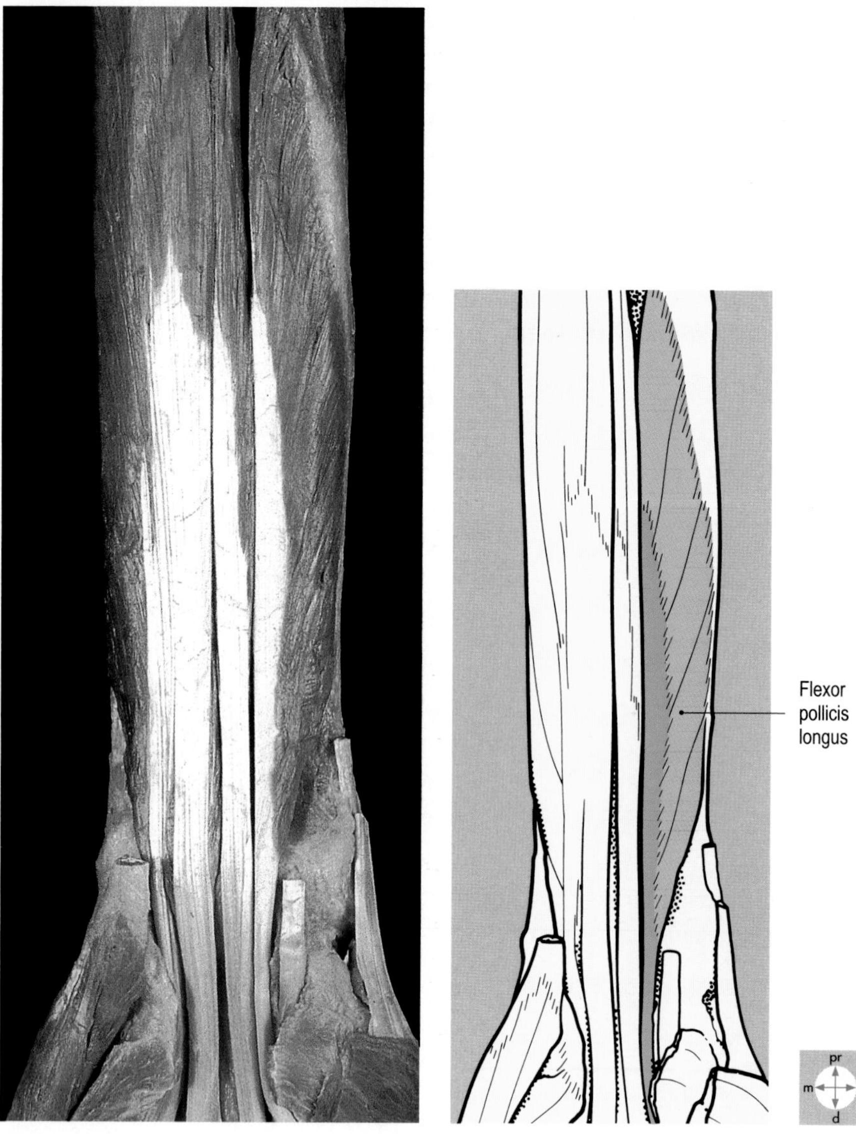

Fig. 1.13 Flexor pollicis longus is a unipennate muscle.

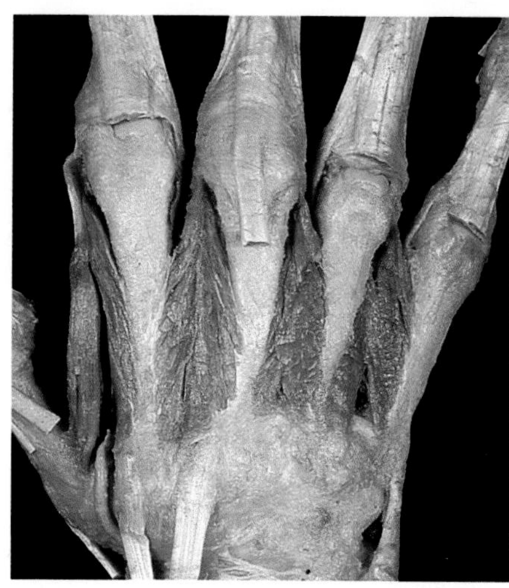

Fig. 1.14 Dorsal interossei are bipennate muscles.

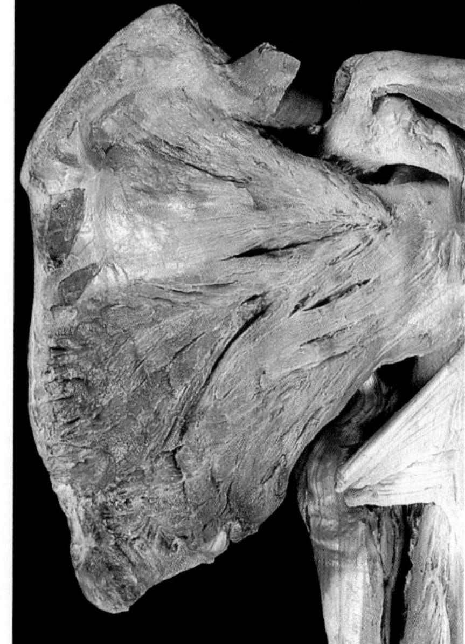

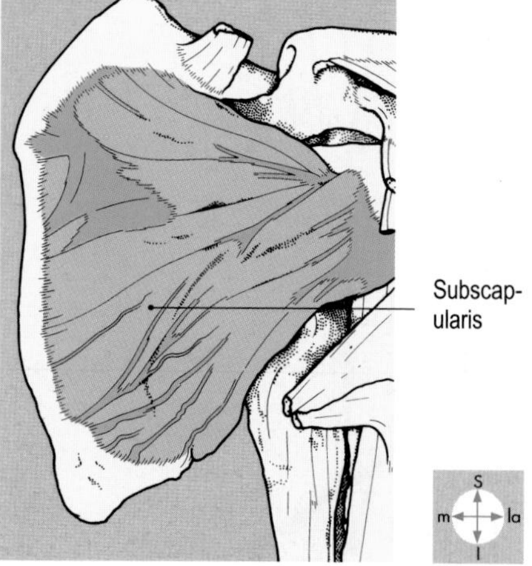

Fig. 1.15 Subscapularis is a multipennate muscle.

Pennate muscles are characterized by fibres that run obliquely. Unipennate muscles (for example flexor pollicis longus, Fig. 1.13) have fibres running from their origin to attach along only one side of the tendon of insertion. In bipennate muscles (such as dorsal interossei, Fig. 1.14) the fibres are anchored to both sides of the tendon of insertion.

Multipennate muscles (for example subscapularis, Fig. 1.15) have several tendons of origin and insertion with muscle fibres passing obliquely between them. Some muscles, for instance digastric, have two fleshy parts (bellies) connected by an intermediate tendon.

Most tendons are thick and round or flattened in cross-section, although some form thin sheets called aponeuroses (see Fig. 1.10). When tendons cross projections or traverse confined spaces they are often enveloped in a double layer of synovial membrane to minimize friction. Where they cross joints, tendons are often held in place by bands of thick fibrous tissue, which prevent 'bowstringing' when the joints are moved. Examples include the retinacula at the wrist and ankle joints, and tendon sheaths in the fingers and toes (Figs 1.16 & 1.17).

The nerve supply to a skeletal muscle contains both motor and sensory fibres, which usually enter the fleshy part of the muscle. Groups of muscles with similar actions tend to be supplied by nerve fibres derived from the same spinal cord segments.

As very metabolically active tissue, muscle has a rich arterial blood supply, usually carried by several separate vessels. The contraction and relaxation of muscles in the limbs compresses the veins in each compartment. As the veins contain unidirectional valves, this 'muscle pump' action assists the return of venous blood from the limbs to the trunk.

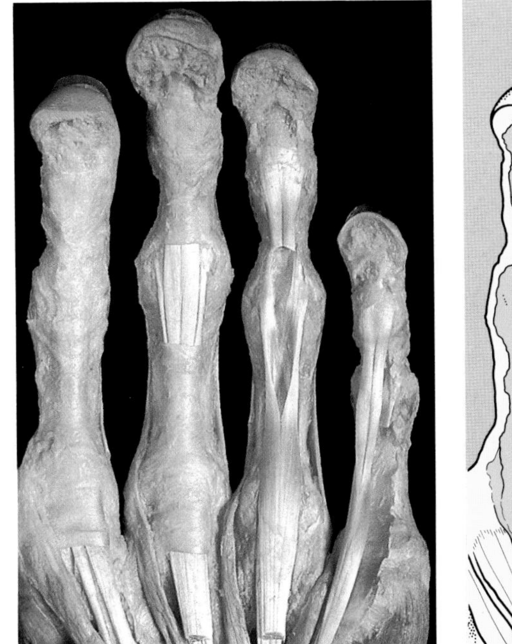

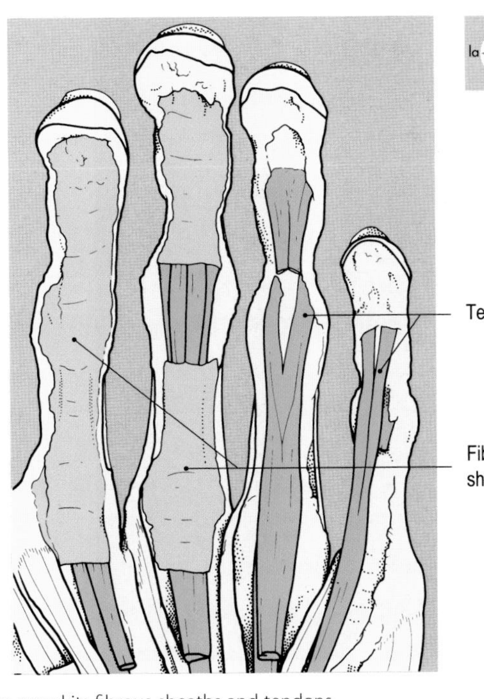

Fig. 1.16 Anterior view of the left hand, dissected to reveal its fibrous sheaths and tendons.

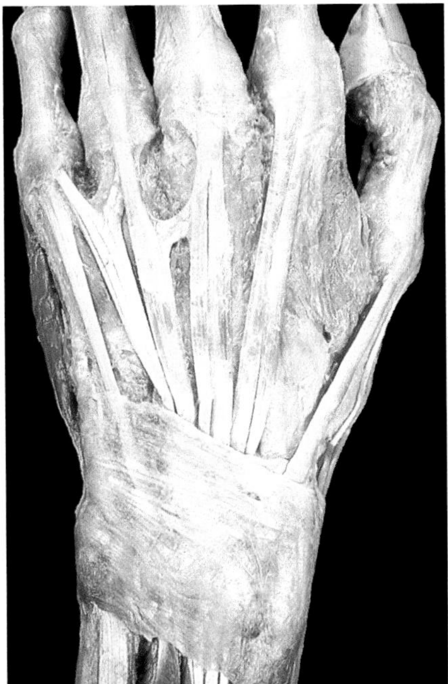

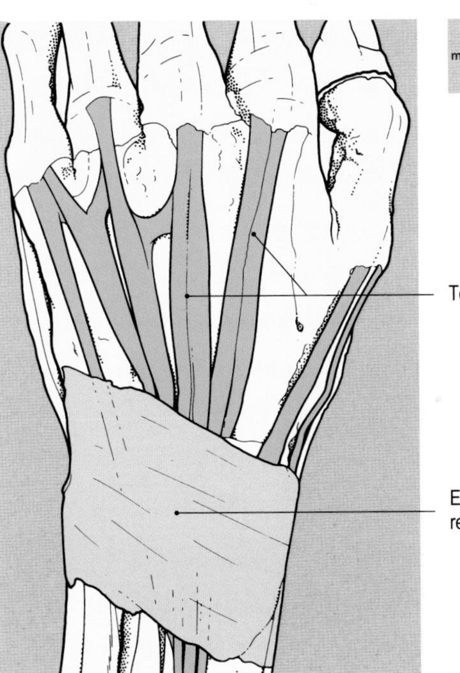

Fig. 1.17 Posterior view of the left hand, dissected to show the extensor retinaculum at the wrist.

Cartilage

Cartilage is a variety of hard connective tissue which gains its nutrition by diffusion from blood vessels in the surrounding tissues. It is classified by its histological structure into hyaline cartilage, fibrocartilage and elastic cartilage.

Hyaline cartilage occurs in costal cartilages (see Fig. 1.11), the cartilages of the larynx and trachea, and in developing bones. In synovial joints (see Fig. 1.23) it forms the glassy, smooth articular surfaces which reduce friction during movement. Articular cartilage is partly nourished by diffusion from the synovial fluid in the joint cavity.

The inclusion of tough inelastic collagen fibres in the matrix constitutes fibrocartilage, which is stronger and more flexible than the hyaline type. Fibrocartilage is found in intervertebral discs (see Fig. 1.22), the pubic symphysis, the manubriosternal joint, and as articular discs in some synovial joints (for example, knee and temporomandibular).

Elastic cartilage, which occurs in the external ear and epiglottis, is the most flexible form of cartilage. It contains predominantly elastic fibres and has a yellowish appearance.

Cartilage may become calcified in old age, becoming harder and more rigid.

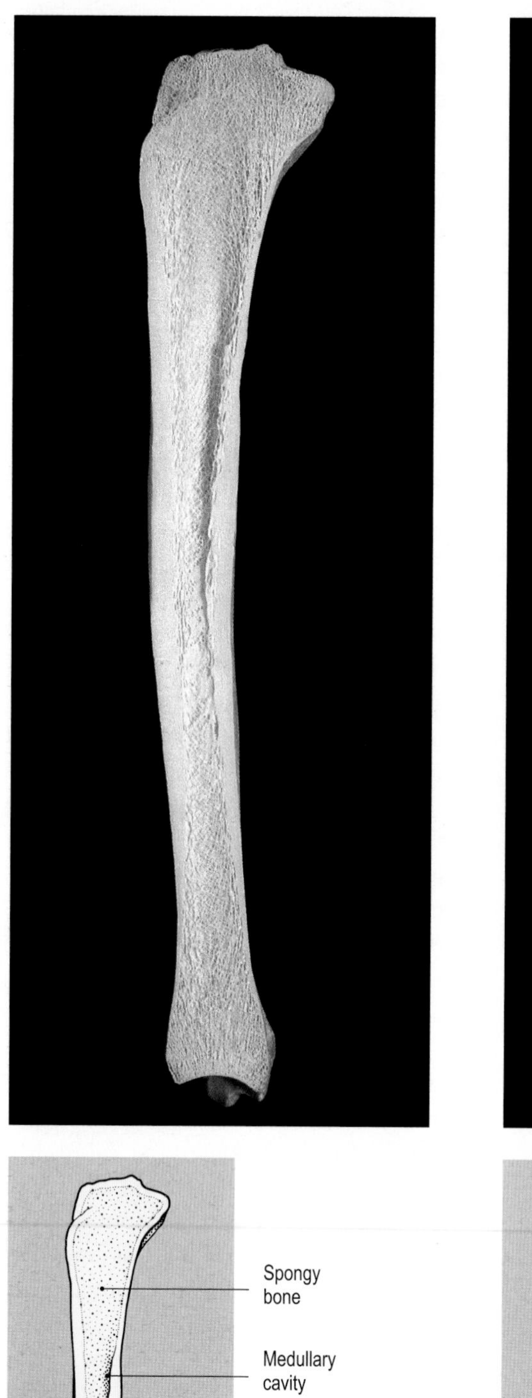

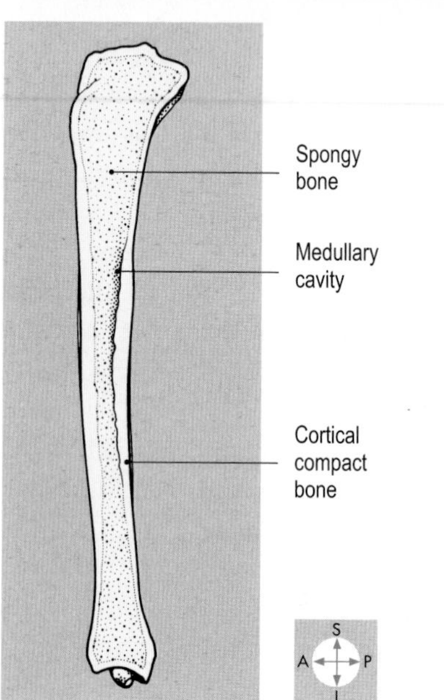

Fig. 1.18 Longitudinal section of an adult tibia.

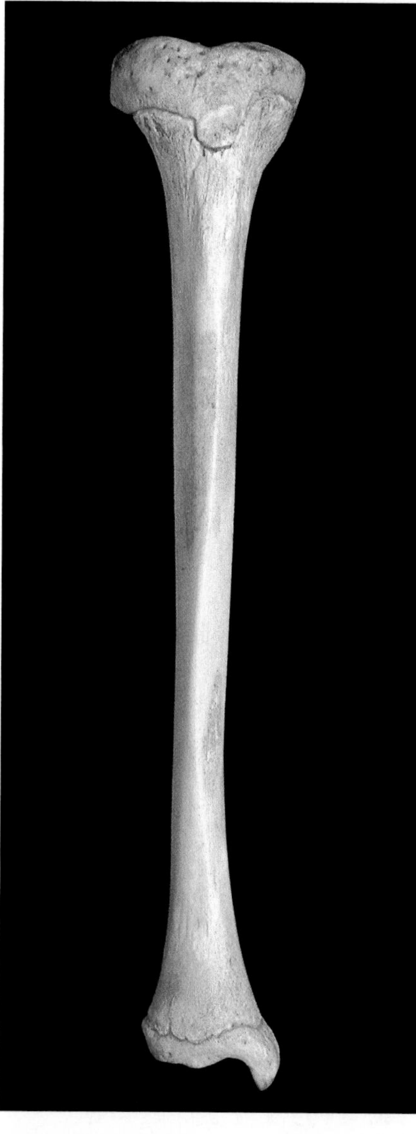

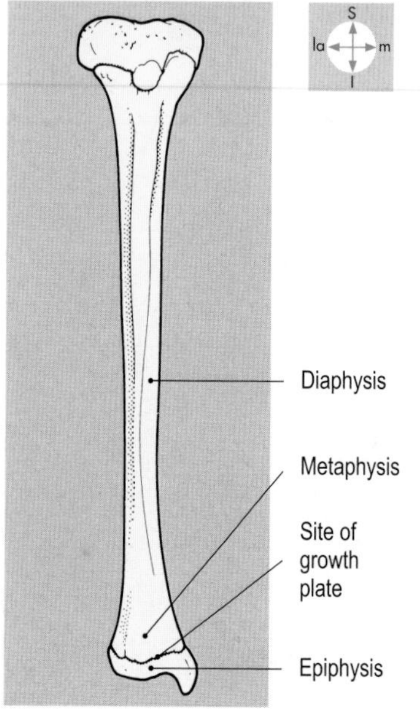

Fig. 1.19 Anterior view of a child's tibia.

Bone

Bone forms the basis of the skeleton and is characterized by a hard, calcified matrix which gives rigidity. In most bones two zones are visible. Near the surface the outer cortical layer of bone appears solid and is called compact bone, whereas centrally the bone is known as spongy (cancellous) bone. Many bones contain a cavity (medulla) occupied by the bone marrow, a potential site of blood cell production (Fig. 1.18).

The numerous bones comprising the human skeleton vary considerably in shape and size, and are classified into long bones (for example, femur), short bones (bones of the carpus), flat bones (parietal bone of skull), irregular bones (maxilla of skull) and sesamoid bones (patella). Sesamoid bones develop in tendons, generally where the tendon passes over a joint or bony projection. Some bones are described as pneumatized because of their air-filled cavities (for instance, ethmoid).

Bone is enveloped by a thin layer of fibrous tissue called periosteum (see Fig. 1.9) which provides anchorage for muscles, tendons and ligaments. Periosteum is a source of cells for bone growth and repair and is richly innervated and exquisitely sensitive to pain.

Bone has a profuse blood supply which is provided partly via the periosteal vessels and partly by nutrient arteries, which enter bones via nutrient foramina and also supply the marrow. Fractured bones often bleed profusely from damaged medullary and periosteal vessels.

Several names are given to the different parts of a long bone in relation to its development (Fig. 1.19). The shaft (or diaphysis) ossifies first and is separated by growth plates from the secondary centres of ossification (or epiphyses) which usually lie at the extremities of the bone. The part of a diaphysis next to a growth plate is called a metaphysis and has a particularly rich blood supply. When increase in bone length ceases, the growth plates disappear and the epiphyses fuse with the diaphysis.

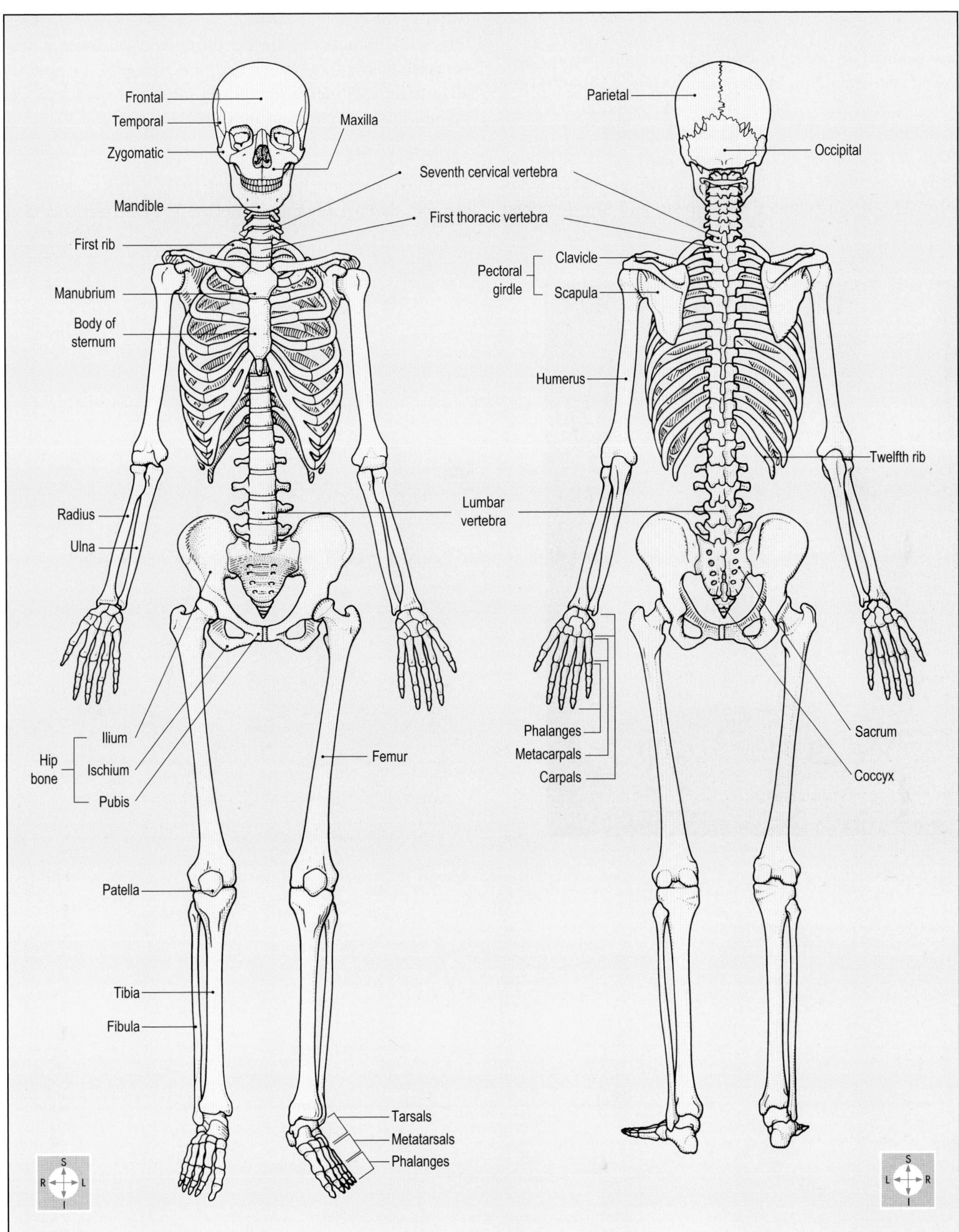

Fig. 1.20 Anterior and posterior views of the skeleton.

Skeleton

The skeleton (Fig. 1.20) is composed of bones and cartilages held together by joints, and gives rigidity and support to the body. It has axial and appendicular components. The axial component includes the skull, vertebral column, ribs, costal cartilages and sternum. The appendicular skeleton comprises the bones of the upper and lower limbs and their associated girdles. In this book, individual bones are described in the appropriate regions.

Joints

Joints are classified according to their structure into fibrous, cartilaginous and synovial types. In fibrous joints (Fig. 1.21) which are relatively immobile, the two bones are joined by fibrous tissue (for example, sutures seen between the bones of the skull).

Cartilage is interposed between bone ends in cartilaginous joints. Primary cartilaginous joints contain hyaline cartilage, are usually capable of only limited movement, and are described between the ribs and sternum. In secondary cartilaginous joints (Fig. 1.22), fibrocartilage unites the bone ends. These joints, which generally allow more movement than those of the primary type, all lie in the midline. Examples include the intervertebral discs, the manubriosternal joint and the pubic symphysis.

Synovial joints

The most common type of joint is the synovial joint, which is complex and usually highly mobile. They are classified according

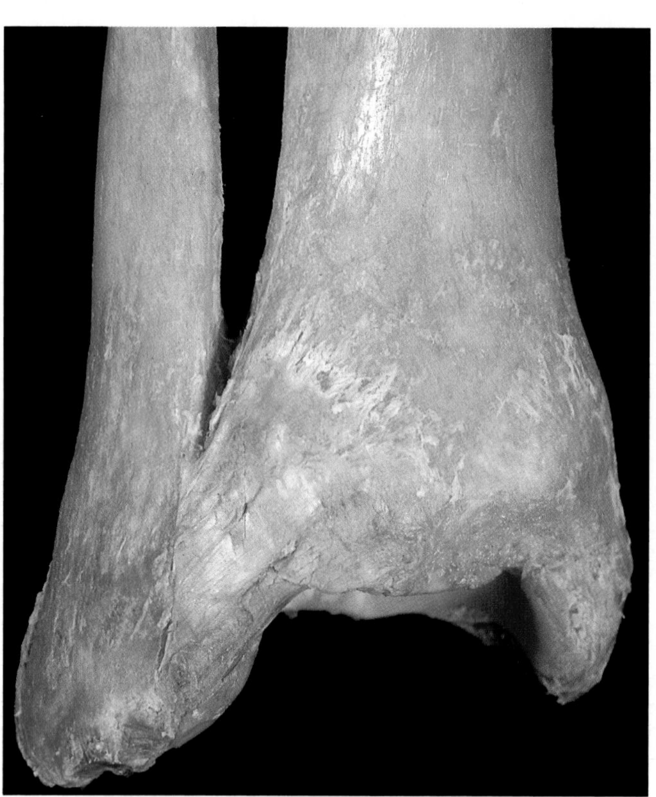

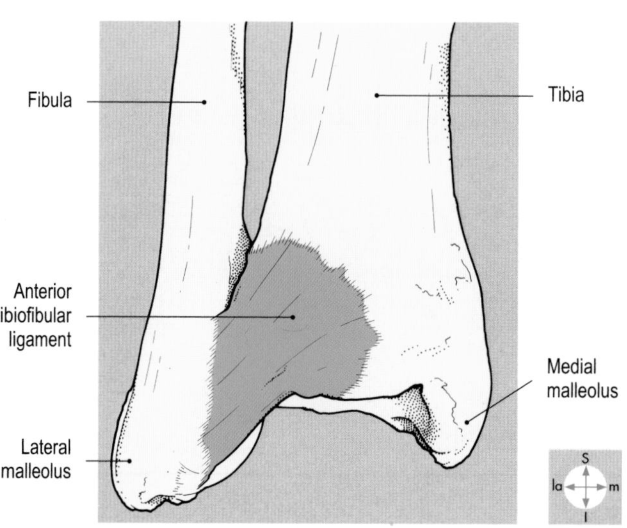

Fig. 1.21 The inferior tibiofibular joint is an example of a fibrous joint.

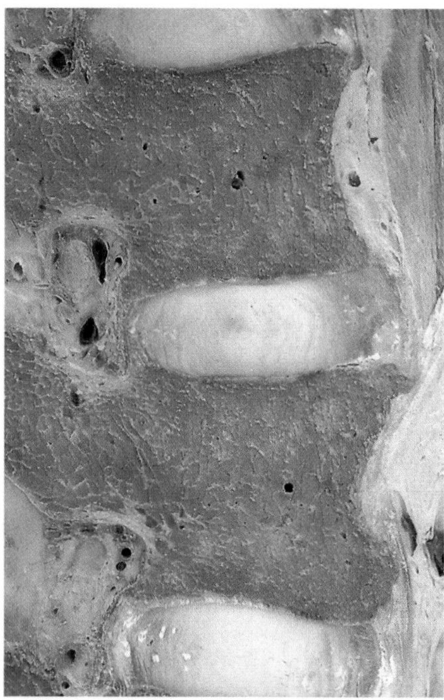

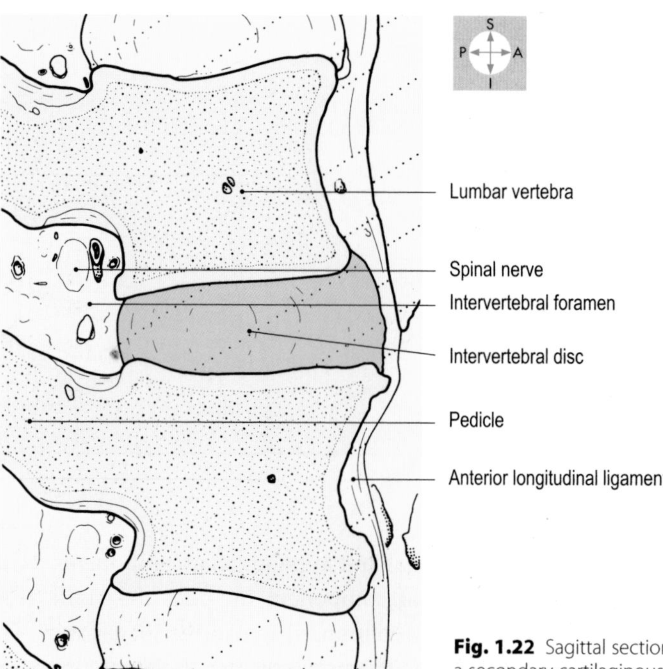

Fig. 1.22 Sagittal section to show an intervertebral disc, a secondary cartilaginous joint.

to the shape of the joint surfaces (such as plane, saddle, ball-and-socket) or by the type of movement they permit (such as sliding, pivot, hinge). In a typical synovial joint (Fig. 1.23) the articulating surfaces are coated with hyaline cartilage and the bones are joined by a fibrous capsule, a tubular sleeve which is attached around the periphery of the areas of articular cartilage. In every synovial joint, all of the interior (except for intra-articular cartilage) is lined with synovial membrane. This thin vascular membrane secretes synovial fluid into the joint space, providing nutrition for the cartilage and lubrication for the joint.

The capsule is usually thickened to form strengthening bands known as capsular ligaments (for example, the pubofemoral ligament). In addition, fibrous bands, discrete from the capsule, may form extracapsular ligaments (such as the costoclavicular ligament). In some joints there are intracapsular ligaments (for instance, the ligament of the head of the femur) which are covered by synovial membrane. Tendons sometimes fuse with the capsule (as in the rotator cuff) or they may run within the joint, covered by synovial membrane, before gaining their bony attachment (for example, biceps brachii at the shoulder joint; Fig. 1.24).

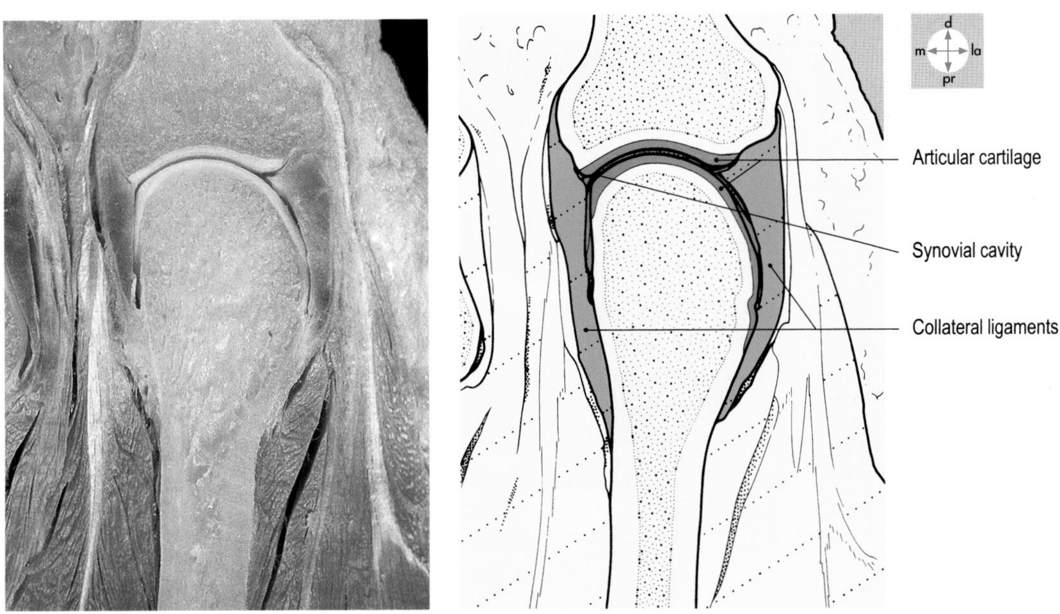

Fig. 1.23 Coronal section through a metacarpophalangeal joint, a synovial joint. The collateral ligaments are thickenings of the joint capsule.

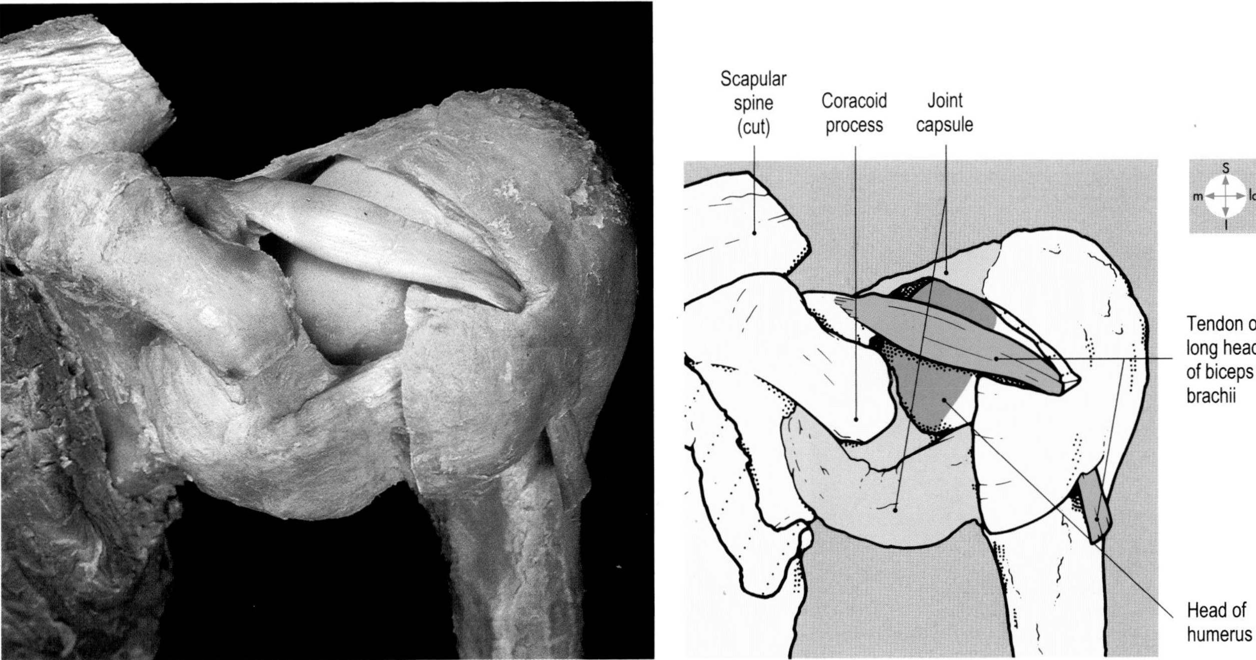

Fig. 1.24 Removal of part of the shoulder joint capsule reveals the intracapsular but extrasynovial tendon of the long head of biceps brachii.

Fluid-containing sacs of synovial membrane called bursae (Fig. 1.25) separate some tendons and muscles from other structures. Bursae which lie close to joints may communicate with the cavity of the joint through a small opening in the capsule (as does the subscapularis bursa).

In some joints (for example, the knee) a disc of cartilage is interposed between the articular cartilage covering the bone ends (Fig. 1.26). This provides a matched shape for each bone end, thus allowing freer movement without compromising stability. In addition, different types of movement are permitted in each half of the joint.

Stability varies considerably from one synovial joint to another, as several factors limit excessive movement and contribute to the stability of the joint. These include the shape of the articulating surfaces, the strength of the capsule and associated ligaments, the tone of the surrounding muscles and, where present, intra-articular discs and ligaments. At the hip joint the ligaments and the shape of the bones provide the main stability, whereas the tone of the surrounding muscles is more important in stabilizing the shoulder joint. Lack of stability associated with muscle weakness or trauma may result in dislocation so that the cartilage-covered surfaces no longer articulate. Dislocation may damage adjacent blood vessels and nerves.

Joints, particularly their capsules, receive a rich sensory innervation derived from the nerves supplying the muscles that act on the joint. For instance, the axillary nerve supplies the shoulder joint and deltoid.

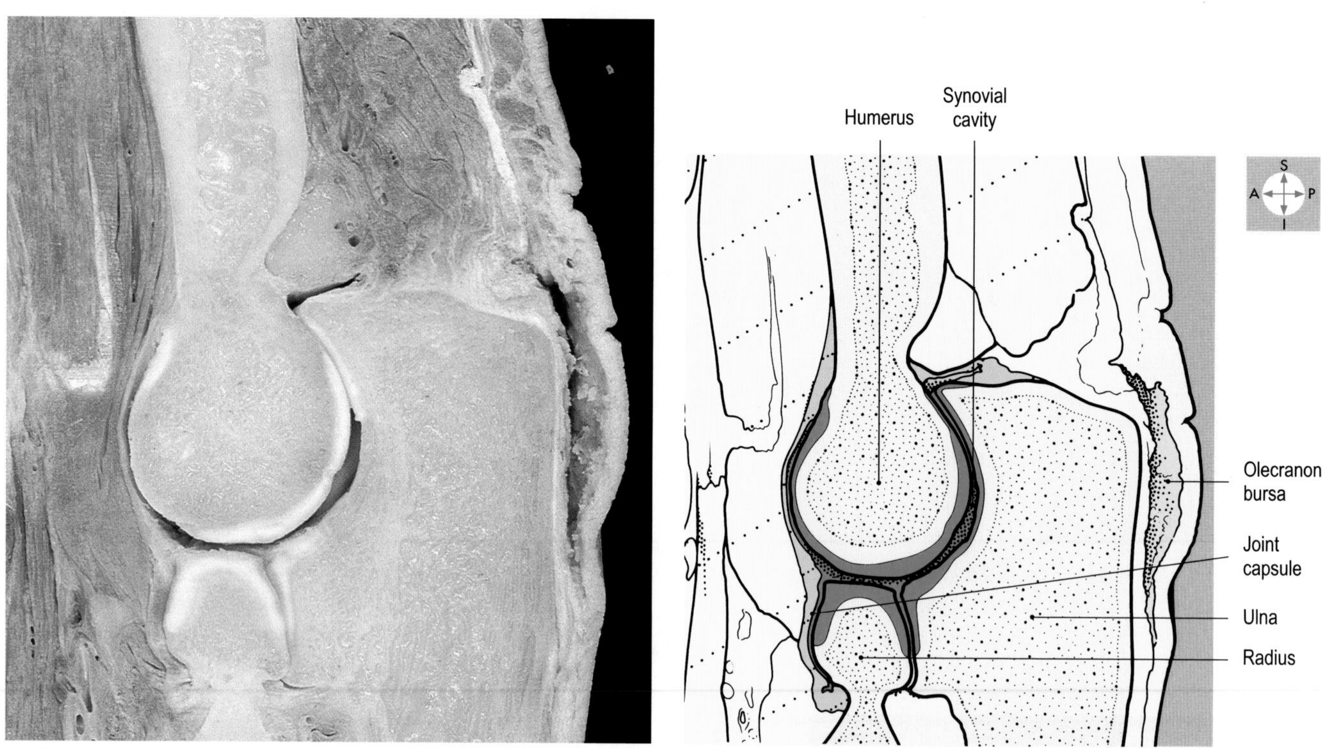

Fig. 1.25 Sagittal section through the elbow joint. The olecranon bursa does not communicate with the joint cavity.

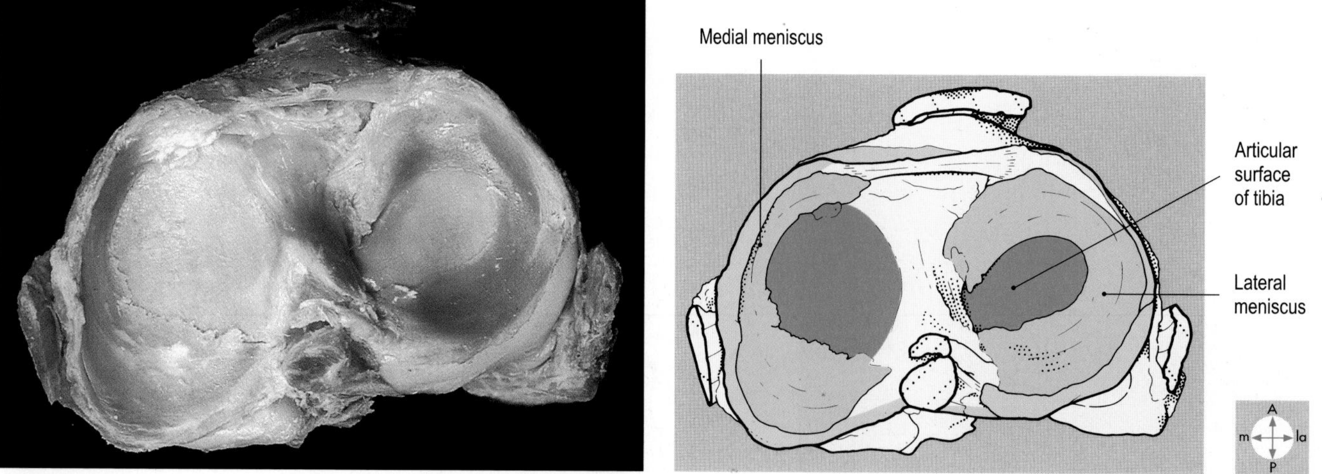

Fig. 1.26 Disarticulated knee joint to show the menisci.

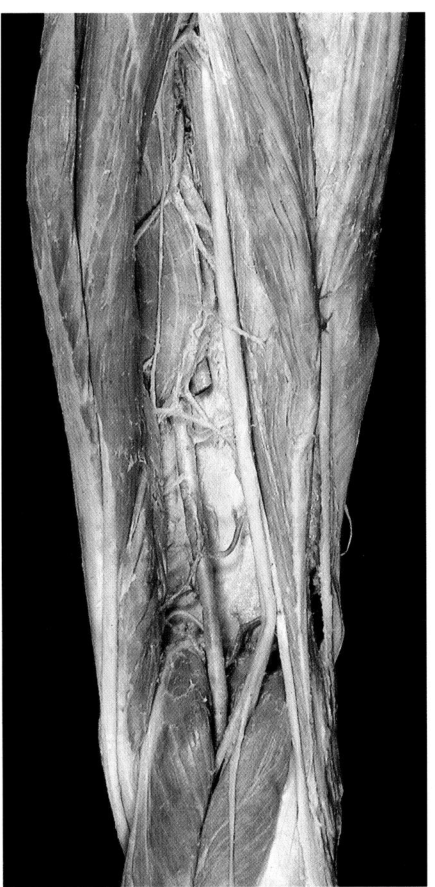

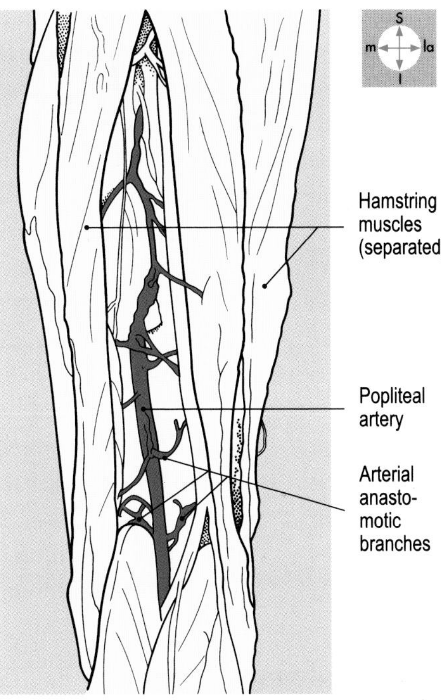

Fig. 1.27 Branches of the popliteal artery anastomose around the knee joint.

Blood vessels around joints frequently take part in rich anastomoses, which allow alternative pathways for blood flow when the joint has moved to a different position and ensure an adequate supply to the synovial membrane (such as in the knee joint; Fig. 1.27).

Serous membranes and cavities

Pericardium, pleura and peritoneum comprise the serous membranes lining the cavities that separate the heart, lungs and abdominal viscera, respectively, from their surrounding structures. Where the membrane lines the outer wall of the cavity it is called parietal, and where it covers the appropriate organ it is called visceral. The parietal and visceral parts are in continuity around the root of the viscus and are separated from each other by a cavity, which normally contains only a thin film of serous fluid. The membranes are in close contact but are lubricated by the intervening fluid, which permits movement between the viscus and its surroundings (Fig. 1.28).

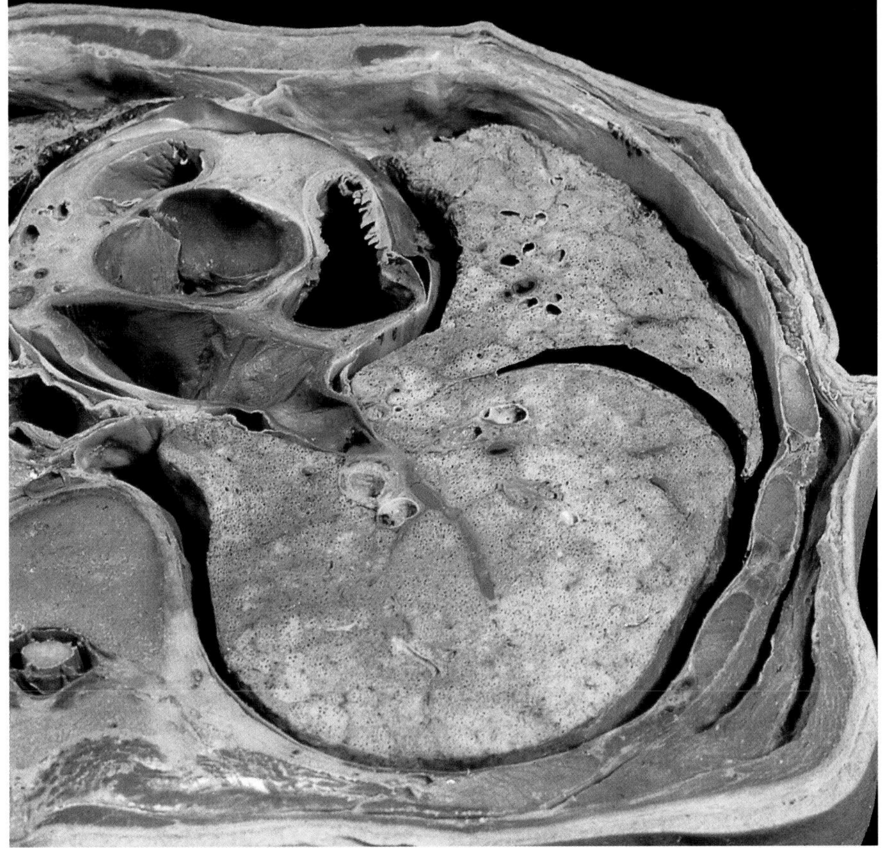

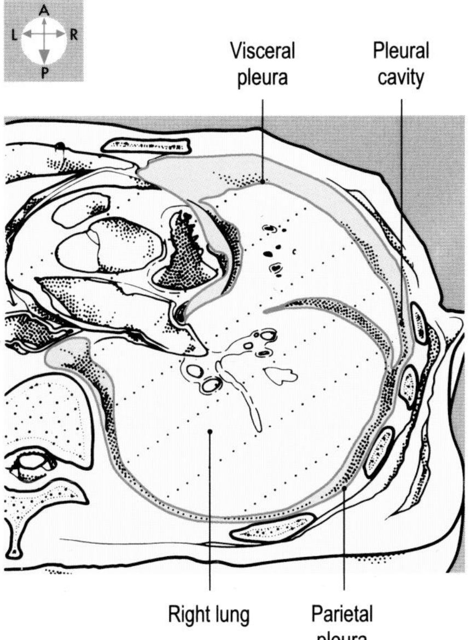

Fig. 1.28 Transverse section through the thorax at the level of T5 showing the right pleural cavity. Superior aspect.

Blood vessels

Blood vessels convey blood around the body and are classified into three main types: arteries, capillaries and veins.

Arteries are relatively thick-walled vessels which convey blood in a branching system of decreasing calibre away from the heart (Fig. 1.31). Some arteries are named after the region through which they pass (such as the femoral artery), while others are named according to the structures they supply (for instance, the renal artery). The largest vessels, such as the aorta, have elastic walls and therefore are called elastic arteries. They give rise to arteries whose walls are more muscular (muscular arteries), such as the radial artery in the forearm. A particularly thick smooth muscle coat is also a feature of the walls of the microscopic arterioles. The tone of arteriolar smooth muscle is under the control of the autonomic nervous system and hormones, and is an important factor in the maintenance of pressure in the arterial system. In general, there are few alternative pathways for arterial blood to reach its destination. However, in some regions (for example, joints and at the base of the brain), arterial supply is provided by more than one vessel (see Fig. 1.27). Such arteries may communicate directly with each other at sites known as arterial anastomoses. Arterial pulses may be felt easily in superficial arteries such as the radial artery at the wrist. Identifying pulses in deeply located arteries such as the abdominal aorta may require firm pressure.

Capillaries link the smallest arteries and the smallest veins and convey blood at low pressure through the tissues. Collectively, these thin-walled microscopic vessels have a very extensive surface area, facilitating gaseous and metabolic exchange between the blood and tissues.

Veins carry blood at low pressure from the capillary bed back to the heart (see Fig. 1.32). They may be deep (accompanying arteries) or superficial (lying in the superficial fascia) (Fig. 1.29) and are usually linked by venous anastomoses. Veins accompanying arteries are often arranged as several interconnecting vessels called venae comitantes. In the limbs the deep veins can be compressed by local muscular action, thus assisting venous return. Many veins (excluding the venae cavae, those draining viscera and those within the cranium) contain unidirectional valves which direct the flow of blood towards the heart (Fig. 1.30). The venous pattern is often variable, and numerous anastomotic connections provide alternative pathways for venous return. In some regions, numerous intercommunicating veins form meshworks called plexuses (such as the pelvic venous plexus). In the cranial cavity, venous blood is carried in special vessels formed by the dura mater lining the interior of the skull. These dural sinuses receive blood from the brain.

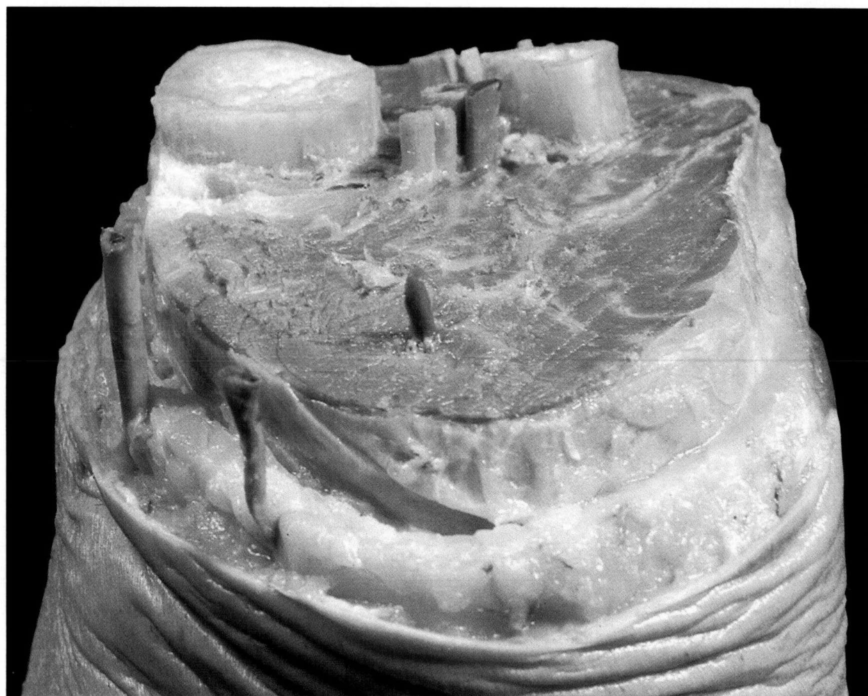

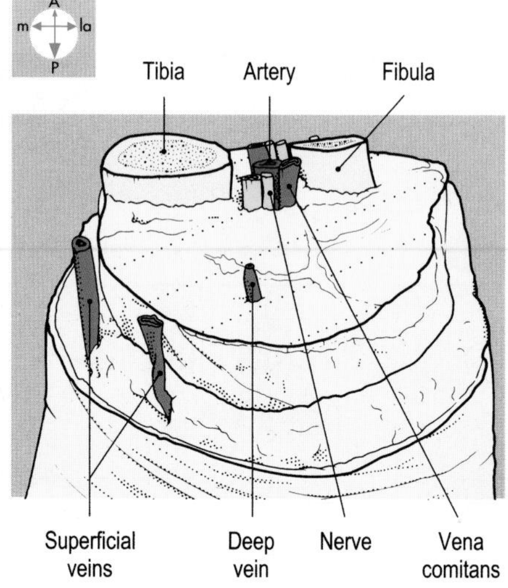

Fig. 1.29 Multilevel 'step' dissection through the right leg showing the blood vessels.

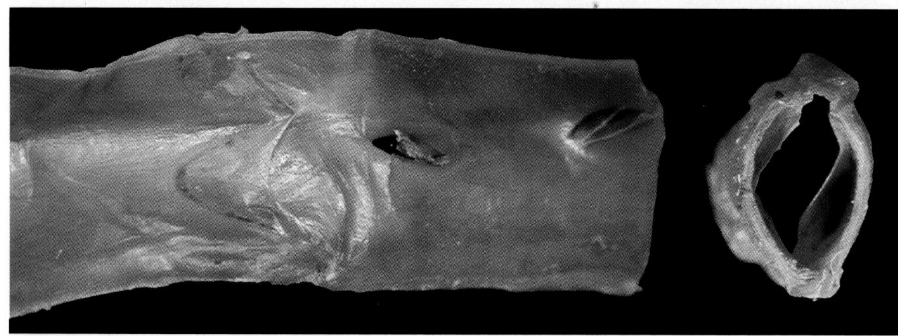

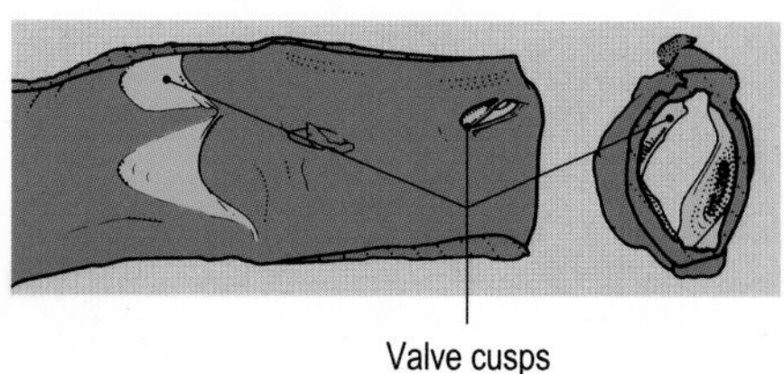

Fig. 1.30 Portion of saphenous vein opened longitudinally and in cross-section.

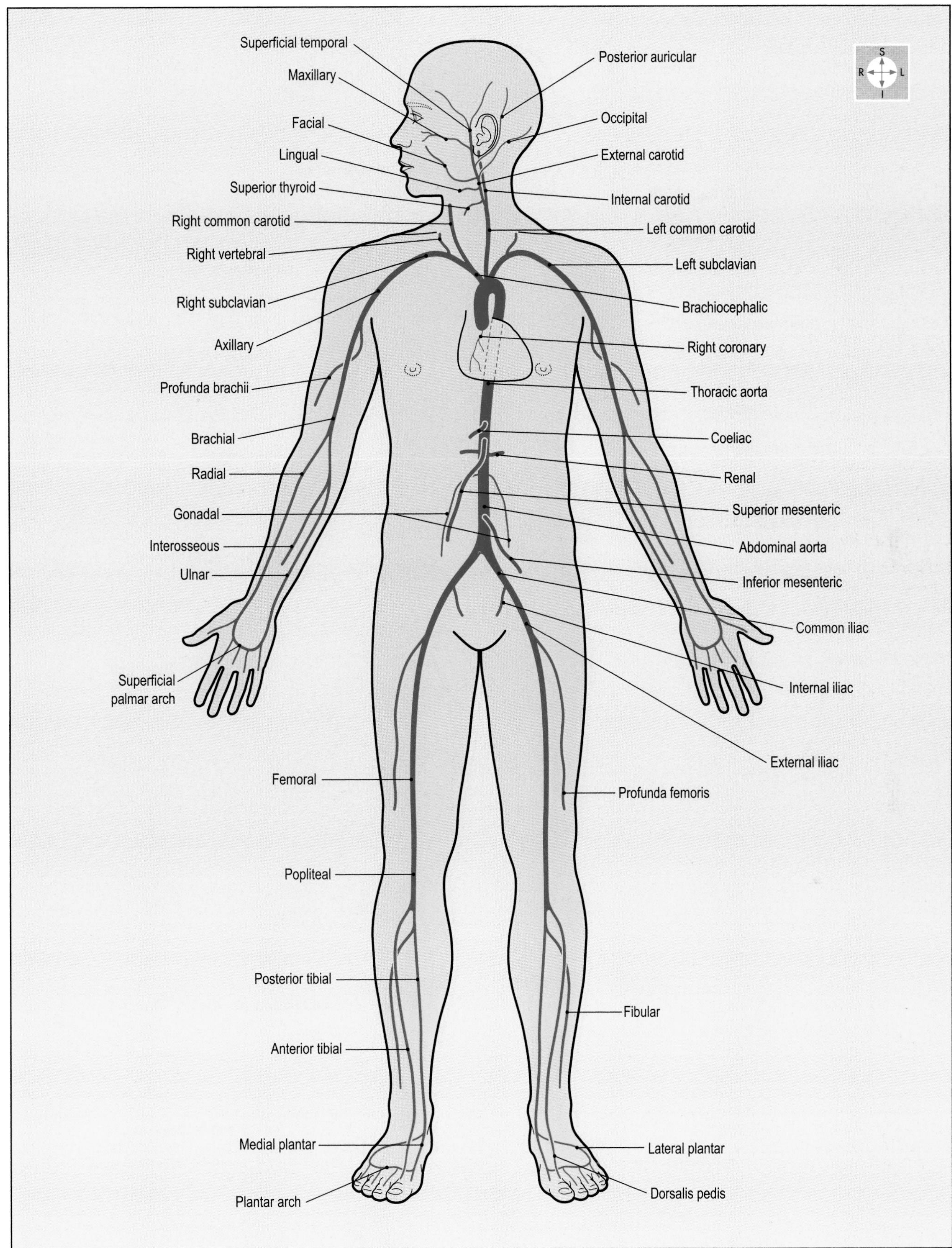

Fig. 1.31 Principal systemic arteries.

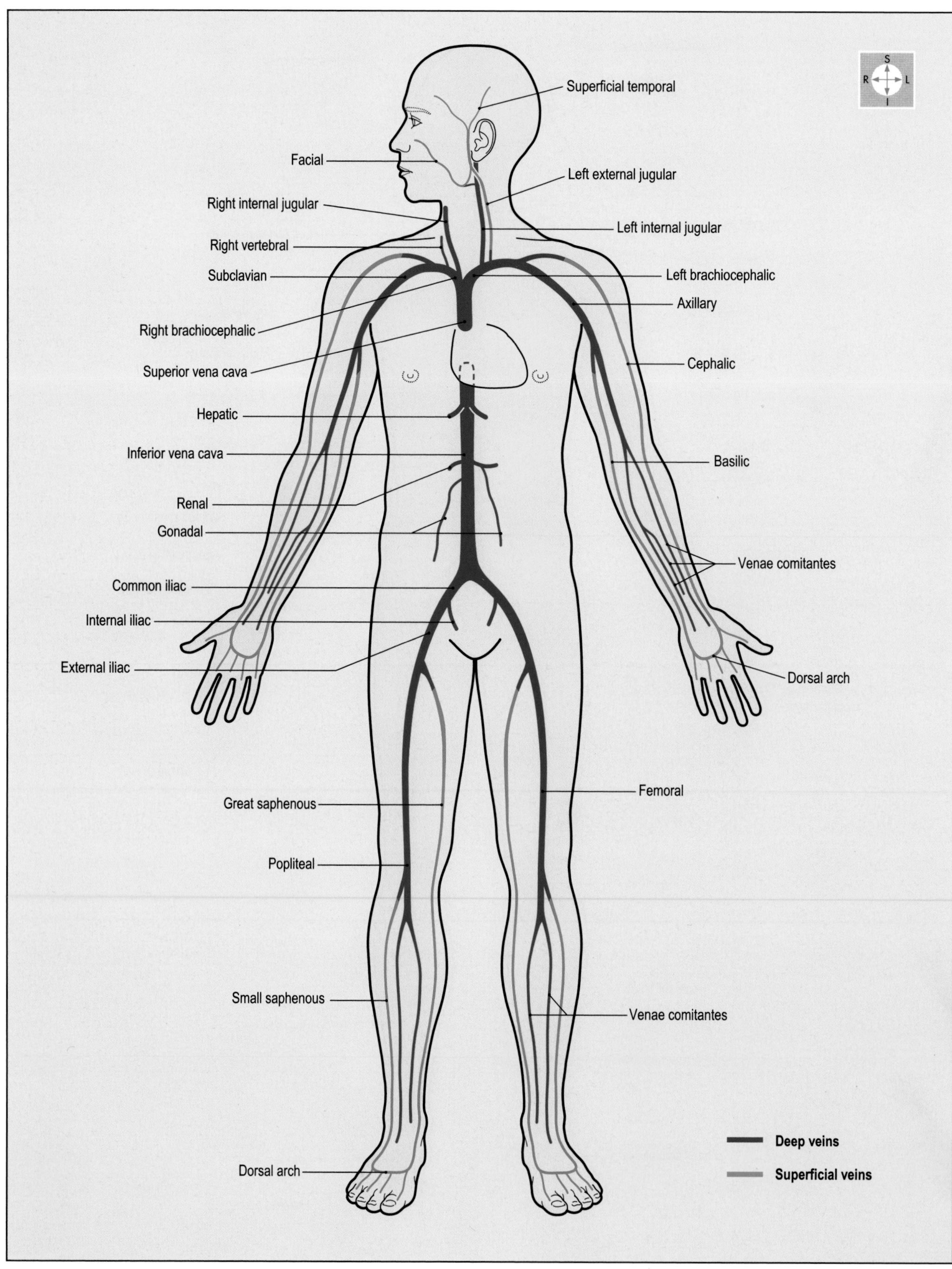

Fig. 1.32 Principal systemic veins.

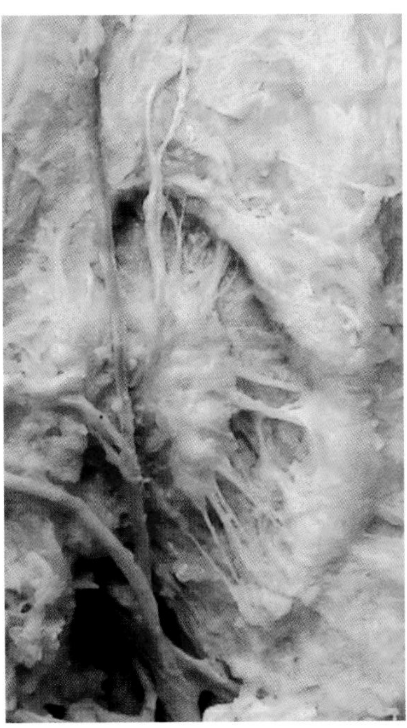

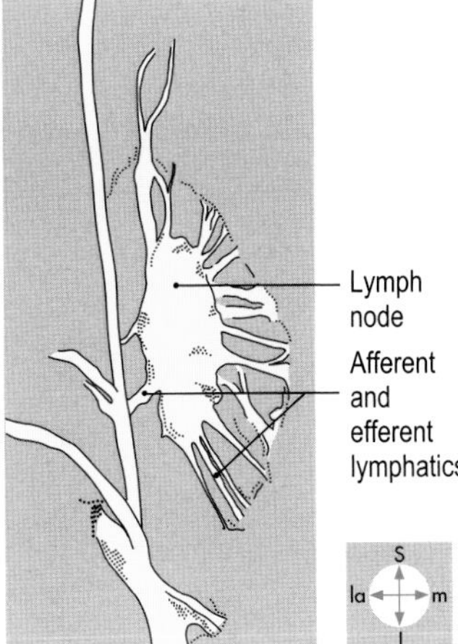

Fig. 1.33 Inguinal lymph node.

Lymphatic vessels and nodes

Tissue fluid is collected by microscopic open-ended channels called lymphatics. From a particular region or organ, these valved lymphatic vessels drain into aggregations of lymphoid tissue (called lymph nodes; Fig. 1.33) which filter lymph. Groups of lymph nodes are often found close to an organ (for example, hilar nodes) or at the root of a limb (for example, axillary lymph nodes). Ultimately, lymph drains into the venous system in the root of the neck through larger lymph channels called the thoracic duct and the right lymphatic trunk (Fig. 1.34).

Because they filter the fluid passing through them, lymph nodes may become involved in the spread of infection or malignancy (for example, cancer). Thus, the surgeon removing a cancerous organ may also excise the lymph nodes draining that organ.

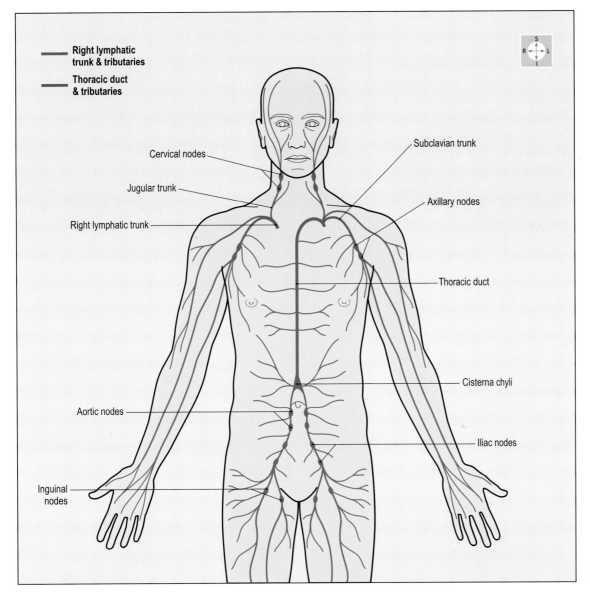

Fig. 1.34 The main lymphatic nodes and vessels.

Nervous tissue

Nervous tissue contains two types of cell: neurones and neuroglia. The neurone is the functional unit responsible for the conduction of nerve impulses. It consists of a cell body and its associated processes. One type of process, of which there is only one per neurone, is the axon. This may be relatively short but sometimes is very long, as in peripheral nerves where axons comprise the individual nerve fibres. The neuroglia undertake supporting roles and include Schwann cells, which provide the myelin sheaths around axons. These sheaths insulate the axons, increasing their speeds of conduction.

The nervous system consists of central and peripheral parts. The brain and spinal cord comprise the central nervous system.

The peripheral nervous system consists of spinal, cranial and autonomic nerves, and their associated ganglia. Bundles of nerve cell processes and their supporting Schwann cells form peripheral nerves. Several nerve processes, bound together by connective tissue, form a nerve bundle; numerous bundles, surrounded by a fibrous sheath (epineurium), constitute the complete peripheral nerve. Nerve cell bodies also form part of the peripheral nervous system and are usually grouped together into ganglia. The peripheral nervous system is divided into somatic and autonomic parts.

Somatic nerves

In general, the somatic nerves innervate skeletal muscle and transmit sensation from all parts of the body except the viscera. Twelve pairs of cranial nerves are attached to the brain and are named: olfactory (I), optic (II), oculomotor (III), trochlear (IV), trigeminal (V), abducens (VI), facial (VII), vestibulocochlear (VIII), glossopharyngeal (IX), vagus (X), accessory (XI), hypoglossal (XII). Most of these nerves supply structures in the head and neck, but the vagus nerve also supplies thoracic and abdominal viscera.

Spinal nerves are also in pairs and each is attached to a specific segment of the spinal cord by anterior and posterior roots. There are eight cervical (C1–C8), twelve thoracic (T1–T12), five lumbar (L1–L5), five sacral (S1–S5), and one or two coccygeal (Co) spinal nerves (see Fig. 1.35).

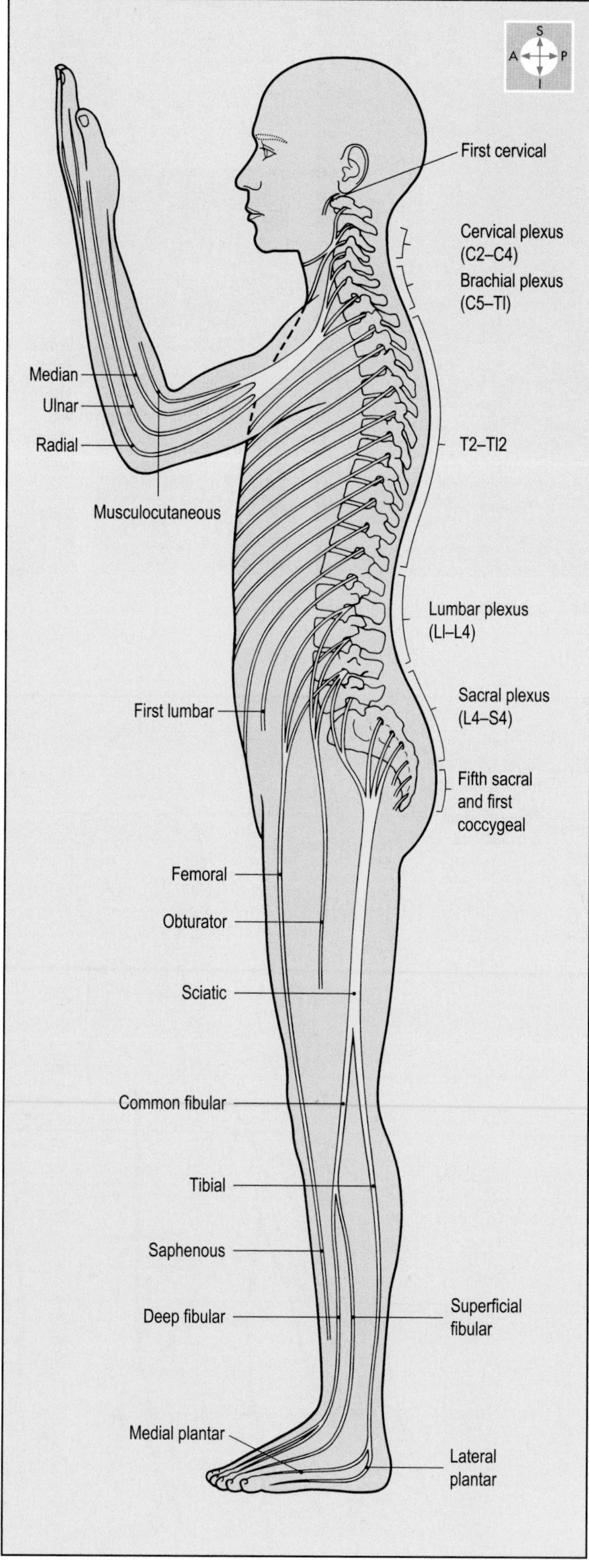

Fig. 1.35 Lateral view of the distribution of the anterior rami of the spinal nerves.

Thoracic spinal nerves illustrate the typical segmental pattern of distribution to the body wall (Fig. 1.36). The area of skin supplied by one spinal (or cranial) nerve is called a dermatome (Figs 1.37 & 1.38). In the trunk the dermatome pattern involves substantial overlap between adjacent areas. Similarly, all the muscles supplied by a single spinal (or cranial) nerve comprise a myotome.

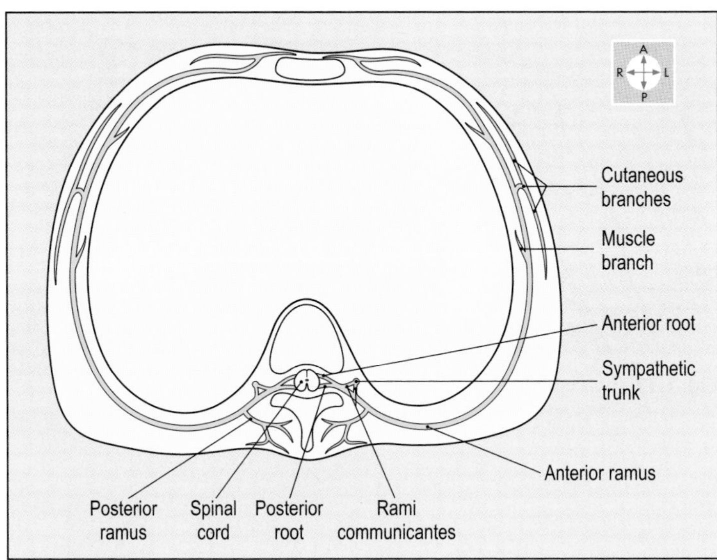

Fig. 1.36 Course and distribution of a typical thoracic spinal nerve. Inferior aspect.

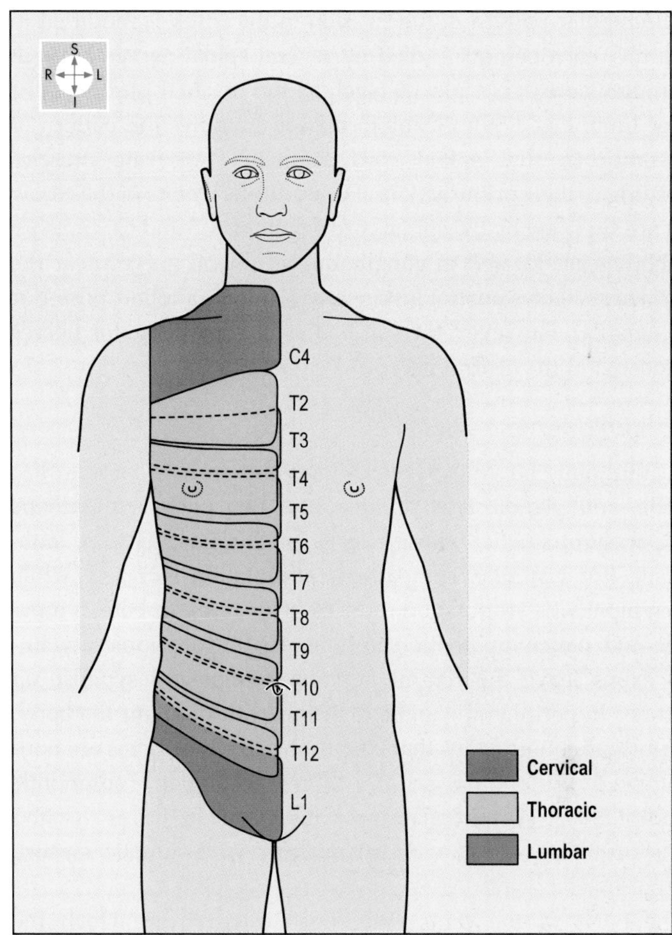

Fig. 1.37 Dermatomes of the trunk.

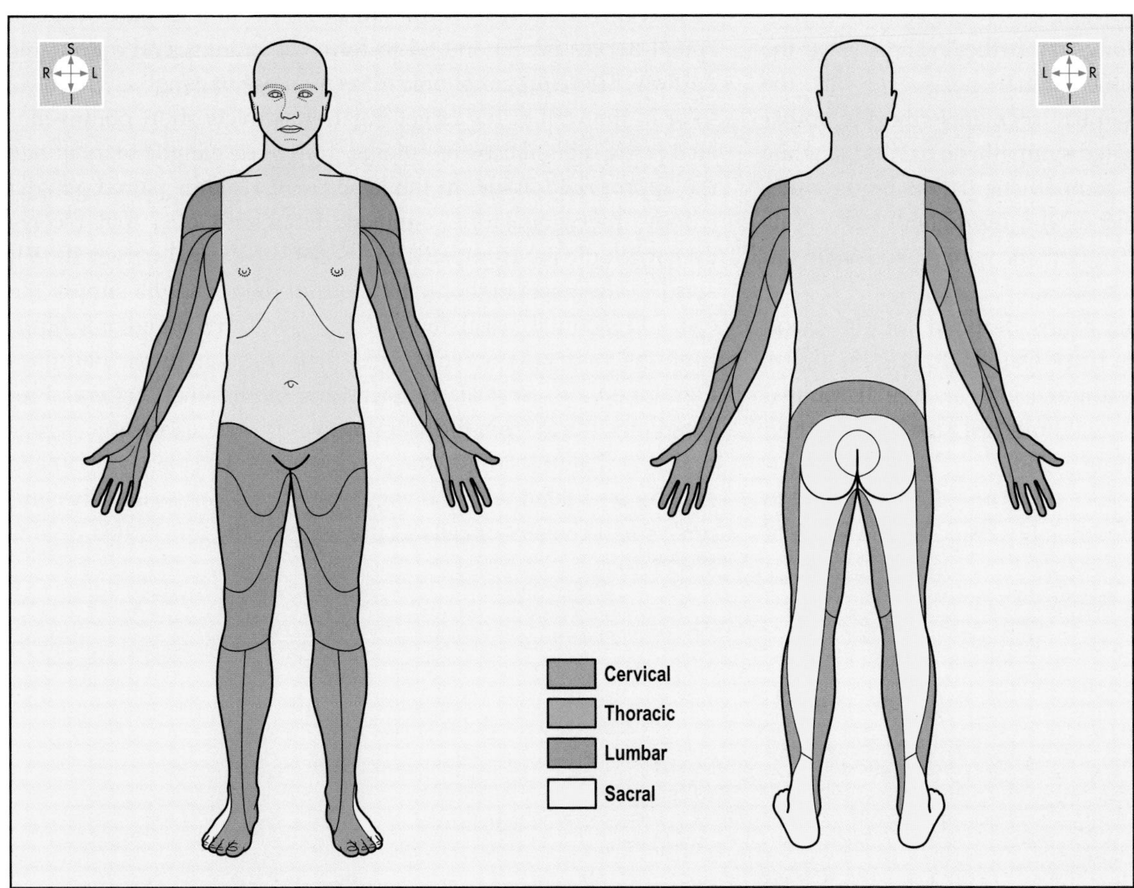

Fig. 1.38 Dermatomes of the limbs.

The regular pattern of innervation in the trunk is modified in the limbs, each being supplied by several spinal nerves through a complex network, a plexus (such as the brachial plexus of the upper limb; Fig. 1.39). Plexus formation modifies the pattern of myotomes so that spinal cord segments innervate muscles according to their prime actions. For example, flexors of the elbow joint are supplied by the spinal cord segments C5 and C6. Sensory cell bodies are located in ganglia on peripheral nerves near the central nervous system (for instance, trigeminal ganglion, posterior root ganglia). However, the cell bodies of somatic motor nerves are located in the central nervous system.

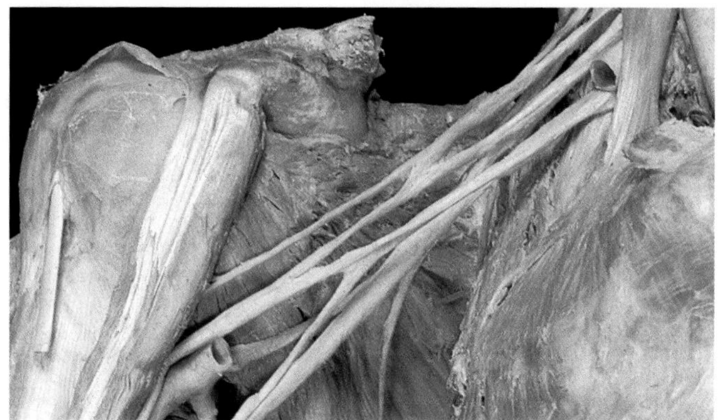

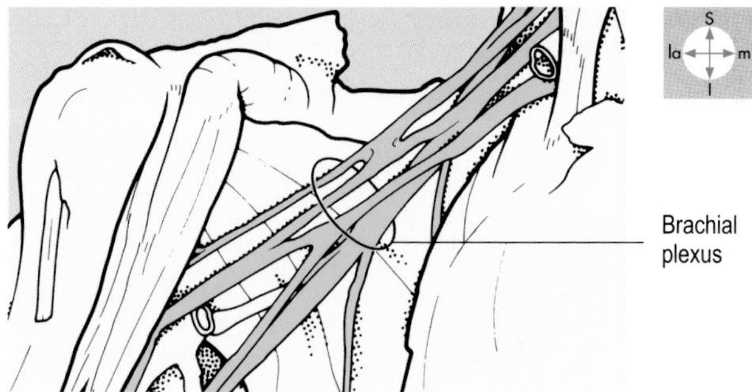

Fig. 1.39 The axilla has been dissected to show the brachial plexus.

Autonomic nerves

The autonomic nervous system innervates smooth and cardiac muscle, and glands. It is divided into two parts, sympathetic and parasympathetic, whose effects for the most part are antagonistic (for example, sympathetic stimulation increases while parasympathetic stimulation reduces heart rate). In both sympathetic and parasympathetic components, preganglionic myelinated axons leave the central nervous system and synapse on neurones in peripheral ganglia distributed throughout the body. The postganglionic axons that pass to the effector organs are nonmyelinated. Autonomic sensory fibres accompany autonomic efferent fibres in peripheral nerves but their cell bodies are located in the posterior root ganglia in company with somatic sensory neurones.

The parts of the central nervous system from which the autonomic nerves emerge differ for the sympathetic and parasympathetic components (Fig. 1.40).

Sympathetic nerves Preganglionic sympathetic fibres leave the central nervous system in the spinal nerves of all the thoracic and the upper two lumbar segments (thoracolumbar outflow) and enter the ganglionated sympathetic trunks via white rami communicantes. The two sympathetic trunks lie on either side of the vertebral column and extend throughout most of its length. Each trunk consists of sympathetic ganglia and interconnecting nerve trunks.

Unmyelinated postganglionic axons destined for the blood vessels and sweat glands of the body wall, including the limbs, leave the ganglia by grey rami communicantes and are distributed by the spinal nerves. Special visceral branches pass directly from the trunks to reach the appropriate organ.

Postganglionic sympathetic nerve fibres are often conveyed to their destinations as plexuses intimately related to the walls of arteries.

Parasympathetic nerves In the parasympathetic system, myelinated preganglionic fibres leave the central nervous system as part of cranial nerves III, VII, IX and X and as part of sacral spinal nerves S2, S3 and S4 to form the craniosacral autonomic outflow. These preganglionic fibres synapse in ganglia lying close to or in the wall of the target organ. Relatively short nonmyelinated postganglionic axons emerge from these ganglia to innervate the appropriate tissue. In the head there are four paired ganglia (ciliary, pterygopalatine, submandibular and otic) that receive preganglionic parasympathetic fibres from cranial nerves III, VII and IX. The postganglionic fibres from these ganglia supply the eye, and lacrimal, nasal and salivary glands. Preganglionic fibres from the vagus (X) nerve synapse with postganglionic neurones that innervate cervical, thoracic and abdominal viscera. Preganglionic fibres from the sacral nerves (pelvic splanchnic nerves or nervi erigentes) supply the pelvic organs. The parasympathetic ganglia associated with the vagus and sacral nerves usually comprise small clusters of cells in the walls of the innervated organs (Fig. 1.40).

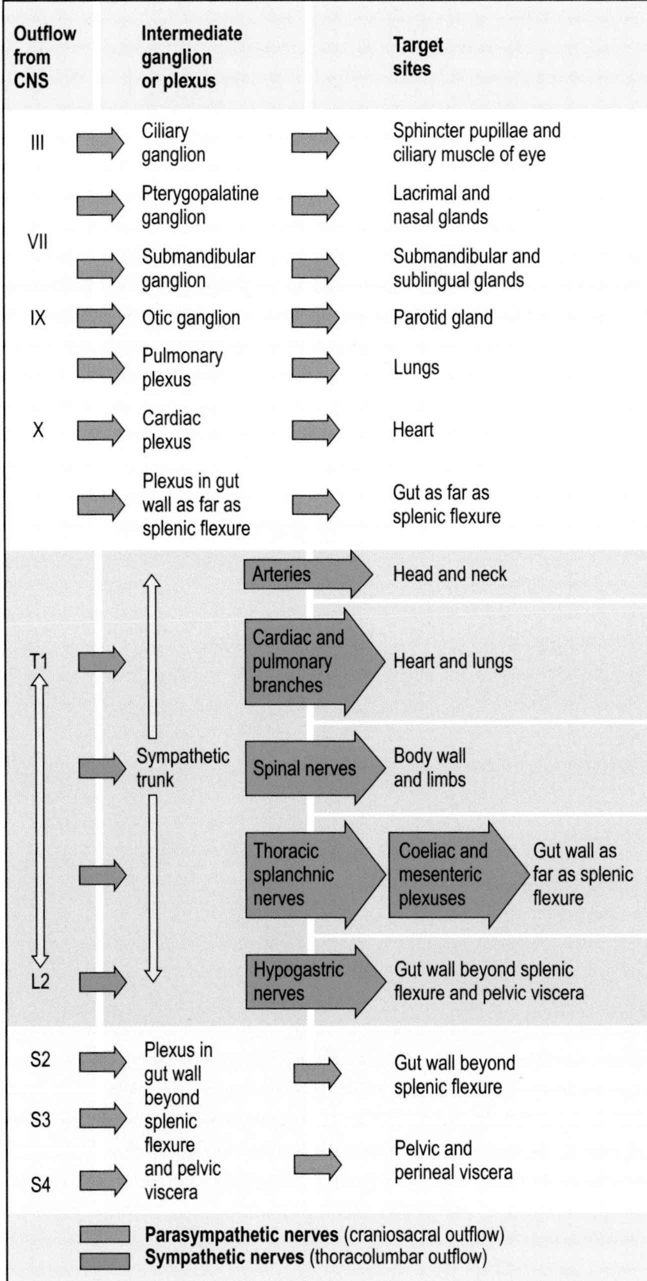

Fig. 1.40 Pattern of innervation in the parasympathetic and sympathetic autonomic nervous systems.

Thorax

CHAPTER 2

Introduction

The thorax is the region of the trunk that includes the sternum, costal cartilages, ribs and thoracic vertebrae, together with the structures they enclose. Superiorly the thorax is limited by the upper surfaces of the first ribs and their costal cartilages, the manubrium of the sternum and the first thoracic vertebra. The space bounded by these structures is the superior thoracic aperture (thoracic inlet) (Fig. 2.1), which allows structures to pass between the root of the neck and the thorax. Space-occupying tumours in this location may compress adjacent structures, leading to the clinical condition called thoracic outlet syndrome. Inferiorly the cavity of the thorax is separated from the abdominal contents by a fibromuscular sheet called the diaphragm. The oesophagus and other intrathoracic structures pass through the diaphragm to gain or leave the abdomen. Since the diaphragm is convex superiorly, some of the organs within the abdomen are covered by the lower ribs and costal cartilages.

The ribs, costal cartilages and sternum form a semi-rigid framework that provides attachment for several muscles; some connect adjacent ribs and costal cartilages, others attach to the

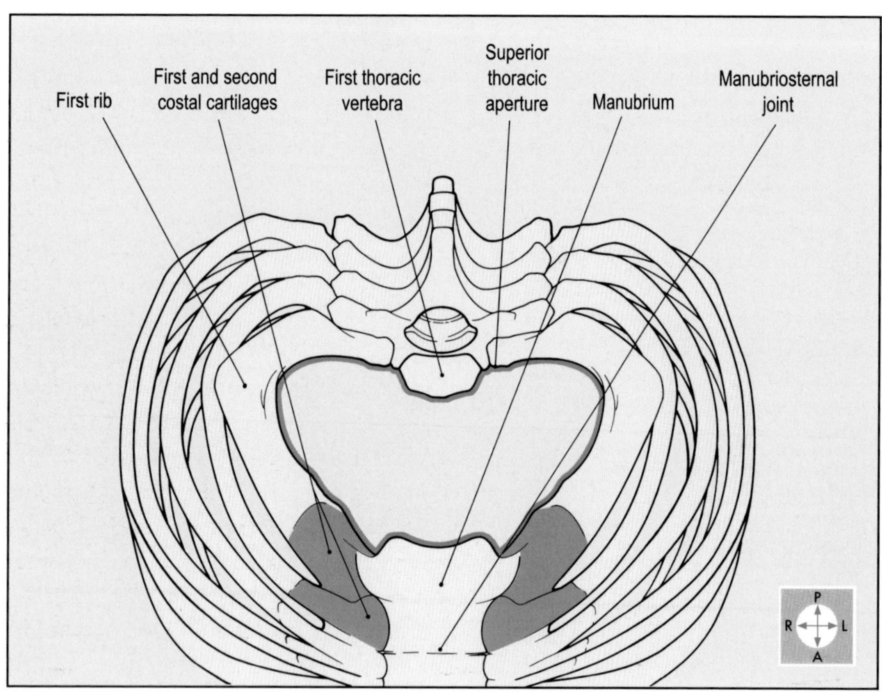

Fig. 2.1 The boundaries of the superior thoracic aperture (pink line).

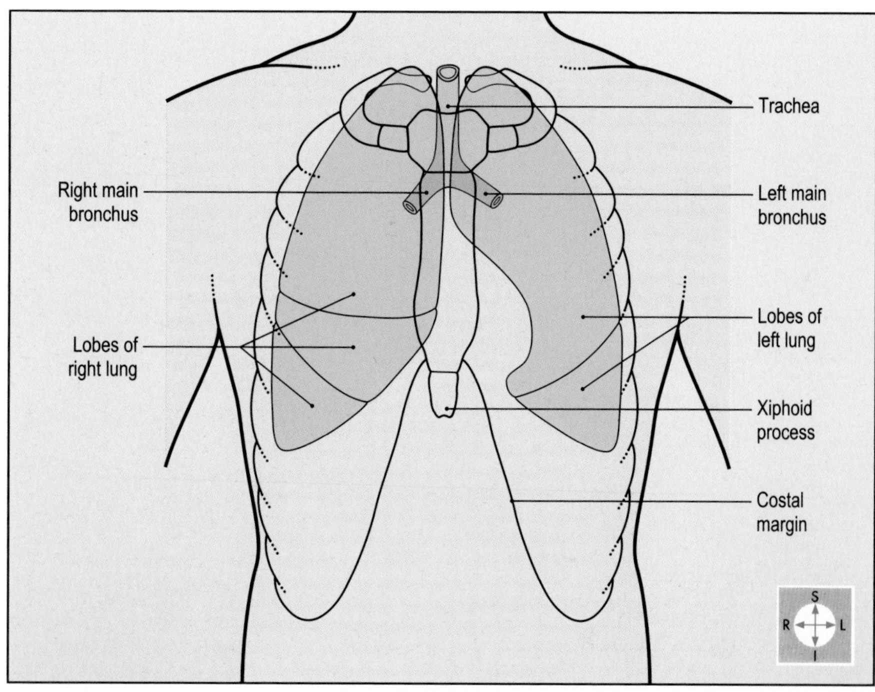

Fig. 2.2 The trachea, bronchi and lungs.

pectoral girdle or humerus or descend from the thorax to contribute to the musculature of the abdominal wall. The medial ends of the clavicles articulate with the upper border of the manubrium and flank the jugular (suprasternal) notch. The manubrium articulates with the body of the sternum at the manubriosternal joint (sternal angle, angle of Louis), which usually forms a horizontal ridge. This is a useful landmark during clinical examination because the second costal cartilages meet the sternum at this level. It is normal practice to count ribs starting at the second costal cartilages as the first ribs are obscured by the clavicles. Inferiorly the thoracic wall is limited by the costal margin, which is formed by the costal cartilages of the lower ribs. The costal margin (subcostal angle) extends upwards and medially as far as the lower end of the sternum and forms the upper boundary of the abdominal wall. The inferior portion of the sternum, the xiphoid process, can usually be identified in the midline between the costal margins. The space between adjacent ribs and costal cartilages is occupied by intercostal muscles, which are active during respiratory movements of the thoracic wall. Intercostal vessels and nerves run between these muscles in each space and give branches to adjacent tissues and the overlying skin. In both sexes, the nipples are surface features, the anatomical locations of which vary depending upon the build of the individual. The glandular components of the breast lie deep to the nipple, embedded in the fat of the subcutaneous tissues that cover the muscles of the chest wall. Posteriorly, the upper ribs are covered by the scapulae and their muscles.

The space contained within the thoracic wall is occupied by several important organs. Some of these are confined to the thorax (e.g., heart) whilst others traverse the region, passing from the neck into the abdomen (e.g. oesophagus). On each side, the lung occupies a large proportion of the thoracic cavity (Fig. 2.2) and is surrounded by a serous sac called the pleura. Each membrane forms a closed cavity that usually contains a thin film of serous fluid enabling the lungs and thoracic wall to move freely over one another. Each pleural cavity is separated from its neighbour by a midline partition called the mediastinum. The mediastinum is the term used to describe all the structures that occupy this central portion, including the heart and its great vessels (Figs 2.3 & 2.4) and the intrathoracic parts of the trachea and oesophagus.

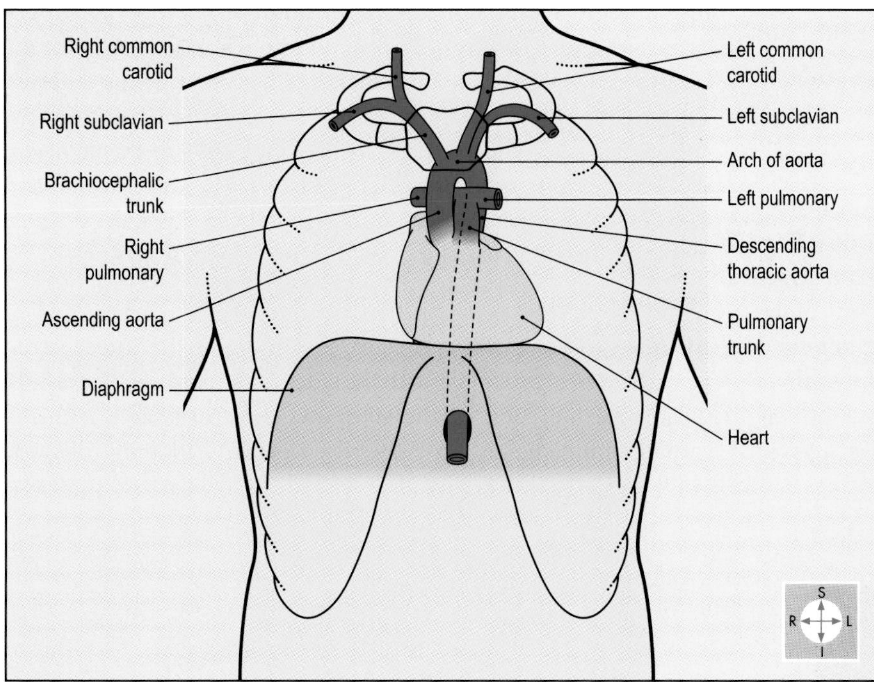

Fig. 2.3 The heart and great arteries.

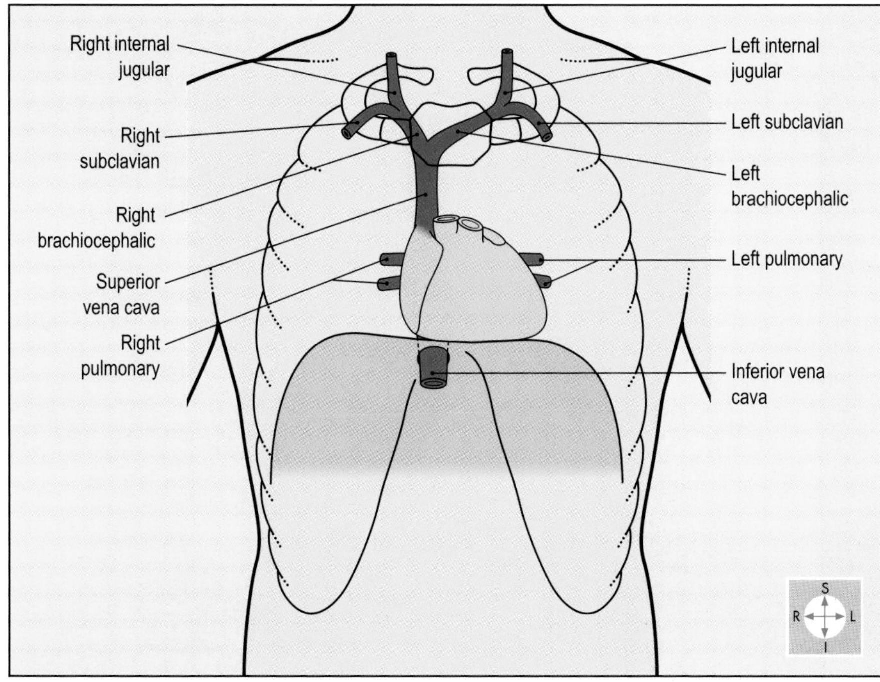

Fig. 2.4 The heart and great veins.

Skeleton of Thorax

The skeleton of the thorax consists of 12 thoracic vertebrae, the 12 pairs of ribs and their costal cartilages, and the sternum (Fig. 2.5). Structures in continuity between the root of the neck and the upper part of the thoracic cavity pass through the superior thoracic aperture (thoracic inlet), which is bounded by the first thoracic vertebral body, the first pair of ribs and costal cartilages and the upper border of the sternum. The inferior thoracic aperture (thoracic outlet) through which structures pass between the thoracic and abdominal cavities is formed by the twelfth thoracic vertebral body, the twelfth and eleventh ribs and the costal margin (the fused costal cartilages of the seventh to the tenth ribs inclusive).

Ribs

Although the ribs differ in size and shape, most (3–9 inclusive) have features in common and are described as 'typical ribs' (Fig. 2.6). Each typical rib consists of a head, neck, tubercle, shaft, upper and lower borders and inner and outer surfaces. The heads of the ribs are those parts which articulate with the thoracic vertebral bodies. The lower part of the head forms a synovial joint with its own vertebral body whilst the upper part articulates with the vertebra above. The intermediate part of the head lies against the intervertebral disc. The neck of the rib connects the head and the tubercle and lies in front of the transverse process. The tubercle of the rib faces posteriorly and the medial part of its surface forms a synovial joint with the articular facet on the transverse process of the corresponding vertebra. The shaft forms the remainder of the rib and ends anteriorly at a shallow depression, which receives the costal cartilage. Passing laterally from the tubercle, the shaft slopes downwards and backwards before turning forwards and outwards to form the angle. Lateral to the angle, the shaft possesses a sharp lower border, which bounds the costal groove.

The first rib is atypical. Its head possesses an articular facet solely for its own vertebral body. The shaft is short and broad and has superior and inferior surfaces. In addition, its superior surface carries a ridge that forms a projection on the inner border of the rib, the scalene tubercle, to which is attached scalenus anterior. Two grooves lie across the shaft, one in front of the ridge (for the subclavian vein) and the other behind (for the subclavian artery and lowest trunk of the brachial plexus). The tenth, eleventh and twelfth ribs are also atypical, in that each head possesses a single facet and the rib is usually devoid of a tubercle or an angle.

Costal cartilages

All ribs possess costal cartilages, and those of the upper seven pairs (true ribs) articulate with the sides of the sternum. Pairs 8–12 (false ribs) fall short of the sternum. These articulate with the cartilage immediately above, whilst 11 and 12 (floating ribs) are

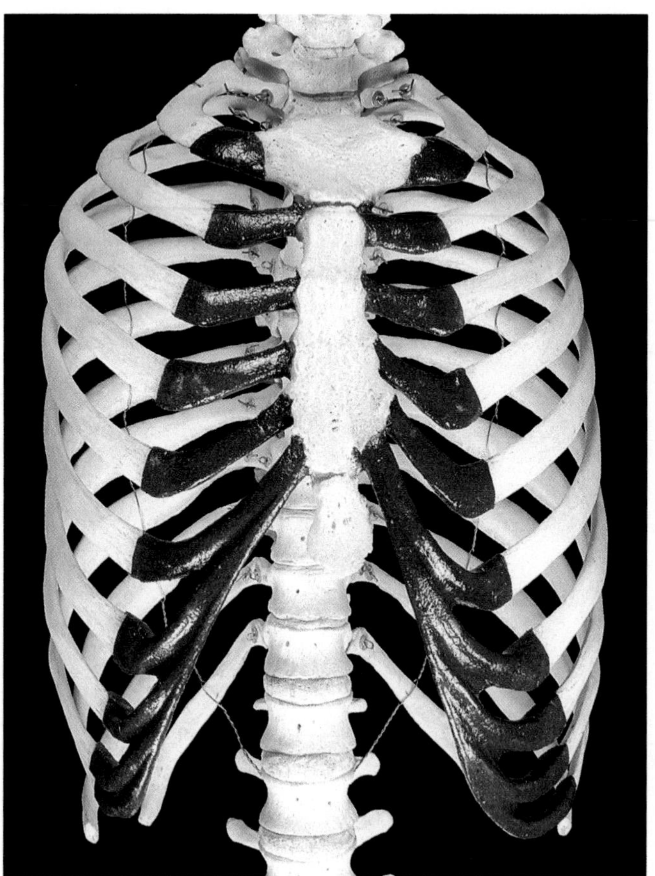

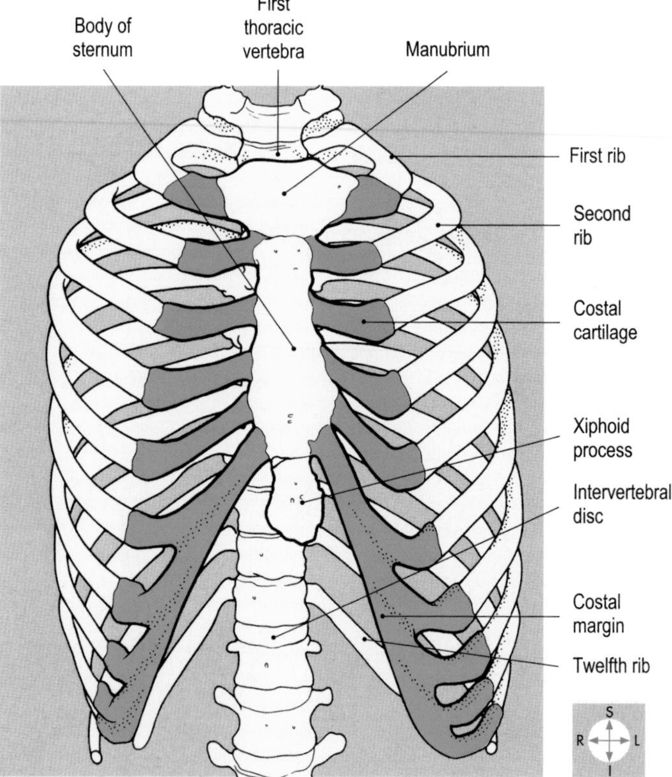

Fig. 2.5 Articulated bones of the thorax showing the relationships between the vertebral column, ribs, costal cartilages and sternum.

pointed and end freely in the muscle of the abdominal wall.

Sternum

The sternum is a flat bone and consists of the manubrium, the body (Fig. 2.7) and the xiphoid process. The manubrium articulates with the medial end of each clavicle at the sternoclavicular joint and with the first costal cartilage. Its upper margin includes the jugular notch, which forms part of the superior thoracic aperture. A palpable secondary cartilaginous joint (the manubriosternal joint) unites the manubrium and body and forms a useful guide to the second costal cartilage, which abuts the sternum at the lateral margin of the joint. The lateral margins of the body of the sternum are indented by the medial ends of the second to the seventh costal cartilages. The xiphoid process lies in the subcostal angle and projects downwards and backwards from the body of the sternum.

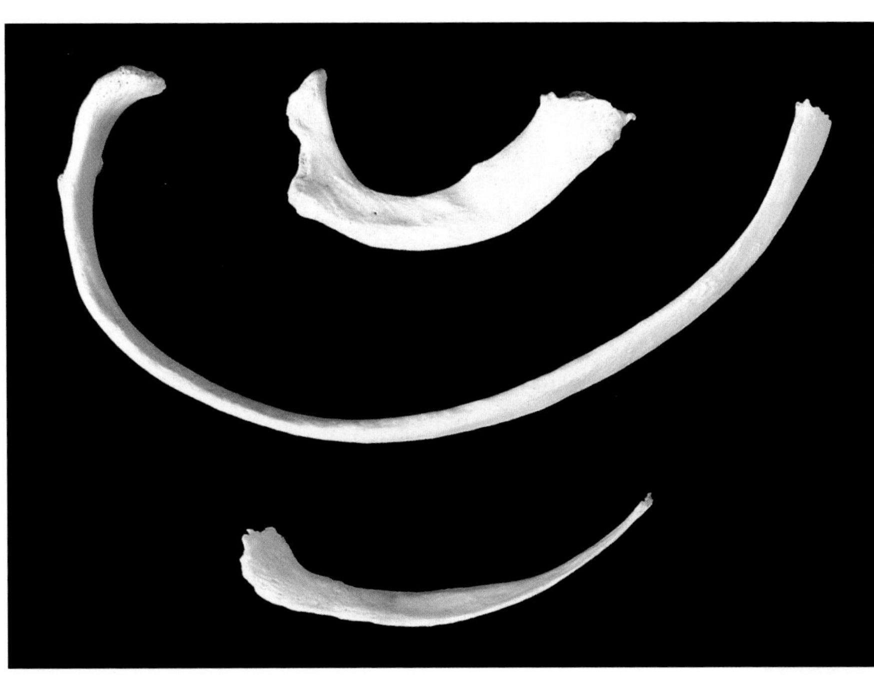

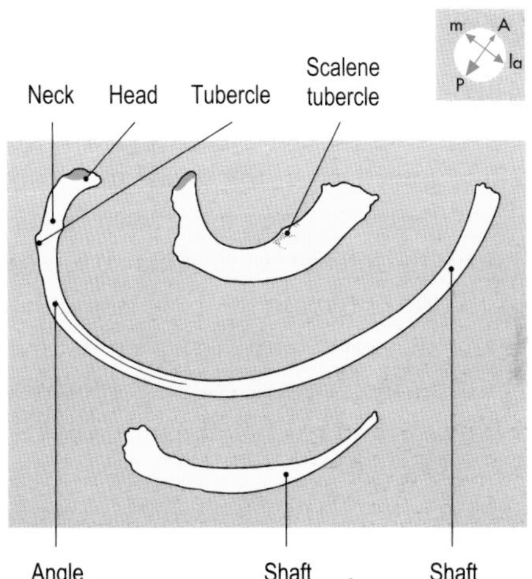

Fig. 2.6 The first, seventh and twelfth ribs showing their surface features and relative sizes.

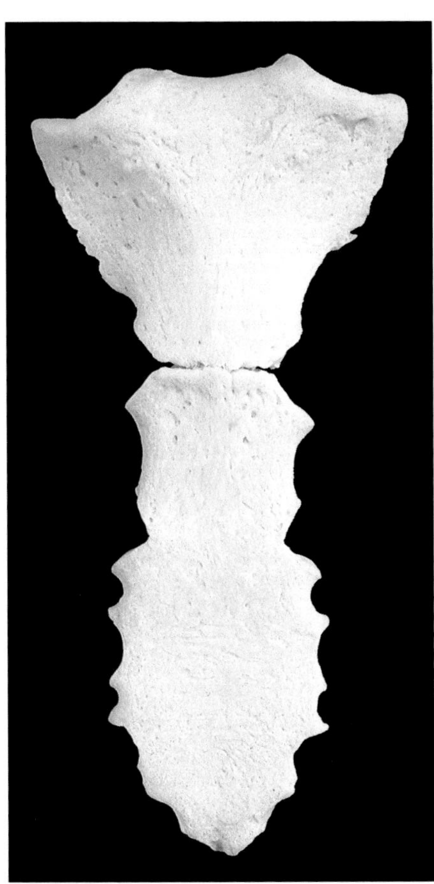

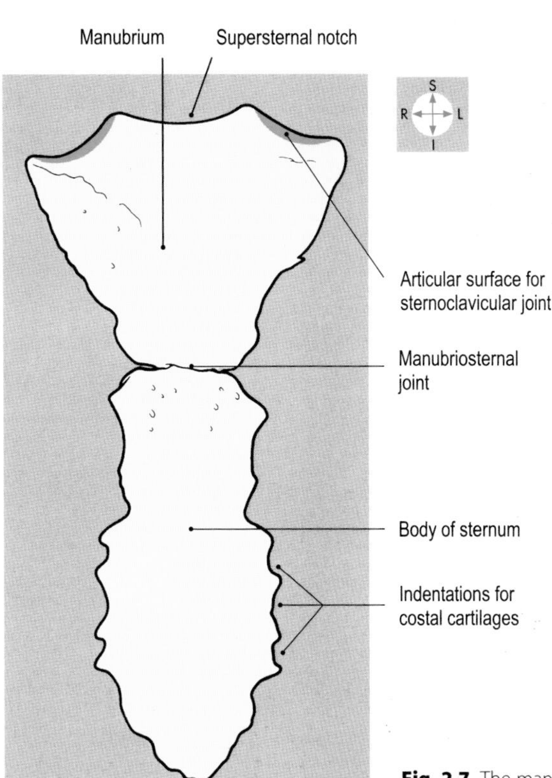

Fig. 2.7 The manubrium and the body of the sternum. The xiphoid process is absent.

Thoracic Wall

Skin

The skin covering the thorax receives its nerve supply from lower cervical and upper thoracic spinal nerves. Above the level of the manubriosternal joint, C4 gives cutaneous innervation, whilst thoracic nerves T2–T11 provide the dermatomes for the remainder of the thoracic wall. The first thoracic nerve does not contribute to the cutaneous nerve supply of the thorax but innervates some of the skin of the upper limb (see Fig. 1.35).

Breast

The breast (Fig. 2.8) consists of glandular tissue and a quantity of fat embedded in the subcutaneous tissue of the anterior chest wall. In the male and immature female the gland is rudimentary. Although the size and shape of the breast in the adult female are variable, the base (the part lying on the deep fascia covering pectoralis major, serratus anterior and rectus abdominis) is constant in position. In the adult female the base is roughly circular and extends between the second and sixth ribs. Medially, the gland overlies the lateral border of the sternum. Part of the breast extends upwards and laterally and reaches the anterior fold of the axilla. This is the axillary tail (process) and is the only part of the breast to penetrate beneath the deep fascia. During clinical palpation of the breast it is essential that the axillary tail is included as part of the physical examination.

The glandular elements consist of 15–20 lobes arranged radially, each draining into a lactiferous duct. These ducts open independently onto the surface of the nipple. The nipple is surrounded by an area of pink skin, the areola, which may develop brown pigmentation during pregnancy.

The gland is traversed by fibrous septa (ligaments of Astley Cooper) (Fig. 2.8), which subdivide the lobes and loosely attach the skin of the breast to the deep fascia covering the chest wall. In certain type of breast carcinoma, these fibrous septa may produce characteristic dimpling of the skin over the lesion. Normally, the breast is freely mobile over the underlying muscles. However, lack of mobility when pectoralis major is contracted indicates that breast pathology has fixed the gland to the underlying chest wall muscles.

Blood supply

The fat and glandular elements of the breast receive blood from arteries that also supply the deeper structures of the chest wall. These vessels include perforating branches from the internal thoracic artery (internal mammary artery) and the second, third and fourth intercostal arteries. The lateral thoracic and thoracoacromial arteries arising from the axillary artery also supply the breast. The gland is drained by veins which accompany the arteries.

Lymph drainage

Within the substance of the breast the lymphatic vessels form a system of interconnecting channels that collect lymph from all parts of the organ. The superior and lateral aspects of the breast usually drain into central and apical axillary nodes via infraclavicular and pectoral nodes. It is therefore important to palpate axillary lymph nodes in suspected cases of malignant breast disease. The medial and inferior parts of the breast drain deeply into glands along the internal thoracic vessels and thence via the bronchomediastinal lymph trunk into the confluence of lymphatic vessels in

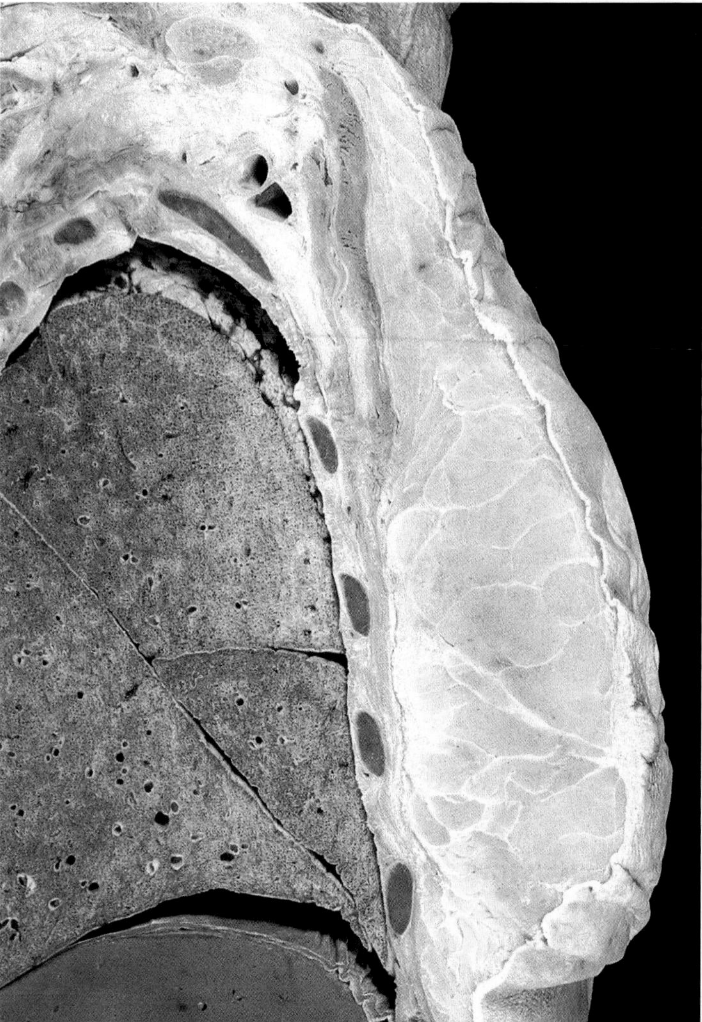

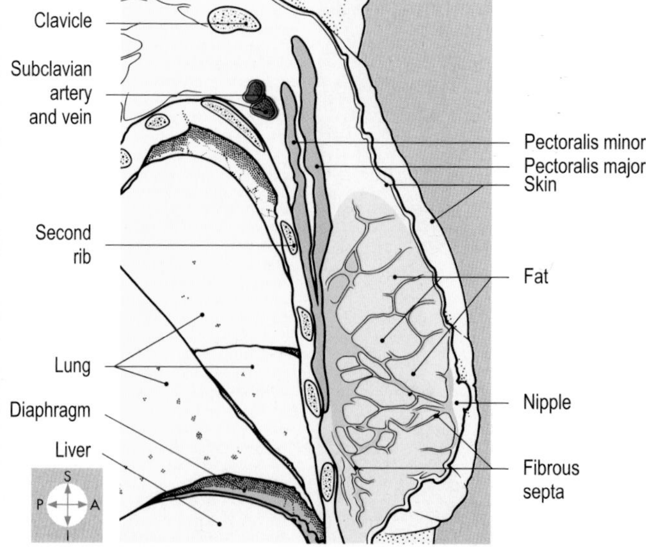

Fig. 2.8 Sagittal section through the right breast and underlying chest wall. In this dissection, the glandular structure of the breast cannot be distinguished.

the root of the neck (see p. 328). Lymphatics may also cross the midline to communicate with vessels in the opposite breast.

Muscles

The outer surfaces of the ribs, costal cartilages and sternum give attachment to muscles involved in movements of the upper limb and the scapula, namely pectoralis major, pectoralis minor and serratus anterior. In addition, the external surfaces of the lower ribs provide attachment for rectus abdominis and the external oblique muscles of the anterior abdominal wall (see pp 141, 143).

Pectoralis major

This large fan-shaped muscle (Fig. 2.9) attaches to the clavicle, sternum and upper costal cartilages and forms the bulk of the anterior wall of the axilla. The clavicular head is attached to the anterior surface of the medial half of the clavicle. The sternocostal head is anchored to the manubrium and body of the sternum, and to the upper six costal cartilages. Laterally, both parts of the muscle attach to the humerus along the lateral lip of the intertubercular sulcus (see p. 77).

Pectoralis major is supplied by the medial and lateral pectoral nerves from the brachial plexus. Functionally, it is a powerful adductor and flexor of the arm at the shoulder joint and also produces medial rotation of the humerus. When the upper limb is fixed, the sternocostal part may act as an accessory muscle of inspiration by elevating the ribs.

Pectoralis minor

This small muscle (Fig. 2.10) lies deep to pectoralis major and is usually attached to the third, fourth and fifth ribs. The muscle converges on the medial border of the coracoid process of the scapula. Pectoralis minor is supplied by the medial and lateral pectoral nerves and assists in movements of protraction and rotation of the scapula.

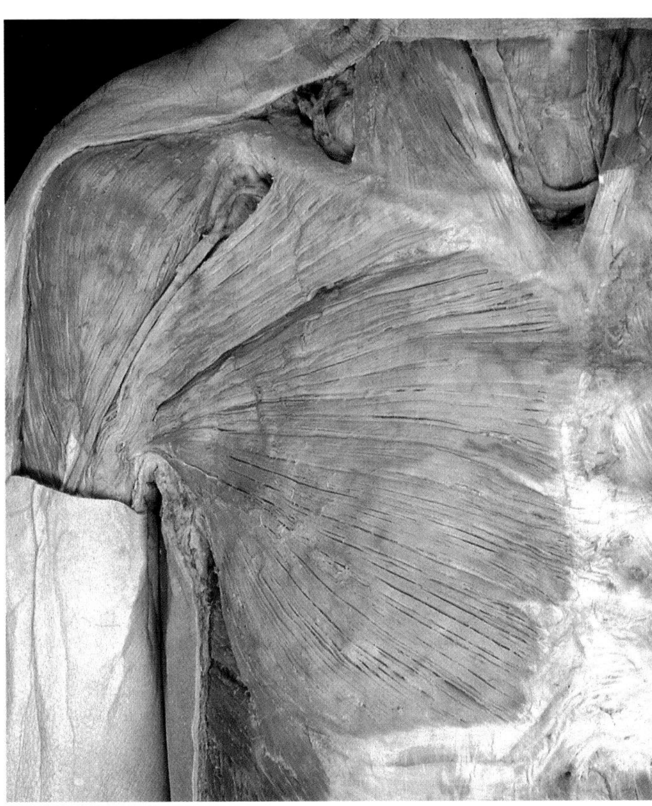

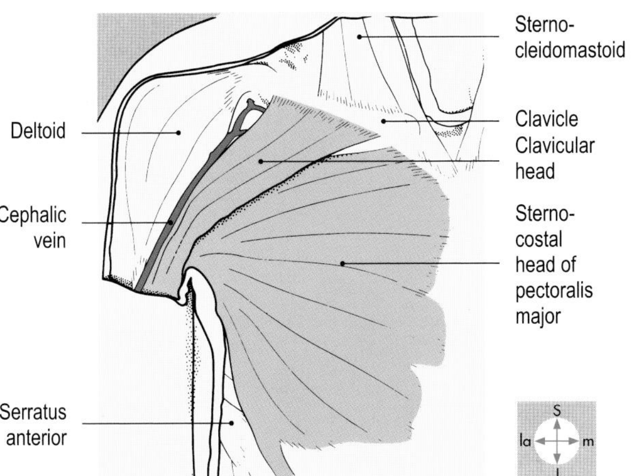

Fig. 2.9 Pectoralis major, revealed by removal of the skin, the subcutaneous tissue and deep fascia.

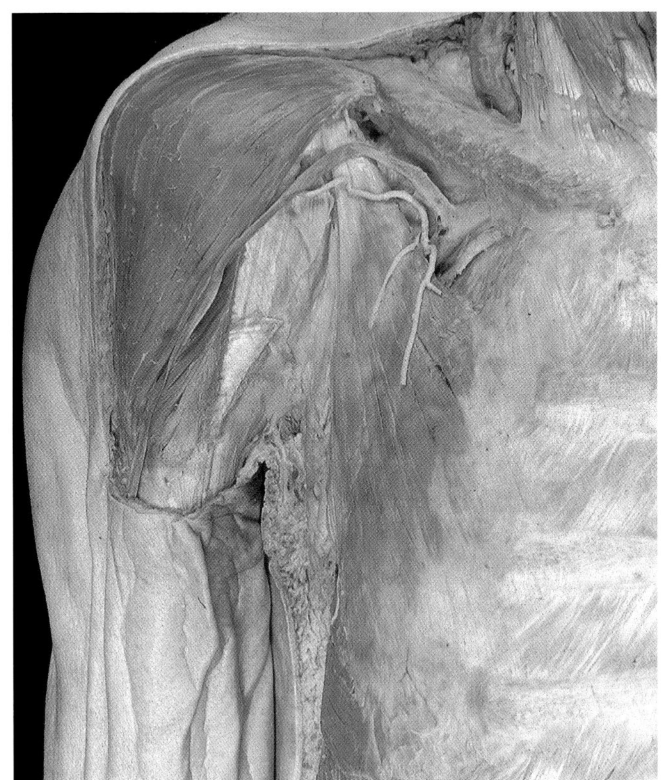

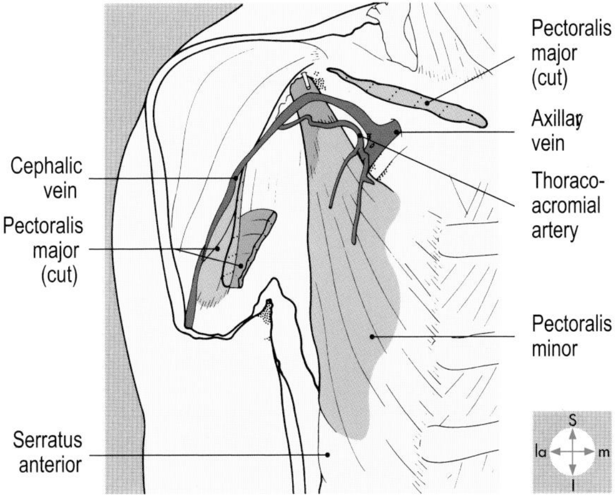

Fig. 2.10 Pectoralis minor, exposed by removal of pectoralis major.

Serratus anterior

This large muscle lies between the scapula and chest wall and attaches to the lateral aspects of the upper eight ribs (Fig. 2.11), forming part of the medial wall of the axilla. The muscle fibres from the upper four ribs attach to the superior angle and to the costal surface of the medial border of the scapula. The fibres from ribs 5–8 converge on the costal surface of the inferior angle of the scapula.

Innervation is provided by the long thoracic nerve arising in the neck from the upper three roots (C5, C6 & C7) of the brachial plexus. The muscle is a powerful protractor of the scapula and assists trapezius in producing scapular rotation during abduction of the upper limb. In addition, the muscle helps to stabilize the scapula during movements of the upper limb.

Intercostal spaces

The interval between two adjacent ribs is called an intercostal space. On each side of the thorax there are 11 such spaces, numbered from above and occupied by muscles, membranes, nerves and vessels. The number given to each intercostal space and its neurovascular structures corresponds to that of the rib which limits the space superiorly. The nerves and vessels immediately inferior to the twelfth ribs are termed the subcostal nerves and vessels. The intercostal nerves and vessels supply the intercostal muscles and

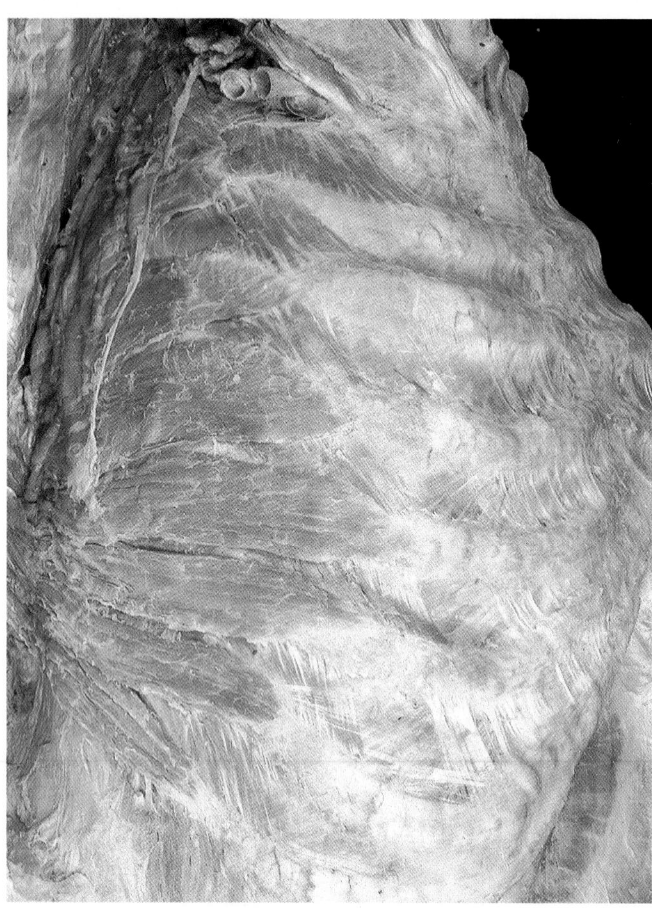

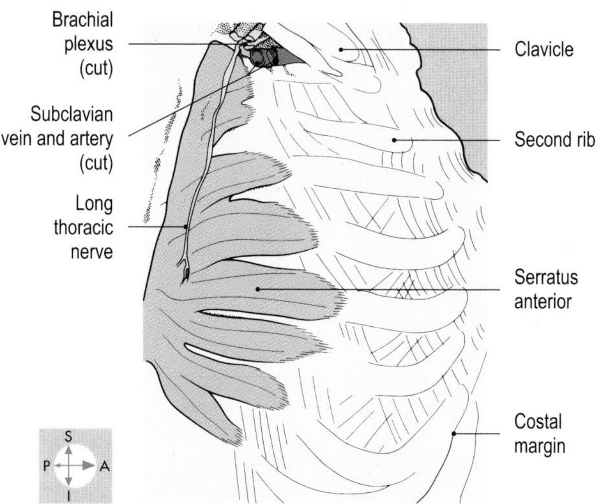

Fig. 2.11 Serratus anterior seen after removal of the pectoral muscles and displacement of the scapula backwards.

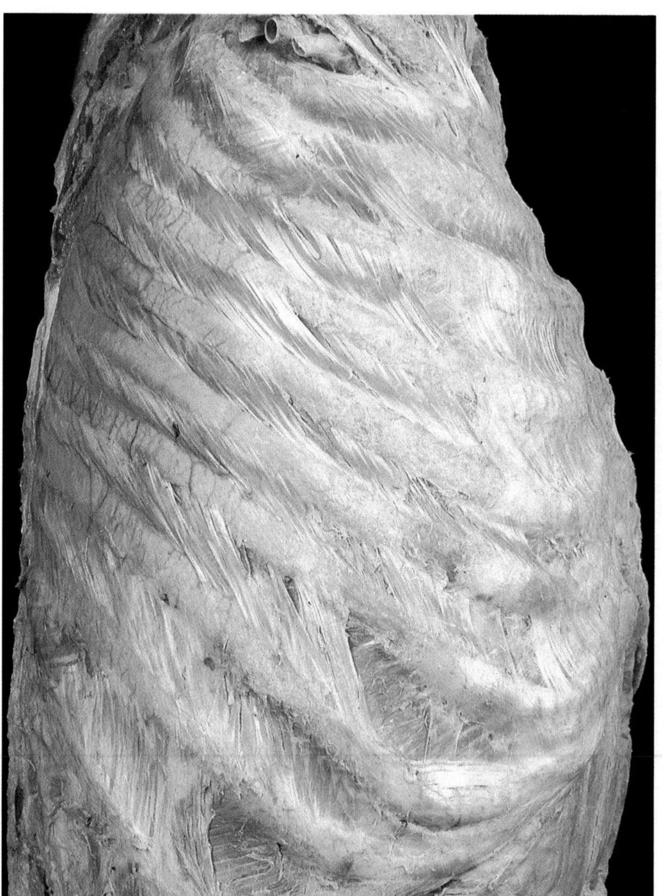

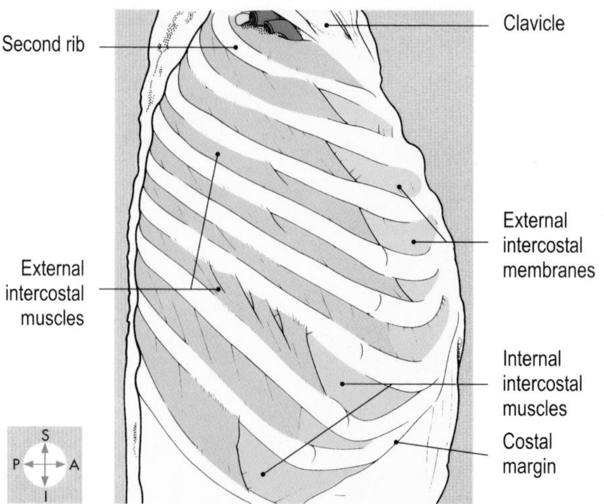

Fig. 2.12 External intercostal muscles, exposed by removal of the upper limb and serratus anterior.

the parietal pleura deep to each space. Branches from these vessels also supply the overlying muscles of the body wall, the superficial fascia and skin. Most intercostal nerves have cutaneous branches that supply the skin covering the chest and abdominal walls.

Intercostal muscles

There are three layers of intercostal muscles, which lie superficial, intermediate and deep. These are named the external, the internal and the innermost intercostal muscles.

External intercostal muscles

The fibres of the external intercostal muscles slope downwards and forwards from the lower border of one rib to the upper border of the subjacent rib (Fig. 2.12). The muscle extends from the tubercle of the rib posteriorly to the junction of the rib and its costal cartilage anteriorly. Between costal cartilages the muscle fibres are replaced by a thin fascial sheet, the external intercostal membrane, which reaches the lateral border of the sternum (Fig. 2.13).

Internal intercostal muscles

The internal intercostal muscles (Fig. 2.14) lie immediately deep to the external intercostal muscles. The fibres of the two muscles are mutually at right angles, those of the internal intercostal muscles running downwards and backwards from the lower border of one rib to the upper border of the subjacent rib. Anteriorly, each muscle continues between the costal cartilages to reach the lateral border of the sternum (Fig. 2.13). Posteriorly, each muscle extends only to the angles of the ribs, where it is replaced by the internal intercostal membrane, which continues as far as the tubercles of the ribs.

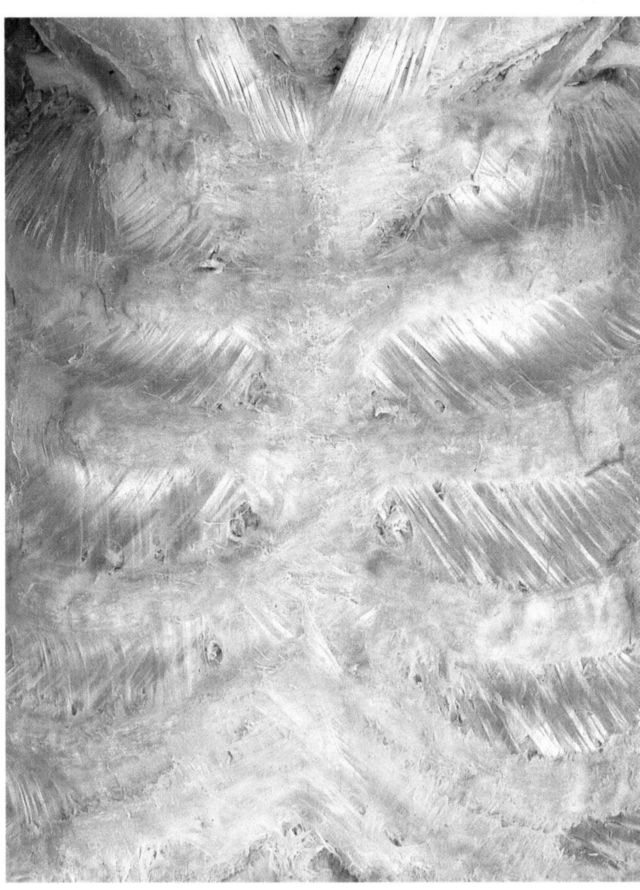

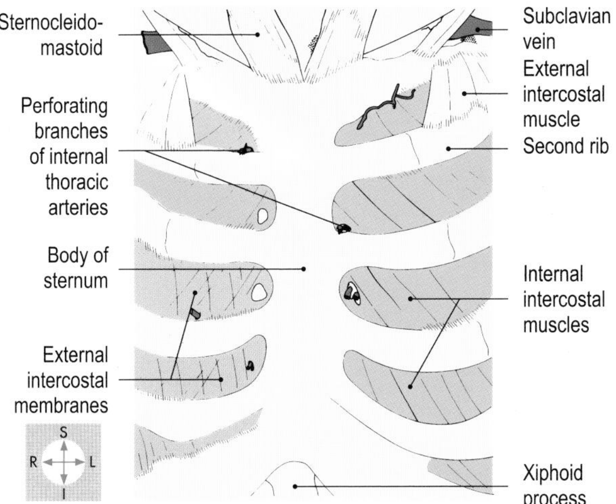

Fig. 2.13 External intercostal membranes and the anterior fibres of the internal intercostal muscles.

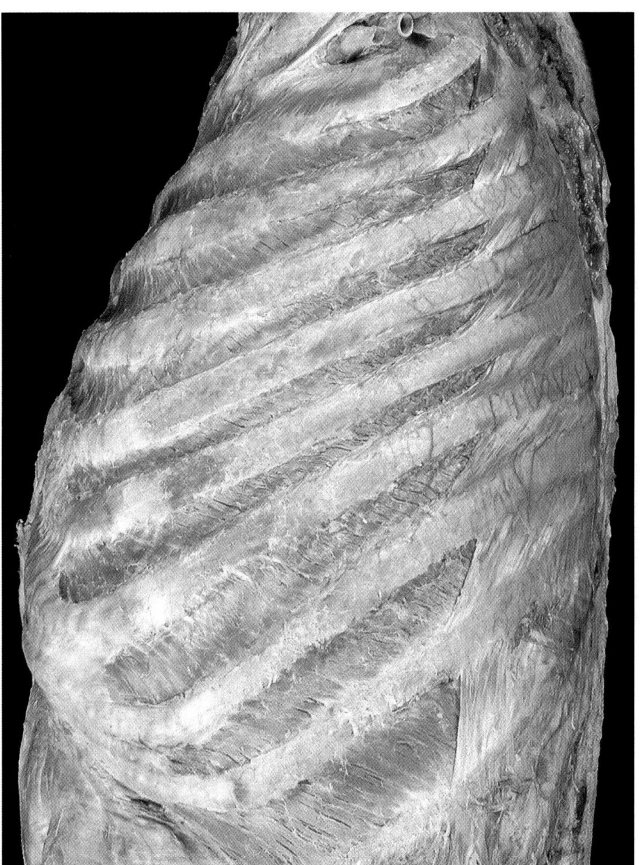

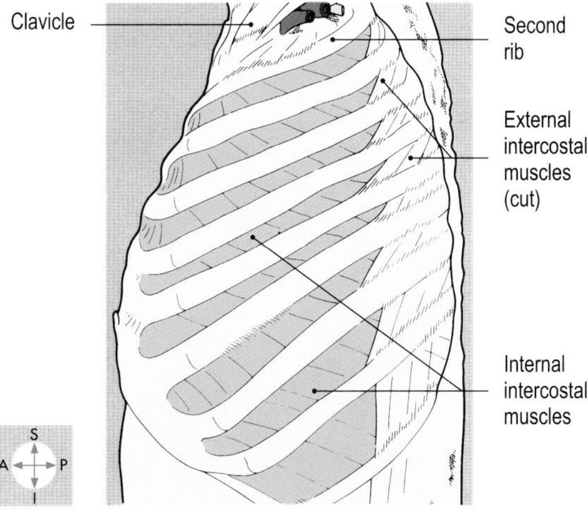

Fig. 2.14 Internal intercostal muscles, exposed by removal of the anterior parts of the external intercostal muscles.

Innermost intercostal muscles

These muscles lie on a plane deep to that of the internal intercostal muscles (Fig. 2.15). They form the lateral part of an incomplete layer of muscle which includes the transversus thoracis (sternocostalis) anteriorly (Fig. 2.16) and subcostalis posteriorly. The innermost intercostal muscles connect the inner surface of each rib to that of its neighbours.

Nerve supply

All the intercostal muscles in a particular intercostal space are supplied by the corresponding intercostal nerve.

Actions

Although the main role of the intercostal muscles is in ventilation of the lungs, it must be emphasized that during normal, quiet breathing the muscles of the thoracic wall make only a small contribution. Inspiration is usually brought about mainly by the diaphragm, whose descent increases the vertical diameter of the thorax. The transverse and anteroposterior diameters of the thorax are increased, especially in deep inspiration, by the external intercostal muscles, which incline the ribs outwards, upwards and forwards so that the intercostal spaces are widened. During quiet breathing, expiration is largely due to the 'elastic' recoil of the lungs and thoracic wall and involves minimal activity by the intercostal muscles. Even when expiration is 'forced', for example during vigorous physical exertion or when coughing, the main muscular effort is provided by the muscles of the abdominal wall rather than the chest wall. However, the internal intercostal muscles contribute to forced expiration by drawing the ribs downwards and inwards, thereby narrowing the intercostal spaces.

Intercostal vessels and nerves

Each intercostal space has a principal artery, vein and nerve, which collectively form the neurovascular bundle (Fig. 2.15). This bundle lies in the neurovascular plane between the internal and innermost intercostal muscles and runs along the upper part of the intercostal space, occupying the costal groove of the rib. Usually, the vein lies superiorly and the nerve inferiorly in the bundle. A collateral nerve and collateral vessels arise posteriorly from the neurovascular bundle and run forwards along the lower border of the intercostal space to supply the intercostal muscles.

Intercostal arteries

Intercostal arteries enter from both anterior and posterior ends of the intercostal space. Anteriorly, the internal thoracic arteries (internal mammary arteries) (Fig. 2.16) arising from the subclavian arteries in the root of the neck (see p. 328) provide branches that run laterally to supply the upper six pairs of intercostal spaces. On each side, the lower five spaces receive anterior intercostal arteries from the musculophrenic artery, one of the terminal branches of the internal thoracic artery. These anterior arteries anastomose end-to-end with the posterior intercostal arteries.

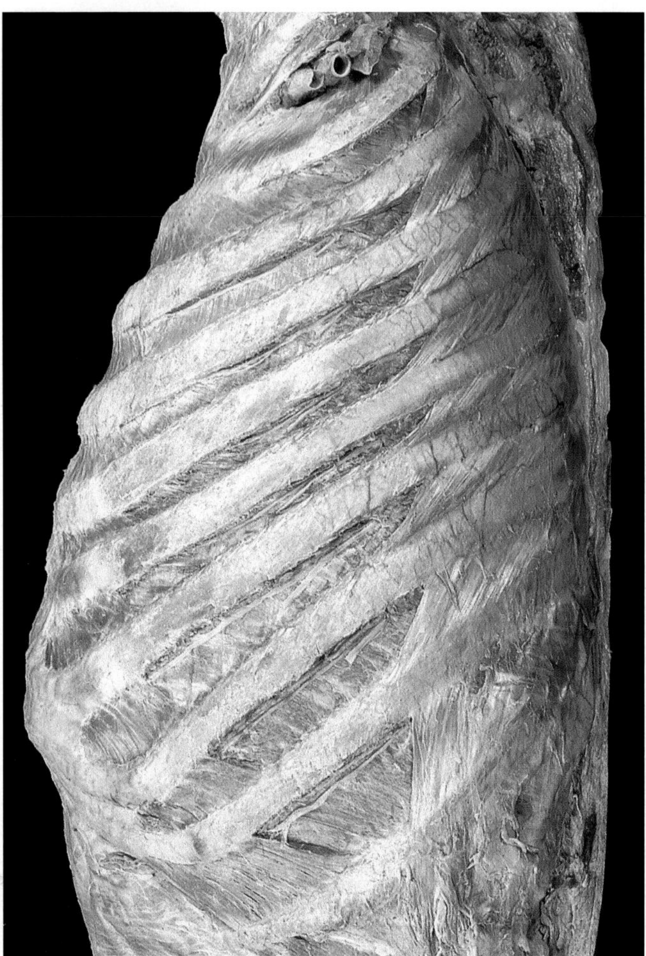

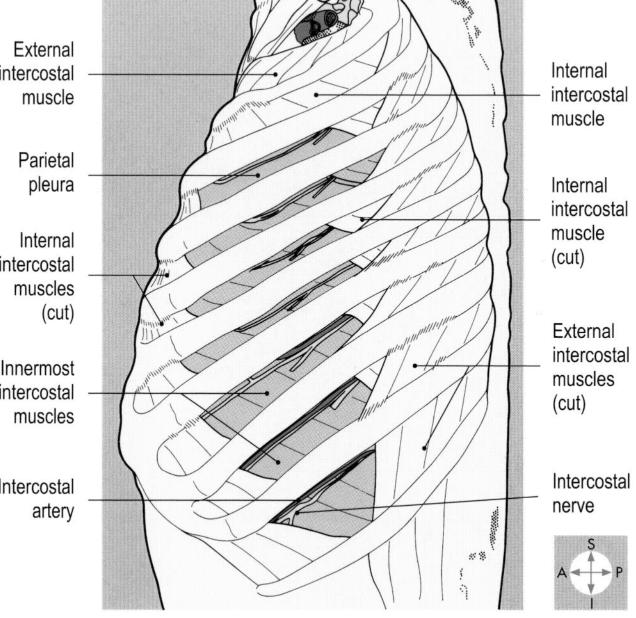

Fig. 2.15 Innermost intercostal muscles and intercostal nerves exposed after removing parts of the internal intercostal muscles. In the third intercostal space the innermost intercostal muscle has been removed to expose the parietal pleura.

Posterior intercostal arteries to the lower nine intercostal spaces arise as direct branches from the descending thoracic aorta (see Fig. 2.63). For the first and second spaces, the posterior intercostal arteries are derived from the intercostal branch of the costocervical trunk. This trunk arises from the subclavian artery (see p. 329) and its intercostal branch enters the thorax by crossing the neck of the first rib. The anastomoses between anterior and posterior intercostal arteries and between the scapular arteries and posterior intercostals are important because they enable blood to reach the descending aorta when the aortic arch is abnormally narrowed (coarctation of the aorta).

Intercostal veins

Anteriorly, the intercostal veins from the lower five intercostal spaces drain into the musculophrenic veins. The upper six intercostal veins and the musculophrenic veins drain into the internal thoracic veins, which themselves are tributaries of the brachiocephalic veins in the root of the neck. Posteriorly, the intercostal veins drain into the azygos venous system. On the right those in the lower eight spaces terminate directly in the azygos vein (see Fig. 2.63). The veins from the second and third spaces combine into a single vessel, the right superior intercostal vein, which drains into the arch of the azygos vein. The first posterior intercostal vein (supreme intercostal vein) leaves the thorax to terminate in the root of the neck, usually in the right vertebral vein.

On the left the lower eight posterior intercostal veins enter either the hemiazygos or accessory hemiazygos veins (see Fig. 2.64). The left superior intercostal vein drains the second and third spaces and crosses the left side of the arch of the aorta to terminate in the left brachiocephalic vein. As on the right the first posterior intercostal vein (supreme intercostal vein) leaves the thorax to terminate usually in the vertebral, but occasionally in the brachiocephalic, vein.

Intercostal nerves

The intercostal nerves comprise the anterior rami of the upper 11 thoracic spinal nerves. Each intercostal nerve enters the neurovascular plane posteriorly (see Fig. 2.64) and gives a collateral branch that supplies the intercostal muscles of the space. Except for the first, each intercostal nerve gives off a lateral cutaneous branch near the midaxillary line which pierces the overlying muscle (see Fig. 1.35). This cutaneous nerve divides into anterior and posterior branches, which supply the adjacent skin. The intercostal nerves of the second to the sixth spaces enter the superficial fascia near the lateral border of the sternum and divide into medial and lateral cutaneous branches.

Most of the fibres of the anterior ramus of the first thoracic spinal nerve join the brachial plexus for distribution to the upper limb (see p. 80). The small first intercostal nerve is the collateral branch and supplies only the muscles of the intercostal space, not the overlying skin.

The intercostal nerves of the lower five spaces continue in the neurovascular plane beyond the costal margin to supply the muscles and skin of the abdominal wall (see p. 145).

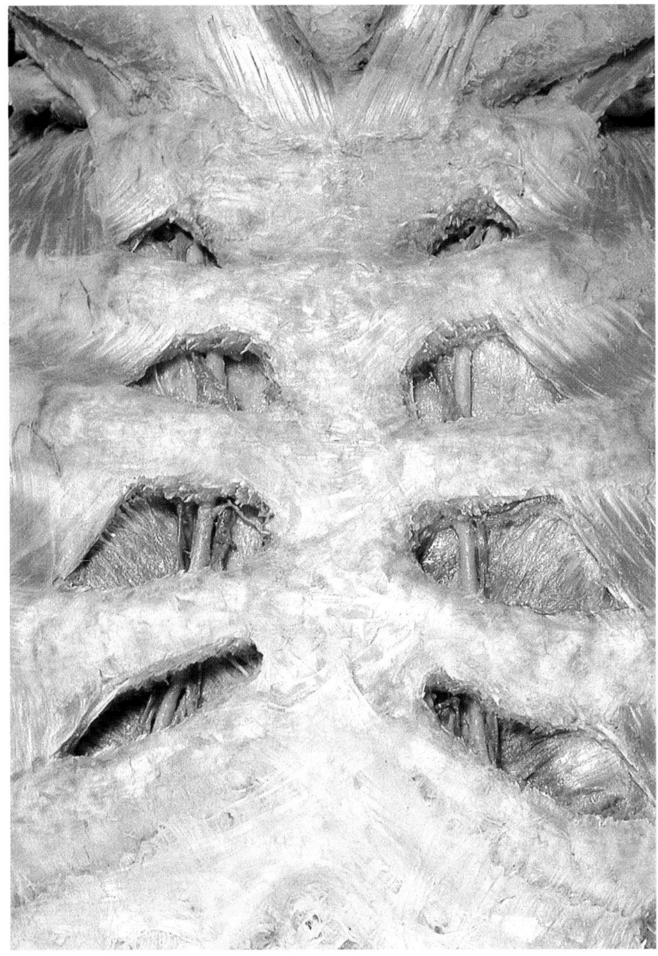

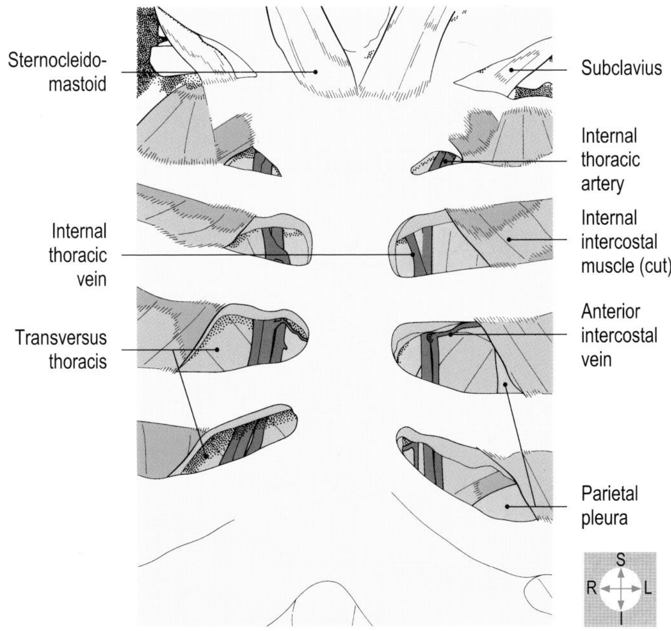

Fig. 2.16 Internal thoracic vessels, revealed by removal of the anterior parts of the intercostal muscles.

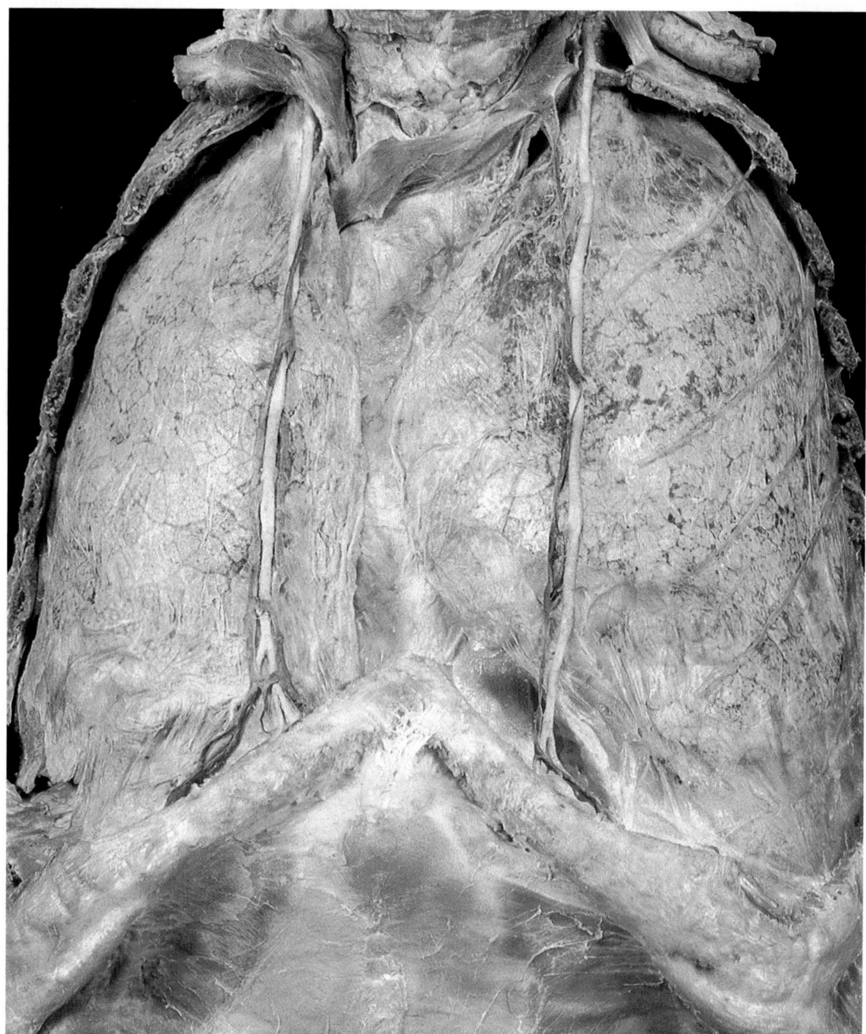

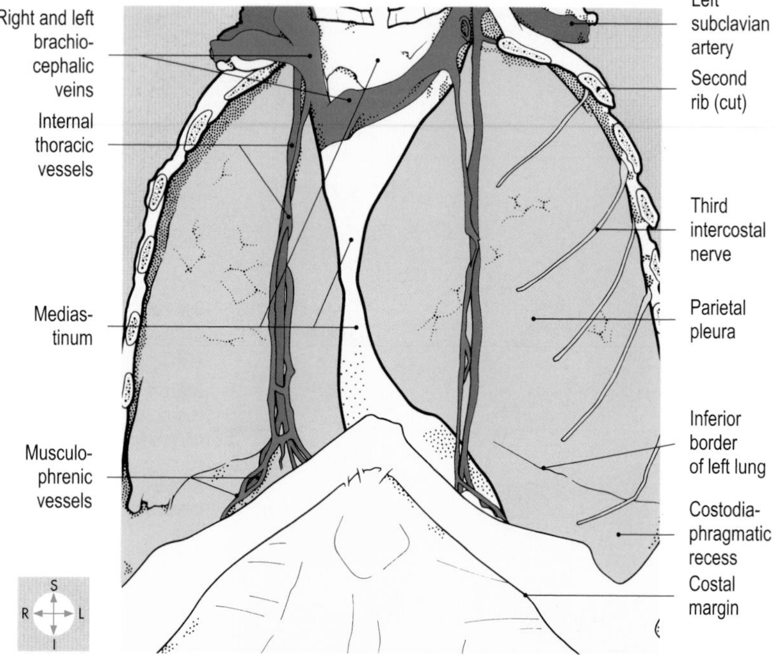

Fig. 2.17 Removal of the anterior chest wall has exposed the internal thoracic vessels and costal part of the parietal pleura, through which the lungs are visible.

Pleura

The thoracic cavity lies within the walls of the thorax and is separated from the abdominal cavity by the diaphragm. The cavity contains the right and left lungs, each surrounded by a serous membrane called the pleura. Between the lungs is a central partition, the mediastinum, which includes the heart and great vessels, the trachea and the oesophagus. Superiorly numerous mediastinal structures enter or leave the root of the neck through the superior thoracic aperture (see pp 328–329). Inferiorly important structures including the aorta, inferior vena cava and oesophagus pass between the mediastinum and the abdomen through openings in the diaphragm (see p. 203).

The pleura surrounds the lungs and lines the walls of the thoracic cavity and is subdivided into visceral and parietal parts. The visceral layer covers the surface of the lung and is continuous with the parietal layer around the mediastinal attachment of the lung at the lung root. The parietal layer covers the lateral aspect of the mediastinum, the upper surface of the diaphragm and the inner aspect of the chest wall (Fig. 2.17). Although the parietal and visceral layers are normally in contact, a space, the pleural cavity (Fig. 2.18), exists between them and contains a thin film of serous fluid. The fluid ensures close apposition of the two pleural surfaces and reduces friction during respiratory movements. Injury or disease may produce an accumulation of air (pneumothorax) or fluid (pleural effusion) within the pleural cavity, causing the lung to collapse.

Parietal pleura

The parietal pleura is named according to the surfaces it covers. Thus, the mediastinal pleura conforms to the contours of the structures forming the lateral surface of the mediastinum and is innervated by sensory branches of the phrenic nerve. Inferiorly the diaphragmatic pleura clothes the upper surface of the diaphragm. The central portion receives sensory branches from each phrenic nerve, whilst the periphery is innervated by lower intercostal nerves. The pleura covering the inner surface of the thoracic wall is called the costal pleura and is innervated segmentally by the intercostal nerves (Fig. 2.17).

The periphery of the diaphragm slopes steeply downwards towards its attachment to the thoracic wall, creating a narrow gutter, the costodiaphragmatic recess. Within this recess, which is particularly deep laterally and posteriorly, the costal and diaphragmatic parts of the parietal pleura lie in mutual contact (see Fig. 4.104).

The parietal pleura extending into the root of the neck is called the cervical pleura and is innervated by the first intercostal nerve. It is applied to the undersurface of a firm fascial layer, the suprapleural membrane, which prevents upward movement of the apex of the lung and pleura during ventilation (see Fig. 7.15).

Surface markings of the parietal pleura

Because the parietal pleura is reflected from the thoracic wall onto both the mediastinum and the diaphragm, a line of pleural reflection can be mapped out on the body surface. Traced from its upper limit, approximately 2.5 cm above the medial third of the clavicle, this line descends behind the sternoclavicular joint and approaches the midline at the level of the manubriosternal joint. On the right the pleural reflection descends vertically to the level of the sixth costal cartilage, while on the left the heart displaces the pleura laterally (Fig. 2.17) so that from the fourth to the sixth costal cartilages the line of reflection lies just lateral to the edge of the sternum. This displacement exposes part of the pericardium underlying the medial ends of the fourth and fifth intercostal spaces. Traced laterally from the sixth costal cartilage, the surface marking is the same on each side, crossing the eighth rib in the midclavicular line and the tenth rib in the midaxillary line.

Posteriorly, the parietal pleura continues horizontally, crosses the twelfth rib 5 cm from the midline and continues medially for a further 2.5 cm. Thus, a small area of parietal pleura lies below the level of the twelfth rib.

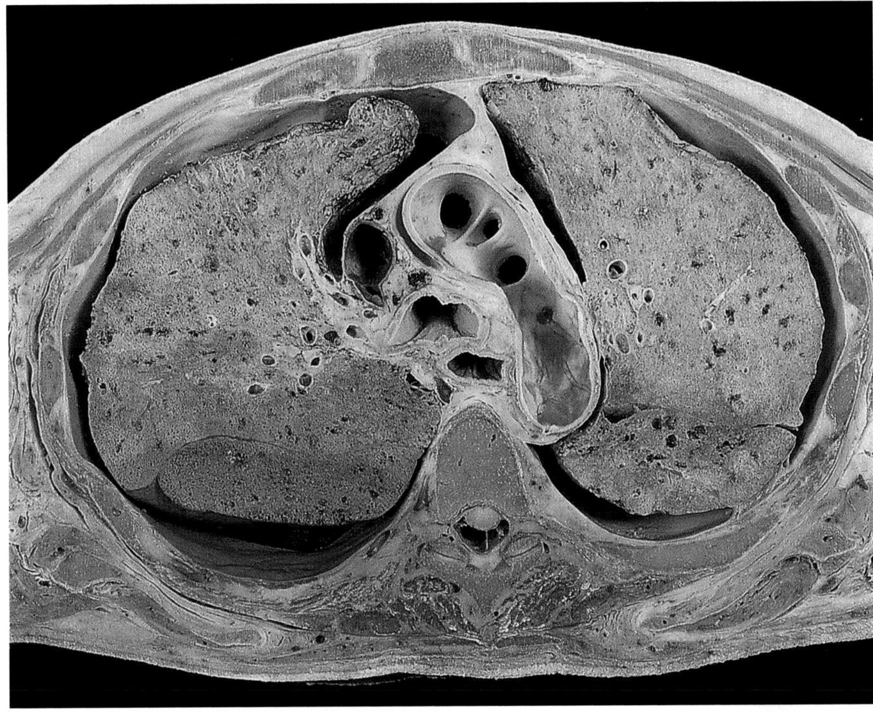

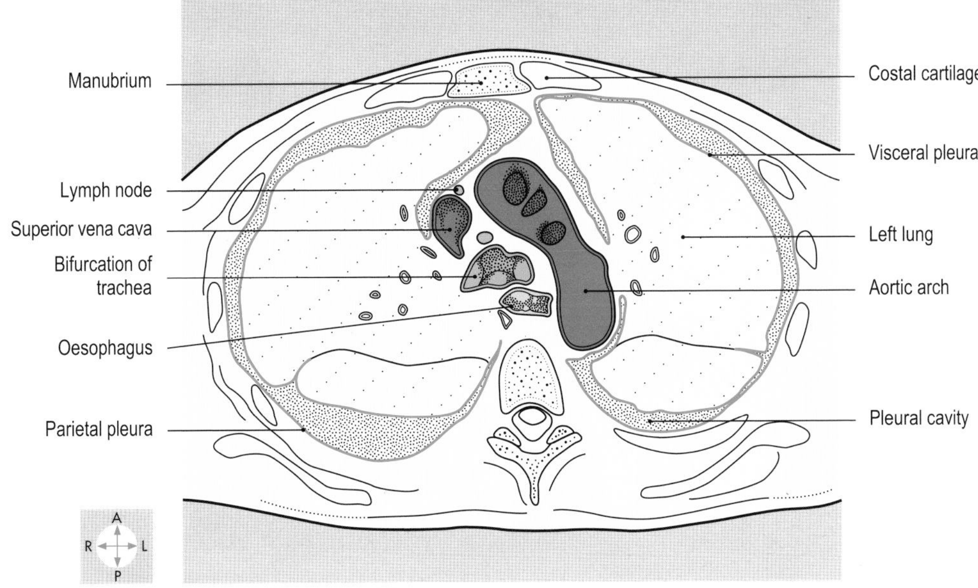

Fig. 2.18 Transverse section at the level of the fourth thoracic vertebra showing the arch of the aorta and the bifurcation of the trachea. Inferior aspect. Compare Fig. 2.67.

Visceral pleura

The visceral pleura (Fig. 2.18) is continuous with the mediastinal parietal pleura around the root of the lung. Structures entering or leaving the lung occupy the upper part of this pleural sleeve, the lower part consisting of an empty fold of pleura, the pulmonary ligament (see Fig. 2.25). The visceral pleura firmly adheres to the surface of the lung and extends into the depths of the fissures. Unlike the parietal layer, visceral pleura does not have a somatic innervation.

Surface markings of the visceral pleura

Since the visceral pleura covers the surface of the lung, its surface markings coincide with those of the lung (see p. 41).

Lungs

The two lungs lie in the thoracic cavity and are separated by the structures in the mediastinum (Fig. 2.19). Although the lungs of infants are pink, those of older individuals may have a mottled appearance due to deposits of inhaled carbon. Living lungs are elastic, enabling their volumes to change during ventilation, in contrast to embalmed lungs, which are rigid and often bear the imprints of adjacent structures. Each lung is covered in visceral pleura and is cone-shaped with the base or diaphragmatic surface directed downwards and the apex upwards. The costal surface is smoothly convex while the mediastinal surface is irregular and bears the hilum of the organ. Fissures are usually present, and divide each lung into lobes (usually three lobes on the right and two on the left). Most of the lung consists of the peripheral part of the respiratory tract and the associated pulmonary vascular system. Having entered the lung, the bronchi and pulmonary vessels subdivide extensively (see Fig. 2.26).

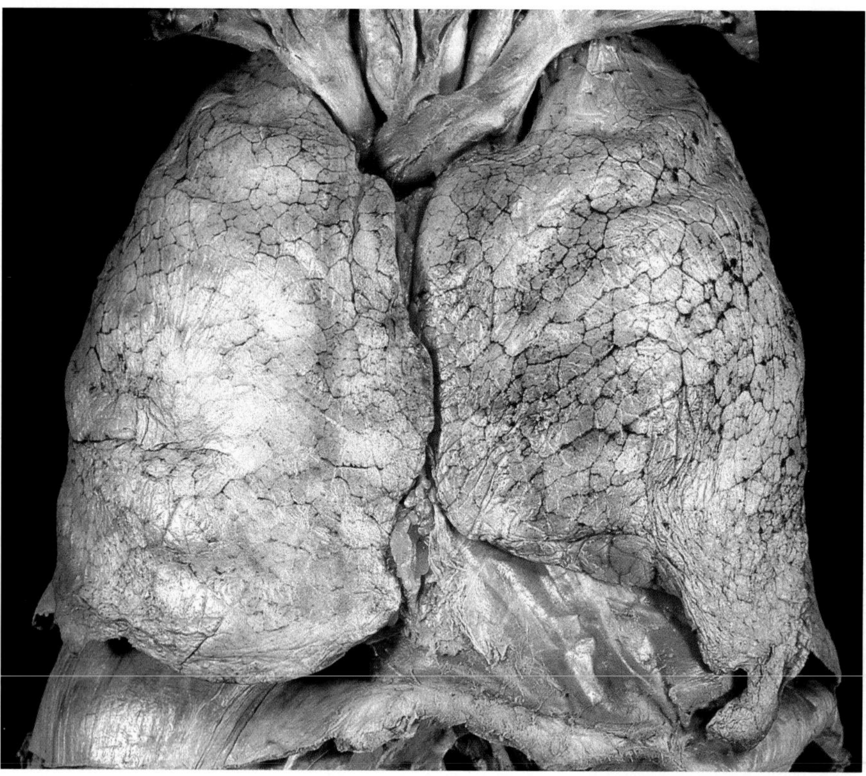

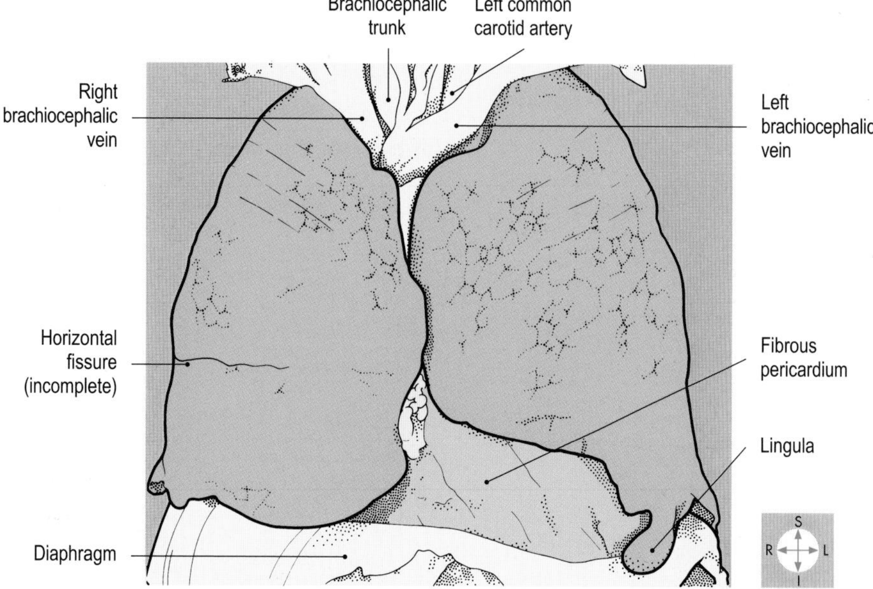

Fig. 2.19 Lungs, after removal of the anterolateral thoracic wall and parietal pleura. In this specimen the lungs overlie more of the mediastinum than is usual.

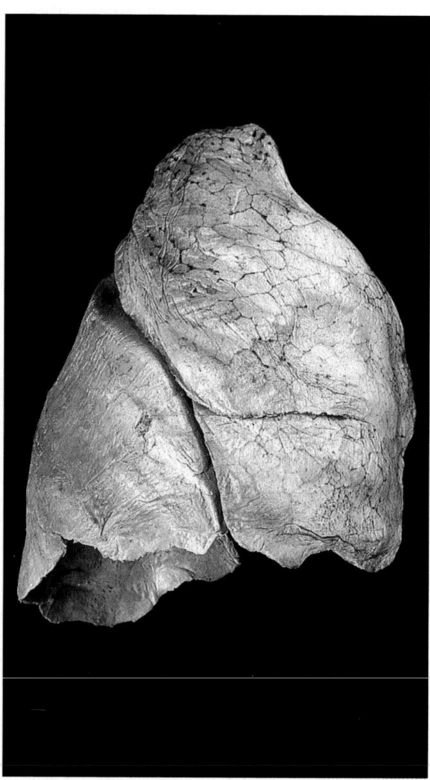

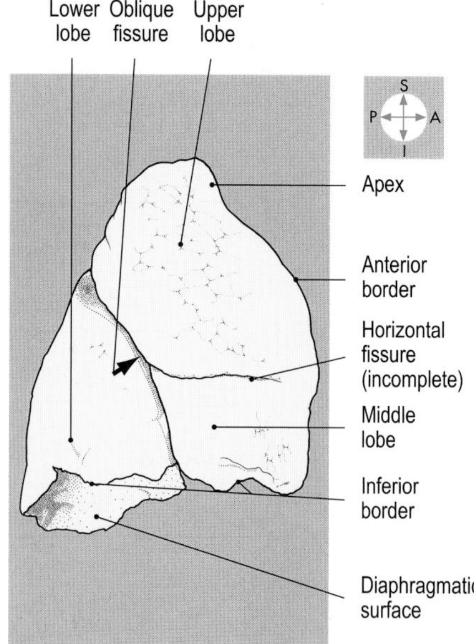

Fig. 2.20 Costal surface of the right lung, showing oblique and horizontal fissures and the upper, middle and lower lobes.

Fissures

Although variations occur, each lung is usually divided into upper and lower lobes by an oblique fissure. On the right the upper lobe is further subdivided by the horizontal fissure (Fig. 2.20), which runs from the anterior border of the lung into the oblique fissure and demarcates the middle lobe. On the left the horizontal fissure is usually absent and the middle lobe is represented by the lingula (Fig. 2.21).

Surfaces, borders and relations

The costal surface is convex and extends upwards into the cervical part of the pleura to form the apex of the lung, which is closely related to the corresponding subclavian artery and vein. The inferior surface (base) is markedly concave (Figs 2.22 & 2.23), conforming to the upward convexity of the dome of the diaphragm. The costal and diaphragmatic surfaces meet at the sharp inferior border. The anterior border is also sharp and is formed where the costal and mediastinal surfaces are in continuity. In contrast, the posterior border is rounded and rather indistinct.

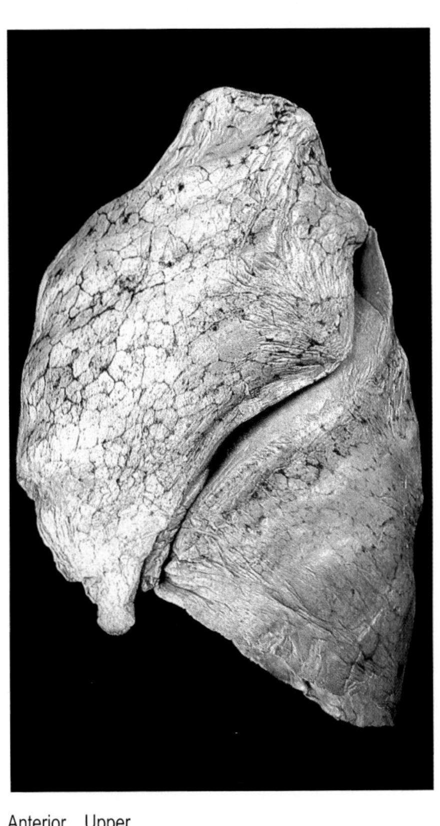

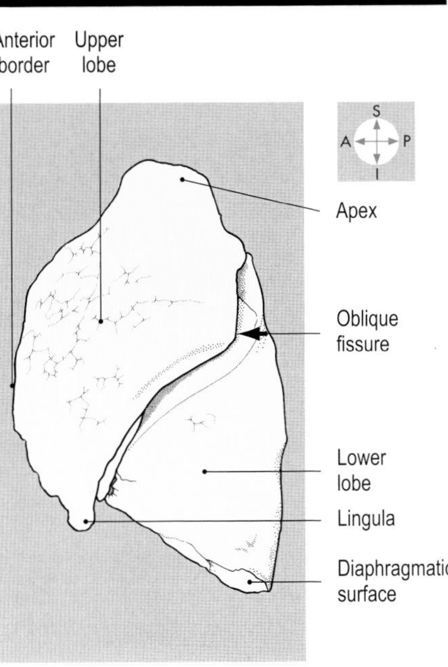

Fig. 2.21 Costal surface of the left lung showing the oblique fissure and upper and lower lobes.

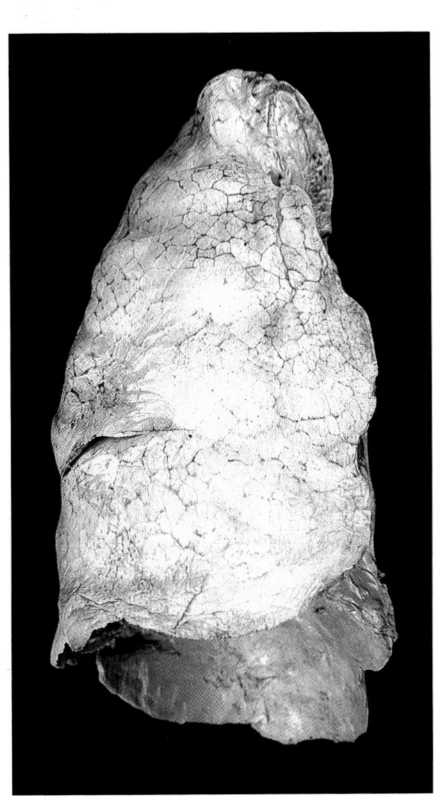

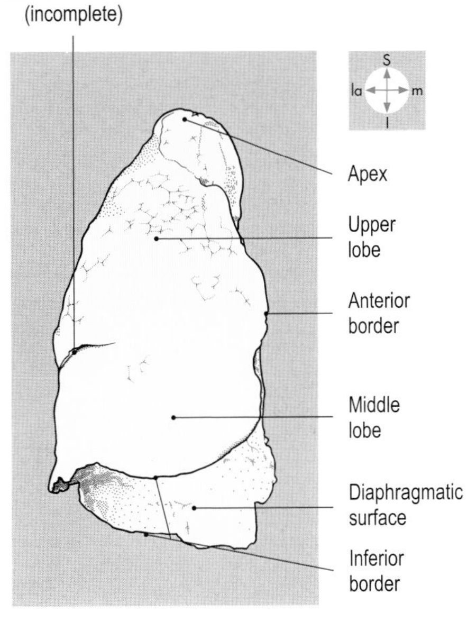

Fig. 2.22 Right lung, showing its concave inferior surface and sharp anterior and inferior borders.

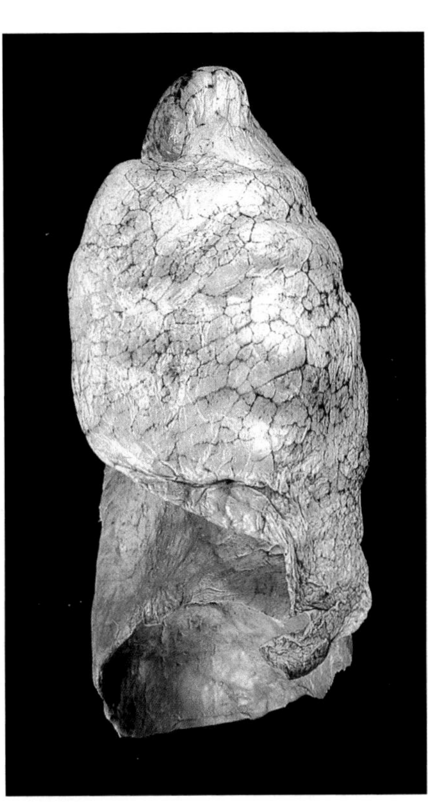

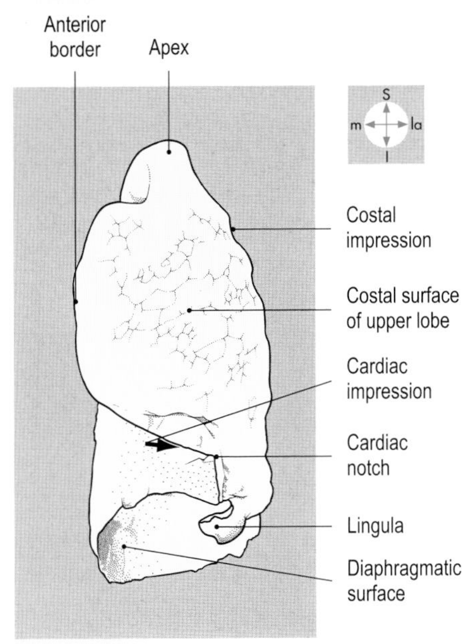

Fig. 2.23 Left lung, showing the cardiac notch and lingula, both of which are particularly obvious in this specimen.

Each lung is attached to the mediastinum by the lung root, the principal components of which are the pulmonary vessels and the bronchi. These structures, accompanied by bronchial vessels, lymphatics and autonomic nerves, enter or leave the lung through the hilum. Usually two pulmonary veins emerge from each lung, the inferior vein being the lowest structure in the hilum (Figs 2.24 & 2.25). The bronchi and pulmonary arteries are adjacent as they pass through the hilum, and on the left the main bronchus lies anterior to the pulmonary artery. However, on the right, the main bronchus frequently divides into two branches, the upper and lower lobe bronchi, before reaching the lung, and each bronchus is accompanied by a branch of the pulmonary artery. The hila of both lungs often contain lymph nodes, which are recognizable by their acquired dark coloration (see Fig. 2.27).

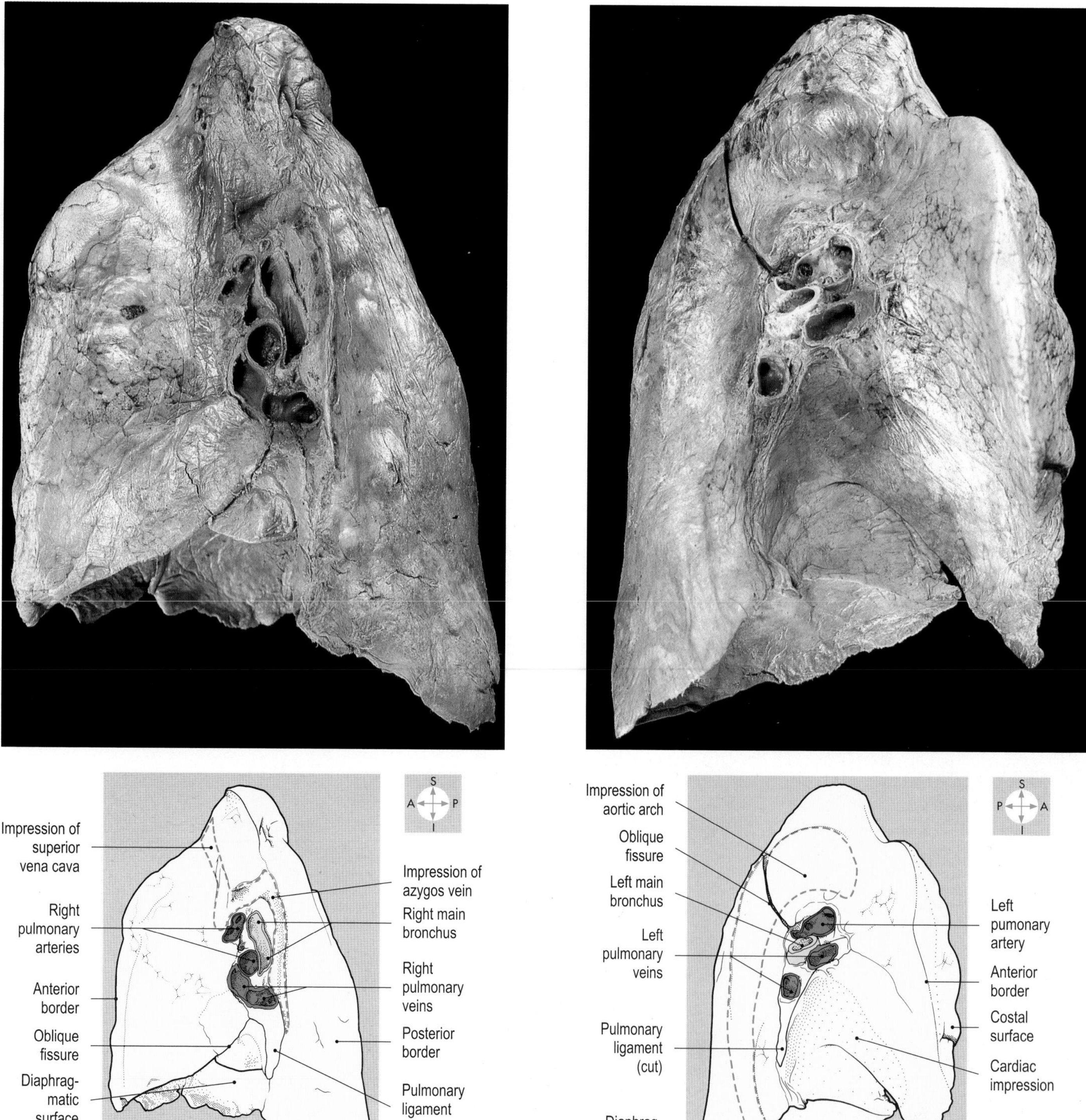

Fig. 2.24 Mediastinal surface of the right lung.

Fig. 2.25 Mediastinal surface of the left lung.

The two lungs have different medial relations. On the right the anterior part of the mediastinal surface of the lung is related to the right brachiocephalic vein, the superior vena cava and the pericardium covering the right atrium of the heart. Intervening between these structures and the mediastinal pleura is the right phrenic nerve, which descends in front of the hilum to reach the diaphragm. The upper part of the hilum is related to the azygos vein (Fig. 2.24), which arches forwards to terminate in the superior vena cava. The trachea and accompanying right vagus nerve are related to the right upper lobe.

On the left, the mediastinal surface of the lung bears distinct impressions produced by the fibrous pericardium and the heart (Fig. 2.25). The left phrenic nerve is related to the mediastinal pleura and passes in front of the hilum as it descends across the pericardium. The aorta creates an obvious groove (Fig. 2.25) where it arches over the lung root and descends behind the hilum as the descending thoracic aorta.

Surface markings

The apex of each lung rises above the medial third of the clavicle. From here the anterior border of the lung follows the reflection of the parietal pleura, passing behind the sternoclavicular and manubriosternal joints. On the right the border descends vertically, close to the midline from the level of the second to the sixth costal cartilages (see Fig. 2.2). On the left the heart displaces the lung and parietal pleura so that the pericardium is exposed behind the medial ends of the fourth and fifth intercostal spaces. This location is sometimes used to insert a needle into the pericardial cavity or heart. On both sides, the inferior border of the lung crosses the sixth rib in the midclavicular line, the eighth rib in the midaxillary line and the tenth rib 5 cm from the midline posteriorly. The lower border of the lung lies at a higher level than the line of pleural reflection; this part of the pleural cavity not occupied by lung is called the costodiaphragmatic recess (see Fig. 4.105) and may be fluid filled in pleural effusion.

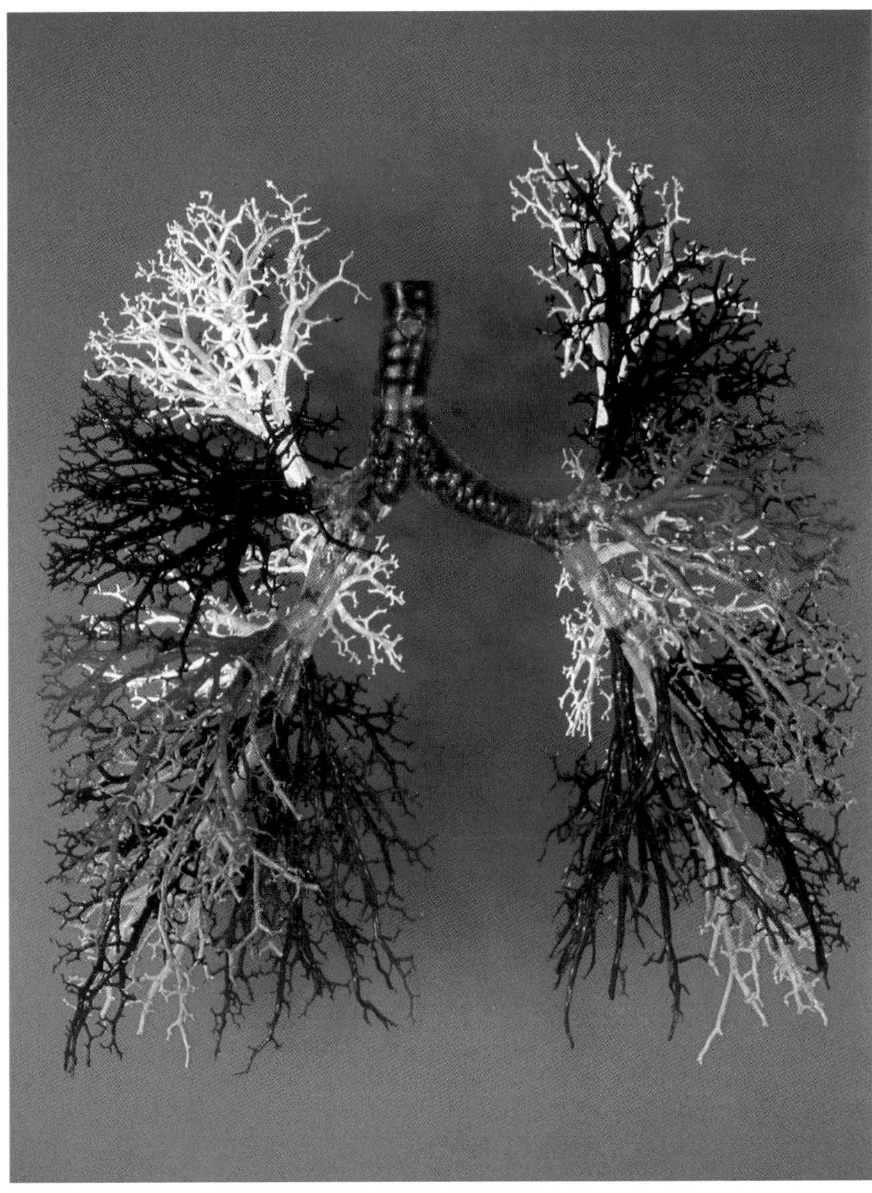

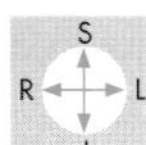

Fig. 2.26 Resin corrosion cast of the lower trachea and the bronchial tree. The amber portions of the specimen relate to the trachea, the main (primary) bronchi and the lobar (secondary) bronchi, while the coloured portions are the segmental (tertiary) bronchi and their branches.

Bronchi

The bifurcation of the trachea in the mediastinum gives rise to the right and left main (principal) bronchi (see Fig. 2.26).

The right main bronchus is wider and more steeply inclined than the left (Fig. 2.27). The main bronchi give rise to lobar (secondary) bronchi, which are confined to their respective lobes. On the right the upper lobe bronchus arises outside the hilum in the lung root, whereas on the left the lobar bronchi arise entirely within the lung. In each lobe, further subdivision occurs into segmental (tertiary) bronchi, which are constant in position and supply specific portions of lung called bronchopulmonary segments. Each lobe consists of a definite number of these segments. Within individual segments the bronchi further sub-divide into bronchioles, then respiratory bronchioles, which in turn lead into the alveolar ducts and alveoli. Bronchial arteries derived from the descending thoracic aorta accompany and supply the major bronchi. Venous return from the bronchi is through bronchial veins that terminate in the azygos venous system (see p. 62).

Pulmonary vessels

The right and left pulmonary arteries divide into branches that correspond to and accompany the subdivisions of the bronchi within the lungs. The bronchi and pulmonary arteries lie centrally in the bronchopulmonary segments. The arteries ultimately give rise to pulmonary capillaries in the alveolar walls. Oxygenated blood drains from these capillaries into tributaries of the pulmonary veins that occupy intersegmental positions. These vessels empty into two pulmonary veins, which usually emerge separately through each hilum (see Figs 2.24 & 2.25) and drain into the left atrium.

Autonomic nerves

The pulmonary plexus, most of which lies behind the lung root, contains both sympathetic and parasympathetic fibres, which accompany the bronchi into the lung. Sympathetic nerves originate in the upper thoracic ganglia of the sympathetic trunk and supply smooth muscle in the walls of the bronchi and pulmonary blood vessels. The parasympathetic fibres are derived from the vagus nerves and supply bronchial smooth muscle and mucous glands.

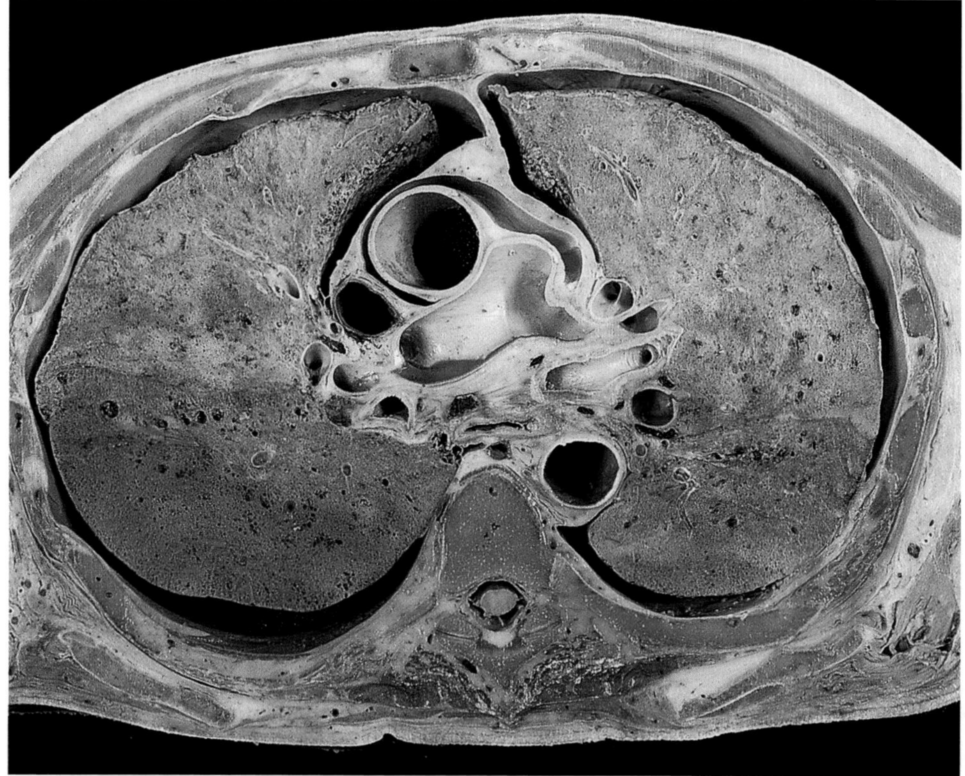

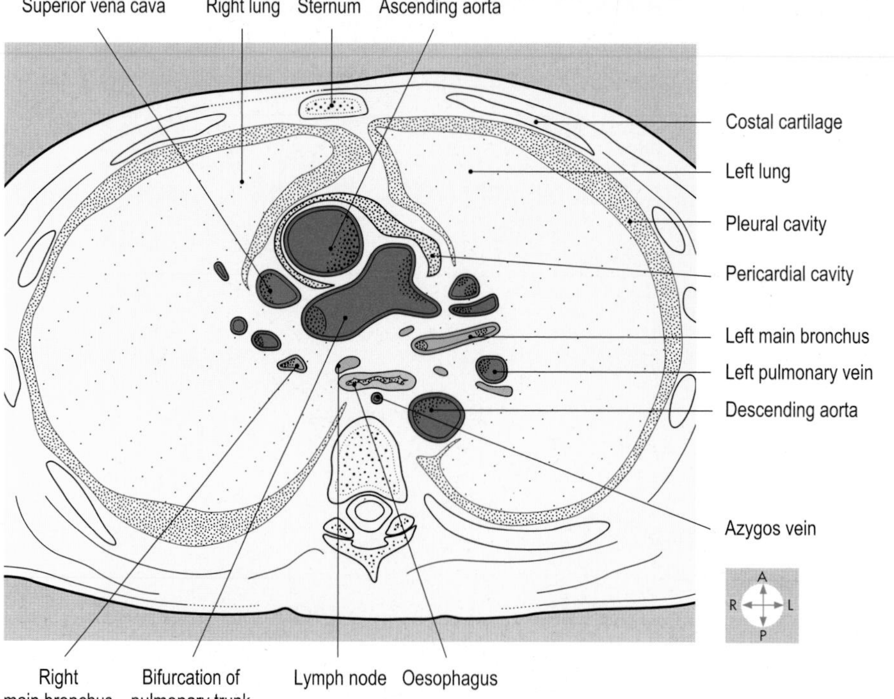

Fig. 2.27 Transverse section at the level of the fifth thoracic vertebra showing the bifurcation of the pulmonary trunk. Inferior aspect. Compare Fig. 2.68.

Mediastinum

The central part of the thorax between the two pleural cavities contains a group of structures collectively termed the mediastinum. These include the heart and great vessels, the trachea and the oesophagus. The mediastinum extends from the superior thoracic aperture above to the diaphragm below and from the sternum in front to the thoracic vertebral bodies behind (Fig. 2.28). By convention, the mediastinum is divided into superior and inferior parts by an imaginary horizontal plane passing through the manubriosternal joint and the lower part of the fourth thoracic vertebra. The superior mediastinum lies between this plane and the superior thoracic aperture and contains the superior vena cava and its tributaries, the arch of the aorta and its branches and the trachea. Also passing through this region are the oesophagus, the thoracic duct and the right and left vagus and phrenic nerves.

The inferior mediastinum lies between the imaginary plane and the diaphragm and consists of three compartments. The largest of these is the middle mediastinum, containing the heart and its covering of fibrous pericardium. In front of the middle mediastinum lies the anterior mediastinum, consisting of a small amount of fat and the remnants of the thymus gland. Behind the fibrous pericardium lies the posterior mediastinum, traversed by the descending thoracic aorta, the oesophagus and the thoracic duct. The sympathetic trunks run alongside the thoracic vertebral bodies.

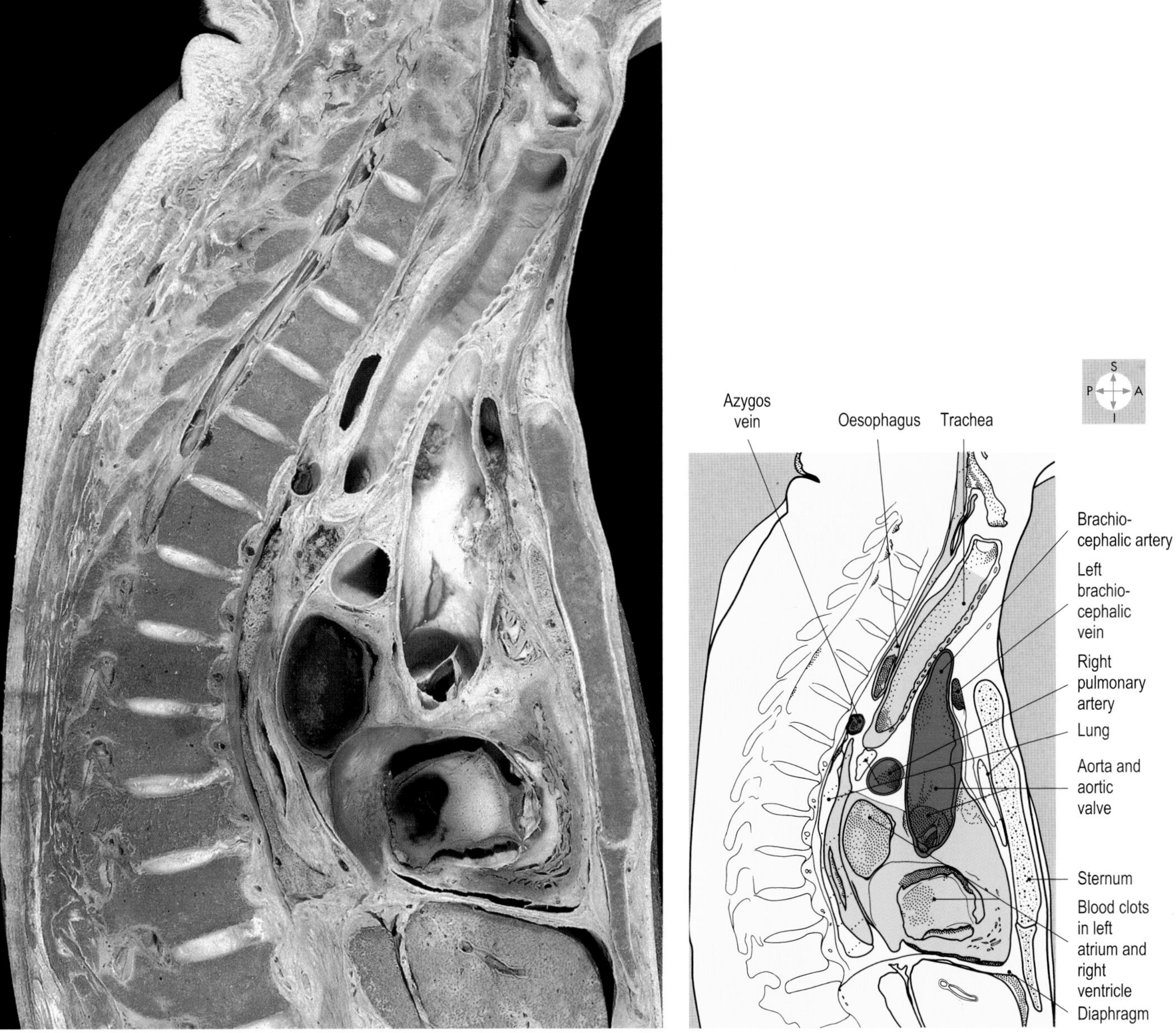

Fig. 2.28 Near-midline sagittal section through the thorax showing some mediastinal structures.

Pericardium

Fibrous pericardium

The fibrous pericardium is a sac of dense connective tissue surrounding the heart. In addition to the heart, it encloses the roots of the great arteries and veins and is covered on its inner surface by serous pericardium (see below). The broad base of the fibrous pericardium is attached to the central tendon of the diaphragm (Fig. 2.29) and is pierced by the inferior vena cava.

Superiorly the sac fuses with the adventitial layers of the aorta, pulmonary trunk and superior vena cava. On each side, the posterior part of the sac blends with the walls of the pulmonary veins.

The anterior aspect of the fibrous pericardium is related to the anterior parts of the two lungs and the anterior reflections of the pleura. Between the pleural reflections, the pericardium lies close to the body of the sternum and to the medial ends of the adjacent fourth and fifth left costal cartilages and associated intercostal structures. During infancy and childhood the thymus (most of which lies in the superior mediastinum) is related to the anterior surface of the pericardium, but after puberty the thymus regresses and is gradually replaced by fat.

Laterally, the pericardium is covered by mediastinal pleura and is crossed by the right and left phrenic nerves as they descend to the diaphragm. These nerves supply sensory fibres to the fibrous pericardium, the parietal serous pericardium and the mediastinal pleura. Most of the blood supply to the fibrous pericardium is provided by the internal thoracic arteries and veins via pericardiacophrenic vessels that accompany the phrenic nerves.

Behind the fibrous pericardium lie the oesophagus, the descending thoracic aorta and the thoracic duct (see p. 61–62).

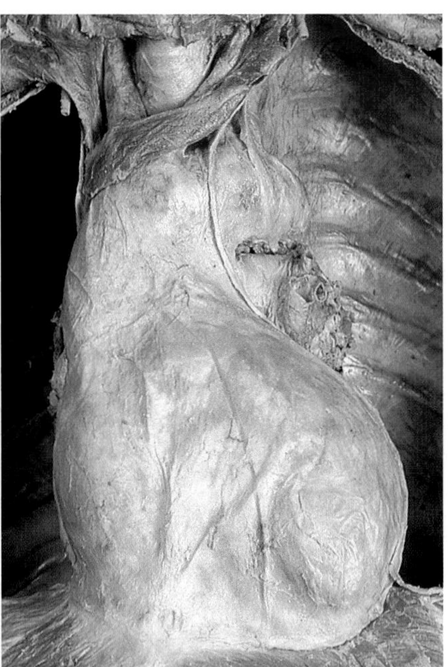

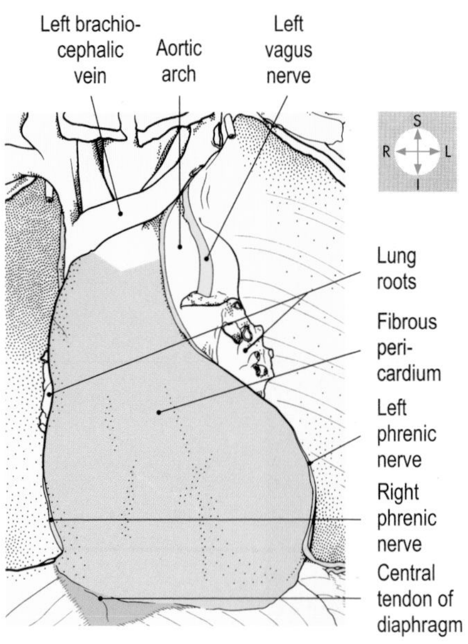

Fig. 2.29 The fibrous pericardium and phrenic nerves revealed after removal of the lungs.

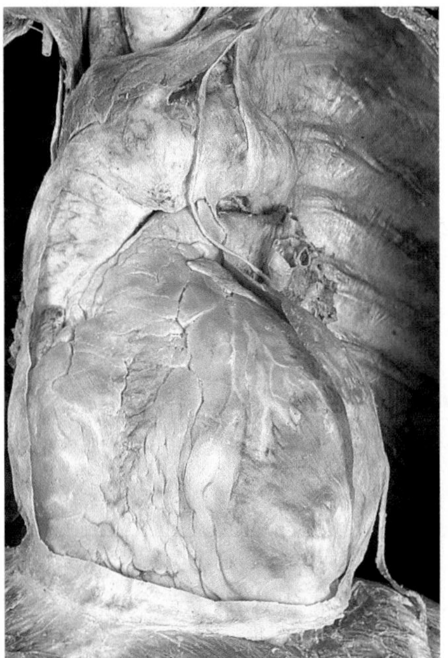

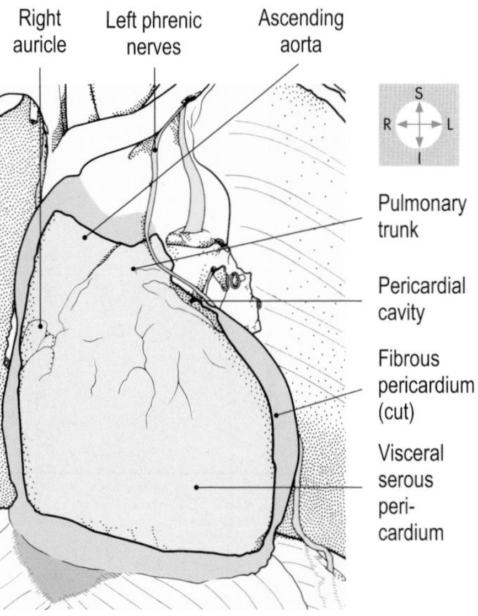

Fig. 2.30 The fibrous pericardium has been opened to expose the visceral pericardium covering the anterior surface of the heart.

Serous pericardium

Deep to the fibrous pericardium lies the serous pericardium, consisting of parietal and visceral layers. Between the two layers is the pericardial cavity, a narrow space containing a thin film of serous fluid. The parietal layer lines the inner surface of the fibrous pericardium, to which it is firmly attached. The visceral layer covers the outer surface of the heart and the roots of the great vessels (Fig. 2.30).

These two layers slide freely against each other and are in continuity where the great vessels pierce the fibrous pericardium. The reflections between the parietal and visceral layers form two sleeves. One sleeve surrounds the ascending aorta and pulmonary trunk; the second is more extensive and surrounds the superior and inferior venae cavae and pulmonary veins. The two pericardial sleeves lie adjacent to each other and the narrow intervening channel is called the transverse pericardial sinus (see Fig. 2.40). A second sinus lies behind the left atrium of the heart. This is the oblique pericardial sinus, which is limited superiorly by the pericardial reflection around the pulmonary veins and superior vena cava (see Fig. 2.35). An accumulation of fluid (e.g. blood) within the pericardial cavity may compromise venous return to the heart and therefore reduce cardiac output.

Heart

External features

The heart, enclosed in pericardium, occupies the middle mediastinum. It is roughly cone-shaped and lies behind the sternum with its base facing posteriorly and its apex projecting inferiorly, anteriorly and to the left, producing the cardiac impression in the left lung.

The heart consists of four chambers, namely the right and left atria and the right and left ventricles (Fig. 2.31). A fat-filled groove, the coronary or atrioventricular sulcus, separates the surfaces of the atria from the ventricles and carries the right and left coronary arteries and the coronary sinus. The right atrium receives the superior and inferior venae cavae and the coronary sinus. The right and left pulmonary veins drain into the left atrium. The right ventricle is continuous with the pulmonary trunk while the left ventricle opens into the ascending aorta.

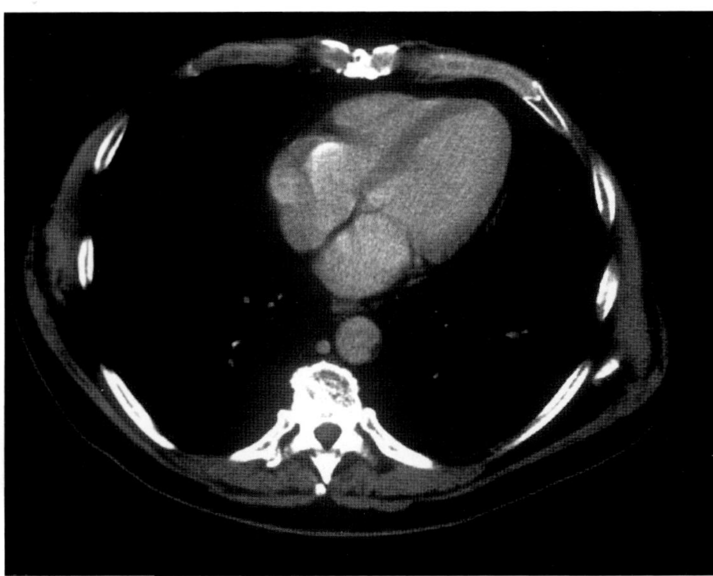

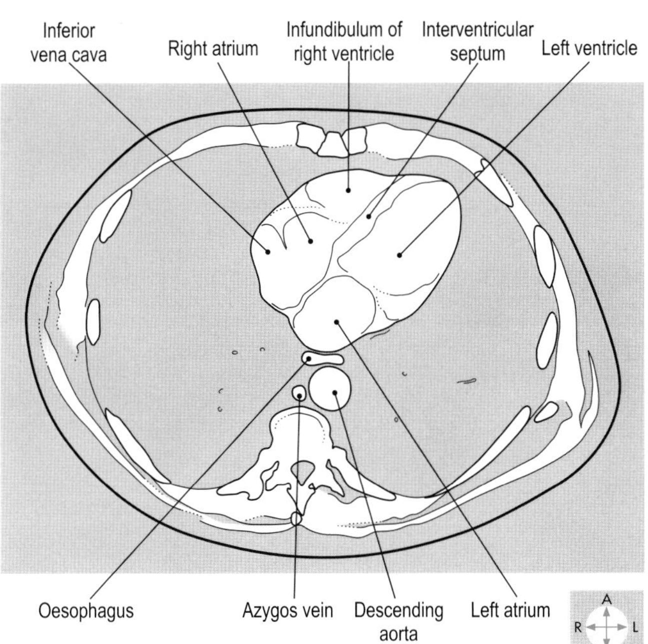

Fig. 2.31 Transverse CT image at the level of the eighth thoracic vertebra. Compare Fig. 2.71.

Borders

It is useful in clinical practice to represent the outline of the heart as a projection onto the anterior chest wall. When represented in this way the heart has right, inferior and left borders (Fig. 2.32). The right border is formed by the right atrium and runs between the third and sixth right costal cartilages approximately 3 cm from the midline. The inferior border is formed mainly by the right atrium and right ventricle. At its left extremity, the border is completed by that part of the left ventricle which forms the apex of the heart. The inferior border runs from the sixth right costal cartilage approximately 3 cm from the midline to the apex, which usually lies behind the fifth left intercostal space, 6 cm from the midline. In the living, the apex usually produces an impulse (apex beat) palpable on the anterior chest wall. The left ventricle together with the left auricle (left atrial appendage) form the left border of the heart, which slopes upwards and medially from the apex to the second left intercostal space, approximately 3 cm from the midline.

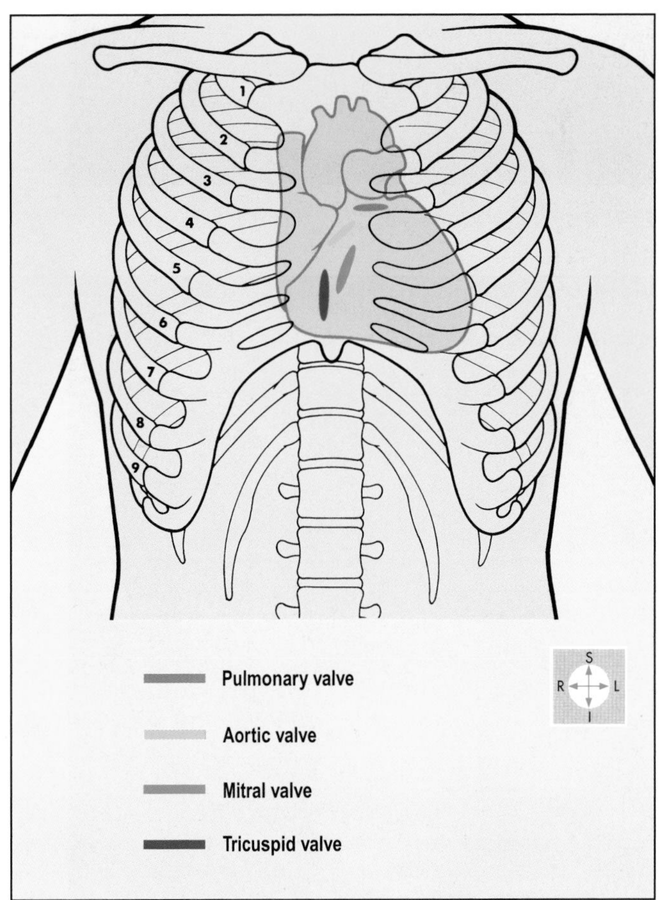

Fig. 2.32 Borders and valves of the heart and their relationships to the anterior chest wall.

Surfaces

Most of the anterior surface of the heart consists of the right atrium and right ventricle (Fig. 2.33). The left ventricle contributes a narrow strip adjacent to the left border of the heart. The anterior surface is completed by the right and left auricles. The coronary sulcus descends more or less vertically across the anterior surface and contains the right coronary artery surrounded by fat. The anterior surfaces of the right and left ventricles are separated by the anterior interventricular artery (left anterior descending artery).

Most of the inferior (diaphragmatic) surface of the heart (Fig. 2.34) consists of the two ventricles, the left usually contributing the greater area. The posterior interventricular vessels mark the boundary between these two chambers. The surface is completed by a small portion of the right atrium adjacent to the termination of the inferior vena cava.

The posterior surface or base of the heart (Fig. 2.35) consists mostly of the left atrium together with a small part of the right atrium.

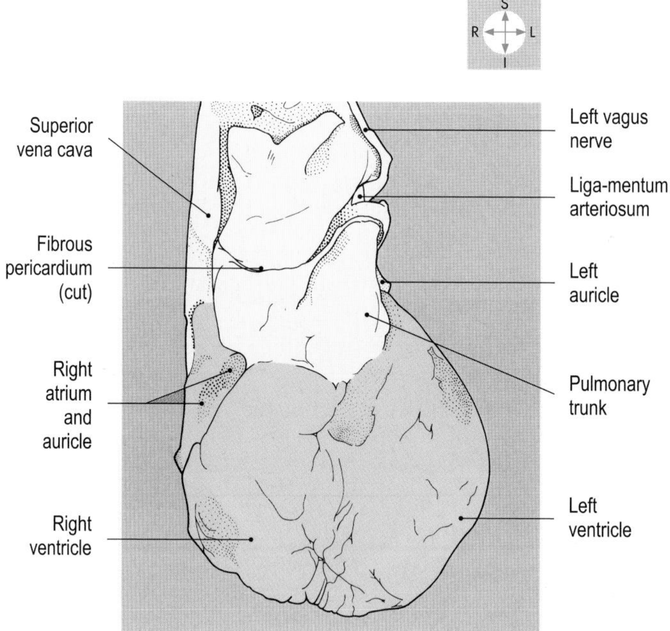

Fig. 2.33 Anterior surface of the heart.

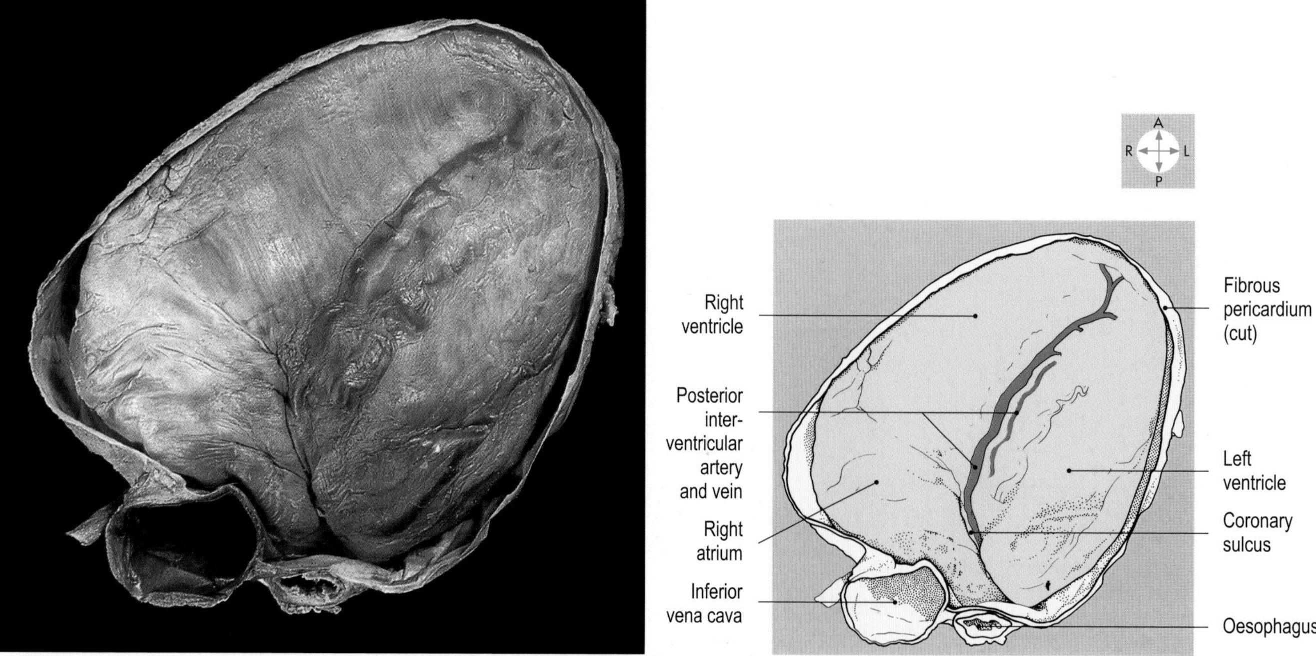

Fig. 2.34 Inferior surface of the heart. The inferior part of the fibrous pericardium has been removed with the diaphragm.

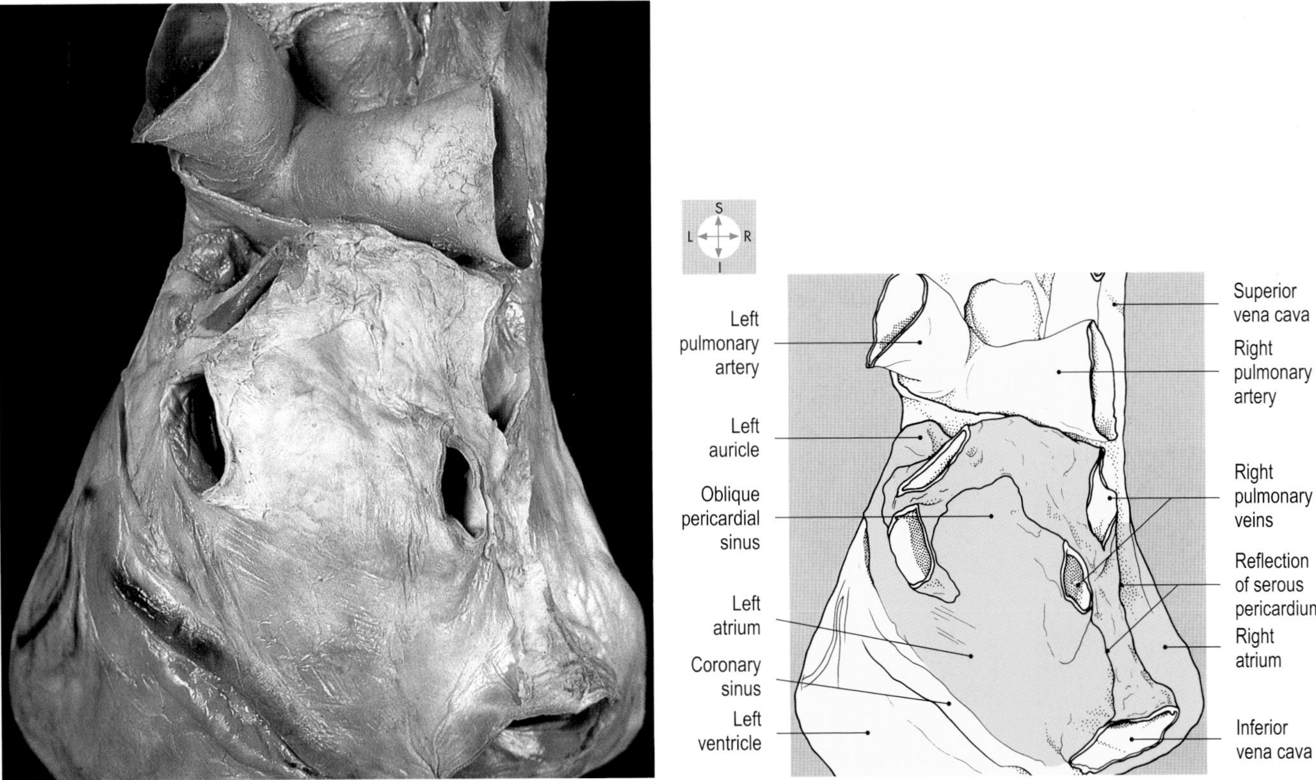

Fig. 2.35 The posterior surface of the heart showing the reflection of the serous pericardium and the site of the oblique pericardial sinus.

Chambers and valves

The cavities of the right and left atria are continuous with those of their respective ventricles through the atrioventricular orifices. Each orifice possesses an atrioventricular valve, which prevents backflow of blood from the ventricle into the atrium. The myocardium of the atria is separated from that of the ventricles by connective tissue, which forms a complete fibrous ring around each atrioventricular orifice. Interatrial and interventricular septa separate the cavities of the atria and ventricles. Valves, each with three semilunar cusps, guard the orifices between the right ventricle and pulmonary trunk (pulmonary valve) and the left ventricle and ascending aorta (aortic valve). All these valves close passively in response to differential pressure gradients.

Right atrium

The right atrium receives blood from the superior and inferior venae cavae and from the coronary sinus and cardiac veins which drain the myocardium. The superior vena cava enters the upper part of the chamber. Adjacent to its termination is a broad triangular prolongation of the atrium, the auricle (atrial appendage), which overlaps the ascending aorta (Fig. 2.36).

Internally, the anterior wall of the right atrium possesses a vertical ridge, the crista terminalis (Fig. 2.36). From the crista, muscular ridges (musculi pectinati) run to the left and extend into the auricle. The posterior (septal) wall is relatively smooth but possesses a well-defined ridge surrounding a shallow depression named the fossa ovalis. This fossa is the site of the foramen ovale, which, in the fetus, allows blood to pass directly from the right to the left atrium. The coronary sinus empties into the chamber close to the atrioventricular orifice. Inferiorly the right atrium receives the inferior vena cava immediately after the vessel has pierced the central tendon of the diaphragm. A fold called the valve of the inferior vena cava (Fig. 2.36) projects into the chamber and is the remnant of a fetal structure that directed the flow of blood across the right atrium towards the foramen ovale.

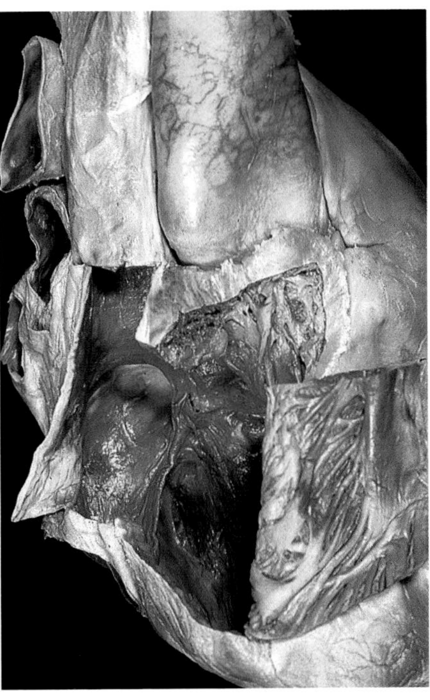

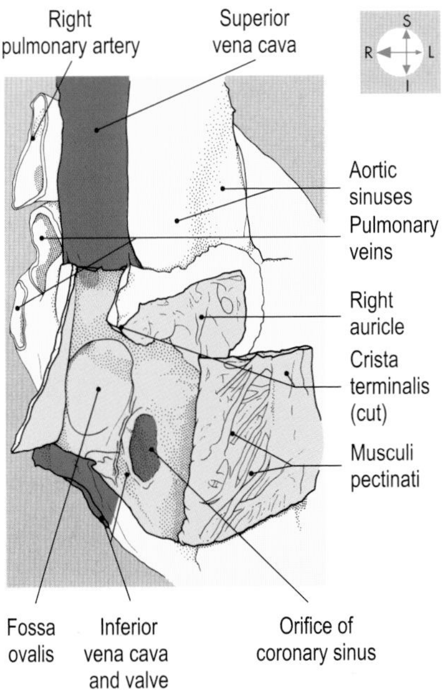

Fig. 2.36 Interior of the right atrium and auricle, exposed by reflection and excision of part of the anterior atrial wall.

Tricuspid valve

From the right atrium blood flows into the right ventricle through the right atrioventricular orifice, which is guarded by the tricuspid valve (Fig. 2.37). The valve possesses three cusps, the bases of which attach to the margins of the atrioventricular orifice while their free borders project into the cavity of the right ventricle (Fig. 2.38), where they are anchored by fibrous strands (chordae tendineae) to the papillary muscles of the ventricle. During ventricular contraction (systole) the papillary muscles pull on the chordae, preventing eversion of the valve cusps and reflux of blood into the atrium. The valve lies in the midline behind the lower part of the body of the sternum (see Fig. 2.32) and its sounds are heard best by auscultation over the xiphisternum.

Right ventricle

The right ventricle has the right atrium on its right and the left ventricle both behind and to its left. The chamber forms parts of the anterior and inferior surfaces of the heart and narrows superiorly at the infundibulum, which leads into the pulmonary trunk (Fig. 2.38). The walls of the right ventricle are thicker than those of

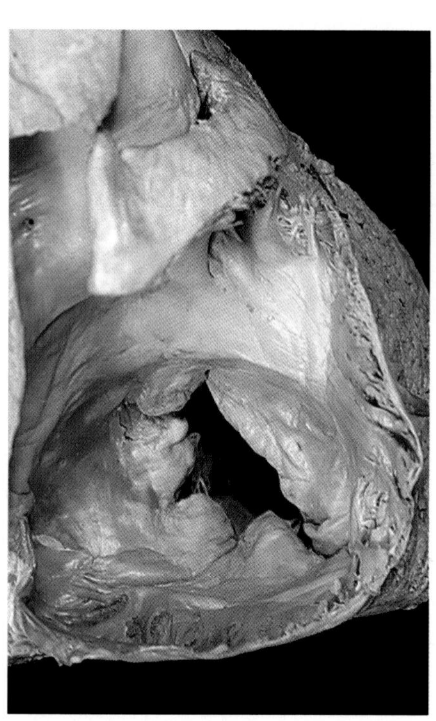

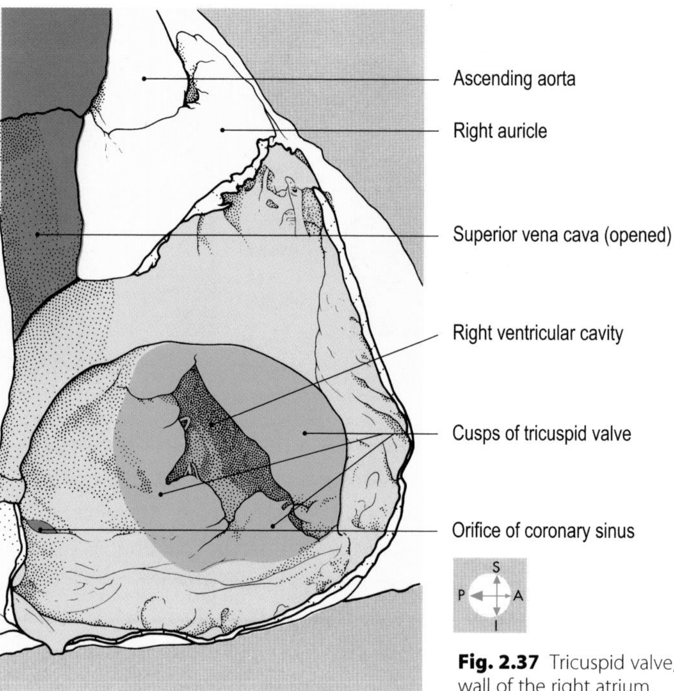

Fig. 2.37 Tricuspid valve, revealed after removal of the lateral wall of the right atrium.

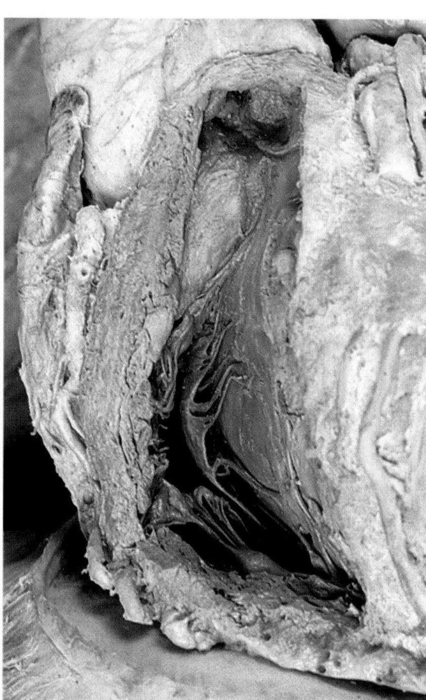

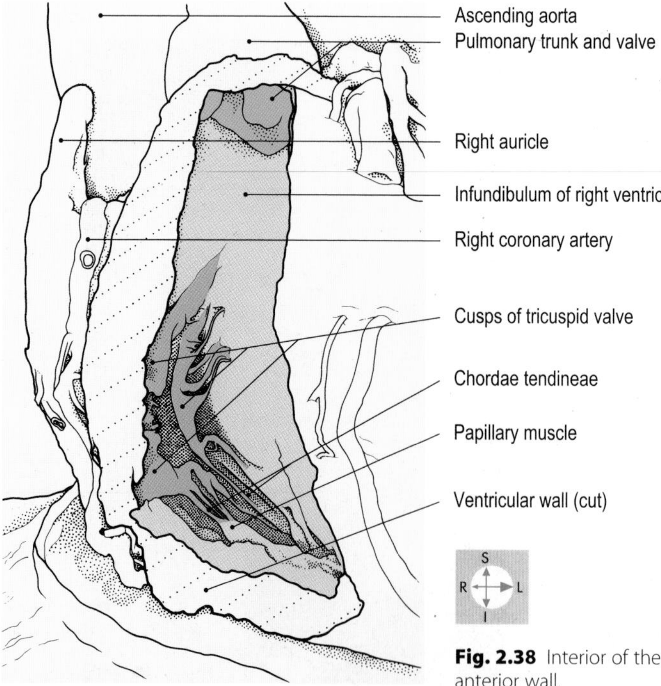

Fig. 2.38 Interior of the right ventricle seen after removal of its anterior wall.

the right atrium and internally possess numerous muscular ridges called trabeculae carneae (see Fig. 2.43). One of these, the moderator band (see Fig. 2.54), often bridges the cavity of the chamber, connecting the interventricular septum to the anterior ventricular wall. When present, it carries the right branch of the atrioventricular bundle of conducting tissue (see p. 56). Projecting from the ventricular walls into the interior of the chamber are processes of myocardium, the papillary muscles, each attached at its apex to several chordae tendineae. The right ventricle is separated from the left ventricle by the interventricular septum, which is muscular inferiorly and membranous superiorly (see Figs 2.43, 2.46).

Pulmonary valve

The pulmonary orifice lies between the infundibulum and the pulmonary trunk and is guarded by the pulmonary valve (Figs 2.39 & 2.40), which consists of three semilunar cusps. The valve closes during ventricular relaxation (diastole), preventing backflow of blood from the pulmonary trunk into the right ventricle. The valve lies behind the left border of the sternum at the level of the third costal cartilage (see Fig. 2.32). Sounds generated by this valve are loudest over the anterior end of the second left intercostal space.

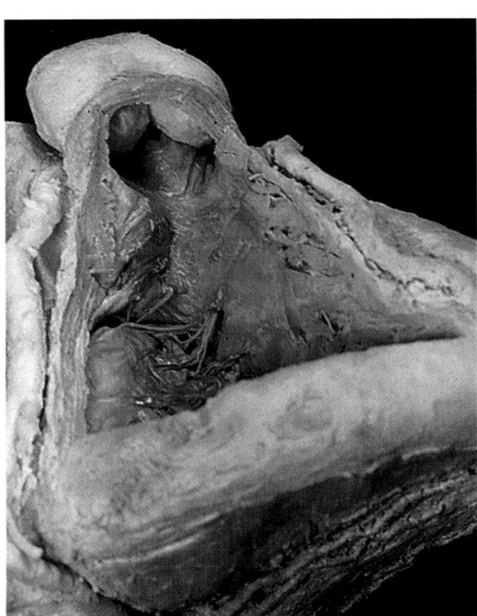

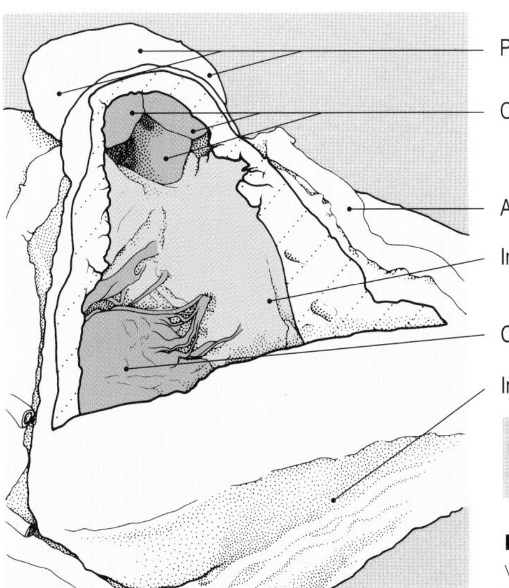

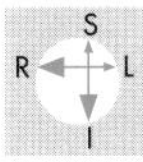

Fig. 2.39 Ventricular surfaces of the cusps of the pulmonary valve seen after removal of part of the anterior wall of the right ventricle.

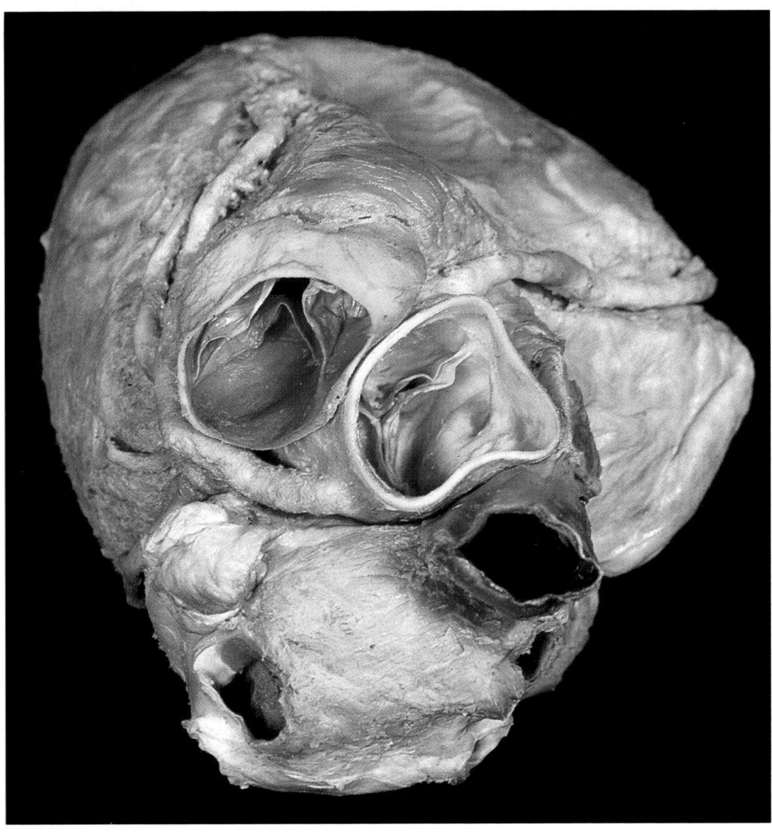

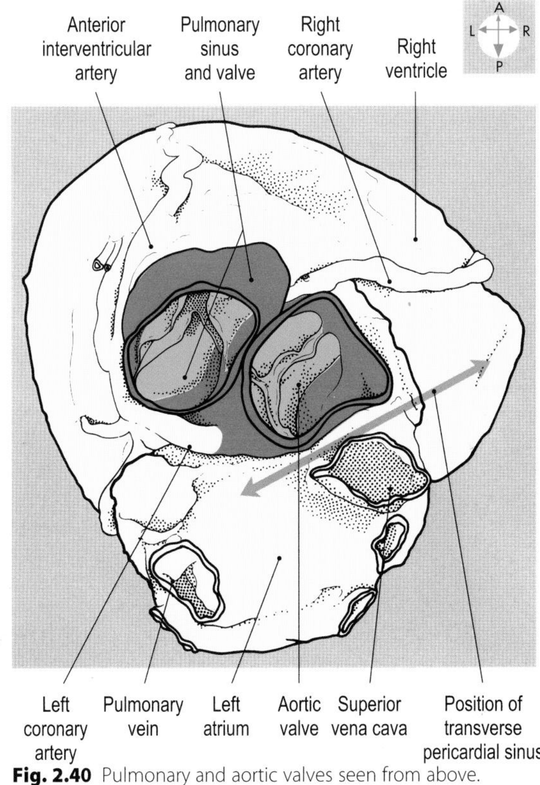

Fig. 2.40 Pulmonary and aortic valves seen from above.

Left atrium

The left atrium lies behind the right atrium and forms the base of the heart. It possesses a hook-like auricle (left atrial appendage), which projects forwards to the left of the pulmonary trunk and infundibulum. The chamber receives superior and inferior pulmonary veins from each lung (see Fig. 2.35). The four pulmonary veins, together with the two venae cavae, are all enclosed in a sleeve of serous pericardium, forming the superior limit of the oblique pericardial sinus. The left atrium forms the anterior wall of this sinus, which separates the chamber from the fibrous pericardium and oesophagus. Most of the inner surface of the left atrium is smooth (Fig. 2.41), although musculi pectinati are present in the auricle.

Mitral (bicuspid) valve

The left atrium communicates anteroinferiorly with the left ventricle through the left atrioventricular orifice, which is guarded by the mitral valve. This valve possesses two cusps, whose bases attach to the margins of the atrioventricular orifice (Fig. 2.41) while their free borders and cusps are anchored by chordae tendineae to the papillary muscles within the left ventricle (Fig. 2.42). The valve prevents reflux during ventricular contraction. Although it lies in the midline at the level of the fourth costal cartilages (see Fig. 2.32), the sounds of the mitral valve are best heard over the apex of the heart.

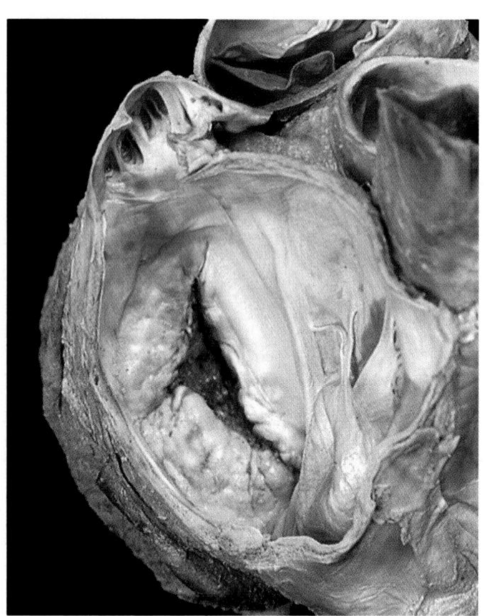

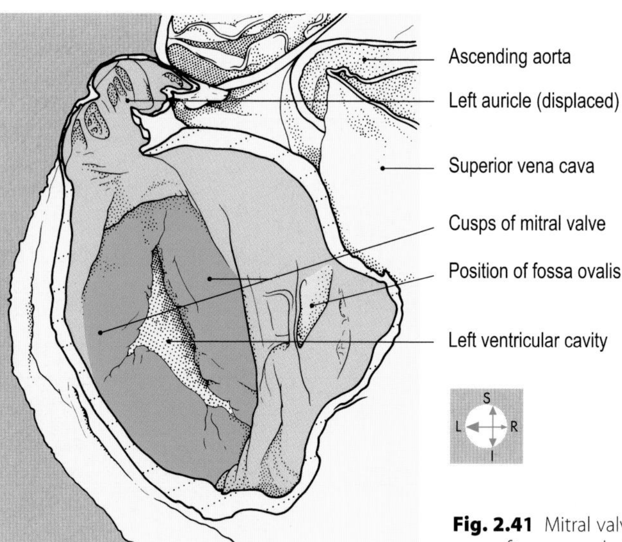

Fig. 2.41 Mitral valve and interior of the left atrium and auricle seen after removal of the posterior wall of the chamber.

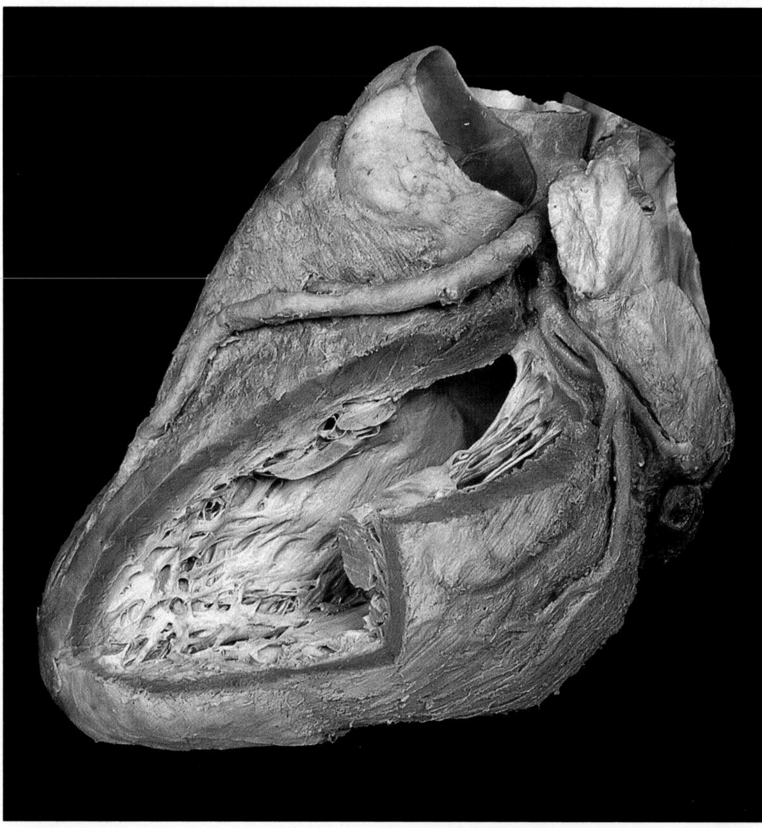

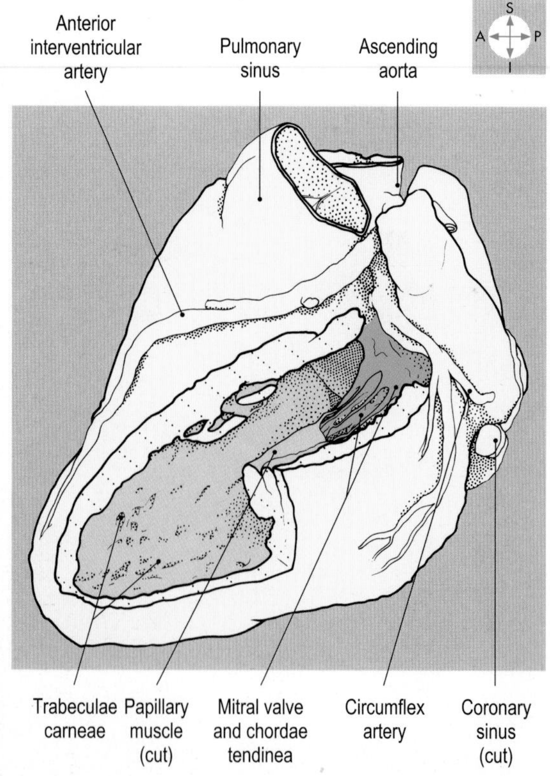

Fig. 2.42 Interior of the left ventricle seen after removal of part of its wall.

Left ventricle

From the left atrioventricular orifice the left ventricle extends forwards and to the left as far as the apex. The thickness of the wall of the chamber is normally three times that of the right ventricle (Fig. 2.43). Internally, there are prominent trabeculae carneae and papillary muscles (see Fig. 2.46). The chamber narrows as it passes upwards and to the right behind the infundibulum to form the aortic vestibule (Fig. 2.44), the part of the ventricle that communicates with the ascending aorta through the aortic orifice.

Aortic valve

The aortic valve consists of three semilunar cusps (see Fig. 2.45), which prevent backflow of blood from the ascending aorta during ventricular diastole. The valve lies behind the sternum to the left of the midline at the level of the anterior end of the third left intercostal space (see Fig. 2.32). However, its sounds are best heard over the medial ends of the first and second right intercostal spaces.

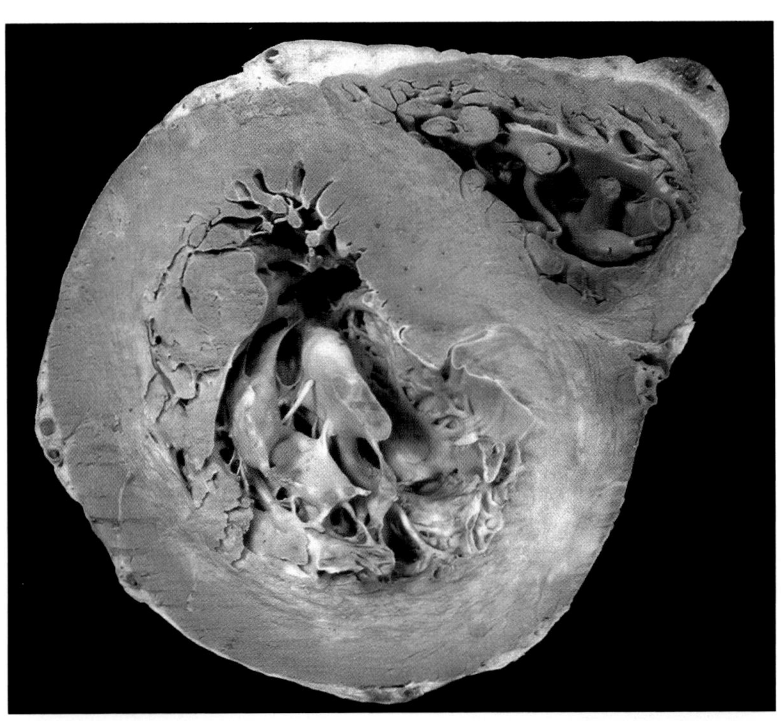

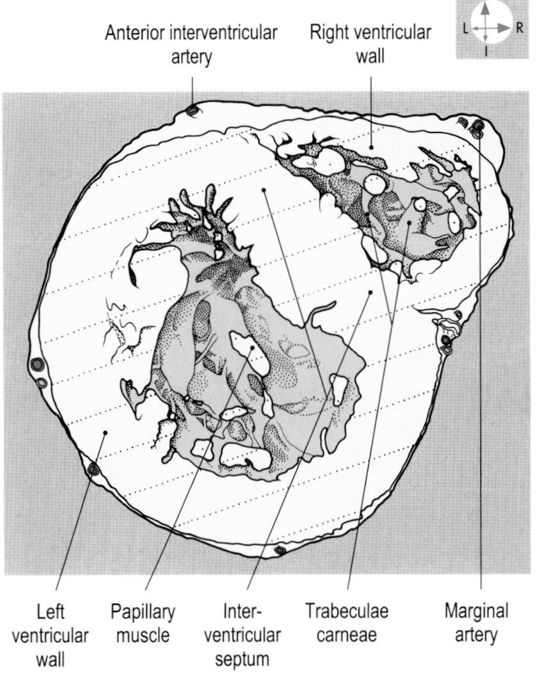

Fig. 2.43 Section through the heart showing the apical portions of the left and right ventricles.

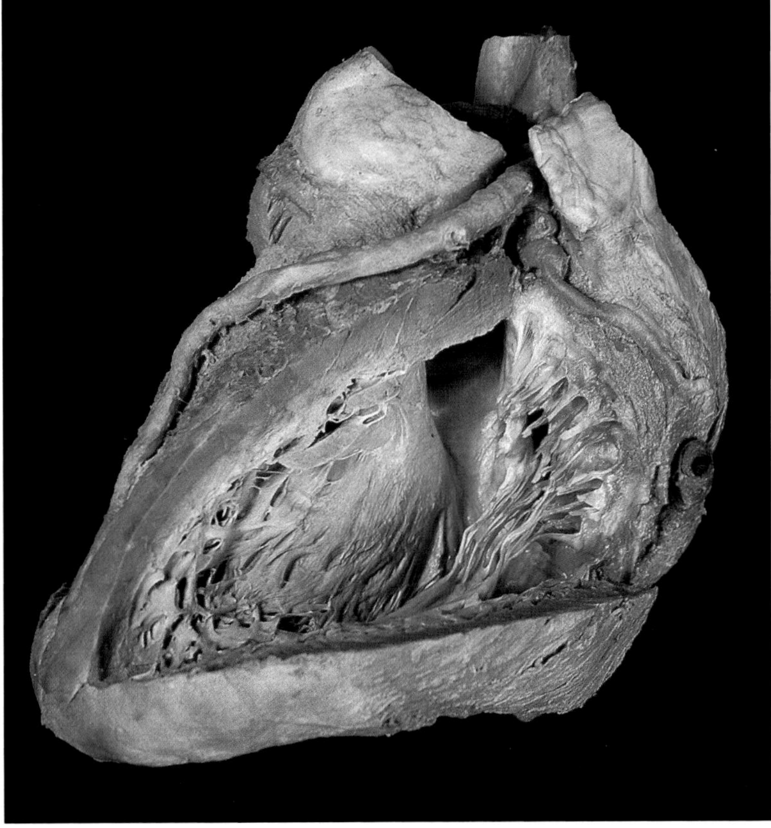

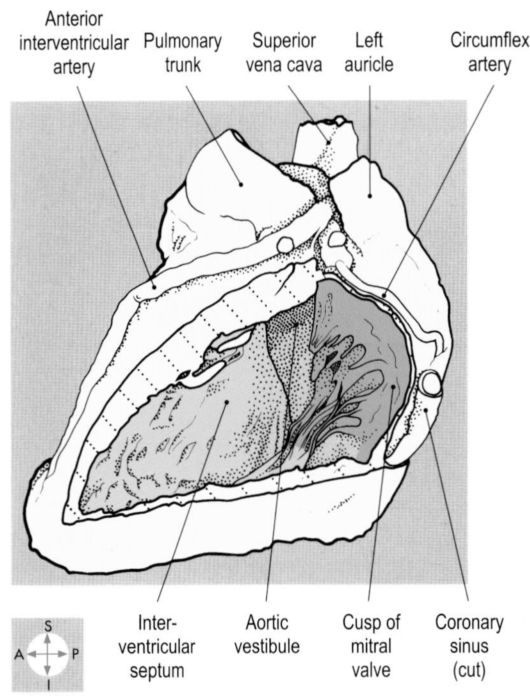

Fig. 2.44 Mitral valve and aortic vestibule, exposed by removal of part of the left ventricular wall.

Pulmonary trunk and ascending aorta

The pulmonary trunk and the ascending aorta lie within the fibrous pericardium, enclosed together in a sleeve of serous pericardium anterior to the transverse pericardial sinus (see Fig. 2.40). The pulmonary trunk extends upwards and backwards while the ascending aorta initially lies behind it and passes upwards and forwards, overlapped by the right auricle. At the origin of each vessel are three dilatations or sinuses (see Fig. 2.45), one immediately above each of the cusps of the pulmonary and aortic valves. When ventricular contraction ceases, blood flows into the sinuses, thus pushing against the cusps and closing the valves. Two of the aortic sinuses give rise to the right and left coronary arteries.

The pulmonary trunk emerges from the pericardium and divides into right and left pulmonary arteries in the concavity of the aortic arch, anterior to the bifurcation of the trachea at the level of the fourth thoracic vertebra. As the ascending aorta pierces the fibrous pericardium, it turns backwards and to the left, becoming the arch of the aorta.

Connecting the aortic arch to the pulmonary trunk (or to the commencement of the left pulmonary artery) is the ligamentum arteriosum (Fig. 2.46), the remnant of the fetal ductus arteriosus which conveyed blood from the pulmonary trunk to the aorta, bypassing the pulmonary circulation. Occasionally, the ductus remains patent after birth, giving rise to serious circulatory abnormalities.

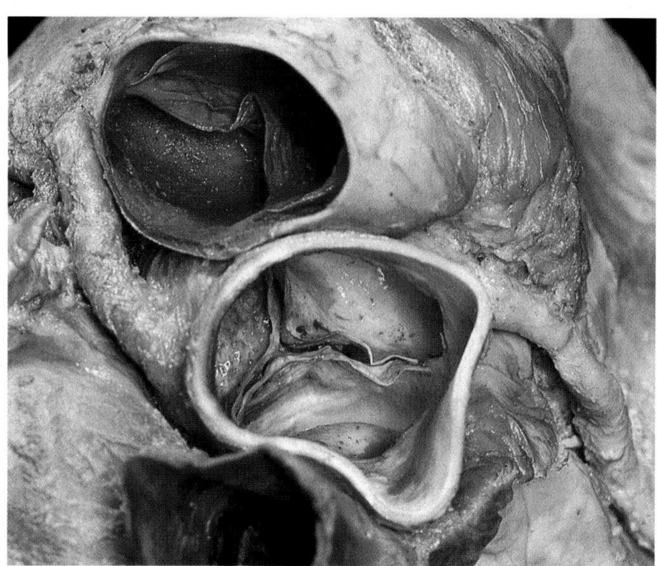

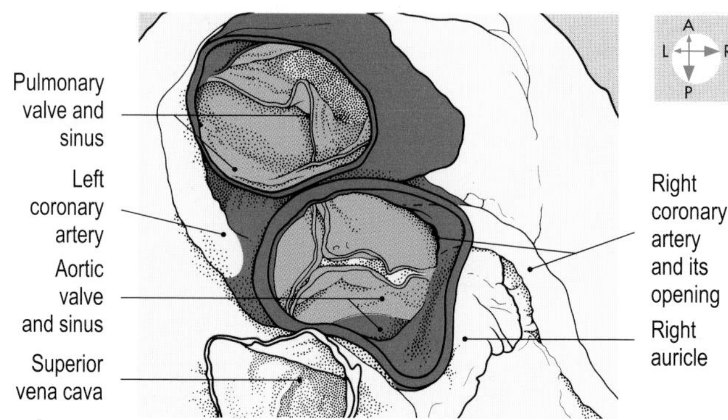

Fig. 2.45 Aortic and pulmonary valves viewed obliquely from above.

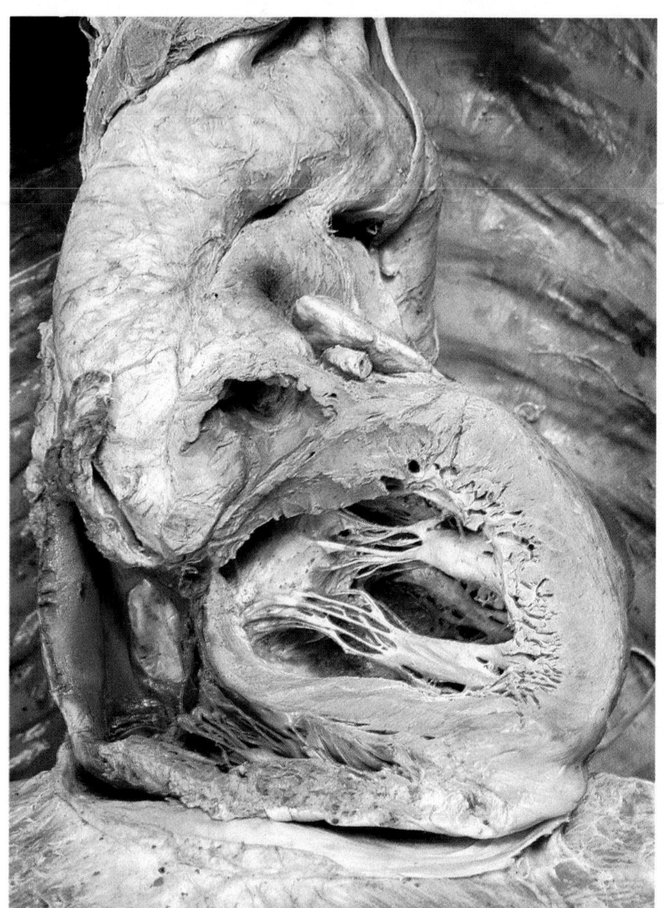

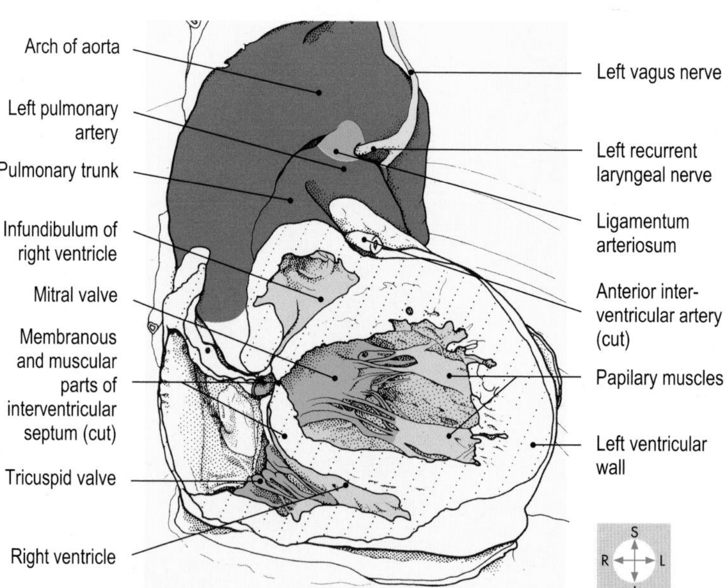

Fig. 2.46 Anterior view of the aorta, pulmonary trunk and ligamentum arteriosum. Most of the muscular part of the interventricular septum has been removed to show the interior of the left ventricle.

Blood vessels

The arterial supply to the heart is provided by the right and left coronary arteries, which arise from the ascending aorta just above the aortic valve (Fig. 2.47). They supply the myocardium, including the papillary muscles and conducting tissue. The principal venous return is via the coronary sinus and the cardiac veins.

Right coronary artery

This vessel arises from the anterior aspect of the root of the aorta and descends in the anterior coronary sulcus (Figs 2.47 & 2.48). At the inferior border it gives off a marginal branch, which runs to the left towards the apex of the heart. The right coronary artery continues on the inferior surface in the coronary sulcus (see Fig. 2.49) and terminates by anastomosing with the left coronary artery. On the inferior surface, the posterior (inferior) interventricular artery arises from the right coronary artery (occasionally the left coronary artery) and runs in the posterior interventricular groove towards the apex. When the posterior interventricular artery arises from the right coronary artery, the heart is described as right dominant. The right coronary artery and its branches supply the anterior surface of the right atrium, the lower part of the left atrium, most of the right ventricle and parts of the left ventricle and interventricular septum. In addition, branches from this artery usually supply most of the conducting tissue of the heart (see p. 56).

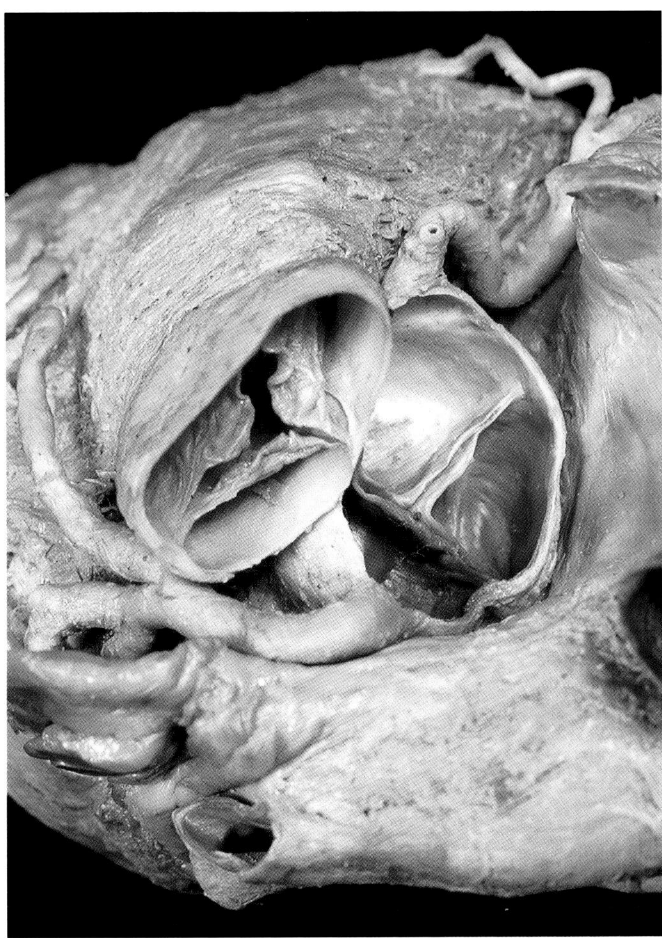

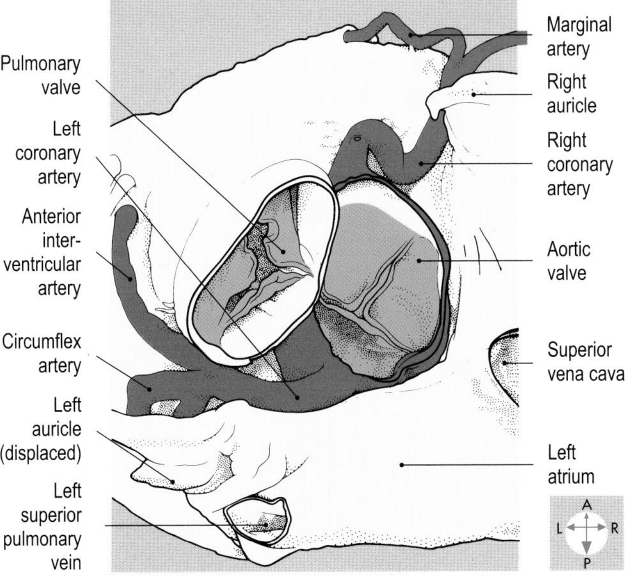

Fig. 2.47 Origins of the right and left coronary arteries from the root of the ascending aorta seen from above.

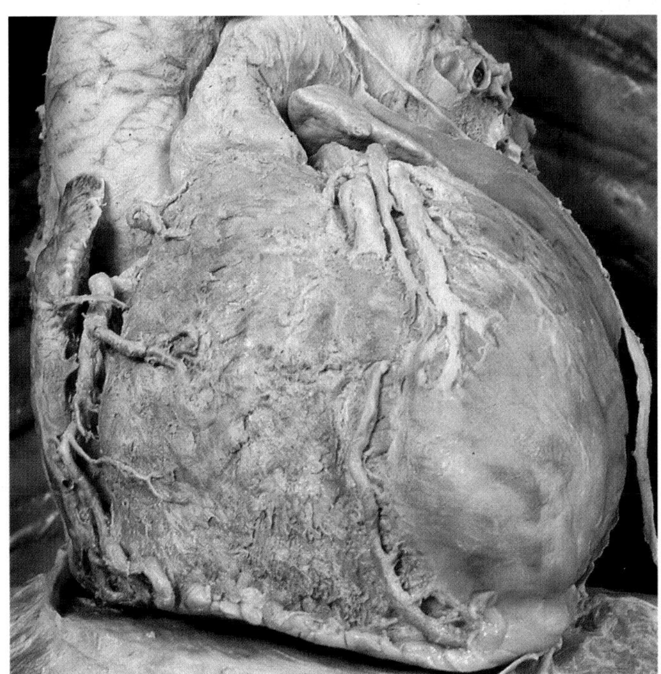

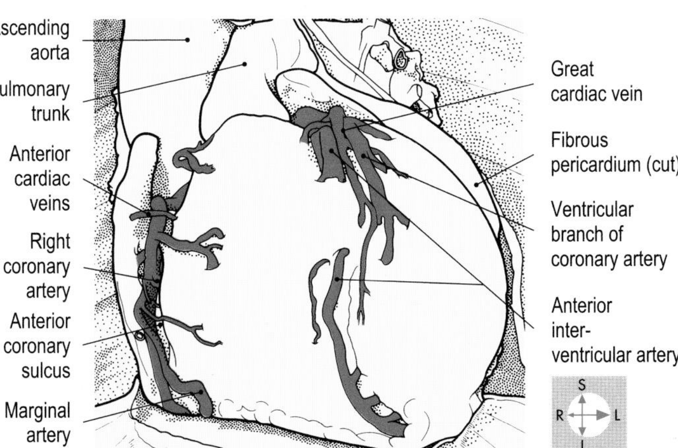

Fig. 2.48 Right and left coronary arteries and their branches on the anterior surface of the heart.

Left coronary artery

This artery takes origin from the posterior aspect of the root of the ascending aorta and runs to the left behind the pulmonary trunk where its major branch, the anterior interventricular artery, arises (Figs 2.47 & 2.50). The latter vessel descends in the anterior interventricular groove towards the apex of the heart. The left coronary artery continues as the circumflex artery in the posterior part of the coronary sulcus and terminates by anastomosing with the right coronary artery. The vessel supplies the posterior wall of the left atrium and auricle, most of the left ventricle and parts of the right ventricle and interventricular septum.

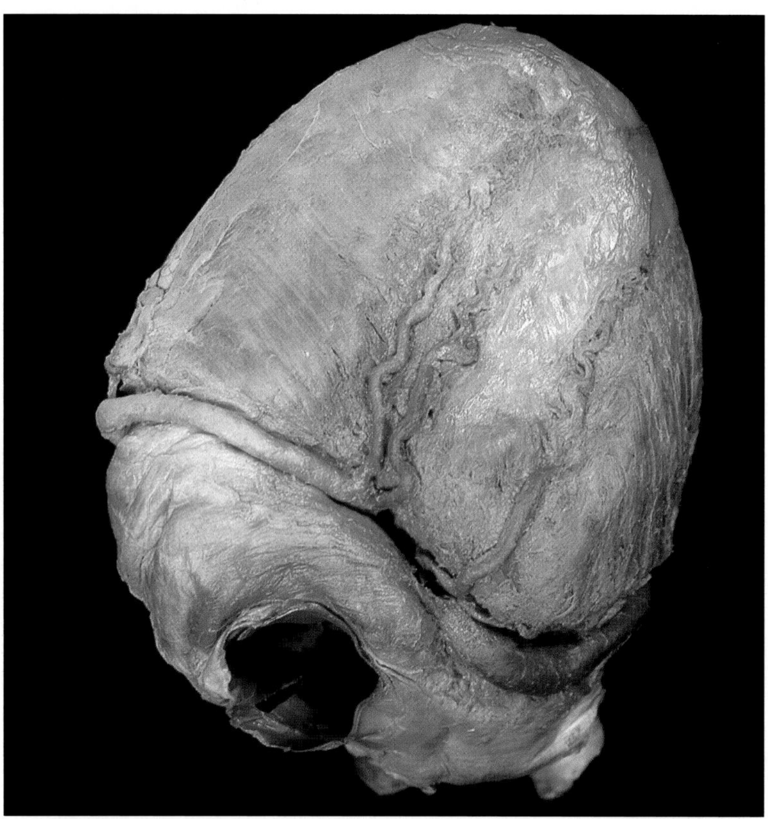

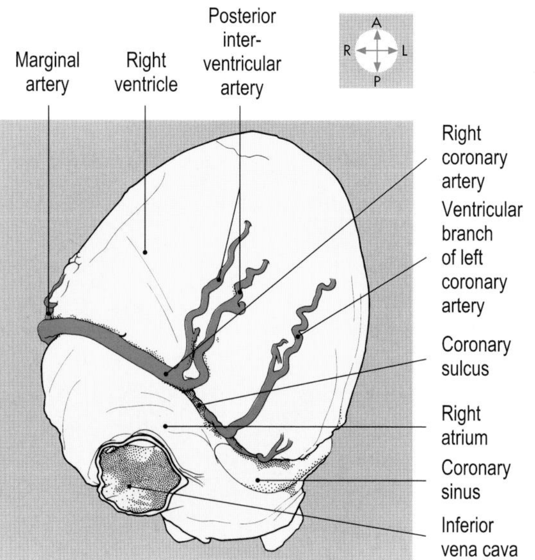

Fig. 2.49 Right and left coronary arteries and their branches on the inferior surface of the heart. The posterior interventricular artery is duplicated in this specimen.

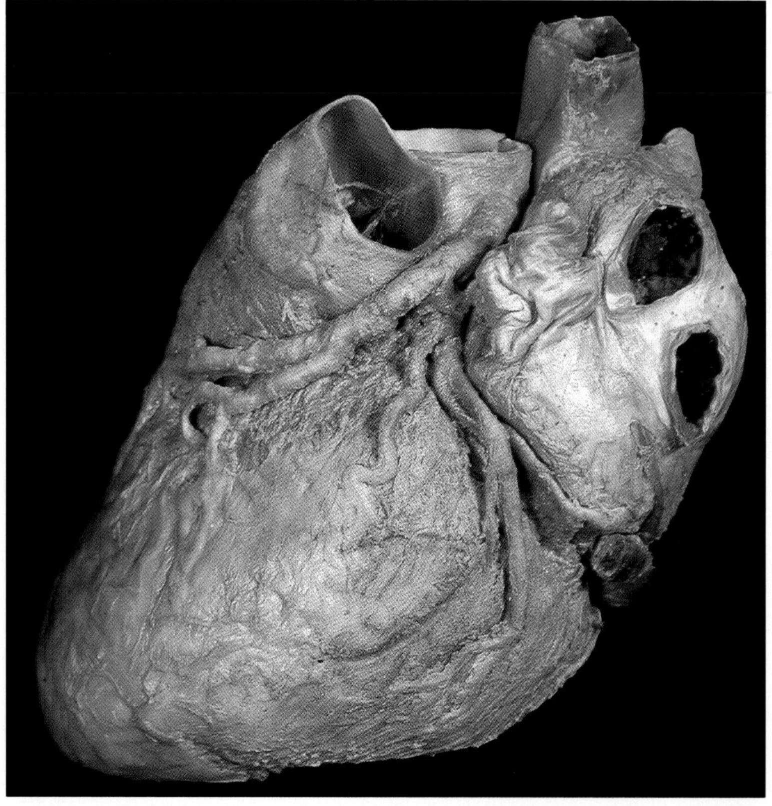

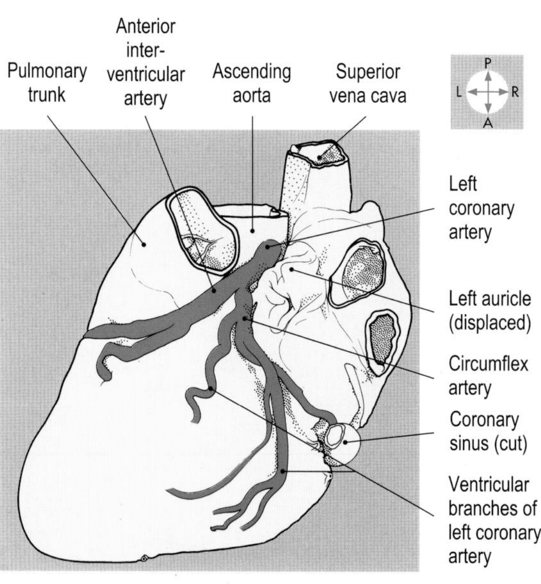

Fig. 2.50 Left coronary artery and its branches, viewed from the left.

Coronary sinus and cardiac veins

Most of the venous return from the heart is carried by the coronary sinus, which runs along the posterior part of the coronary sulcus and terminates in the right atrium. The coronary sinus is formed near the left border of the heart by the union of the posterior vein of the left ventricle and the great cardiac vein (Fig. 2.51), which accompanies the anterior interventricular artery. Other veins enter the coronary sinus, including the middle cardiac vein (Fig. 2.52), which accompanies the posterior interventricular artery. Some cardiac veins enter the right atrium independently (see Fig. 2.48).

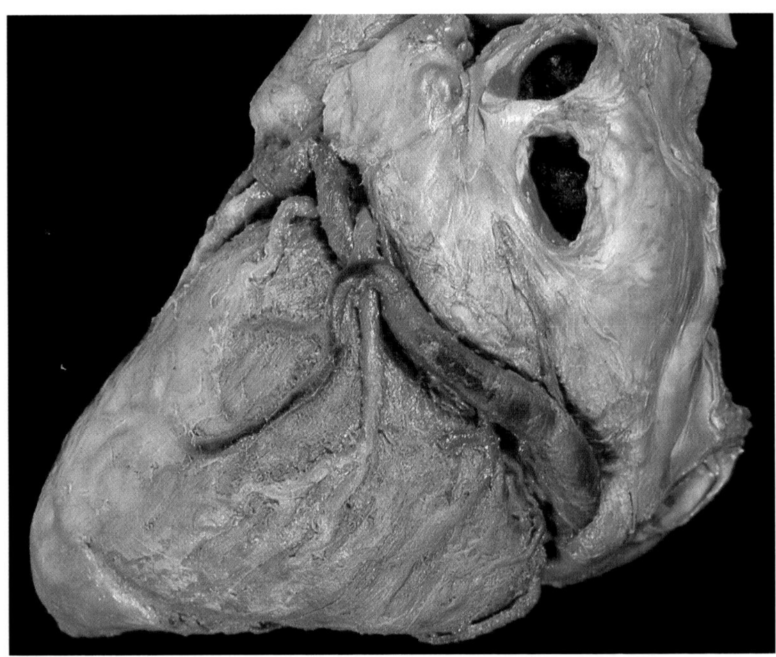

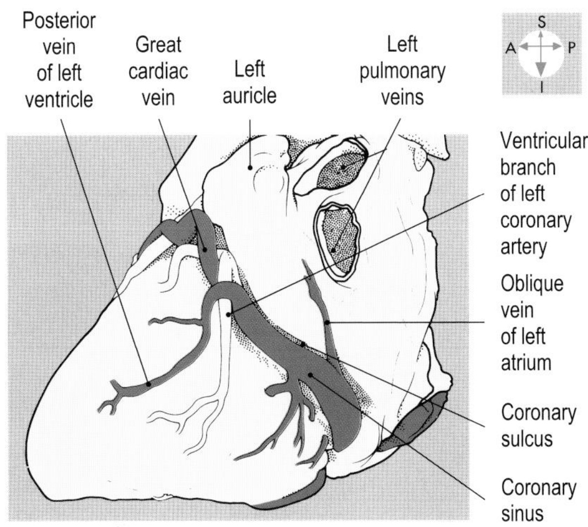

Fig. 2.51 Oblique view of the coronary sinus lying in the coronary sulcus.

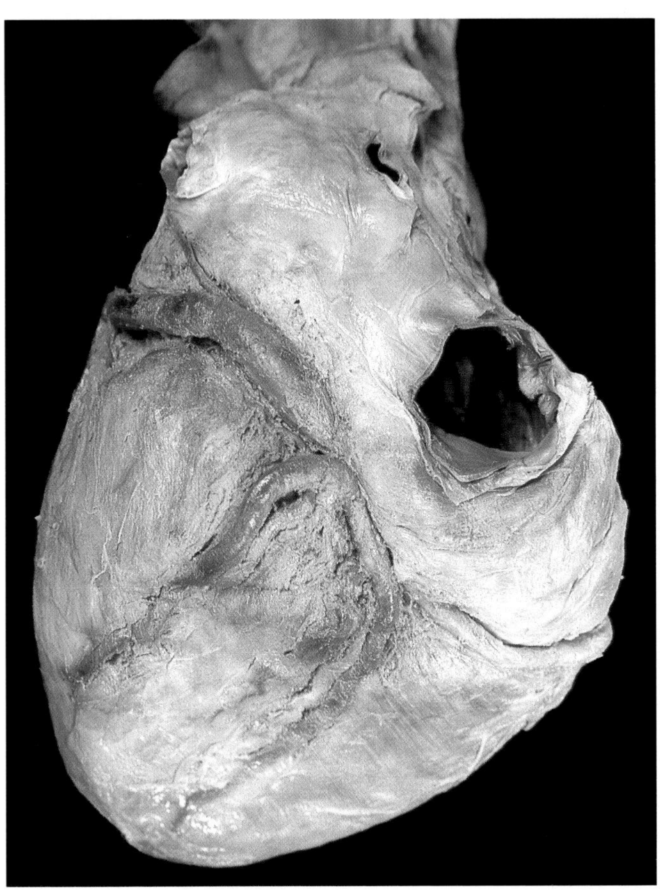

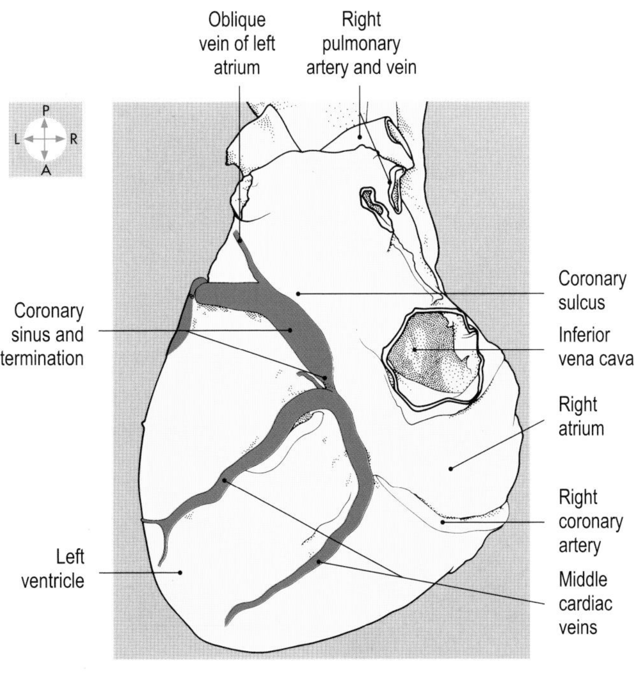

Fig. 2.52 Posteroinferior view of the termination of the coronary sinus in the right atrium.

Conducting system

Coordinated contraction of the myocardium is controlled by specialized conducting tissues, consisting of the sinuatrial (SA) node, the atrioventricular (AV) node, the atrioventricular bundle (of His) and its right and left branches (Fig. 2.53).

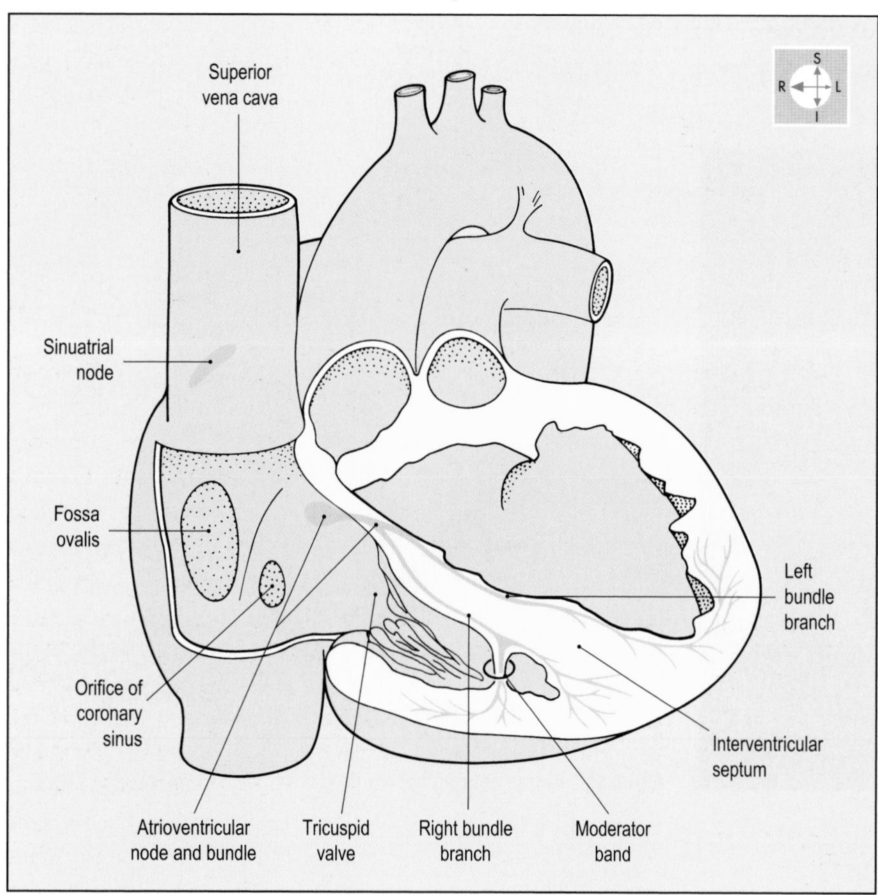

Fig. 2.53 Location of the conducting tissues.

The sinuatrial node lies in the anterior wall of the right atrium close to the termination of the superior vena cava. It occupies part of the root of the auricle and the upper end of the sulcus terminalis. Numerous autonomic nerves supply the node and modify its rate of discharge. The SA node usually receives blood from an atrial branch of either the right or left coronary artery. From the SA node the cardiac excitation wave passes through the atrial myocardium to reach the AV node.

The AV node lies in the interatrial septum anterosuperior to the termination of the coronary sinus. It is continuous with the atrioventricular bundle, which passes through the fibrous ring separating the atria and ventricles. The bundle gains the upper part of the interventricular septum and promptly divides into right and left branches. The AV node and bundle are supplied by branches of the posterior interventricular artery. Interruption of the arterial supply to the conducting tissues may result in cardiac arrhythmias.

Lying beneath the endocardium, the right branch of the atrioventricular bundle descends in the interventricular septum and often passes in the moderator band (Fig. 2.54) to ramify within the anterior wall of the right ventricle. The left branch runs on the left side of the interventricular septum. Both branches divide repeatedly at the ventricular apices and spread out into the myocardium of the respective ventricles.

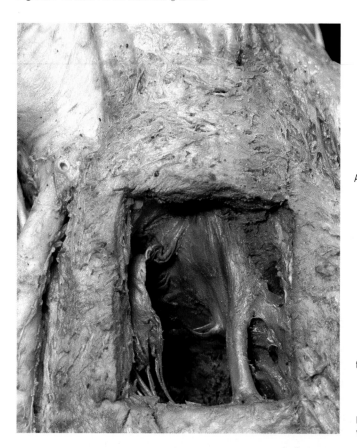

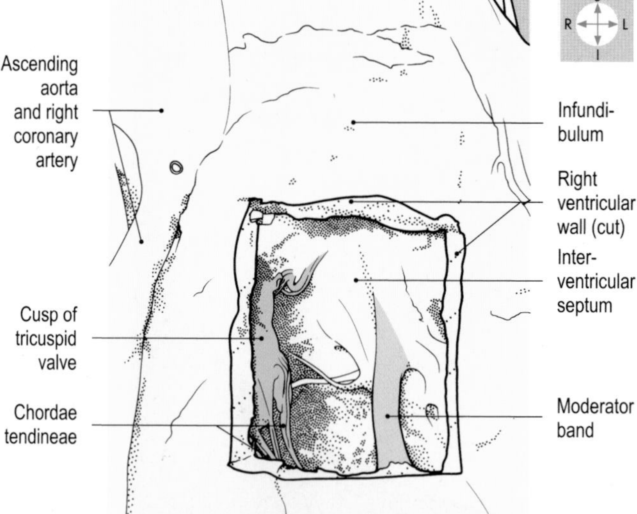

Fig. 2.54 Moderator band, seen through a window cut in the anterior wall of the right ventricle.

Mediastinal Structures

Brachiocephalic veins

On each side, the brachiocephalic vein is formed in the root of the neck by the union of the internal jugular and subclavian veins. At its origin the vein lies behind the sternoclavicular joint and in front of the first part of the subclavian artery.

The right brachiocephalic vein runs a short vertical course in the superior mediastinum to unite with the left brachiocephalic vein (Fig. 2.55) behind the medial end of the first right costal cartilage. It receives the right vertebral and internal thoracic veins, together with the right jugular and subclavian lymph trunks and the right lymph duct. The vessel is accompanied by the right phrenic nerve.

The left brachiocephalic vein enters the thorax and runs obliquely to the right, passing behind the manubrium. The vessel lies in front of the origin from the arch of the aorta of the left common carotid artery and the brachiocephalic trunk. At its commencement the vein is joined by the termination of the thoracic duct and, along its course, receives the left vertebral, internal thoracic and superior intercostal veins and, usually, the inferior thyroid veins.

Superior vena cava

Formed by the union of the two brachiocephalic veins, this large vessel descends vertically (Fig. 2.55) and terminates in the right atrium of the heart. It lies to the right of the ascending aorta and to the left of the right phrenic nerve and receives the azygos vein before piercing the fibrous pericardium.

Arch of aorta and branches

The arch of the aorta lies within the superior mediastinum, in continuity with the ascending aorta. The vessel curves backwards and to the left to reach the left side of the fourth thoracic vertebral body, where it becomes the descending aorta. The arch possesses a concavity inferiorly, left and right sides, and a superior convexity.

The concavity is related to the bifurcation of the pulmonary trunk and the left main bronchus. The ligamentum arteriosum attaches the pulmonary trunk (or left pulmonary artery) to the concavity of the aortic arch and is closely related to the left recurrent laryngeal nerve (see Figs 2.46 & 2.57).

The left side of the aortic arch is crossed by the left phrenic and vagus nerves (see Fig. 2.56) and covered by mediastinal pleura. The phrenic nerve lies in front of the vagus and passes onto the fibrous pericardium in front of the lung root. The vagus nerve inclines backwards to pass behind the lung root, having given off the left recurrent laryngeal nerve. The left superior intercostal vein passes forwards across the arch and usually terminates in the left brachiocephalic vein.

The right side of the arch is related, from in front backwards, to the superior vena cava, trachea, left recurrent laryngeal nerve, oesophagus and thoracic duct. These structures lie between the aorta and the right mediastinal pleura.

The convexity of the arch gives rise to the brachiocephalic trunk, left common carotid and left subclavian arteries (see Fig. 2.57), which ascend into the root of the neck. The brachiocephalic trunk is the first branch of the arch of the aorta and arises behind the left brachiocephalic vein. The trunk slopes upwards and to the right across the anterior surface of the trachea, leaving the thorax to the right of the trachea to divide in the root of the neck into the right subclavian and right common carotid arteries.

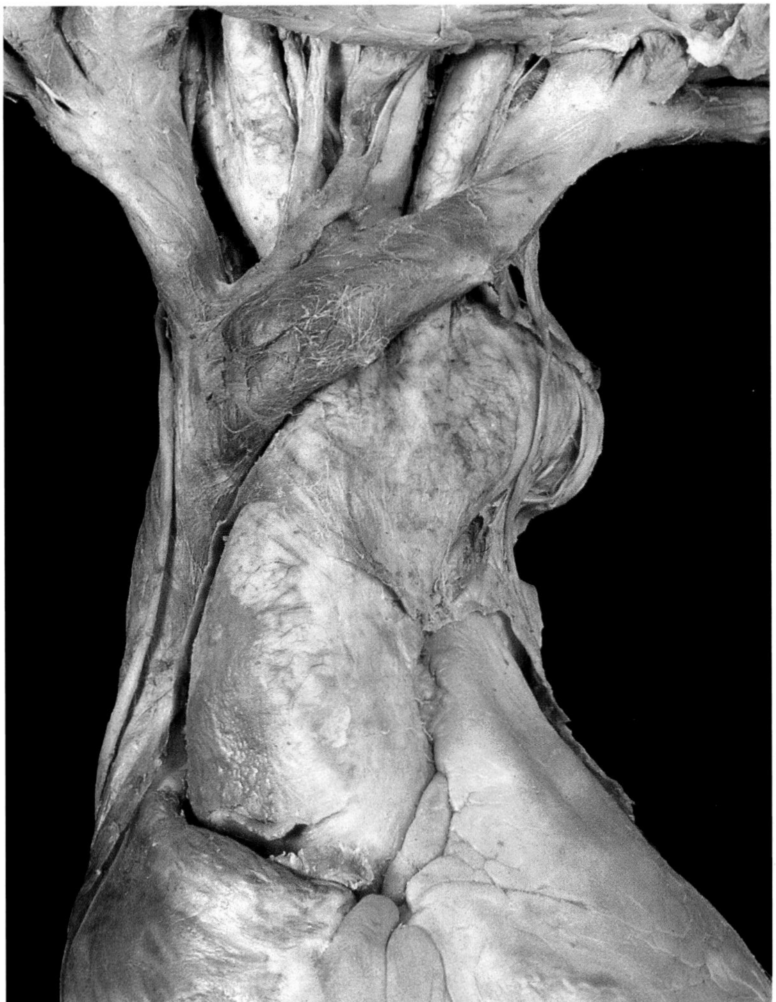

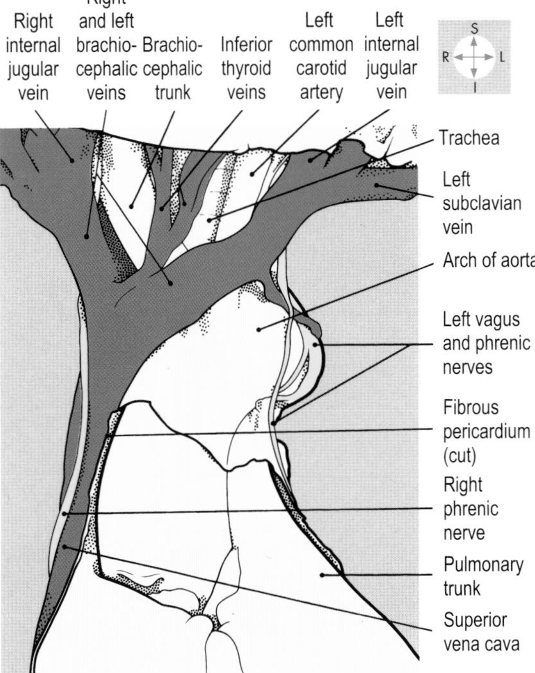

Fig. 2.55 Relationships of the brachiocephalic veins to the great arteries arising from the aortic arch.

The left common carotid artery arises behind the brachiocephalic trunk and ascends, in company with the left phrenic and vagus nerves, through the superior mediastinum on the left of the trachea into the root of the neck (Fig. 2.57).

The left subclavian artery is the most posterior artery arising from the aortic arch and lies immediately behind the left common carotid artery. It runs upwards and laterally, closely related to the pleura covering the apex of the left lung, entering the root of the neck behind the sternoclavicular joint.

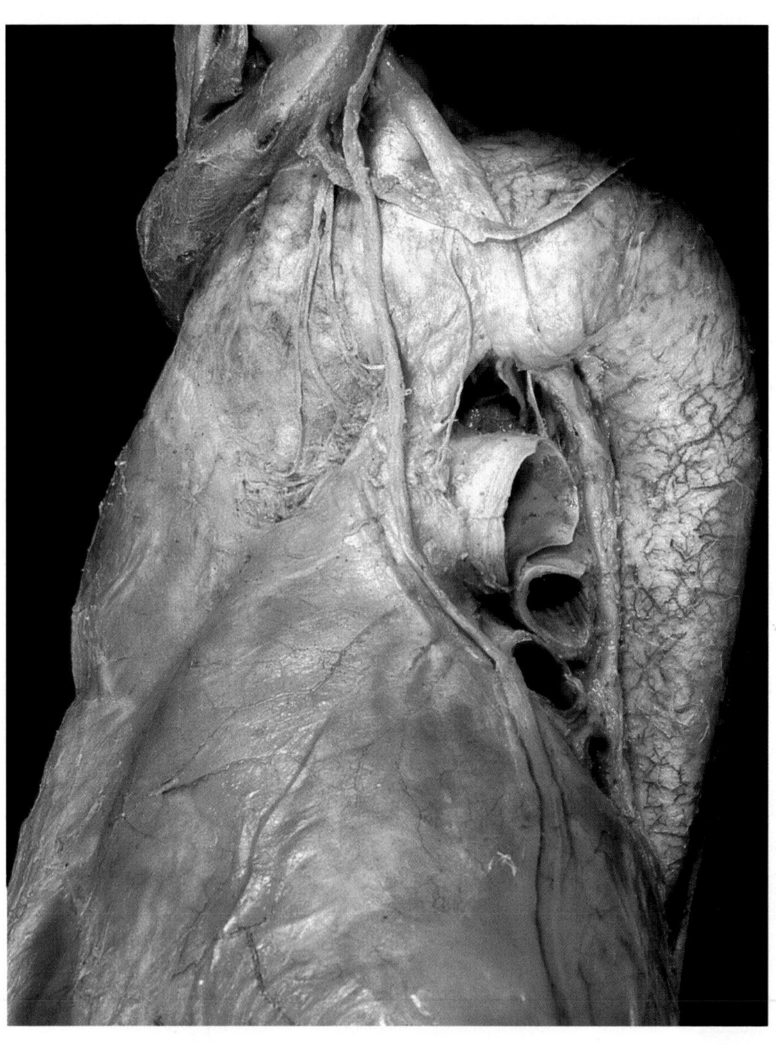

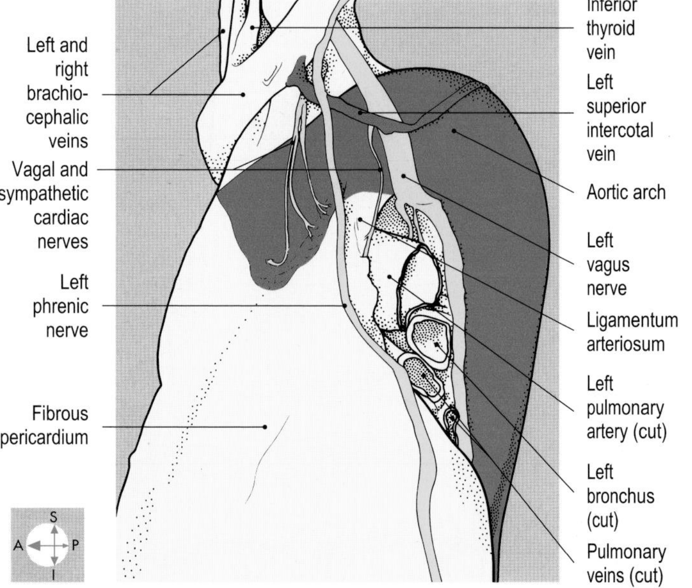

Fig. 2.56 Oblique view of the arch of the aorta showing the courses of the left vagus and phrenic nerves.

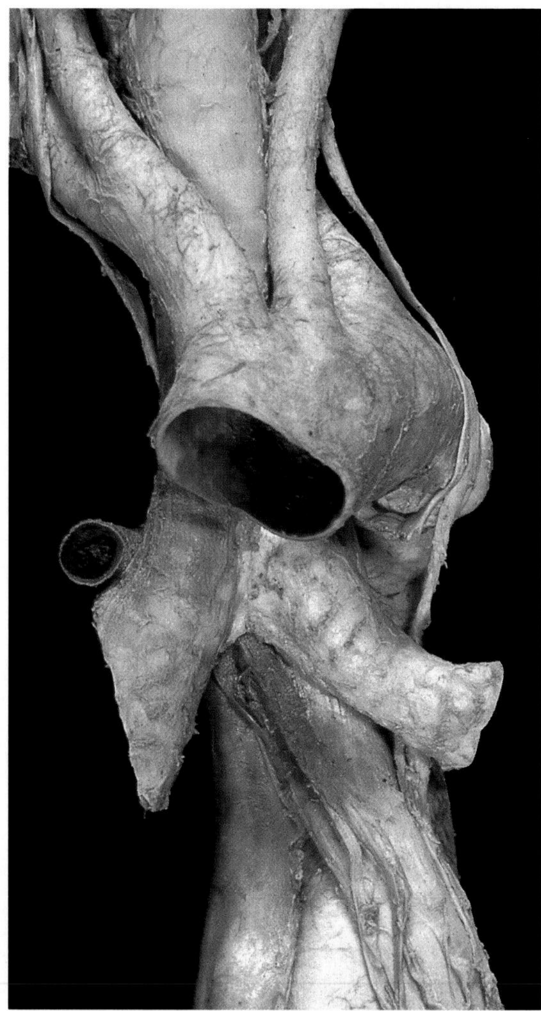

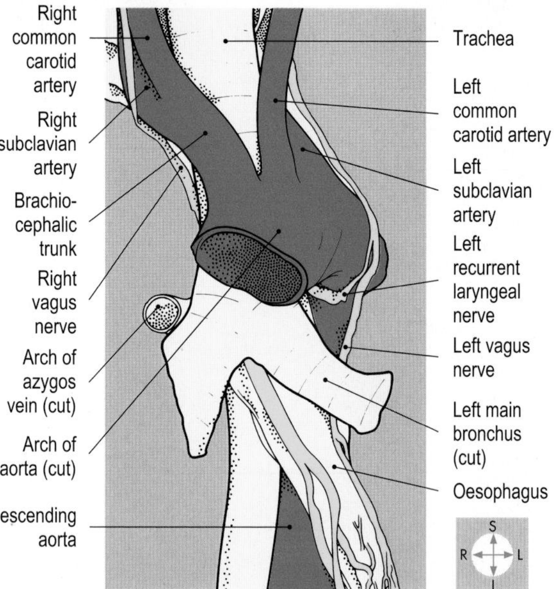

Fig. 2.57 Arch of the aorta and its branches viewed anteriorly.

Phrenic nerves

The right and left phrenic nerves (C3, C4 & C5) pass through the superior thoracic aperture behind the respective subclavian veins. Owing to the asymmetry of the mediastinal organs, the intrathoracic courses of the two nerves differ. The right phrenic nerve, covered by mediastinal pleura, accompanies the right brachiocephalic vein and the superior vena cava in front of the root of the right lung (Fig. 2.58). It descends vertically across the fibrous pericardium covering the right atrium and pierces the diaphragm alongside the inferior vena cava.

The left phrenic nerve, also covered by mediastinal pleura, lies lateral to the left common carotid artery and crosses the left side of the aortic arch to gain the fibrous pericardium in front of the left lung root (Fig. 2.56). The nerve then descends across the pericardium as far as the apex of the heart, where it pierces the diaphragm (see Fig. 2.59).

The phrenic nerves supply the muscle of the diaphragm, excluding the crura. They give sensory fibres to the fibrous and parietal serous pericardium and the mediastinal and diaphragmatic pleura, and sensory branches to the peritoneum covering the inferior surface of the diaphragm (see pp 36, 205).

Trachea

The trachea descends through the neck, where normally it is palpable, and enters the thorax in the midline, immediately behind the upper border of the manubrium. It runs vertically through the superior mediastinum and, at the level of the aortic arch, divides into right and left main bronchi (see Fig. 2.60).

The right main bronchus is wider than the left and inclines steeply downwards to enter the right lung root. The right upper lobar bronchus often arises outside the hilum of the lung. The left main bronchus runs obliquely to the left within the concavity of the arch of the aorta, passing behind the left pulmonary artery to gain the left lung root.

The thoracic part of the trachea is crossed anteriorly by the brachiocephalic trunk and the left brachiocephalic vein (Fig. 2.58). In addition, the trachea is overlapped by the anterior margins of the pleura and lungs and the thymus (or its remnants). The trachea is related on the left to the arch of the aorta and left common carotid and subclavian arteries, on the right to the superior vena cava, the termination of the azygos vein, the right vagus nerve and the mediastinal pleura, and posteriorly to the oesophagus and the left recurrent laryngeal nerve. (The right recurrent laryngeal nerve does not enter the thorax but passes around the right subclavian artery in the root of the neck; see p. 329.)

The vascular supply of the trachea is from the inferior thyroid arteries and veins. The recurrent laryngeal nerves supply sensory and parasympathetic secretomotor fibres to the mucous membrane and motor fibres to the smooth muscle (trachealis).

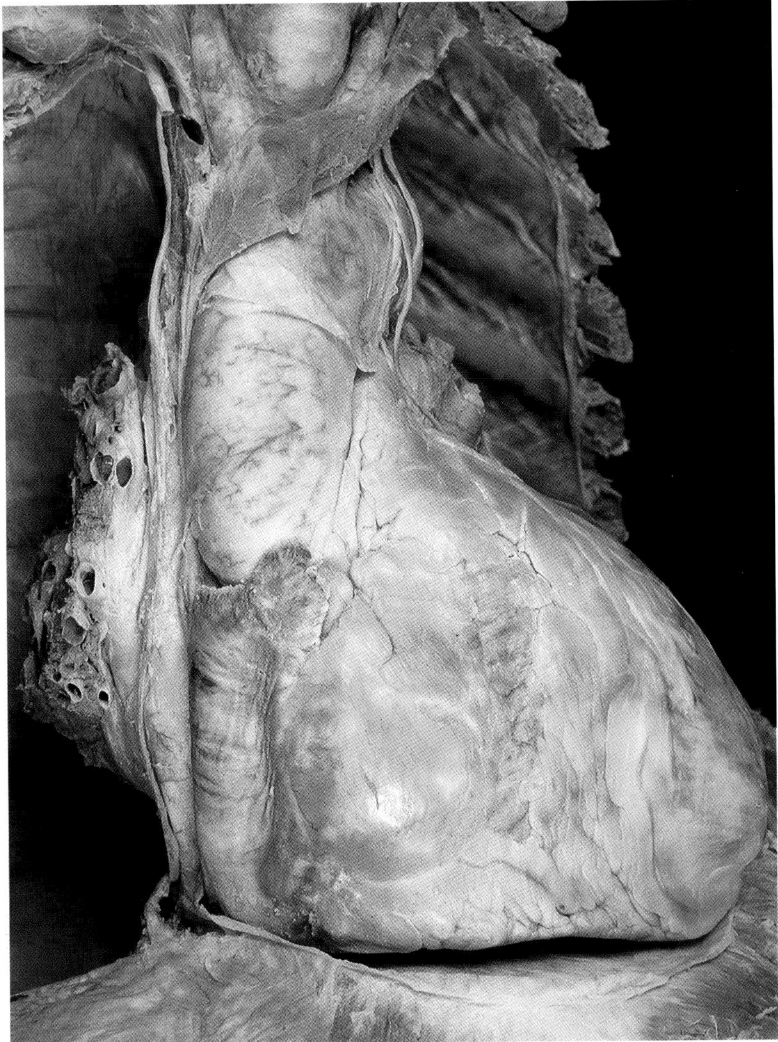

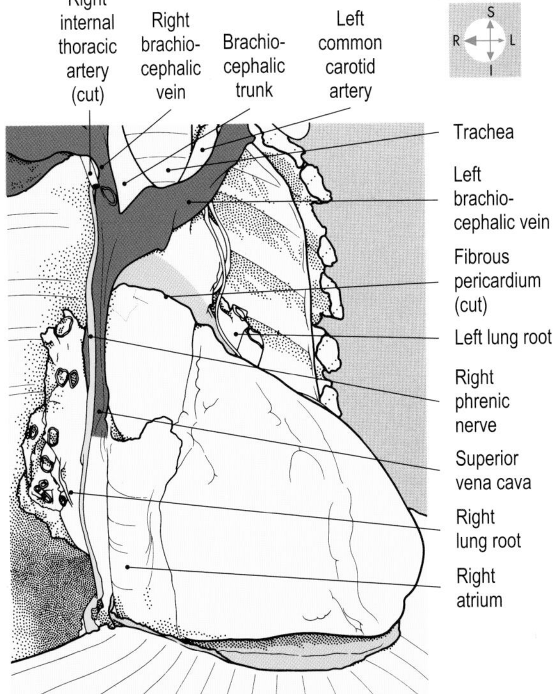

Fig. 2.58 Oblique view showing the course of the right phrenic nerve.

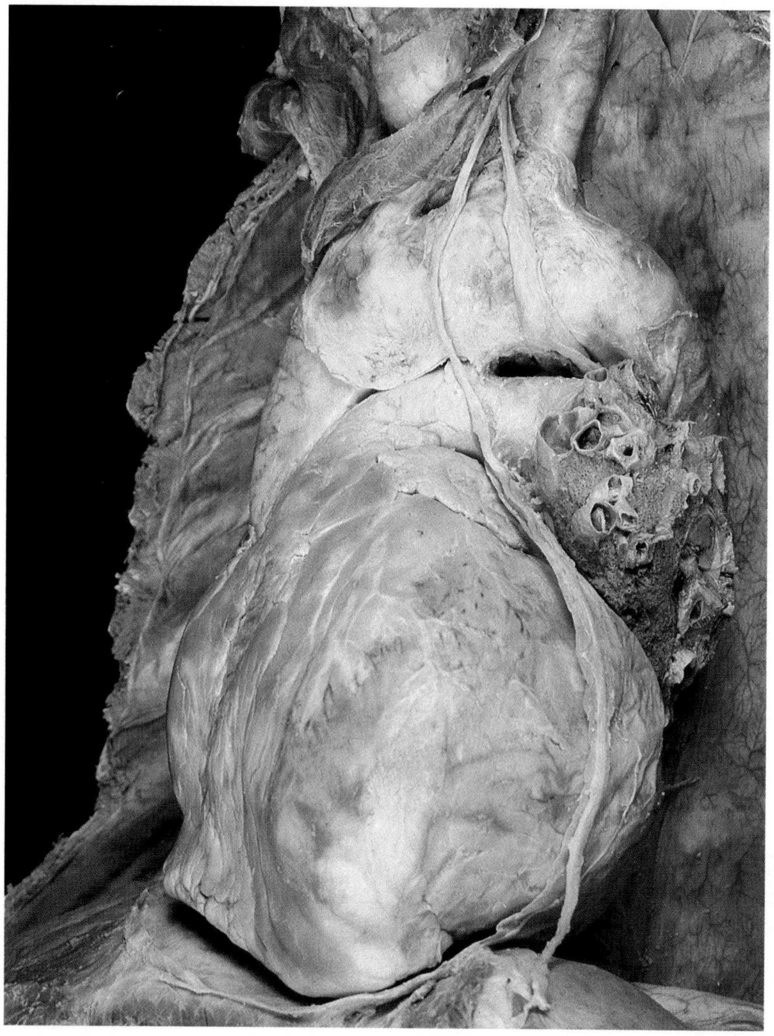

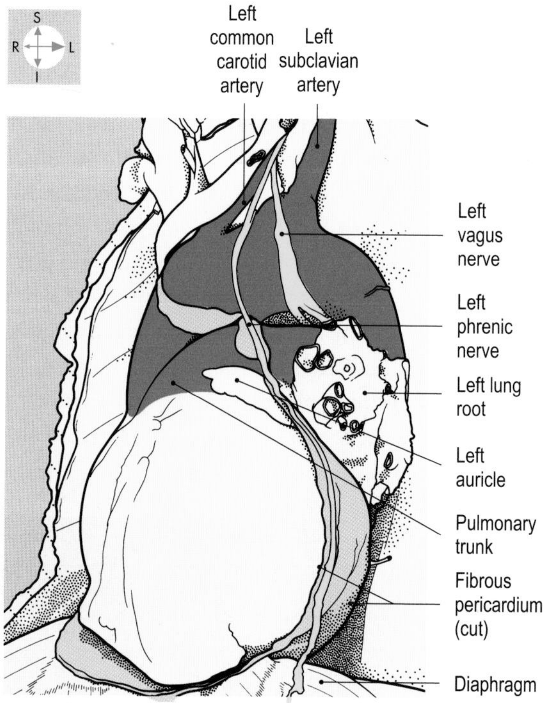

S
R
L
I
Left common carotid artery
Left subclavian artery
Left vagus nerve
Left phrenic nerve
Left lung root
Left auricle
Pulmonary trunk
Fibrous pericardium (cut)
Diaphragm

Fig. 2.59 Oblique view of the intrathoracic course of the left phrenic nerve.

Right vagus nerve
Right common carotid artery
Trachea
S
R
L
I
Arch of azygos vein (cut)
Arch of aorta (cut)
Left vagus and recurrent laryngeal nerves
Right main bronchus (cut)
Left main bronchus (cut)
Oesophagus

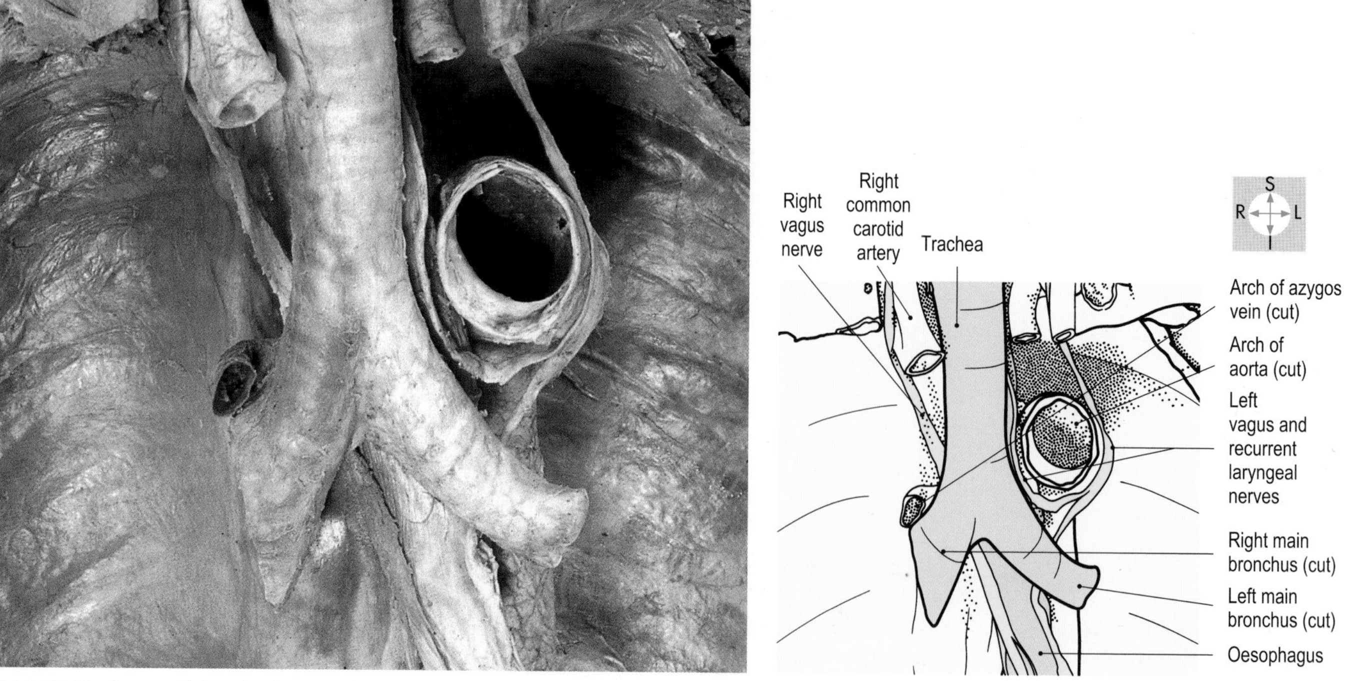

Fig. 2.60 Trachea and left and right main bronchi, exposed after removal of the anterior part of the aortic arch.

Oesophagus

The oesophagus descends through the root of the neck and traverses the superior thoracic aperture behind the trachea. In the superior mediastinum the oesophagus lies in front of the upper four thoracic vertebral bodies and behind the trachea, the left main bronchus and left recurrent laryngeal nerve. The aortic arch and the thoracic duct are on its left while the azygos vein arches forwards on its right (Fig. 2.61).

The oesophagus continues into the posterior mediastinum in front of the fifth thoracic vertebra accompanied by the right and left vagus nerves. It descends behind the fibrous pericardium and inclines to the left to cross in front of the descending aorta. On its right side the oesophagus is covered by mediastinal pleura. On the left, once anterior to the descending aorta, it is related to pleura as far as the diaphragm. Accompanied by branches of the vagus nerves (see below), the oesophagus passes through the diaphragm at the level of the tenth thoracic vertebra.

The oesophagus is supplied by branches from the inferior thyroid arteries and from the descending thoracic aorta. Its lower part receives branches from the left gastric artery that ascend through the oesophageal opening in the diaphragm. Radicles of the left gastric vein (a tributary of the portal vein) anastomose with veins that drain venous blood from the oesophagus into the azygos system (see portacaval anastomoses; p. 185). The upper part of the oesophagus is drained by the brachiocephalic veins. Sensory and parasympathetic motor fibres to the oesophagus are provided by the vagi and their recurrent laryngeal branches.

Vagus (X) nerves

In the superior mediastinum the relationships of the right and left vagi differ. The right vagus nerve (Fig. 2.61) enters the thorax behind the bifurcation of the brachiocephalic artery and on the right of the trachea. The nerve, covered by mediastinal pleura, inclines backwards and passes behind the right lung root to gain the oesophagus. The left vagus nerve descends behind the left common carotid artery to cross the left side of the aortic arch, gives off the left recurrent laryngeal nerve, and continues behind the left lung root to reach the oesophagus.

The left recurrent laryngeal nerve (Fig. 2.61) passes around the arch of the aorta adjacent to the ligamentum arteriosum and ascends in the interval between the trachea and oesophagus. In the posterior mediastinum the right and left vagus nerves divide on the surface of the oesophagus to form a network, the oesophageal plexus. The terminal branches of the plexus (the anterior and posterior vagal trunks) enter the abdomen with the oesophagus (see p. 197).

Descending thoracic aorta and branches

The descending aorta (Fig. 2.62) is continuous with the aortic arch and initially lies to the left of the fifth thoracic vertebral body. As it traverses the posterior mediastinum it inclines forwards and to the right, gaining the midline anterior to the twelfth thoracic vertebra. On the right the upper part of the descending aorta is related to the thoracic vertebral bodies and the oesophagus. The lower part and all of its left side are covered by mediastinal pleura. The thoracic duct and the azygos vein lie to the right of the aorta, and anteriorly it is crossed by the oesophagus sloping obliquely from the midline to the left. The descending aorta leaves the thorax in front of the twelfth thoracic vertebra and behind the median arcuate ligament of the diaphragm with the thoracic duct and azygos vein (see Fig. 2.64).

Posterior intercostal arteries from the descending aorta supply the third to the eleventh intercostal spaces on both sides. They anastomose with the anterior intercostal arteries derived from either the internal thoracic or the musculophrenic arteries. Other branches from the aorta supply the right and left bronchi and the oesophagus.

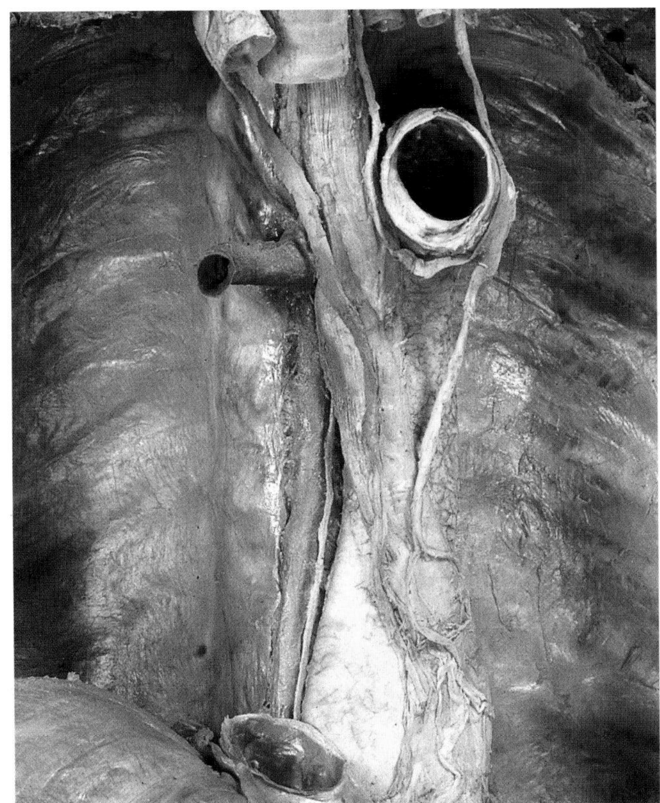

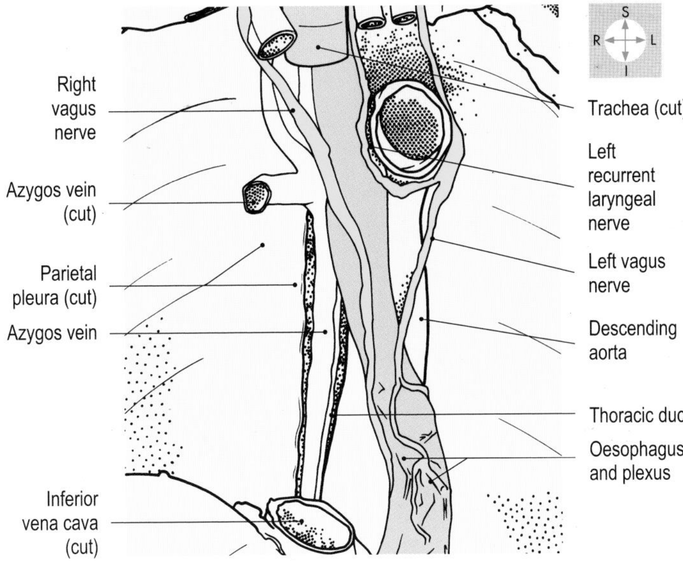

Fig. 2.61 Intrathoracic part of the oesophagus and accompanying vagus nerves after removal of the main bronchi and the lower part of the trachea.

Thoracic duct

Arising from the upper part of the cisterna chyli (see p. 196), the thoracic duct passes into the thorax, lying between the azygos vein and descending aorta, and with these structures (Figs 2.61 & 2.62) ascends through the posterior mediastinum to gain the superior mediastinum on the left of the oesophagus. The duct then curves forwards and to the left, crossing the apex of the left lung to enter the root of the neck where it terminates in the confluence of the left internal jugular and subclavian veins.

Azygos venous system

This system of veins drains blood from most of the posterior thoracic wall and from the bronchi, the pericardium and part of the intrathoracic oesophagus. The azygos vein enters the thorax through the aortic opening and receives posterior intercostal veins from the lower eight spaces on the right (Fig. 2.63). Veins from the second and third spaces drain into the right superior intercostal vein, which terminates in the azygos vein as it arches over the right lung root to join the superior vena cava. The venous

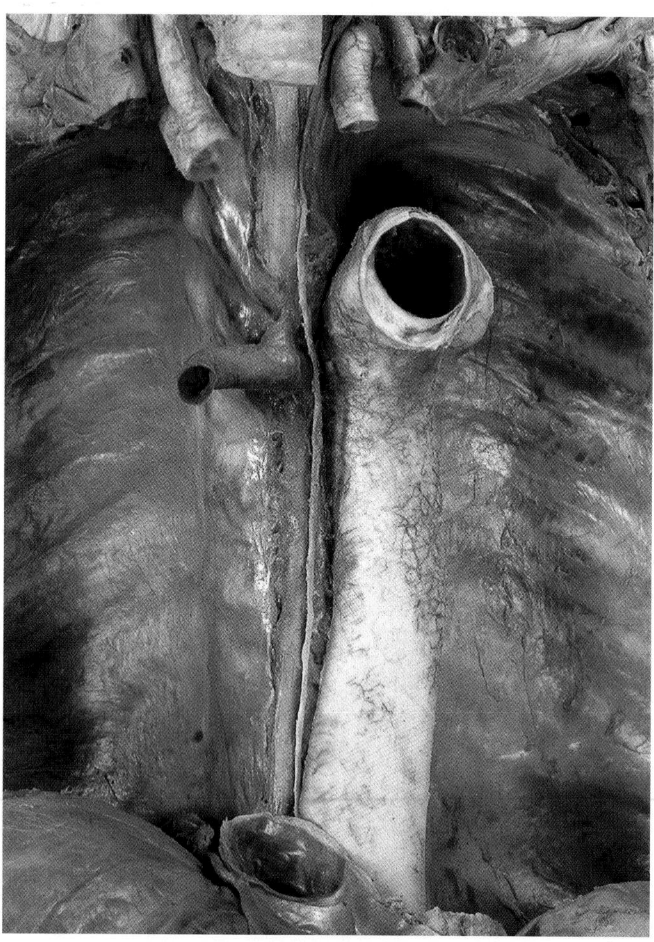

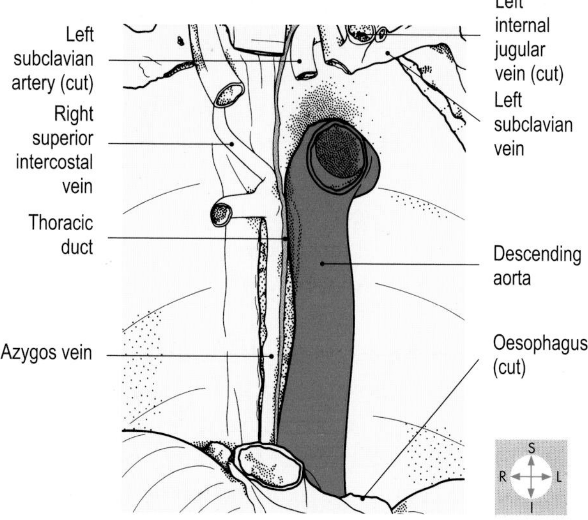

Fig. 2.62 Descending aorta and thoracic duct, exposed after removal of the thoracic part of the oesophagus.

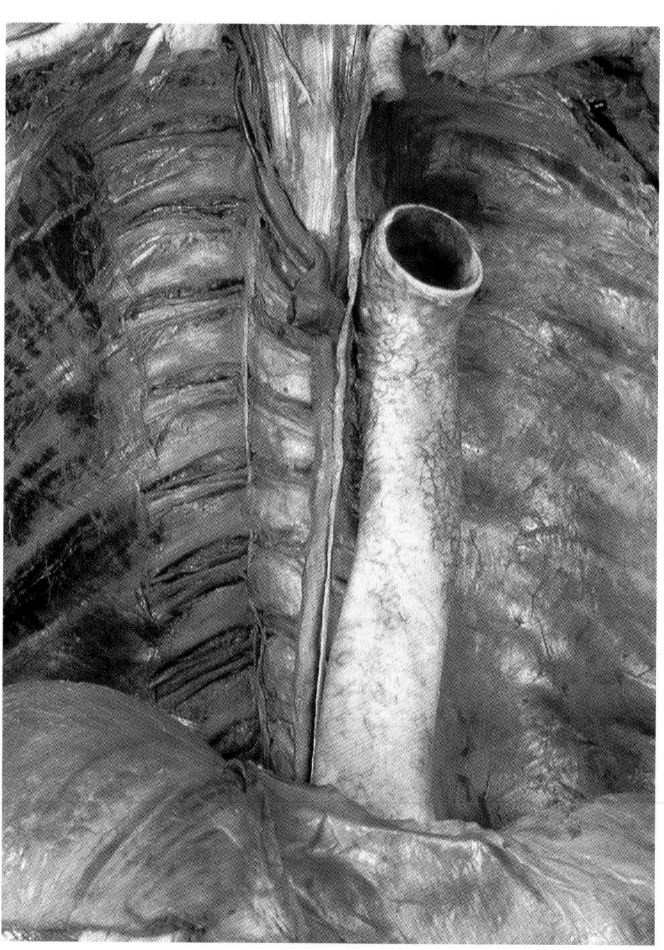

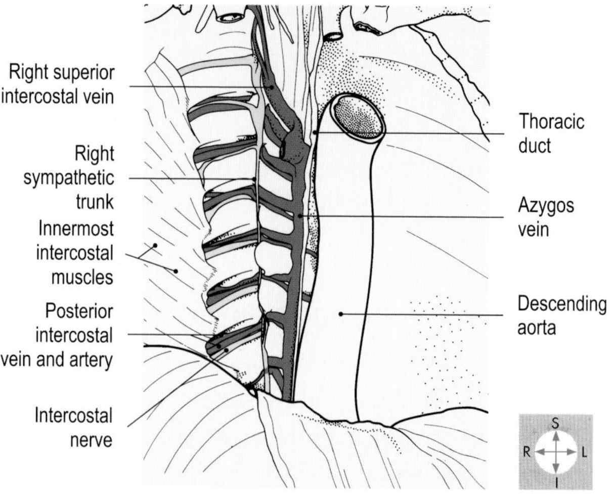

Fig. 2.63 Azygos vein, right intercostal nerves and posterior intercostal vessels, exposed after removal of the parietal pleura.

return from the first space drains into the right brachiocephalic vein. The azygos vein also receives the hemiazygos veins.

The hemiazygos and accessory hemiazygos veins drain the lower eight posterior intercostal spaces on the left side. The lowermost four spaces usually empty into the hemiazygos vein, which crosses the midline to terminate in the azygos vein (Fig. 2.64). Veins from the next four intercostal spaces usually join to form the accessory hemiazygos vein, which also crosses the midline to end in the azygos. Sometimes, the hemiazygos and accessory hemiazygos veins drain into the azygos vein by a single vessel. The second and third spaces on the left are drained by the left superior intercostal vein (see Fig. 2.56), which crosses the aortic arch to end in the left brachiocephalic vein. The first left intercostal space drains into the corresponding brachiocephalic vein.

Thoracic sympathetic trunk

The thoracic part of the sympathetic trunk (chain) runs along the lateral aspects of the thoracic vertebral bodies (Figs 2.64 & 2.65). In continuity with the cervical and abdominal parts, the thoracic sympathetic trunk consists of a series of interconnected enlargements (ganglia) occurring at intervals along its length. Usually, each thoracic spinal nerve is connected to its own ganglion by two branches, a white (preganglionic) and a grey (postganglionic) ramus communicans. Not infrequently, adjacent ganglia fuse together and, most often, the inferior cervical and first thoracic ganglia fuse to form the stellate ganglion.

Branches

Fine nerve filaments running from the sympathetic trunk contribute to the autonomic prevertebral plexuses supplying the thoracic organs, including the heart (cardiac plexuses), lungs (pulmonary plexuses) and the oesophagus (oesophageal plexus). The lower thoracic ganglia give rise to a collection of autonomic fibres that form the greater (Fig. 2.65), lesser and least splanchnic nerves, destined to supply intra-abdominal structures which are gained by piercing the crura of the diaphragm. All thoracic spinal nerves receive from the grey rami communicantes sympathetic postganglionic fibres, which are distributed to various structures of the body wall (for example, blood vessels, hair follicles and sweat glands) by the segmental spinal nerves.

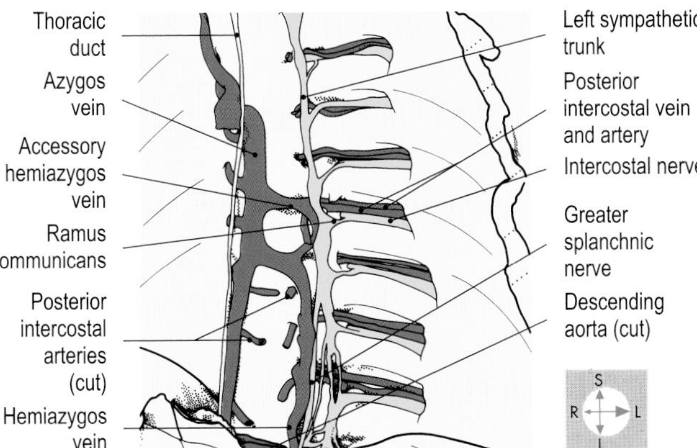

Fig. 2.64 Oblique view of left sympathetic trunk, hemiazygos vein, intercostal nerves and posterior intercostal vessels after removal of the descending aorta and parietal pleura on the left side of the midline.

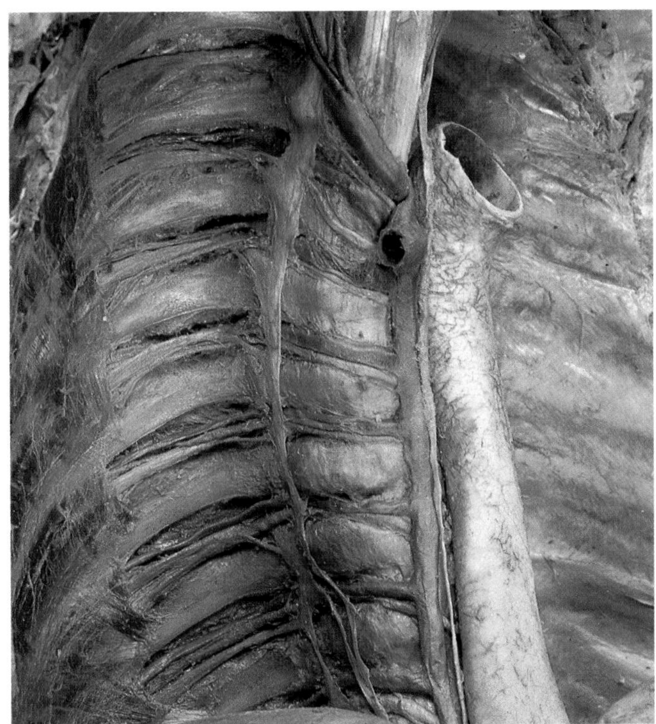

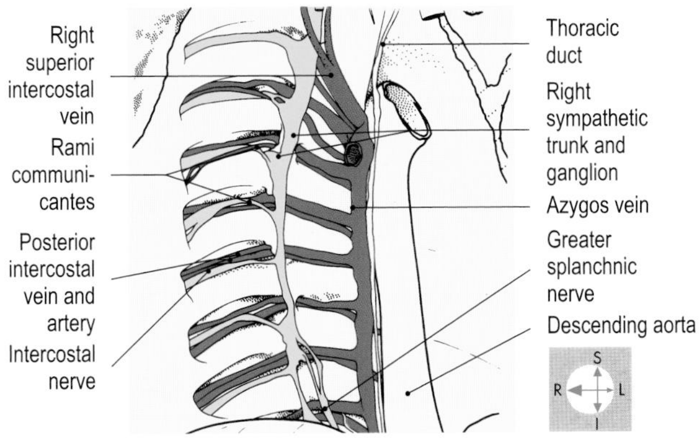

Fig. 2.65 Oblique view of right sympathetic trunk and posterior intercostal vessels and intercostal nerves after removal of the parietal pleura.

Exam Skills

Each of the incomplete statements below is followed by five suggested answers or completions. Decide which are true and which are false. The answers are supplied on page 415.

1. In the right atrium features visible on the interatrial septum include:

a) the orifice of the coronary sinus.
b) the valve of the inferior vena cava.
c) the fossa ovalis.
d) the crista terminalis.
e) musculi pectinati.

2. In the mediastinum:

a) the left brachiocephalic vein passes behind the left common carotid artery.
b) the brachiocephalic trunk arises from the aortic arch.
c) the left vagus nerve crosses the aortic arch.
d) the ligamentum arteriosum connects the aortic arch to the left pulmonary artery.
e) the oesophagus lies anterior to the descending thoracic aorta.

3. The right lung:

a) possesses a transverse fissure.
b) is in contact with the pericardium overlying the right ventricle.
c) possesses an oblique fissure separating the lower from the middle lobe.
d) has an impression of the azygos arch on its medial surface.
e) receives a rich somatic sensory innervation.

4. A typical rib:

a) articulates with the transverse process of the thoracic vertebra of the same number.
b) possesses a head which articulates with the body of the same numbered vertebra.
c) is attached by a costal cartilage to the sternum.
d) is attached to the rib below by fibres of external intercostal muscle.
e) has parietal pleura in contact with its deep surface.

5. The oesophagus:

a) passes through the right crus of the diaphragm.
b) receives innervation from the phrenic nerve.
c) is indented by the arch of the aorta.
d) is closely related to the right recurrent laryngeal nerve in the thorax.
e) has veins draining into the hepatic portal vein.

6. The trachea:

a) has the right brachiocephalic vein anteriorly.
b) divides at the level of the fourth thoracic vertebra.
c) has the aortic arch on its left.
d) has a sensory supply from the phrenic nerves.
e) is closely related to the recurrent laryngeal nerves.

7. The right coronary artery:

a) lies in the coronary sulcus.
b) anastomoses directly with the anterior interventricular artery.
c) supplies the SA node.
d) has a right marginal branch.
e) supplies most of the left ventricle.

8. In the thorax, the right vagus:

a) is closely related to the trachea.
b) gives rise to the right recurrent laryngeal nerve.
c) is crossed by the azygos arch.
d) lies anterior to the root of the right lung.
e) contributes to the formation of the oesophageal plexus.

9. The arch of the aorta:

a) is crossed by the left recurrent laryngeal nerve.
b) is crossed by the left vagus.
c) is covered by parietal pleura of the left lung.
d) is crossed by the left phrenic nerve.
e) is located within the superior mediastinum.

10. In the thorax, the sympathetic chains:

a) connect with the intercostal nerves.
b) give rise to splanchnic nerves.
c) leave in company with the descending thoracic aorta.
d) are covered by parietal pleura.
e) are closely related to the oesophagus.

11. The left brachiocephalic vein:

a) lies partly within the middle mediastinum.
b) lies anterior to the brachiocephalic trunk.
c) usually receives the thoracic duct.
d) terminates in the superior vena cava.
e) receives inferior thyroid veins.

12. The fibrous pericardium:

a) is innervated by intercostal nerves.
b) is firmly attached to the diaphragm.
c) is closely related to the phrenic nerves.
d) is closely related to the oesophagus.
e) is lined by parietal serous pericardium.

13. The left main bronchus:

a) lies within the concavity of the arch of the aorta.
b) is closely related to the oesophagus.
c) is usually wider than the right main bronchus.
d) lies posterior to the left vagus nerve.
e) receives branches from the internal thoracic artery.

14. Concerning respiratory movements:

a) the diaphragm descends during expiration.
b) the lung extends into the costodiaphragmatic recess during inspiration.
c) intercostal muscles contract during inspiration.
d) expiration is assisted by contraction of pectoralis major.
e) elasticity of the lungs contributes to expiration.

15. The thoracic duct:

a) enters the thorax in company with the oesophagus.
b) lies in the posterior mediastinum.
c) arches across the apex of the left lung.
d) lies anterior to the trachea in the superior mediastinum.
e) lies to the left of the azygos vein as it enters the thorax.

16. Concerning the cardiac conducting system:

a) the SA node lies in the interatrial septum.
b) specialized conducting tissue connects the SA and AV nodes.
c) the AV node lies close to the termination of the coronary sinus.
d) the AV bundle lies in the interventricular septum.
e) the left coronary artery is commonly the main arterial supply.

Clinical Skills

The answers are supplied on page 416.

Case Study 1

A 51-year-old woman complained to her family practitioner that she had felt very fatigued for several weeks. She had lost 7–10 pounds in weight over the previous month. On physical examination the physician discovered a firm nodular swelling, about 3–4 cm in diameter, in the left breast that was anchored in tissue several centimetres beneath the skin.

Questions:

1. To which additional areas of this woman's body should the physician direct special attention during the physical examination and why?
2. Which muscle should be caused to contract in order to demonstrate the fixation of the swelling?
3. Following surgical removal of the swelling and exploration of the axilla, the patient is found to have a winged scapula. How has this occurred?
4. Following surgery, she noted a swollen left arm - why?

Case Study 2

A 67-year-old man developed a worsening cough over several months and, when the sputum began to show streaks of blood, he consulted a physician. The patient gave a history of smoking cigarettes for 40 years and recently had noted that his voice had become hoarse. An X-ray of the chest revealed an irregularly shaped density in the hilar region of the left lung.

Questions:

1. How might the hoarseness relate to the location of the density?
2. Which other structures are situated in the vicinity of the hilar region of the lung?
3. What is the nerve supply of the mediastinal pleura against which the density lies?
4. If the density obstructed the left upper lobe bronchus, what would the effect be?

Case Study 3

While playing golf, a 74-year-old man felt tingling down the medial side of his left arm. He continued to play but 10 minutes later began to have difficulty breathing and became dizzy. He sat down on a nearby bench but soon complained of severe chest pain and then lapsed into unconsciousness.

He was rushed to hospital where an electrocardiogram showed irregularities in the heart's electrical activity. Some minutes later he deteriorated markedly, and his blood pressure dropped dramatically. He lapsed into a deep coma and died several minutes later. A post-mortem showed total obstruction of the left coronary artery and near-complete obstruction of the right coronary artery.

Questions:

1. What is the cause of the tingling sensation in the left arm?
2. How does coronary artery disease cause irregularities in the cardiac cycle?
3. Which coronary artery is more likely to cause irregularities in rhythm if obstructed?
4. Where do anastomoses occur between the coronary arteries?

Case Study 4

An 8-year-old boy was found to have high blood pressure during a school physical examination. He was referred to his physician, who verified the high blood pressure and noted that his femoral pulses were weak in comparison to the radial and carotid pulses. His feet seemed cool to the touch and the patient said he always had to wear warm socks even in summer. A chest radiograph was remarkable for irregular notches along the lower borders of several of the ribs on both sides of his chest.

Questions:

1. How can unequal pulses in the upper and lower limbs be explained?
2. Which vessels caused the notching along the ribs, and in which direction was blood flowing through them?
3. Rib notching was absent from the upper two ribs. Why?
4. Would auscultation of the thorax reveal any abnormal sounds?

Observation Skills

Identify the structures indicated. The answers are supplied at the foot of the page.

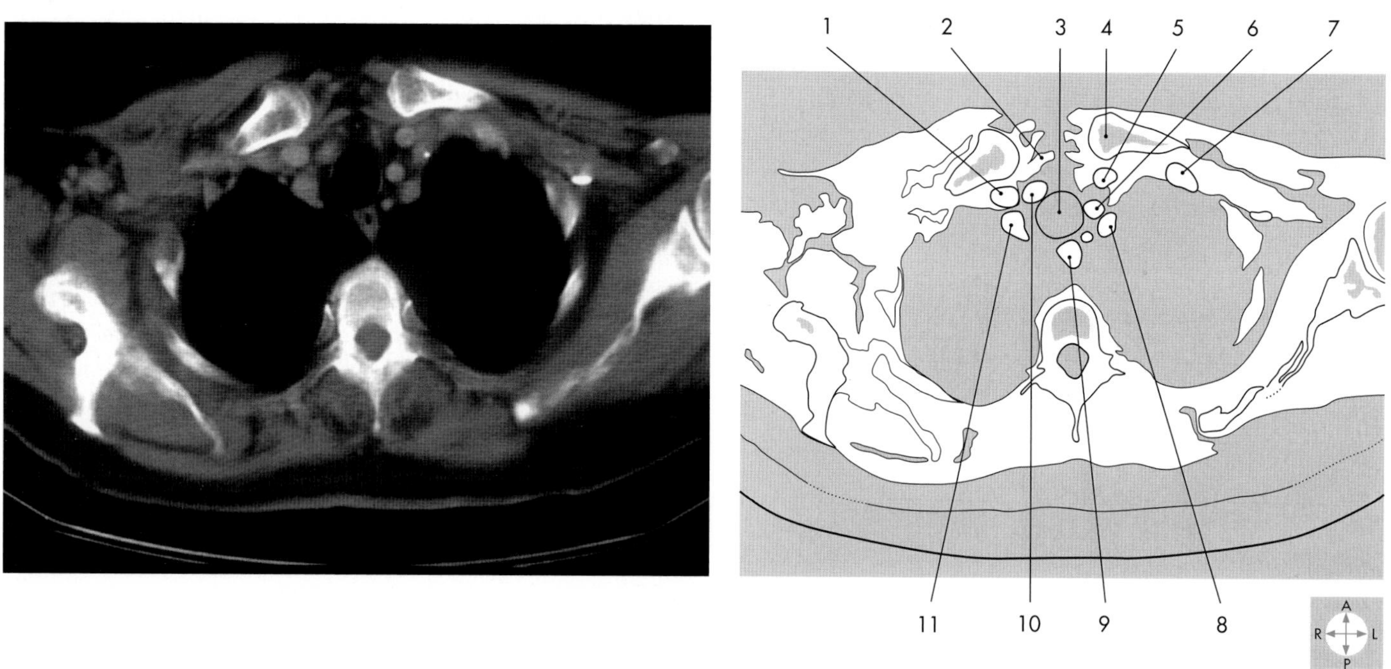

Fig. 2.66 Transverse CT image at the level of the second thoracic vertebra. Compare Fig. 2.70.

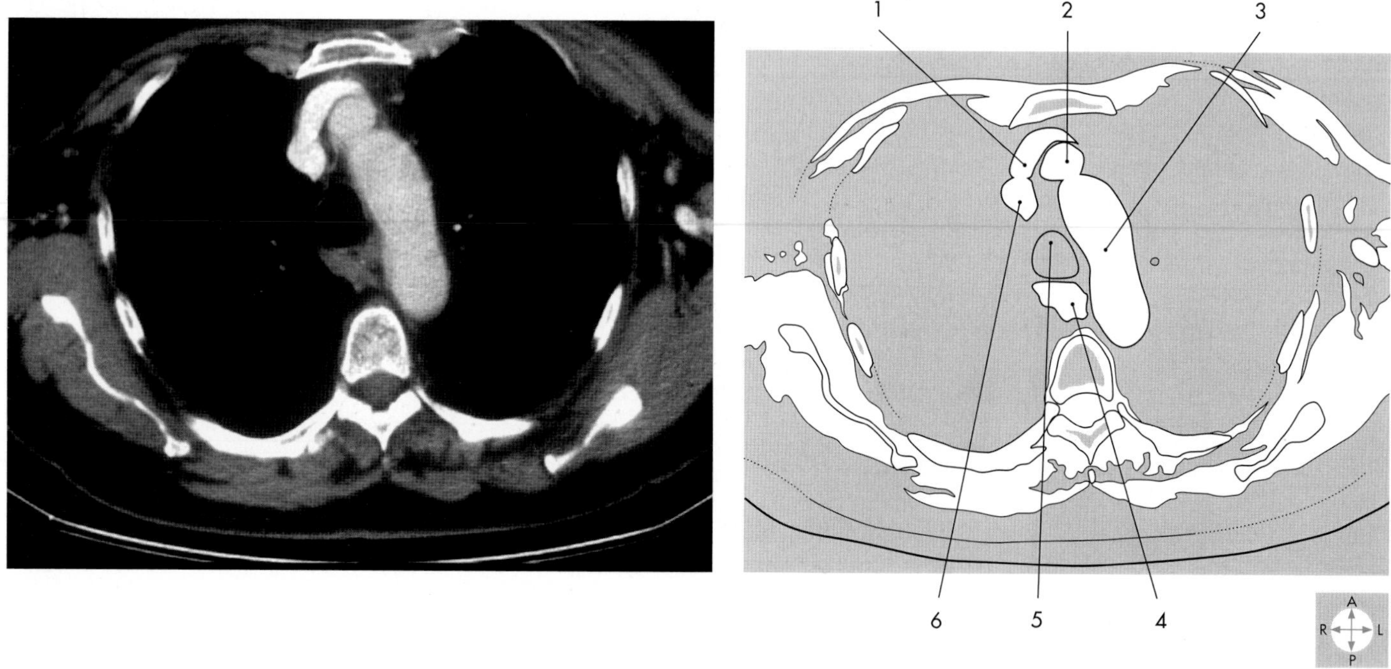

Fig. 2.67 Transverse CT image at the level of the fourth thoracic vertebra. Compare Fig. 2.18.

Answers

Fig. 2.66 1 = right internal jugular vein; 2 = infrahyoid strap muscle; 3 = trachea; 4 = medial end of left clavicle; 5 = left internal jugular vein; 6 = left common carotid artery; 7 = left subclavian vein; 8 = left subclavian artery; 9 = oesophagus; 10 = right common carotid artery; 11 = right subclavian artery.

Fig. 2.67 1 = left brachiocephalic vein; 2 = brachiocephalic trunk arising from arch of aorta; 3 = aortic arch; 4 = oesophagus; 5 = trachea; 6 = termination of right brachiocephalic vein.

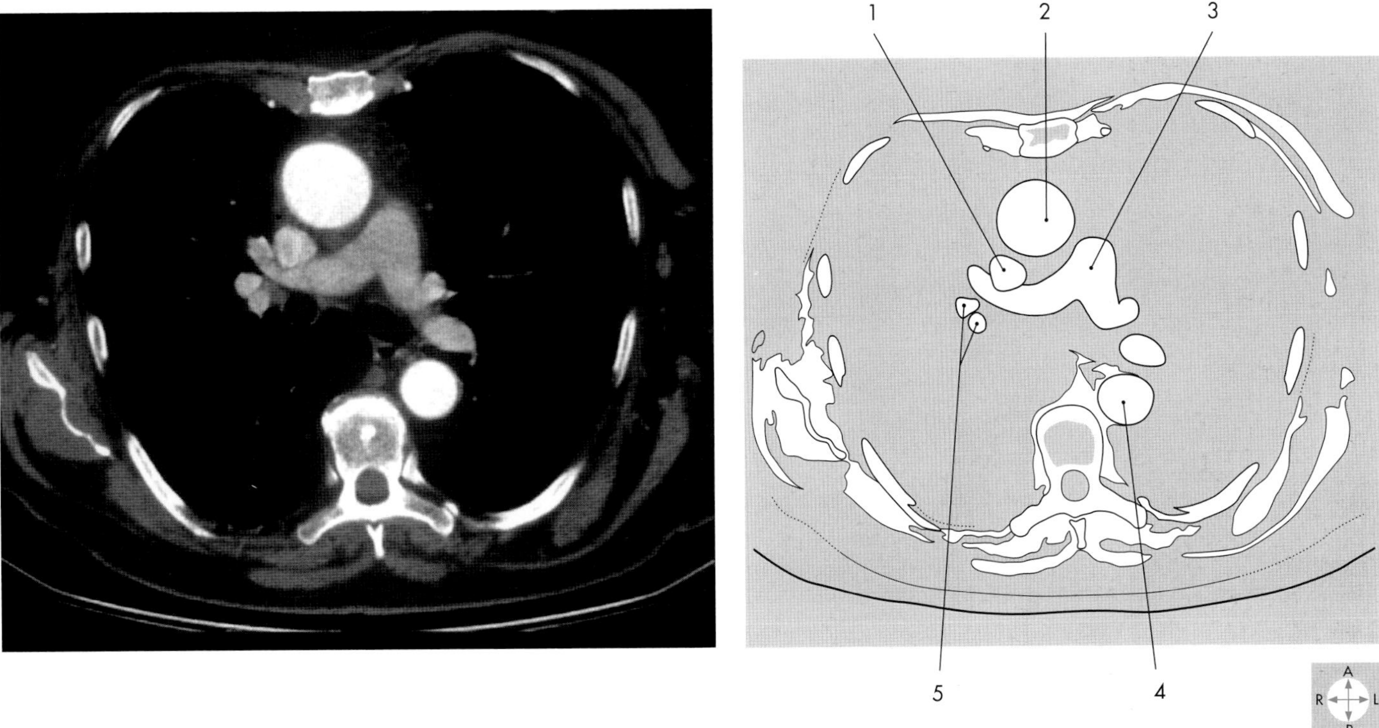

Fig. 2.68 Transverse CT image at the level of the fifth thoracic vertebra. Compare Fig. 2.27.

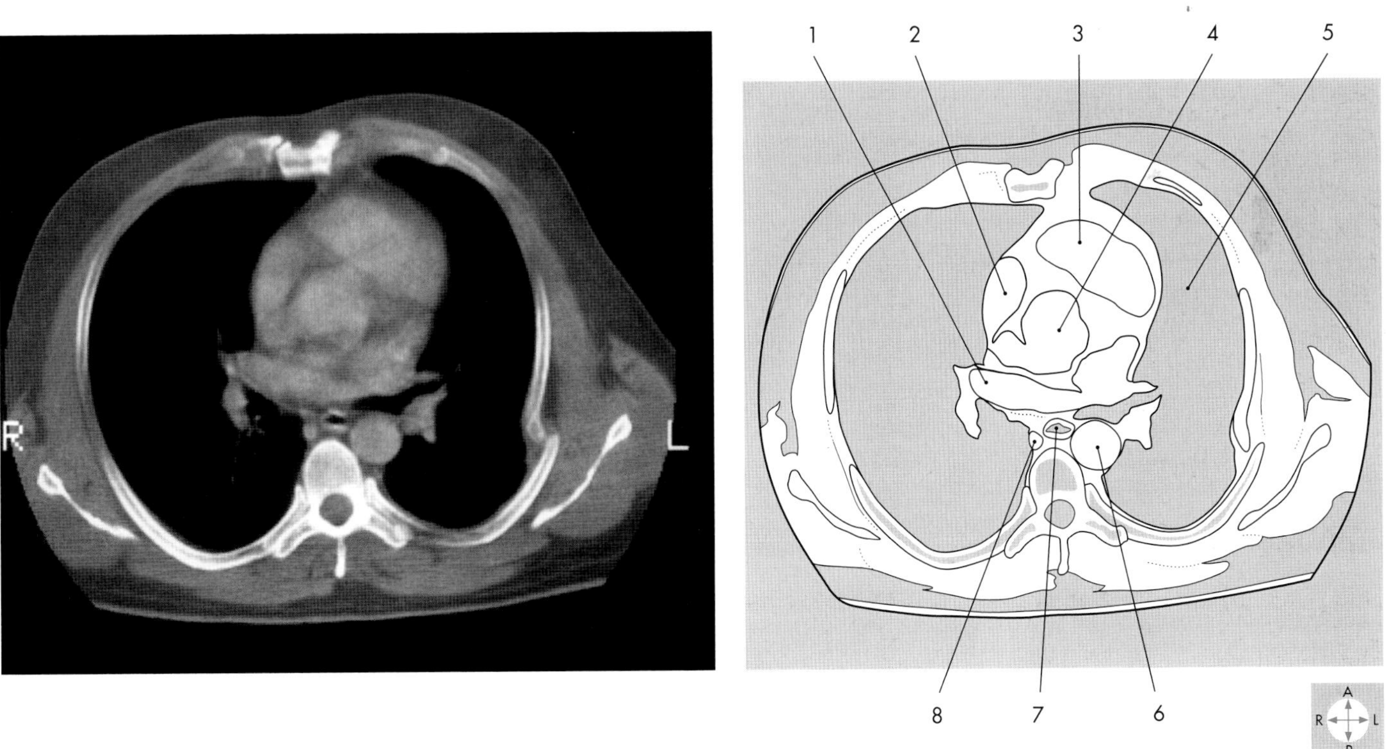

Fig. 2.69 Transverse CT image at the level of the seventh thoracic vertebra. Compare Fig. 1.5.

Answers

Fig. 2.68 1 = superior vena cava; 2 = ascending aorta; 3 = bifurcation of pulmonary trunk into right and left pulmonary arteries; 4 = descending aorta; 5 = pulmonary veins.

Fig. 2.69 1 = right pulmonary vein entering left atrium; 2 = right atrium; 3 = right ventricle; 4 = infundibulum of left ventricle; 5 = left lung; 6 = descending aorta; 7 = oesophagus; 8 = azygos vein.

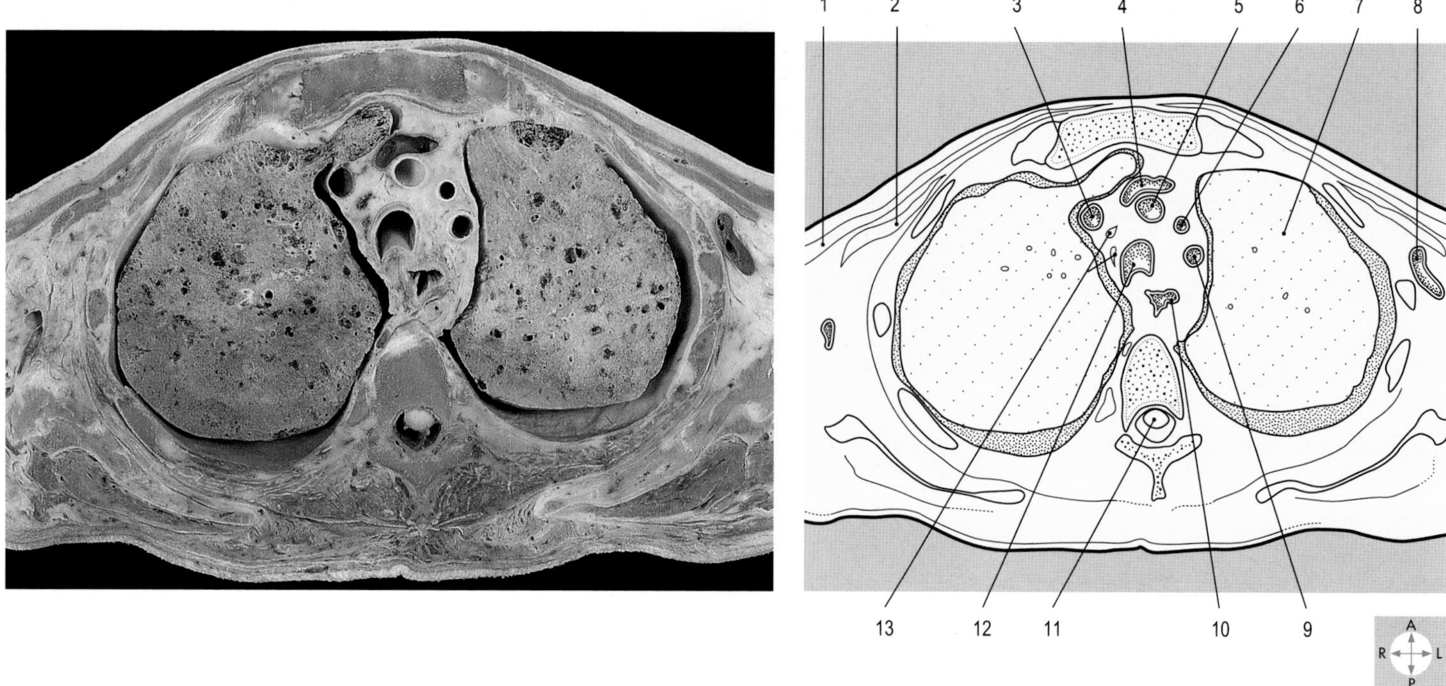

Fig. 2.70 Transverse section at the level of the third thoracic vertebra. Inferior aspect. Compare Fig. 2.66.

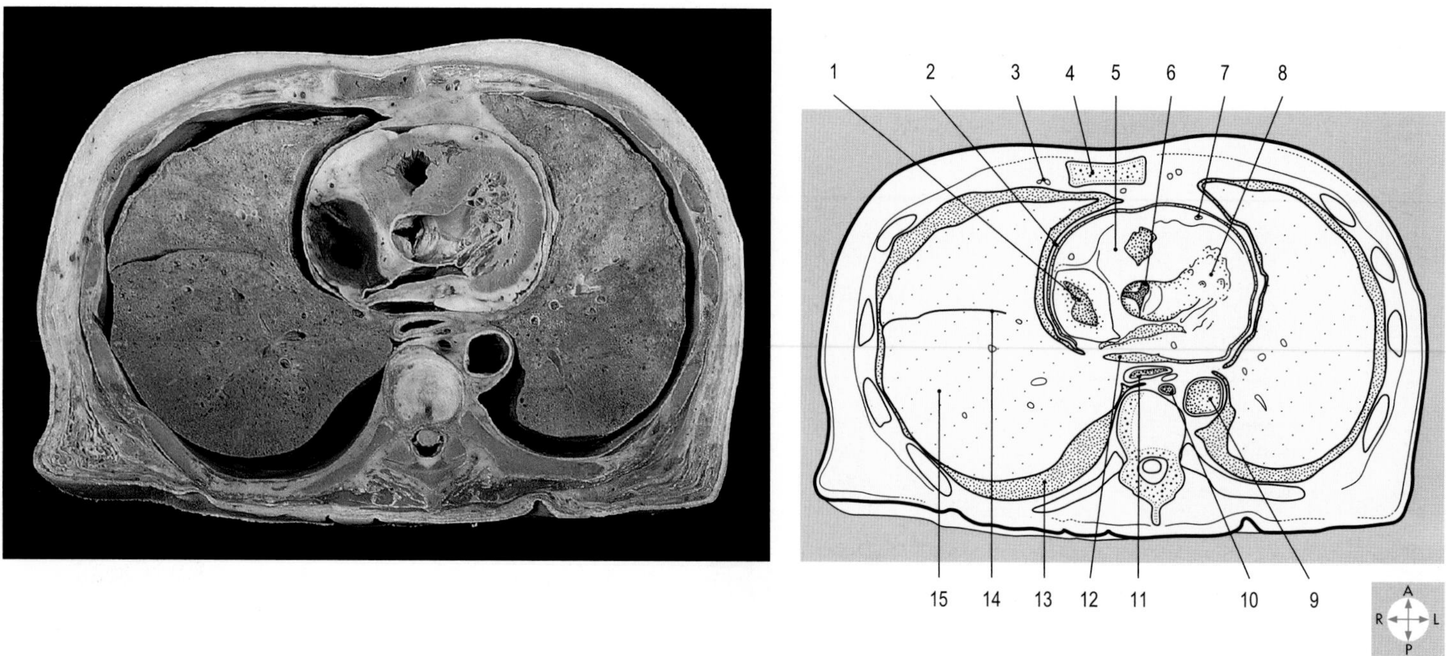

Fig. 2.71 Transverse section at the level of the sixth thoracic vertebra. Inferior aspect. Compare Fig. 2.31.

Answers

Fig. 2.70 1 = pectoralis major; 2 = pectoralis minor; 3 = right brachiocephalic vein; 4 = left brachiocephalic vein; 5 = brachiocephalic trunk; 6 = left common carotid artery; 7 = left lung; 8 = left axillary vein; 9 = left subclavian artery; 10 = oesophagus; 11 = thoracic spinal cord; 12 = trachea; 13 = lymph nodes.

Fig. 2.71 1 = right atrium; 2 = fibrous pericardium; 3 = internal thoracic vessels; 4 = sternum; 5 = right ventricle; 6 = aortic valve; 7 = anterior interventricular artery; 8 = left ventricle; 9 = descending aorta; 10 = azygos vein; 11 = oesophagus; 12 = pericardial cavity; 13 = pleural cavity; 14 = oblique fissure; 15 = lower lobe of right lung.

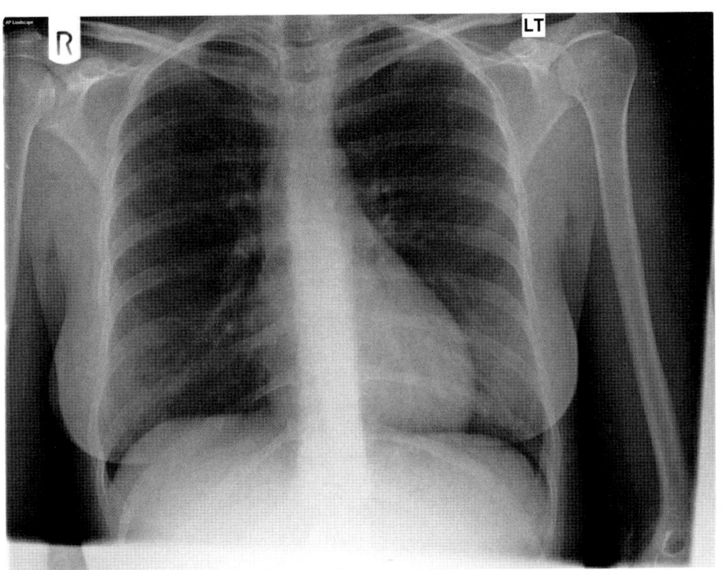

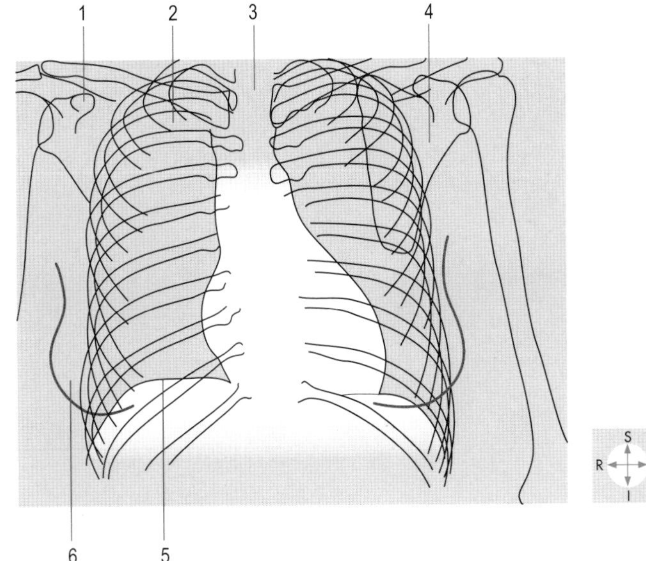

Fig. 2.72 Posteroanterior chest radiograph.

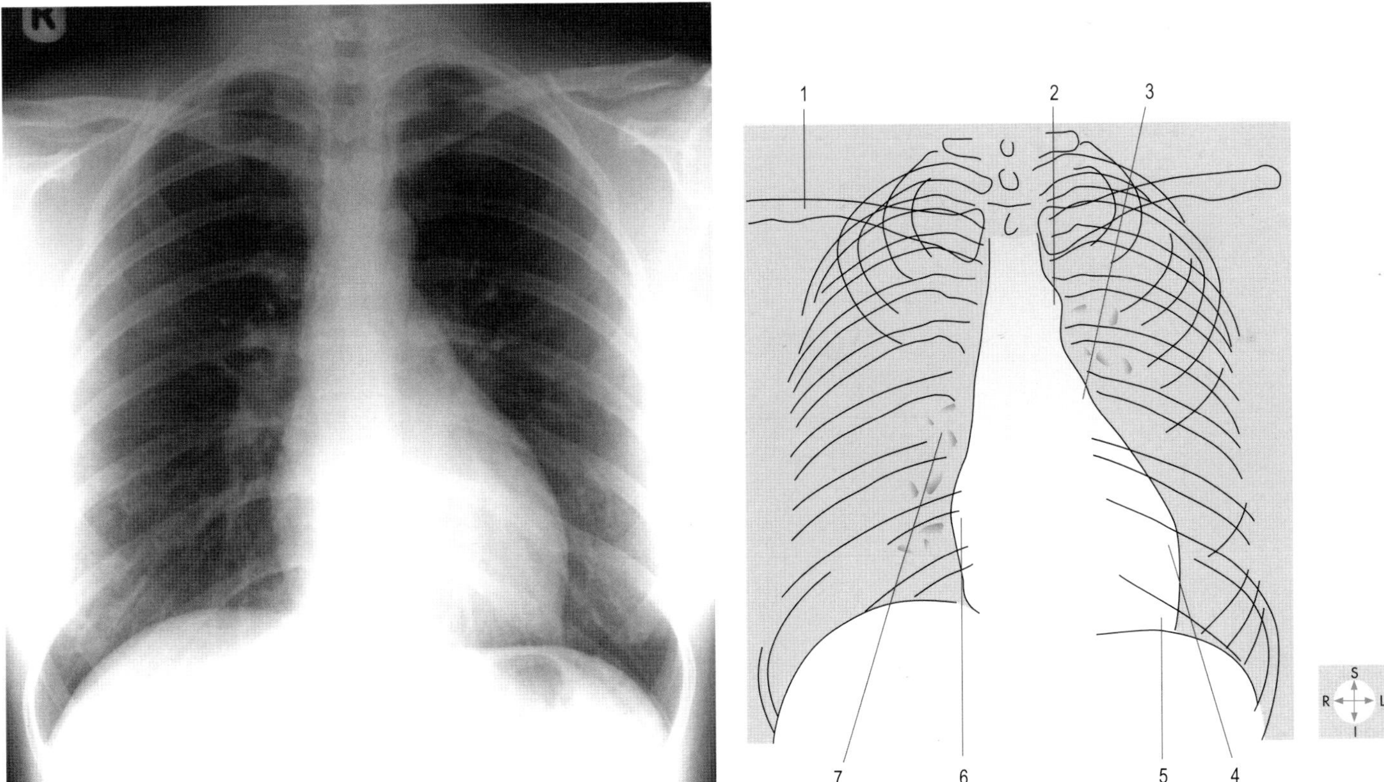

Fig. 2.73 Posteroanterior chest radiograph.

Answers

Fig. 2.72 1 = coracoid process; 2 = first rib; 3 = trachea; 4 = blade of scapula; 5 = diaphragm; 6 = breast.

Fig. 2.73 1 = clavicle; 2 = arch of aorta; 3 = pulmonary trunk; 4 = left ventricle; 5 = apex; 6 = right atrium; 7 = hilar markings.

Upper limb

CHAPTER 3

Introduction

The upper limb (extremity) comprises several bones and their joints (Fig. 3.1), clothed by soft tissues. For descriptive purposes the limb is divided into regions (Fig. 3.2), each enveloped by fascia and containing muscles with nerve and vascular supplies. The scapula with its associated muscles and soft tissues comprise the scapular region, the muscles attaching between the front of the chest wall and the upper limb (together with the overlying fascia, breast and skin) constitute the pectoral region. The scapula and the clavicle, which together form the pectoral girdle, articulate at the acromioclavicular joint. The clavicle articulates with the trunk at the sternoclavicular joint and the scapula with the humerus at the glenohumeral (shoulder) joint.

Between the proximal part of the limb and the chest wall is the axilla, a region traversed by the principal nerves and vessels passing between the upper limb and the root of the neck.

The arm is that part of the upper limb between the shoulder and the elbow. The muscles of the arm are disposed in anterior (flexor) and posterior (extensor) compartments, separated by the humerus and the medial and lateral intermuscular septa (Fig. 3.3). In front of the elbow joint (at which the humerus, radius and ulna articulate) lies the cubital fossa, a region traversed by vessels and nerves passing between the arm and the forearm.

The forearm lies between the elbow and the wrist, and its muscles are arranged in anterior (flexor) and posterior (extensor) compartments, separated by the radius, ulna, and interosseous membrane (Fig. 3.4). Rotation at the proximal and distal radioulnar joints permits the hand to function in any position between the extremes of supination (palm facing up), and pronation (palm facing down).

The forearm articulates with the carpus at the wrist (radiocarpal) joint. Together with the flexor retinaculum, the bones of the carpus form the carpal tunnel, which links the anterior compartment of the forearm and the palm of the hand. The structures of the palm lie anterior to the metacarpals, while posteriorly is the dorsum of the hand. The digits are named, from lateral to medial, the thumb and the index, middle, ring and little fingers.

The skin and subcutaneous tissue of the shoulder region are supplied by supraclavicular nerves, whereas the cutaneous supply of the remainder of the upper limb is derived from

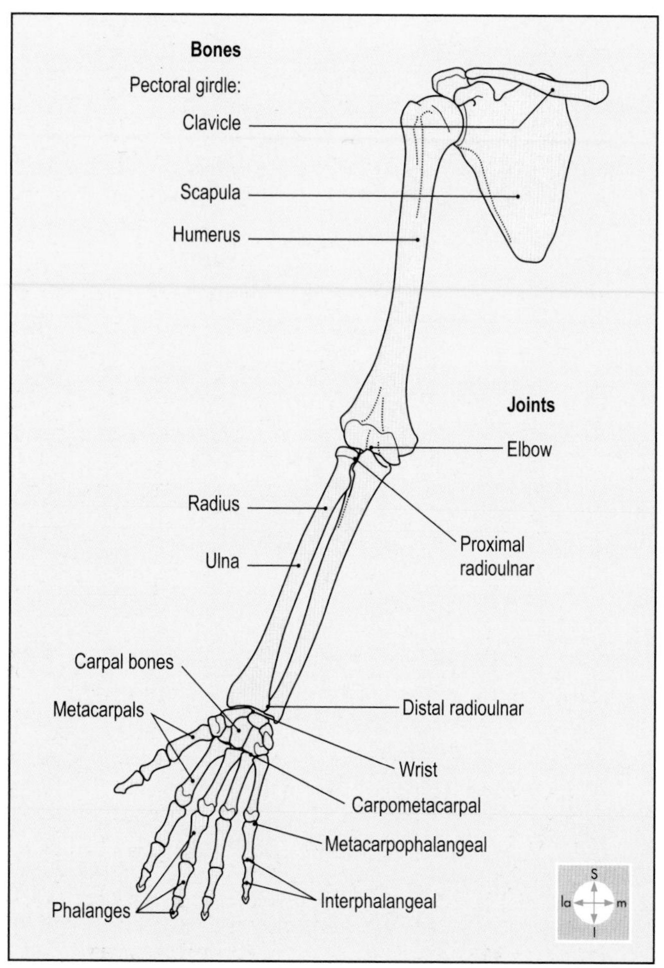

Fig. 3.1 Bones and joints of the upper limb.

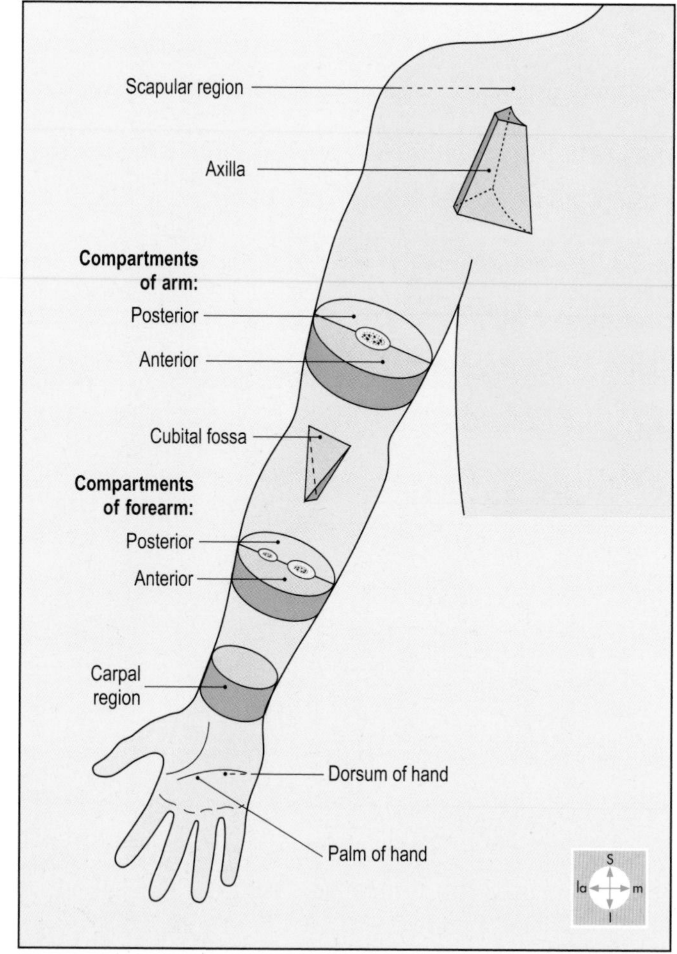

Fig. 3.2 Parts of the upper limb.

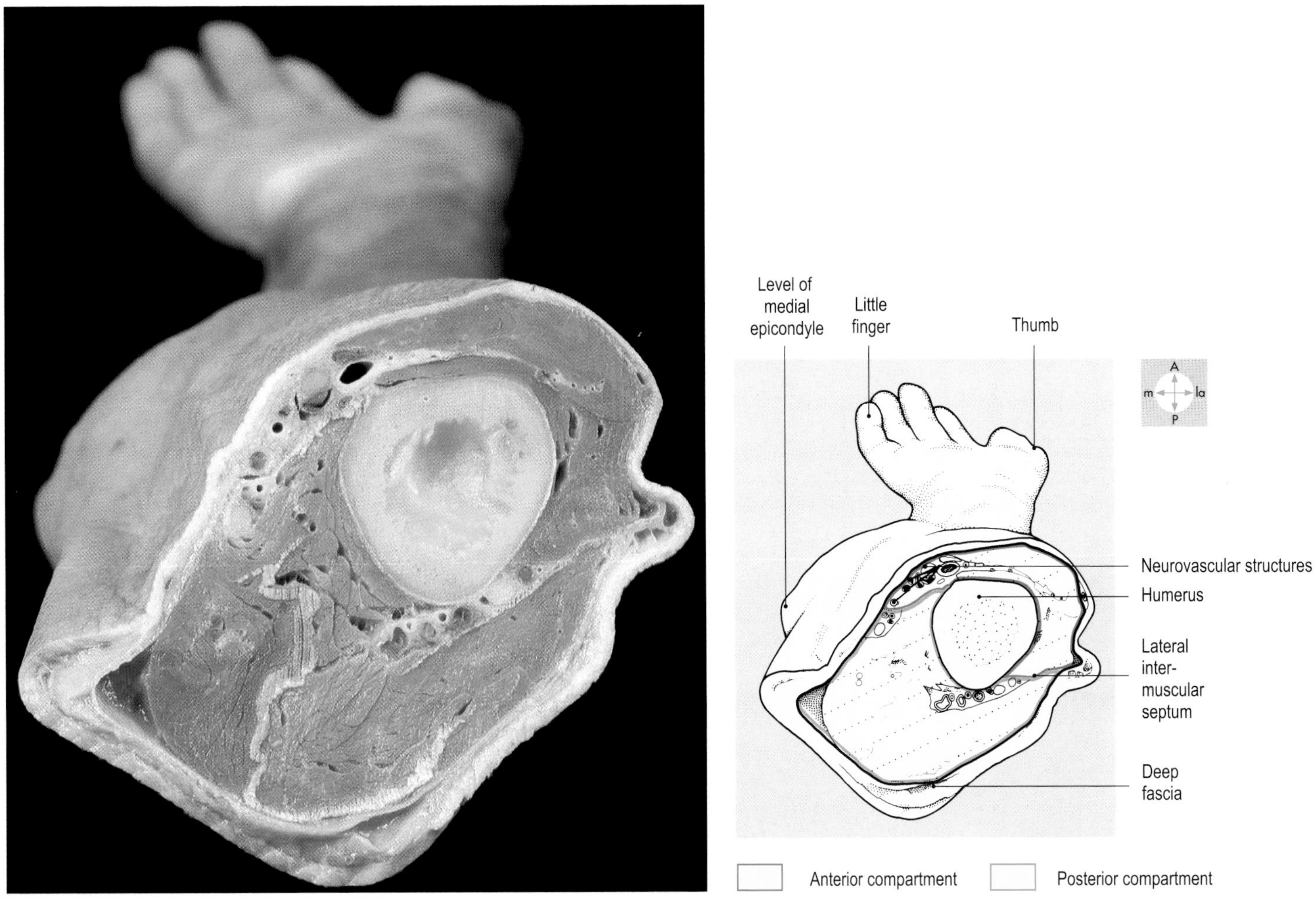

Level of medial epicondyle
Little finger
Thumb
A
m
la
P
Neurovascular structures
Humerus
Lateral inter-muscular septum
Deep fascia
Anterior compartment
Posterior compartment

Fig. 3.3 Transverse section midway between glenohumeral and elbow joints to show the compartments of the arm.

Superficial vein
Little finger
Inter-osseous membrane
A
m
la
P
Thumb
Deep fascia
Radius
Intermuscular septa
Ulna
Anterior compartment
Posterior compartment

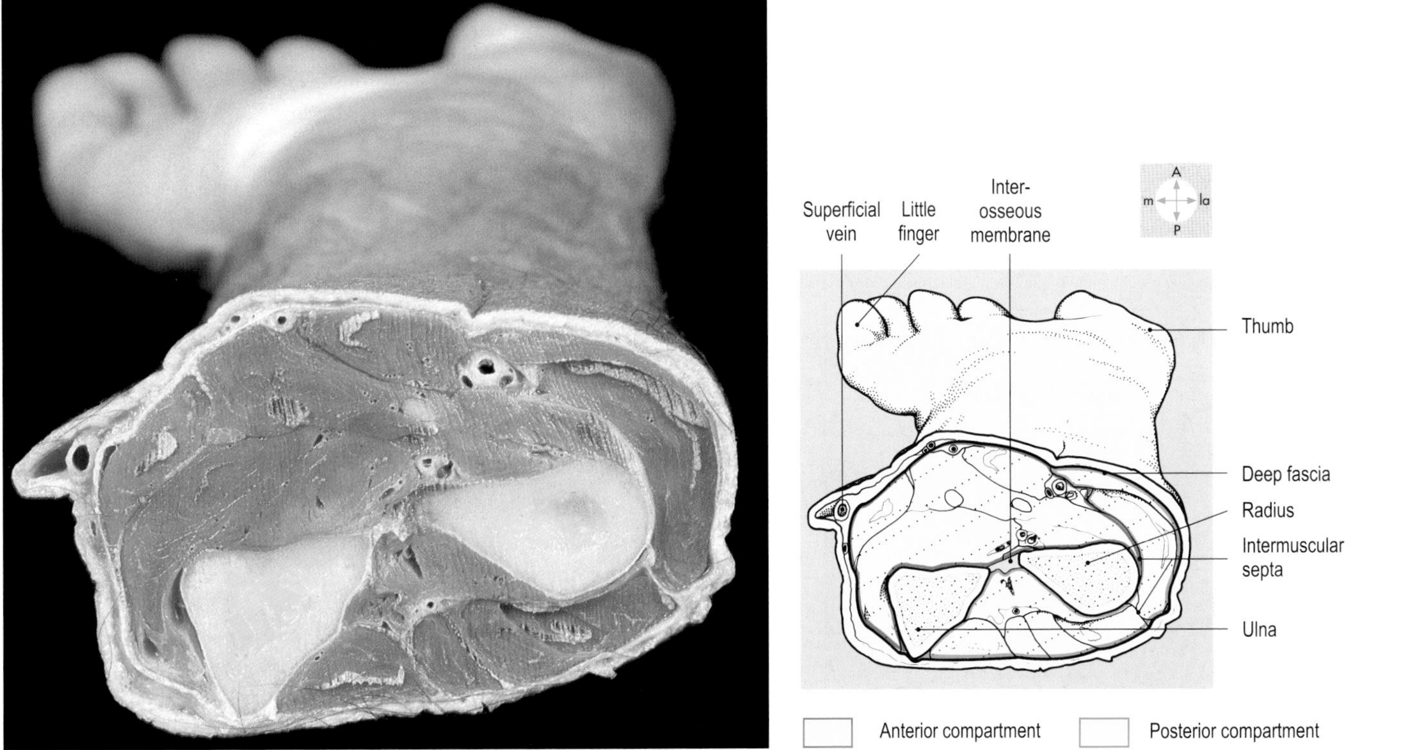

Fig. 3.4 Transverse section midway between elbow and wrist joints to show the compartments of the forearm.

the brachial plexus (Fig. 3.5). Each of the anterior (ventral) rami contributing to this plexus supplies a specific area of skin (dermatome; Fig. 3.6). Each dermatome and the area supplied by each individual superficial nerve may vary somewhat from one person to another. There is overlapping of innervation by adjacent superficial nerves, and therefore damage to a single nerve produces anaesthesia over an area smaller than that supplied by the nerve.

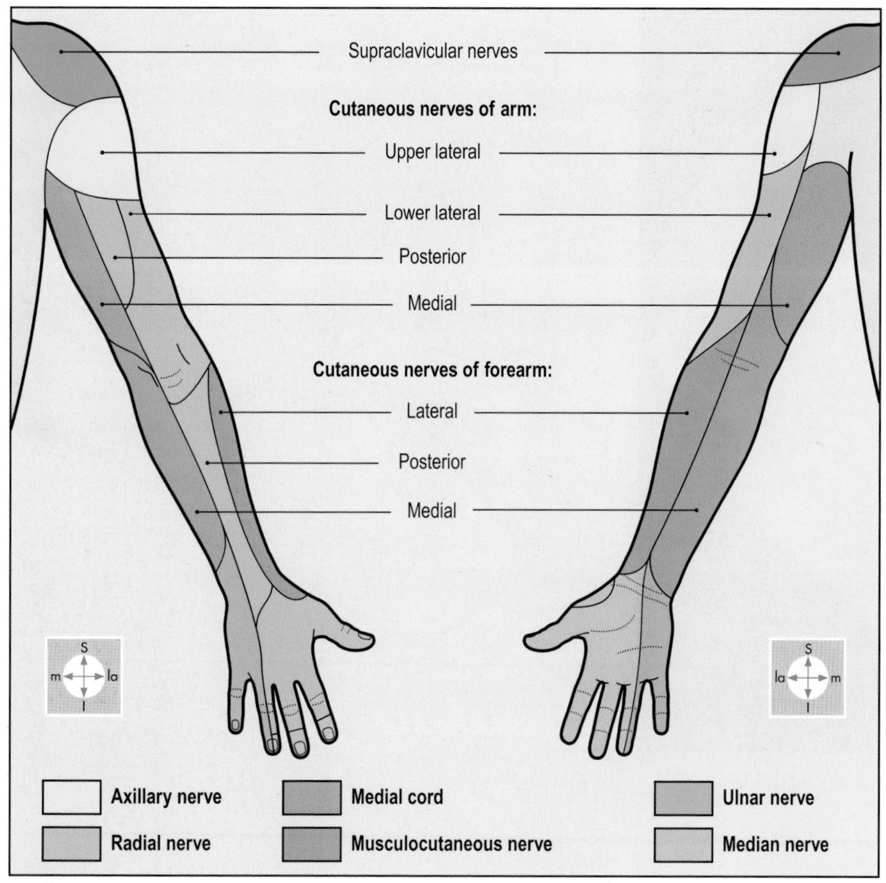

Fig. 3.5 Typical distribution of cutaneous nerves in the upper limb.

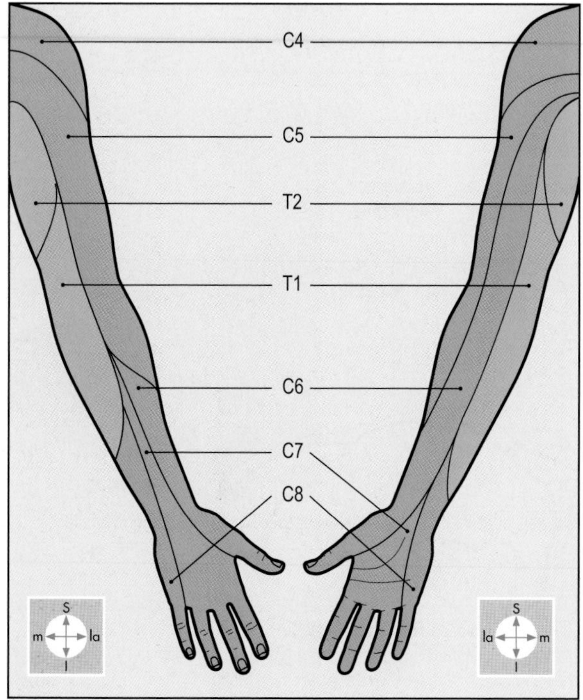

Fig. 3.6 Typical arrangement of dermatomes of upper limb. There may be considerable overlap of areas supplied.

The courses of the principal arteries are shown in Figure 3.7. In the root of the neck the axillary artery is continuous with the subclavian artery which derives from the brachiocephalic trunk on the right, but directly from the arch of the aorta on the left side. In the axilla and arm there is a single main arterial channel, which terminates in the forearm by dividing into radial and ulnar arteries.

There are deep and superficial veins in the upper limb (Fig. 3.8). Deep veins accompany the arteries in the forearm and hand and consist of interconnecting networks of venae comitantes. The brachial artery may be accompanied by either one or two veins, but there is usually a single axillary vein which drains via the subclavian into the brachiocephalic vein. The superficial veins, lying outside the muscle compartments, are often visible through the skin and those on the forearm and back of the hand are often used for venepuncture. The veins contain valves which prevent backflow of blood. The smaller superficial veins, and on occasion the main veins of the limb, are subject to considerable variation, even between the right and left sides of the same individual.

Most superficial lymphatics of the upper limb drain to the axillary nodes (see p. 81), although lymph from the medial aspect of the forearm first traverses a small group of nodes near the medial aspect of the cubital fossa. In the shoulder region some lymph may pass through supra- or infraclavicular nodes. The deep lymphatics of the limb also drain to the axillary lymph nodes. From here, lymph passes into the subclavian trunk and then into either the right lymphatic duct or, on the left, the thoracic duct (see Fig. 1.34).

Figure 3.9 illustrates the important sites at which the principal nerves of the limb are closely related to bone: axillary nerve to the neck of the humerus; radial nerve to the midshaft of the humerus; ulnar nerve to the medial epicondyle; posterior interosseous nerve to the neck of the radius. Injury to one of these bones may damage the adjacent nerve. The main parts of the brachial plexus in the axilla, the cords, are continuous via the divisions and trunks in the lower part of the neck with the anterior (ventral) rami of spinal nerves C5, C6, C7, C8 and T1, which form the roots of the plexus.

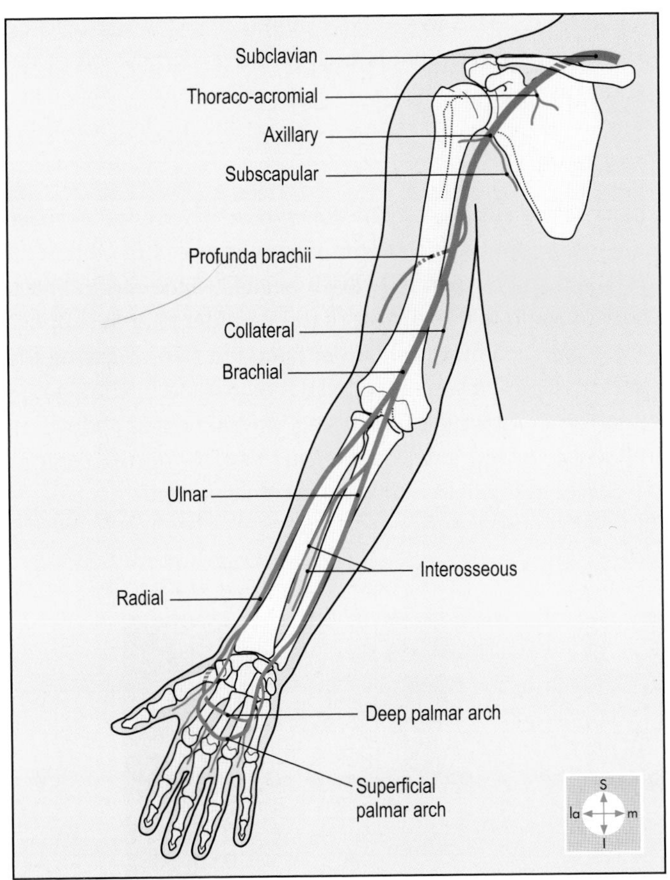

Fig. 3.7 Principal arteries of the upper limb. No muscular branches are shown.

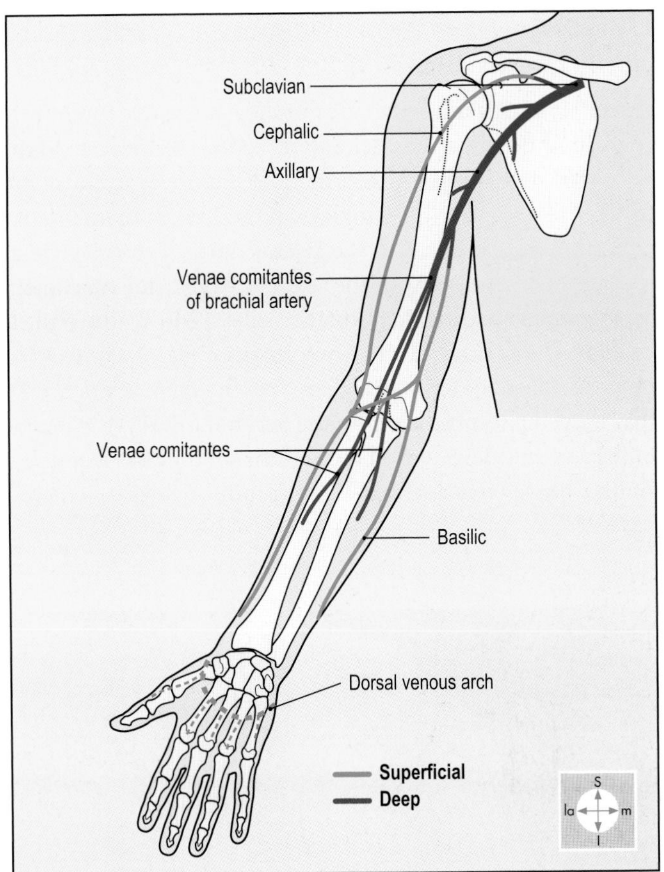

Fig. 3.8 Typical arrangement of the principal veins of the upper limb. For clarity, venae comitantes are illustrated as single channels.

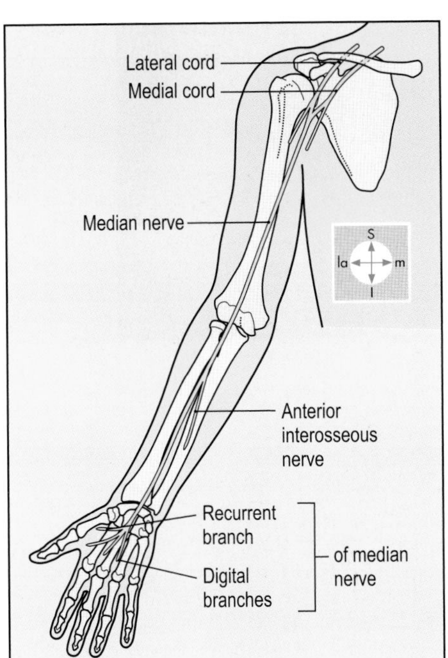

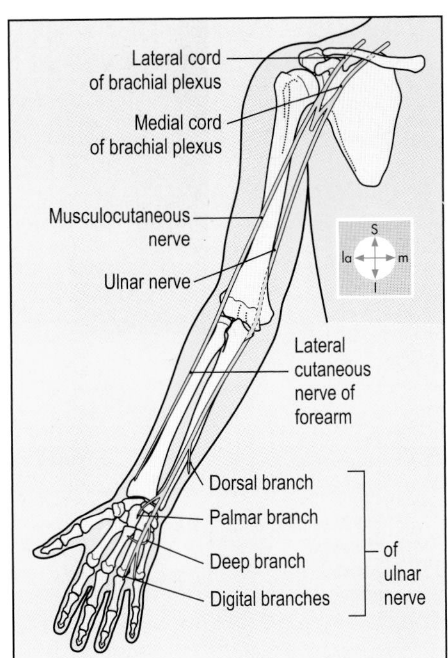

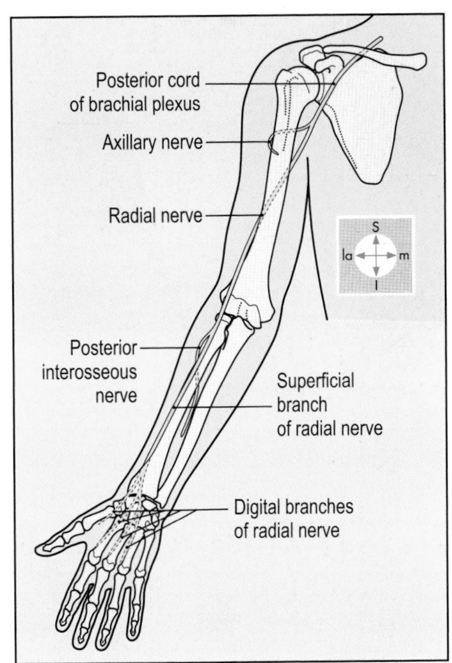

Fig. 3.9 Courses of the principal nerves of the upper limb. From left to right: median nerve, musculocutaneous and ulnar nerves, radial and axillary nerves.

Deltoid

Deltoid is a large multipennate muscle responsible for the rounded contour of the shoulder region (Fig. 3.10). The muscle overlies the shoulder joint and the attachments of the short scapular muscles to the upper end of the humerus (Fig. 3.11). Proximally, it has a continuous attachment to the lateral third of the clavicle and to the acromion and spine of the scapula. The distal attachment is to a roughened area, the deltoid tuberosity, midway down the lateral surface of the shaft of the humerus (see Fig. 3.23). Deltoid acts only on the shoulder joint, where it is the main abductor. During this movement, produced by the acromial fibres, the joint is stabilized by the clavicular fibres and those from the scapular spine. Acting alone, the anterior fibres produce flexion, whereas the posterior fibres extend the shoulder joint. Deltoid is supplied by the axillary nerve, a terminal branch of the posterior cord of the brachial plexus.

Axillary nerve

The axillary nerve leaves the axilla through the quadrangular space (see Fig. 3.64) accompanied by the posterior circumflex humeral artery. In its course the nerve is closely related to the surgical neck of the humerus and to the capsule of the shoulder joint. It supplies deltoid and teres minor, the shoulder joint and skin overlying the lower part of deltoid. Damage to the nerve may occur during dislocation of the shoulder joint, resulting in weakness of abduction, impaired sensation and, subsequently, in loss of the normal contour of the shoulder as the deltoid muscle becomes wasted.

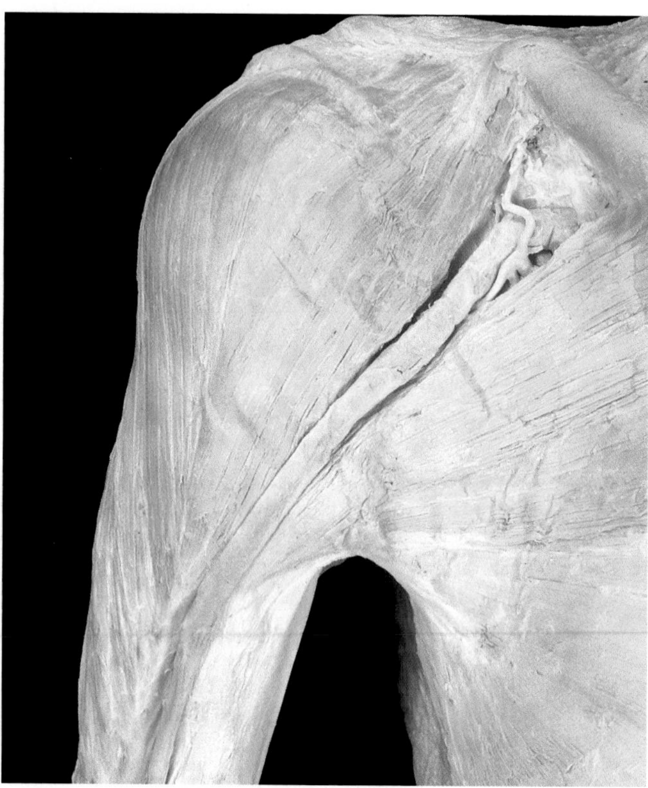

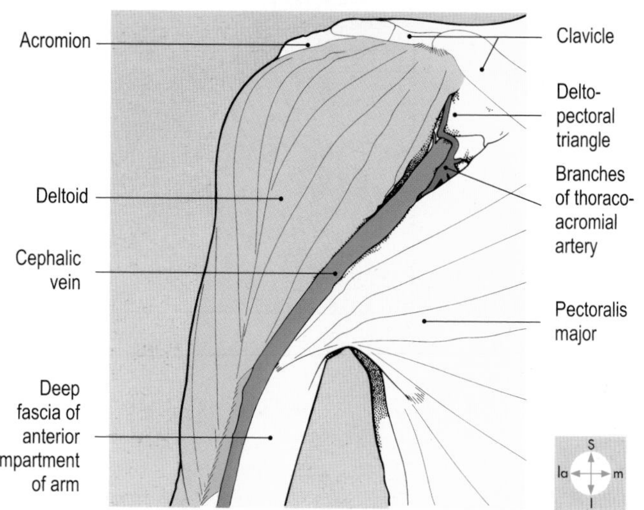

Fig. 3.10 Anterior view of deltoid. The cephalic vein lies in the deltopectoral groove. Deformity of the clavicle is due to a healed fracture.

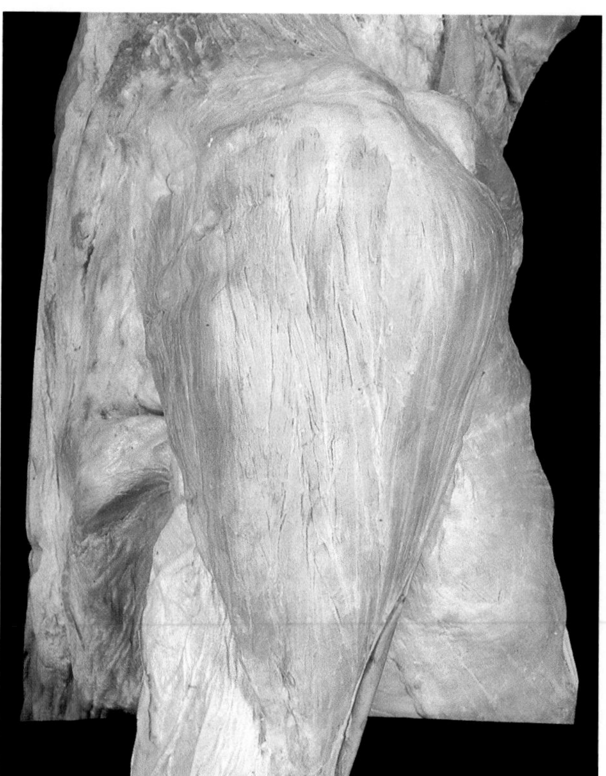

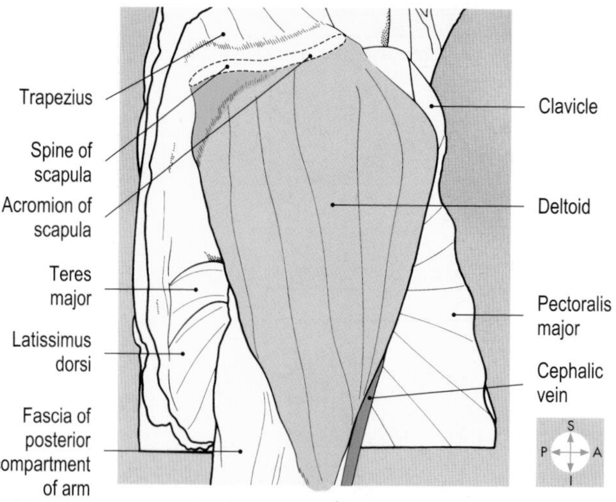

Fig. 3.11 Lateral view. Deltoid has a continuous proximal attachment to the spine and acromion of the scapula and the lateral part of the clavicle.

Axilla

The axilla is the space between the root of the upper limb and the chest wall. It is traversed by the principal vessels and nerves that pass between the upper limb and the root of the neck. The shape and size of the axilla vary according to the position of the shoulder joint but when the limb is in the anatomical position the axilla is shaped like a truncated pyramid with a narrow apex (inlet) superiorly, a broad base and three walls (Fig. 3.12).

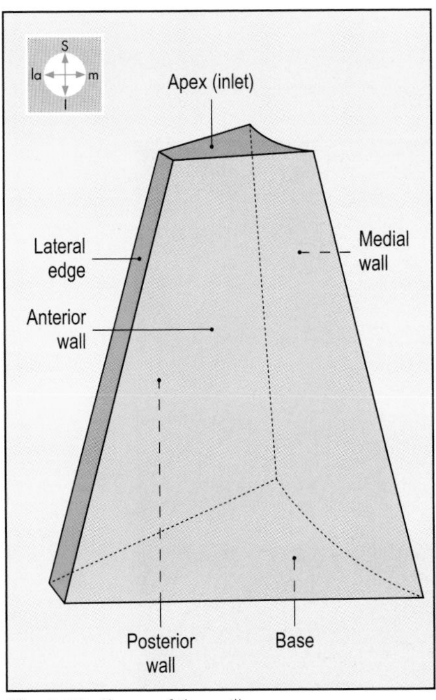

Fig. 3.12 Shape of the axilla.

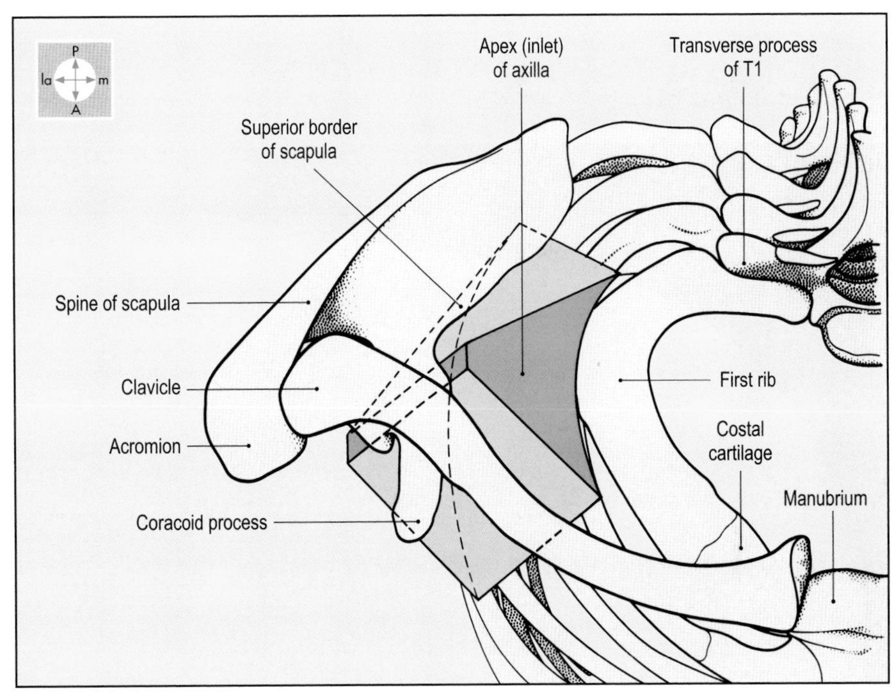

Fig. 3.13 Axilla from above, showing the boundaries of its apex.

Walls

The upper ribs and intercostal spaces, covered by serratus anterior, form the medial wall (see Fig. 3.15), which is convex laterally. The anterior wall consists of pectoralis major overlying pectoralis minor and subclavius (Fig. 3.14; see Fig. 3.16) while the posterior wall is formed by subscapularis, teres major and latissimus dorsi. The muscles of the anterior and posterior walls converge on the humerus (see Fig. 3.15) so that the axilla is limited laterally by the narrow intertubercular sulcus of the humerus. The base of the axilla, convex upwards, is formed by fascia passing between the inferior margins of the anterior and posterior walls. The triangular apex of the axilla provides continuity between the root of the neck and the upper limb and is bounded by the clavicle, the superior border of the scapula and the first rib (Fig. 3.13).

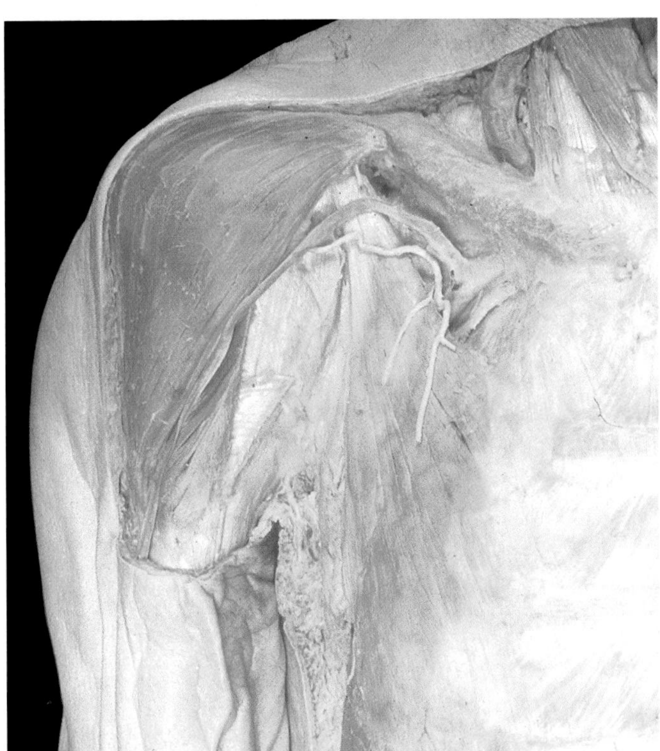

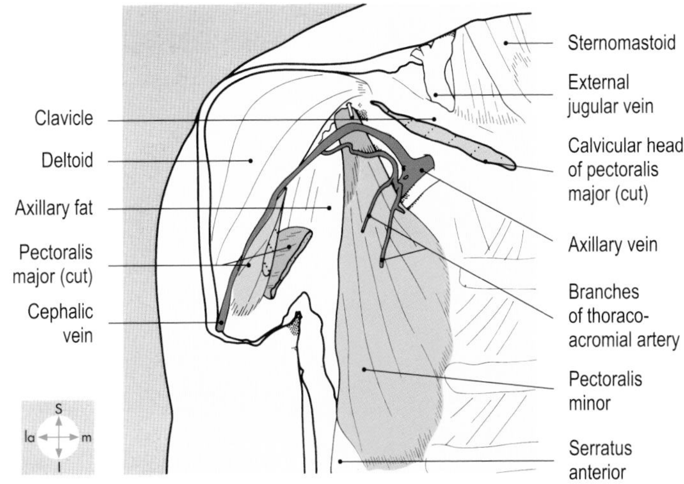

Fig. 3.14 Structures that pass above pectoralis minor in the anterior wall of the axilla. Pectoralis major and fascia around pectoralis minor have been removed.

Contents

The axilla contains the axillary artery and its branches, the axillary vein and its tributaries, parts of the brachial plexus and the axillary lymph nodes.

Coracobrachialis and the short and long heads of biceps brachii traverse the axilla. In addition, the tail of the breast usually enters the axilla. All these structures are embedded in loose fatty connective tissue (Fig. 3.15).

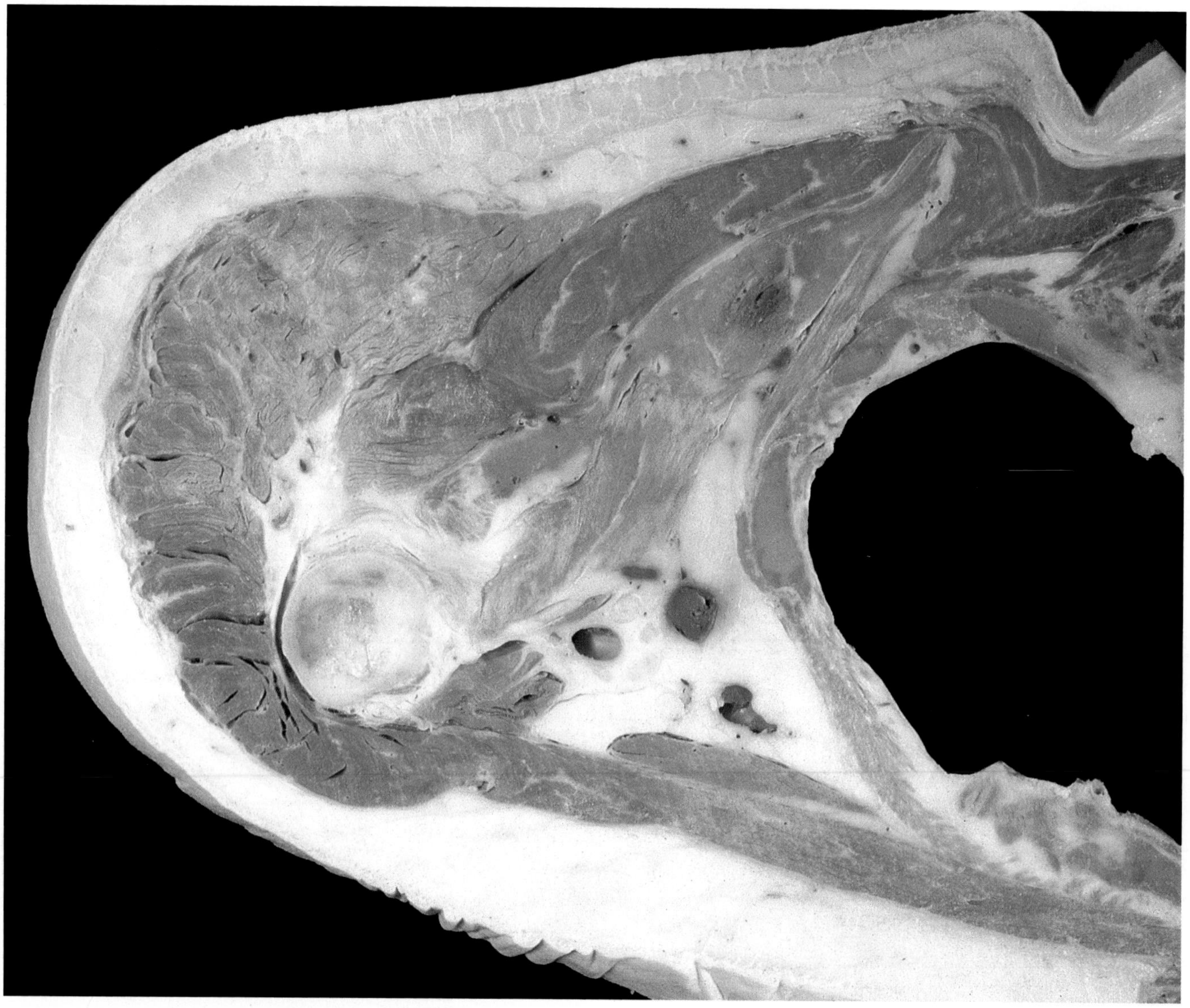

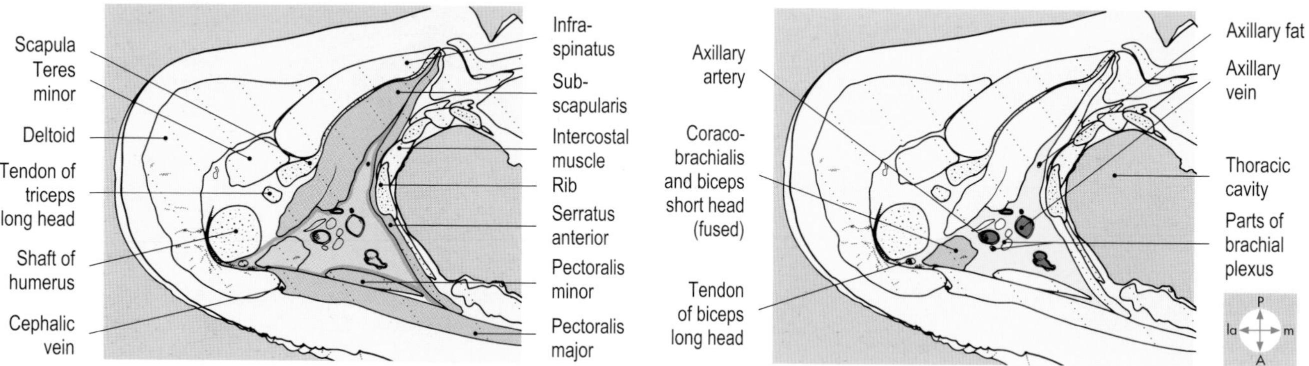

Fig. 3.15 Transverse section showing (left) the walls and (right) the contents of the axilla. Superior aspect. The lung has been removed.

Axillary artery

The subclavian artery continues as the axillary artery beyond the lateral edge of the first rib. Near the inlet the axillary artery lies posterior to the axillary vein (Figs 3.16 & 3.17) but more distally the artery lies lateral to the vein close to the humerus. The axillary artery and parts of the brachial plexus that surround it are bound together by a fibrous layer called the axillary sheath. Local anaesthetic injected inside the sheath will spread to produce a brachial plexus nerve block. Coracobrachialis and the short head of biceps brachii lie lateral to the artery while pectoralis minor crosses it anteriorly. By convention, the axillary artery is described in parts which lie above, behind and below pectoralis minor. Distal to the lower border of teres major, the vessel continues into the arm as the brachial artery (see Fig. 3.18).

Branches of the axillary artery supply the walls of the axilla and adjacent structures. The thoracoacromial artery (see Fig. 3.14) supplies the anterior wall while the superior thoracic and lateral

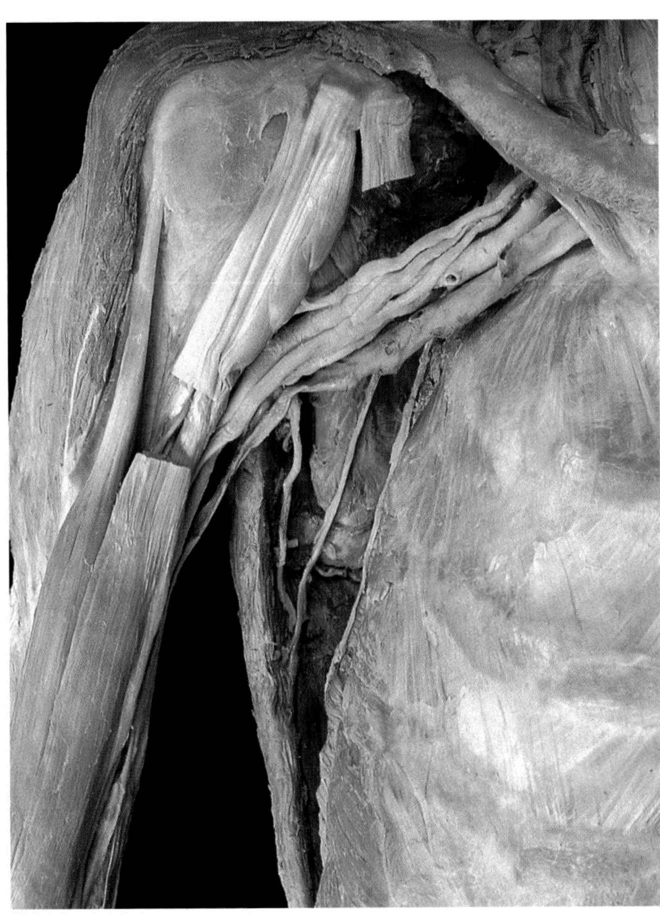

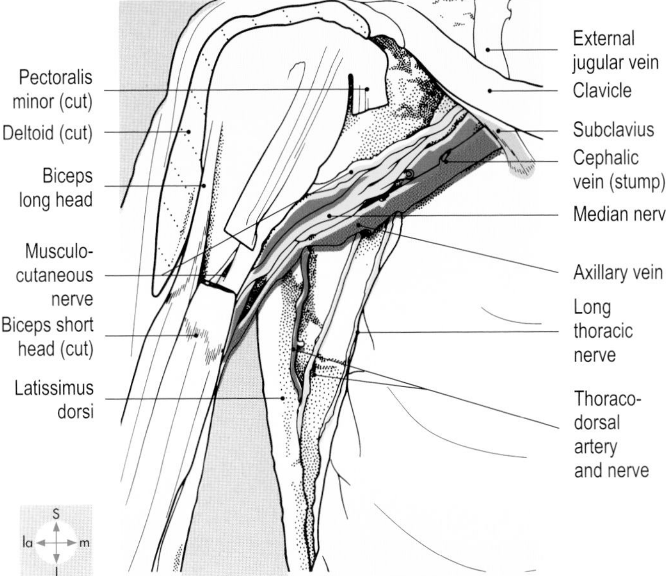

Fig. 3.16 Axillary neurovascular bundle, exposed by removal of the pectoral muscles and axillary fat.

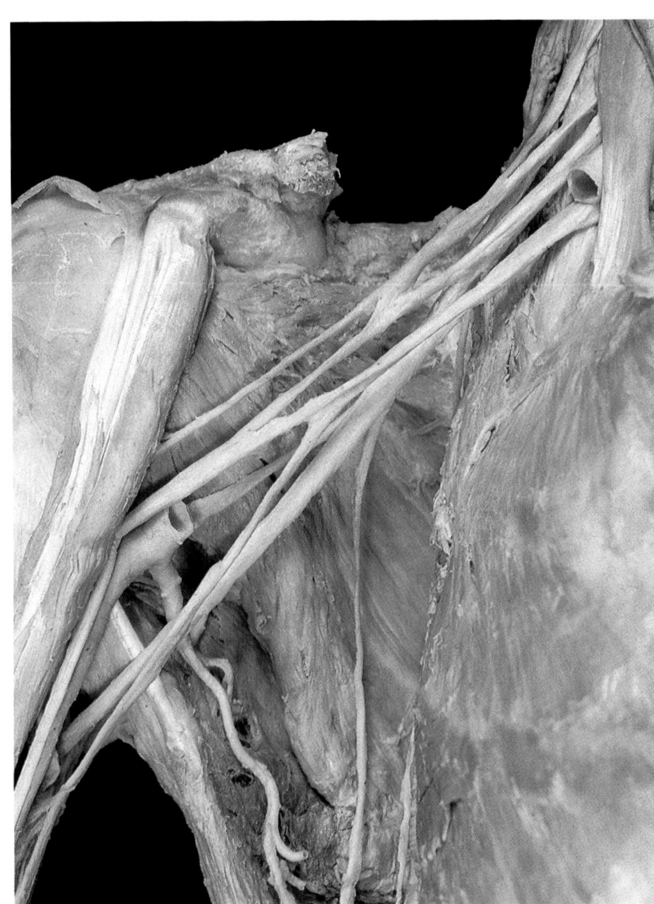

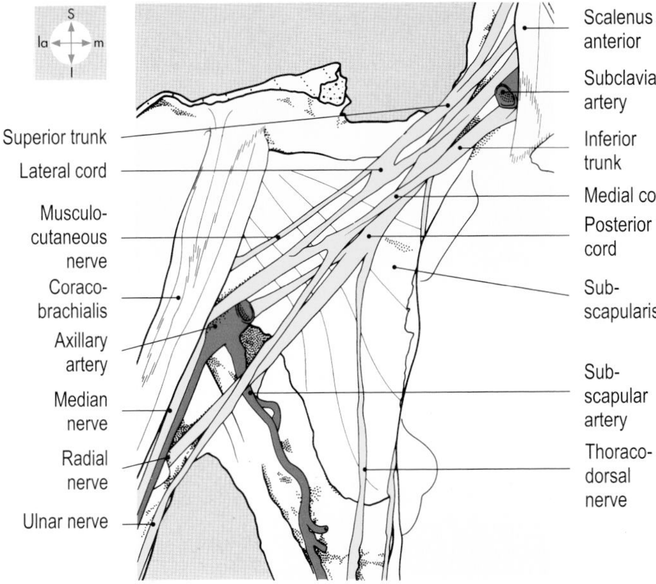

Fig. 3.17 Components of the brachial plexus. The clavicle and the veins and most of the axillary artery have been removed.

thoracic arteries supply the medial and anterior walls. The thoracoacromial and lateral thoracic arteries also supply part of the breast. The posterior wall is supplied by the subscapular artery. The anterior and posterior circumflex humeral arteries (Fig. 3.18) pass laterally and encircle the surgical neck of the humerus, supplying the shoulder joint and the upper part of the arm. An important collateral circulation, the scapular anastomosis, is formed by communications between the circumflex scapular branch of the subscapular artery and the suprascapular branch from the thyrocervical trunk, a branch of the subclavian artery.

Axillary vein

The venae comitantes of the brachial artery unite with the basilic vein in the upper part of the arm and continue as the axillary vein above the inferior border of teres major. The vein ascends medial to the axillary artery (see Fig. 3.16), passing behind pectoralis minor, and crosses the lateral edge of the first rib to continue as the subclavian vein, lying anterior to its companion artery. A major tributary of the axillary vein is the cephalic vein, which ascends in the groove between deltoid and pectoralis major. Just below the clavicle, it enters the axilla by piercing the fascia above pectoralis minor (see Fig. 3.14). The progress of a catheter inserted proximally along the cephalic vein may be impeded by the acute angulations often present above pectoralis minor or near its termination in the axillary vein. The axillary vein receives other tributaries, which in general correspond to the branches of the axillary artery.

Brachial plexus

The whole plexus will be described here, although only the divisions, cords and certain branches lie within the axilla. The brachial plexus supplies the upper limb and consists of a branching network of nerves derived from the anterior rami of the lower four cervical and the first thoracic spinal nerves. The plexus enables nerve fibres originating in several spinal cord segments to be distributed to each peripheral branch. Knowledge of the segmental arrangement and distribution is necessary for accurate diagnosis in diseases or injuries involving the spinal cord or the brachial plexus. The parts of the plexus are named, from proximal to distal, roots, trunks, divisions and cords (Fig. 3.19). The five roots (anterior rami) give rise to three trunks (superior, middle and inferior), which emerge between scalenus medius and scalenus anterior to lie in the floor of the posterior triangle of the neck (see p. 324). The roots of the plexus lie deep to the prevertebral fascia while the trunks are covered by its lateral extension, the axillary sheath. Each trunk divides into an anterior and a posterior division behind the clavicle, at the apex of the axilla. Within the axilla, the divisions combine to produce the three cords, which are named lateral, medial and posterior according to their relationships to the axillary artery. Each cord ends near the lower

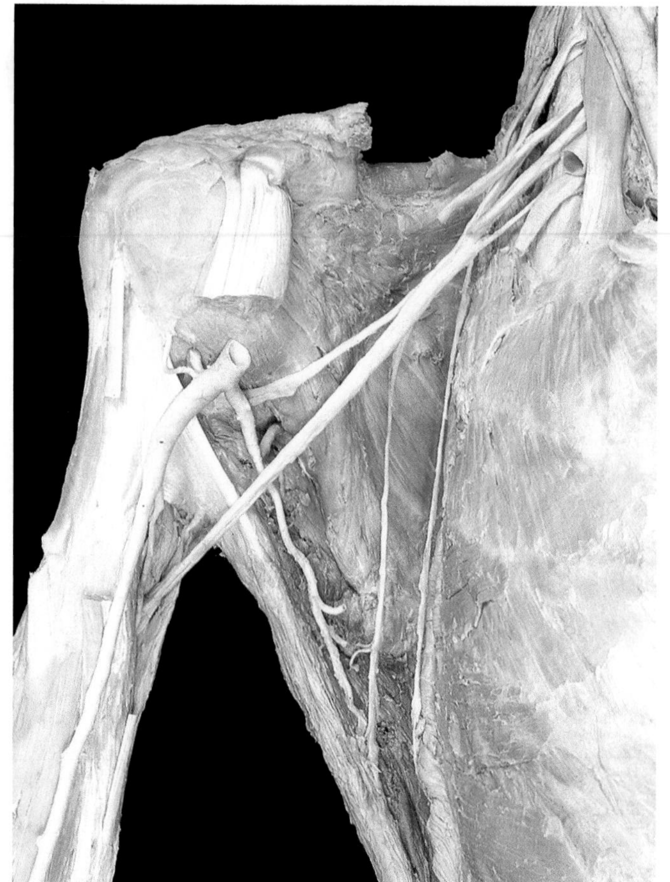

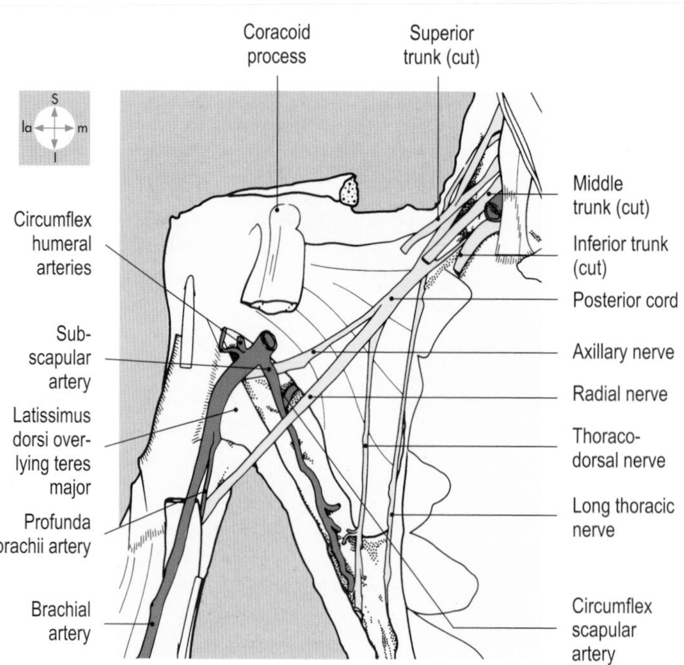

Fig. 3.18 Some posterior branches of the brachial plexus seen after removal of the more anterior parts of the plexus. Biceps brachii and coracobrachialis have been excised.

border of pectoralis minor by dividing into two terminal branches. Other branches of the plexus arise in the neck and axilla directly from the roots, trunks and cords (Fig. 3.20). The anterior divisions form the lateral and medial cords (see Fig. 3.17), whose branches supply the flexor muscles of the arm, forearm and hand and the skin overlying the flexor compartments. The three posterior divisions unite to form the posterior cord (Fig. 3.18), whose branches supply the extensor musculature of the shoulder, arm and forearm and the skin of the posterior surface of the limb.

Axillary lymph nodes

The axillary lymph nodes receive lymph not only from the upper limb but also from the superficial tissues of the trunk above the level of the umbilicus, including the breast.

The nodes are described in groups according to their positions in the axilla. Anteriorly lies the pectoral group, which drains the lateral and anterior aspects of the body wall including the breast. Laterally, along the axillary vessels, is the humeral (lateral) group of nodes, which receives most of the lymph from the upper limb. Posteriorly the subscapular nodes receive lymph from the dorsal aspect of the body wall. Within the axilla, efferent lymph channels drain centrally and then proximally to apical nodes from which a subclavian lymph trunk arises; this terminates in the root of the neck by joining, on the right, the right lymphatic duct or, on the left, the thoracic duct. Sometimes the lymph trunks join the subclavian vein directly (see p. 328).

The principal vessels and nerves entering or leaving the axilla are listed in Table 3.1.

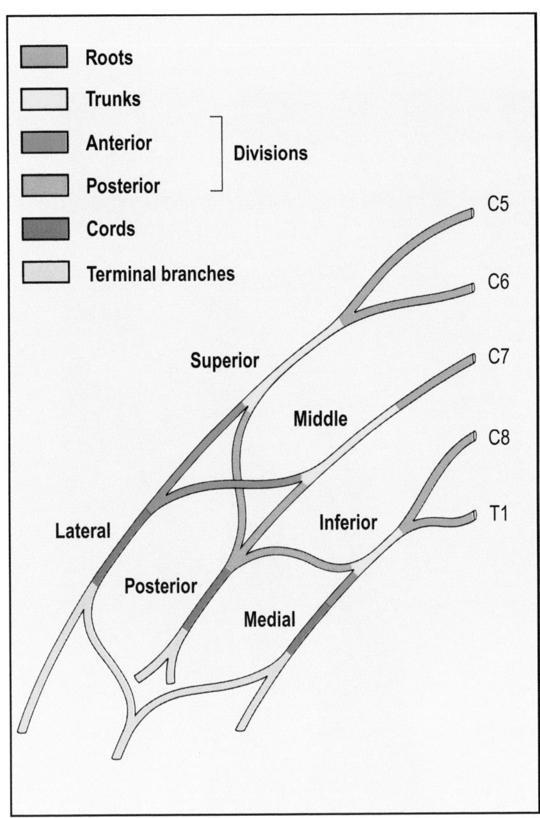

Fig. 3.19 Main components of the brachial plexus in their usual arrangement.

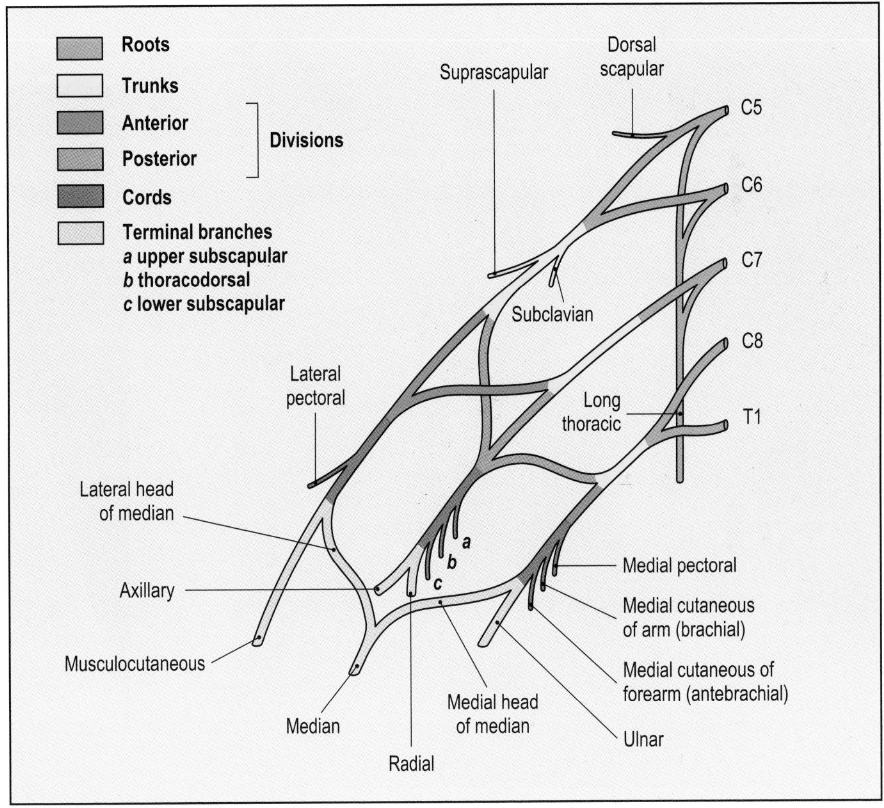

Fig. 3.20 Branches of the brachial plexus. The arrangement of these nerves may vary considerably.

Between Axilla and Root of Neck (Via Inlet of Axilla)	Between Axilla and Arm (Lateral to Fascia of Axillary Floor)	Through Anterior Wall (Via Interval Between Clavicle and Pectoralis Minor)	Through Posterior Wall (Via Triangular and Quadrangular Intermuscular Spaces)
Subclavian/axillary artery	Axillary/brachial artery	Thoracoacromial artery	Circumflex branch of subscapular artery
Axillary/subclavian vein	Brachial/axillary vein	Cephalic vein	Axillary nerve C5, C6 with posterior circumflex humeral artery
Trunks/divisions of brachial plexus	Median nerve C6, C7, C8, T1	Pectoral nerves C5, C6, C7, C8, T1	
Subclavian lymph trunk	Musculocutaneous nerve C5, C6, C7	Deltopectoral lymphatics	
	Ulnar nerve C8, T1		
	Radial nerve C5, C6, C7, C8		
	Brachial lymphatics		

Table 3.1 Principal vessels and nerves entering or leaving the axilla

Anterior Compartment of Arm

The anterior compartment of the arm contains three muscles (biceps brachii, coracobrachialis and brachialis), the brachial artery with its venae comitantes, and three nerves (the median, ulnar and musculocutaneous nerves).

Muscles

The three muscles of the compartment are supplied by the musculocutaneous nerve. The two heads of biceps separate proximally (Fig. 3.21) and have tendinous attachments to the scapula. The short head lies medially and attaches to the tip of the coracoid process. The tendon of the long head attaches to the supraglenoid tubercle, leaves the shoulder joint deep to the transverse humeral ligament and continues distally in the intertubercular sulcus deep to the tendon of pectoralis major. The muscle bellies fuse and are attached by a tendon (see Fig. 3.27) to the tuberosity of the radius and by the bicipital aponeurosis, which fuses with deep fascia on the medial side of the forearm. Biceps is a strong flexor of the elbow and supinator of the forearm at the radioulnar joints, and a weak flexor of the shoulder joint.

Coracobrachialis attaches to the coracoid process with the short head of biceps. The muscle attaches distally to the medial side of the shaft of the humerus near its midpoint (Fig. 3.23). Coracobrachialis is pierced by the musculocutaneous nerve (Fig. 3.22) and functions as a weak flexor and adductor of the shoulder joint.

Brachialis lies deeply and has an extensive attachment to the anterior surface of the distal half of the shaft of the humerus

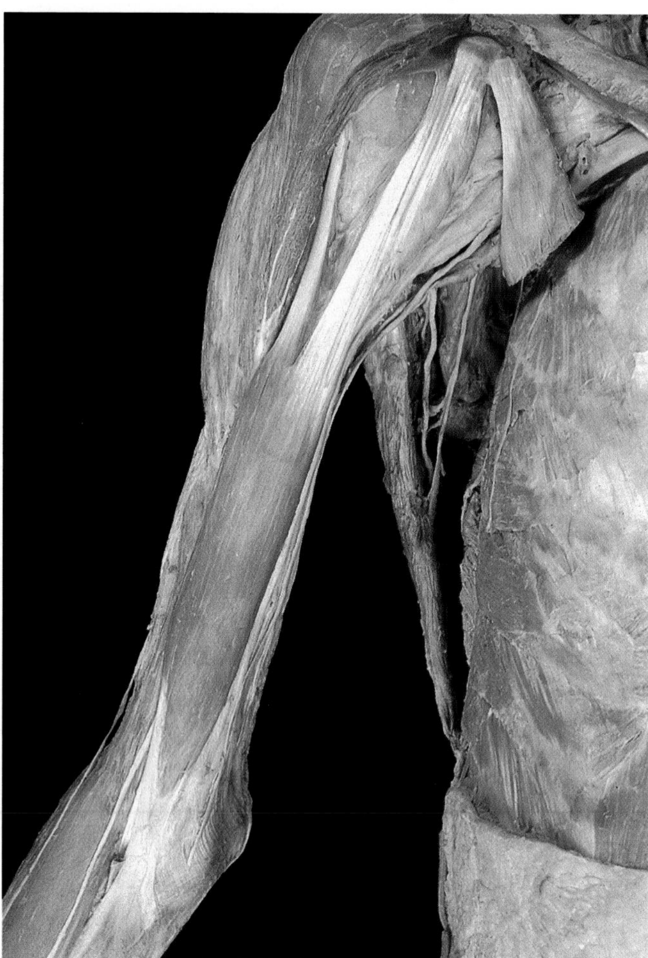

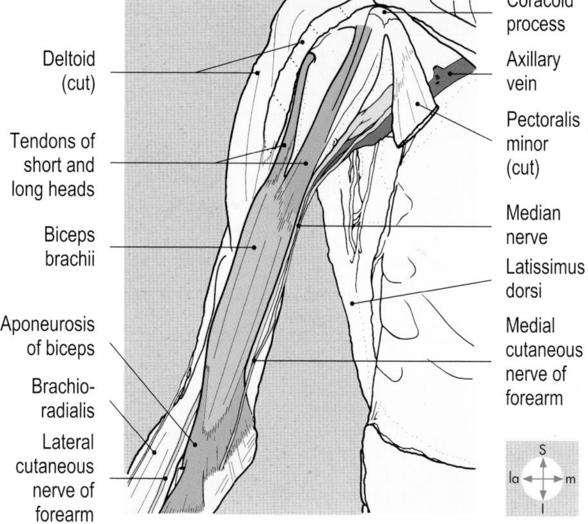

Fig. 3.21 Anterior view of biceps brachii after removal of deep fascia and anterior fibres of deltoid.

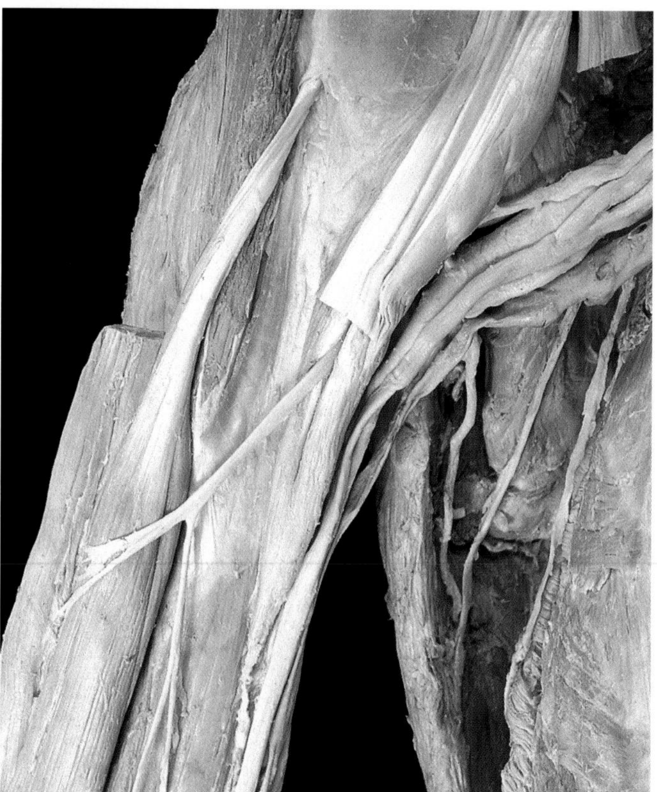

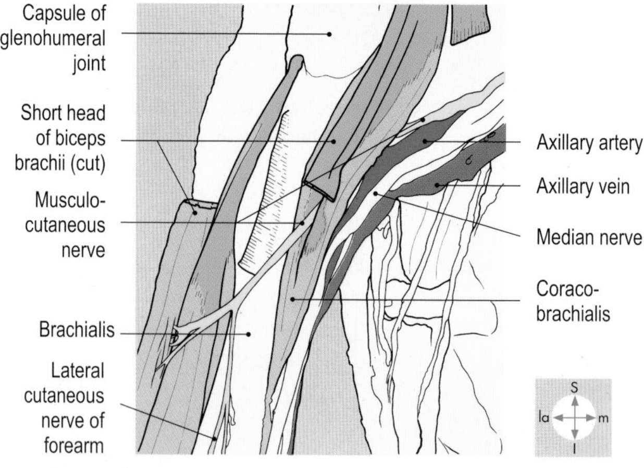

Fig. 3.22 The musculocutaneous nerve piercing coracobrachialis. The short head of biceps brachii has been divided and the muscle reflected laterally.

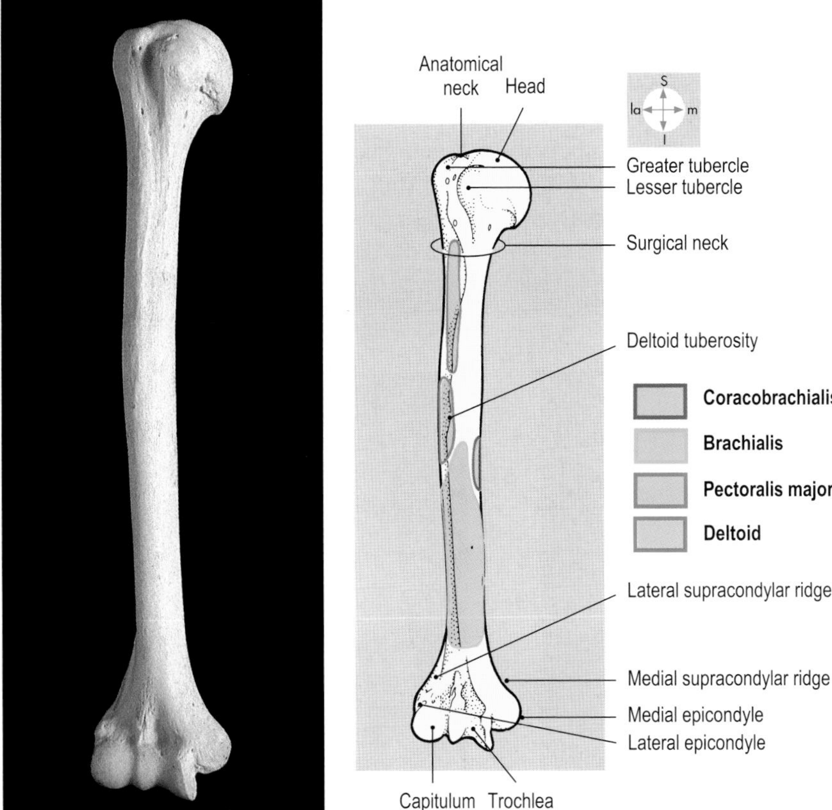

Fig. 3.23 Anterior aspect of humerus.

(Fig. 3.23) and adjacent intermuscular septa. The muscle passes to the coronoid process of the ulna (see Fig. 3.34) and acts as a powerful flexor of the elbow joint.

Vessels

The brachial artery is the continuation of the axillary artery distal to teres major. In the upper part of the arm the brachial artery with its venae comitantes is accompanied by the median and ulnar nerves (Fig. 3.24) and the medial cutaneous nerve of forearm. The artery passes distally and laterally, lying medial to biceps and anterior to coracobrachialis and brachialis. An important branch, the profunda brachii artery (see p. 107), supplies the posterior compartment of the arm. Division of the brachial artery into its terminal radial and ulnar branches usually occurs in the cubital fossa but may occur more proximally.

Venae comitantes, ascending from the cubital fossa, accompany the brachial artery and are joined by the basilic vein after it has pierced the deep fascia at about midarm level. At the lower border of the axilla the venous channels usually combine to form a single axillary vein.

Nerves

The musculocutaneous nerve (see Fig. 3.23) is a terminal branch of the lateral cord. It pierces coracobrachialis and lies between biceps and brachialis, supplying each of these muscles. The nerve continues distally

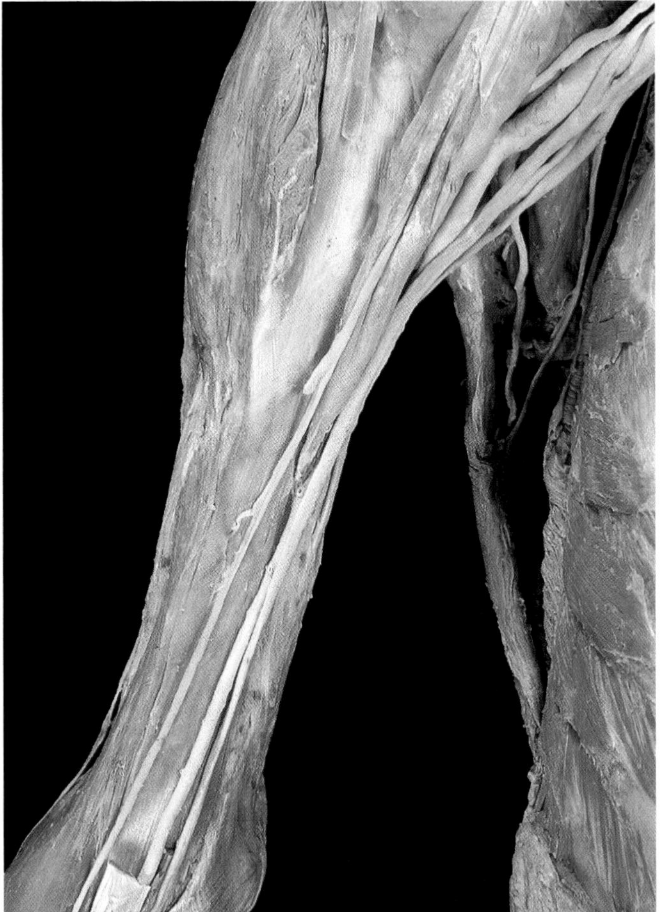

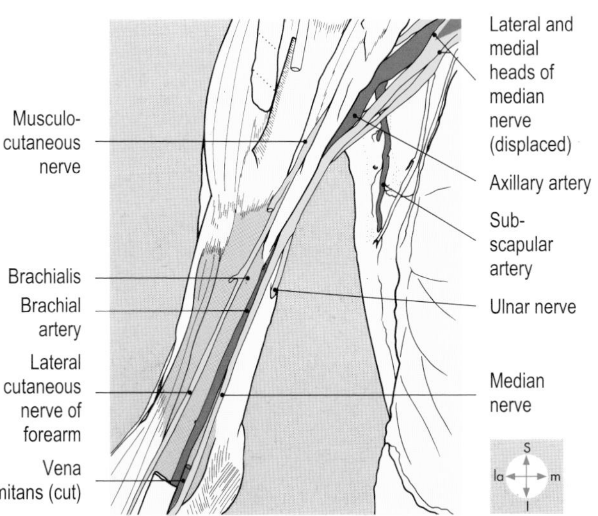

Fig. 3.24 Brachialis, the brachial artery and the nerves of the compartment. Biceps brachii and most veins have been excised.

as the lateral cutaneous nerve of forearm, which pierces the deep fascia between biceps and brachioradialis to lie superficially over the cubital fossa (Fig. 3.26).

The median and ulnar nerves traverse the entire length of the arm, but neither gives any branches above the elbow joint. The median nerve arises by lateral and medial heads, which are terminal branches of the lateral and medial cords. In the upper part of the arm the nerve lies lateral to the brachial artery but at midarm level it crosses anterior to the vessels and finally lies medial to the artery (see Fig. 3.24), a position retained in the cubital fossa. The ulnar nerve is a terminal branch of the medial cord and, together with the medial cutaneous nerve of forearm, initially lies medial to the brachial artery but leaves the artery at midarm level (see Fig. 3.24). It then pierces the medial intermuscular septum and enters the posterior compartment to lie between the septum and the medial head of triceps.

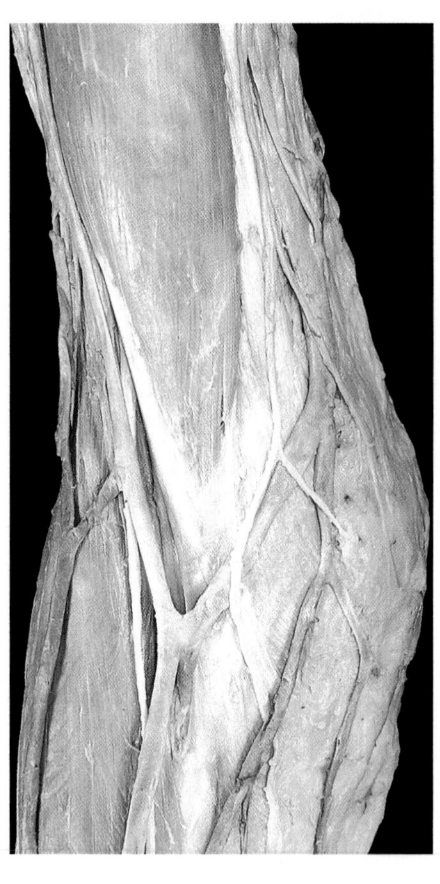

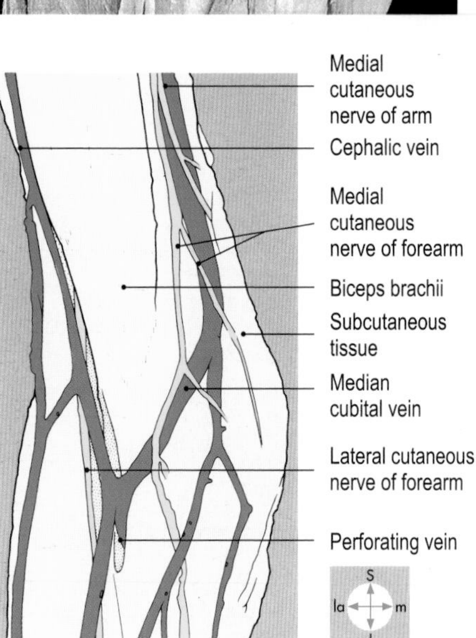

Fig. 3.25 Cutaneous nerves and superficial veins overlying the right cubital fossa. Subcutaneous tissue has been retained medial to the basilic vein.

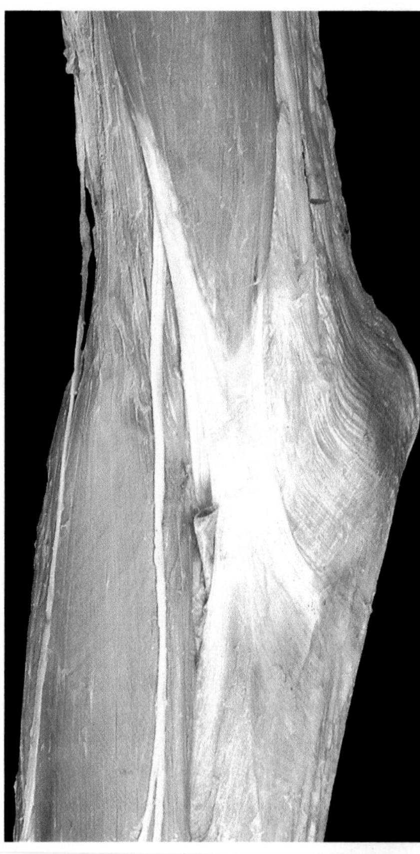

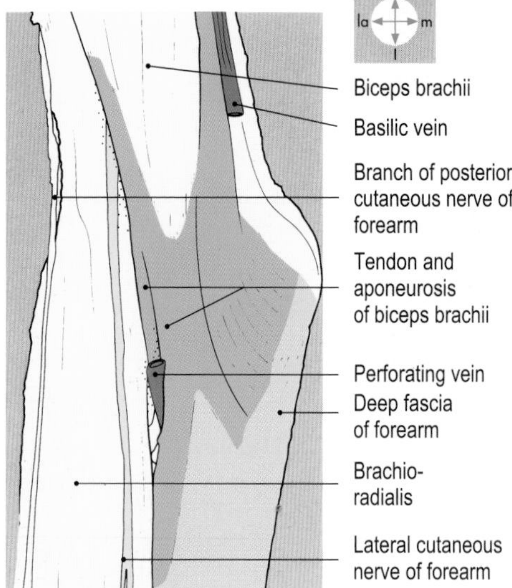

Fig. 3.26 Roof of the cubital fossa after removal of subcutaneous tissue, veins and nerves. A perforating vein communicates with deep veins by passing through the deep fascia.

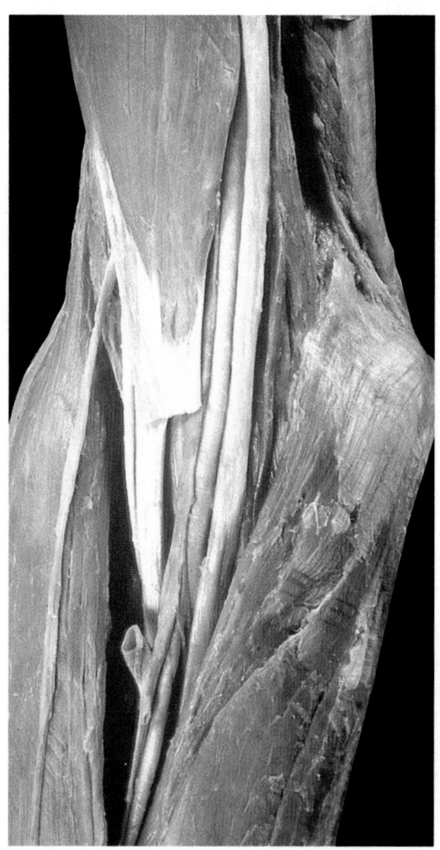

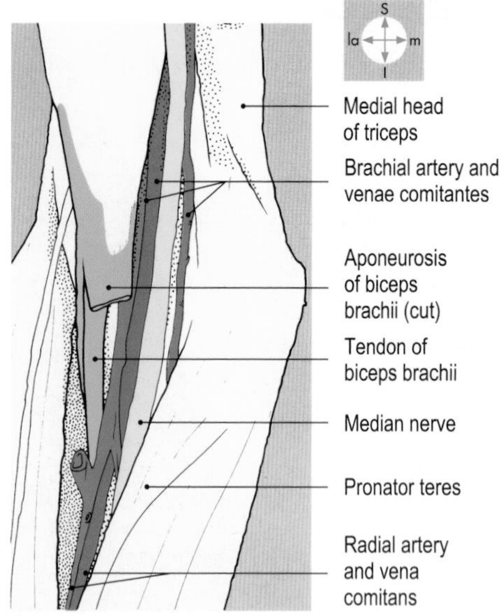

Fig. 3.27 Contents of the cubital fossa. The aponeurosis of biceps brachii and deep fascia have been removed.

Cubital Fossa

The cubital fossa is a triangular space in front of the elbow joint, bounded laterally by brachioradialis and medially by pronator teres (Fig. 3.28). By convention, the fossa is limited proximally by an imaginary line drawn between the two humeral epicondyles. The roof is formed by deep fascia, reinforced by the aponeurosis of biceps (Fig. 3.26). The subcutaneous tissue overlying the roof contains branches of the lateral and medial cutaneous nerves of forearm and superficial veins such as the median cubital vein, which links the cephalic and basilic veins (Fig. 3.25). The arrangement of these superficial veins, which are often punctured to obtain samples of blood for laboratory analysis, may vary considerably between individuals.

The fossa is traversed by nerves and vessels passing between the arm and the forearm. Its contents (Figs 3.27 & 3.29), embedded in fatty connective tissue, are, from medial to lateral, the median nerve, the brachial artery and its venae comitantes, the tendon of biceps and the radial nerve. Distally, the terminal branches of the radial nerve, the superficial and deep radial (posterior interosseous) nerves, and the terminal branches of the brachial artery (namely the radial and ulnar arteries) also lie within the fossa. The floor of the cubital fossa (Fig. 3.29) is formed by supinator and brachialis overlying the capsule of the elbow joint.

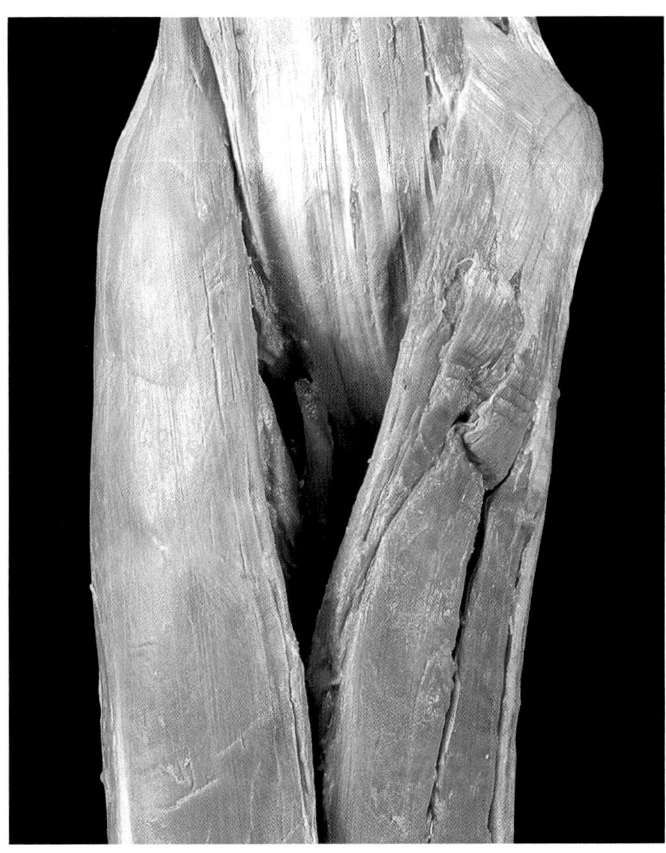

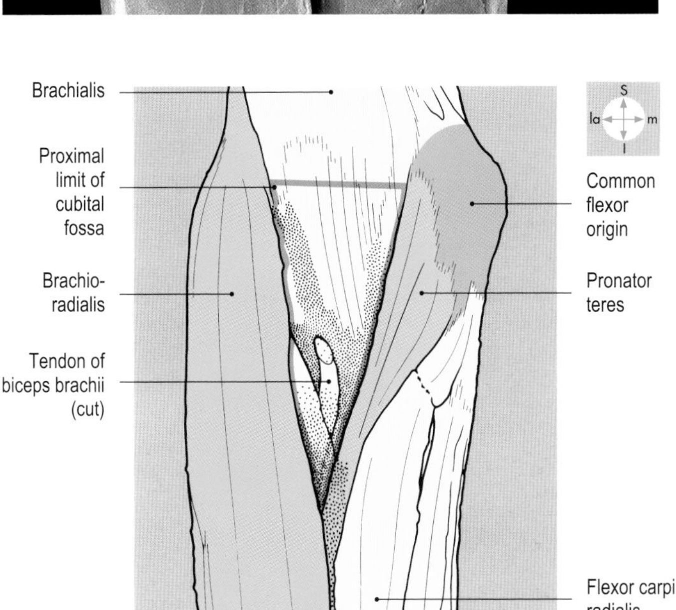

Fig. 3.28 Boundaries of the cubital fossa after removal of the roof and contents.

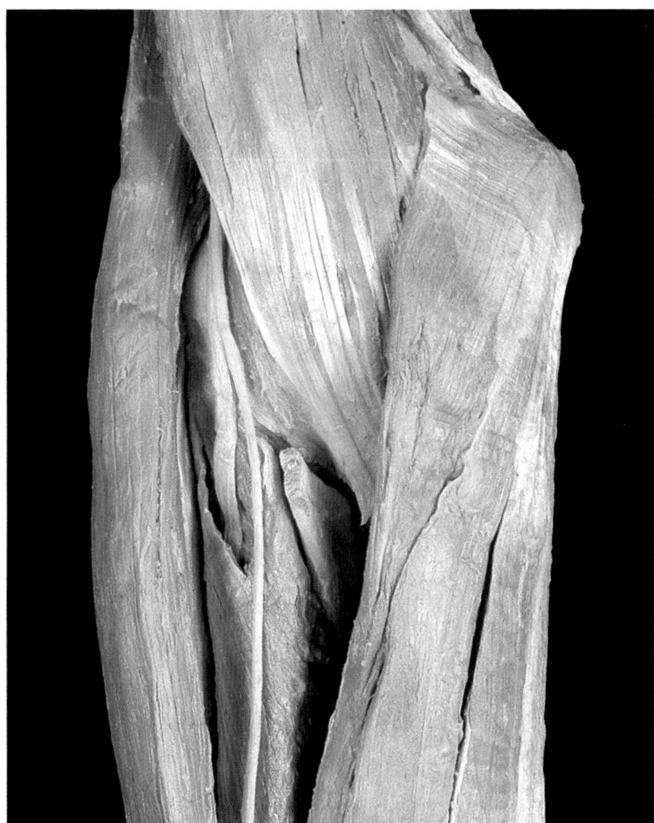

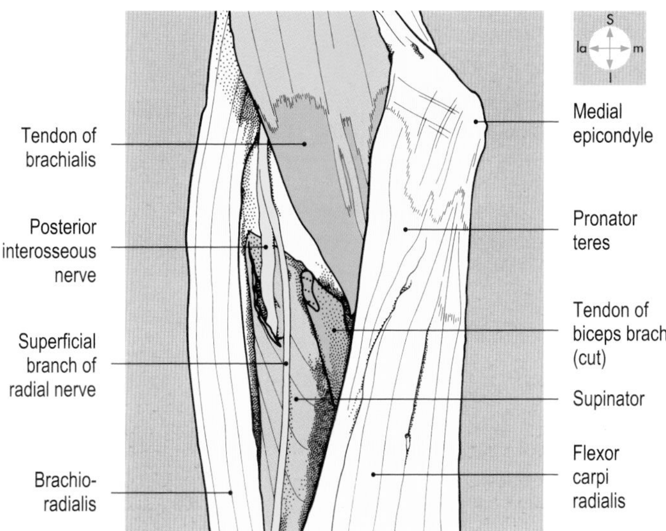

Fig. 3.29 Brachioradialis and pronator teres have been retracted to reveal the floor of the cubital fossa and expose the radial nerve.

Anterior Compartment of Forearm

The anterior compartment of the forearm (see Fig. 3.4) contains a superficial and a deep group of muscles, which include flexors of the wrist, fingers and thumb, and two muscles that act as pronators. The compartment is traversed by the median and ulnar nerves and by the radial and ulnar arteries with their venae comitantes. A layer of deep fascia continuous with a similar layer on the posterior aspect of the limb encloses the compartment and provides additional attachment for the superficial muscles. In front of the carpus, deep fascia forms the flexor retinaculum (Fig. 3.30), which lies anterior to tendons in the carpal tunnel (see p. 124). Subcutaneous tissue overlying the compartment contains cutaneous nerves and tributaries of the cephalic and basilic veins. Branches of the medial and lateral cutaneous nerves of the forearm may continue distal to the wrist over the carpal region of the hand.

Superficial muscles

The superficial muscles are, from lateral to medial, pronator teres, flexor carpi radialis, palmaris longus and flexor carpi ulnaris (Fig. 3.31). Flexor digitorum superficialis is also included in this group but is partly covered by the other muscles.

All the superficial muscles attach proximally to the common flexor origin on the front of the medial epicondyle of the humerus (see Fig. 3.34). In addition, pronator teres attaches to the medial side of the coronoid process of the ulna, and flexor carpi ulnaris attaches to the medial border of the olecranon and the adjacent part of the subcutaneous border of the ulna. Flexor digitorum superficialis has an additional attachment to the ulnar collateral ligament of the elbow, the coronoid process and the anterior oblique line of the radius.

Distally, pronator teres attaches halfway along the lateral aspect of the shaft of the radius and forms the medial border of the cubital fossa. The muscle pronates the forearm. Flexor carpi radialis attaches to the bases of the second and third metacarpal

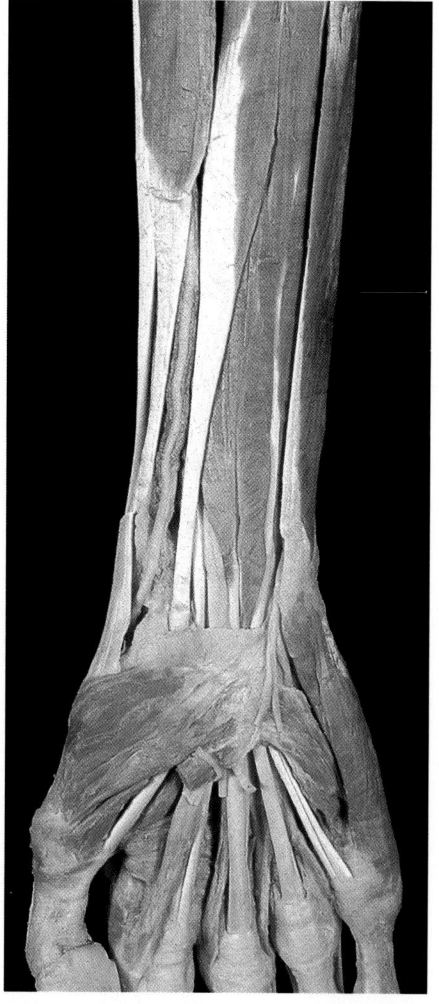

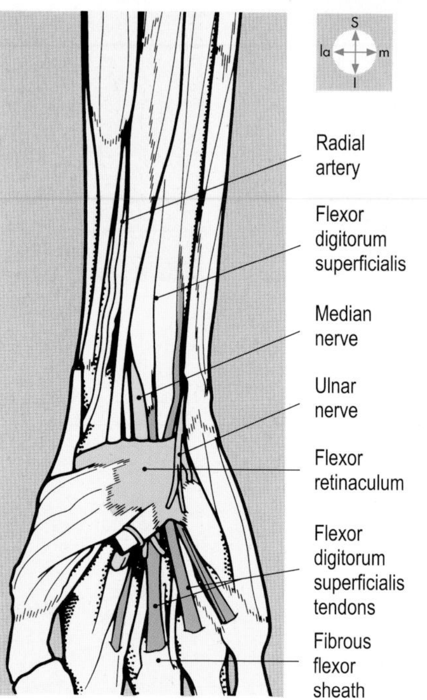

Fig. 3.30 Flexor retinaculum revealed by removal of subcutaneous tissue and most of the deep fascia. The retinaculum is partly obscured by some of the intrinsic muscles of the hand.

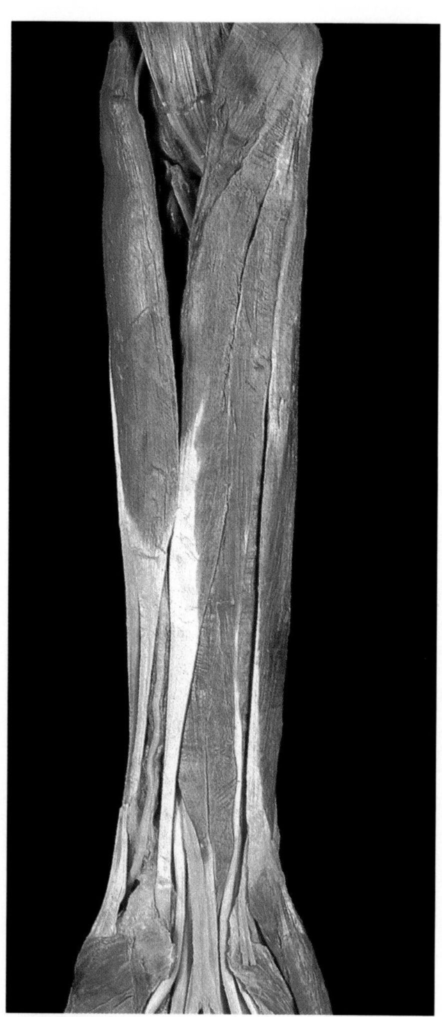

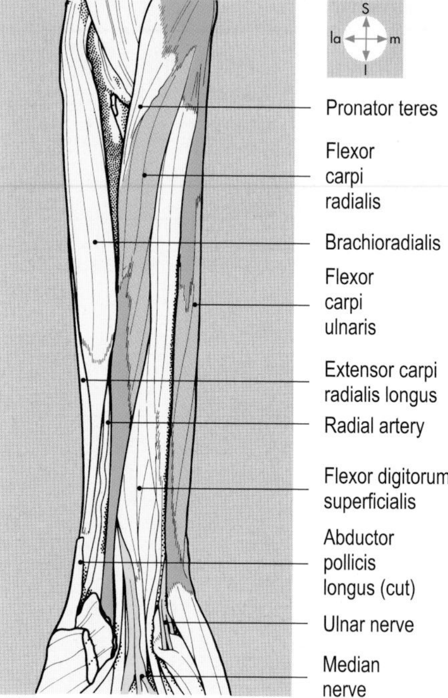

Fig. 3.31 Flexor carpi radialis and flexor carpi ulnaris seen after removal of deep fascia and the flexor retinaculum. This specimen lacks palmaris longus.

bones (see Fig. 3.37). It is a flexor and abductor of the wrist joint. Palmaris longus, a vestigial muscle that may be absent, has a long thin tendon, which attaches to the palmar aponeurosis. The muscle is a weak flexor of the wrist joint. Flexor carpi ulnaris attaches distally to the pisiform and, via ligaments from the pisiform, to the hook of the hamate and the base of the fifth metacarpal (see Fig. 3.47). It is the most medial of the superficial muscles and is a flexor and adductor of the wrist.

Flexor digitorum superficialis (Fig. 3.32) is relatively large and is the deepest of this group of muscles. Distally, it gives rise to four tendons, one for each finger, which pass into the hand deep to the flexor retinaculum. In the carpal tunnel the tendons have a characteristic grouping (Fig. 3.32). Within each finger the tendon forms two slips, which pass around the profundus tendon and then partly reunite before attaching to the sides of the middle phalanx (see Fig. 3.37). The muscle flexes the wrist and the metacarpophalangeal and proximal interphalangeal joints of the fingers.

The superficial muscles all pass anterior to the elbow and therefore act as weak flexors of that joint in addition to their roles in the movements of the wrist and hand. Collectively, the carpal flexors and extensors stabilize the wrist joint during movements of the fingers and thumb.

All the superficial muscles are innervated by the median nerve, except flexor carpi ulnaris, which is supplied by the ulnar nerve.

Deep muscles

The deep muscles are flexor pollicis longus, flexor digitorum profundus and pronator quadratus. Their attachments to the radius and ulna are illustrated in Figure 3.34. Distally the flexor pollicis longus tendon (see Fig. 3.35) passes through the carpal tunnel and attaches to the base of the distal phalanx of the thumb. The muscle flexes the interphalangeal and metacarpophalangeal joints of the thumb. Flexor digitorum profundus (see Fig. 3.35) gives rise to four tendons, which traverse the carpal tunnel deep to the tendons of flexor digitorum superficialis (see Fig. 3.40). In the palm the tendons diverge, one entering each finger.

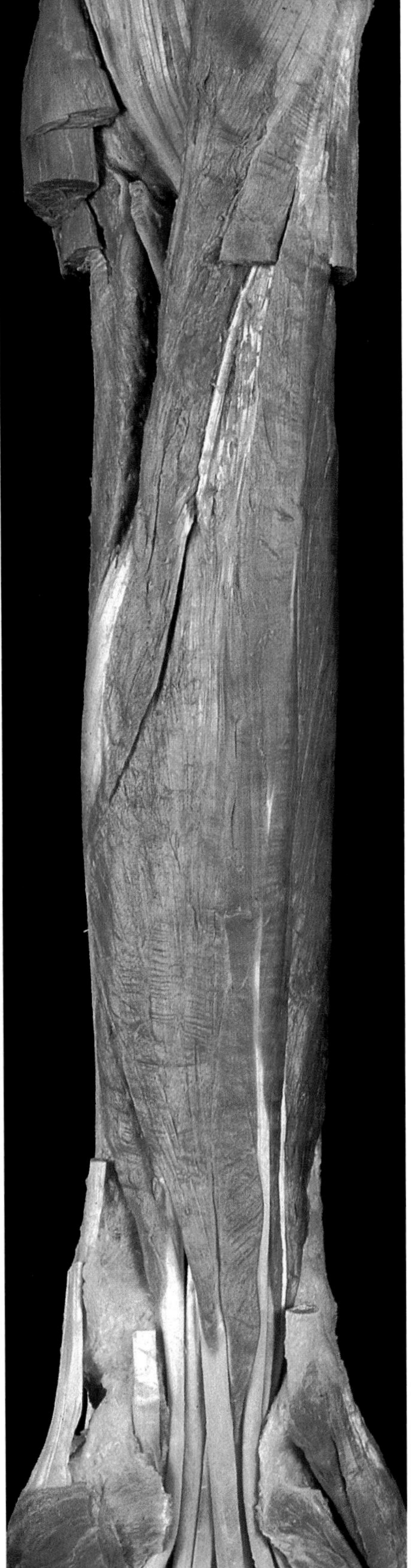

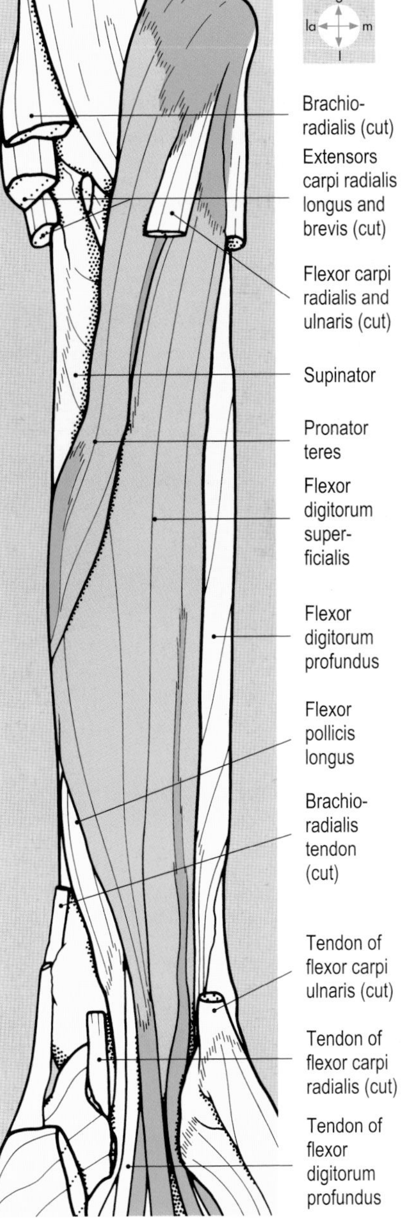

Fig. 3.32 Flexor digitorum superficialis and pronator teres revealed by division of flexors carpi ulnaris and radialis, and of brachioradialis. The vessels and nerves in the forearm have been removed.

Each tendon passes between the slips of the corresponding superficialis tendon, continuing distally to attach to the base of the terminal phalanx. The muscle is a flexor of the fingers and of the wrist joint. Pronator quadratus, a small rectangular muscle lying transversely between the anterior surfaces of the shafts of the radius and ulna (Fig. 3.33), pronates the forearm.

The deep muscles are innervated by the anterior interosseous nerve, except for the medial part of flexor digitorum profundus, which is supplied by the ulnar nerve.

Vessels

The brachial artery usually divides into the radial and ulnar arteries in the cubital fossa (see Fig. 3.36). The radial artery passes distally, under brachioradialis, lying on the flexor muscles. In the lower forearm the vessel is accompanied by the superficial branch of the radial nerve and, near the

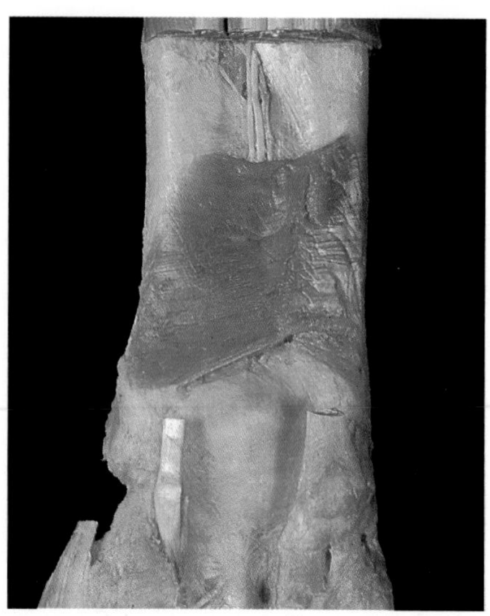

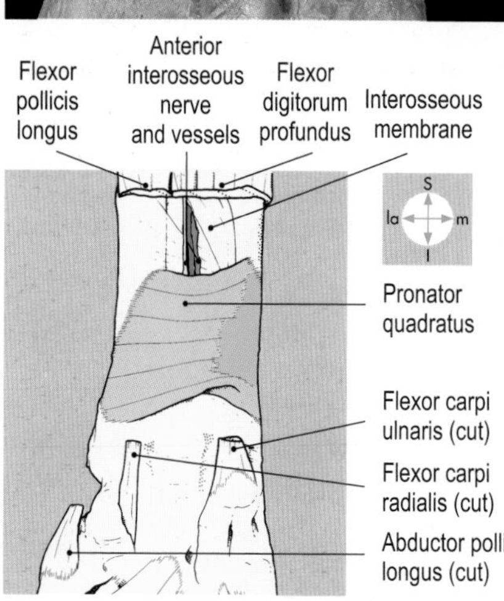

Fig. 3.33 Pronator quadratus exposed by division of flexor pollicis longus and flexor digitorum profundus.

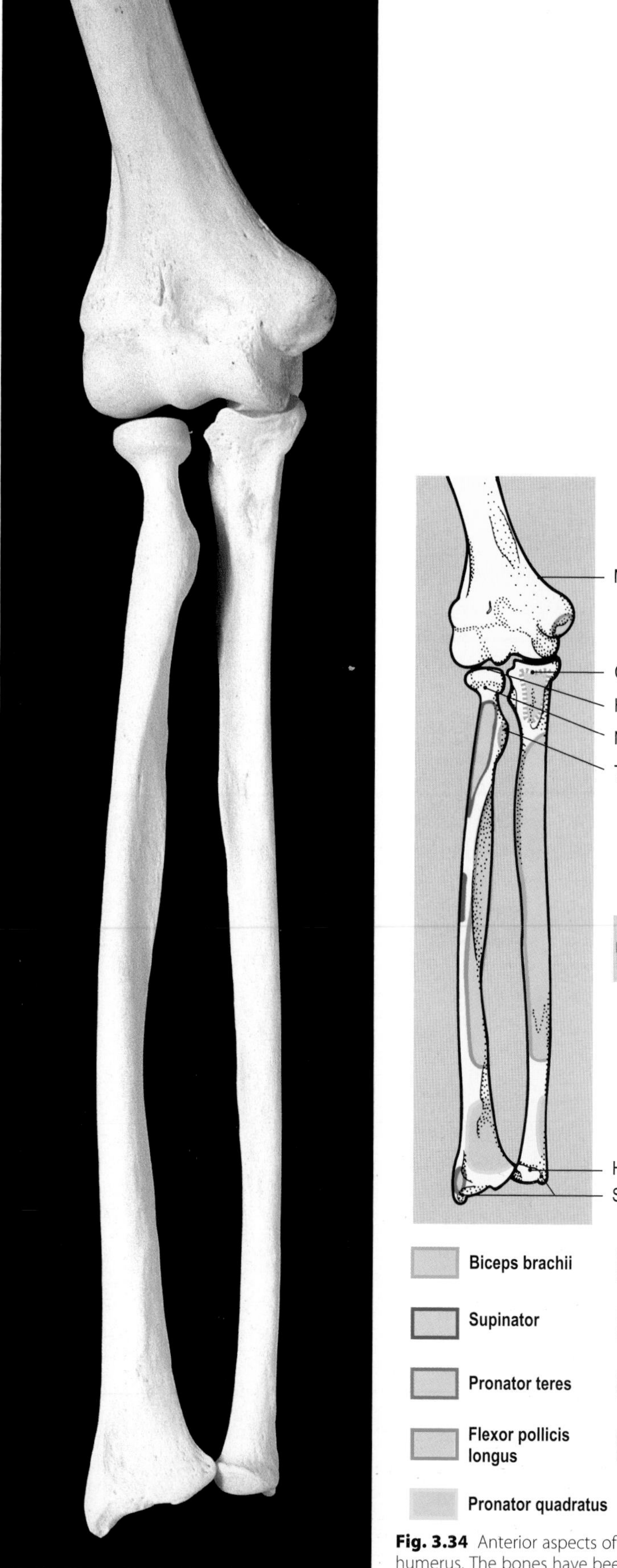

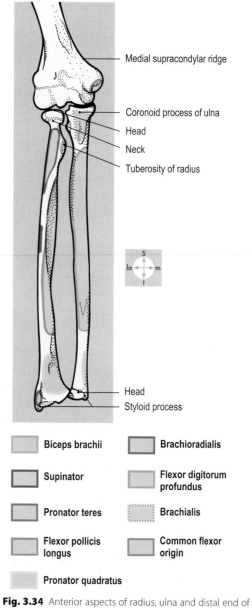

Biceps brachii
Brachioradialis
Supinator
Flexor digitorum profundus
Pronator teres
Brachialis
Flexor pollicis longus
Common flexor origin
Pronator quadratus

Fig. 3.34 Anterior aspects of radius, ulna and distal end of humerus. The bones have been separated slightly.

wrist, is subcutaneous and palpable against the anterior surface of the radius. The artery winds round the lateral aspect of the wrist, traverses the 'anatomical snuff box' and subsequently enters the palm to form the deep palmar arch (see Fig. 3.54). In the forearm the artery gives branches to muscles and contributes to anastomoses around the elbow and wrist joints.

The ulnar artery passes deep to the arch formed by the radial and ulnar attachments of flexor digitorum superficialis and continues between the superficial and deep flexor muscles. In the distal part of the forearm the artery is accompanied on its medial side by the ulnar nerve. It lies beneath flexor carpi ulnaris but at the wrist emerges to lie lateral to the tendon of this muscle, where its pulse can be palpated. The ulnar artery crosses superficial to the flexor retinaculum and, as it enters the hand, divides into superficial and deep palmar branches. The ulnar artery gives branches to the muscles of the anterior compartment and to the anastomoses around the elbow and wrist joints. Its largest branch, the common interosseous artery (see Fig. 3.36), arises near the origin of the ulnar artery and promptly divides into posterior and anterior interosseous branches. The posterior interosseous artery enters the posterior compartment of the forearm (see Fig. 3.77). The larger anterior interosseous artery passes distally in the anterior compartment, lying on the interosseous membrane, accompanied by the anterior interosseous nerve. The vessel supplies the deep flexor muscles and gives nutrient branches to the radius and ulna. Distally, it penetrates the interosseous membrane to assist in the anastomoses around the wrist.

Venae comitantes accompany the arteries of the anterior compartment and drain proximally into veins around the brachial artery.

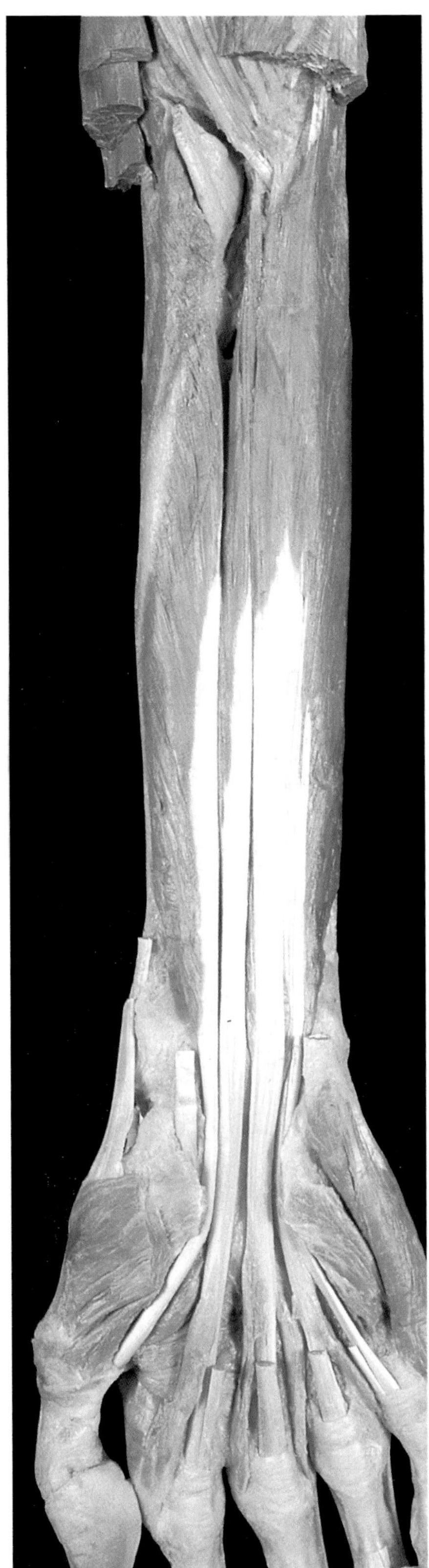

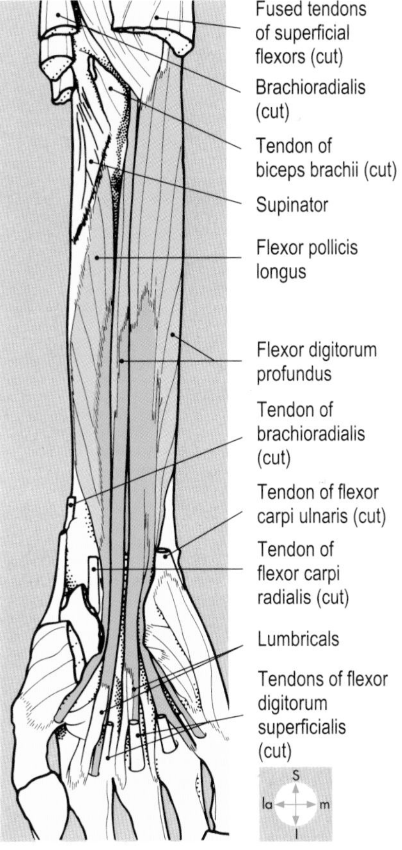

Fig. 3.35 Flexor digitorum profundus and flexor pollicis longus exposed by removal of the superficial flexors. As in this specimen, the index component of flexor digitorum profundus is often separate from the rest of the muscle.

Nerves

The median nerve enters the forearm from the cubital fossa between the two heads of pronator teres. It crosses anterior to the ulnar artery (see Fig. 3.36) and descends between the superficial and deep flexors. At the wrist the median nerve is remarkably superficial, lying medial to the tendon of flexor carpi radialis and just deep to the palmaris longus tendon. The median nerve passes through the carpal tunnel into the hand, where it divides into terminal branches (see Fig. 3.52). The nerve supplies all the superficial muscles of the anterior compartment except flexor carpi ulnaris. The anterior interosseous branch of the median nerve (see Fig. 3.36) supplies all the deep muscles of the compartment except the medial part of flexor digitorum profundus. This branch lies between flexor digitorum profundus and flexor pollicis longus and passes behind pronator quadratus to supply the wrist (Fig. 3.33). In the forearm the median nerve also gives a palmar cutaneous branch, which crosses superficial to the flexor retinaculum and supplies skin of the lateral part of the palm. Superficial lacerations near the wrist may damage the palmar cutaneous branches but leave the median and ulnar nerves intact. Testing digital sensation alone will miss injuries to these nerves supplying the palm.

The ulnar nerve passes behind the medial epicondyle and enters the forearm between the two heads of flexor carpi ulnaris. Lying on flexor digitorum profundus and covered by flexor carpi ulnaris, it traverses the medial side of the anterior compartment, accompanied in the lower part of the forearm by the ulnar artery. Near the wrist the ulnar nerve emerges lateral to the flexor carpi ulnaris tendon and crosses superficial to the flexor retinaculum with the ulnar artery on its lateral side. The nerve terminates in the hand by dividing into superficial and deep branches (see p. 95). The ulnar nerve supplies the elbow joint and gives branches to flexor carpi ulnaris and the medial part of flexor digitorum profundus. It also provides a palmar cutaneous nerve supplying skin on the medial aspect of the palm, and dorsal cutaneous branches that innervate the medial part of the dorsum of the hand (see Fig. 3.78).

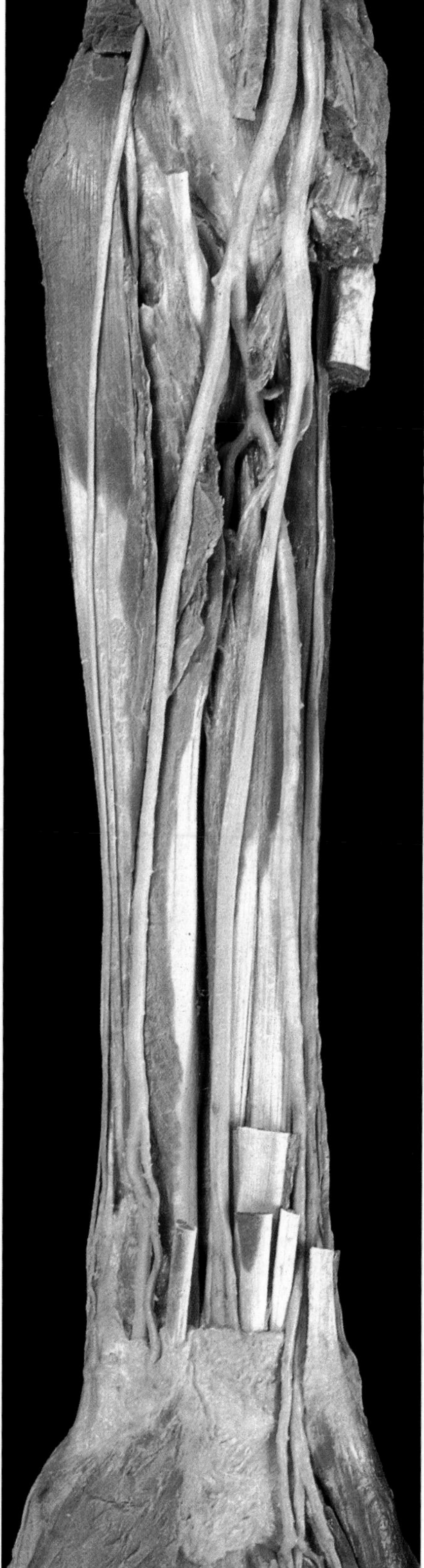

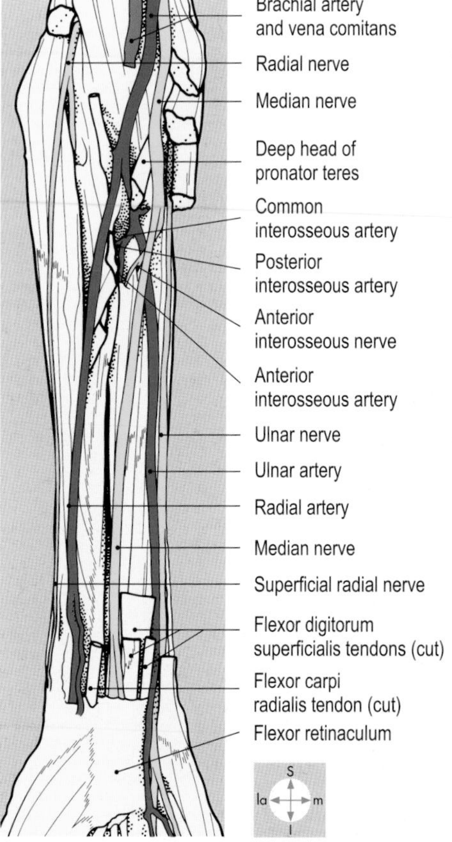

Fig. 3.36 Vessels and nerves of the anterior compartment of the forearm. The superficial flexor muscles and brachioradialis have been divided and most of the venae comitantes have been removed.

Palm and Digits

The hand comprises the wrist (carpus), the palm (metacarpus) and the digits (Figs 3.37 & 3.38). The palm of the hand (see Fig. 3.39) contains the palmar aponeurosis, intrinsic muscles, tendons originating from muscles in the anterior compartment of the forearm, and palmar vessels and nerves. The intrinsic muscles comprise the thenar and hypothenar groups, the lumbricals and interossei, and adductor pollicis. The tendons enter the palm through the carpal tunnel (see Fig. 3.98) deep to the flexor retinaculum. The skin of the anterior surface of the hand is thick, devoid of hair and contains many sweat glands. It is firmly bound to the underlying deep fascia, producing characteristic creases.

Deep fascia of palm

The deep fascia of the palm is thickened centrally to form the triangular palmar aponeurosis (see Fig. 3.39) and is thinner at each side where it covers the thenar and hypothenar muscles. Proximally, the palmar aponeurosis attaches to the flexor retinaculum and is continuous with the tendon of palmaris longus. Distally, the aponeurosis gives rise to four pairs of digital slips, which cross the metacarpophalangeal joints and

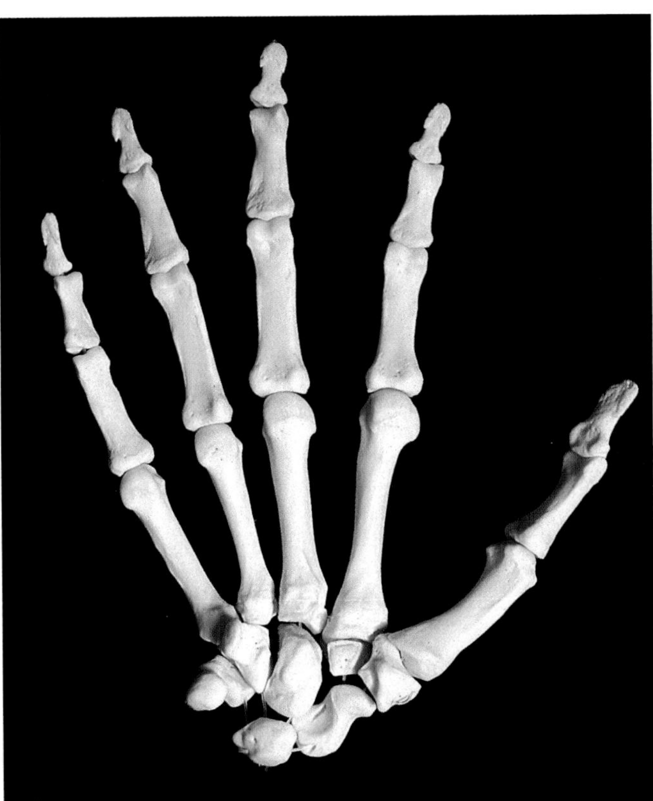

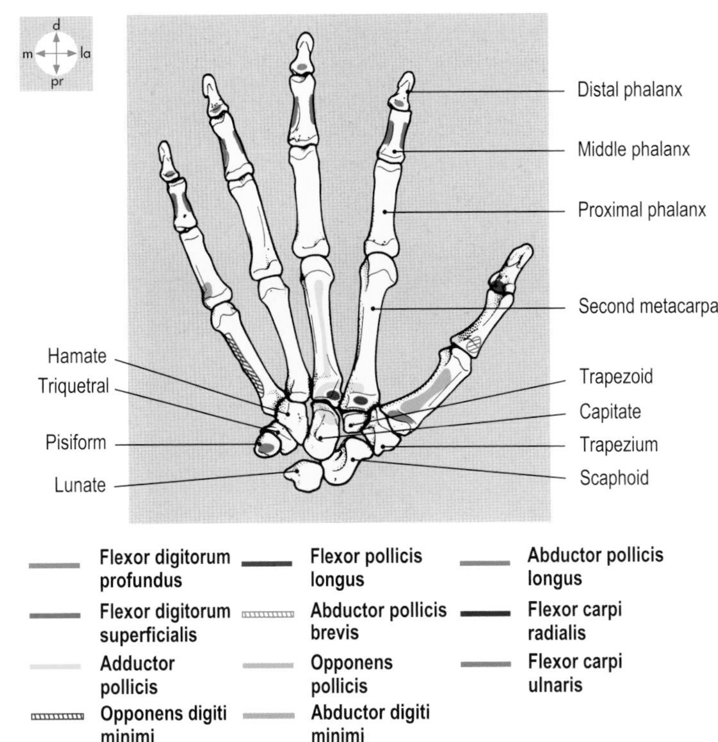

Fig. 3.37 Bones of the hand. The distal attachments of the forearm flexor muscles and of the thenar and hypothenar muscles and the attachments of adductor pollicis are indicated.

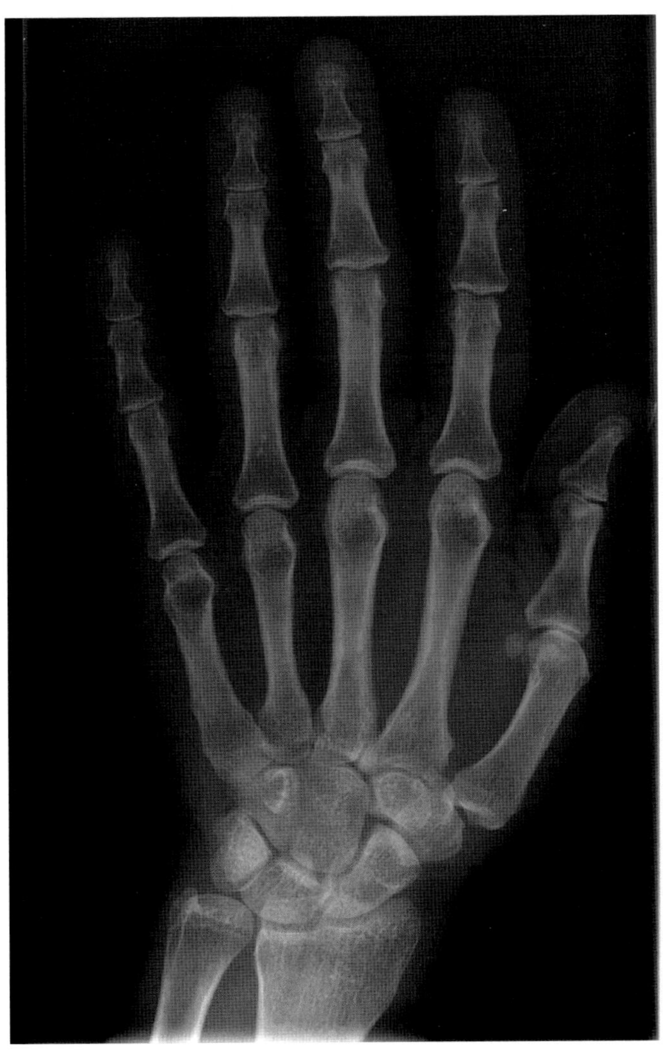

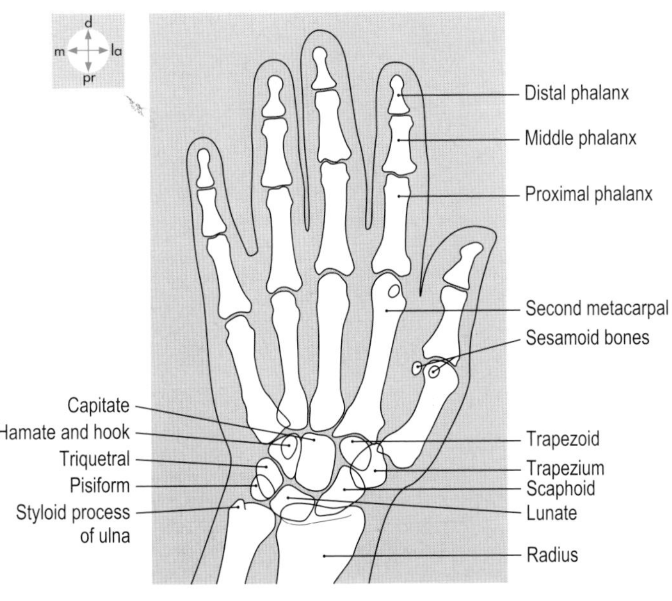

Fig. 3.38 Radiograph of an adult hand. Compare Fig. 3.97.

attach to the proximal phalanges of the fingers via the fibrous flexor sheaths. The aponeurosis covers the superficial palmar arch, the median nerve and the tendons of the long flexors of the digits.

Lateral and medial septa pass from the edges of the palmar aponeurosis to the first and fifth metacarpal bones respectively. These septa separate the thenar and hypothenar muscles from a 'central palmar space', which is traversed by the palmar digital vessels and nerves and by the tendons of the long flexor muscles of the fingers.

The subcutaneous tissue of the medial side of the palm usually contains palmaris brevis (Fig. 3.39), a small muscle attaching to the overlying skin and to the palmar aponeurosis.

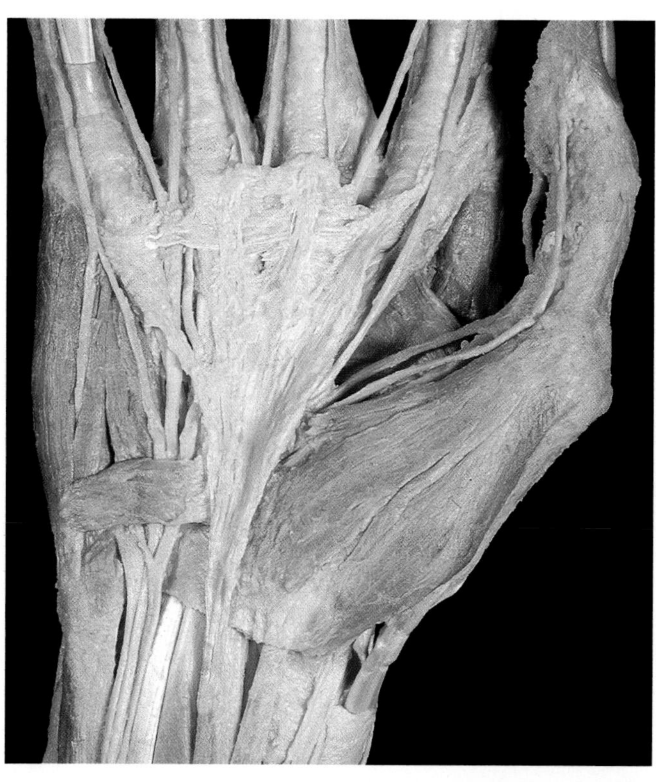

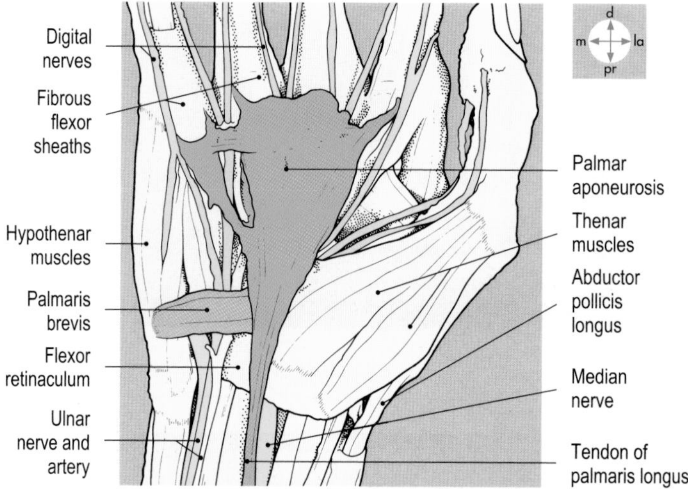

Fig. 3.39 Palmar aponeurosis exposed by removal of skin and subcutaneous tissue.

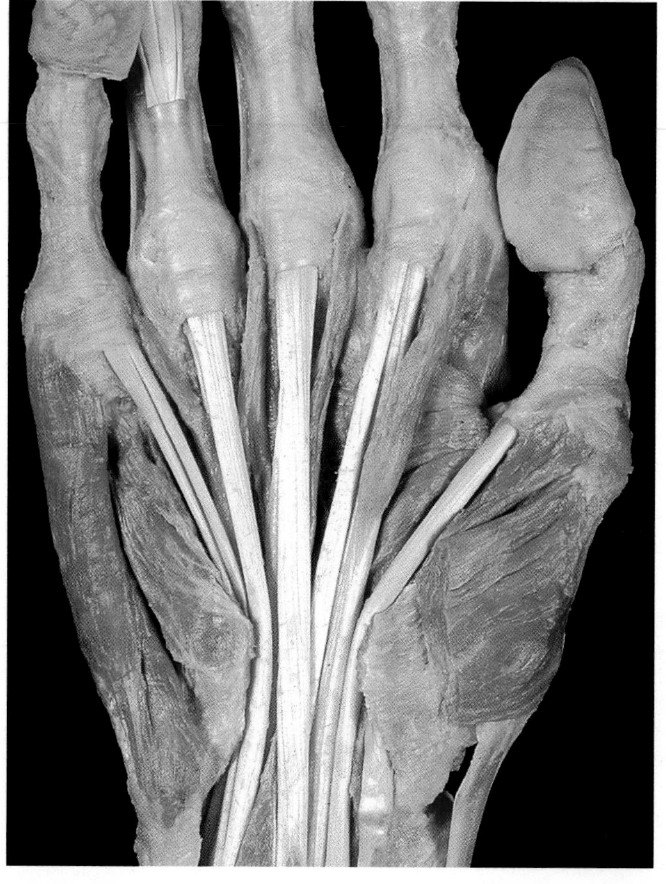

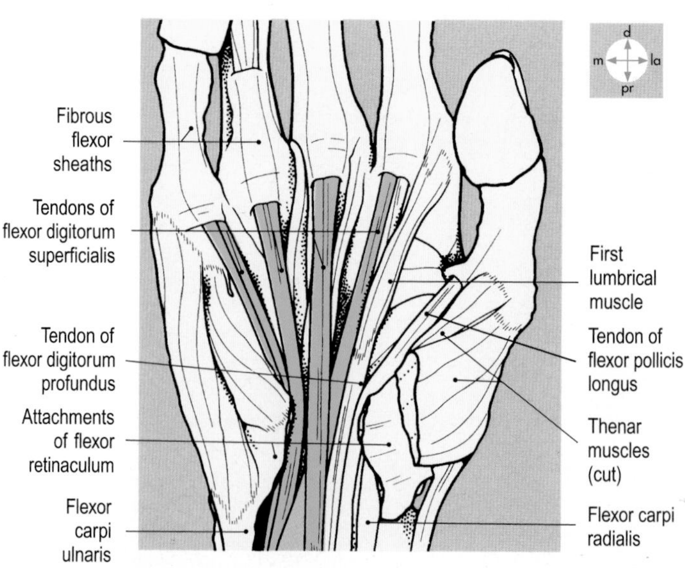

Fig. 3.40 Tendons of flexor digitorum superficialis in the palm. The palmar aponeurosis, flexor retinaculum and palmar vessels and nerves have been removed.

Flexor tendons in the hand

The tendons of flexor pollicis longus, flexor digitorum profundus and flexor digitorum superficialis enter the hand deep to the flexor retinaculum (see Fig. 3.99). On reaching the appropriate digit each tendon traverses a tunnel formed by the fibrous flexor sheath and the phalanges (Fig. 3.40). The fibrous sheath is attached to the edges of the anterior surfaces of the phalanges (Fig. 3.41) and continues as far as the distal phalanx (Fig. 3.42). The sheath is thinner and more flexible in front of the interphalangeal joints, allowing flexion of the digit without 'bowstringing' of the tendons and thus facilitating gripping. Within the flexor sheaths the tendons are invested by synovial membrane and receive vincula tendinum, small folds of synovium that convey blood vessels to the tendons.

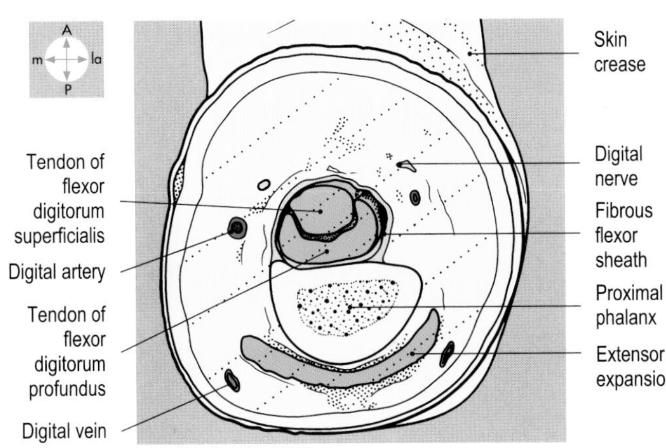

Fig. 3.41 Transverse section through the index finger at the level of the proximal phalanx.

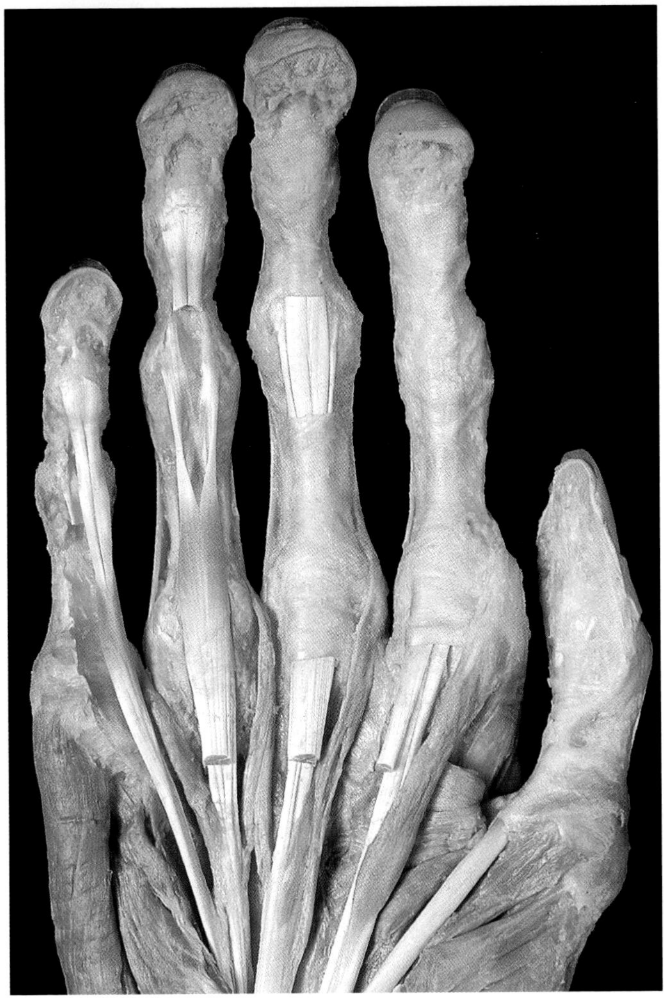

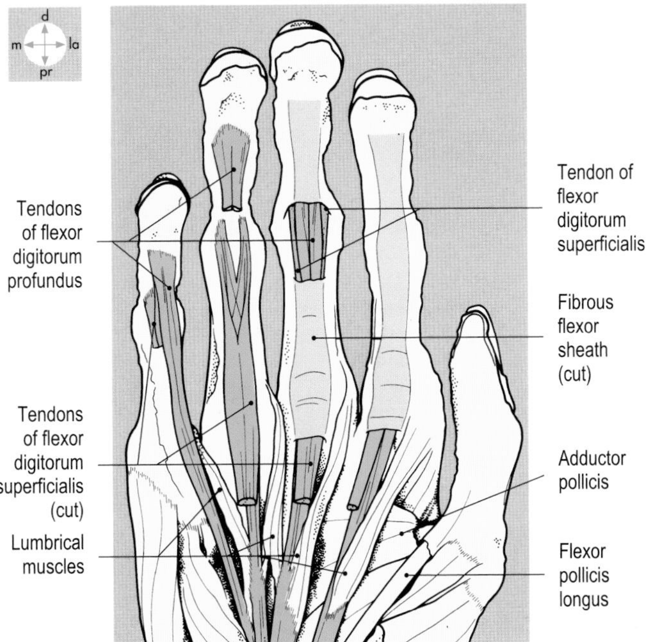

Fig. 3.42 Digital fibrous flexor sheaths. The partially cut away sheath of the middle finger exposes the tendons of flexor digitorum superficialis and profundus, whose phalangeal attachments are revealed on the ring and little fingers.

Thenar muscles

Abductor pollicis brevis, flexor pollicis brevis and opponens pollicis form the thenar eminence on the lateral side of the palm. They attach proximally to the trapezium and scaphoid and to the lateral part of the flexor retinaculum (see Fig. 3.37).

Abductor pollicis brevis (Fig. 3.43) lies superficial to the other thenar muscles and passes from the scaphoid to the base of the proximal phalanx of the thumb. The muscle abducts the thumb, moving the digit anteriorly at right angles to the plane of the palm.

Flexor pollicis brevis, lying deep and medial to the abductor, passes from the trapezium to the proximal phalanx of the thumb. The muscle flexes the carpometacarpal and metacarpophalangeal joints, drawing the thumb across the palm (maintaining the thumbnail at right angles to the palmar plane).

Opponens pollicis (Fig. 3.44), the deepest of the thenar muscles, attaches proximally to the trapezium and distally to the shaft of the first metacarpal. The muscle produces opposition of the thumb, allowing pulp-to-pulp contact with the fingers. This movement combines flexion, adduction and rotation of the first metacarpal at its carpometacarpal joint.

The thenar muscles are supplied by the recurrent branch of the median nerve (Figs 3.43 & 3.44). Injury to this nerve may be assessed by palpating the thenar muscles while the subject attempts abduction of the thumb.

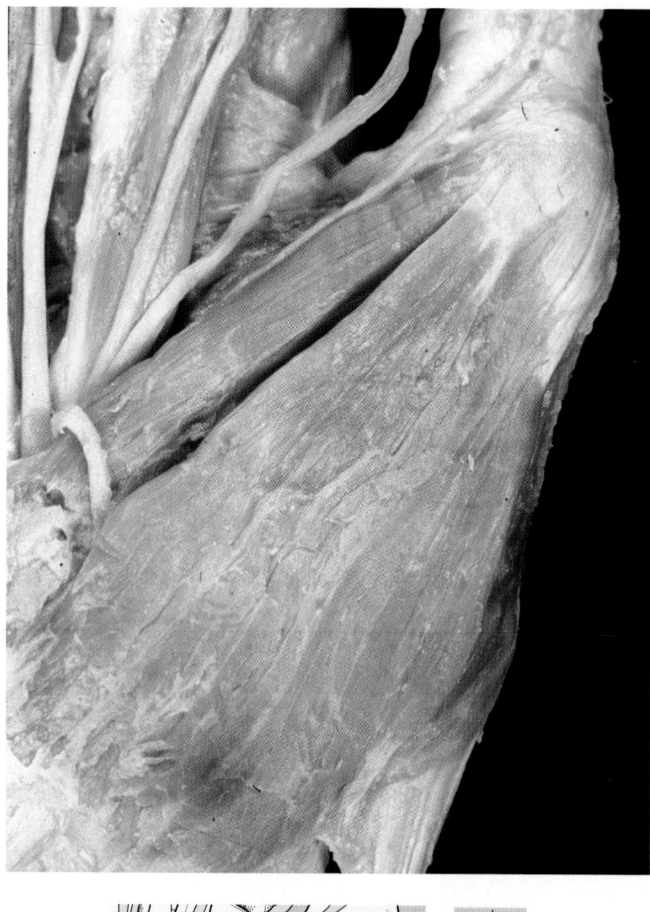

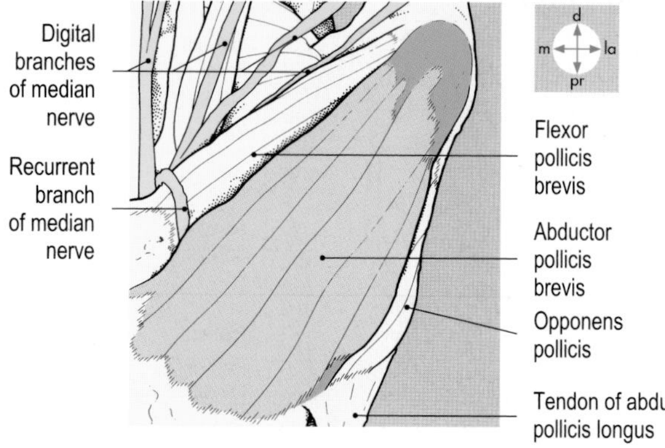

Fig. 3.43 Muscles of the thenar eminence exposed by removal of deep fascia. Abductor pollicis brevis is superficial to flexor pollicis brevis and opponens pollicis.

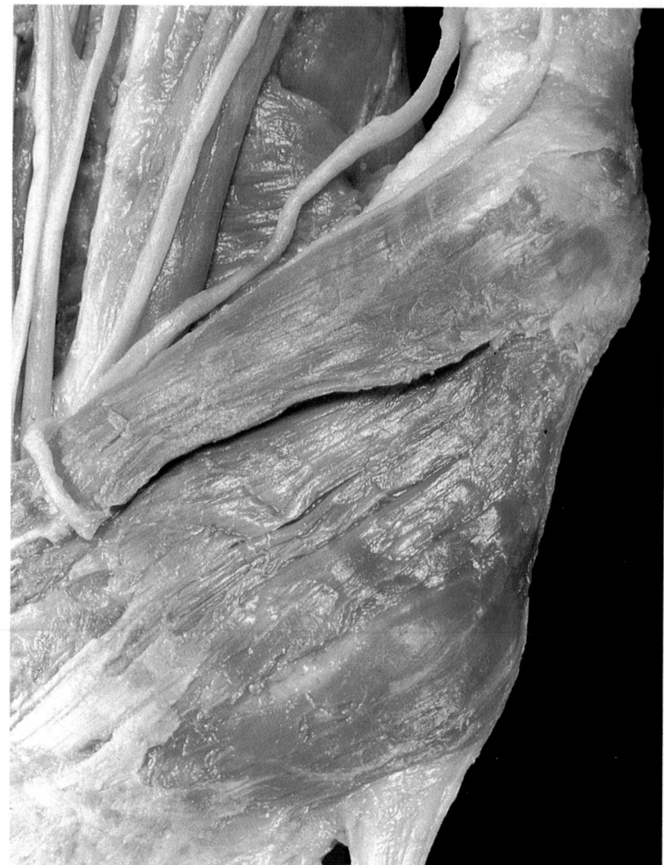

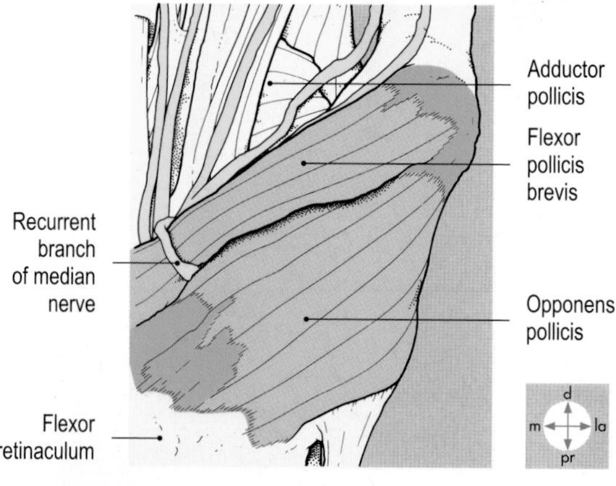

Fig. 3.44 Opponens pollicis and flexor pollicis brevis exposed by removal of abductor pollicis brevis.

Hypothenar muscles

Abductor digiti minimi, flexor digiti minimi brevis and opponens digiti minimi (Fig. 3.45) form the hypothenar eminence and attach proximally to the pisiform, the hook of the hamate and the adjacent part of the flexor retinaculum. Abductor digiti minimi passes from the pisiform to the base of the proximal phalanx of the little finger and abducts the digit, moving it medially in the plane of the palm. Flexor digiti minimi brevis attaches between the hamate and base of the proximal phalanx of the little finger and flexes the metacarpal and proximal phalanx of the little finger. Opponens digiti minimi passes from the hamate to the shaft of the fifth metacarpal and on contraction deepens the hollow of the palm.

The hypothenar muscles are supplied by the deep branch of the ulnar nerve (Fig. 3.45).

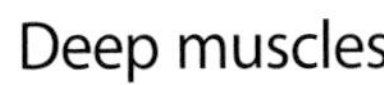

Deep muscles

The deep muscles of the hand consist of adductor pollicis, the palmar and dorsal interossei, and the lumbricals.

Adductor pollicis (Fig. 3.46) has transverse and oblique heads. The transverse

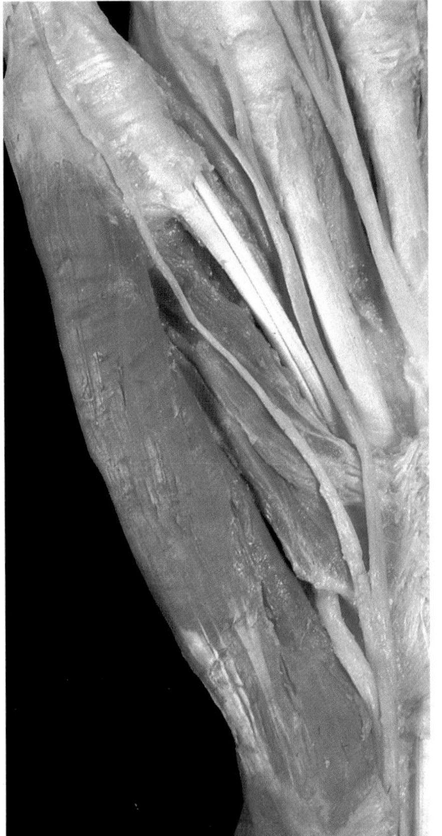

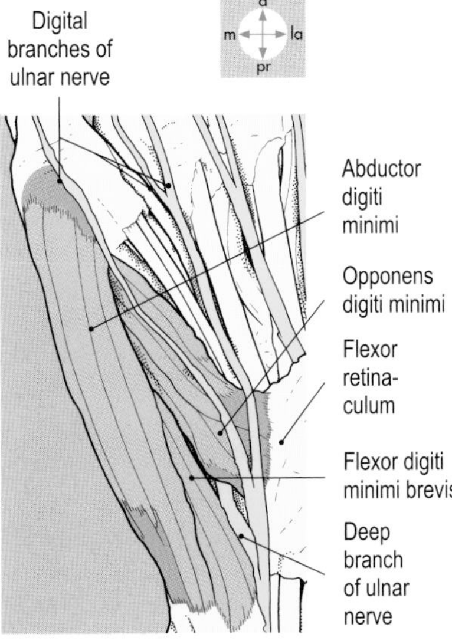

Fig. 3.45 Hypothenar muscles exposed by removal of the deep fascia.

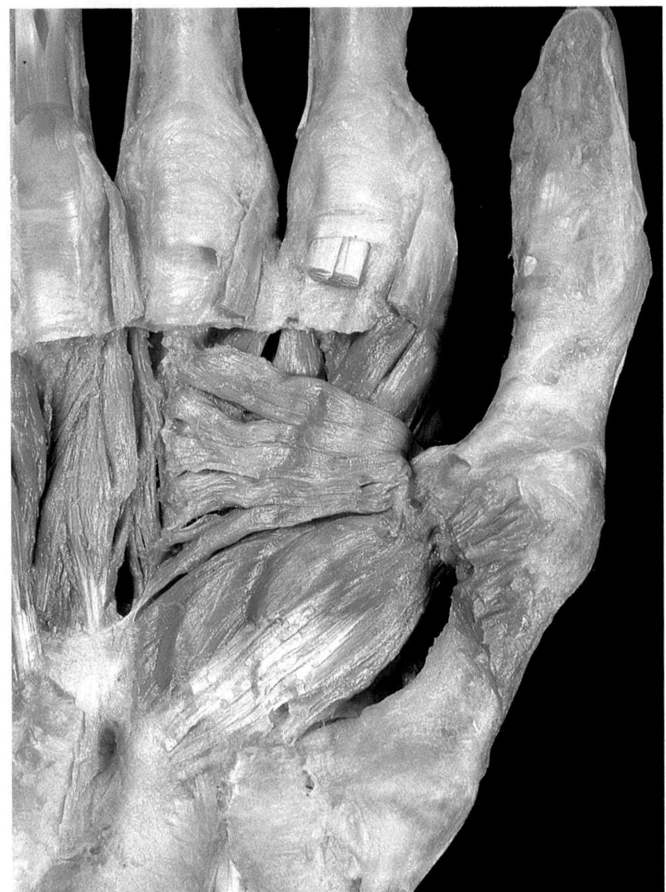

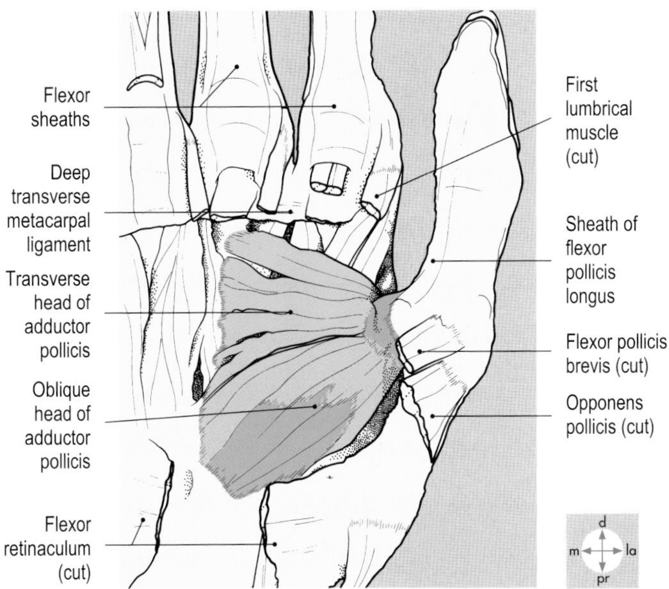

Fig. 3.46 Adductor pollicis. The muscles of the thenar eminence, long flexor tendons, and palmar and digital vessels and nerves have been removed.

head attaches to the shaft of the third metacarpal bone, and the oblique head to the trapezoid, capitate and bases of the second and third metacarpals. Both heads pass laterally to attach to the base of the proximal phalanx of the thumb by a common tendon which usually contains a sesamoid bone (see Fig. 3.38). The muscle adducts and flexes the thumb at its carpometacarpal and metacarpophalangeal joints and is supplied by the deep branch of the ulnar nerve (see Fig. 3.54).

The interossei consist of three palmar and four dorsal muscles (Fig. 3.47). Each palmar interosseous muscle (Fig. 3.48) arises by a single head from the anterior border of the shaft of the second, fourth or fifth metacarpal. Each dorsal interosseous muscle

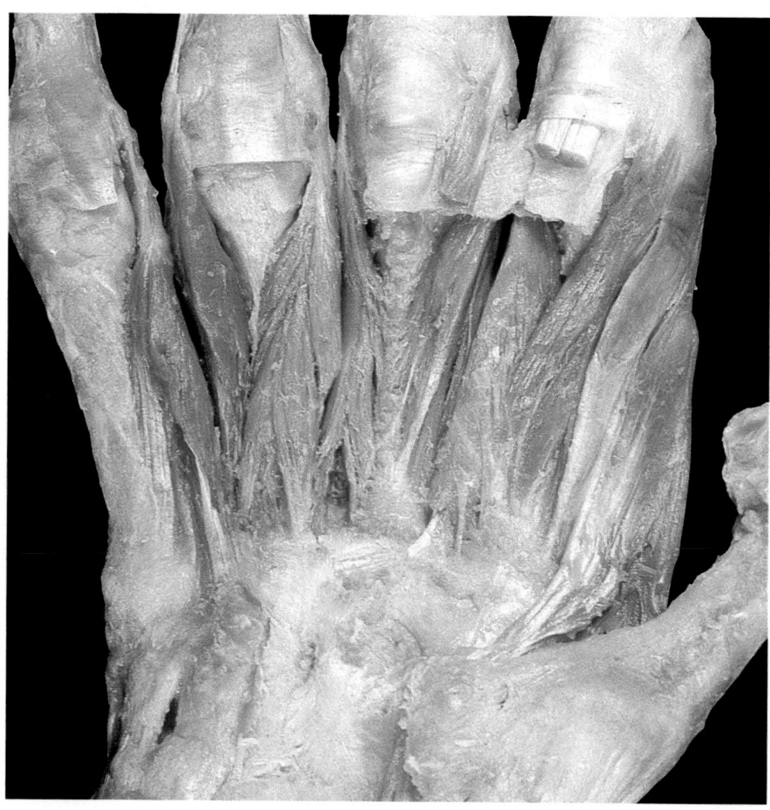

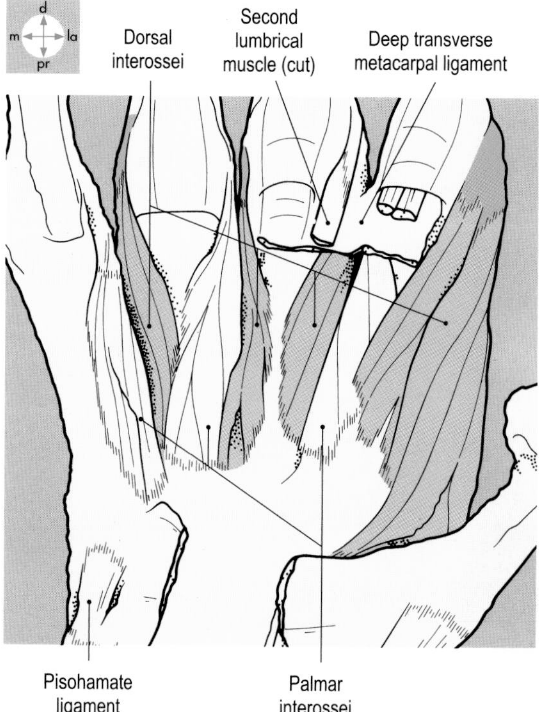

Fig. 3.47 Palmar and dorsal interossei exposed by removal of the long flexor tendons and adductor pollicis. The dorsal interossei have much more bulk than the palmar interossei.

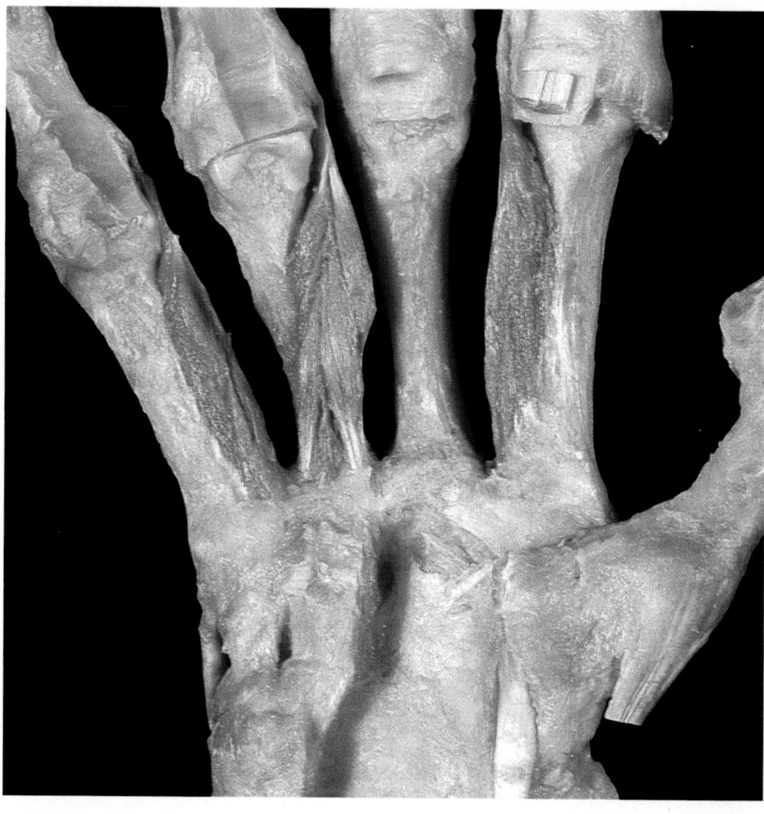

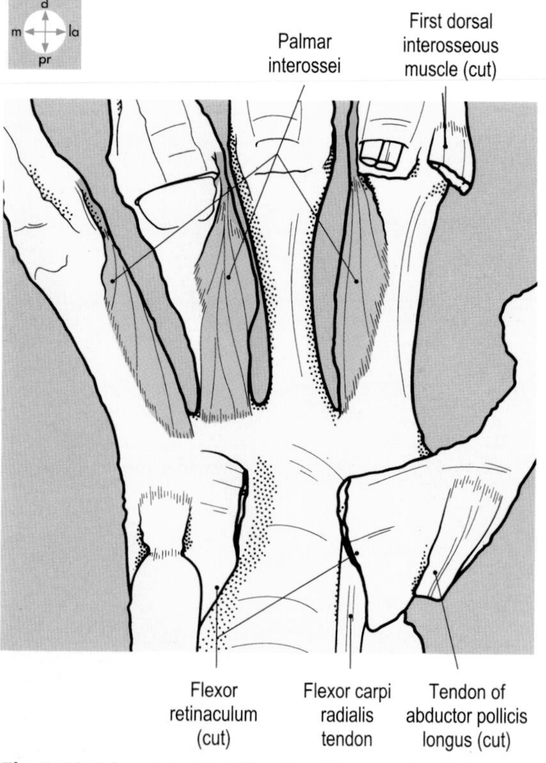

Fig. 3.48 Palmar interossei. The dorsal interossei and deep transverse metacarpal ligaments have been excised.

(Fig. 3.49) arises by two heads from the contiguous sides of the shafts of the adjacent metacarpals. Distally the tendon of each interosseous muscle attaches to the base of the proximal phalanx and to the extensor expansion of the appropriate digit (see Fig. 3.51). The interossei move the fingers in the plane of the palm (coronal plane); movement of a finger away from the long axis of the middle finger is called abduction while movement towards the middle finger is adduction. The palmar interossei adduct and the dorsal interossei abduct the fingers. In addition, the interossei flex the metacarpophalangeal joints and extend the interphalangeal joints. All the interossei are supplied by the deep branch of the ulnar nerve (see Fig. 3.54).

The lumbricals are four small muscles attaching proximally to the tendons of flexor digitorum profundus (Fig. 3.50). Distally, each lumbrical attaches to the radial side of the extensor expansion of the appropriate finger. The muscles extend the interphalangeal joints and flex the metacarpophalangeal joints. The first and second lumbricals usually have only one head each and are supplied by the median nerve, whereas the third and fourth (medial) usually have two heads and are supplied by the ulnar nerve.

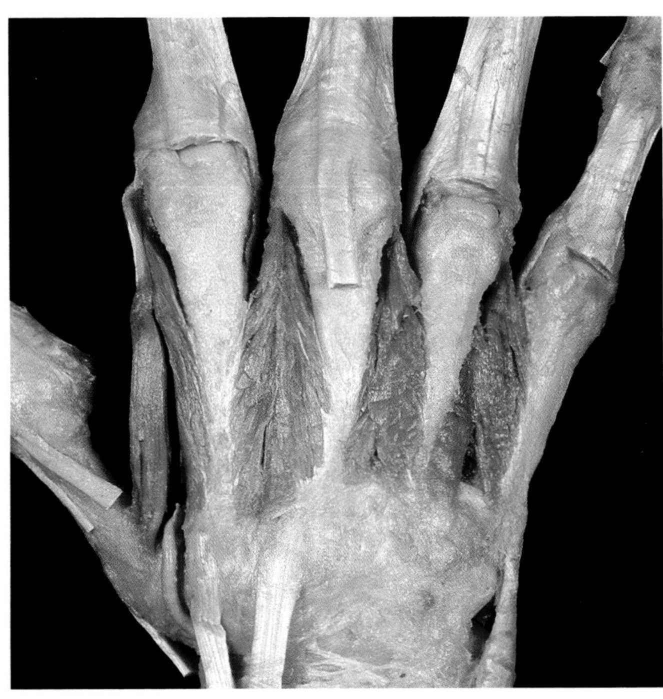

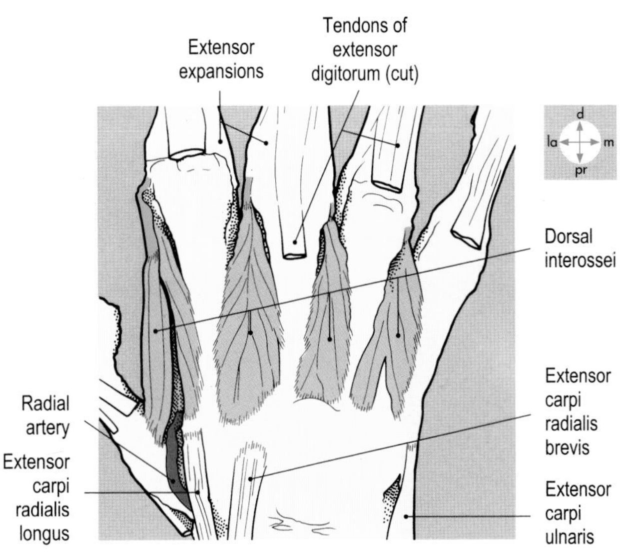

Fig. 3.49 Dorsal interossei exposed by removal of deep fascia and tendons of extensor digitorum.

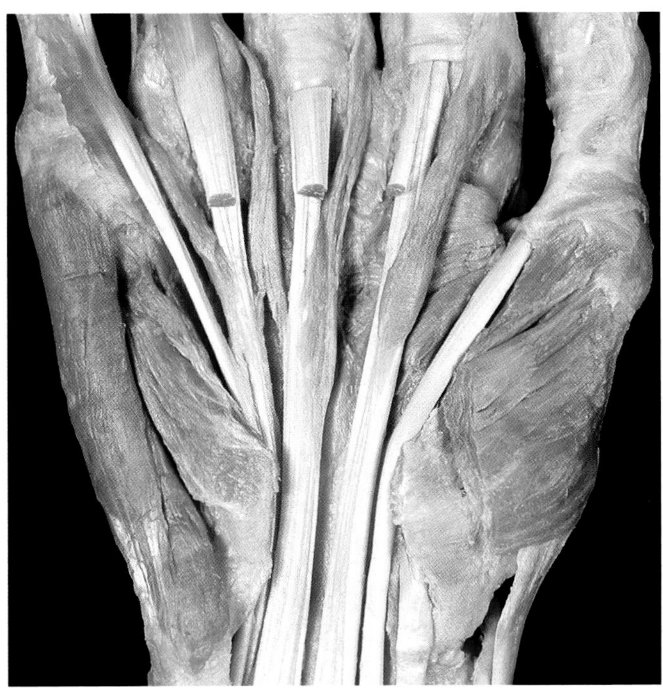

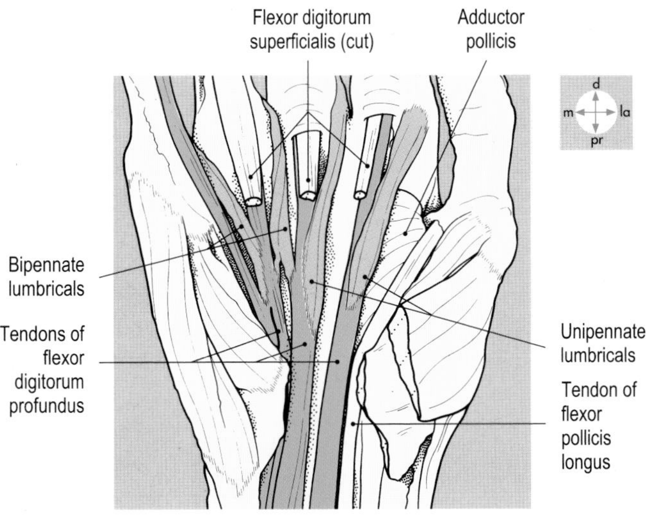

Fig. 3.50 Removal of the tendons of flexor digitorum superficialis has revealed the attachments of the lumbrical muscles to the tendons of flexor digitorum profundus.

Digital extensor expansions

Each finger possesses an extensor expansion or hood (Fig. 3.51) which receives the tendons of the appropriate long extensor muscle(s), interossei and lumbricals. The broad proximal part of the expansion overlies the metacarpophalangeal joint. Distally, the expansion tapers and attaches by a central slip to the base of the middle phalanx and by two marginal slips to the base of the distal phalanx.

Blood vessels

The arterial supply to the hand is derived from branches of the ulnar and radial arteries, which form superficial and deep palmar arches linking the two main arteries and ensuring a rich blood supply to the palm and fingers.

The ulnar artery enters the hand superficial to the flexor retinaculum and gives a deep branch that accompanies the deep branch of the ulnar nerve. The main artery continues as the superficial palmar arch (Fig. 3.52), which passes distally to the level of the thumb web, lying deep to the palmar aponeurosis but anterior to the digital nerves and flexor tendons. The superficial palmar arch gives four palmar digital branches, which supply the adjacent sides of the fingers (Fig. 3.53) and medial side of the little finger, and is completed laterally by a branch of the radial artery.

The radial artery enters the palm from the dorsum of the hand between the two heads of the first dorsal interosseous muscle (see Fig. 3.49). The artery gives branches to the thumb and index finger and continues as the deep palmar arch (Fig. 3.54), which lies over the bases of the metacarpal bones, deep to the flexor tendons, and is about 1 cm proximal to the superficial arch. The deep arch provides perforating branches, which anastomose with dorsal metacarpal arteries, and three palmar metacarpal arteries, which anastomose with the palmar digital arteries of the superficial arch. The deep arch is completed medially by the deep branch of the ulnar artery. Other vessels such as dorsal metacarpal arteries from the dorsal carpal arch may provide an important supply of blood to the hand. The anastomoses between branches of arteries supplying the hand usually provide an adequate blood supply even if one artery is blocked.

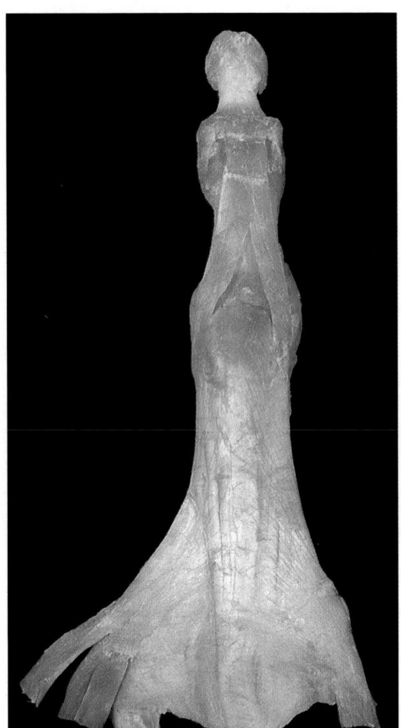

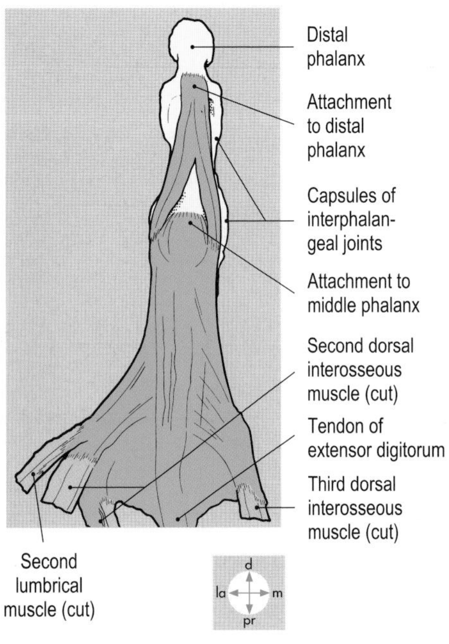

Fig. 3.51 Dorsal view of the digital expansion of the middle finger. The expansion has been flattened proximally to show the attachments of lumbrical and interosseous muscles.

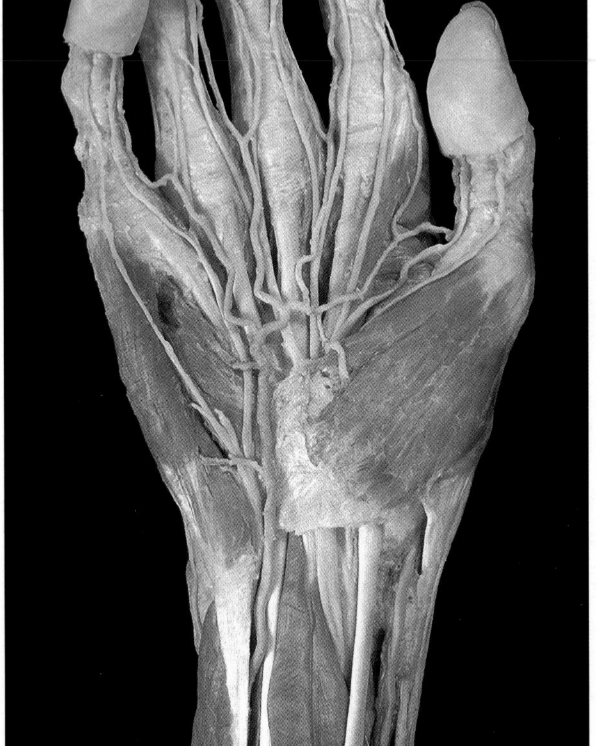

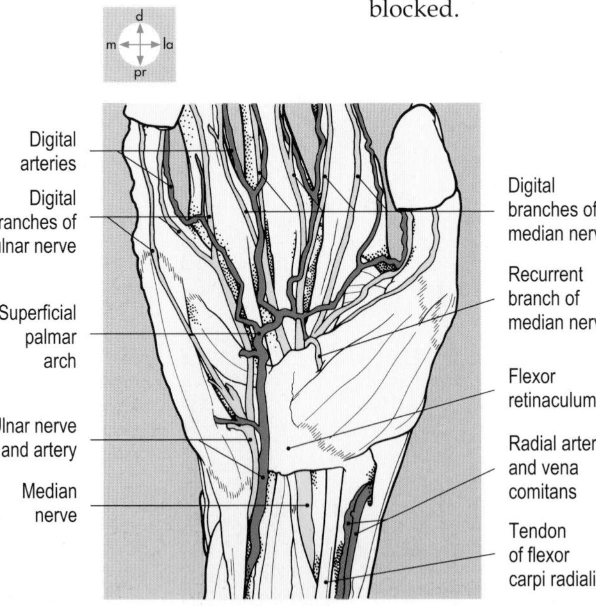

Fig. 3.52 Superficial vessels and nerves of the palm. Skin, subcutaneous tissue and the palmar aponeurosis have been removed.

Most venous blood from the fingers and palm drains into superficial veins on the dorsum of the hand to enter the cephalic or basilic veins.

Nerves

Innervation of the anterior aspect of the hand is shared by the ulnar and median nerves. The ulnar nerve supplies more intrinsic muscles than the median nerve, which supplies a larger area of skin.

The ulnar nerve (Fig. 3.52) enters the palm superficial to the flexor retinaculum and terminates as superficial and deep branches. The superficial branch supplies digital branches to the skin of the medial one-and-one-half digits. A corresponding area of the palm is supplied by palmar branches that arise from the ulnar nerve in the forearm. The deep branch of the ulnar nerve (Fig. 3.54) accompanies the deep palmar arch and supplies the three hypothenar muscles, the medial two lumbricals, all the interossei and adductor pollicis. The ulnar nerve also supplies palmaris brevis. Injury to the ulnar nerve produces marked wasting (atrophy) of the muscles between the first and second metacarpal bones.

The median nerve traverses the carpal tunnel and terminates as digital and recurrent branches. The digital branches (Fig. 3.52) supply skin of the lateral three-and-one-half digits and usually the lateral two lumbricals. A corresponding area of the palm is supplied by palmar branches arising from the median nerve in the forearm. The recurrent branch of the median nerve (see Fig. 3.43) supplies the three thenar muscles.

In the palm the digital branches of the ulnar and median nerves lie deep to the superficial palmar arch (Fig. 3.52), but in the fingers they lie anterior to the digital arteries arising from the superficial arch (Fig. 3.53). Although there may be variability of innervation of the ring and middle fingers, the skin on the anterior surface of the thumb is always supplied by the median nerve and that of the little finger by the ulnar nerve. The palmar digital branches of the median and ulnar nerves also supply the nail beds of their respective digits.

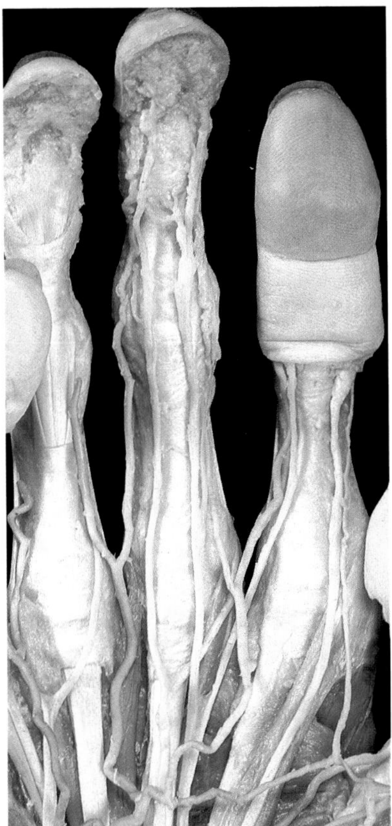

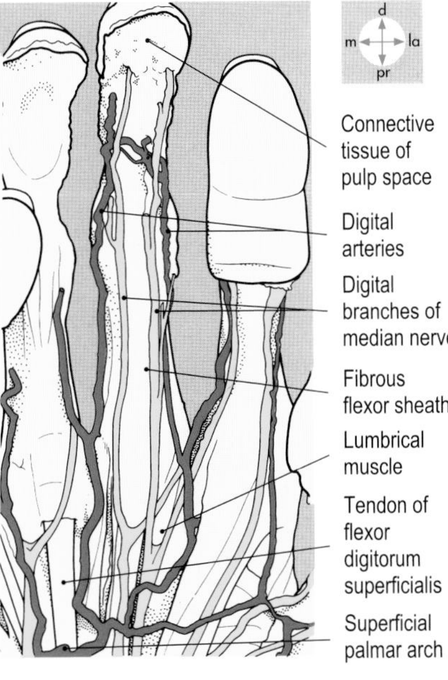

Fig. 3.53 Palmar digital arteries and nerves of the fingers.

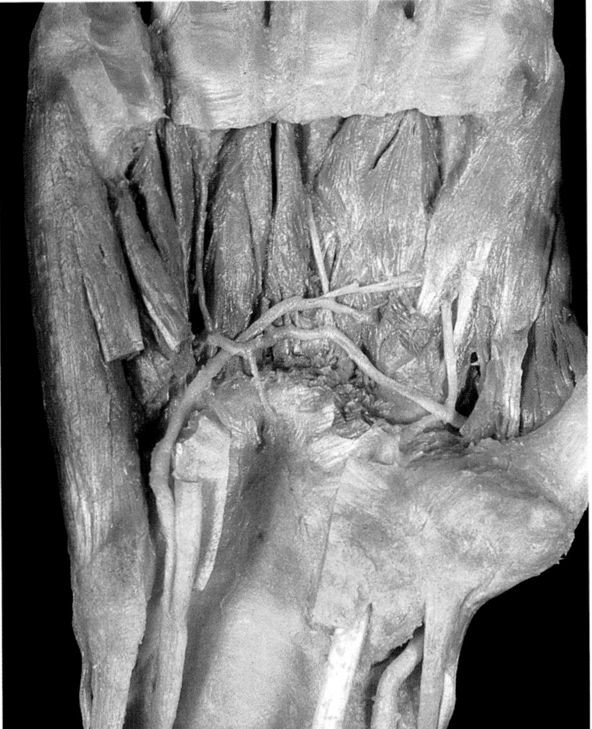

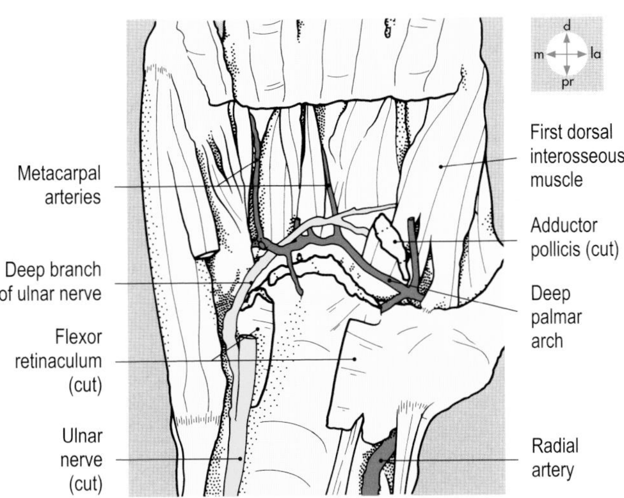

Fig. 3.54 Deep palmar arch and deep branch of ulnar nerve. The long flexor tendons and muscles of the thenar eminence have been removed, and adductor pollicis and the hypothenar muscles divided.

Muscles Attaching Upper Limb to Trunk

Three muscles connect the root of the upper limb to the chest wall and are usually dissected with the thorax. For this reason, pectoralis major and minor and serratus anterior are described with the thoracic wall (see p. 31). Only the posterior group of muscles attaching the limb and its girdle to the vertebral column are described here: trapezius, latissimus dorsi, levator scapulae and the rhomboids (Fig. 3.55).

Trapezius

Trapezius (Fig. 3.56) is a large superficial muscle overlying the dorsum of the neck and thorax. Its upper fibres attach to the ligamentum nuchae, the external occipital protuberance and the superior nuchal line and pass downwards and laterally to the acromion of the scapula and the lateral part of the clavicle. These fibres produce elevation of the scapula as in shrugging the shoulder. When the scapula is fixed they produce lateral flexion of the neck. The middle fibres of trapezius run horizontally from the ligamentum nuchae and upper thoracic spinous processes to the acromion and spine of the scapula and retract the scapula. Fibres of the lower part of the muscle attach to the lower thoracic spinous processes superficial to latissimus dorsi (Fig. 3.56) and pass upwards and laterally to the spine of the scapula. These fibres depress the scapula. Acting together, the upper and lower parts of trapezius produce rotation of the scapula, turning the glenoid fossa superiorly to permit full abduction of the limb (see p. 117). In the neck the anterior edge of the muscle forms the posterior boundary of the posterior triangle. The accessory nerve crosses the triangle (see Fig. 7.9) and supplies the trapezius from its deep surface.

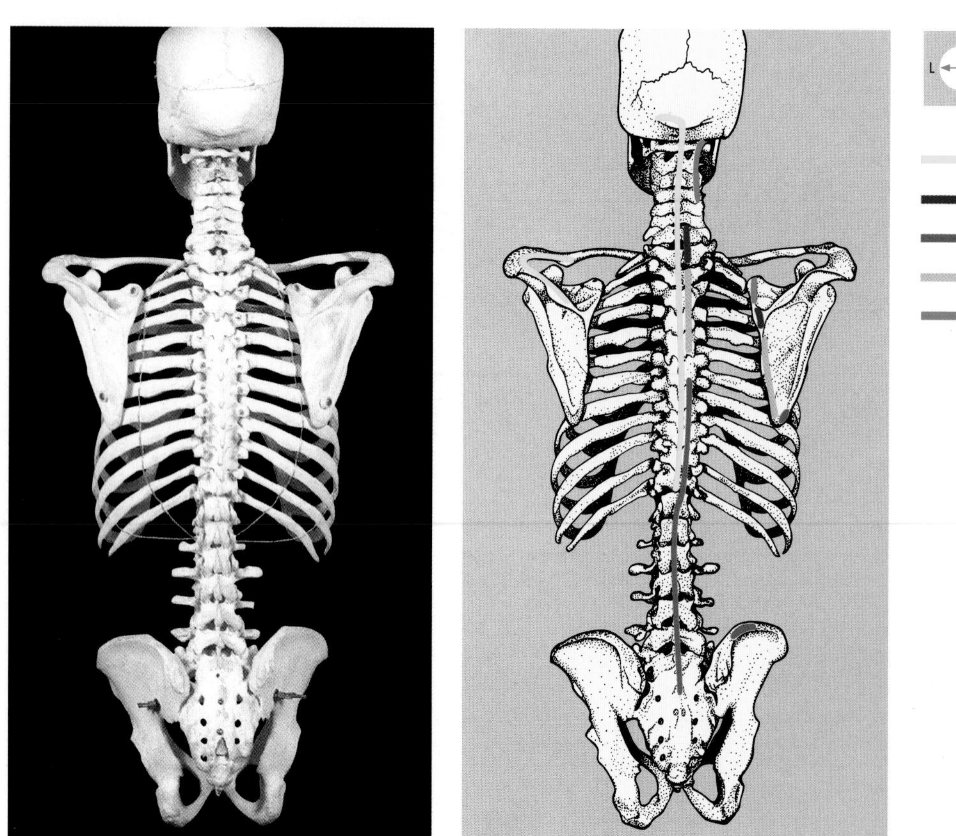

Fig. 3.55 Attachments of trapezius, rhomboid major and minor, levator scapulae and latissimus dorsi.

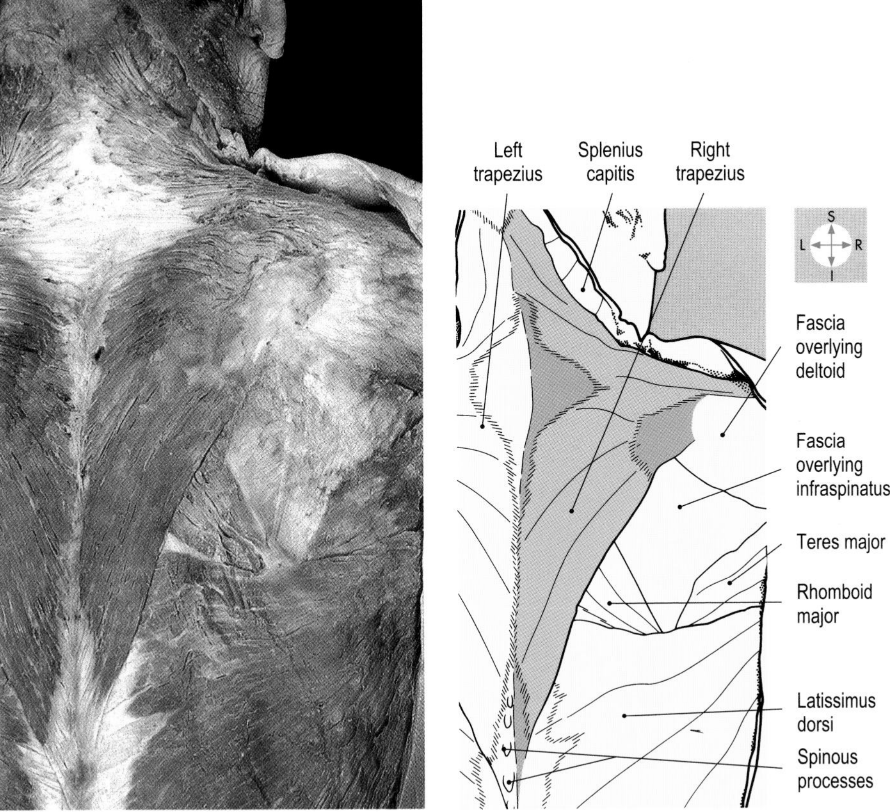

Fig. 3.56 The trapezius muscles have fascial attachments to the cervical and thoracic spinous processes and, in this dissection, are asymmetric inferiorly.

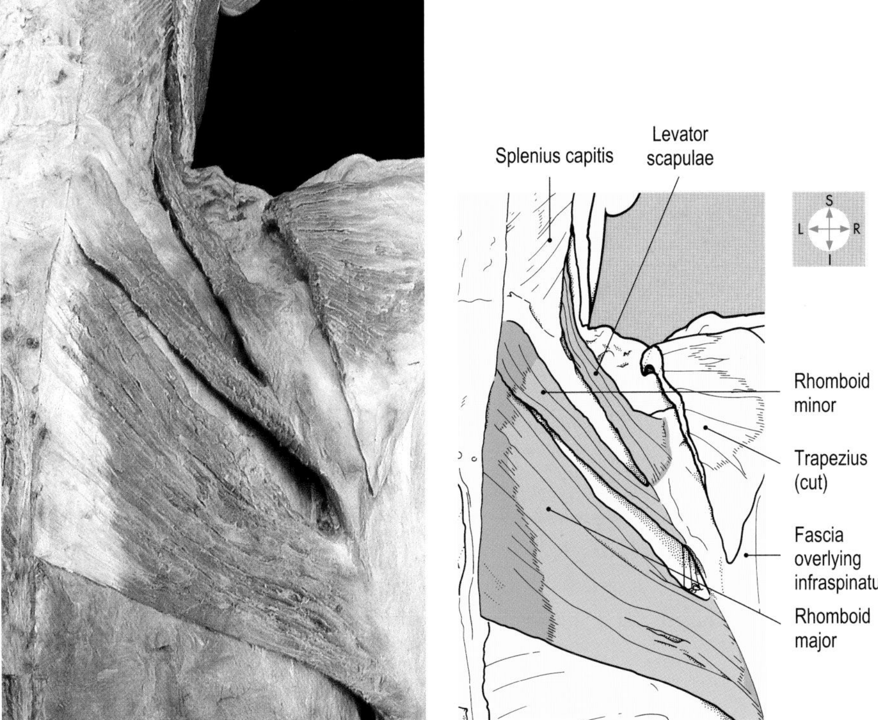

Fig. 3.57 Levator scapulae and rhomboids exposed by removal of trapezius.

Levator scapulae and rhomboids

These three muscles are covered by trapezius. Levator scapulae (Fig. 3.57) ascends from the medial border of the scapula above the root of the spine to the transverse processes of the upper four cervical vertebrae. The fibres of the rhomboids incline upwards and medially (Fig. 3.57). Rhomboid minor attaches to the medial border of the scapula at the root of its spine and to the spinous processes of the seventh cervical and first thoracic vertebrae. Rhomboid major passes between the remainder of the medial border of the scapula and the spines of the second to fifth thoracic vertebrae.

All three muscles elevate the scapula and assist in scapular rotation during adduction of the upper limb. The dorsal scapular nerve from the brachial plexus (C5) supplies the rhomboids and may innervate levator scapulae, which is also supplied by branches from the cervical plexus (C3 & C4).

Latissimus dorsi

Latissimus dorsi (Fig. 3.58) is a large triangular muscle overlying much of the dorsal aspect of the trunk. The muscle attaches to the spinous processes of the lower six thoracic vertebrae and through the lumbar fascia to the spines of the lumbar vertebrae and the sacrum. The most inferior fibres attach to the posterior part of the iliac crest. Fibres also attach to the lower four ribs and to the inferior angle of the scapula. All the fibres converge on a narrow tendon in the posterior fold of the axilla. The tendon winds round the lower border of teres major to attach to the intertubercular sulcus of the humerus.

The muscle is a powerful adductor and extensor of the humerus at the shoulder joint, particularly when the upper limb is abducted and flexed. Latissimus dorsi is also a medial rotator at the shoulder joint and assists with rotation and retraction of the scapula. In movements such as rising from an armchair, if the humerus is fixed, both muscles contract to raise the trunk. This action is particularly important in patients with paralysed lower limbs. Latissimus dorsi is supplied by a single neurovascular bundle which contains the thoracodorsal nerve (a branch of the posterior cord of the brachial plexus; see Fig. 3.18) and the thoracodorsal vessels, which are branches of the subscapular vessels. In reconstructive surgery, the muscle and its overlying skin may be mobilized on this neurovascular pedicle to provide a large myocutaneous flap.

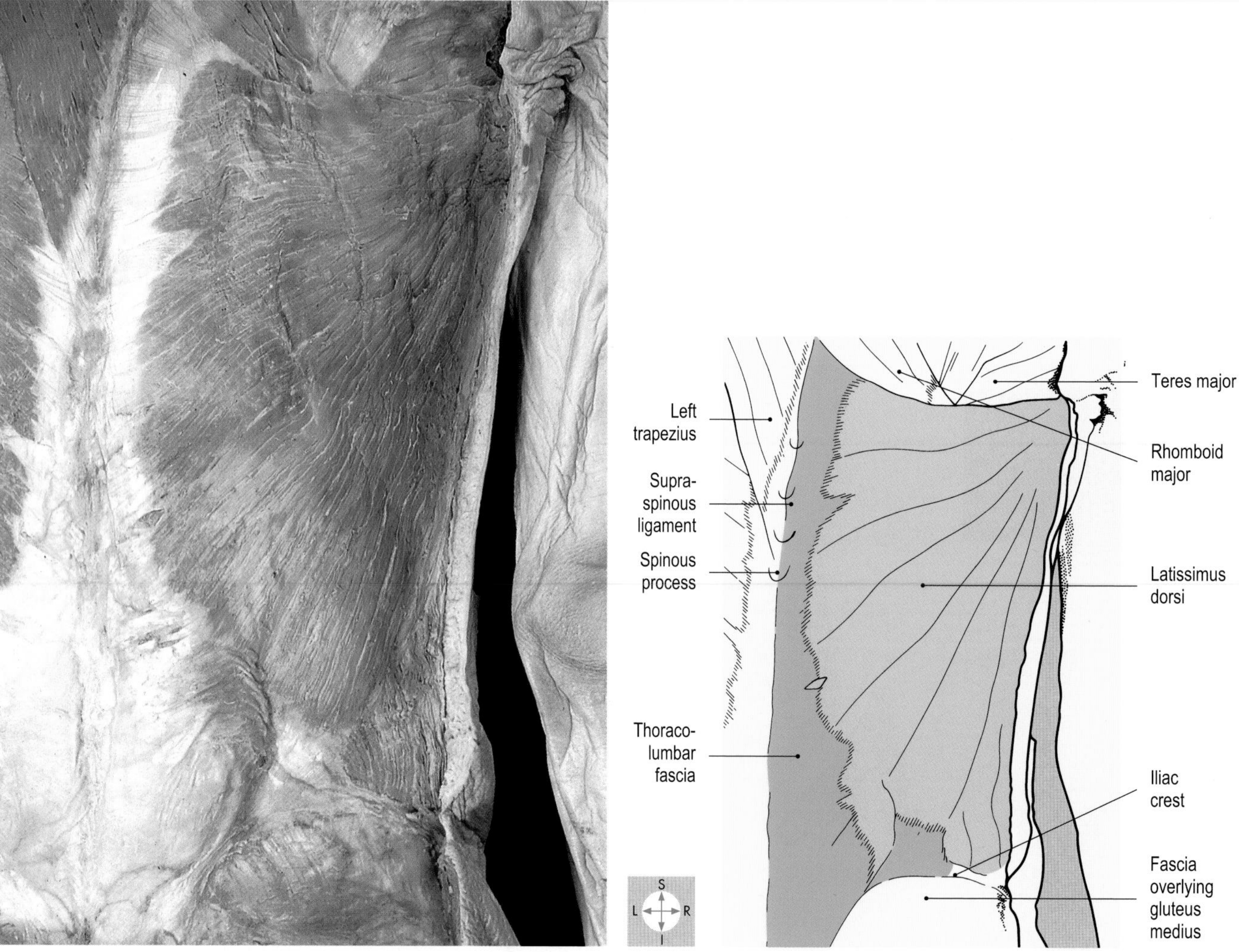

Fig. 3.58 Latissimus dorsi. The anterior border lies parallel to the cut skin edge, and the thoracic attachment has been exposed by removal of trapezius.

Short Scapular Muscles

These short muscles, the four rotator cuff muscles and teres major, span the shoulder (glenohumeral) joint, attaching to the scapula and to the proximal part of the humerus (Fig. 3.59 and see Fig. 3.62).

Rotator cuff muscles

This important group of muscles, namely subscapularis, supraspinatus, infraspinatus and teres minor, is intimately related to the shoulder joint. By attaching not only to the tubercles of the humerus but also to the capsule of the joint they hold the humeral head firmly in the glenoid fossa and help stabilize the joint.

Subscapularis

Subscapularis (Fig. 3.60) attaches proximally to the medial part of the costal surface of the scapula. Its tendon, separated from the neck of the scapula by the subscapular bursa, is attached to the lesser tubercle of the humerus. The muscle is supplied by the subscapular nerves from the posterior cord of the brachial plexus. Subscapularis produces medial rotation of the arm at the shoulder joint.

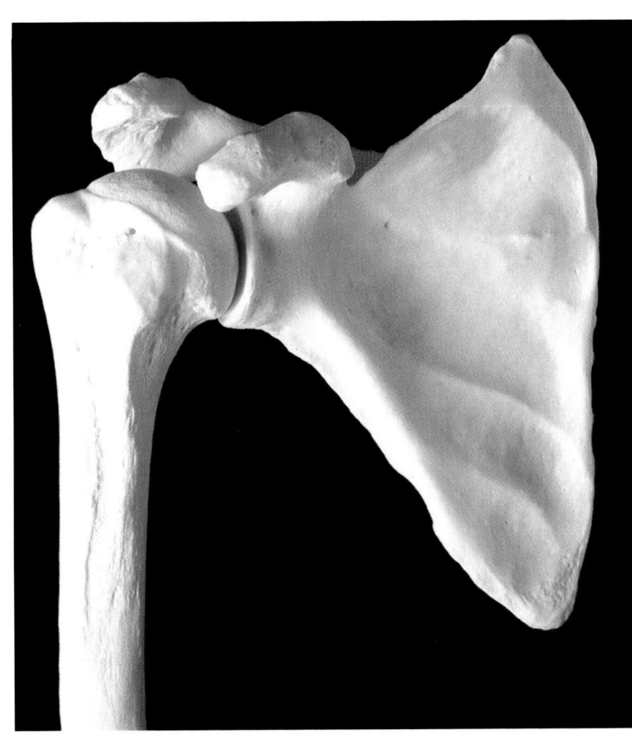

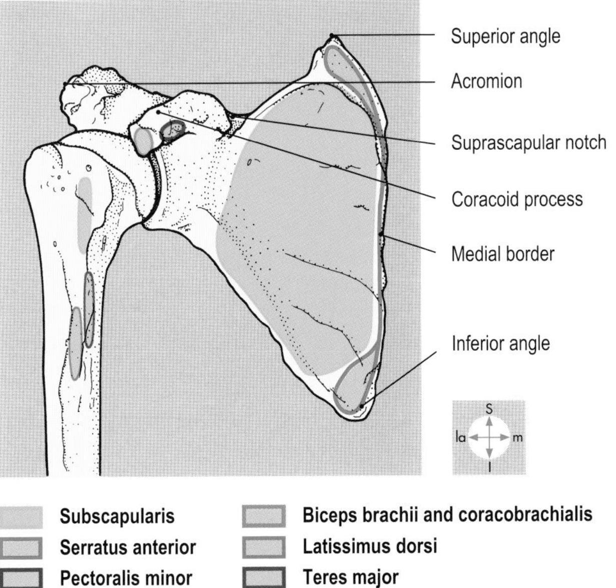

Fig. 3.59 Anterior aspects of scapula and proximal end of humerus. The head of the humerus is partly obscured by the overlying coracoid process of the scapula.

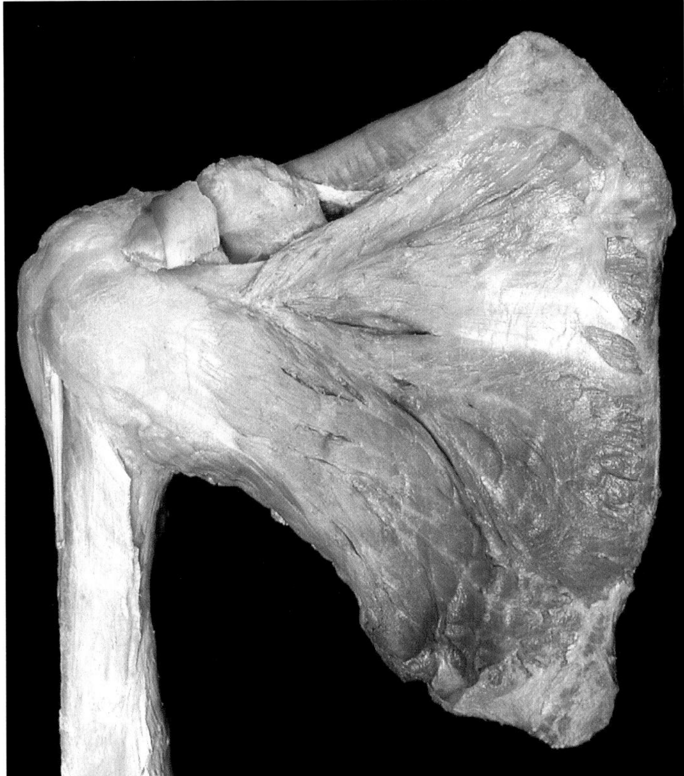

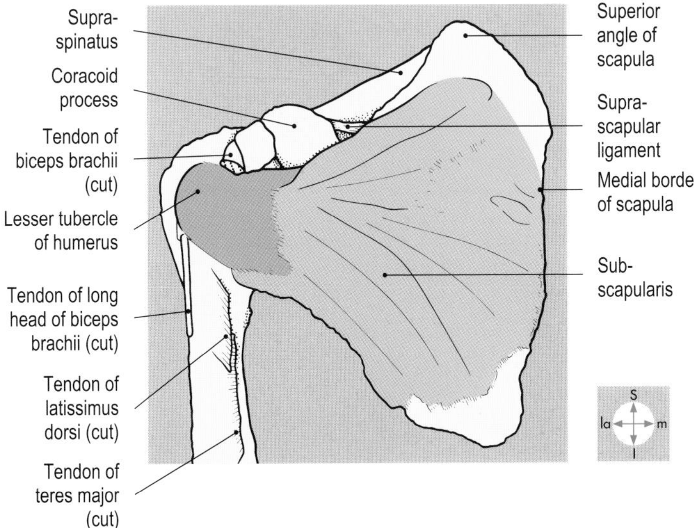

Fig. 3.60 Anterior view of subscapularis. The attachment of serratus anterior to the medial border of the scapula has been excised.

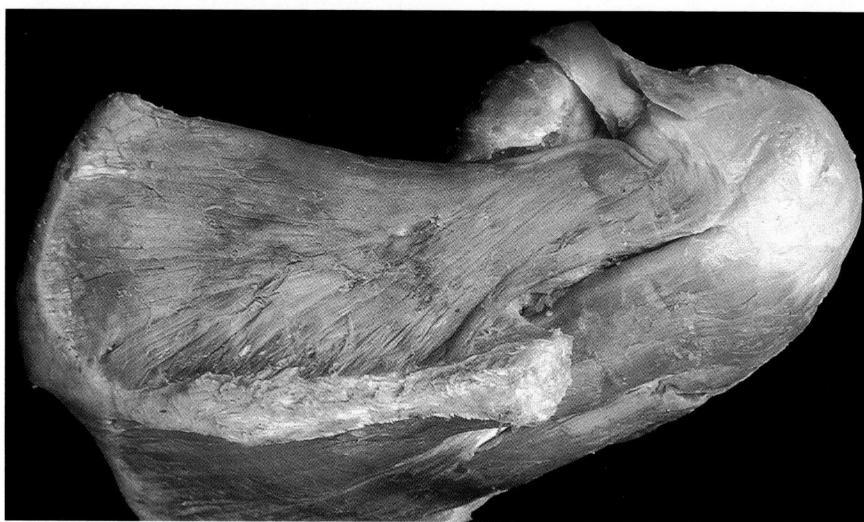

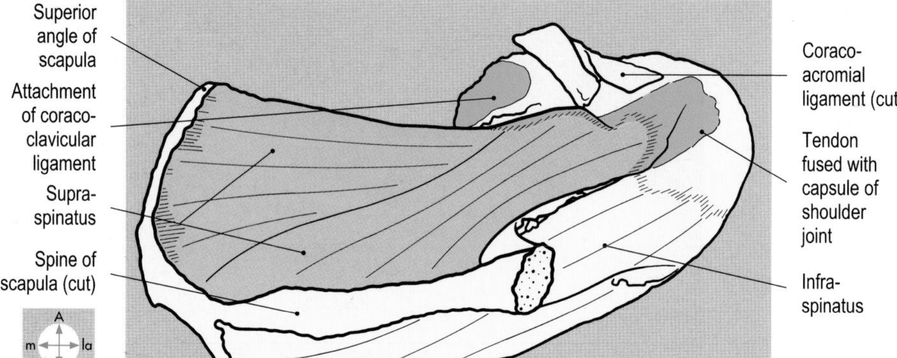

Fig. 3.61 Superior view of supraspinatus after removal of the acromion of the scapula.

Supraspinatus

Supraspinatus (Fig. 3.61) attaches to the supraspinous fossa of the scapula and to the superior facet of the greater tubercle of the humerus (Fig. 3.62). The subacromial bursa lies above the tendon of supraspinatus, separating the tendon and the capsule of the shoulder joint from the coracoacromial arch. The muscle initiates abduction of the shoulder joint, and damage to its tendon produces pain during the early stages of this movement.

Infraspinatus

Infraspinatus (Fig. 3.63) arises from the infraspinous fossa and its tendon inserts into the middle facet of the greater tubercle of the humerus. The muscle is covered by a strong fascial membrane. A bursa sometimes separates the tendon from the neck of the scapula.

Supraspinatus and infraspinatus are supplied by the suprascapular nerve which

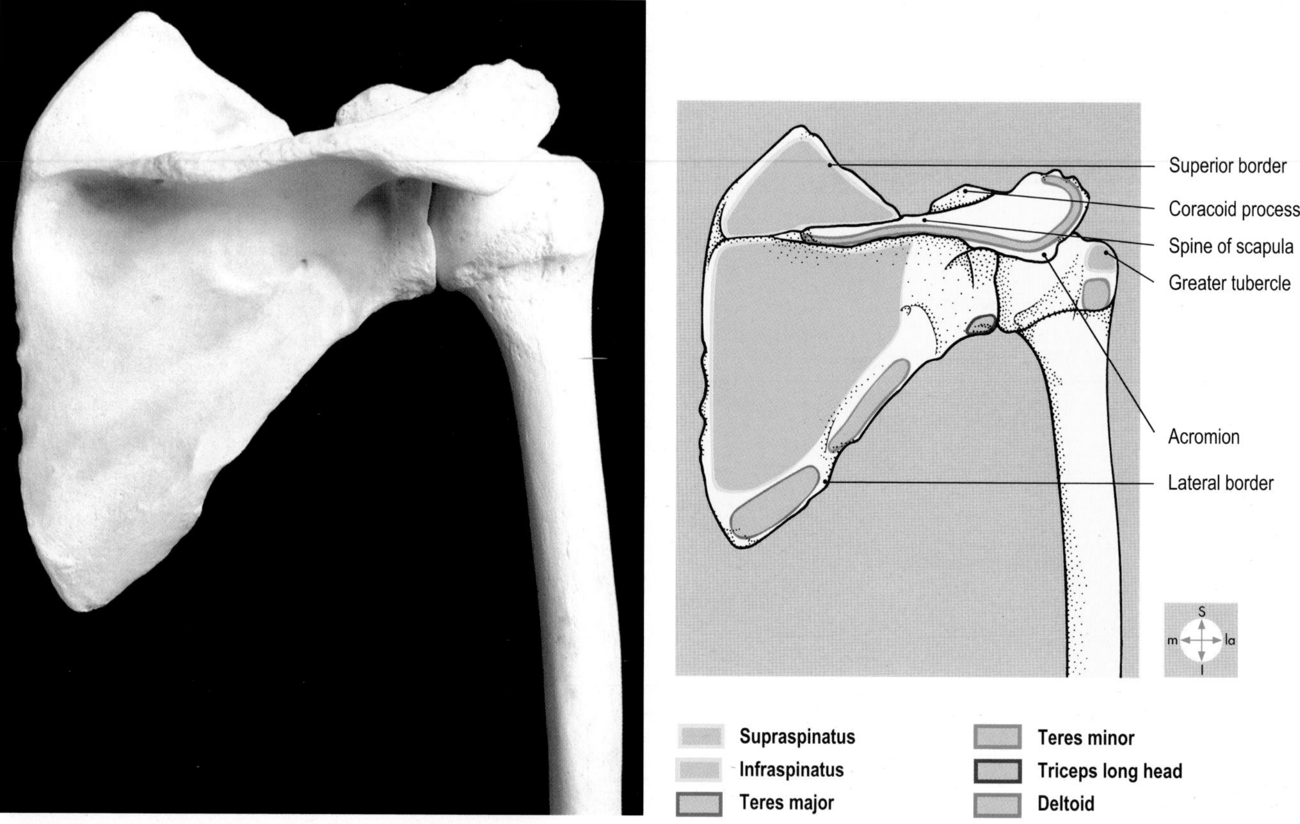

Fig. 3.62 Posterior aspects of scapula and proximal end of humerus. The head of the humerus is partly obscured by the overlying acromion of the scapula.

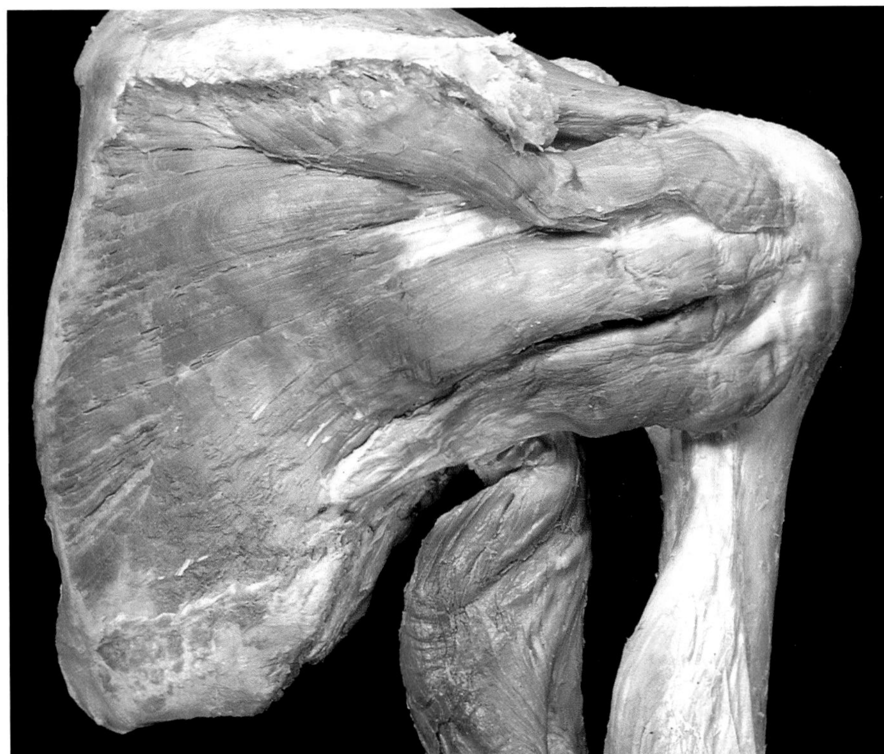

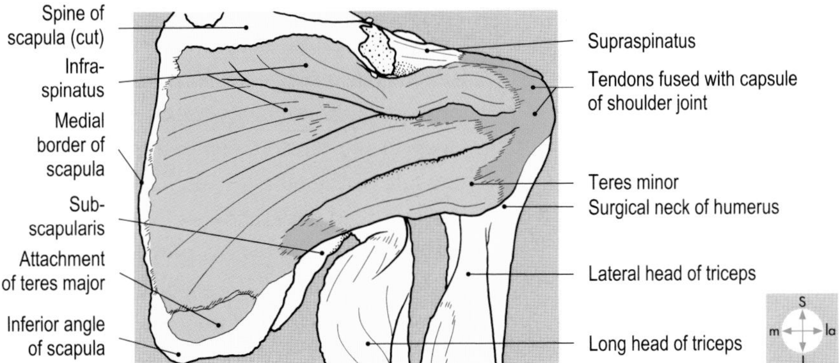

Fig. 3.63 Posterior view of infraspinatus and teres minor. Teres major has been removed.

arises from the upper trunk of the brachial plexus and passes beneath the suprascapular ligament (see Fig. 3.59).

Teres minor

Teres minor (Fig. 3.63) attaches to the posterior surface of the scapula along the upper part of the lateral edge and to the inferior facet of the greater tubercle of the humerus. It is supplied by the axillary nerve.

Both infraspinatus and teres minor laterally rotate the humerus at the shoulder joint.

Teres major

Teres major (Fig. 3.64) is a short bulky muscle which attaches to the lower part of the posterior surface of the scapula. Laterally, the muscle attaches below the lesser tubercle of the humerus to the medial lip of the intertubercular sulcus (see Fig. 3.59). Teres major is supplied by the lower subscapular nerve and adducts and medially rotates the humerus at the shoulder joint.

The axillary nerve and posterior circumflex humeral vessels pass between the teres minor and major muscles, lateral to the long head of triceps, through the quadrangular space (Fig. 3.64).

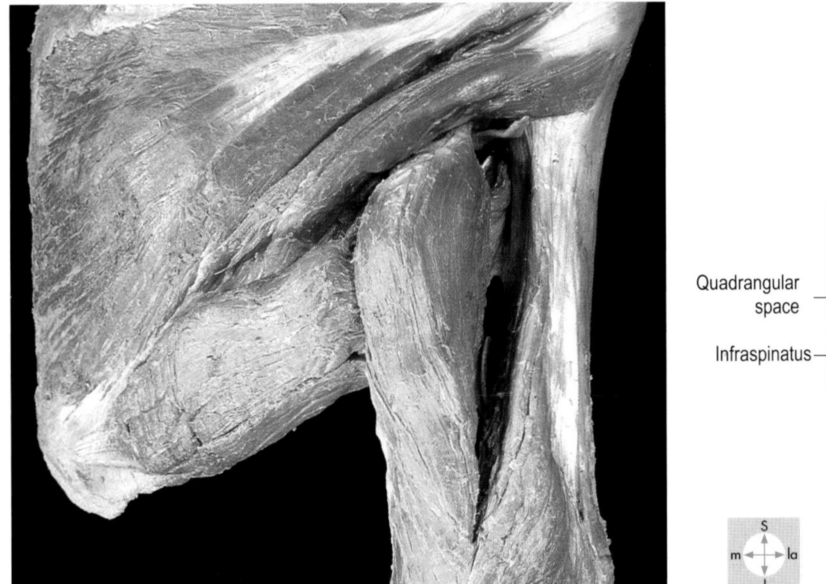

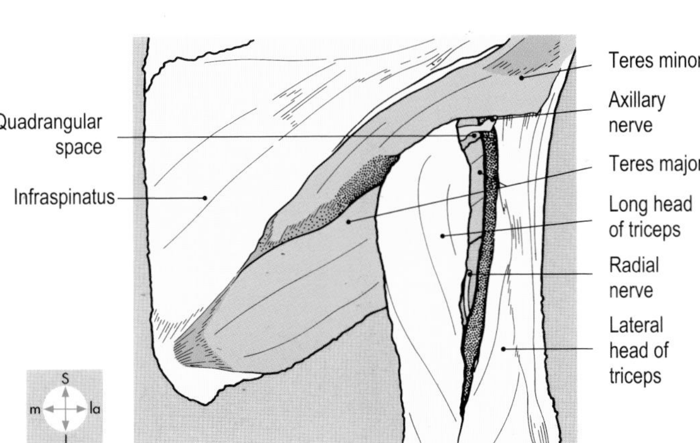

Fig. 3.64 Teres major and minor. The axillary nerve passes above teres major while the radial nerve lies below the muscle. Both nerves pass medial to the long head of triceps.

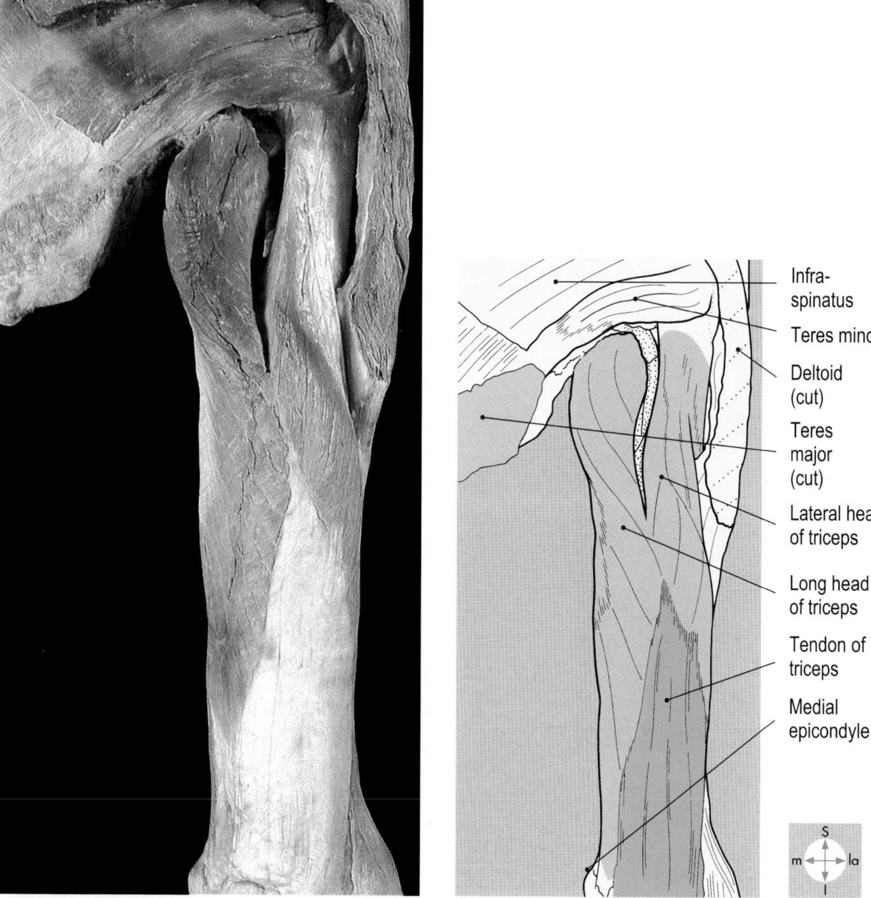

Fig. 3.65 Posterior aspect of triceps. Teres major and the posterior fibres of deltoid have been excised.

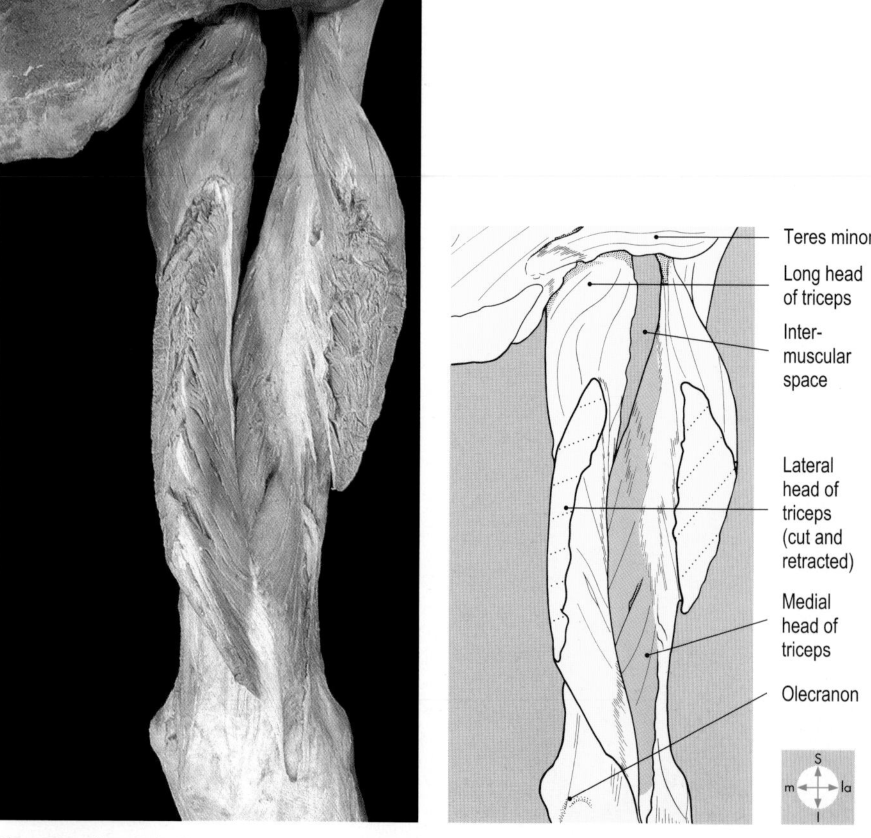

Fig. 3.66 The medial head of triceps has been exposed by removal of deltoid and division and retraction of the lateral head.

Posterior Compartment of Arm

The posterior compartment of the arm contains triceps brachii, the radial nerve accompanied by the profunda brachii artery with its venae comitantes, and the ulnar nerve.

Triceps brachii

Proximally, this muscle attaches to the scapula and the humerus by three heads. The tendon of the long head (Fig. 3.65) attaches to the infraglenoid tubercle of the scapula, and the lateral head attaches to the posterior aspect of the shaft of the humerus above the radial groove (spiral groove, sulcus of the radial nerve) (Fig. 3.67). Both the long and lateral heads lie superficial to the medial head (Fig. 3.66), which has an extensive origin from the lateral and medial intermuscular septa and from the shaft of the humerus below the radial groove. Distally, the three heads fuse, and triceps attaches by a single tendon to the olecranon process of the ulna. Frequently, a bursa lies deep to the tendon, separating it from the capsule of the elbow joint. The three heads are supplied separately by branches of the radial nerve. Triceps is a powerful extensor of the elbow joint. The long head alone spans the shoulder joint and may assist in stabilizing that joint, particularly in full abduction.

Vessels and nerves

Radial nerve

The radial nerve, a terminal branch of the posterior cord, leaves the axilla by passing below teres major and between the humerus and the long head of triceps (see Fig. 3.64). In the posterior compartment the nerve passes between the medial and lateral heads of triceps and in the radial groove is intimately related to the shaft of the humerus (Fig. 3.68). It then leaves the posterior compartment by piercing the lateral intermuscular septum to reach the lateral part of the cubital fossa in front of the elbow joint (see Fig. 3.29). In the arm, the radial nerve gives muscular branches to the medial and lateral heads of triceps and to brachioradialis and extensor carpi radialis longus, and cutaneous branches to the lateral aspect of the arm and the posterior aspect of the forearm. The branch to

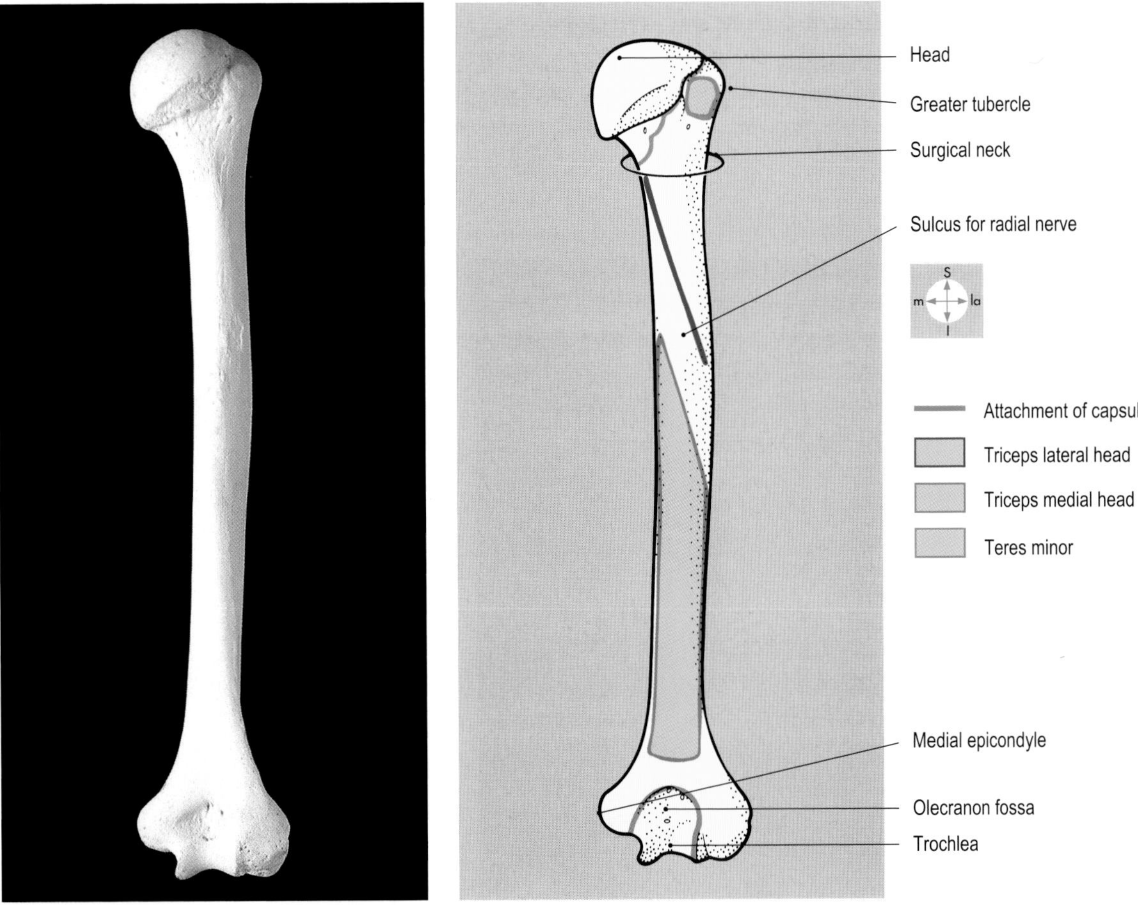

Fig. 3.67 Posterior aspect of humerus.

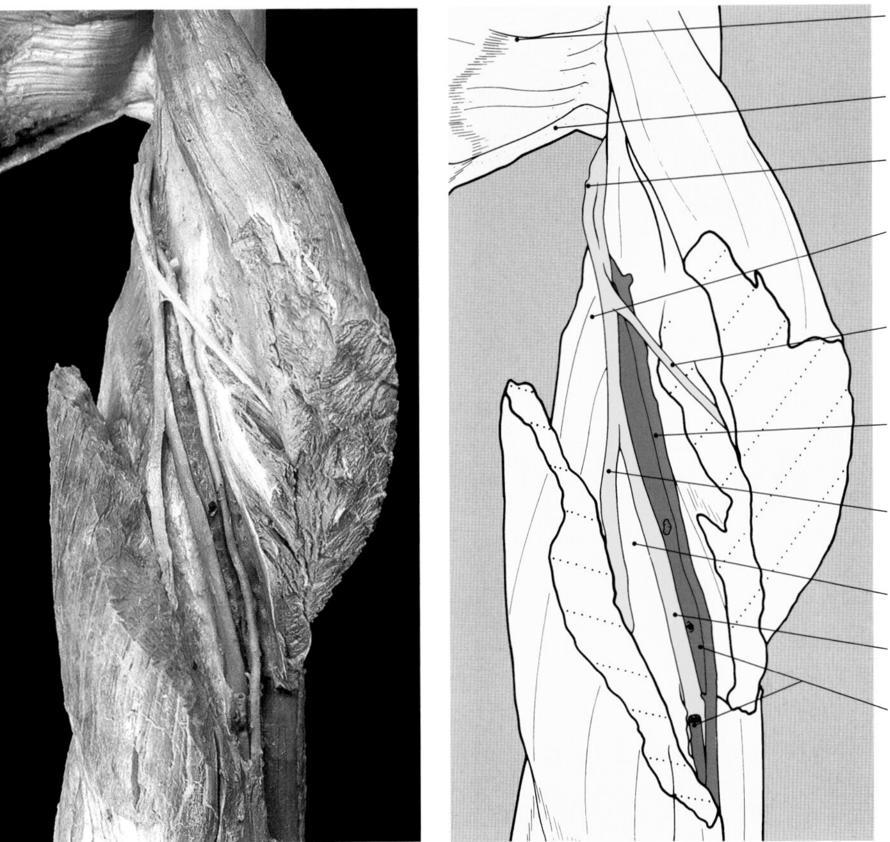

Fig. 3.68 The radial nerve and profunda brachii artery in the radial groove, seen after retraction of the cut lateral head of triceps. The long head has been excised.

the long head of triceps usually arises in the axilla. The radial nerve may be damaged in the radial groove by fracture of the shaft of the humerus (see p. 113).

Profunda brachii artery

The profunda brachii artery, a proximal branch of the brachial artery (see Fig. 3.18), supplies the posterior compartment and accompanies the radial nerve in the radial groove of the humerus (Fig. 3.68). It gives muscular branches and contributes to the anastomosis around the elbow joint. The venae comitantes of the profunda brachii artery drain into the axillary vein.

Ulnar nerve

The ulnar nerve passes from the anterior to the posterior compartment by piercing the medial intermuscular septum at about midarm level (see Fig. 3.24), and descends between the septum and the medial head of triceps. At the elbow it passes posterior to the medial epicondyle of the humerus, medial to the joint, and enters the forearm between the humeral and ulnar heads of flexor carpi ulnaris. The nerve gives no branches in the arm.

Posterior Compartment of Forearm

The posterior compartment of the forearm lies behind the radius and ulna and the intervening interosseous membrane. It contains the extensor muscles of the wrist and fingers, the extensors and long abductor of the thumb, and also brachioradialis, supinator and anconeus. The muscles are supplied by the posterior interosseous artery and nerve (deep branch of the radial nerve), assisted by the radial nerve itself. The compartment is enclosed by a layer of deep fascia which attaches to the posterior

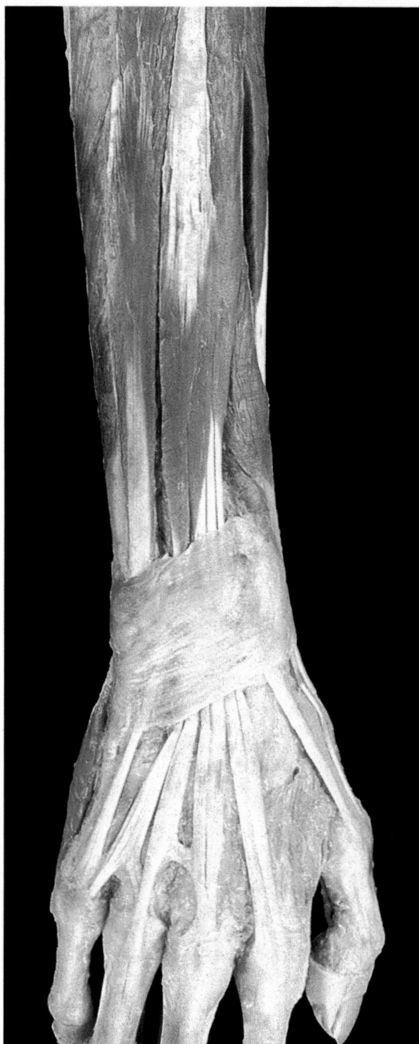

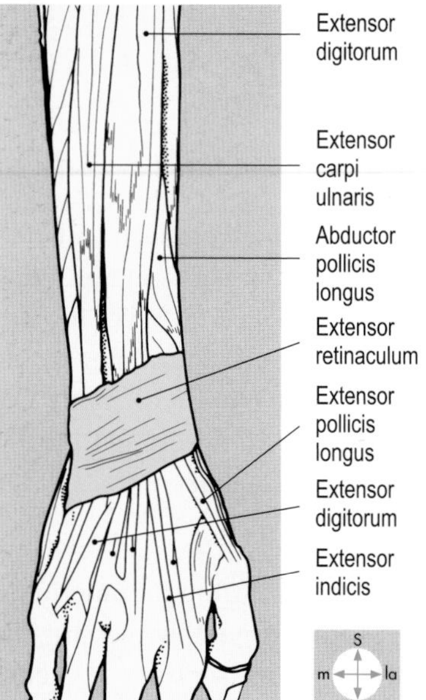

Fig. 3.69 Extensor retinaculum exposed by removal of subcutaneous tissue and deep fascia. The fibres of the retinaculum run obliquely, passing medially and inferiorly from the radius towards the hamate and pisiform bones.

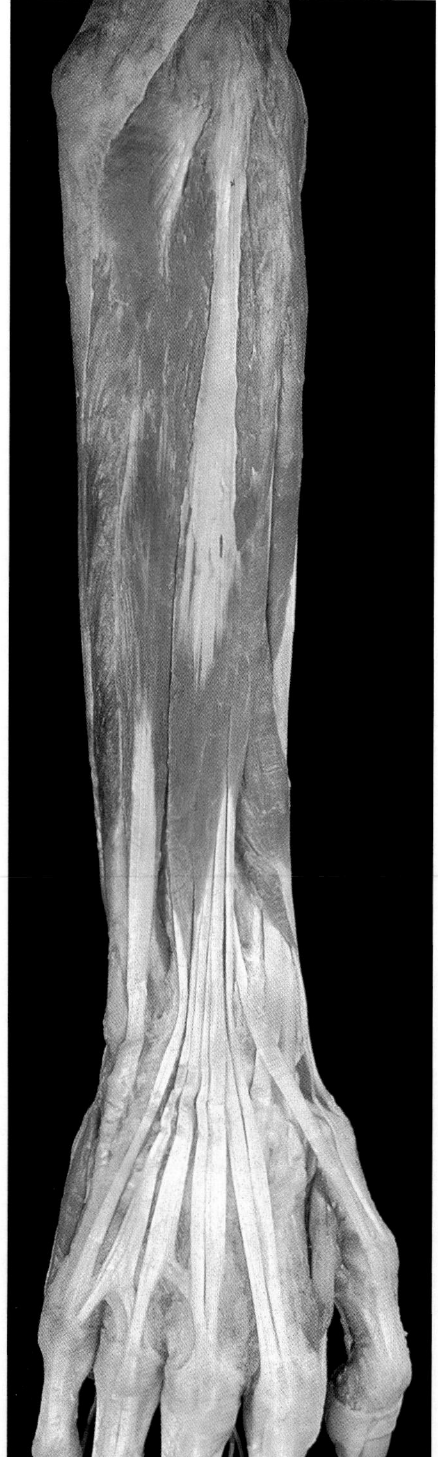

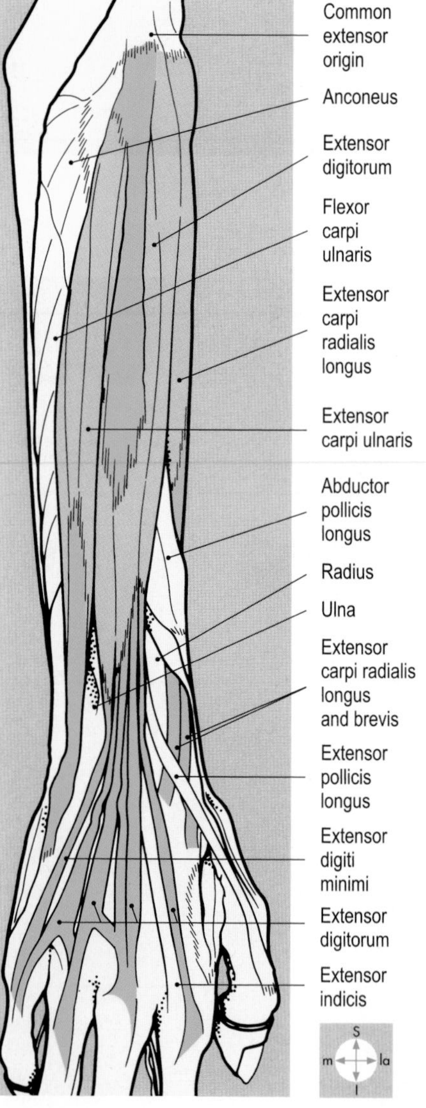

Fig. 3.70 Superficial muscles of the posterior compartment exposed by removal of deep fascia and the extensor retinaculum. Flexor and extensor carpi ulnaris lie edge-to-edge along the subcutaneous border of the ulna.

(subcutaneous) border of the ulna. In the region of the wrist the fascia is thickened to form the extensor retinaculum (Fig. 3.69). The extensor tendons, invested by synovial sheaths, pass deep to the retinaculum and enter the hand.

Superficial muscles

Four superficial extensors attach proximally to the anterior surface of the lateral humeral epicondyle at the common extensor origin (Fig. 3.70). Extensor carpi radialis brevis (Fig. 3.71) passes distally to the base of the third metacarpal and is an extensor and abductor of the wrist. Extensor digitorum (Figs 3.69 & 3.70) has four tendons which pass to the fingers and form the dorsal expansions or extensor hoods (see Fig. 3.51). On the dorsum of the hand these tendons are interconnected by fibrous bands. The muscle is an extensor of the fingers and the wrist joint. Extensor digiti minimi (Fig. 3.70) attaches via two tendons to the dorsal expansion of the little finger and assists extension of this finger. Extensor carpi ulnaris (Fig. 3.70) attaches proximally to both the common extensor origin and the posterior surface of the ulna. Distally, it attaches to the base of the fifth metacarpal bone. The muscle is an extensor and adductor of the wrist. These four superficial extensors span the elbow but, since their attachments are close to the axis of movement, do not act effectively on that joint. They are innervated by the posterior interosseous (deep branch of the radial) nerve.

Two other superficial muscles, brachioradialis and extensor carpi radialis longus, arise from the lateral supracondylar ridge of the humerus and are innervated directly from the main trunk of the radial nerve. Brachioradialis (Figs 3.71 & 3.72) arises from the upper two-thirds of the ridge and attaches distally

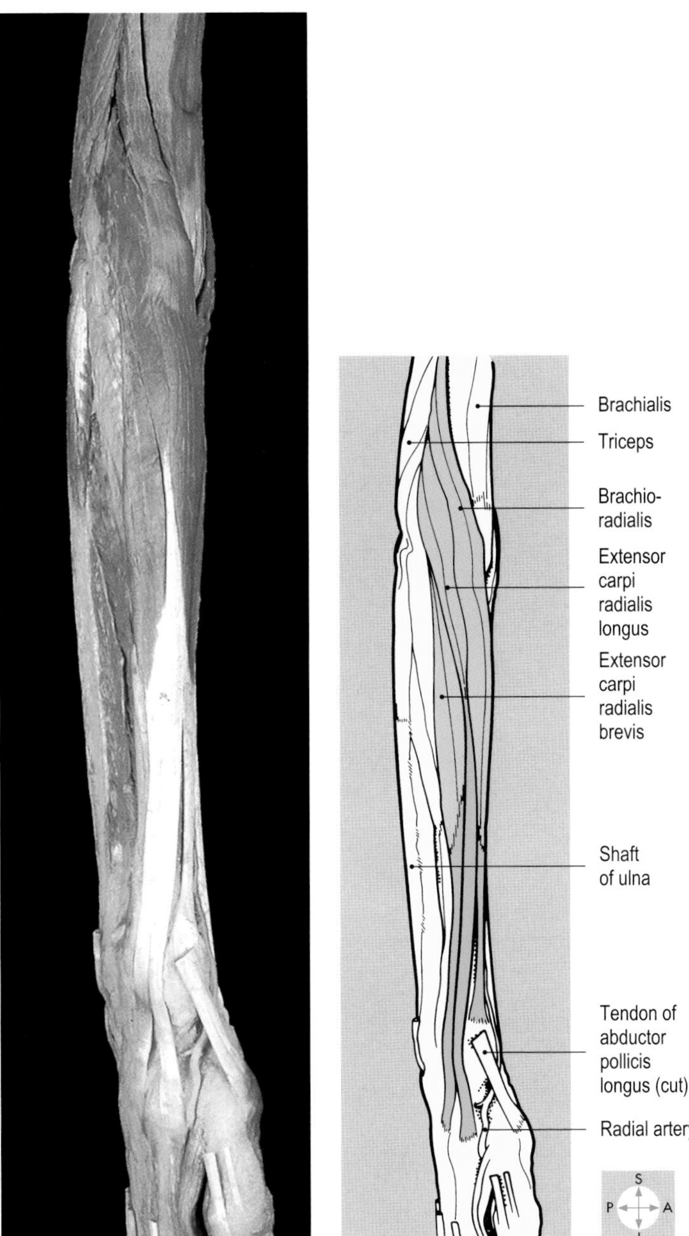

Fig. 3.71 Extensors carpi radialis longus and brevis, and brachioradialis after removal of abductor pollicis longus and extensors pollicis longus and brevis.

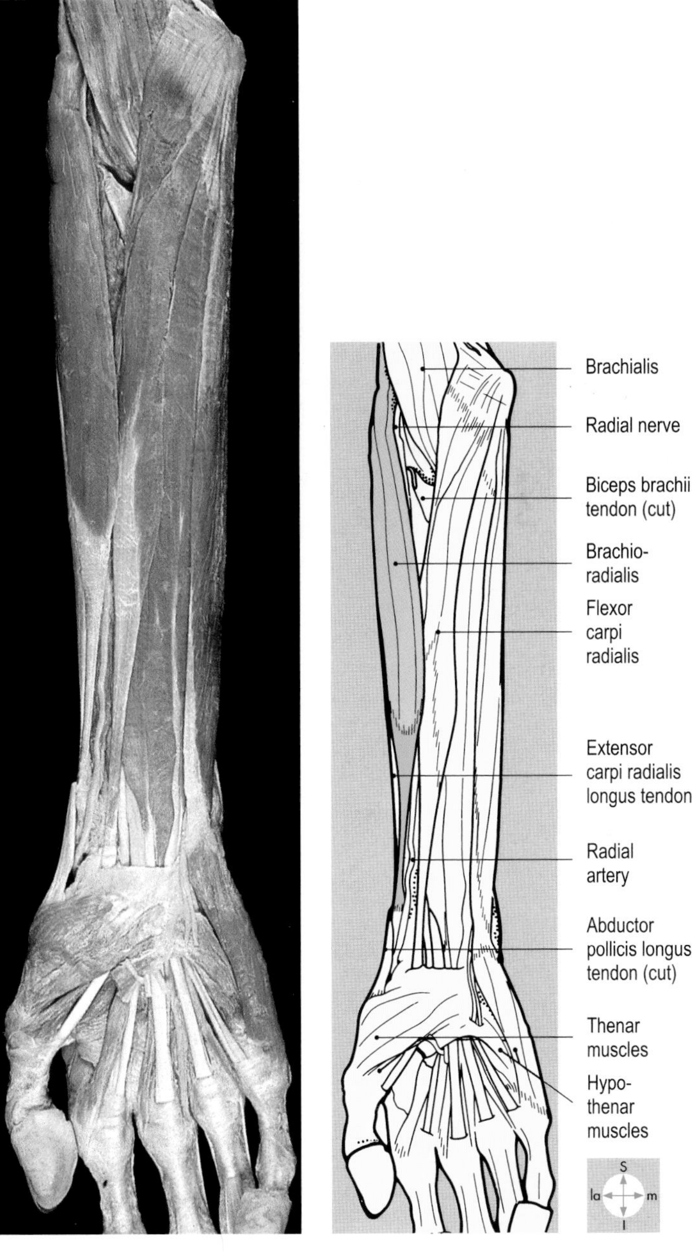

Fig. 3.72 Brachioradialis (anterior aspect). The muscle forms the lateral boundary of the cubital fossa and covers the radial artery and the superficial branch of the radial nerve in the forearm.

to the radial styloid process. The muscle is a flexor of the elbow joint and rotates the forearm from full pronation or supination into an intermediate position. Extensor carpi radialis longus (see Figs 3.70 & 3.71) arises from the lower third of the supracondylar ridge and attaches distally to the base of the second metacarpal bone. The muscle is an extensor and abductor of the wrist joint.

In addition to their primary roles, the three carpal extensors provide an essential contribution to the power grip by fixing the wrist in an optimum position while the long flexors act on the fingers. Overuse of the muscles attaching to the lateral epicondyle may produce inflammation near the attachment with pain during extension of the wrist and fingers (epicondylitis or 'tennis elbow').

Deep muscles

The proximal attachments of four of the deep muscles are illustrated in Figure 3.73. The tendon of extensor indicis (Fig. 3.74) passes distally, medial to that of extensor digitorum, and attaches to the extensor expansion of the index finger. The extensor pollicis longus tendon passes distally around the ulnar (medial) side of the

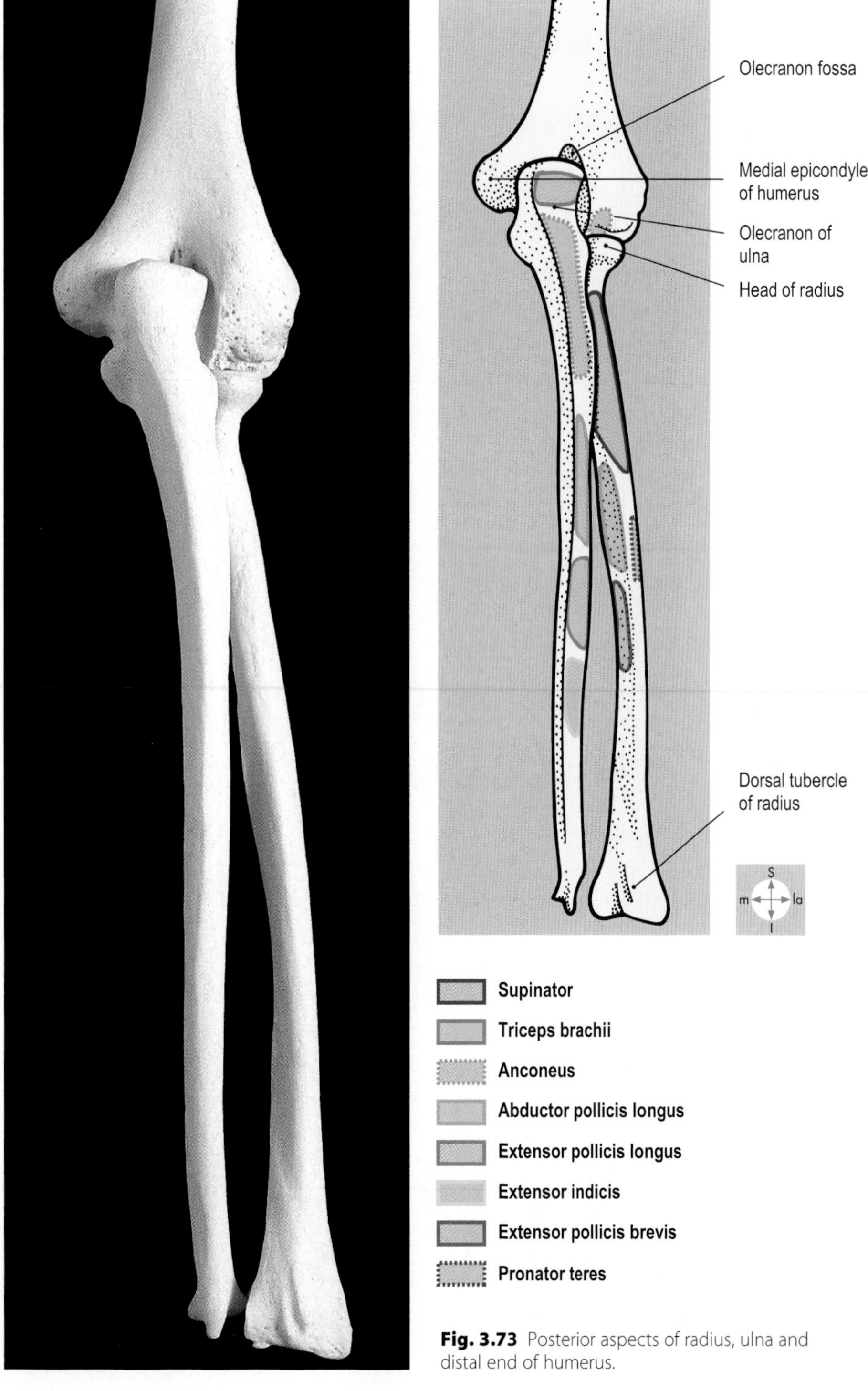

Fig. 3.73 Posterior aspects of radius, ulna and distal end of humerus.

dorsal tubercle of the radius (Fig. 3.74), then crosses the radial extensors of the carpus to attach to the base of the distal phalanx of the thumb (see Fig. 3.75). The muscle extends the thumb and its carpometacarpal joint. The tendons of extensor pollicis brevis and abductor pollicis longus (see Fig. 3.75) lie together as they cross the radial carpal extensors and brachioradialis. Extensor pollicis brevis attaches to the base of the proximal phalanx of the thumb, which it extends. Abductor pollicis longus attaches to the base of the first metacarpal bone, which it extends and abducts.

Although these four deep muscles act primarily on the joints of the hand, they also span the wrist joint; but their actions here are weak. They are all innervated by the posterior interosseous (deep branch of the radial) nerve.

Extension of the thumb creates a hollow on the posterolateral aspect of the wrist called the 'anatomical snuff box' (see Fig. 3.75). It is limited anteriorly by the tendons of abductor pollicis longus and extensor pollicis brevis and posteriorly by extensor pollicis longus. Superficial to the snuff box lie the origin of the cephalic vein and branches of the superficial radial nerve supplying the dorsum of the hand. The branches can be palpated where they cross superficial to the tendon of extensor pollicis longus. The tendons of the two radial carpal extensors and the radial artery pass through the snuff box. The bony floor comprises the radial styloid process, scaphoid, trapezium and base of the first metacarpal bone. Fracture of the scaphoid bone often produces pain, swelling and tenderness in the snuff box.

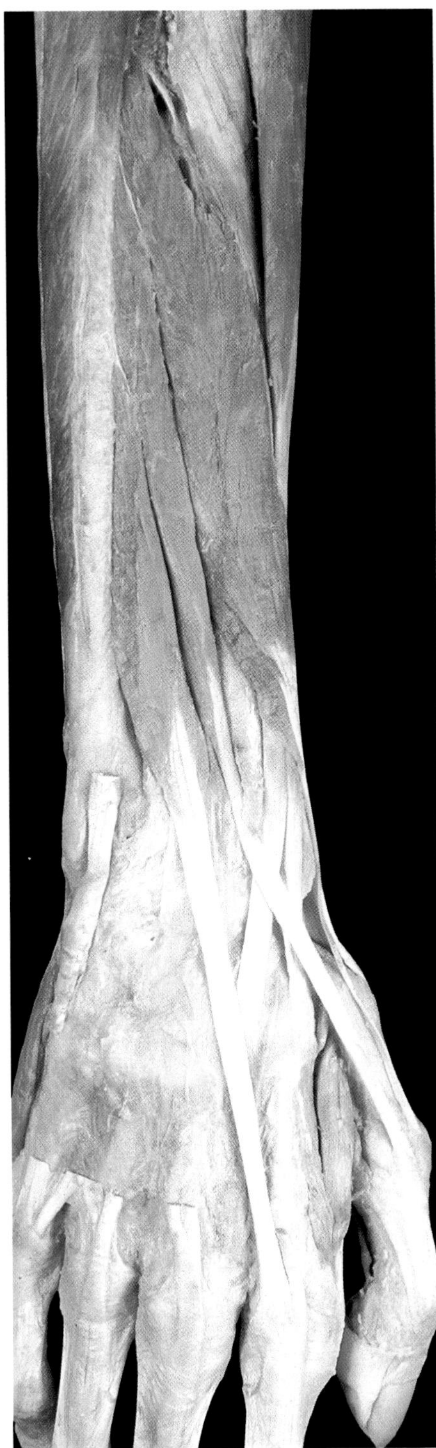

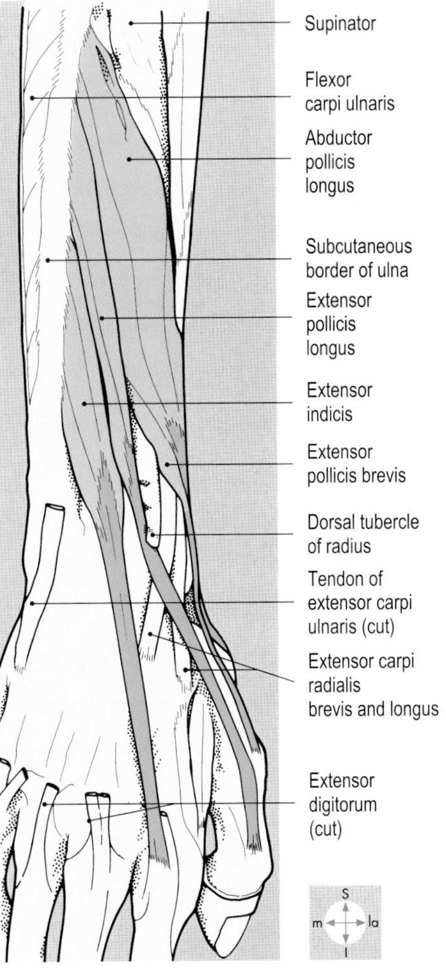

Fig. 3.74 Extensor indicis and extensors pollicis longus and brevis, after division of extensor digitorum. The tendon of extensor indicis lies on the ulnar (medial) side of the index tendon of extensor digitorum.

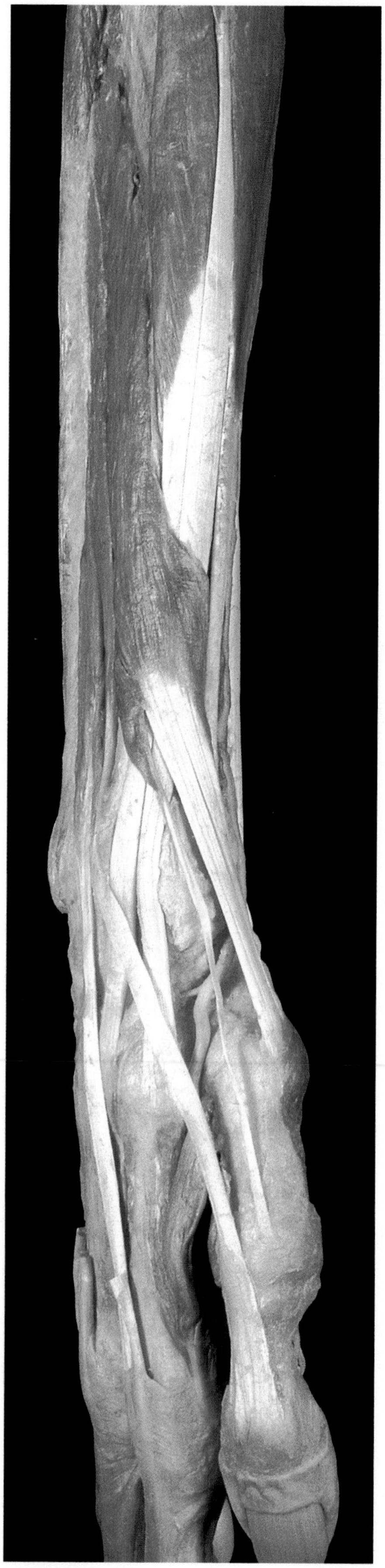

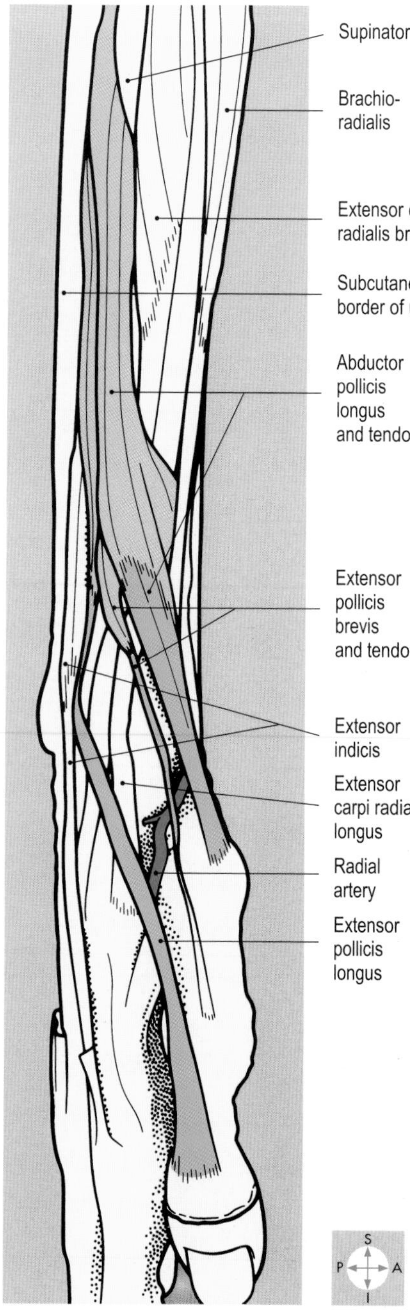

Supinator

Brachio-
radialis

Extensor carpi
radialis brevis

Subcutaneous
border of ulna

Abductor
pollicis
longus
and tendon

Extensor
pollicis
brevis
and tendon

Extensor
indicis

Extensor
carpi radialis
longus

Radial
artery

Extensor
pollicis
longus

S
P A
I

Fig. 3.75 Abductor pollicis longus and extensors pollicis longus and brevis. At the wrist, the radial carpal extensors are crossed by the tendons of these three muscles passing to the thumb.

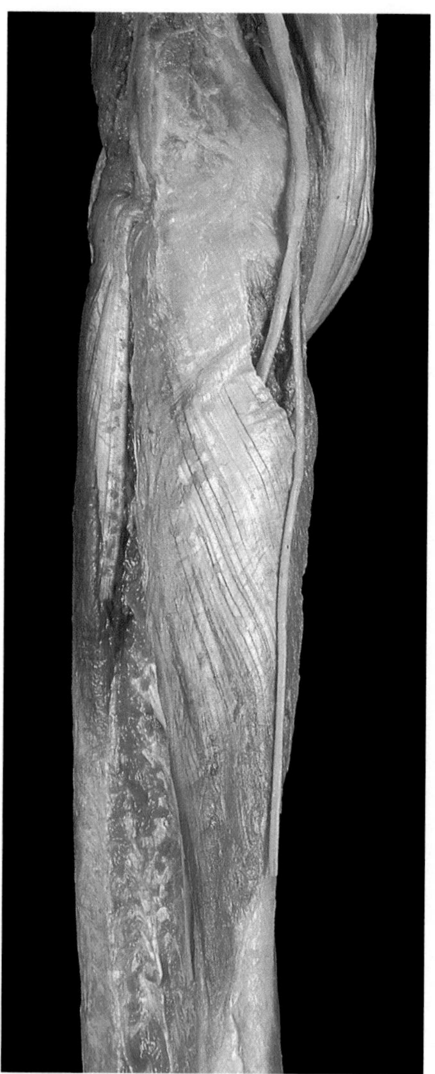

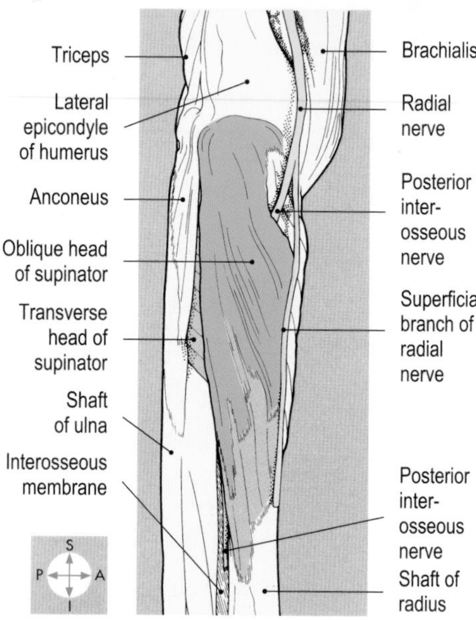

Fig. 3.76 Supinator, revealed by removal of the other muscles of the posterior compartment. The posterior interosseous nerve passes between the transverse and oblique heads of the muscle.

Supinator, also a deep muscle, consists of oblique and transverse heads (Fig. 3.76). The oblique head attaches to the lateral epicondyle and collateral ligament, while the transverse head is attached to the supinator crest of the ulna. Both heads wind laterally around the proximal part of the radius and attach to its anterior surface (see Fig. 3.73). The muscle supinates the forearm and is supplied by the deep branch of the radial nerve (posterior interosseous nerve), which passes between the two heads of the muscle (Fig. 3.77).

Vessels

In the cubital fossa the common interosseous branch of the ulnar artery divides into larger anterior and smaller posterior interosseous arteries, which pass distally into their respective compartments of the forearm. The posterior interosseous artery (Fig. 3.77) lies between and supplies the superficial and deep groups of muscles. Near the wrist a branch of the anterior interosseous artery penetrates the interosseous membrane to assist in the supply of the distal part of the posterior compartment. In addition, muscles on the lateral aspect of the compartment may receive blood from branches of the radial artery. The arteries of the compartment are accompanied by venae comitantes that drain into veins accompanying the brachial artery.

On the dorsum of the wrist the radial artery enters the anatomical snuff box from the anterior compartment of the forearm deep to the tendons of abductor pollicis longus and extensor pollicis brevis. The artery crosses the floor of the snuff box and leaves the dorsum of the hand by penetrating the first dorsal interosseous muscle to enter the palm.

Nerves

The posterior compartment of the forearm is supplied by the radial nerve, which leaves the arm by penetrating the lateral intermuscular septum. Anterior to the elbow the nerve lies between brachialis and brachioradialis and divides into superficial and deep branches (Fig. 3.76). The superficial branch continues distally through the forearm covered by brachioradialis, leaving its posterior border near the wrist and crossing the snuff box to terminate as cutaneous branches on the dorsum of the hand (Fig. 3.78). The deep branch, the posterior interosseous nerve, arises from the radial nerve at the level of the neck of the radius and enters the posterior compartment by passing between the two heads of supinator (Fig. 3.77). Initially, it accompanies the posterior interosseous artery but distally lies more deeply on the interosseous membrane. The posterior interosseous nerve gives branches to the elbow, radioulnar and wrist joints, and supplies most of the posterior compartment muscles. Brachioradialis and extensor carpi radialis longus are supplied directly by the radial nerve from branches arising in the arm, and anconeus is supplied by the branch of the radial nerve to the medial head of triceps. Damage to the radial nerve or to its posterior interosseous branch may weaken the extensor muscles of the wrist and fingers so that they are unable to overcome gravity, causing 'wrist drop'.

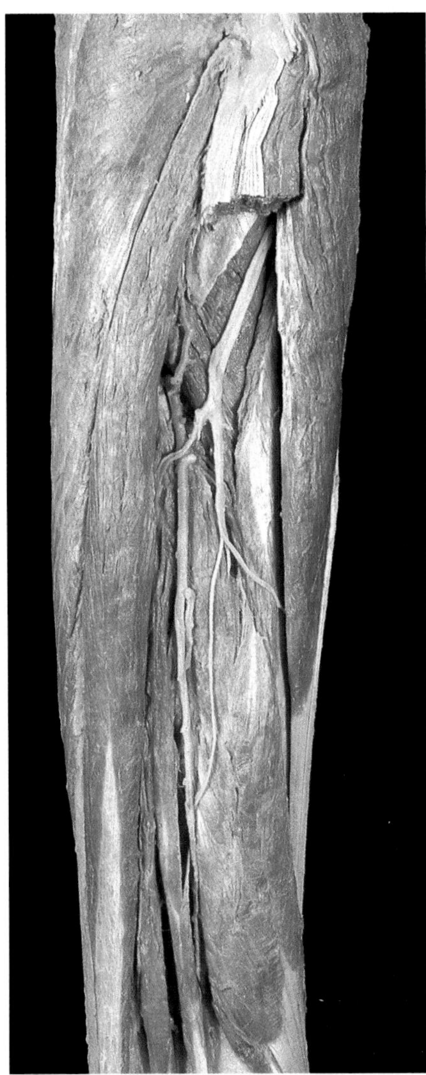

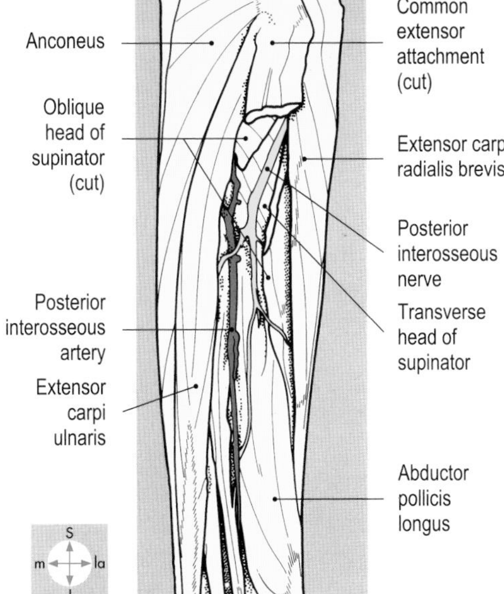

Fig. 3.77 Posterior interosseous artery and nerve, exposed by division of extensor digitorum. The specimen is partly pronated, so the radial border of the forearm faces anteriorly.

Dorsum of Hand

The dorsum of the hand is innervated by branches of the radial and ulnar nerves (Fig. 3.78). The superficial branch of the radial nerve usually supplies the skin of the lateral three and one-half digits (excluding the nail beds) and a corresponding part of the dorsum of the hand. Skin of the dorsal aspect of the first web space is usually supplied exclusively by the radial nerve and is tested when radial nerve injury is suspected. The skin over the remainder of the posterior aspect of the hand and the medial one and one-half fingers (excluding the nail beds) is supplied by dorsal branches of the ulnar nerve that arise in the anterior compartment and pass around the medial aspect of the wrist.

Much of the venous blood from the digits and the palm drains into a network of vessels that often forms a superficial venous arch on the dorsum of the hand.

At the wrist the tendons of extensor digitorum lie deep to the extensor retinaculum (Fig. 3.79), invested by a single synovial sheath. On the dorsum of the hand the tendons diverge to reach the fingers.

Skin on the dorsum of the hand is elastic and freely mobile on the underlying loose connective tissue: infection or injury of the hand frequently results in swelling of these lax tissues.

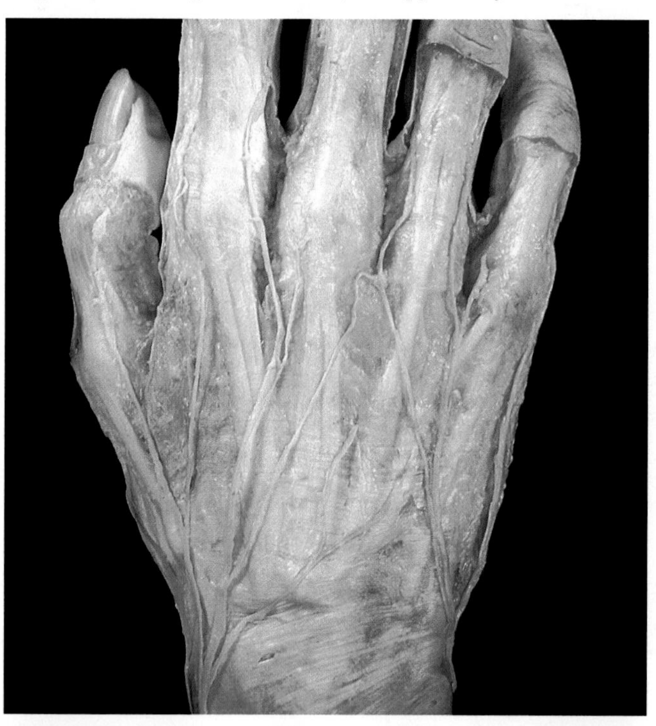

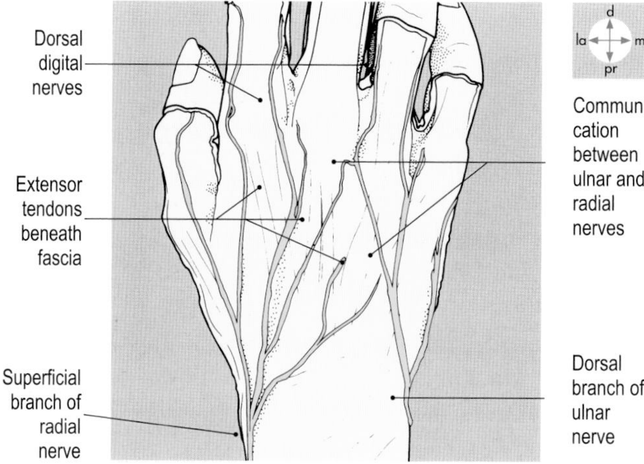

Fig. 3.78 Cutaneous branches of the radial and ulnar nerves on the dorsum of the hand after removal of the superficial veins.

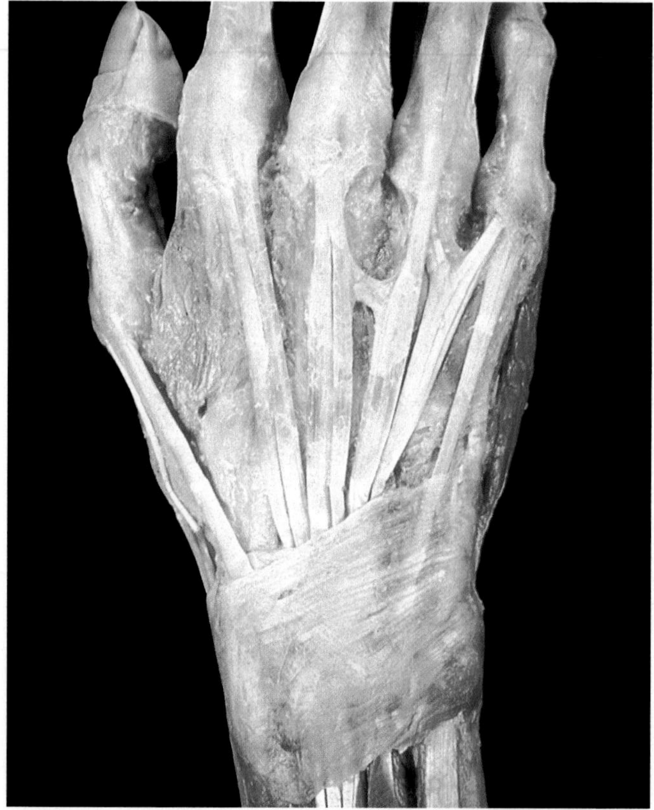

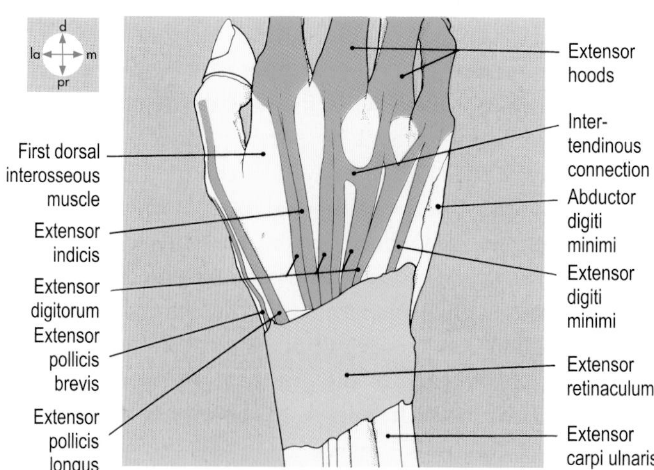

Fig. 3.79 Extensor retinaculum and extensor tendons, exposed by removal of subcutaneous tissue. The tendons pass through fibro-osseous tunnels deep to the retinaculum and are enveloped by synovial sheaths (here removed), which continue beyond the edges of the retinaculum.

Clavicular and Shoulder Joints

Three joints contribute to the considerable mobility of the arm; movement occurs between the humerus and the scapula at the shoulder (glenohumeral) joint, and the scapula moves on the chest wall through the joints at each end of the clavicle. Although few muscles attach to the clavicle, the numerous muscles attached to the scapula and upper humerus all contribute to movement at the clavicular joints. Indeed, movement at the shoulder joint is almost always associated with movement at the sternoclavicular and acromioclavicular joints.

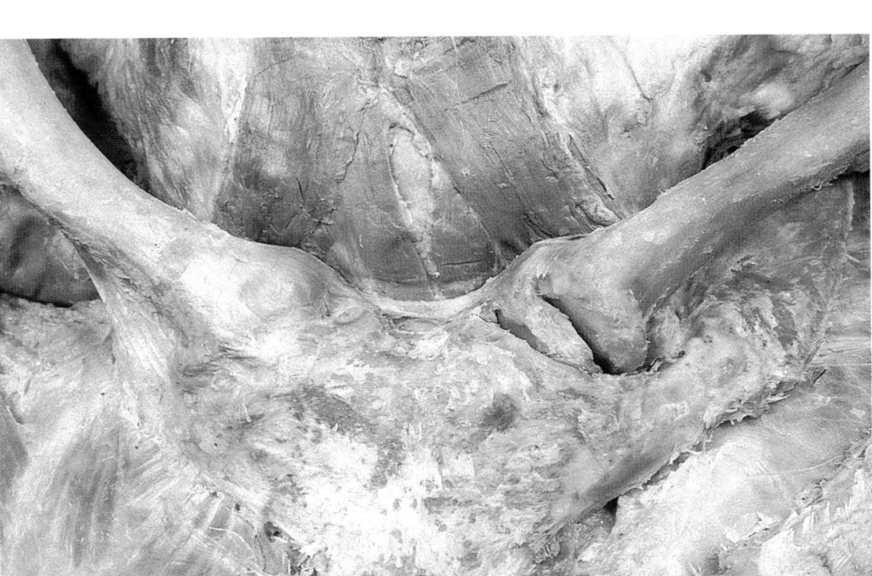

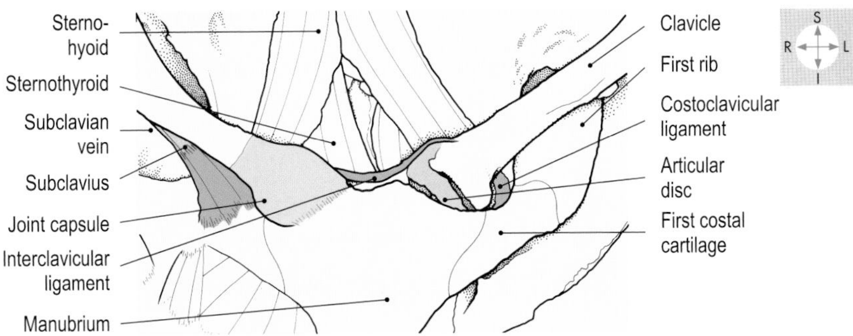

Fig. 3.80 Sternoclavicular joints. On the left, the joint capsule and subclavius have been excised to reveal the cartilaginous disc and costoclavicular ligament. Pleura is exposed in the first left intercostal space.

Clavicular joints

The sternoclavicular and acromioclavicular joints are subcutaneous and easily palpable in the living subject. Each has a tubular capsule lined by synovial membrane.

At the sternoclavicular joint (Fig. 3.80), the medial end of the clavicle articulates with the notch on the upper border of the manubrium and with the first costal cartilage. The joint is partitioned by an intracapsular disc of fibrocartilage that attaches superiorly to the clavicle, inferiorly to the first costal cartilage and around its periphery to the capsule. There are two accessory ligaments. Above the capsule is the interclavicular ligament which joins the medial ends of the clavicles. Just lateral to the joint is the costoclavicular (rhomboid) ligament, which attaches the clavicle firmly to the first costal cartilage. Stability depends on the disc and accessory ligaments, which limit both medial displacement and elevation of the medial end of the clavicle. The sternoclavicular joints are separated from the origins of the brachiocephalic veins and other structures in the root of the neck by the sternohyoid and sternothyroid muscles.

At the acromioclavicular joint (Fig. 3.81) the lateral end of the clavicle articulates with the medial aspect of the acromion of the scapula. The joint capsule attaches to the edges of the articular surfaces that lie obliquely, the clavicular facet facing

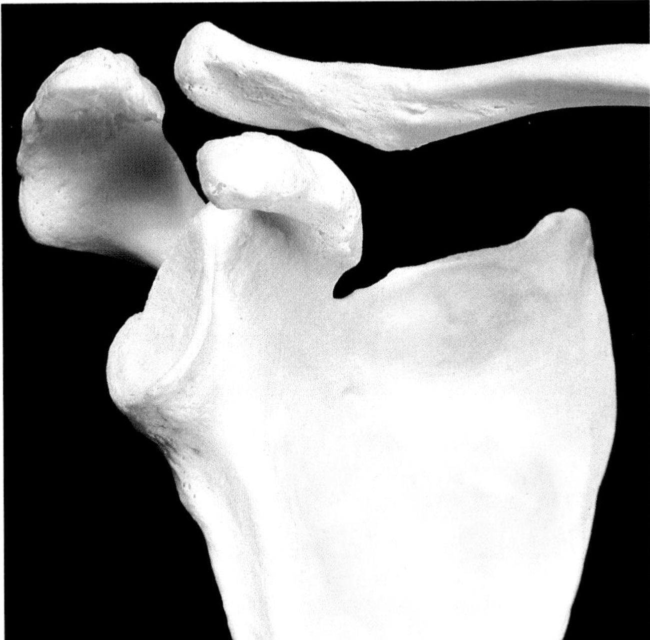

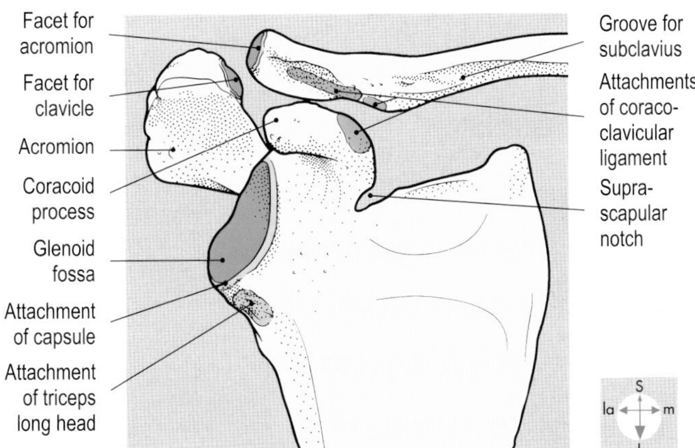

Fig. 3.81 Oblique anterior view of scapula and lateral part of clavicle. The bones have been separated to show the articular surfaces of the acromioclavicular joint and the sites of attachment of the coracoclavicular ligament.

laterally and inferiorly. Stability of the joint is provided mostly by the strong coracoclavicular ligament linking the coracoid process and the undersurface of the clavicle near its lateral end. This ligament consists of conoid and trapezoid parts.

Both the sternoclavicular and acromioclavicular joints are supplied by branches of the supraclavicular nerves (C3 & C4).

The lateral end of the clavicle may be elevated or depressed and drawn forwards or backwards. The axes of these movements occur at the costoclavicular and coracoclavicular ligaments rather than through the clavicular joints. Thus, the medial end of the clavicle is elevated during depression of the scapula and moves posteriorly when the scapula is protracted. Full abduction of the upper limb requires rotation of the scapula so that the glenoid fossa tilts upwards. Rotation of the clavicle through 40° at the sternoclavicular joint supplements the 20° of movement available at the acromioclavicular joint, permitting the scapula to rotate through about 60°. The principal muscles of scapular rotation are trapezius and serratus anterior. Protraction is produced by pectoralis minor and serratus anterior and retraction by trapezius and the rhomboids.

The clavicle forms a strut that supports the scapula against the medial pull of muscles such as pectoralis major and latissimus dorsi. The clavicular joints are stabilized by their accessory ligaments which are so strong that trauma, such as falling onto the outstretched limb, is more likely to fracture the clavicle than rupture the ligaments. The lateral part of a fractured clavicle tends to be displaced inferiorly by the weight of the limb and medially by spasm of pectoralis major and latissimus dorsi muscles.

Shoulder joint

The shoulder (glenohumeral) joint is synovial, of the ball-and-socket type, and is capable of a wide range of movement. The hemispherical head of the humerus is directed medially and backwards and articulates with the much smaller glenoid fossa of the scapula (Fig. 3.82). The fossa faces anterolaterally and is slightly deepened by the glenoid labrum, a cartilaginous lip round its edge.

The joint capsule (Fig. 3.83) forms a loose sleeve attaching medially to the glenoid labrum. Its humeral attachment is around

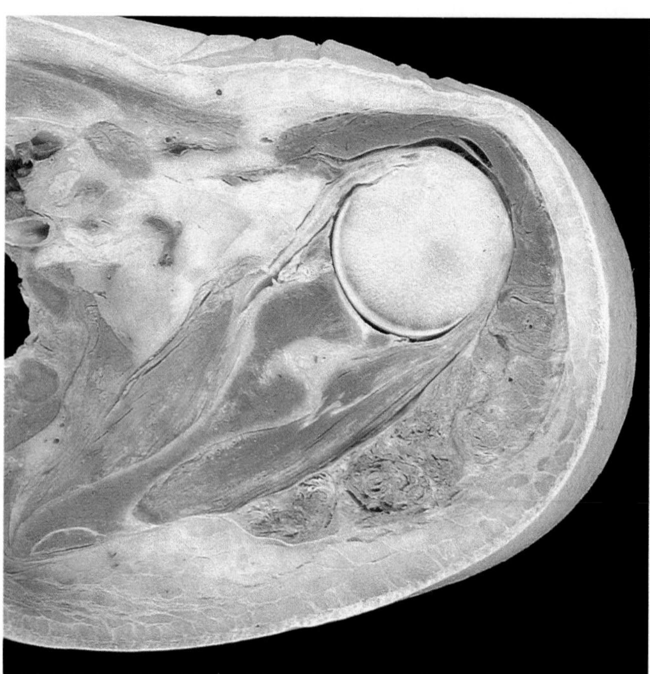

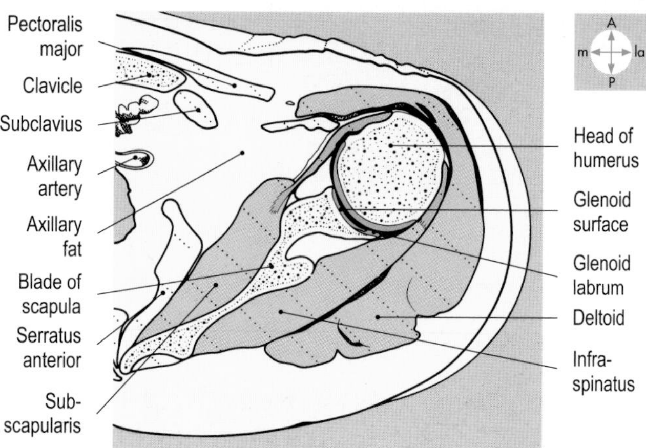

Fig. 3.82 Transverse section at the level of the humeral head showing the relations of the shoulder joint. Superior aspect.

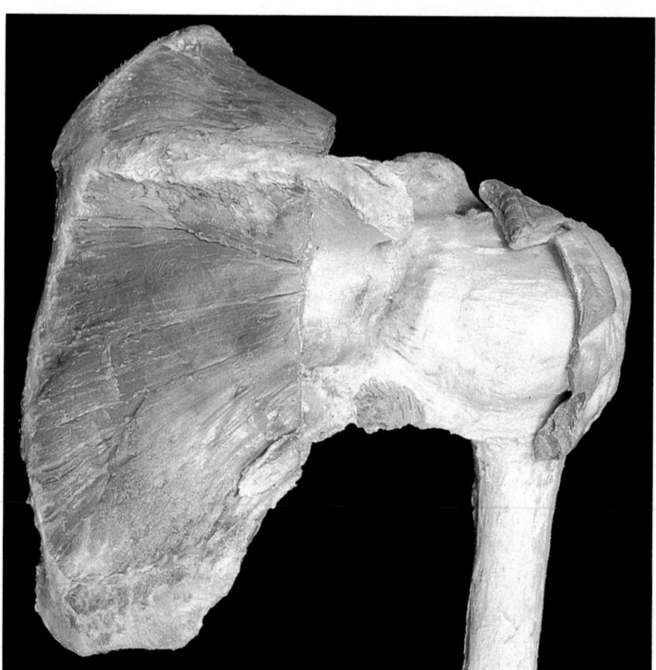

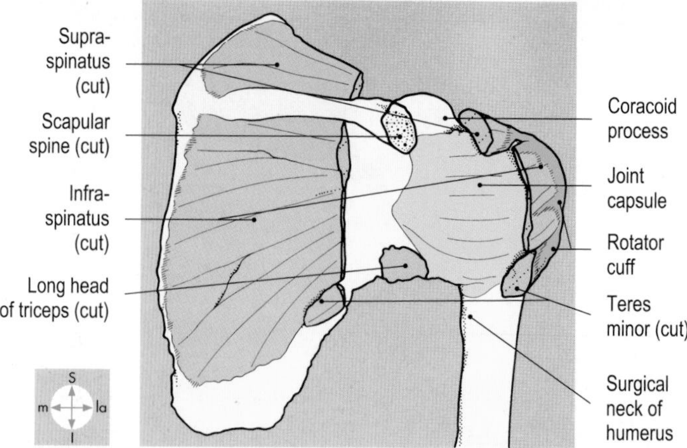

Fig. 3.83 Posterior aspect of the shoulder joint. The acromion and parts of the rotator cuff muscles have been excised to reveal the joint capsule.

the anatomical neck except inferiorly on the medial side, where it descends to the level of the surgical neck.

Synovial membrane lines the fibrous capsule and covers the intracapsular part of the humeral shaft (Fig. 3.84). The cavity of the joint usually communicates with the subscapular bursa through a deficiency in the anterior part of the capsule. Indistinct thickenings in the capsule form the glenohumeral ligaments. Between the greater and lesser tubercles (Fig. 3.85) the capsule forms the transverse humeral ligament beneath which the tendon of the long head of biceps enters the joint from the intertubercular groove. The tendon is surrounded by a tubular sheath of synovial membrane as it passes over the humeral head to attach to the supraglenoid tubercle (see Fig. 3.86).

The joint is intimately related to subscapularis, supraspinatus, infraspinatus and teres minor (see Figs 3.86 & 3.87) whose tendons fuse with the capsule to form the rotator cuff (Fig. 3.83). Above the joint is the coracoacromial arch formed by the coracoid process, the acromion and the intervening coracoacromial ligament. The arch is separated from supraspinatus by the subacromial bursa.

Articular nerves are derived from the suprascapular and subscapular nerves and also from the axillary nerve which passes very close to the joint. As this nerve leaves the axilla through the quadrangular space (see Fig. 3.64), it lies immediately inferior to the capsule. The vascular supply is provided by branches of the circumflex humeral and suprascapular arteries.

Flexion of the shoulder joint (up to 180°) is produced mainly by the clavicular fibres of pectoralis major and the anterior fibres of deltoid. Extension (limited to about 45°) is produced by latissimus dorsi and the posterior fibres of deltoid. At the shoulder joint itself, about 120° of abduction is possible, produced by supraspinatus and deltoid; simultaneous rotation of the scapula through 60°

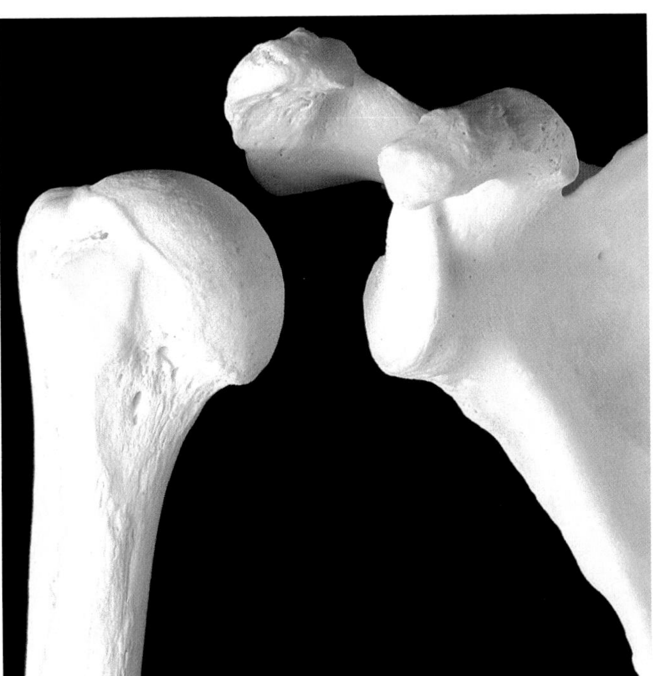

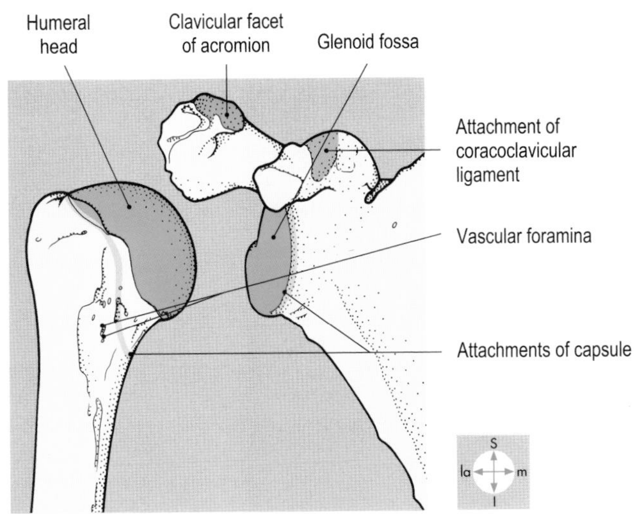

Fig. 3.84 The bones that form the shoulder joint have been separated to reveal their articular surfaces.

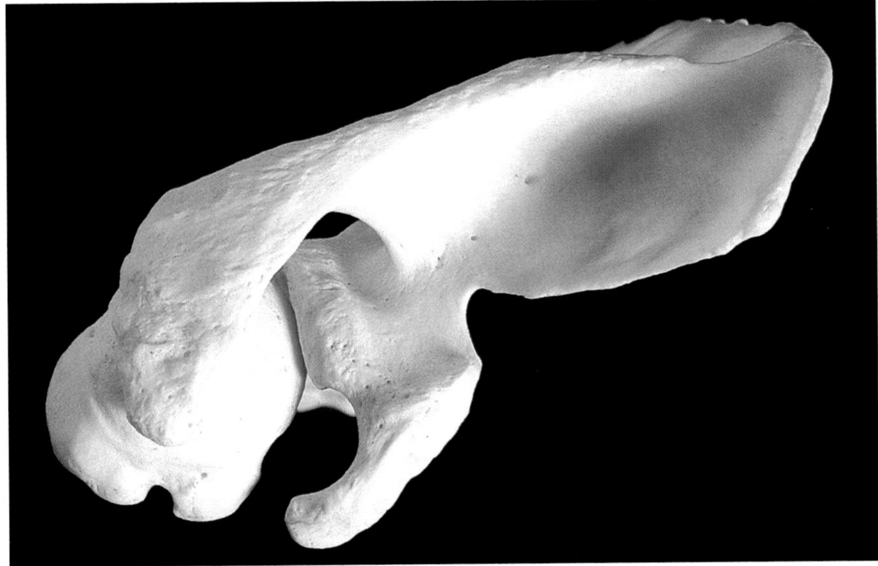

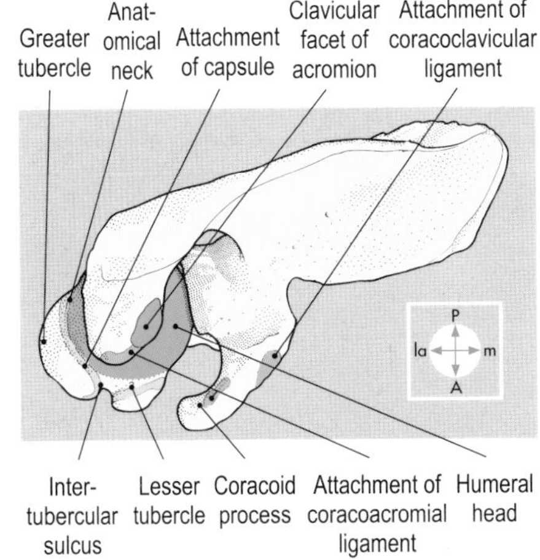

Fig. 3.85 Superior view of scapula and upper end of humerus. The acromion and coracoacromial ligament prevent upward displacement of the humeral head.

permits full elevation of the arm above the head. Adduction, produced by teres major, latissimus dorsi and pectoralis major, is limited by the area of the articular surface of the humerus. Medial rotation is produced by pectoralis major, subscapularis, teres major and the anterior fibres of deltoid, and lateral rotation by infraspinatus, teres minor and the posterior fibres of deltoid.

Although the coracoacromial arch prevents upward displacement of the humerus, stability of the shoulder joint relies principally on the rotator cuff muscles that hold the humeral head firmly in the glenoid fossa. Despite the labrum, the glenoid fossa is a shallow socket. The capsular ligaments are lax in most positions and tighten only near the extremes of movement. Dislocation of the joint, usually with inferior displacement of the head of the humerus, associated with trauma or weakness of the rotator cuff muscles, is relatively common and may result in damage to the axillary nerve.

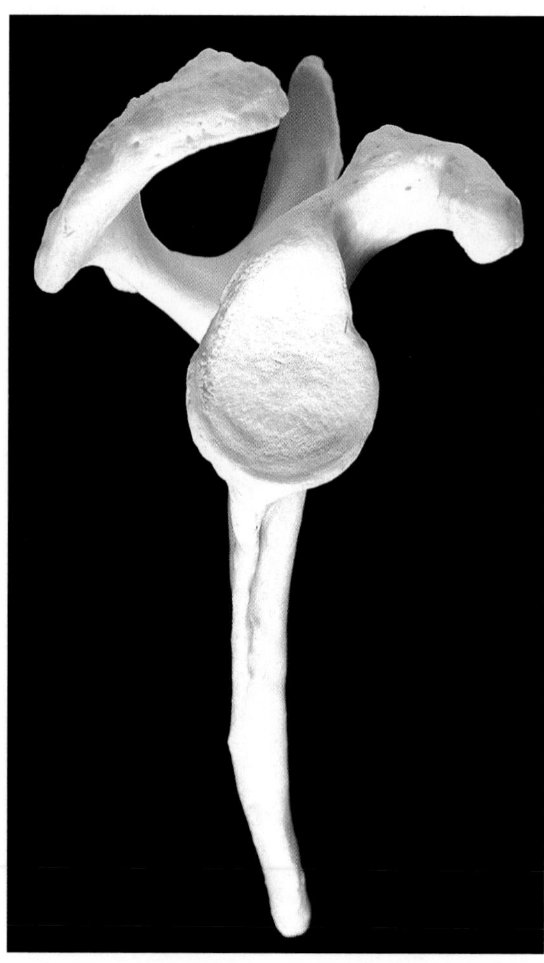

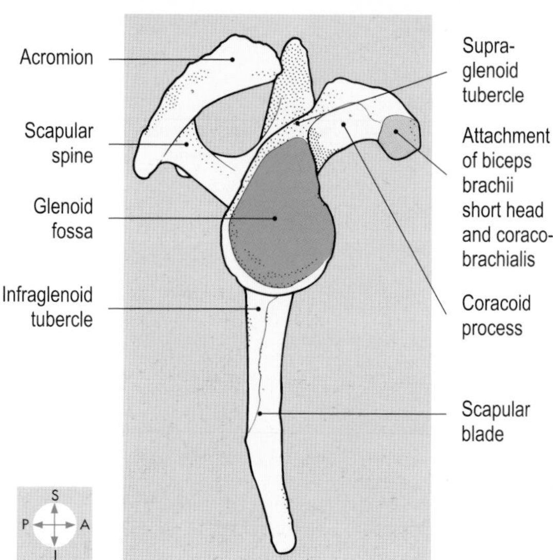

Fig. 3.86 Lateral aspect of scapula showing the pear-shaped glenoid fossa. The positions of supraspinous, infraspinous and subscapular fossae can be appreciated.

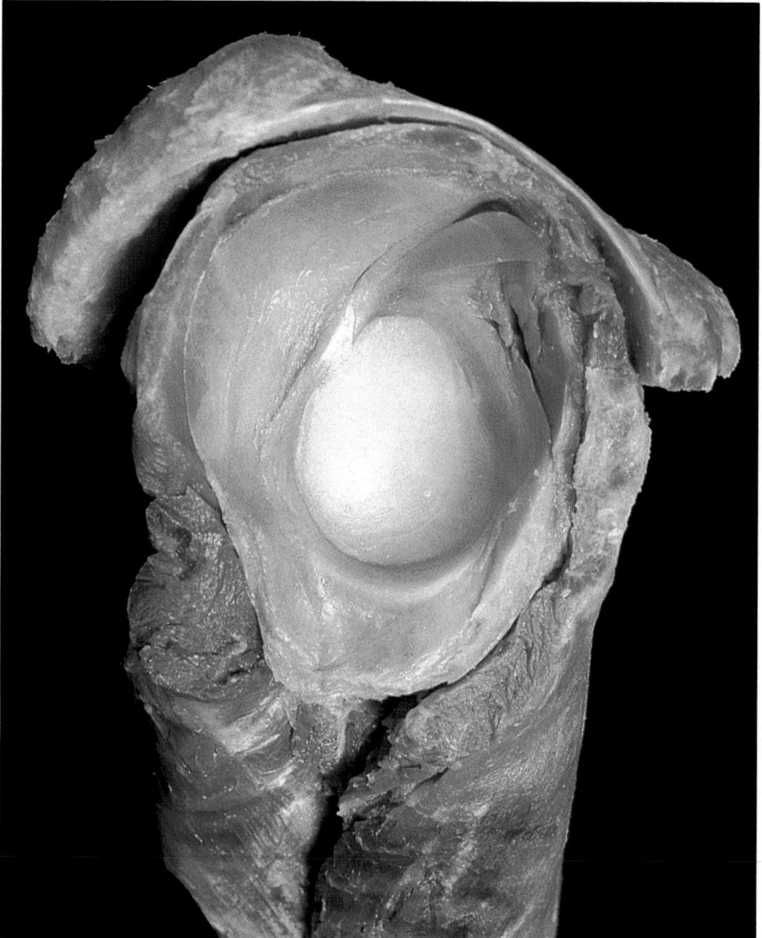

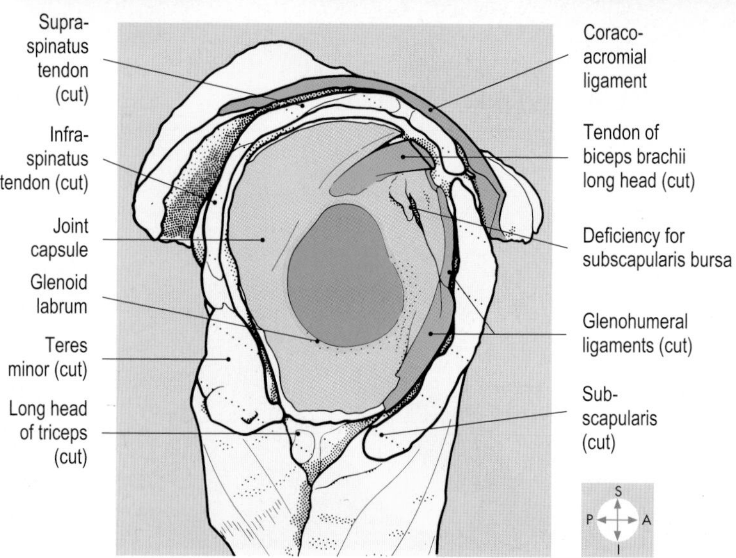

Fig. 3.87 The scapular component of a disarticulated shoulder joint showing the relations and internal features of the joint.

Elbow Joint

The elbow is a synovial hinge joint between the distal end of the humerus and the proximal ends of the radius and ulna (Fig. 3.88). Laterally, the capitulum of the humerus articulates with the slightly concave upper surface of the head of the radius. Medially, the trochlea of the humerus articulates with the deep trochlear notch of the ulna. In the anatomical position (in which the elbow is extended and the forearm is supinated) the orientation of the joint surfaces produces a 'carrying angle' which displaces the hand somewhat laterally. This angle between the long axes of the arm and the forearm disappears when the forearm is pronated.

The joint capsule (Fig. 3.89 & see Fig. 3.90) attaches proximally to the shaft of the humerus above the radial and coronoid fossae anteriorly, and to the margins of the olecranon fossa posteriorly. Distally, it attaches to the anular ligament of the proximal radioulnar joint and to the margins of the trochlear notch of the ulna. Synovial membrane lines the capsule and clothes the underlying pads of fat that project into the radial, coronoid and olecranon fossae of the humerus. The cavity of the elbow joint is continuous with that of the proximal radioulnar joint.

There are two collateral ligaments (Fig. 3.89 & see Fig. 3.90). The radial (lateral) collateral ligament passes between the lateral epicondyle and the anular ligament. The ulnar (medial) collateral ligament attaches proximally to the medial epicondyle, whilst distally its fibres diverge and attach to the medial aspects of the coronoid and olecranon processes of the ulna. Stability of the joint depends on the integrity of these collateral ligaments, which hold the trochlea of the humerus firmly in the trochlear notch.

Rotation of the ulna is prevented by the shape of the articular surfaces of the

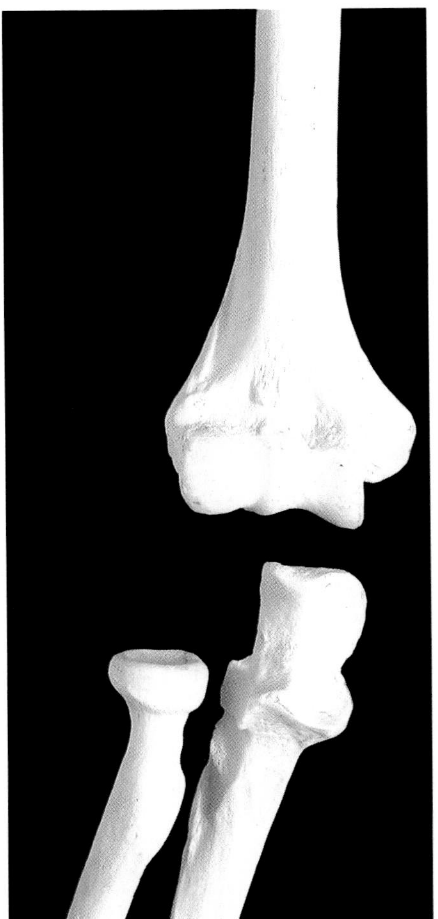

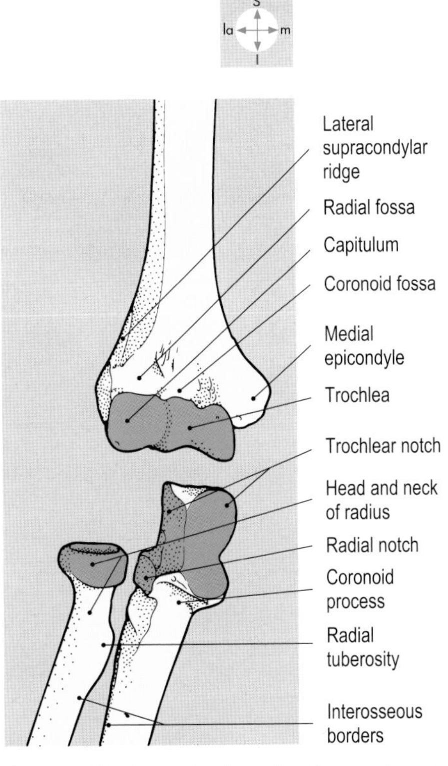

Fig. 3.88 The bones that form the elbow and proximal radioulnar joints have been separated to reveal their articular surfaces.

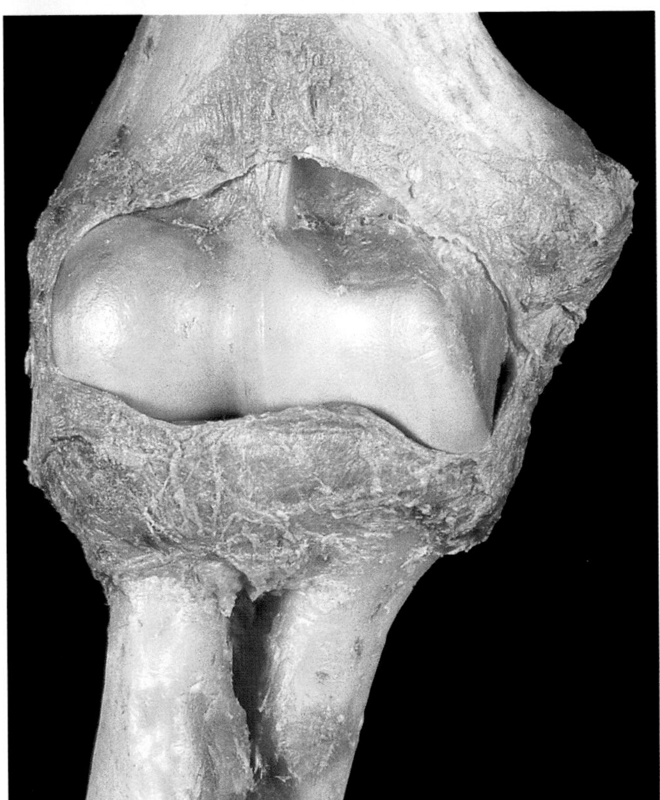

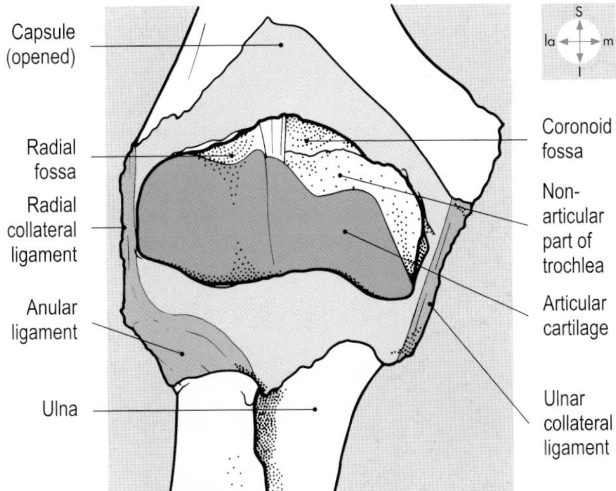

Fig. 3.89 Anterior aspect of elbow joint. The capsule has been opened to expose the interior of the joint.

trochlea. Dislocation of the joint is usually associated with ligamentous or bony injury.

Only flexion and extension occur at the elbow joint. Flexion (about 150°) is produced mainly by biceps and brachialis with a contribution from brachioradialis when the elbow is partially flexed. Flexion is limited by contact between the anterior surfaces of the arm and the forearm. Extension is often assisted by gravity. Active extension is produced by triceps assisted by anconeus. In full extension the olecranon engages in the olecranon fossa of the humerus, limiting the movement and increasing joint stability. The flexors and extensors of the wrist and hand arising from the humerus close to the joint do not contribute significantly to elbow movements.

Behind the elbow joint lies the tendon of triceps (Fig. 3.91). Immediately anterior to the capsule are brachialis and the tendon of biceps in the cubital fossa (see Fig. 3.29). The brachial artery and median nerve are separated from the capsule by brachialis. The ulnar nerve lies behind the medial epicondyle in contact with the ulnar collateral ligament. The vessels and nerves are vulnerable to injury in traumatic dislocation of the joint.

The elbow receives blood from the anastomosis around the joint formed by branches of the brachial, radial and ulnar arteries. The vessels supplying the joint are accompanied by articular nerves derived from branches of the musculocutaneous, radial, ulnar (and sometimes the median) nerves.

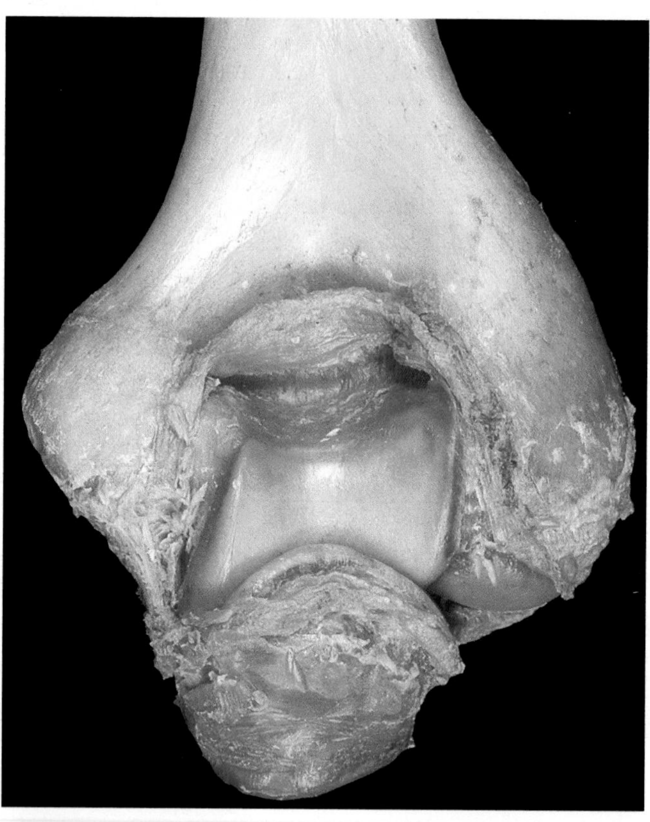

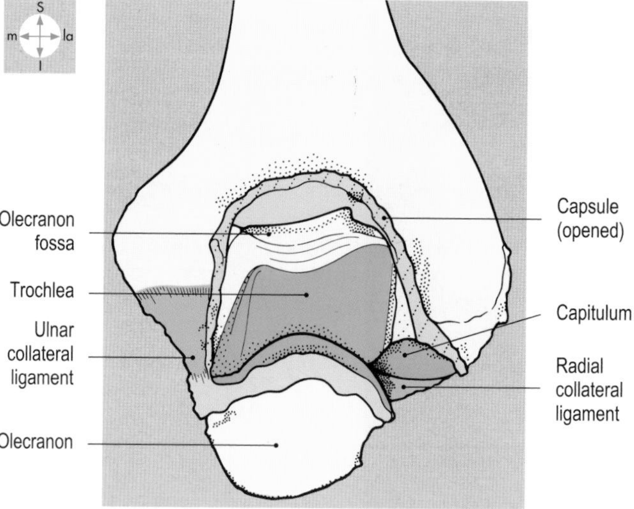

Fig. 3.90 Posterior aspect of flexed elbow joint. The capsule has been opened to reveal the olecranon fossa.

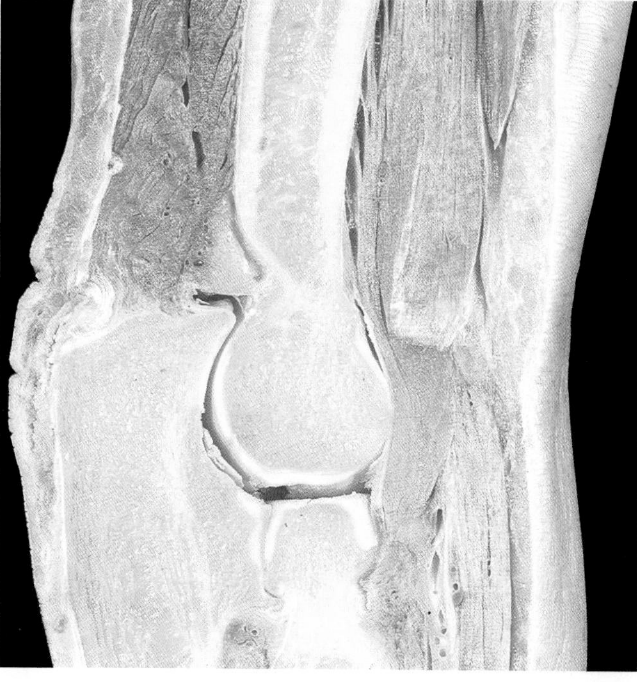

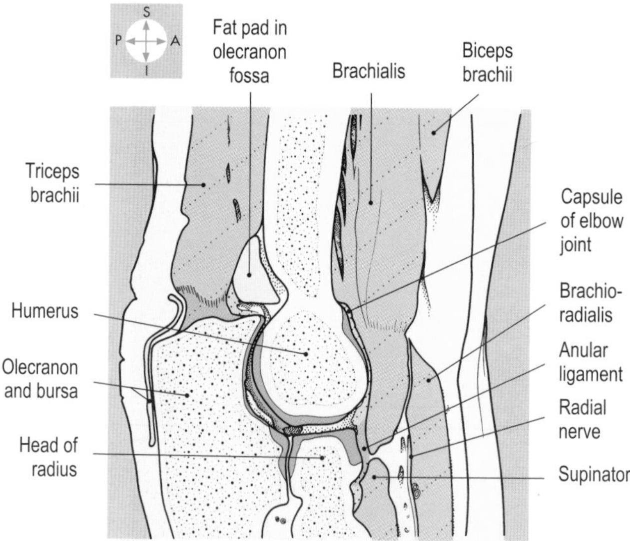

Fig. 3.91 Oblique longitudinal section of elbow (extended) and proximal radioulnar joints showing the articular surfaces and relations of the joints.

Radioulnar Joints

The radius and ulna articulate at the proximal and distal radioulnar joints, which are synovial. At the proximal joint the head of the radius articulates with the radial notch of the ulna (see Fig. 3.88). The head and neck are encircled by the anular ligament, which attaches to the anterior and posterior margins of the notch on the ulna (Fig. 3.92) and blends with the capsule and radial collateral ligament of the elbow. Thus the cavity of the proximal joint is continuous with that of the elbow.

The distal radioulnar joint occurs between the head of the ulna and the ulnar notch of the radius (Fig. 3.93). An articular disc (a triangular cartilage) attaches the ulnar styloid process to the distal end of the radius and separates the cavity of the distal joint from that of the wrist.

The anular ligament of the proximal joint and the articular disc of the distal joint prevent separation of the radius and ulna, yet allow the radius to rotate freely. In addition, the shafts of the bones are joined by the interosseous membrane, whose fibres incline downwards and medially from the interosseous border of the radius to that of the ulna. The membrane may be regarded as a fibrous radioulnar joint.

The movements of supination and pronation occur through approximately 180° at the radioulnar joints. During pronation the radius rotates across the ulna and twists the forearm and hand so that the palm faces posteriorly. Supination returns the limb to the anatomical position. The axis of the movement passes through the head of the radius and the styloid process of the ulna. Supination is the more powerful movement and is produced by biceps and supinator, although biceps is ineffective when the elbow is fully extended. Pronation is produced by pronator teres and pronator quadratus. Also, when the elbow is flexed, brachioradialis rotates the forearm and returns the limb to the midposition from the extremes of supination or pronation. The head of the radius can be felt rotating about 2 cm distal to the lateral epicondyle during these movements.

In a fall onto the hand, the interosseous membrane may transmit force from the radius to the ulna, protecting the radial head from compression against the capitulum of the humerus. However, since the membrane does not oppose distraction, a sudden tug on the hand may dislocate the radial head downwards from within the anular ligament of the proximal radioulnar joint.

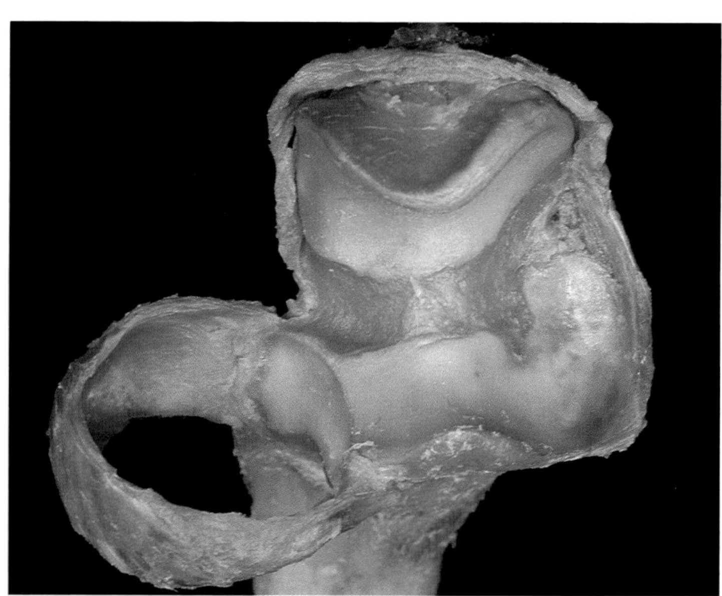

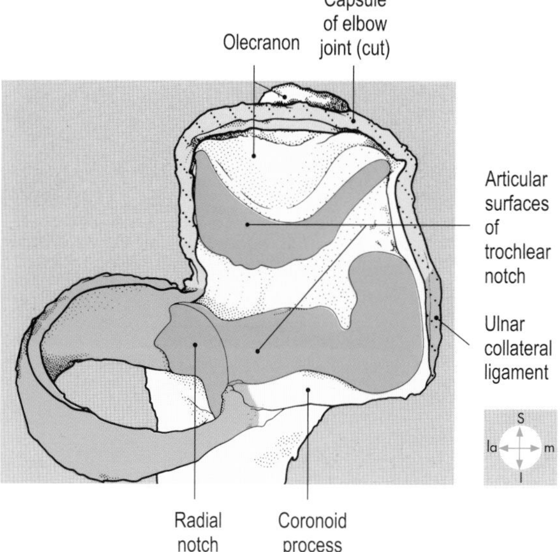

Fig. 3.92 Anterior view of proximal end of ulna with attached anular ligament, showing articular surfaces of trochlear and radial notches.

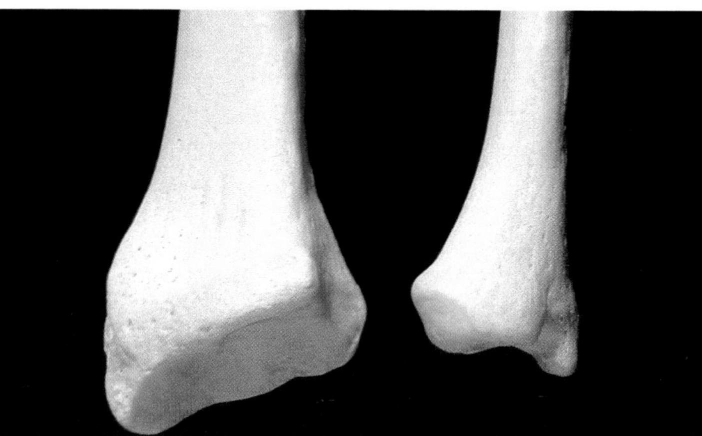

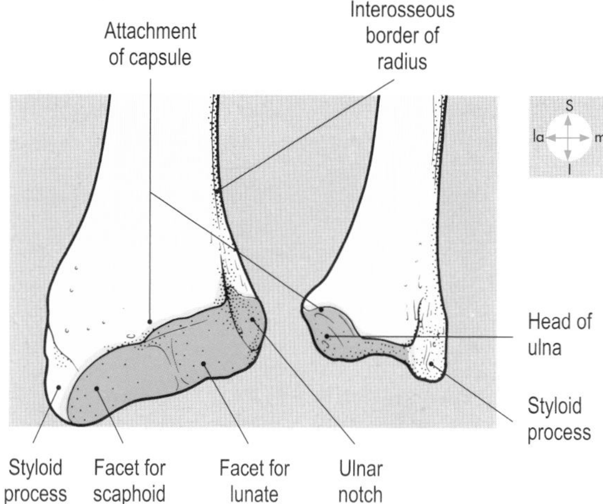

Fig. 3.93 Anterior view of distal ends of radius and ulna. The bones have been separated to reveal the ulnar notch.

Wrist Joint

Mobility of the hand on the forearm is provided by a series of synovial joints. Most of the movement occurs at the radiocarpal (wrist) joint, supplemented by movement between the carpal bones themselves. However, minimal rotation occurs here but is achieved for the hand by pronation and supination.

Radiocarpal joint

At the radiocarpal joint the distal end of the radius and the attached articular disc articulate with the proximal row of carpal bones including, from lateral to medial, the scaphoid, lunate and triquetral (Fig. 3.94). Pisiform does not take part in the wrist joint. The articular disc attaches to the radius and the root of the ulnar styloid process and separates the cavity of the radiocarpal joint from that of the inferior radioulnar joint (Fig. 3.95). The capsule, lined by synovial membrane, attaches to the edges of the articular surfaces and is strengthened by collateral ligaments that pass from the styloid processes of the ulna and radius to the adjacent carpal bones. The movements of this joint are considered on page 123. Function at the wrist may be severely compromised by fracture of the scaphoid across its narrow 'waist'. This injury may deprive part of the bone of its blood supply, resulting in ischaemic necrosis.

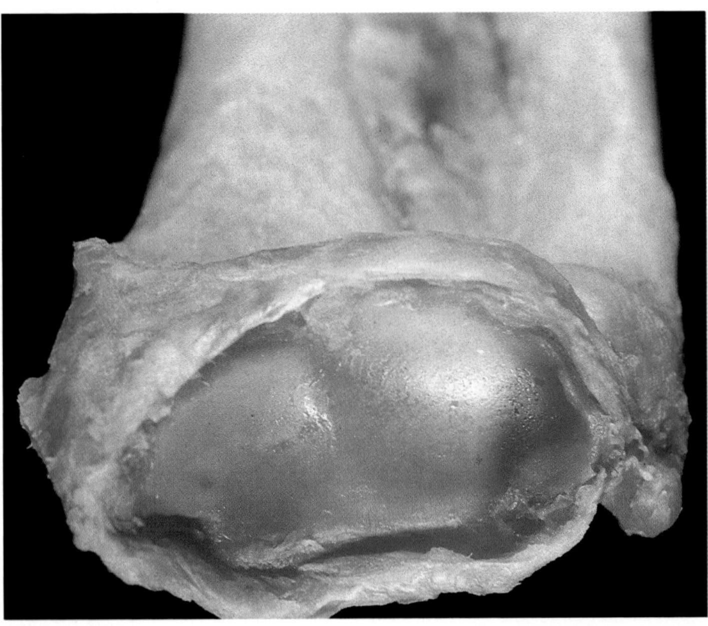

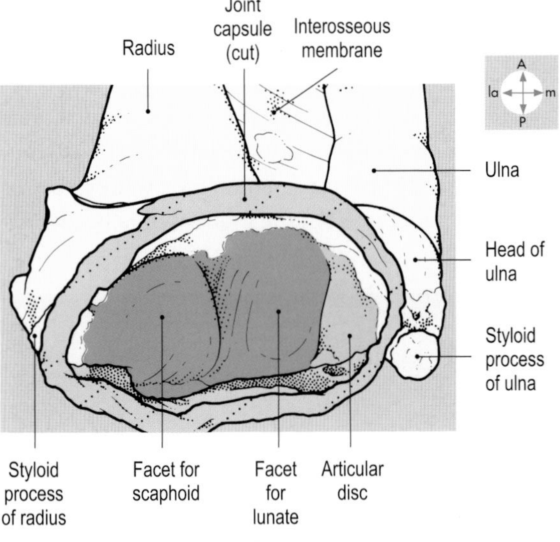

Fig. 3.94 Articular surface of the distal end of the radius and adjacent articular disc.

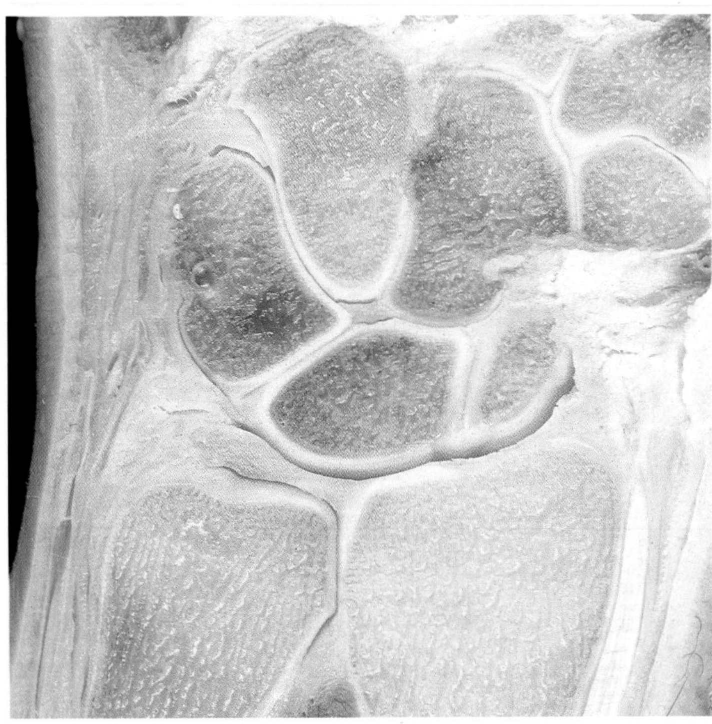

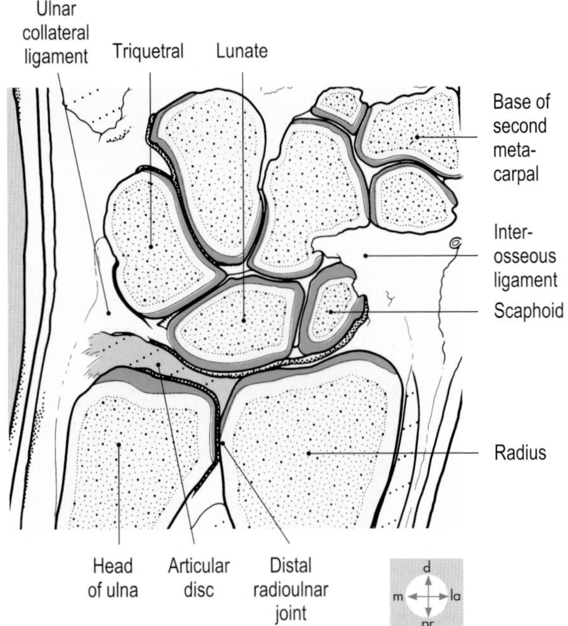

Fig. 3.95 Coronal section of the wrist joint showing articular surfaces and articular disc.

Joints of Carpus

The carpal bones are arranged in two rows: a proximal row, consisting of, from lateral to medial, scaphoid, lunate, triquetral and pisiform; and a distal row consisting of trapezium, trapezoid, capitate and hamate bones (Fig. 3.96).

Intercarpal joints

The joints between the carpal bones are supported by anterior, posterior and interosseous ligaments. The cavities of these joints usually communicate (Fig. 3.96) and function as a single unit called the 'midcarpal joint' (see Fig. 3.97). The joints are most stable in full extension when the anterior ligaments are taut.

The pisiform, a sesamoid bone in the tendon of flexor carpi ulnaris, has a separate joint with the triquetral (see Fig. 3.98), and is firmly anchored distally to the hook of the hamate and base of the fifth metacarpal bone by pisohamate and pisometacarpal ligaments (see Fig. 3.47). The relations of the intercarpal joints are illustrated in Figure 3.98.

Movements

Movements at the radiocarpal and intercarpal joints are complementary, allowing flexion, extension, adduction and abduction of the hand on the forearm. Although the long flexors and extensors of the digits act on the radiocarpal and intercarpal joints, flexion is due principally to the two carpal flexors, and extension to the three carpal extensors. Adduction is produced mainly by the simultaneous contraction of the flexors and extensors on the ulnar side of the forearm and abduction by contraction of the muscles on the radial side.

The radiocarpal and intercarpal joints are stabilized by the extensors and flexors of the wrist during action of the long flexors and/or extensors of the digits. In many activities, movement between the hand and forearm combines extension and abduction, achieved by the two radial carpal extensors.

Carpal tunnel

The carpal tunnel (canal) is a fibro-osseous passage linking the anterior compartment of the forearm with the palm of the hand. The walls of the tunnel consist anteriorly of the flexor retinaculum and posteriorly of the two rows of carpal bones which form a deep groove on their flexor surfaces. The retinaculum (see Fig. 3.99) lies transversely across the anterior aspect of the wrist, attaching to the trapezium and scaphoid laterally, and to the pisiform and hook of the hamate medially. The retinaculum lies in the hand, its proximal border level with the distal skin crease. The tendon of palmaris longus gains partial attachment to the retinaculum and enters the hand in front of the carpal tunnel (see Fig. 3.39). The tendon is accompanied on its medial side by the ulnar artery and nerve which pass lateral to the pisiform and the flexor carpi ulnaris tendon, but medial to the hook of the hamate. However, the median nerve and the other tendons entering the palm pass deep to the flexor retinaculum and traverse the carpal tunnel.

Within the tunnel (see Fig. 3.98) the tendons of flexor digitorum superficialis lie anterior to those of flexor digitorum profundus. These tendons all possess a common synovial sheath, which is usually in continuity with the digital synovial sheath of the little finger but not with those of the other fingers. The tendon of flexor pollicis longus also traverses the tunnel, invested by a separate synovial sheath which continues into the thumb. The tendon of flexor carpi radialis lies laterally in a groove on the trapezium, isolated from the main part of the carpal tunnel.

The median nerve traverses the tunnel immediately deep to the flexor retinaculum, lying approximately at the midpoint of the wrist close to the tendon of palmaris longus, anterior to the tendon of flexor pollicis longus and medial to the flexor carpi radialis tendon. Compression of the median nerve may occur within the carpal tunnel, giving rise to a condition called the 'carpal tunnel syndrome', which may result in weakness of the thenar muscles and altered sensation (paresthesiae or 'pins and needles') felt in the thumb, index and middle fingers. The syndrome may be treated operatively by dividing the flexor retinaculum to decompress the tunnel.

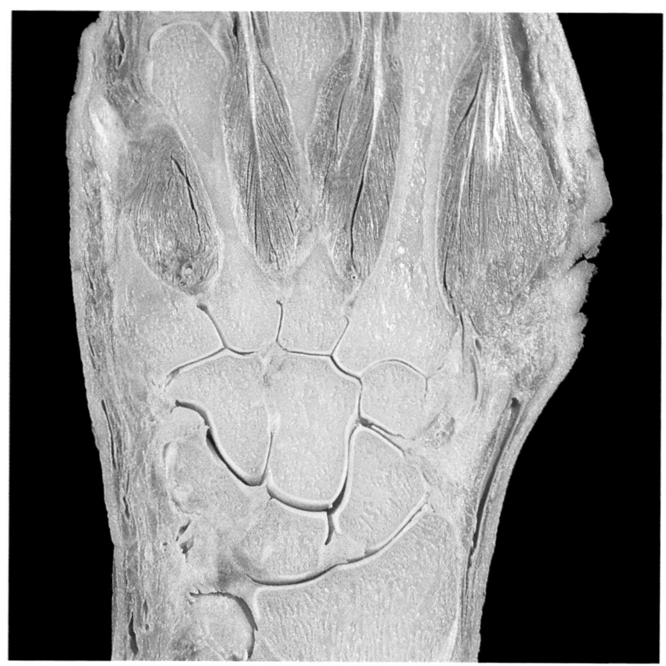

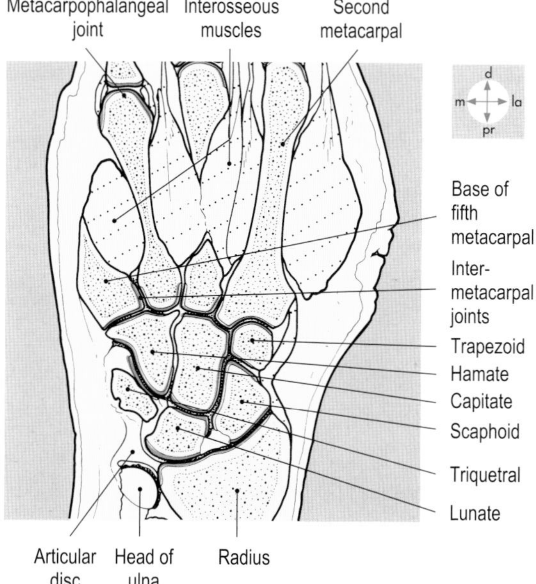

Fig. 3.96 Coronal section of the hand showing the joints of the carpal region. The thumb and little finger lay anterior to the plane of section.

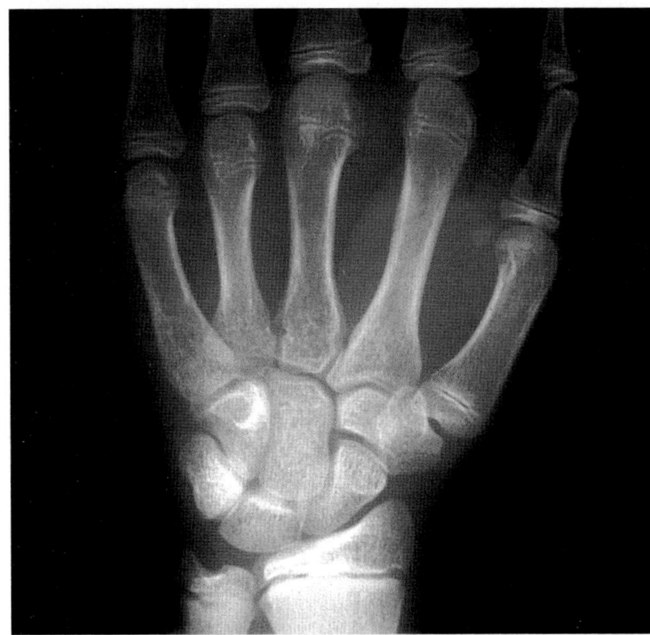

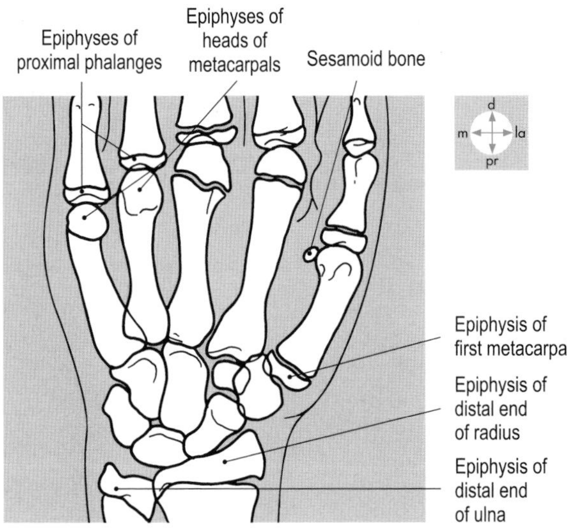

Fig. 3.97 Radiograph of the hand of an adolescent showing metacarpal and carpal bones. Epiphyseal plates are present. Compare Fig. 3.38.

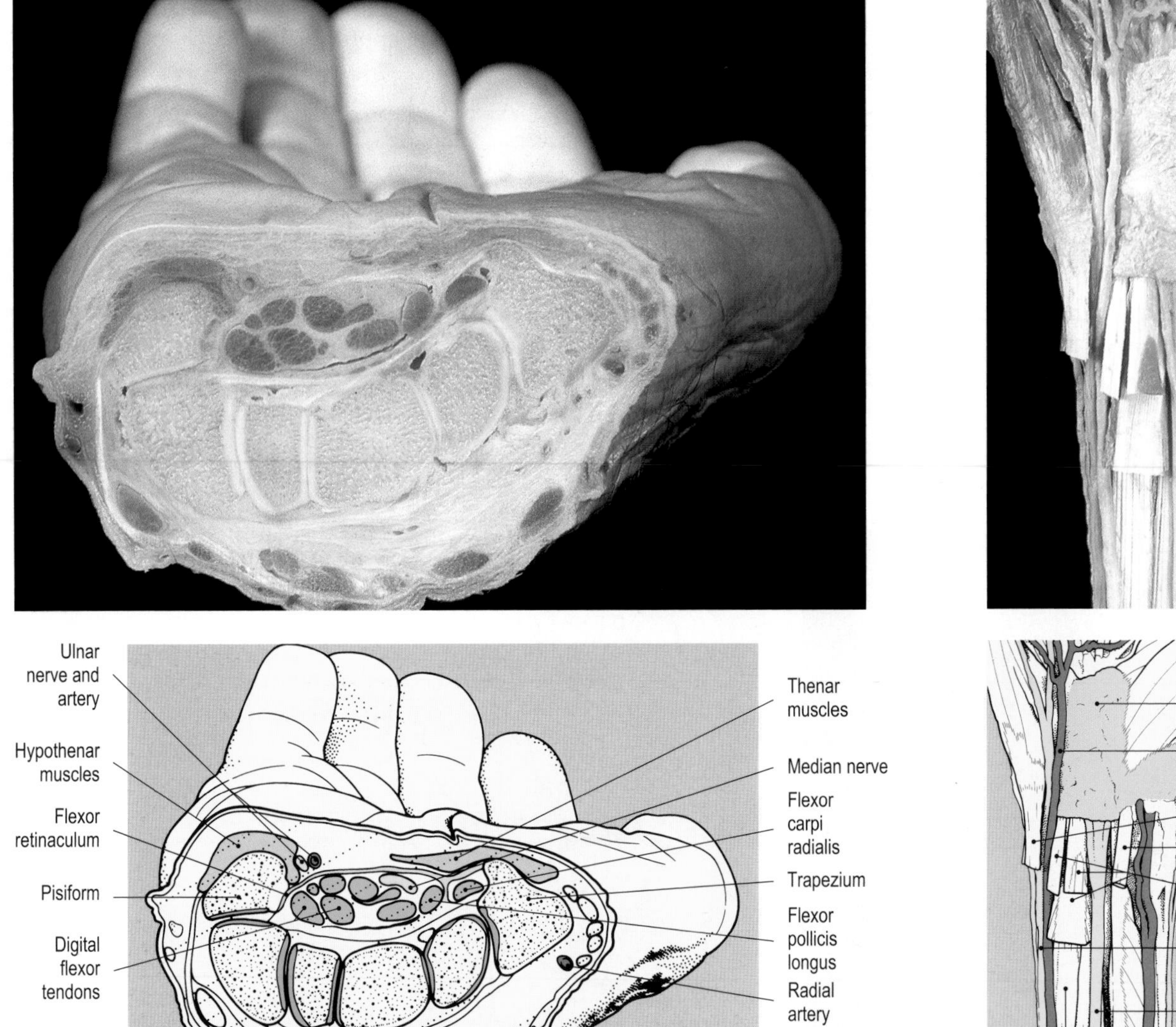

Fig. 3.98 Transverse section through the carpus showing the carpal tunnel and its contents.

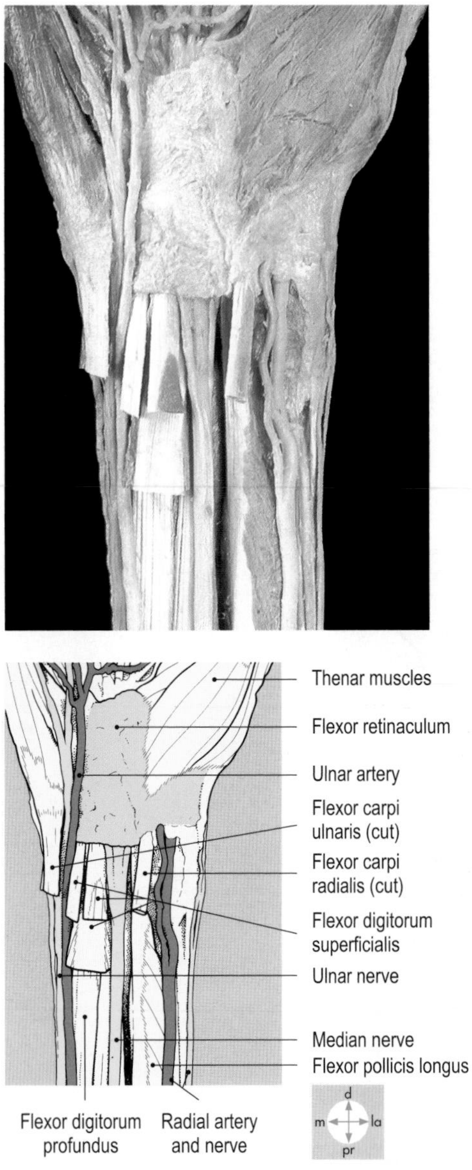

Thenar muscles
Flexor retinaculum
Ulnar artery
Flexor carpi
ulnaris (cut)
Flexor carpi
radialis (cut)
Flexor digitorum
superficialis
Ulnar nerve
Median nerve
Flexor pollicis longus
Flexor digitorum
profundus
Radial artery
and nerve
d
m
la
pr

Fig. 3.99 Flexor retinaculum and the superficial relations and structures entering the carpal tunnel.

Joints of Hand

The carpometacarpal, metacarpophalangeal and interphalangeal joints are synovial and allow the hand to perform its various functions, including the intricate movements involved in gripping objects. The intrinsic muscles perform delicate movements of the fingers: power is provided by contraction of the muscles in the compartments of the forearm.

Carpometacarpal joints

There are three separate carpometacarpal joints, one for the thumb and two for the fingers. The joint between the first metacarpal and trapezium (Fig. 3.100) possesses saddle-shaped articular surfaces and a lax capsule. This joint permits flexion and extension in a plane parallel to that of the palm, and adduction and abduction in a plane at right angles to that of the palm (and in the plane of the thumbnail). During opposition (the combined movements of medial rotation, adduction and flexion), the thumb rotates so that it may touch any of the fingers 'pulp-to-pulp'. This ability is essential in everyday manipulative movements.

The remaining two carpometacarpal joints, those for the fingers, are plane joints and less mobile than the first. Laterally, a joint cavity lies between the second and third metacarpals and the trapezoid and capitate, whilst medially the fourth and fifth metacarpals articulate with the hamate (see Fig. 3.97). These carpometacarpal joints communicate with the three plane (intermetacarpal) joints that lie between the bases of the medial four metacarpals.

Metacarpophalangeal joints

These joints occur between the rounded heads of the metacarpals and concave bases of the proximal phalanges (see Fig. 3.38). Each joint capsule is reinforced at the sides by collateral ligaments and is thickened anteriorly to form a fibrocartilaginous plate. The plates of the medial four digits are interconnected by the deep transverse metacarpal ligament. The joints permit flexion, extension, adduction and abduction. Because the collateral ligaments tighten during flexion, adduction and abduction are possibly only in the extended position.

Interphalangeal joints

Each of these joints possesses a capsule reinforced by collateral ligaments (see Fig. 3.101). However, posteriorly, the capsule is deficient and is replaced by the extensor expansion (see Fig. 3.102). These are hinge joints that allow only flexion and extension.

The carpometacarpal, metacarpophalangeal and interphalangeal joints are supplied by branches of adjacent vessels and nerves traversing the palm and digits.

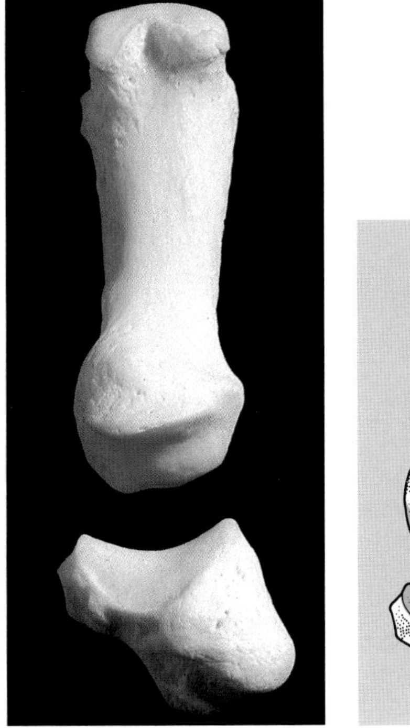

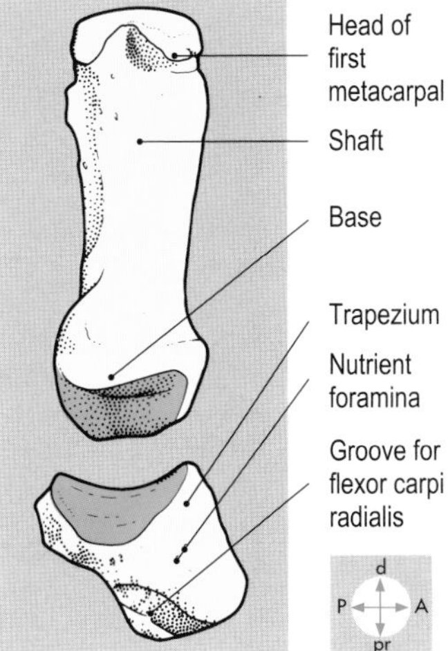

Fig. 3.100 Trapezium and metacarpal of thumb, separated to show the saddle-shaped articular surfaces of the carpometacarpal joint.

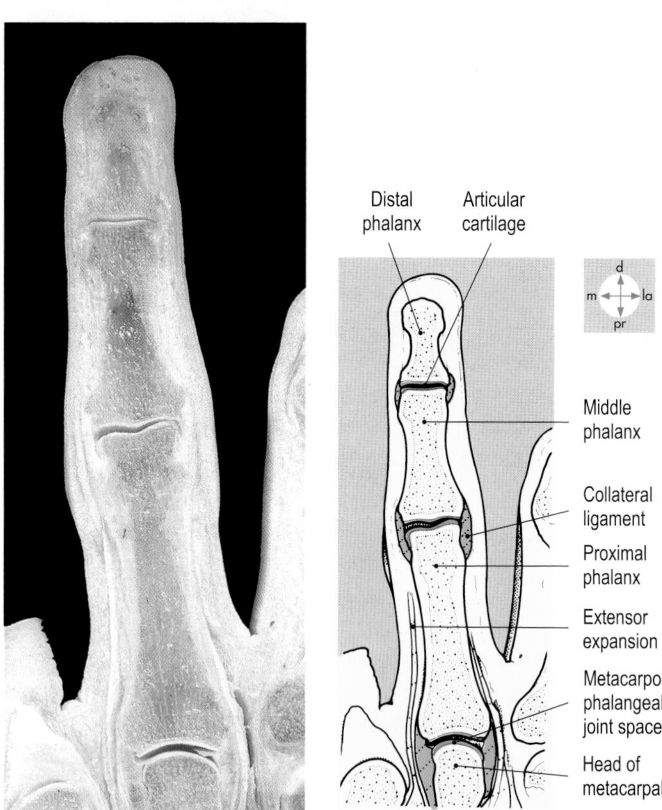

Fig. 3.101 Coronal section of a finger. The joint spaces have been exaggerated by hyperextension of the specimen.

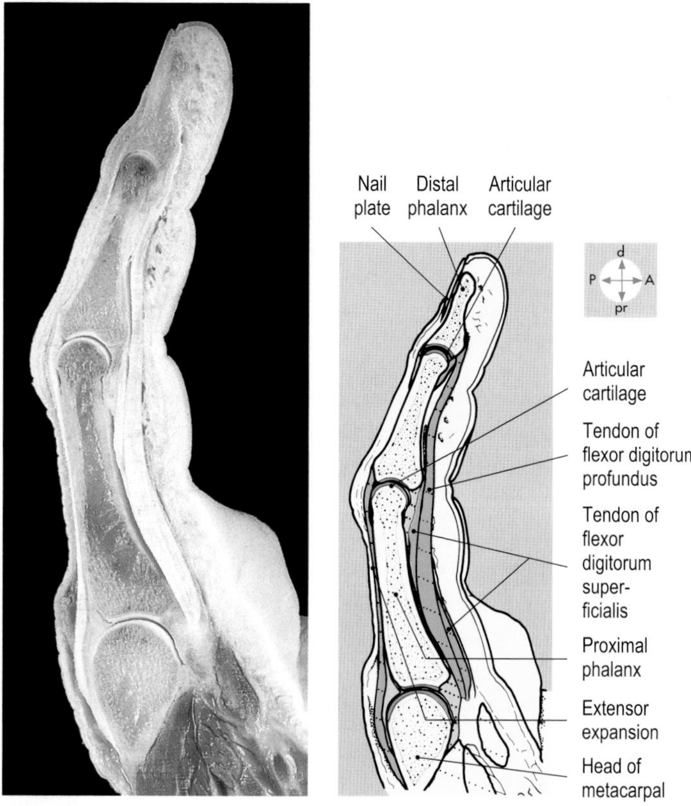

Fig. 3.102 Sagittal section of a finger to show the capsules and relations of the joints.

Exam Skills

Each of the incomplete statements below is followed by five suggested answers or completions. Decide which are true and which are false. The answers are supplied on page 415.

1. The flexor retinaculum:

a) forms part of the carpal tunnel.
b) is crossed superficially by the median nerve.
c) is crossed superficially by the ulnar artery.
d) gives attachment to the thenar muscles.
e) attaches to the trapezium.

2. The following muscles act on the metacarpophalangeal joint of the thumb:

a) opponens pollicis.
b) abductor pollicis brevis.
c) extensor pollicis brevis.
d) the first dorsal interosseous.
e) flexor pollicis brevis.

3. Deltoid:

a) is innervated by the axillary nerve.
b) is usually active against gravity during abduction of the shoulder joint.
c) acts to initiate abduction of the shoulder joint.
d) may suffer damage to its nerve supply during dislocation of the glenohumeral joint.
e) attaches to the lateral surface of the shaft of the humerus.

4. The following lie within the axilla:

a) the cords of the brachial plexus.
b) the tendon of the long head of biceps.
c) coracobrachialis.
d) branches of the axillary artery.
e) lymph nodes.

5. These muscles act as follows:

a) pectoralis major causes flexion at the shoulder.
b) brachialis causes flexion at the elbow.
c) biceps brachii causes supination.
d) pronator teres causes pronation.
e) trapezius causes abduction at the glenohumeral joint.

6. Medial rotation of the humerus at the shoulder joint is produced by:

a) teres minor.
b) supraspinatus.
c) subscapularis.
d) latissimus dorsi.
e) pectoralis major.

7. The following enter and/or leave the cubital fossa:

a) the tendon of biceps brachii.
b) the radial nerve.
c) the cephalic vein.
d) the ulnar nerve.
e) the brachial artery.

8. For part of its course, the brachial artery accompanies the:

a) axillary nerve.
b) median nerve.
c) radial nerve.
d) ulnar nerve.
e) musculocutaneous nerve.

9. The following usually receive fibres from the lateral cord of the brachial plexus:

a) the median nerve.
b) the axillary nerve.
c) the musculocutaneous nerve.
d) the lateral cutaneous nerve of the forearm.
e) the ulnar nerve.

10. Branches of the radial nerve supply:

a) skin of the thumb.
b) skin of the forearm.
c) skin of the hypothenar eminence.
d) no muscle that has flexor actions.
e) no muscle(s) located in the hand.

11. Supination:

a) occurs at the radioulnar joints.
b) causes the ulna to move around the radius.
c) is produced mainly by biceps brachii when the elbow joint is fully extended.
d) is opposed by contraction of brachialis.
e) involves active movement of the elbow joint.

12. Complete division of the ulnar nerve at the elbow will:

a) paralyze flexor digitorum superficialis.
b) paralyze flexor carpi ulnaris.
c) prevent abduction and adduction of the fingers.
d) cause anaesthesia of skin on the palmar surface of the fifth digit.
e) cause wasting of the adductor pollicis.

13. Skin of the dorsum of the hand is innervated by the:

a) lateral cutaneous nerve of the forearm.
b) superficial branch of the radial nerve.
c) ulnar nerve.
d) median nerve.
e) posterior cutaneous nerve of the forearm.

14. Flexor digitorum superficialis:

a) flexes the distal interphalangeal joints.
b) receives innervation from the ulnar nerve.
c) attaches to the medial epicondyle of the humerus.
d) lies superficial to the median nerve through most of the forearm.
e) gives attachment for the lumbricals.

15. The interossei:

a) flex the interphalangeal joints.
b) abduct and adduct the fingers.
c) are innervated by the ulnar nerve.
d) flex the metacarpophalangeal joints of the fingers.
e) attach to the extensor expansions.

16. The radial nerve:

a) is a branch of the posterior cord of the brachial plexus.
b) lies in the radial (spiral) groove of the humerus.
c) enters the forearm anterior to the elbow joint.
d) has a branch which passes through supinator.
e) innervates flexor carpi radialis.

Clinical Skills

The answers are supplied on page 416.

Case Study 1

A frail 90-year-old woman was admitted to sheltered accommodation and soon after arrival complained of pain in her right hand - which was ignored by a care assistant, who gave her sleeping tablets. The visiting physician found the woman had a painful blue right hand. The whole limb was cold, especially below the elbow, and cutaneous sensation was absent in the hand. She could not move her hand or fingers. The doctor could not identify pulses in the right upper limb but palpated a strong, though irregular, left radial pulse. The physician explained that a fragment of blood clot had probably escaped from the heart and been carried in the blood to the right arm where it had blocked the brachial artery as an embolus. Admission to the nearby hospital was organized but unfortunately the elderly patient suffered a major stroke, from which she died 12 hours later.

Questions:

1. Assuming that the clot was atrial in origin, name the pathway it took from the left atrium to reach the brachial artery.
2. What determines the level of an initial arterial blockage?
3. Although the whole limb was poorly perfused (ischaemic) what was a good guide to the severity of the ischaemia?
4. What arterial anastomoses exist between the subclavian and axillary arteries?

Case Study 2

A 50-year-old grandmother with rheumatoid arthritis found that her wrists and the joints in her fingers had become more stiff and painful. She complained of having more difficulty than usual with her right hand and she had dropped several treasured cups. On one occasion while tidying away the broken fragments she cut her thumb but had not noticed until she saw blood on her clothes. She was having difficulty sleeping as she was being woken by pain in her hand and arm - and she volunteered that something similar happened during her pregnancies but resolved spontaneously after the birth of her children. The physician examined her hands and in addition to her usual joint features noticed flattening of her right thenar eminence compared with the left and some loss of cutaneous sensation. After discussing nerve conduction studies, her physician explained that an operation on the front of her wrist with the scar running near the crease lines would probably be needed to help relieve her problems.

Questions:

1. What is the significance of 'flattening' of the thenar muscles? Which nerve supplies these muscles and where is it particularly vulnerable to compression?
2. What had alerted the physician to sensory deficit, and what was found on examination?
3. Why is the skin incision orientated transversely at the wrist?
4. Which nerve(s) may be vulnerable at operations to divide the flexor retinaculum?

Case Study 3

A fit college student fell heavily and injured his right shoulder while playing football. He had dislocated the same shoulder about a year earlier and injured it again several times since. His shoulder felt very painful and he was unable to move his right arm. The hospital doctor noticed that his shoulders were not symmetrical, since there was a hollow below the right acromion, and ordered radiographs of the shoulder region to exclude fractures. The radiographs confirmed the suspicion of dislocation of the right shoulder joint: there were no fractures. The dislocation was reduced easily during a short general anaesthetic and the student was allowed home wearing a collar and cuff support and bandaging that held his right elbow against his chest wall. Subsequently, an orthopaedic specialist noticed that the right deltoid was less well developed than on the left. Surgical exploration of the joint revealed a capsular tear, which was repaired. Postoperatively intensive physiotherapy was instituted to strengthen all the muscles acting at the shoulders and the student has now resumed playing football.

Questions:

1. What anatomical features render the shoulder joint particularly prone to dislocation?
2. Which nerve closely related to the joint is liable to injury by dislocation of the shoulder and how should the doctor have examined for this injury?
3. Why was the upper limb bandaged against the chest wall?
4. What is the probable significance of previous injuries?
5. What is the most important stabilizing influence on the glenohumeral joint?

Case Study 4

A 30-year-old, right-handed teacher decided to repair his wooden garden shed. He purchased new roofing, removed the partly rotten wood without difficulty and began to nail the new timbers in place. As the day progressed the hammer he was using seemed to feel heavier and heavier until just picking it up was an effort and he eventually completed the job using his left hand. That evening the whole of his arm, but especially his elbow, was uncomfortable and even picking up a glass of lager made his elbow sore! He found that squeezing water out of the sponge after taking a shower hurt his elbow. His physician demonstrated exquisite tenderness over the lateral epicondyle of the right humerus and pronounced, 'You've got tennis elbow!' After following his usual activities at work the teacher found that his pain gradually eased and that he could use his arm completely normally after approximately a week.

Questions:

1. Which muscles attach near the lateral epicondyle?
2. Which unaccustomed repetitive action provoked the inflammatory response (give precise movements at the joint)?
3. Which two muscles were likely to be particularly involved?
4. Why did squeezing water from the sponge produce pain?

Observation Skills

Identify the structures indicated. The answers are supplied at the foot of the page.

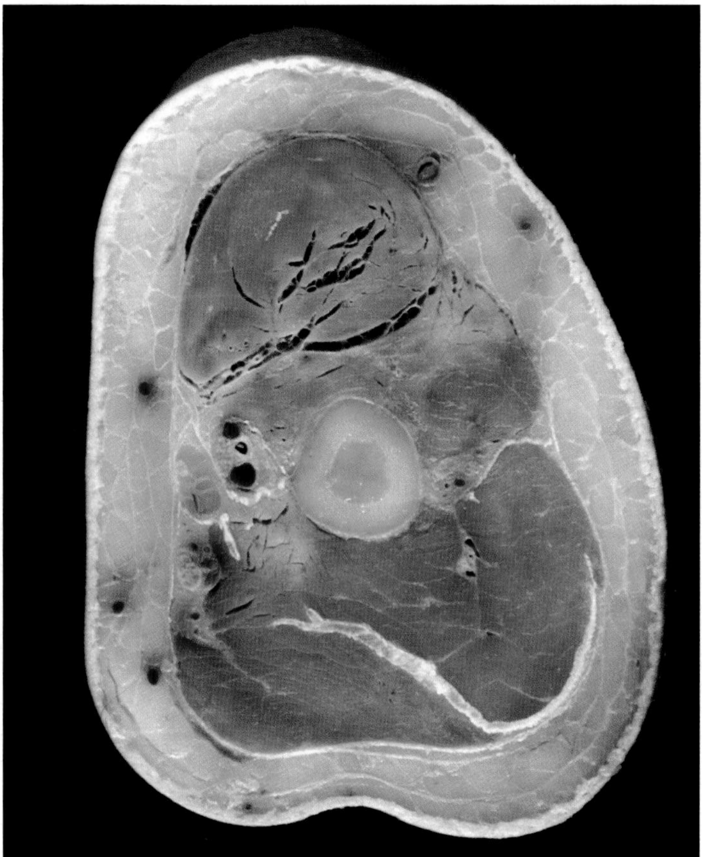

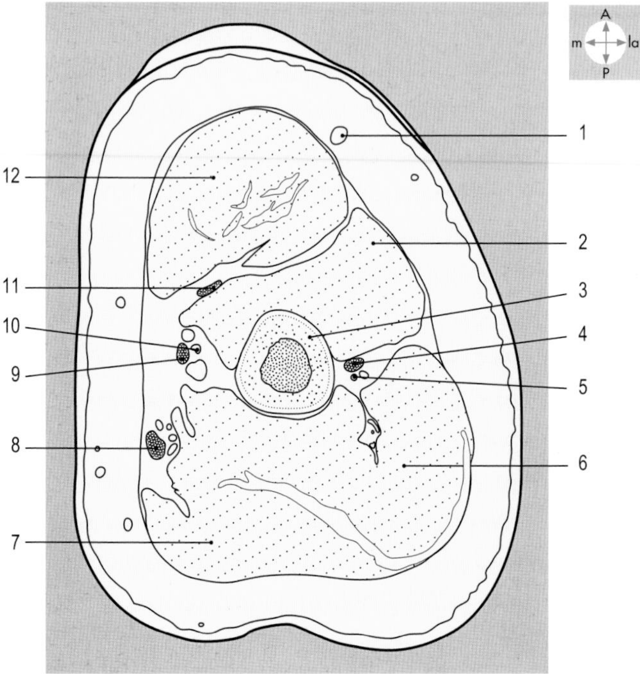

Fig. 3.103 Cross-section through the arm.

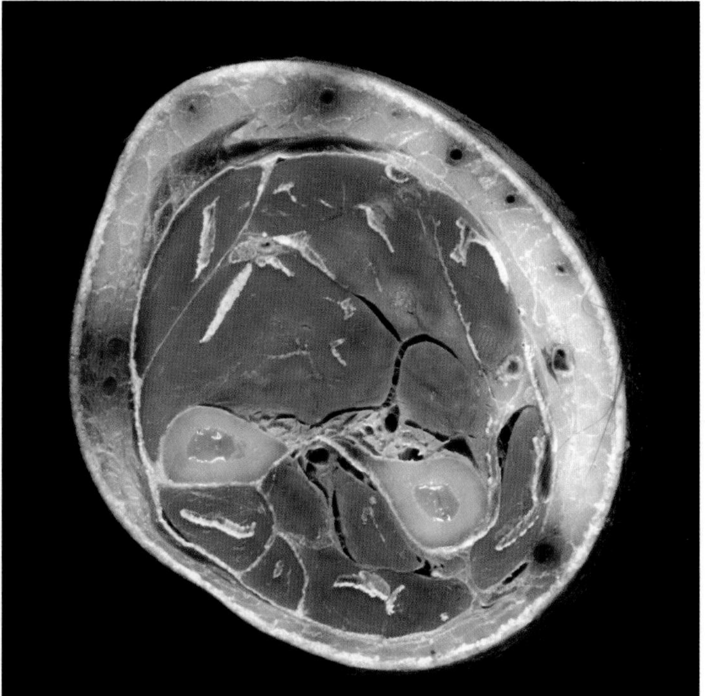

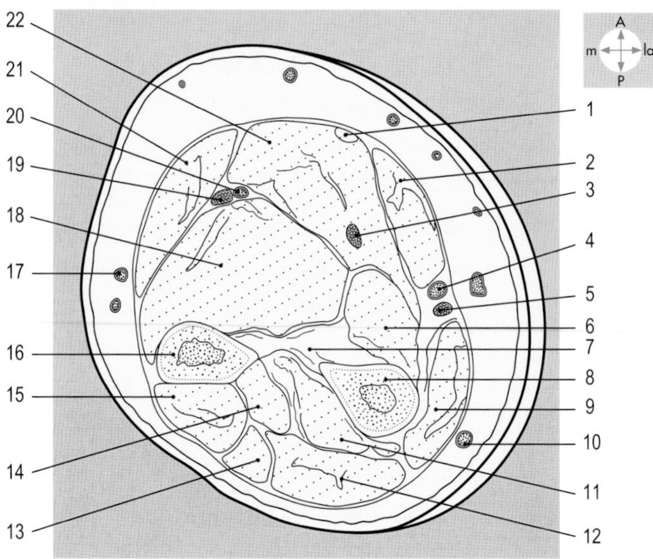

Fig. 3.104 Cross-section through the forearm.

Answers

Fig. 3.103 1 = cephalic vein; 2 = brachialis; 3 = humerus; 4 = radial nerve; 5 = deep branchial artery; 6 = medial head of triceps; 7 = triceps long head; 8 = ulnar nerve; 9 = median nerve; 10 = brachial artery; 11 = musculocutaneous nerve; 12 = biceps brachii.

Fig. 3.104 1 = palmaris longus tendon; 2 = flexor carpi radialis; 3 = median nerve; 4 = radial artery; 5 = radial nerve; 6 = flexor pollicis longus; 7 = interosseous membrane; 8 = radius; 9 = extensor carpi radialis; 10 = cephalic vein; 11 = abductor pollicis longus; 12 = extensor digitorum; 13 = extensor digiti minimi; 14 = extensor pollicis longus; 15 = extensor carpi ulnaris; 16 = ulna; 17 = basilic vein; 18 = flexor digitorum profundus; 19 = ulnar nerve; 20 = ulnar artery; 21 = flexor carpi ulnaris; 22 = flexor digitorum superficialis.

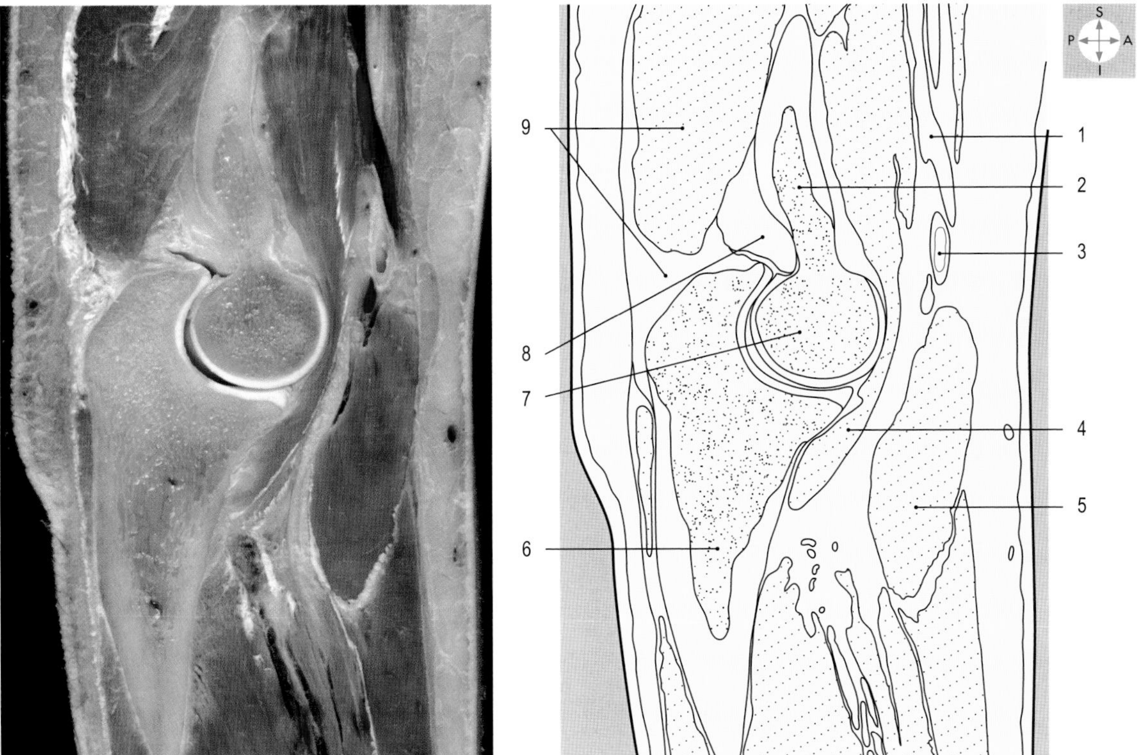

Fig. 3.105 Sagittal section through the elbow and proximal end of ulna.

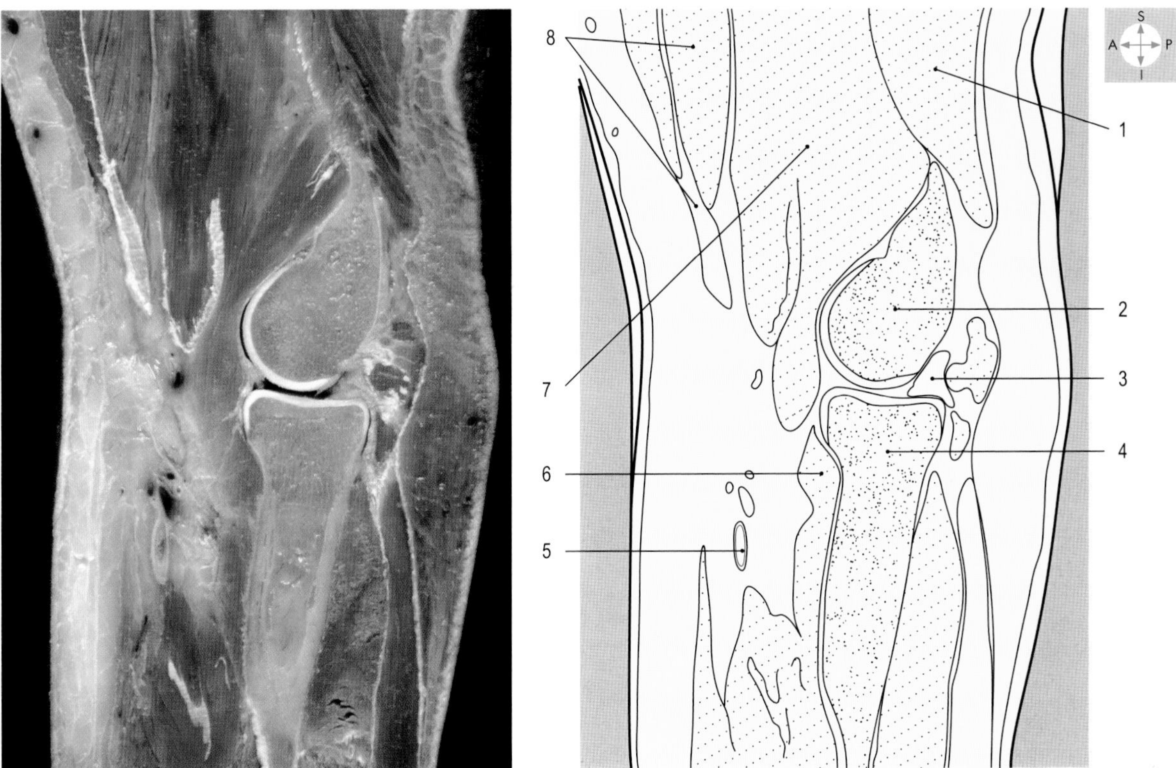

Fig. 3.106 Sagittal section through the elbow and proximal end of radius.

Answers

Fig. 3.105 1 = brachial vein; 2 = humerus; 3 = brachial artery; 4 = brachialis; 5 = fused flexor muscles; 6 = ulna; 7 = trochlea of humerus; 8 = fat pad; 9 = triceps and tendon.
Fig. 3.106 1 = triceps brachii; 2 = capitulum of humerus; 3 = fat pad; 4 = head of radius; 5 = brachial artery; 6 = supinator; 7 = brachialis; 8 = biceps brachii and tendon.

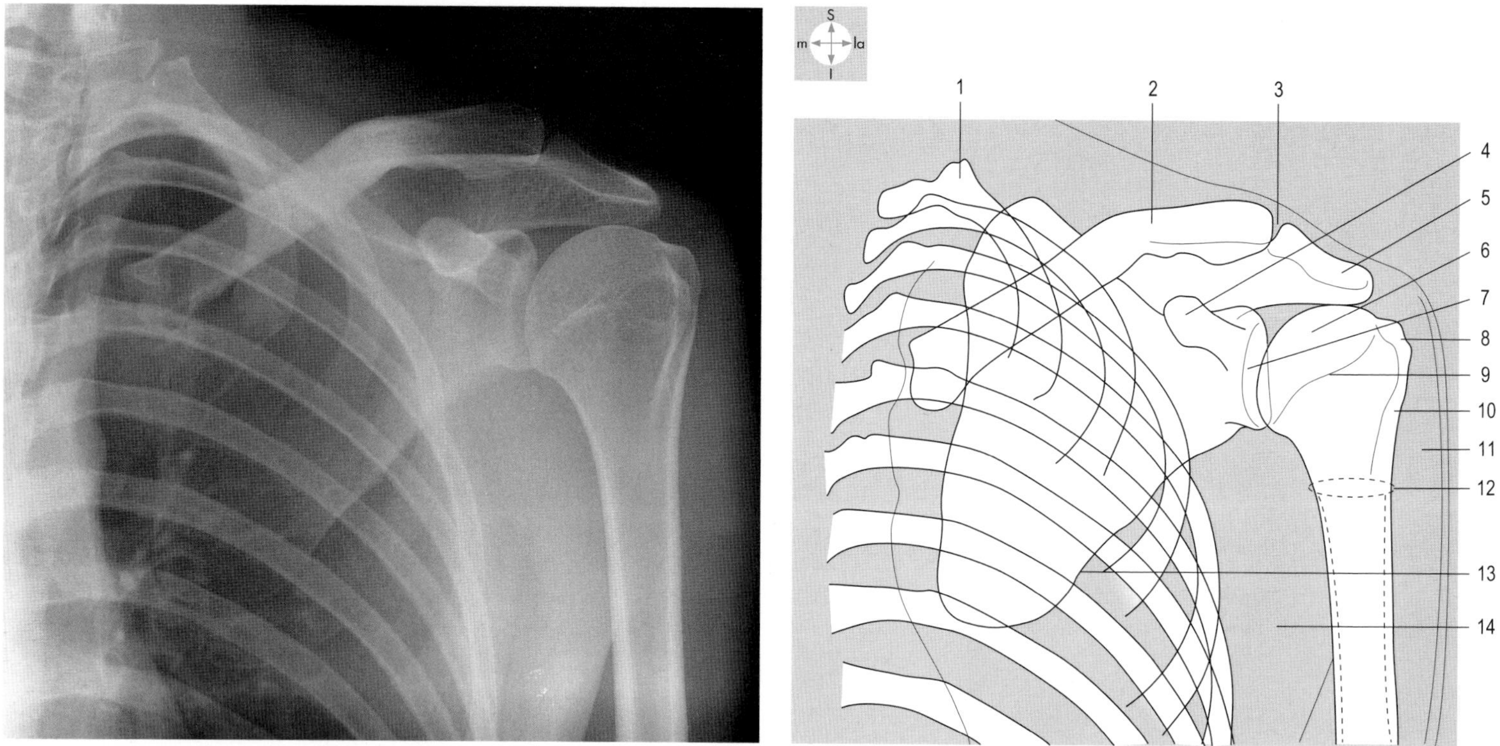

Fig. 3.107 Anteroposterior radiograph of shoulder region.

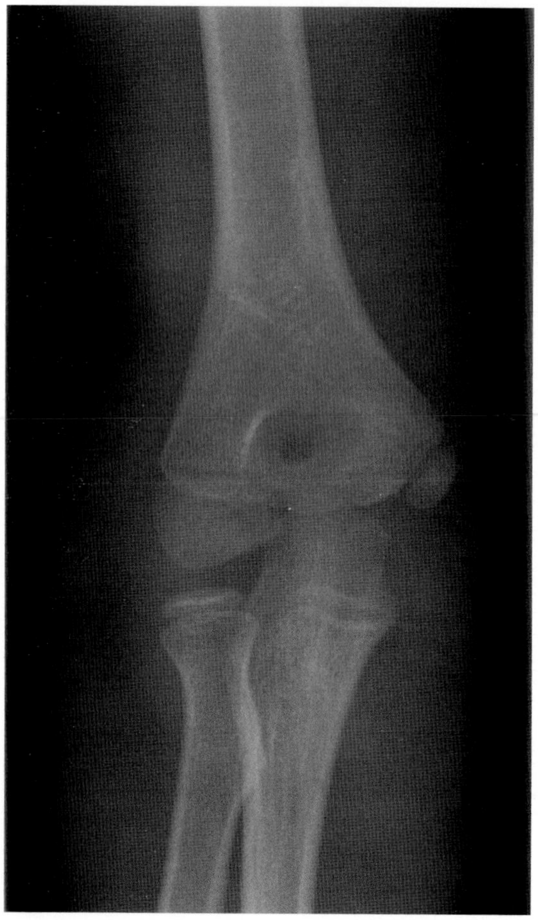

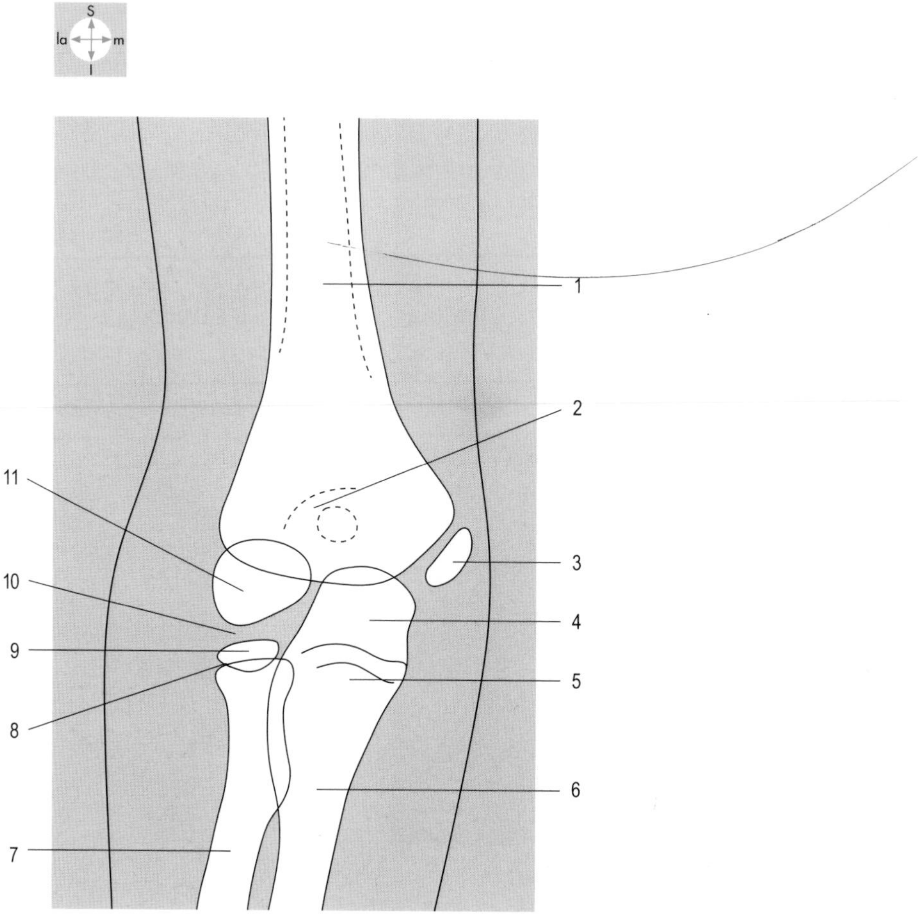

Fig. 3.108 Anteroposterior radiograph of juvenile elbow.

Answers

Fig. 3.107 1 = first rib; 2 = clavicle; 3 = acromioclavicular joint; 4 = coracoid process; 5 = acromion; 6 = head of humerus; 7 = articular surface of glenoid fossa; 8 = greater tubercle; 9 = anatomical neck; 10 = intertubercular groove; 11 = soft tissue shadow of deltoid; 12 = surgical neck; 13 = lateral border of scapula; 14 = soft tissue shadow of muscles of axillary folds.

Fig. 3.108 1 = shaft of humerus; 2 = olecranon fossa; 3 = epiphysis of medial epicondyle; 4 = olecranon process; 5 = coronoid process; 6 = shaft of ulna; 7 = shaft of radius; 8 = epiphyseal cartilage plate; 9 = proximal epiphysis of radius; 10 = radio-humeral joint; 11 = epiphysis of capitulum.

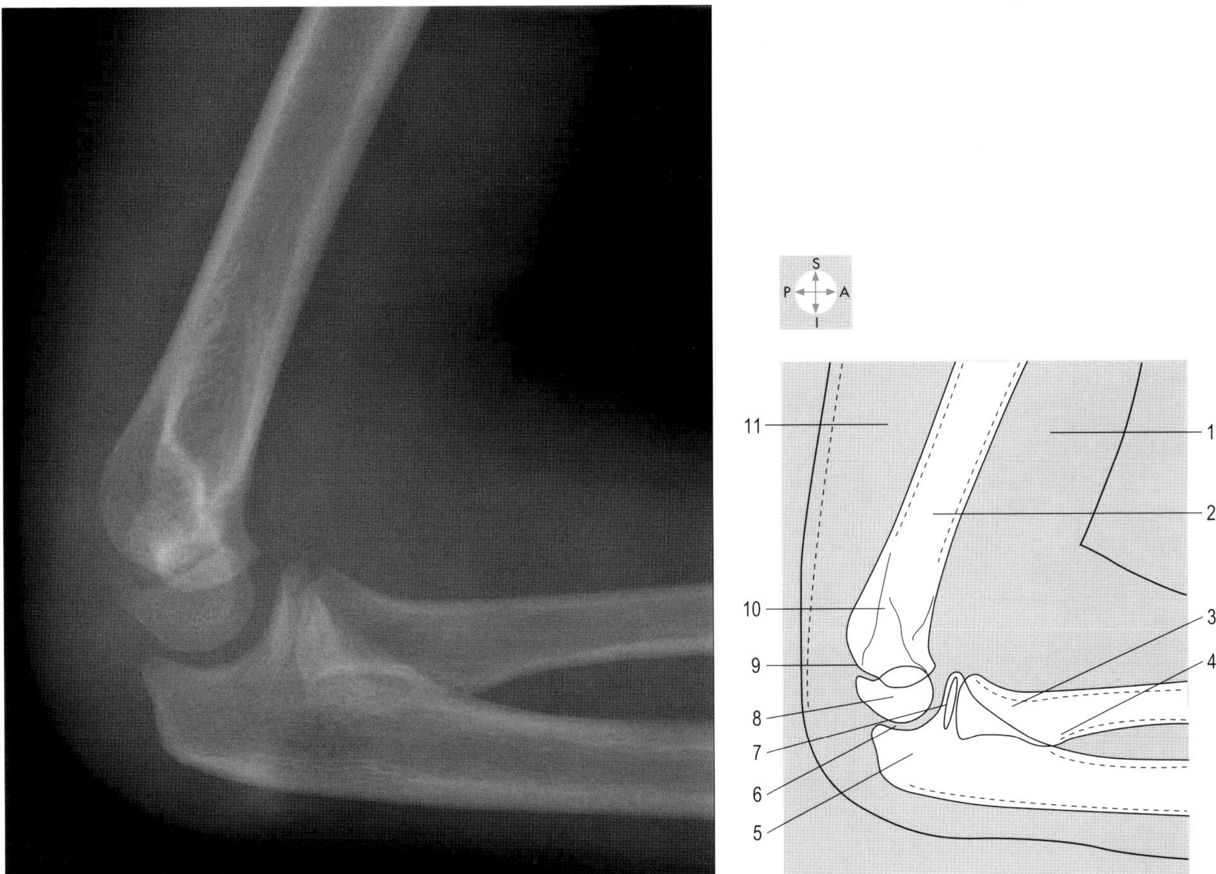

Fig. 3.109 Lateral radiograph of juvenile elbow.

Answers

Fig. 3.109 1 = soft tissue shadow of biceps brachii and brachialis; 2 = shaft of humerus; 3 = neck of radius; 4 = radial tuberosity; 5 = olecranon process; 6 = humero-ulnar joint; 7 = proximal epiphysis of radius; 8 = epiphysis of capitulum; 9 = epiphyseal cartilage plate; 10 = supracondylar ridge; 11 = soft tissue shadow of triceps brachii.

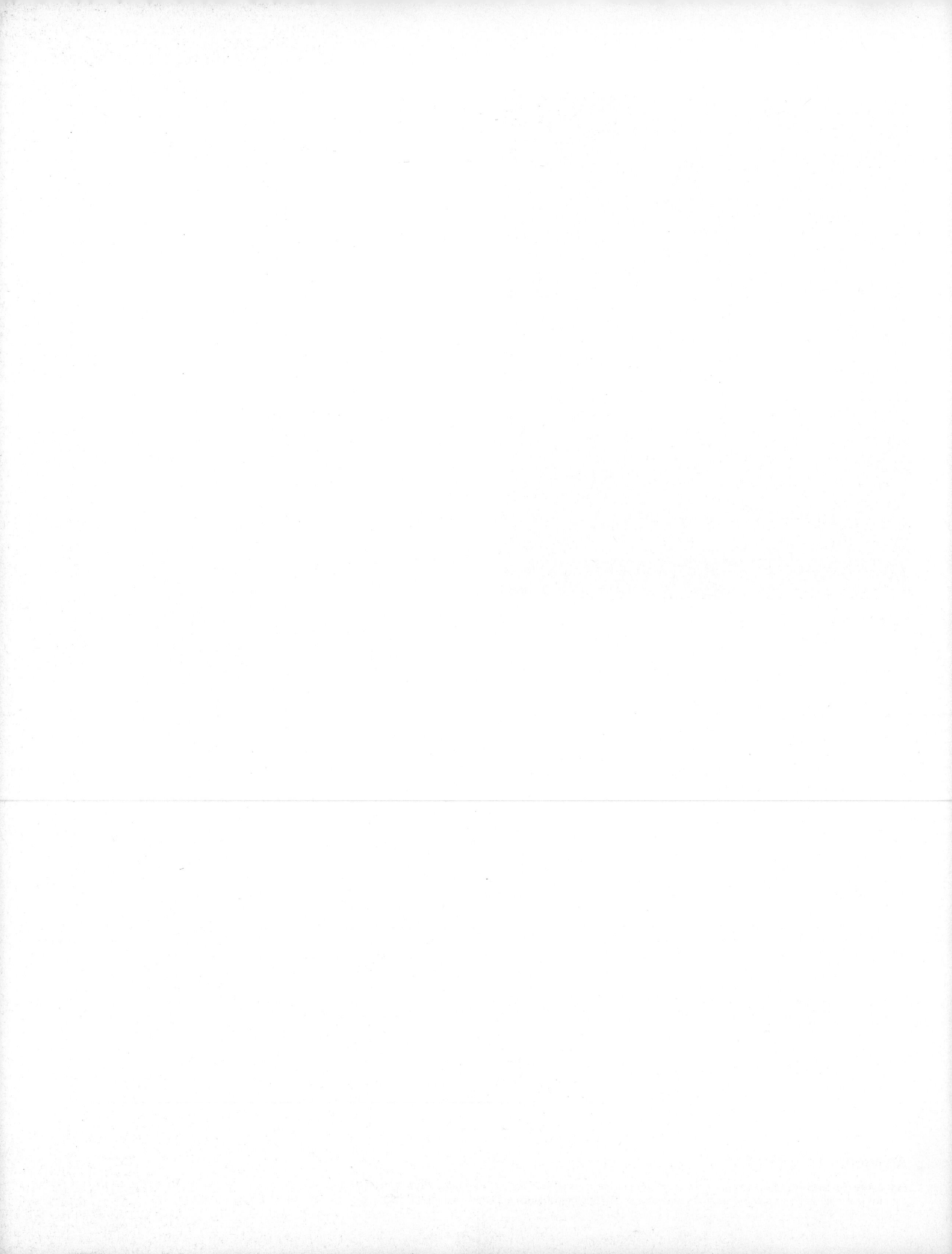

Abdomen

CHAPTER 4

Introduction

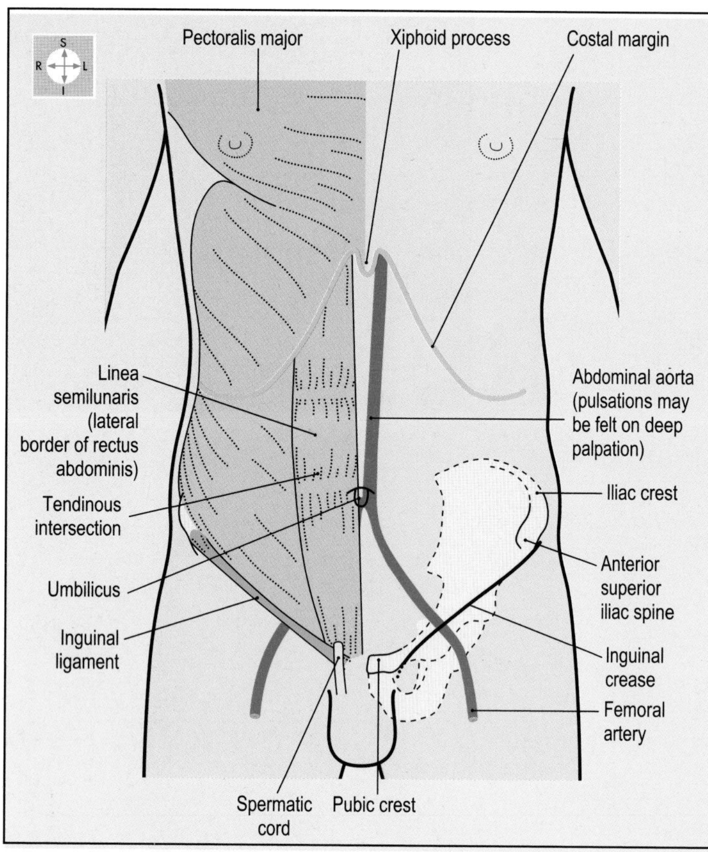

Fig. 4.1 Structures often visible or palpable in the living.

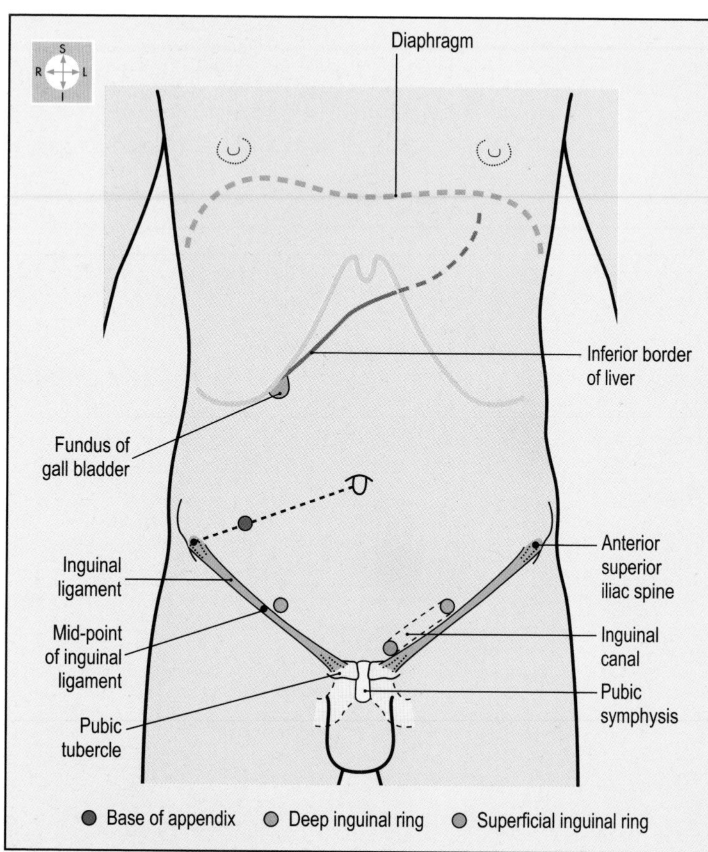

Fig. 4.2 Clinically important structures not usually visible or palpable in the living.

The abdomen is separated from the thorax above by the diaphragm, and below is continuous with the pelvis at the pelvic inlet. Passing through the diaphragm are the aorta, oesophagus and inferior vena cava. Because the diaphragm is strongly convex upwards, the upper abdominal organs lie deep to the lower ribs and costal cartilages. The pelvic inlet is an arbitrary plane sloping downwards and forwards through which run the small and large intestines, the ureters and several vessels and nerves.

The posterior abdominal wall includes muscles that attach to the last rib, the hip bone and the lumbar vertebrae. Laterally, their fasciae merge with the anterolateral abdominal wall whose three layers of muscle broaden out and become aponeurotic before meeting in the midline anteriorly. Close to this median raphe is a vertical strap-like muscle, rectus abdominis, running from the pubis to the anterior chest wall.

The inguinal canal, an oblique passage through the anterolateral abdominal wall, conveys the spermatic cord in the male and the round ligament of the uterus in the female (Figs 4.1 & 4.2).

The nerves and vessels of the abdominal wall run between the muscles and supply all layers from skin to parietal peritoneum. Most of the arteries, and their accompanying veins and lymphatics, arise from the thoracic wall or the inguinal region while the

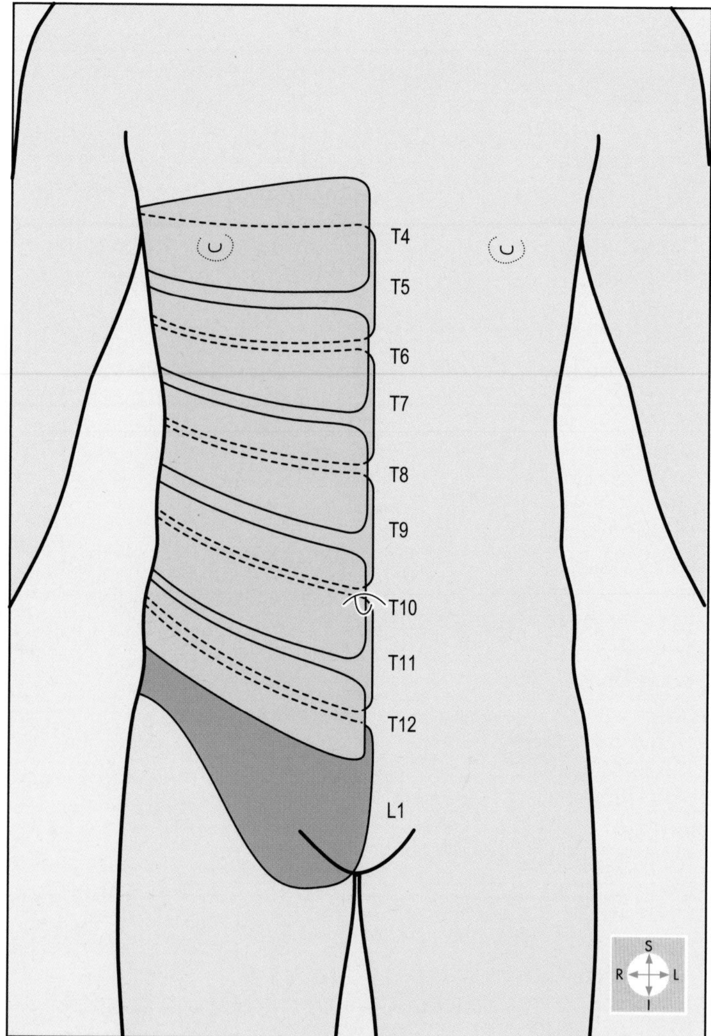

Fig. 4.3 Dermatomes of abdominal wall, showing how they overlap.

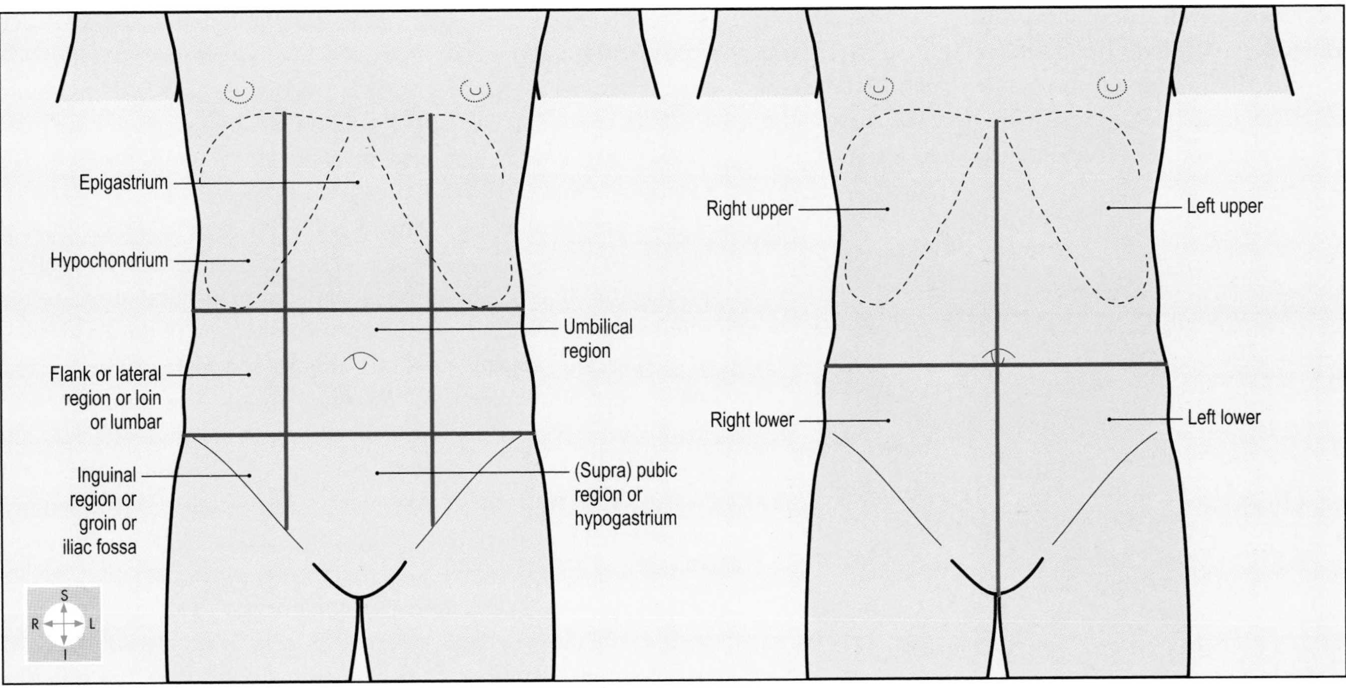

Fig. 4.4 Subdivisions of the abdomen used in clinical practice. Left: 9 regions. Right: 4 quadants.

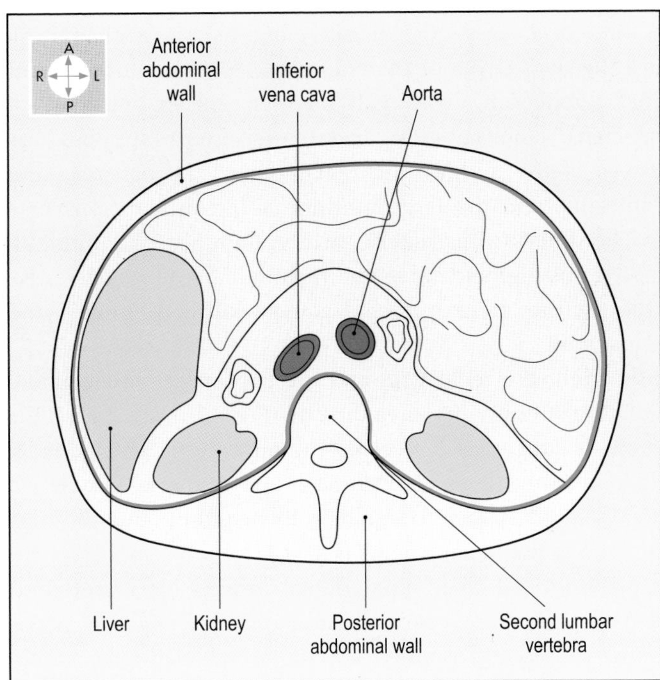

Fig. 4.5 Transverse section through the abdomen to demonstrate the shape of the cavity.

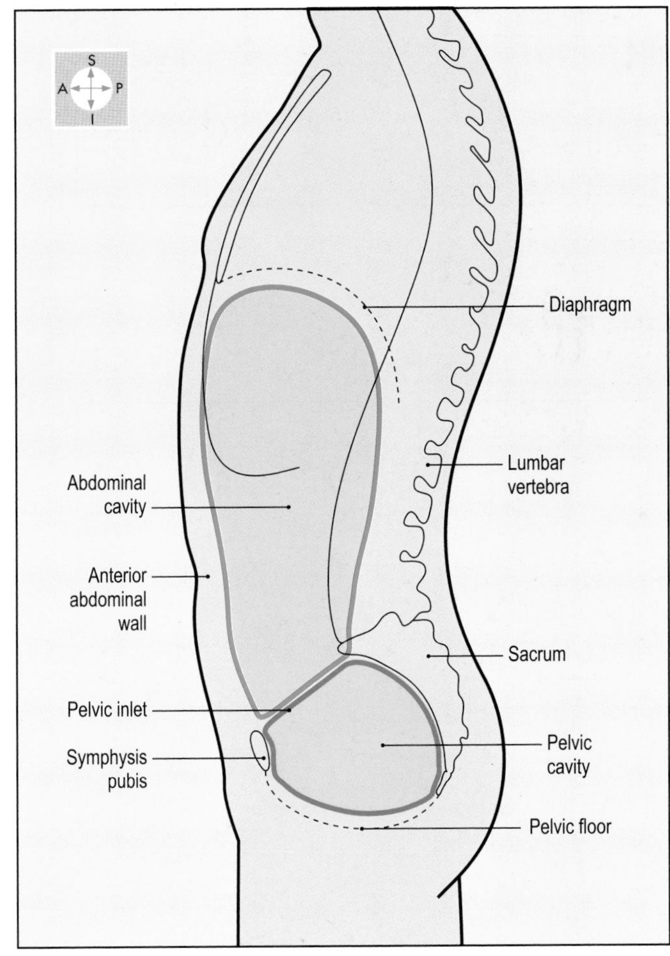

Fig. 4.6 Longitudinal section through the abdomen to show its shape and superior and inferior boundaries.

innervation is provided by spinal nerves. The cutaneous distribution of these nerves displays considerable overlap, as shown in Figure 4.3.

The abdominal wall muscles accommodate to volume changes of the abdominal and pelvic hollow organs, increase intra-abdominal pressure during forced expiration and straining, and produce movements of the lumbar spine.

The shape of the abdominal cavity is shown in Figures 4.4, 4.5 and 4.6. Projecting into the abdomen, the lumbar vertebrae form a substantial midline ridge anterior to which run the aorta and inferior vena cava. On each side of the lumbar vertebrae are deep paravertebral gutters. The liver lies predominantly to the right of the midline while the spleen and most of the stomach lie to the left (Fig. 4.7). The digestive organs, including the duodenum, jejunum, ileum and colon, lie anterior to the suprarenal glands, kidneys and ureters (Fig. 4.8). The abdominal organs vary considerably in their size, shape and relative position, the stomach and intestines expanding and contracting as they accommodate to their contents. The upper abdominal organs move with the diaphragm and in response to changes in body position, for example from upright to lying down.

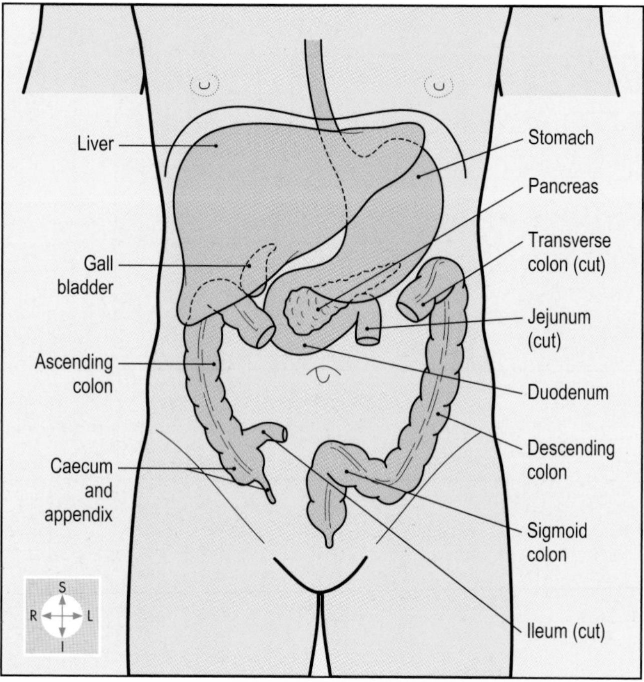

Fig. 4.7 The digestive organs within the abdomen.

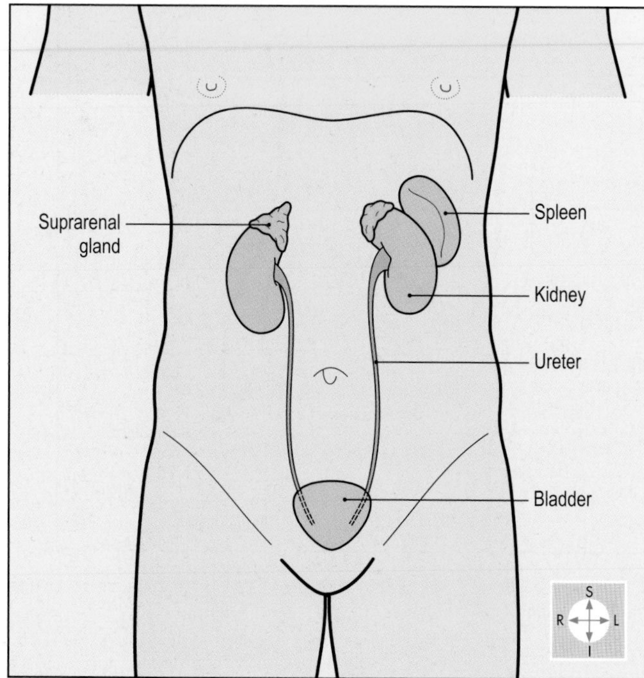

Fig. 4.8 The kidneys and related organs.

The peritoneum is a serous sac with parietal and visceral layers that are normally in close apposition. The parietal peritoneum lines the abdominal wall and the undersurface of the diaphragm, whilst the visceral layer coats many of the abdominal organs. Some organs have an almost complete covering and are termed intraperitoneal, for example the stomach, jejunum, ileum and liver. They are relatively mobile and attached by double layers of peritoneum between which run vessels and nerves. Such folds form mesenteries, for example the mesentery of the small intestine, or ligaments such as the falciform ligament of the liver, or omenta like the greater omentum that hangs like an apron from the stomach. Other organs are retroperitoneal, such as the pancreas and kidneys. They have no mesenteries and only partial coverings of peritoneum, usually on the anterior surface.

The aorta descends in the midline and bifurcates to form the common iliac arteries (Fig. 4.9). From its anterior surface spring three branches to the digestive organs. The coeliac trunk supplies the derivatives of the embryonic foregut: stomach and proximal duodenum, liver, gall bladder, spleen and part of the pancreas. The superior mesenteric artery supplies the derivatives of the midgut: the remainder of the pancreas and small intestine and the large intestine as far as the transverse colon. The inferior mesenteric artery supplies the hindgut: descending and sigmoid colon and rectum. Paired branches arise from the aorta to the suprarenal glands, kidneys, gonads and abdominal wall.

On the right the renal vein and the suprarenal and gonadal veins join the inferior vena cava directly (Fig. 4.10). On the left the renal vein is longer and receives the suprarenal and gonadal veins. Blood from the spleen, stomach and intestines drains via the portal venous system to the liver, thence to the inferior vena cava by way of the hepatic veins (Fig. 4.11).

Lymph from the abdominal organs drains by vessels and nodes that accompany the arterial supply. There are nodes within mesenteries and around the aorta, from which vessels drain upwards to enter the cysterna chyli. The latter gives rise to the thoracic duct carrying lymph upwards through the thorax (see Fig. 1.35).

Most viscera receive autonomic innervation via both sympathetic and parasympathetic plexuses around the blood vessels, particularly the aorta and its branches. The thoracic splanchnic nerves, branches of the thoracic portion of the sympathetic trunk, pierce the diaphragm close to its aortic opening. Parasympathetic fibres travel in the vagus nerve which supplies the stomach, liver and biliary system, the small intestine and the proximal part of the large intestine. The distal portion of the colon is supplied by parasympathetic nerves from sacral segments of the spinal cord.

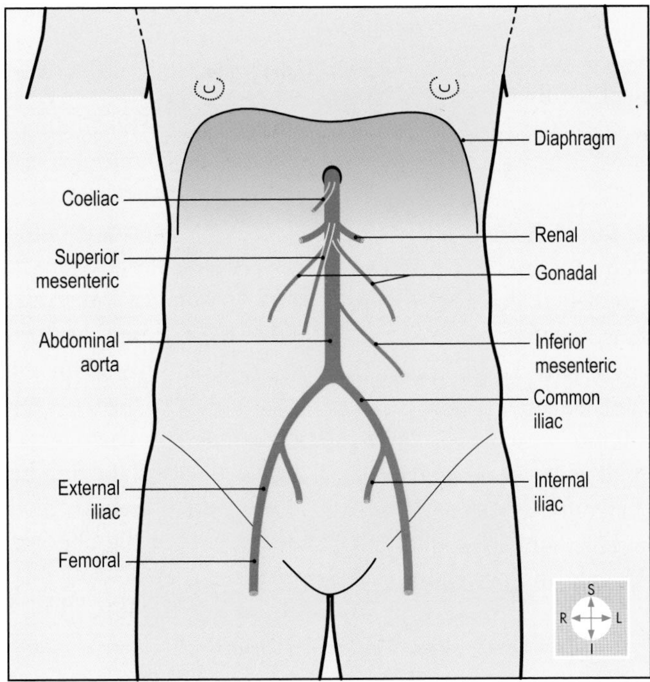

Fig. 4.9 Principal arteries of the abdomen.

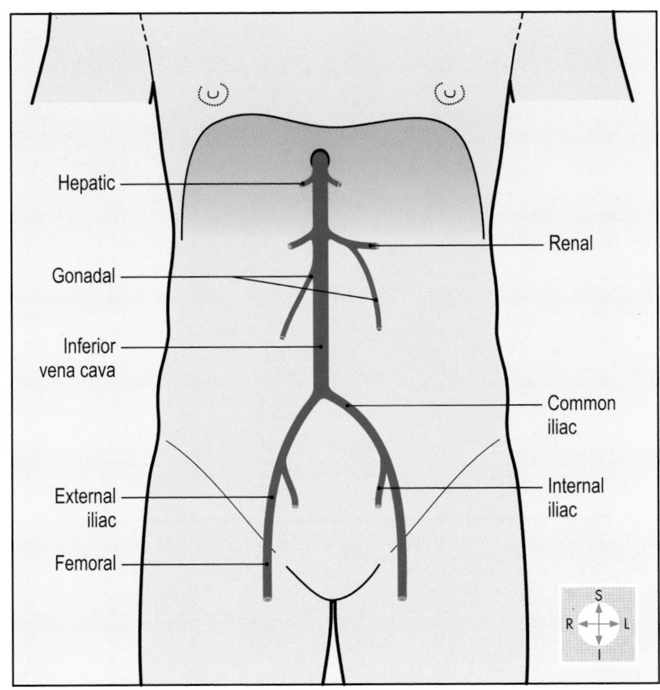

Fig. 4.10 Principal systemic veins of abdomen.

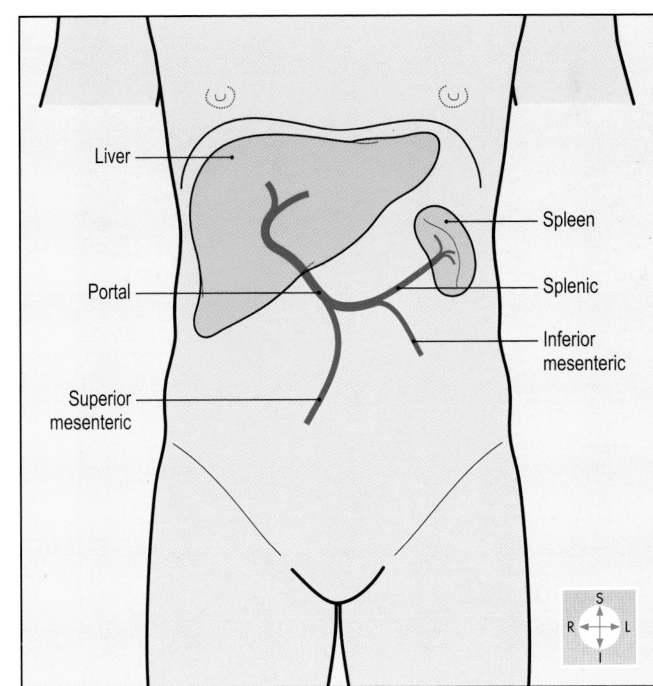

Fig. 4.11 Principal components of the portal venous system.

Anterior Abdominal Wall

The skin and subcutaneous tissue of the anterior abdominal wall overlie four muscles that move the trunk, control intra-abdominal pressure and support the abdominal contents. The main nerves and blood vessels lie in the neurovascular plane, deep to all but one of the muscles. Deep to the muscles are the transversalis fascia, extraperitoneal fat and the parietal peritoneum.

Skin and subcutaneous tissue

The midline umbilicus marks the site of former attachment of the umbilical cord. In a lean person it usually lies midway between the xiphisternum and the symphysis pubis, at the level of the fourth lumbar vertebra, but its position is variable.

The subcutaneous tissue has an outer fatty layer, which is particularly thick in obese individuals, and a deeper membranous layer, which lies on the external oblique muscle (Fig. 4.12). Although thin over most of the abdominal wall, the membranous layer becomes substantial inferiorly. Laterally, it descends into the thigh and attaches to the fascia lata, whilst medially it continues around the external genitalia into the perineum (see p. 244).

The subcutaneous tissue receives its blood from small branches of the arteries that supply the abdominal muscles. The superficial veins drain either upwards towards the axilla or downwards to the groin. The nerve supply to the skin is segmental and is provided by cutaneous branches of the lower thoracic spinal nerves and the first lumbar nerve (see Figs 4.2 & 4.3).

Muscles

On each side of the midline there are four principal muscles. Three of these are flat muscles, arranged in layers in the lateral part of the abdominal wall. External oblique is the most superficial, internal oblique lies deep to it and the deepest layer is transversus abdominis. As each of these muscles is traced anteriorly and medially its fleshy part gives way to an aponeurosis (Fig. 4.12). The aponeuroses of the flat muscles form a sheath around the fourth muscle, rectus abdominis. In the midline the aponeuroses from both sides interdigitate to form the linea alba, whilst inferiorly they attach to the pubic crest. These muscles are innervated by the lower six thoracic nerves and the first lumbar nerve (see p. 145).

Immediately above the groin the inguinal canal traverses the lowest part of the abdominal wall and transmits the spermatic cord in the male and the round ligament of the uterus in the female (see p. 146).

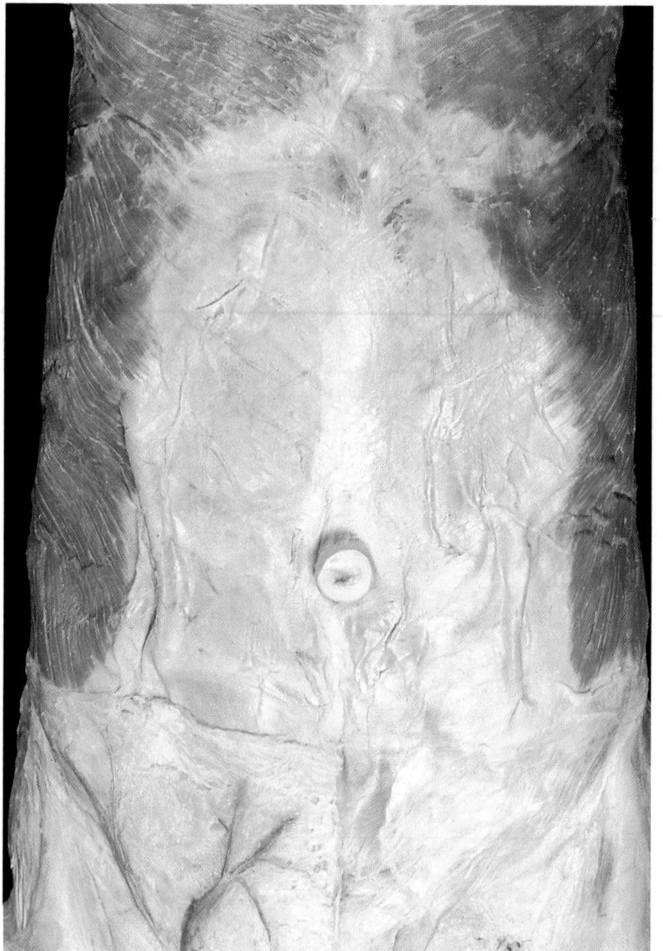

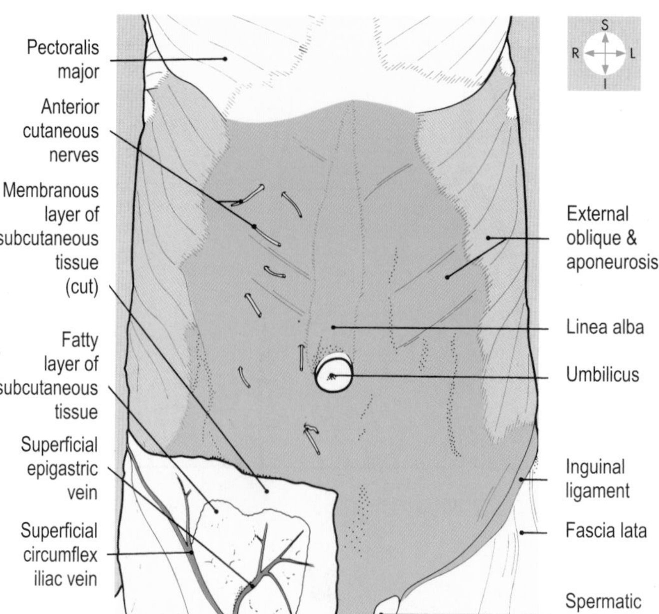

Fig. 4.12 External oblique muscles and aponeuroses. Some subcutaneous tissue, veins and cutaneous nerves have been preserved on one side.

External oblique

The muscle fibres of external oblique slope downwards and forwards (Fig. 4.13). Superiorly a series of fleshy slips attaches to the outer surfaces of the lower eight ribs, the upper slips interdigitating with serratus anterior, the lower ones with latissimus dorsi. The most posterior fibres attach inferiorly to the iliac crest; elsewhere, the fibres give way to the aponeurosis which passes medially in front of rectus abdominis to reach the linea alba. The aponeurosis possesses a free lower border that extends from the anterior superior iliac spine to the pubic tubercle and forms the inguinal ligament (see Figs 4.1 & 4.12), which marks the boundary between the abdominal wall and the anterior aspect of the thigh.

Immediately above the medial end of the inguinal ligament, the external oblique aponeurosis presents an aperture, the superficial inguinal ring, which is the medial opening of the inguinal canal (see p. 146).

Internal oblique

Internal oblique attaches to the lateral two-thirds of the inguinal ligament, to the anterior part of the iliac crest and to the thoracolumbar fascia (Fig. 4.15), through which it is anchored to the lumbar vertebrae. Most of its fibres slope forwards and upwards. The uppermost fibres attach to the costal margin between the ninth and twelfth ribs while the remainder give way to the aponeurosis of the muscle (Fig. 4.14).

Some aponeurotic fibres reach the linea alba by passing anterior to rectus abdominis, whilst others pass behind rectus (see p. 143). The lowest fibres arch medially and downwards, contributing to the roof of the inguinal canal. They unite with the underlying fibres of transversus to form the inguinal falx (conjoint tendon), which descends to the pecten pubis (pectineal line) on the pubic bone.

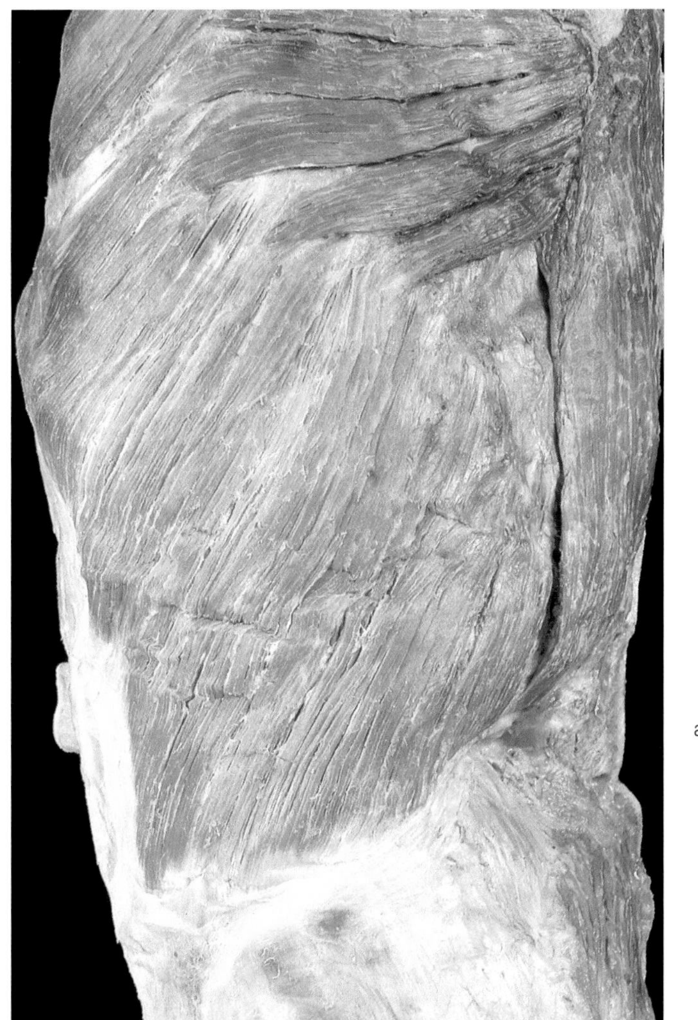

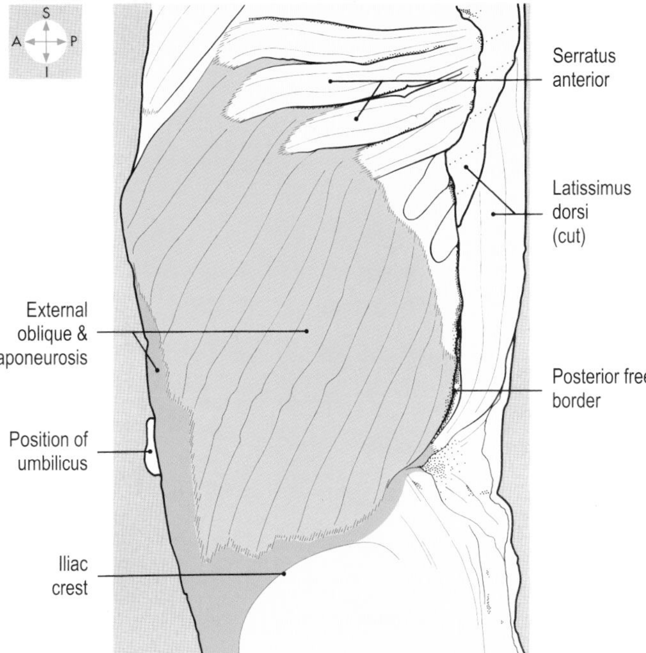

Fig. 4.13 The left external oblique showing its attachments to the lower ribs and the iliac crest.

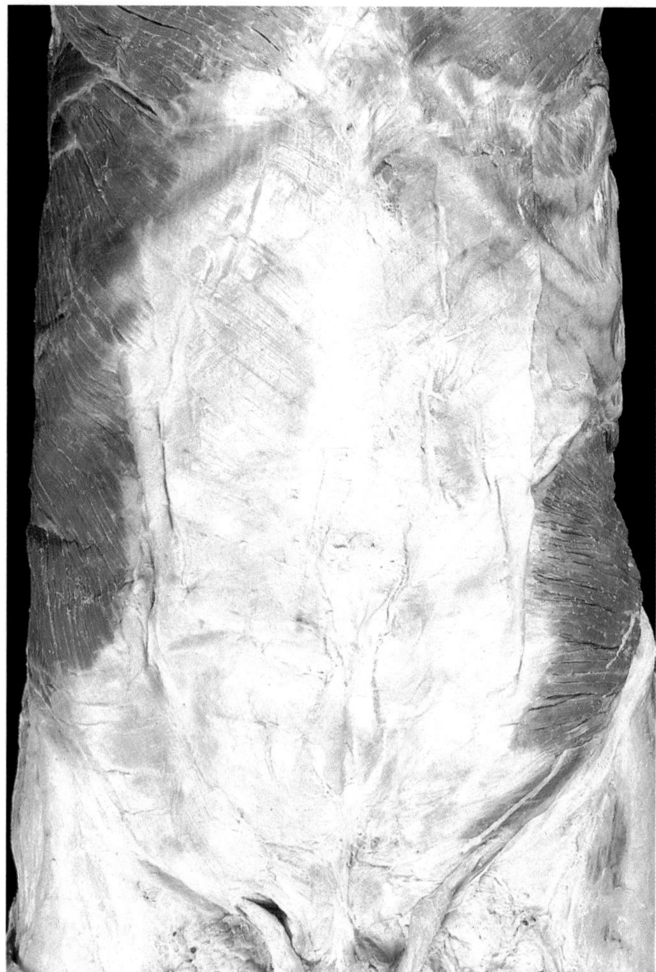

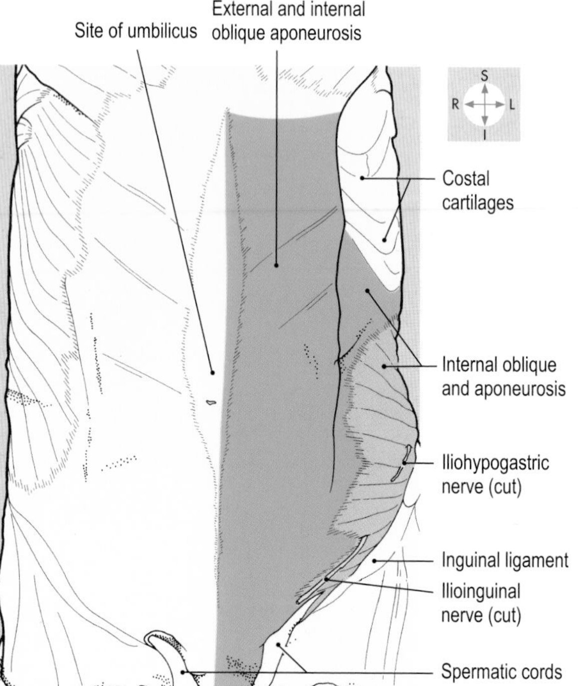

Fig. 4.14 Most of the left external oblique has been excised to reveal the underlying internal oblique muscle.

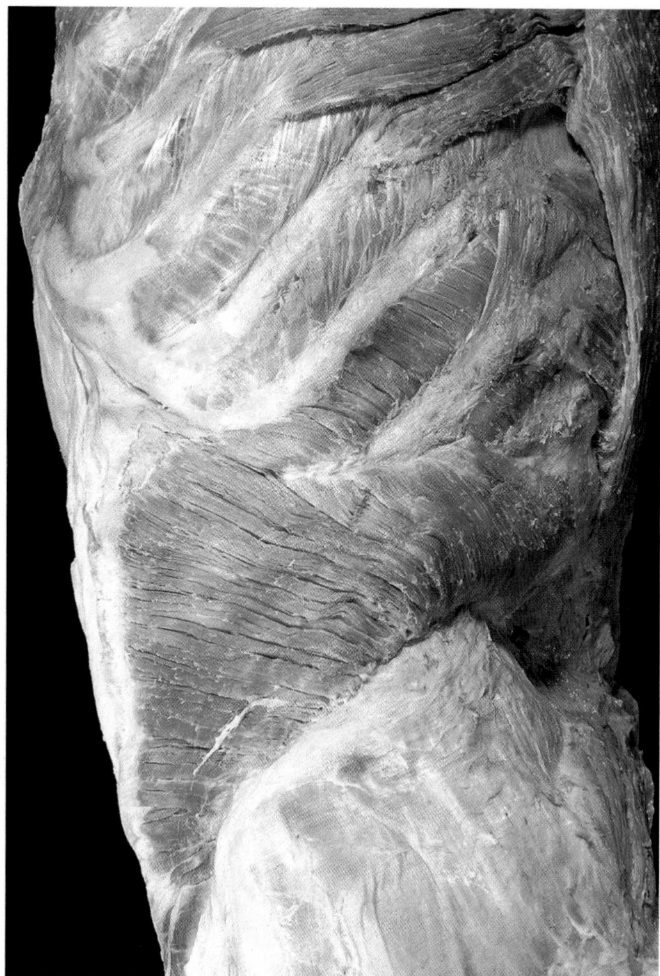

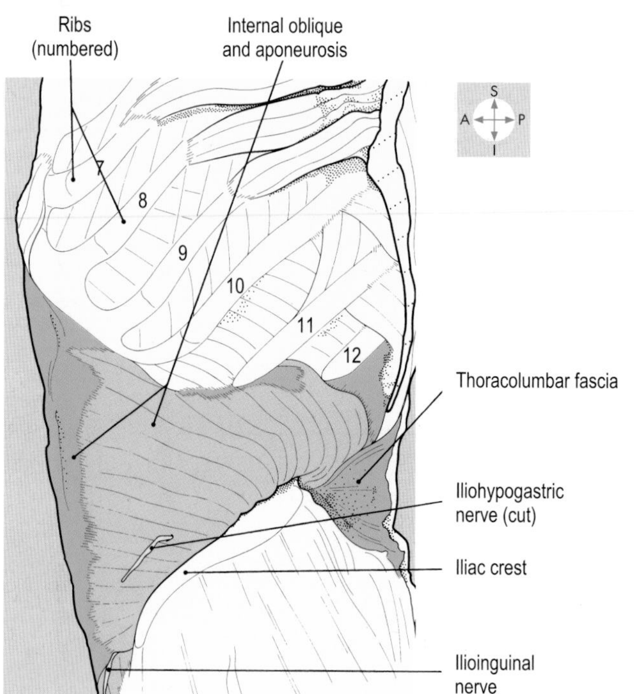

Fig. 4.15 Left internal oblique and attachments, revealed by removal of the external oblique. In this specimen the costal attachments of serratus anterior include the ninth rib.

Transversus abdominis

The upper part of this muscle arises from the inner aspects of the lower six costal cartilages (Fig. 4.17) by fleshy slips which interdigitate with the costal attachments of the diaphragm. The middle part of the muscle fuses with the thoracolumbar fascia while the lowest fibres attach to the iliac crest and the lateral half of the inguinal ligament. Most of the fibres run horizontally forwards and are replaced, near the lateral border of rectus, by an aponeurosis (Figs 4.16 & 4.18). The upper part of the aponeurosis reaches the linea alba by passing posterior to rectus abdominis while the inferior part passes anterior to it (see below).

The lowest fibres of transversus abdominis attach to the lateral part of the inguinal ligament and arch over the inguinal canal and, fusing with those of the overlying internal oblique, contribute to the inguinal falx.

Rectus abdominis

Rectus abdominis runs vertically on each side of the linea alba, from the pubis to the front of the chest wall (Fig. 4.16). The inferior attachment is to the anterior aspect of the pubic symphysis and to the pubic crest. The muscle widens superiorly and attaches to the anterior surfaces of the fifth, sixth and seventh costal cartilages. Its gently convex lateral border forms a surface feature called the linea semilunaris. Rectus abdominis is characterized by transverse tendinous intersections, usually at the levels of the xiphisternum, the umbilicus and midway between the two.

Rectus sheath

Rectus abdominis is enclosed in a sheath formed by the aponeuroses of the flat abdominal muscles. The anterior wall of the sheath, which is anchored to the tendinous intersections, covers the entire length of the muscle (see Fig. 4.14). By contrast, the posterior wall is not attached to the muscle and falls short of its superior and inferior extremities. Superiorly the posterior wall of the sheath terminates at the costal margin, above which rectus is in direct contact with the costal cartilages. Inferiorly the posterior wall continues only a short distance below the umbilicus, where it thins out or ends abruptly. In the latter case, the posterior wall has a recognizable inferior margin, the arcuate line (see Fig. 4.18), below which the posterior surface of rectus is in direct contact with the transversalis fascia.

In addition to rectus abdominis, the rectus sheath contains the small triangular pyramidalis muscle, the superior and inferior epigastric vessels (Figs 4.16 & 4.18) and the terminal parts of the lower six intercostal nerves that supply rectus and the overlying skin.

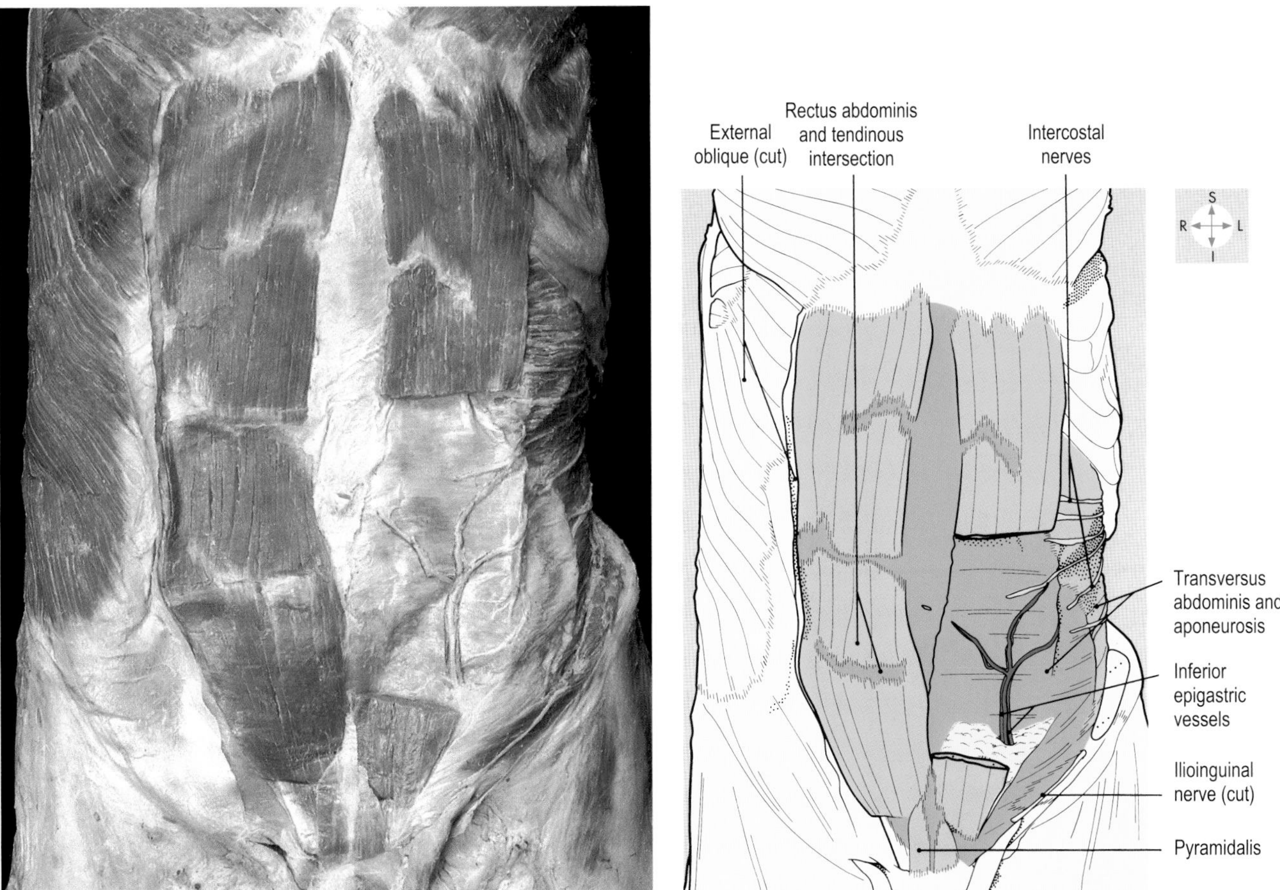

Fig. 4.16 Rectus abdominis muscles and neurovascular plane. The anterior walls of both rectus sheaths, the left oblique muscles and part of the left rectus abdominis have been removed.

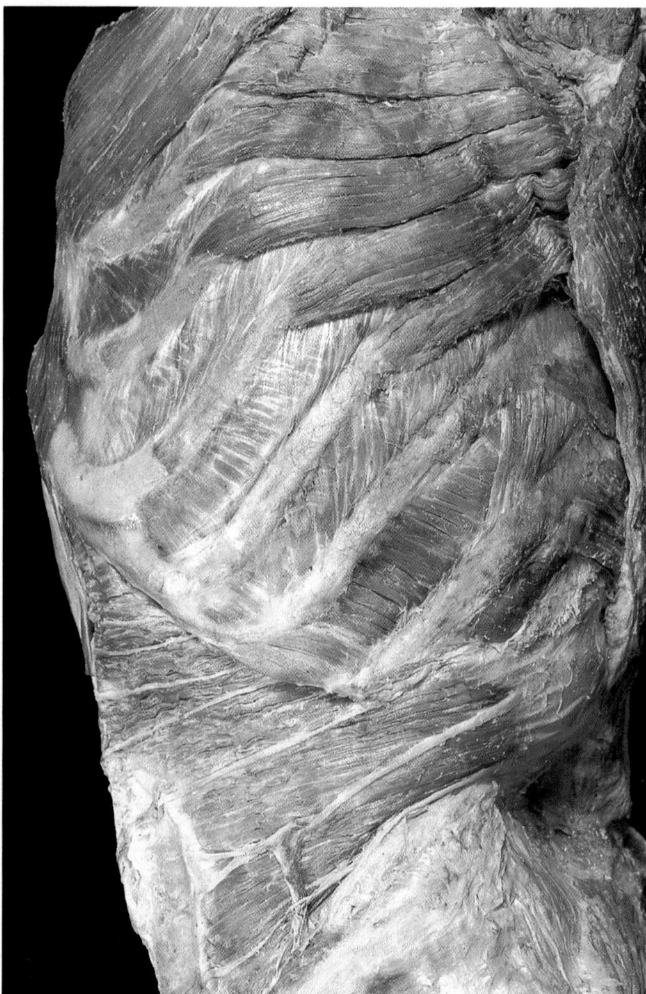

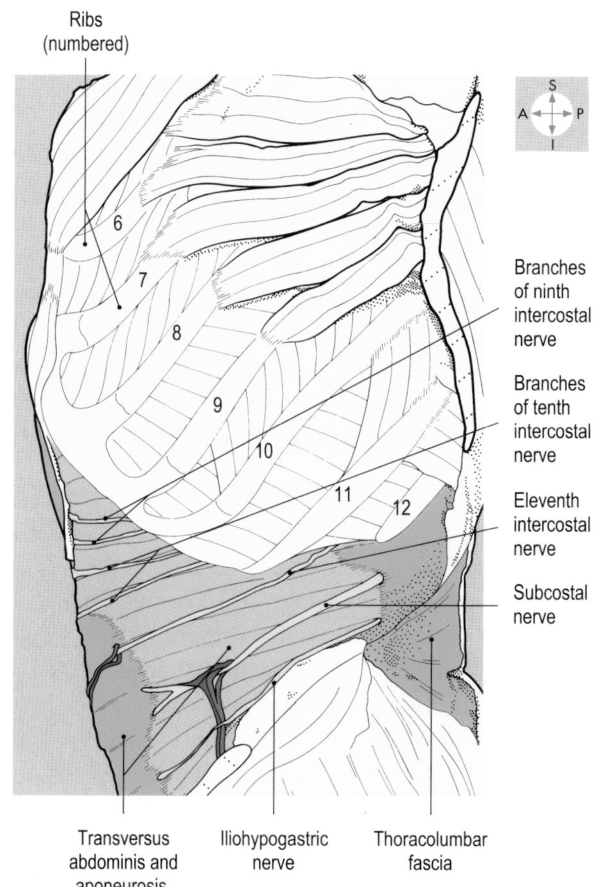

Fig. 4.17 Removal of the external and internal oblique muscles has revealed the transversus abdominis muscle and aponeurosis. Running across its surface are the lower intercostal, subcostal and iliohypogastric nerves.

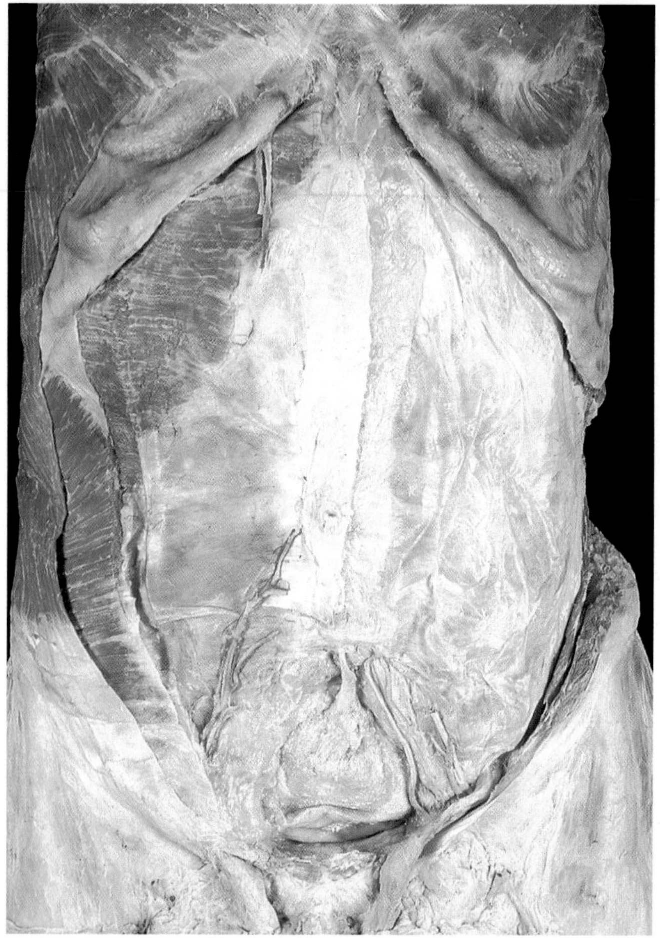

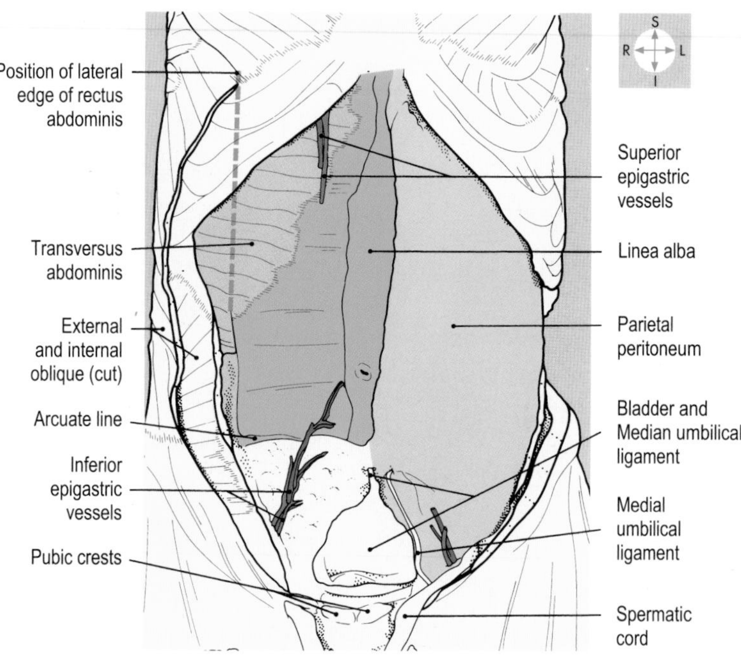

Fig. 4.18 On the right most of the oblique muscles and all of rectus abdominis have been excised to reveal the posterior wall of the rectus sheath. On the left all the muscles have been removed to show the parietal peritoneum. The bladder is enlarged.

Actions of abdominal muscles

The abdominal muscles flex the lumbar spine, rectus abdominis being particularly powerful in this action. Lateral flexion and rotation of the trunk are produced by coordinated contraction of the oblique muscles on both sides of the midline. Acting collectively, the abdominal muscles increase intra-abdominal pressure and, if the respiratory passages are open, the diaphragm is pushed upwards as in forced expiration, sneezing and coughing. Increased abdominal pressure with the airway closed (straining) occurs when lifting heavy objects and during defecation, childbirth and vomiting.

Structures deep to muscles

The deep surfaces of transversus and rectus abdominis are covered by the transversalis fascia, which forms part of a complete fascial sheet lying deep to the muscles surrounding the peritoneal cavity. Several names are given to this continuous fascial sheet and are derived from the muscles to which the fascia relates. For example, the iliac fascia and psoas fascia cover the iliacus and psoas muscles. Above the midpoint of the inguinal ligament an aperture in the transversalis fascia (the deep inguinal ring) forms the lateral opening of the inguinal canal.

Deep to the transversalis fascia is the extraperitoneal fat, which contains four vestigial structures converging on the umbilicus. Descending from the liver is the round ligament of the liver (ligamentum teres hepatis; see Figs 4.30 & 4.59), the remnant of the left umbilical vein. Ascending in the midline from the urinary bladder is the median umbilical ligament or urachus (see Fig. 4.18). Inclining upwards from each side of the pelvis is the occluded part of the umbilical artery.

The deepest layer of the abdominal wall is the parietal peritoneum (see Fig. 4.18). Although the peritoneum and the abdominal musculature are adherent in most areas, they are only loosely attached between the pubis and umbilicus. Therefore, an enlarging bladder intervenes between them and the organ can be approached surgically through the abdominal wall without traversing the peritoneal cavity.

Nerves and vessels

The skin, muscles and parietal peritoneum of the anterior abdominal wall are innervated by the lower six thoracic nerves and the first lumbar nerve.

Lower thoracic nerves

At the costal margin, thoracic nerves seven to eleven leave their intercostal spaces and enter the neurovascular plane of the abdominal wall between transversus abdominis and internal oblique (Fig. 4.17). The seventh and eighth nerves slope upwards, the ninth runs horizontally and the tenth and eleventh incline downwards. The nerves pierce rectus abdominis and the anterior layer of the rectus sheath to emerge as anterior cutaneous branches that supply the overlying skin (see Fig. 4.12).

The subcostal nerve (T12) takes the line of the twelfth rib across the posterior abdominal wall (see p. 201). It continues around the flank in the neurovascular plane and terminates in a similar manner to the lower intercostal nerves.

The seventh to twelfth thoracic nerves give off lateral cutaneous nerves which further divide into anterior and posterior branches. The anterior branches supply skin as far forwards as the lateral edge of rectus abdominis while the posterior branches supply skin overlying latissimus dorsi. The lateral cutaneous branch of the subcostal nerve is distributed to the skin on the side of the buttock.

First lumbar nerve

The first lumbar nerve divides into upper and lower branches, the iliohypogastric and ilioinguinal nerves (see Figs 4.102 & 4.103). The iliohypogastric nerve reaches the neurovascular plane in the loin and divides just above the iliac crest into two terminal branches. The lateral cutaneous branch supplies the side of the buttock and the anterior cutaneous branch supplies the suprapubic region.

The ilioinguinal nerve leaves the neurovascular plane by piercing internal oblique above the iliac crest (see Fig. 4.14). It continues between the two oblique muscles and accompanies the spermatic cord or round ligament of the uterus in the inguinal canal (see Figs 4.21 & 4.24). Emerging from the superficial inguinal ring (Fig 4.20), it gives cutaneous branches to skin on the medial side of the root of the thigh, the proximal part of the penis and front of the scrotum or the mons pubis and the anterior part of the labium majus.

Blood vessels

The blood supply to the abdominal wall is provided by the superior and inferior epigastric arteries, supplemented by the musculophrenic artery and the lower posterior intercostal arteries. The superior epigastric artery descends behind rectus abdominis and may anastomose with the inferior epigastric artery (Fig. 4.18). The latter vessel arises from the external iliac artery immediately above the inguinal ligament and inclines upwards and medially, passing just medial to the deep inguinal ring (Figs 4.18 & 4.23). The inferior epigastric artery enters the rectus sheath by passing in front of its posterior wall at the arcuate line. From the anterior ends of the lower two or three intercostal spaces, posterior intercostal arteries continue forwards in the neurovascular plane.

Venous drainage of the deeper layers of the abdominal wall is via venae comitantes of the respective arteries. Blood from the superficial tissues drains into veins, lying in the subcutaneous tissue, which run towards the axilla and groin. Dilatation of the subcutaneous veins is an important clinical sign in patients with obstruction of venous flow within the abdomen, for example, within the inferior vena cava or the liver.

Lymphatics

Lymph from the abdominal wall above the level of the umbilicus drains upwards. Lymphatics from the skin and subcutaneous tissue accompany the subcutaneous veins and drain into the axillary nodes, whilst those from the deeper tissues follow the course of the superior epigastric artery to the internal thoracic nodes. The superficial lymphatics of the lower half of the abdominal wall pass to the superficial inguinal nodes while the deeper lymph vessels follow the course of the inferior epigastric artery to reach the external iliac nodes.

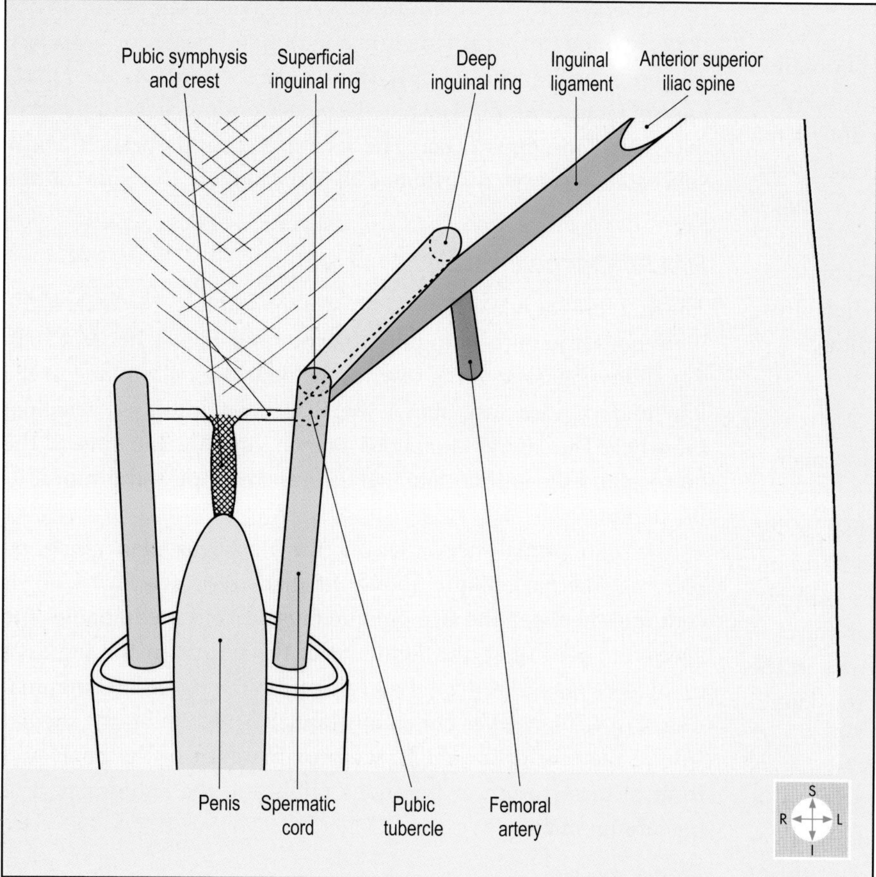

Fig. 4.19 Position of the inguinal canal and its superficial and deep rings in relation to the inguinal ligament.

Inguinal Canal

The inguinal canal is about 4 cm long and passes obliquely through the flat muscles of the abdominal wall just above the medial half of the inguinal ligament (Fig. 4.19). In the male the canal conveys the spermatic cord (comprising the ductus [vas] deferens and the vessels and nerves of the testis). In the female the canal is narrower and contains the round ligament of the uterus.

The lateral end of the canal opens into the abdominal cavity at the midinguinal point, defined as midway between the pubic symphysis and the anterior superior iliac spine. In clinical practice the midinguinal point serves as a guide to the deep inguinal ring and the femoral artery (see p. 136). There may be individual variation in the relative positions of the deep inguinal ring, the femoral artery, and the bony landmarks, and some authors refer to the midinguinal point or the midpoint of the inguinal ligament as appropriate surface markings. The medial end of the canal opens into the subcutaneous tissues at the superficial inguinal ring, an aperture in the external oblique aponeurosis immediately superior to the pubic tubercle (Fig. 4.20). Continuous with the margins of the superficial ring is a thin sleeve surrounding the spermatic cord, the external spermatic fascia (see Fig. 4.21).

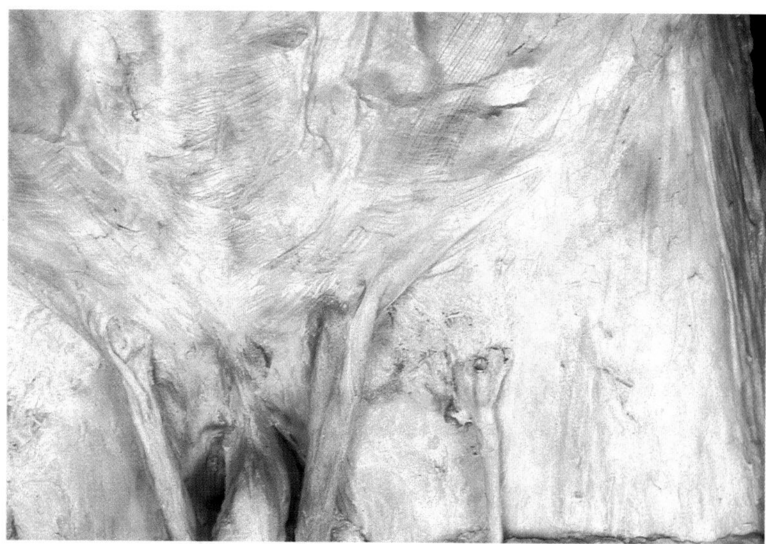

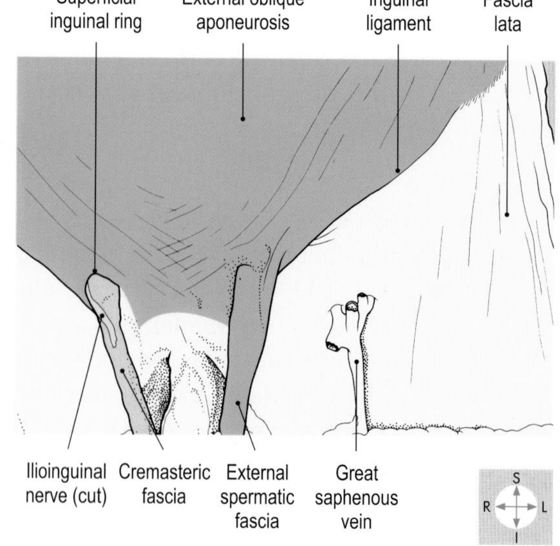

Fig. 4.20 Removal of the skin and subcutaneous tissue reveals both superficial inguinal rings (male specimen). On one side the external spermatic fascia has been removed to show the margins of the superficial ring.

Boundaries

The canal comprises a floor, a roof, and an anterior and a posterior wall. The gutter-shaped floor is formed by the inguinal ligament (see Fig. 4.22), the inturned lower edge of the external oblique aponeurosis. The ligament attaches laterally to the anterior superior iliac spine and medially to the pubic tubercle and the pectineal line of the pubis. The expanded medial end of the inguinal ligament, the lacunar ligament, lies in the floor of the medial end of the canal, and its concave lateral edge forms the medial boundary of the femoral ring (see Fig. 4.23 and p. 147).

The roof is formed by the lowest fibres of internal oblique and transversus abdominis (Fig. 4.22). These fibres arch over the canal and pass medially and downwards to form the inguinal falx (conjoint tendon), which attaches to the crest and pectineal line of the pubis. The anterior wall of the canal is formed by the external oblique aponeurosis, supplemented laterally by fibres of internal oblique. These fibres arise from the lateral part of the inguinal ligament and cover the anterior aspect of the deep ring (Fig. 4.21). The posterior wall is formed by the transversalis fascia, reinforced medially by the conjoint tendon. Deep to the transversalis fascia are the

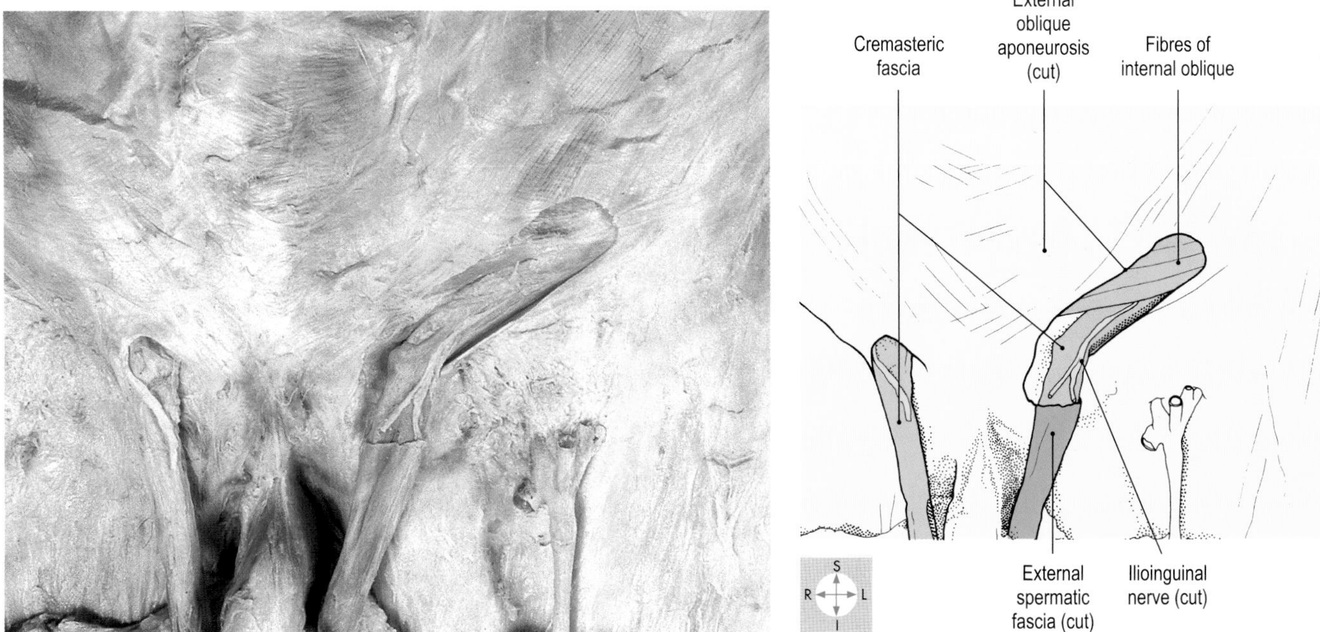

Fig. 4.21 External spermatic fascia and a strip of the external oblique aponeurosis have been removed to show the spermatic cord and ilioinguinal nerve within the canal.

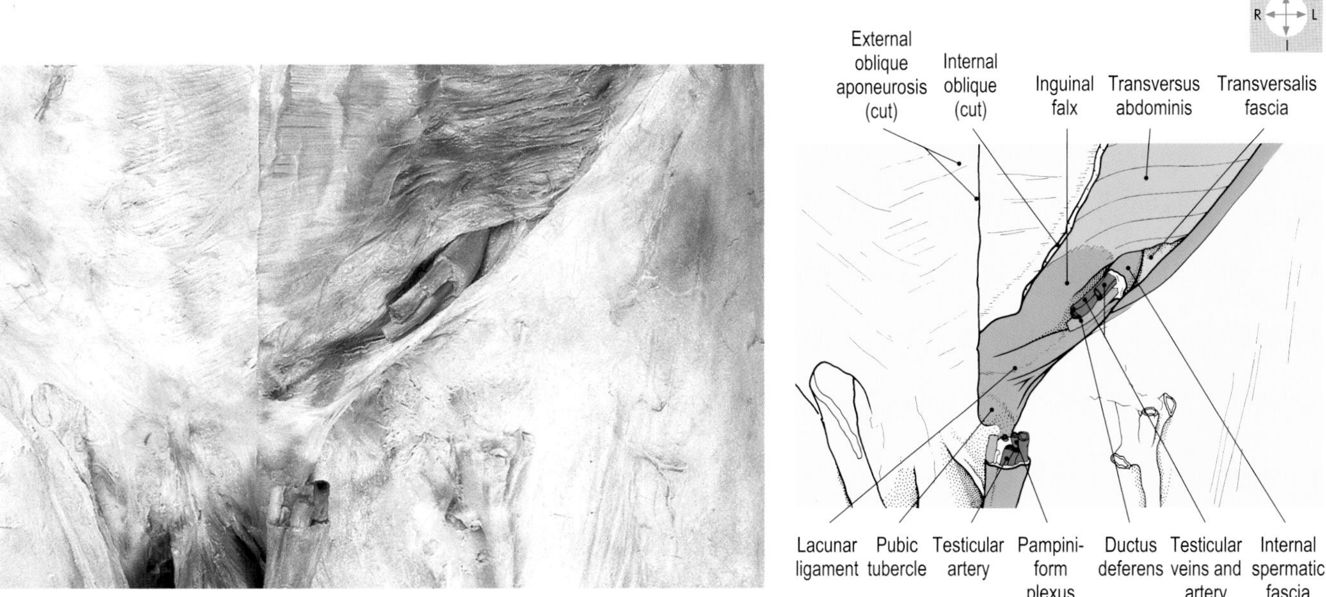

Fig. 4.22 Lower fibres of internal oblique and part of the spermatic cord have been excised to reveal the posterior wall and floor of the canal.

inferior epigastric vessels, which lie just medial to the deep ring (Fig. 4.23).

The inguinal canal is a site of potential weakness in the abdominal wall through which intra-abdominal structures may pass, producing an inguinal hernia (see below). However, several features of the canal's anatomy minimize this weakness. The obliquity of the canal ensures that the superficial and deep inguinal rings do not overlie one another (see Fig. 4.19). Furthermore, the strongest part of the anterior wall lies in front of the deep ring and the strongest part of the posterior wall lies behind the superficial ring. Hence, when pressure within the abdomen rises, the anterior and posterior walls of the canal are firmly opposed. In addition, when the abdominal muscles contract, the canal is compressed by the descent of fibres of internal oblique and transversus abdominis in its roof.

Contents

In the male, the canal contains the spermatic cord (Fig. 4.21). In the female, it transmits the round ligament of the uterus (Fig. 4.24), a fibromuscular cord running from the body of the uterus to the subcutaneous tissues of the labium majus. Lymphatics from part of the body of the uterus accompany the round ligament and terminate in the superficial inguinal nodes (see Fig. 6.11).

In both sexes the ilioinguinal nerve (see Fig. 4.14) lies deep to the external oblique aponeurosis close to the inguinal ligament. The nerve runs medially in the anterior wall of the canal and emerges through the superficial ring (Figs 4.20 & 4.24).

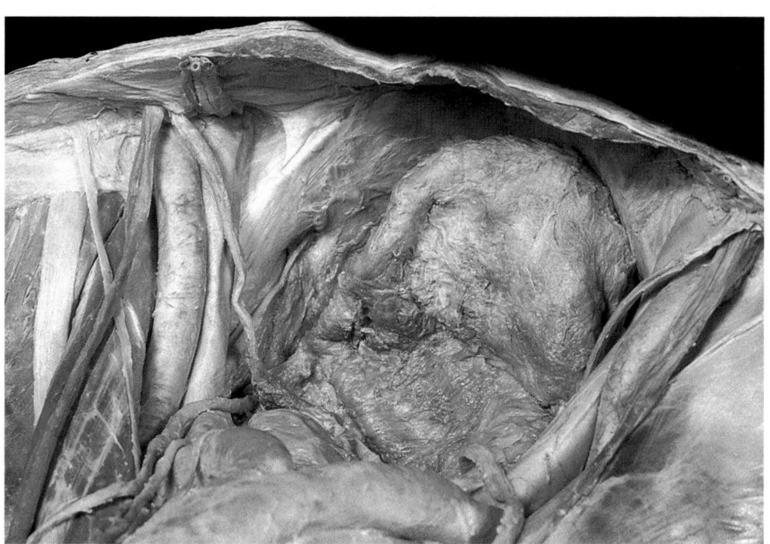

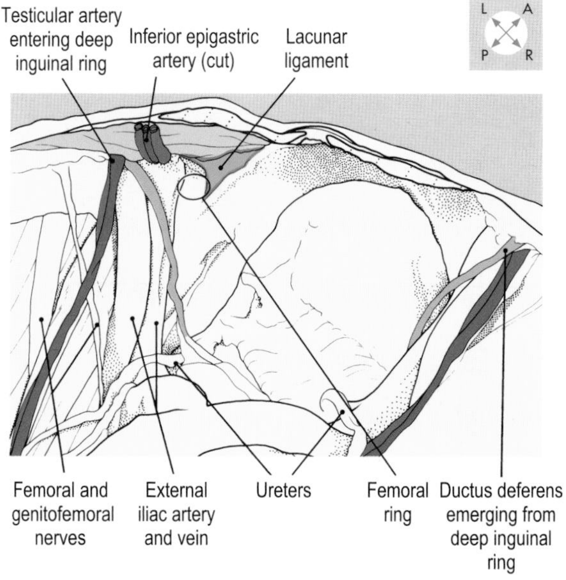

Fig. 4.23 Superior view of the male pelvis to show structures near the deep inguinal ring.

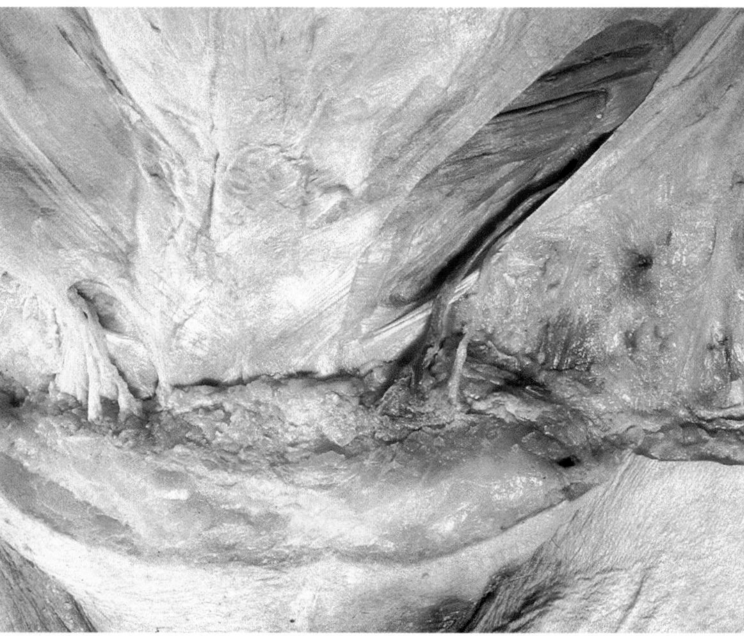

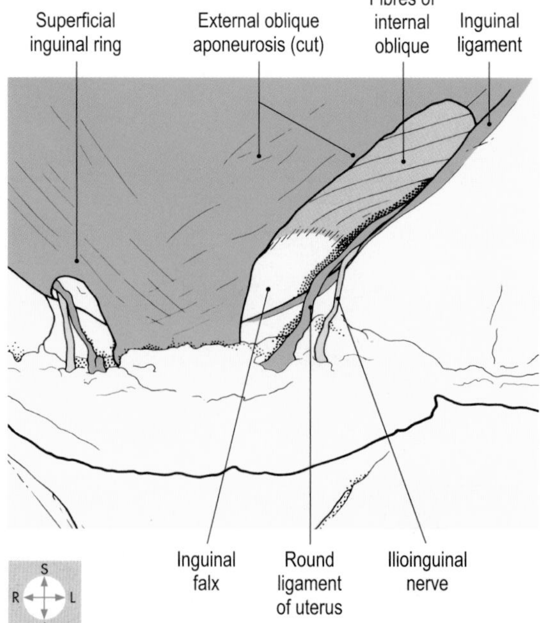

Fig. 4.24 Superficial ring and inguinal canal in the female showing the round ligaments of the uterus.

Inguinal hernias

The inguinal canal is the most common site for an abdominal hernia. Two types of inguinal hernia are recognized. The direct type passes through the inguinal falx into the medial part of the canal. By contrast, the indirect (oblique) type traverses the deep ring and turns medially along the canal. Hernias of both types may emerge through the superficial ring and descend into the scrotum or labium majus. Direct and indirect hernias are distinguished by their relationships to the inferior epigastric vessels. A direct hernia lies on the medial side of these vessels while the indirect type enters the inguinal canal lateral to them.

The processus vaginalis normally closes but may remain patent in infancy, leaving a tubular channel connecting with the peritoneal cavity. Herniation along the patent processus, called an infantile inguinal hernia, is more common in the male child and may extend into the tunica vaginalis around the testis (see p. 151).

Scrotum

The scrotum is a pouch of skin and fascia derived from the anterior abdominal wall and contains the testes, epididymides and the lower parts of the spermatic cords (Fig. 4.25).

Skin and subcutaneous tissue

The skin of the scrotum is supplied anteriorly by the external pudendal vessels and innervated by the ilioinguinal nerve. The remainder of the scrotal skin is supplied by branches of the internal pudendal vessels and branches of the pudendal nerve and posterior cutaneous nerve of thigh. Lymph drains to the superficial inguinal nodes.

Deep to the skin lies the subcutaneous tissue, continuous superiorly with the subcutaneous tissue of the abdominal wall. The scrotal subcutaneous tissue, which contains smooth muscle called dartos, but little fat, forms a median septum, dividing the pouch into right and left sides.

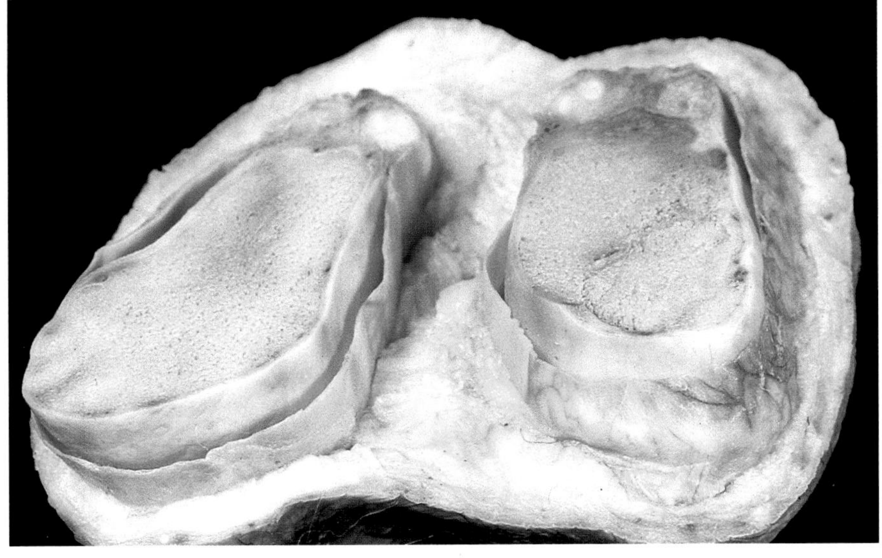

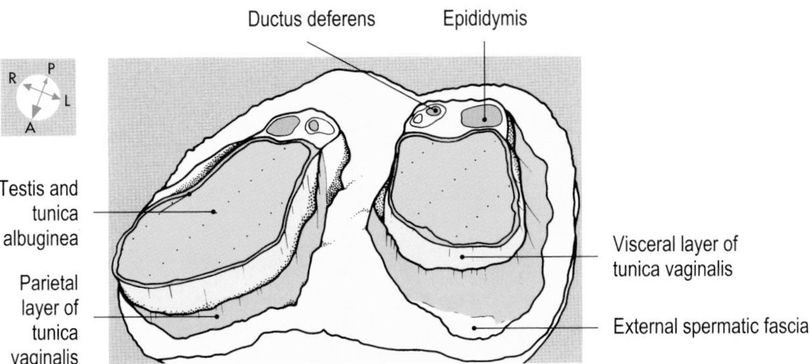

Fig. 4.25 Transverse section through scrotum. The spermatic fasciae are trimmed flush with the subcutaneous tissue.

Spermatic fasciae

Deep to the subcutaneous tissue of each side of the scrotum lie three layers of spermatic fascia (Fig. 4.26). Each layer takes the form of a sleeve derived from one of the layers of the abdominal wall.

The outermost sleeve, the external spermatic fascia, begins at the superficial inguinal ring and is continuous with the external oblique aponeurosis (see Fig. 4.20). The intermediate sleeve is the cremasteric fascia and muscle, continuous within the inguinal canal with the internal oblique muscle (see Fig. 4.21). The transversalis fascia of the abdominal wall (see Fig. 4.22) provides the deepest sleeve, the internal spermatic fascia, which commences at the deep inguinal ring. These three fascial layers surround the components of the spermatic cord and continue downwards to enclose the testis and epididymis.

Spermatic cord

The spermatic cord runs from the deep inguinal ring into the scrotum, terminating posterior to the testis. The cord comprises the ductus (vas) deferens and the vessels and nerves of the testis and epididymis (Fig. 4.27) surrounded by the layers of spermatic fascia (Fig. 4.26).

The principal artery of the spermatic cord is the testicular artery, a branch of the abdominal aorta (see Figs 4.88, 4.89). Also present is the artery to the ductus deferens (Fig. 4.28), usually arising from the superior vesical artery within the pelvic cavity. The

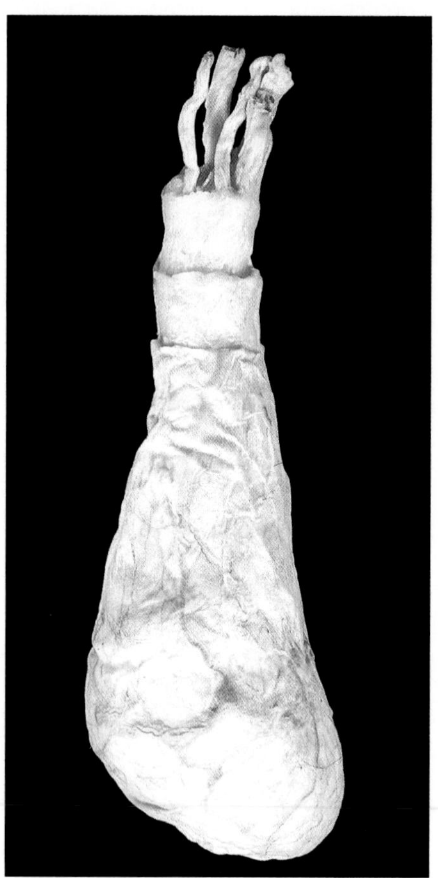

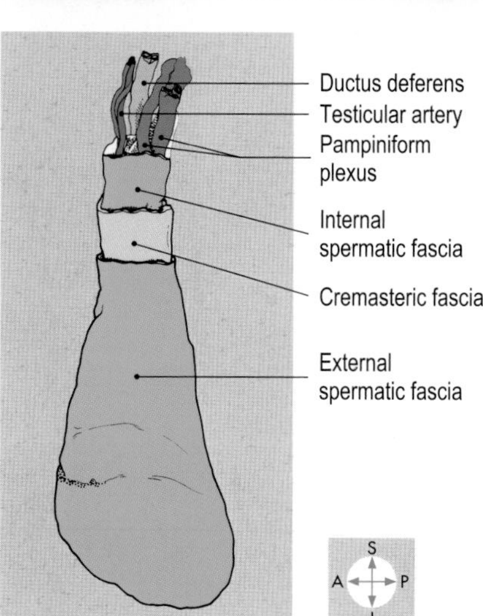

Fig. 4.26 Left testis and spermatic cord within their fascial sleeves.

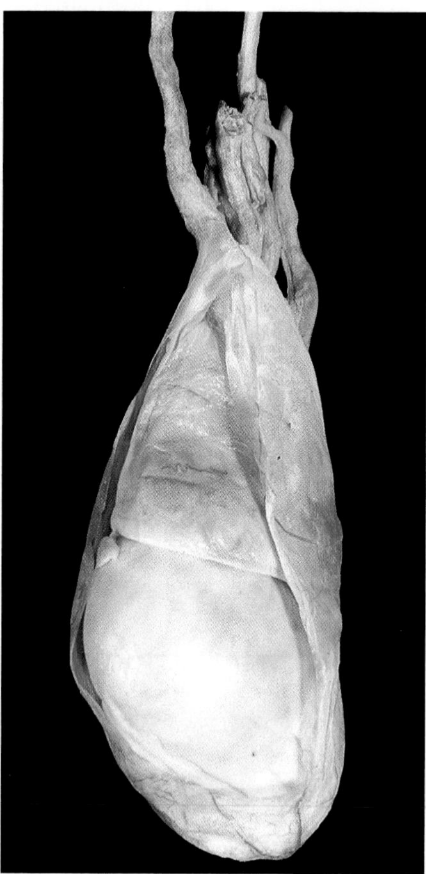

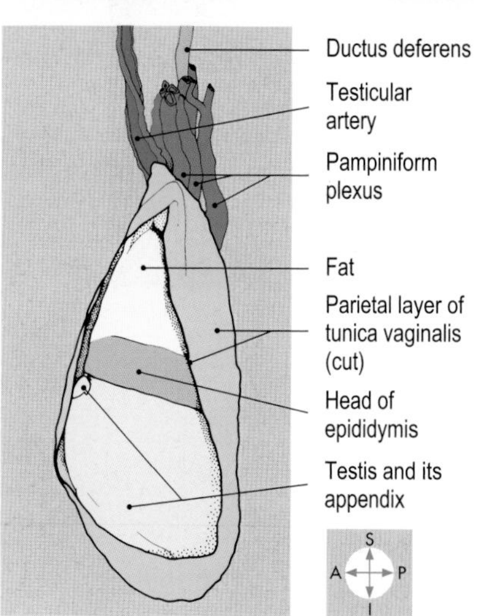

Fig. 4.27 Anterolateral part of the parietal layer of the tunica vaginalis has been removed to reveal the testis and head of the epididymis. This testis bears a vestigial tag, the appendix of the testis.

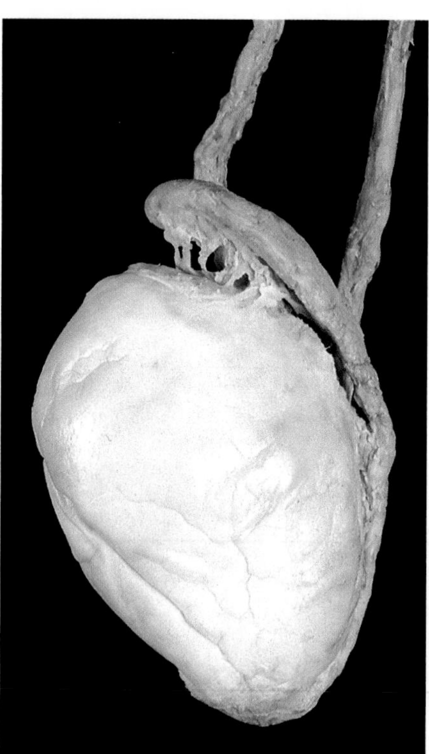

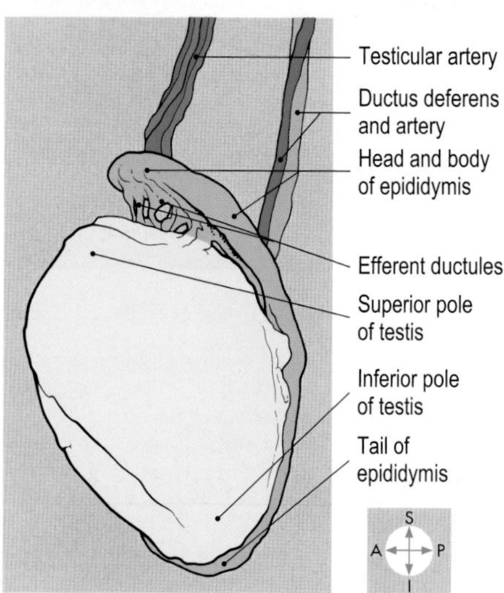

Fig. 4.28 Lateral aspect of testis and epididymis after removal of the tunica vaginalis and pampiniform plexus. The head of the epididymis has been lifted to display the efferent ducts.

veins draining the testis and epididymis form a network, the pampiniform plexus. Occasionally, these veins become dilated, a condition known as a varicocele. From this plexus, one or two veins continue through the deep inguinal ring and ascend the posterior abdominal wall with the testicular artery (see Fig. 4.88). The testicular vessels are accompanied by a plexus of autonomic nerves and by lymph vessels which terminate in the aortic lymph nodes.

Tunica vaginalis

The tunica vaginalis is a closed serous sac which covers the medial, anterior and lateral surfaces of the testis and the lateral aspect of the epididymis (Figs 4.25 & 4.27). Like the peritoneum from which it is derived, the tunica vaginalis has parietal and visceral layers separated by a small quantity of serous fluid. An excessive accumulation of fluid in the sac produces a swelling (hydrocele) anterior to the testis.

In the fetus the processus vaginalis links the tunica vaginalis with the peritoneal cavity. Usually, the processus closes before birth, but occasionally it remains patent.

Testis

The testis is an ovoid organ approximately 5 cm long in the adult, suspended by the spermatic cord in the lower part of the scrotum with its superior pole tilted slightly forwards (Fig. 4.28). The testis has a thick fibrous capsule, the tunica albuginea, which is covered laterally, anteriorly and medially by the visceral layer of the tunica vaginalis (Fig. 4.25). The posterior surface of the organ, devoid of a covering of tunica vaginalis, is pierced by the efferent ductules, branches of the testicular artery and numerous small veins that form the pampiniform plexus (Figs 4.28 & 4.29).

Epididymis

The epididymis consists of a narrow, highly convoluted duct applied to the posterior surface of the testis (Fig. 4.29). Its broad superior part, the head, overhangs the upper pole of the testis, from which it receives several efferent ductules (Fig. 4.28). The body of the epididymis tapers into the tail, which is continuous with the ductus deferens. The epididymis is supplied by branches of the testicular artery and drained by the pampiniform plexus.

Ductus (vas) deferens

The ductus deferens is approximately 25 cm long and connects the tail of the epididymis with the ejaculatory duct in the prostate gland. The ductus ascends behind the testis on the medial side of the epididymis and continues upwards in the cord. When the upper part of the scrotum is palpated, the ductus can be distinguished from the accompanying testicular vessels by its firm consistency.

After traversing the inguinal canal, the ductus runs backwards across the pelvic brim and along the lateral wall of the pelvis (see Fig. 4.23) before terminating in the ejaculatory duct (see p. 229).

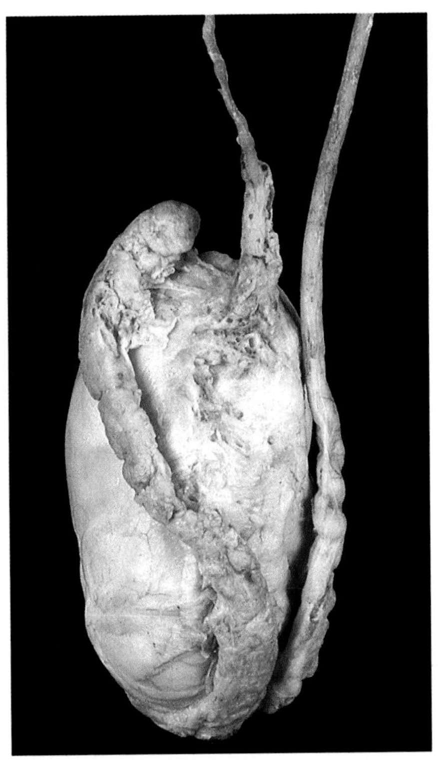

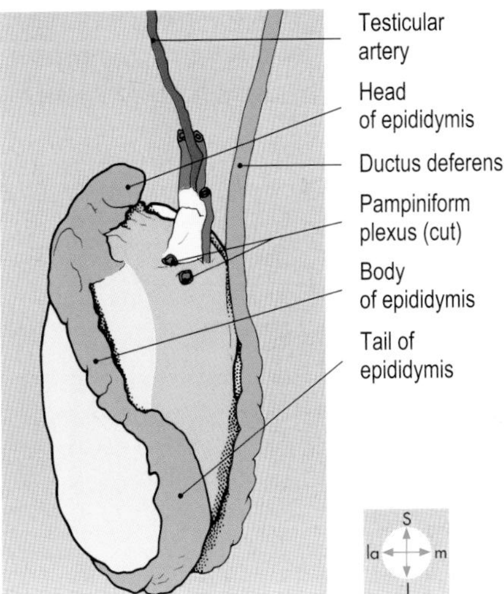

Fig. 4.29 Posterior view of testis, epididymis and ductus deferens.

Peritoneum

The peritoneum is a serous membrane with parietal and visceral layers which encloses a space, the peritoneal cavity. The parietal peritoneum lines the walls of the abdomen and pelvis while the visceral layer covers many of the abdominal and pelvic organs. In the male the peritoneal cavity is a closed sac, but in the female it communicates with the interior of the uterus and vagina via a microscopic channel through each uterine tube. Normally, the peritoneal cavity contains only a few millilitres of serous fluid, but in certain diseases serous fluid can accumulate (ascites), sometimes up to several litres.

The peritoneal cavity comprises the greater and lesser sacs. The greater sac is very extensive and can be traced from the diaphragm above into the pelvic cavity below. The omental bursa (lesser sac) is located in the upper part of the abdomen behind the stomach and communicates with the greater sac through a narrow opening, the omental (epiploic) foramen.

Parietal peritoneum

The parietal peritoneum is applied to the inner aspect of the abdominal and pelvic walls (Fig. 4.30) and continues superiorly across most of the undersurface of the diaphragm. The peritoneum lining the anterior abdominal wall is raised into several folds or ridges. Below the umbilicus the median umbilical ligament often raises a midline ridge (median umbilical fold), on each side of which the occluded part of the umbilical artery (medial umbilical ligament) may produce a further peritoneal fold (medial umbilical fold) (Fig. 4.31). Above the umbilicus the round ligament of the liver (Fig. 4.30) is contained in a large fold of peritoneum, the falciform ligament, which attaches the liver to the anterior abdominal wall and the diaphragm (see Fig. 4.57).

Posteriorly, the peritoneum covers several organs that lie on the muscles of the posterior abdominal wall (Fig. 4.32). These retroperitoneal organs include the ascending and descending parts of the colon, the kidneys, ureters and suprarenal glands, and most of the pancreas and duodenum. Also lying behind the peritoneum are the aorta and its branches, and the inferior vena cava and its tributaries.

Nerve supply

The parietal peritoneum of the abdominal wall is innervated by the lower thoracic and first lumbar nerves. Inflammation spreading from an organ such as the appendix to this peritoneum causes well-localized pain and tenderness, and rigidity of the abdominal muscles. The lower thoracic nerves also innervate the peritoneum covering the periphery of the diaphragm. Inflammation of this peritoneum consequently gives rise to pain in the lower thoracic wall and abdominal wall. By contrast, the peritoneum on the central part of the diaphragm receives sensory branches from the phrenic nerves (C3, C4 & C5) and irritation here may produce pain referred to the region of the shoulder (the fourth cervical dermatome; see Fig 3.6).

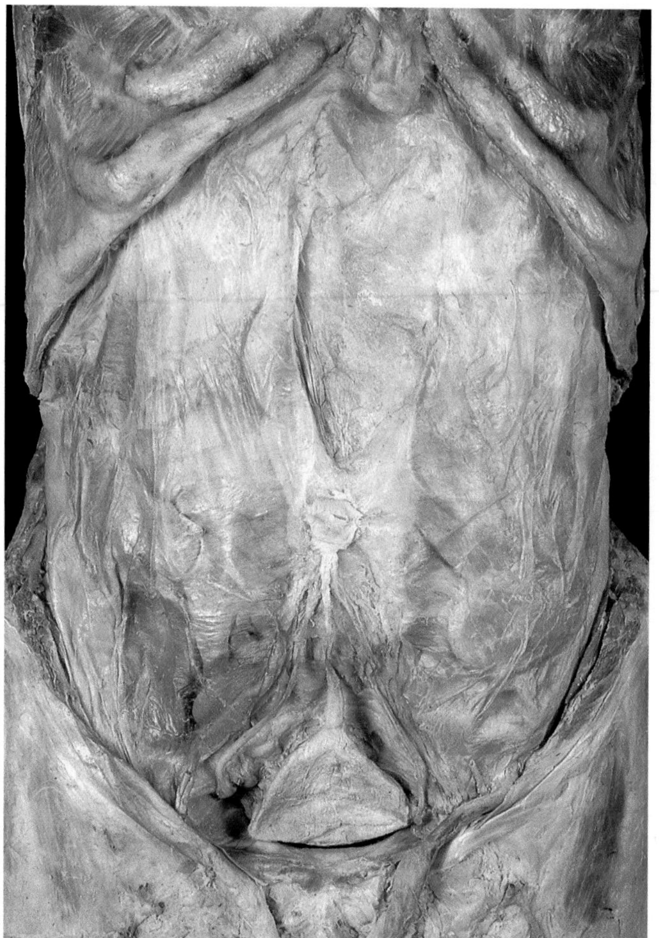

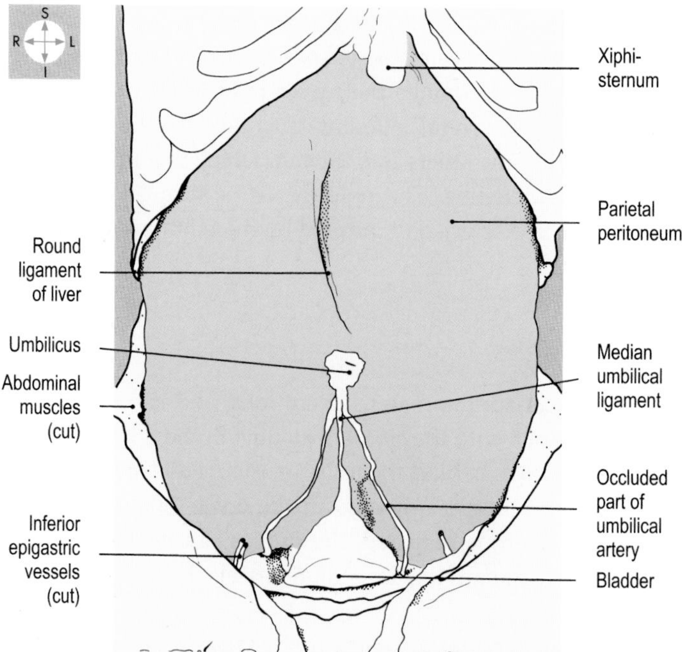

Fig. 4.30 Removal of muscles and fascia of the anterior abdominal wall reveals the parietal peritoneum and extraperitoneal structures.

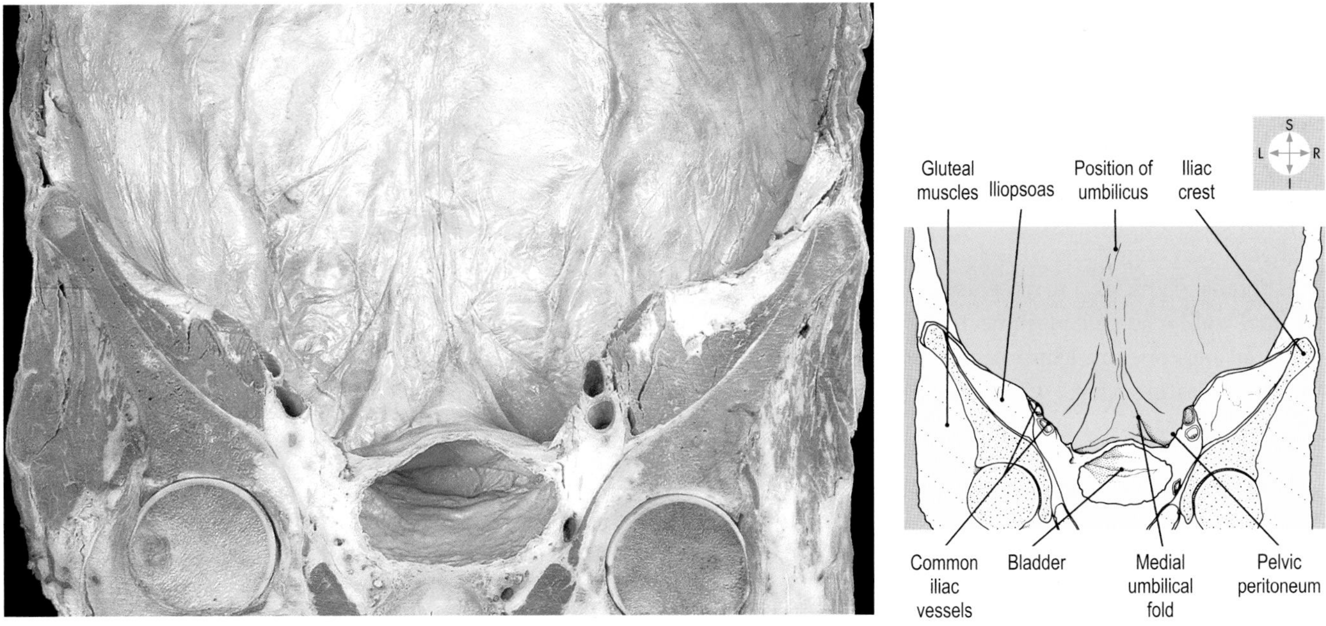

Fig. 4.31 Removal of the abdominal organs from a coronal section shows the parietal peritoneum from within.

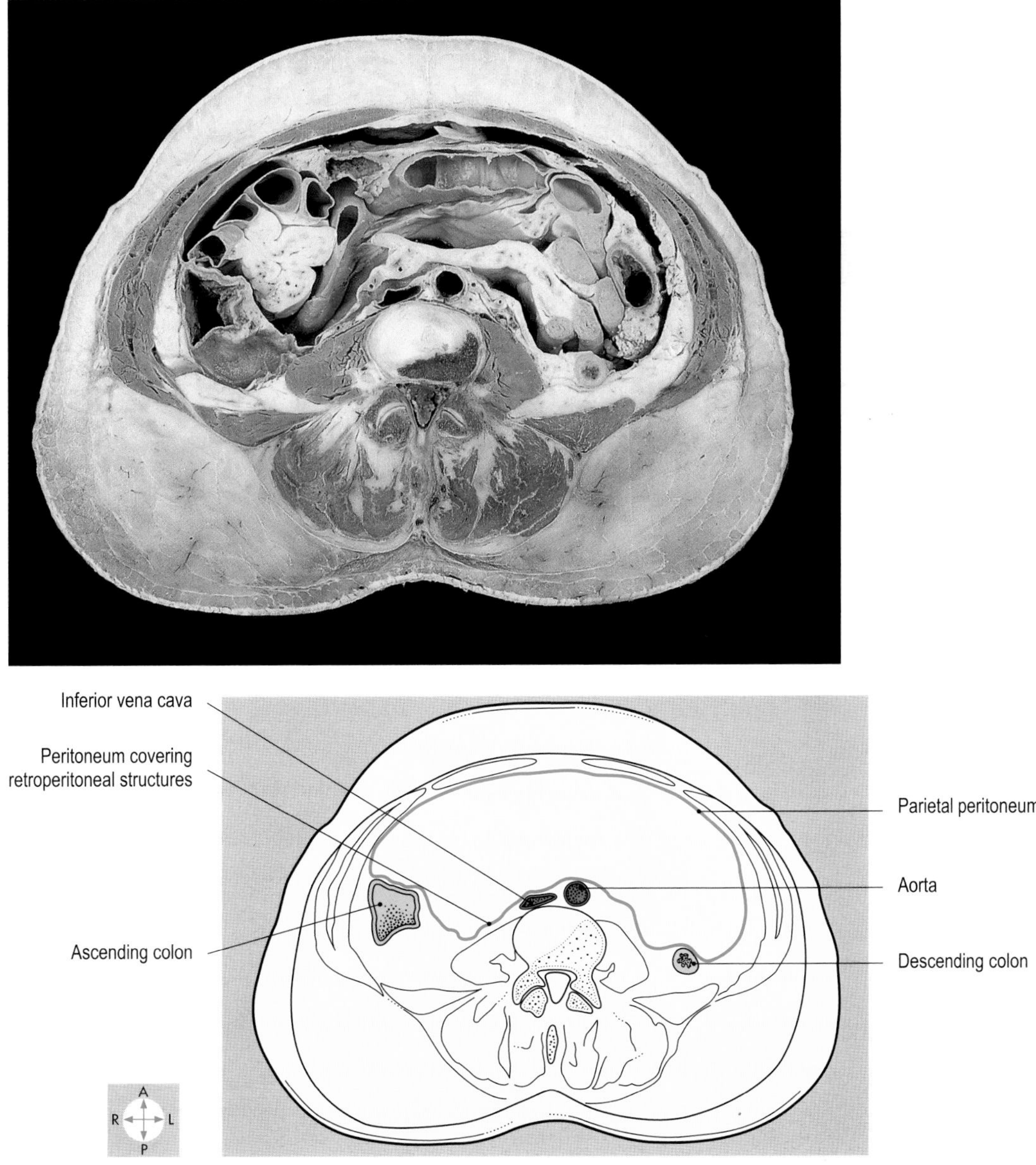

Fig. 4.32 Transverse section at the level of the third lumbar vertebra showing parietal peritoneum and some retroperitoneal structures. Inferior aspect.

Visceral peritoneum and mesenteries

Most of the abdominal organs have a covering of visceral peritoneum and are suspended within the abdominopelvic cavity by mesenteries. Although organs possessing mesenteries are often termed 'intraperitoneal', they do not lie within the peritoneal cavity but merely project into it. Mesenteries consist of double layers of peritoneum containing the vessels and nerves of the 'intraperitoneal' organs. Typically, a mesentery attaches to the posterior abdominal wall, where its peritoneal layers are continuous with the parietal peritoneum. Examples include the mesentery of the small intestine (Fig. 4.35) and the transverse mesocolon.

The mesenteries of the stomach (the omenta) do not attach to the abdominal wall but to other organs. The lesser curvature of the stomach is connected to the liver by the lesser omentum while the upper part of the greater curvature is attached to the spleen by the gastrosplenic ligament (see Figs 4.37 & 4.38). The major portion of the greater curvature gives attachment to the greater omentum.

The greater omentum is an apron-like fold of peritoneum with a free lower border (Fig. 4.33). Hanging behind the anterior abdominal wall and in front of most of the small intestine, this omentum is usually a conspicuous feature when the peritoneal cavity is opened. Superiorly it attaches to both the transverse colon (Fig. 4.34) and the greater curvature of the stomach, enclosing the inferior part of the omental bursa (see below). The free inferior border of the omentum ascends on the right as far as the first part of the duodenum while on the left it merges with the gastrosplenic ligament. The position of the greater omentum is influenced by previous episodes of intra-abdominal disease because it tends to adhere to sites of inflammation such as the appendix or gall bladder.

The transverse mesocolon (Fig. 4.35) has a long horizontal root, attached across the posterior aspect of the abdomen, principally to the pancreas. This mesocolon slopes downwards and forwards into the greater sac, dividing it into supracolic and infracolic compartments. Along its lower margin, close to the anterior abdominal wall, runs the transverse colon.

Infracolic compartment of greater sac

This compartment lies below and behind the transverse mesocolon and is usually covered anteriorly by the greater omentum. The infracolic compartment consists of right and left spaces separated by the mesentery of the small intestine (Fig. 4.35). The root of this mesentery begins to the left of the midline near the transverse mesocolon and slopes downwards into the right iliac fossa. The mesentery is extensively folded and is attached to the jejunum and ileum. The left infracolic space communicates directly with the cavity of the pelvis. By contrast, the right infracolic space is confined inferiorly by the attachment of the lower part of the mesentery.

Behind the peritoneum on either side of the infracolic compartment lie the ascending and descending parts of the colon. Lateral to these are grooves lined by peritoneum, the right and left paracolic gutters (see Fig. 4.68).

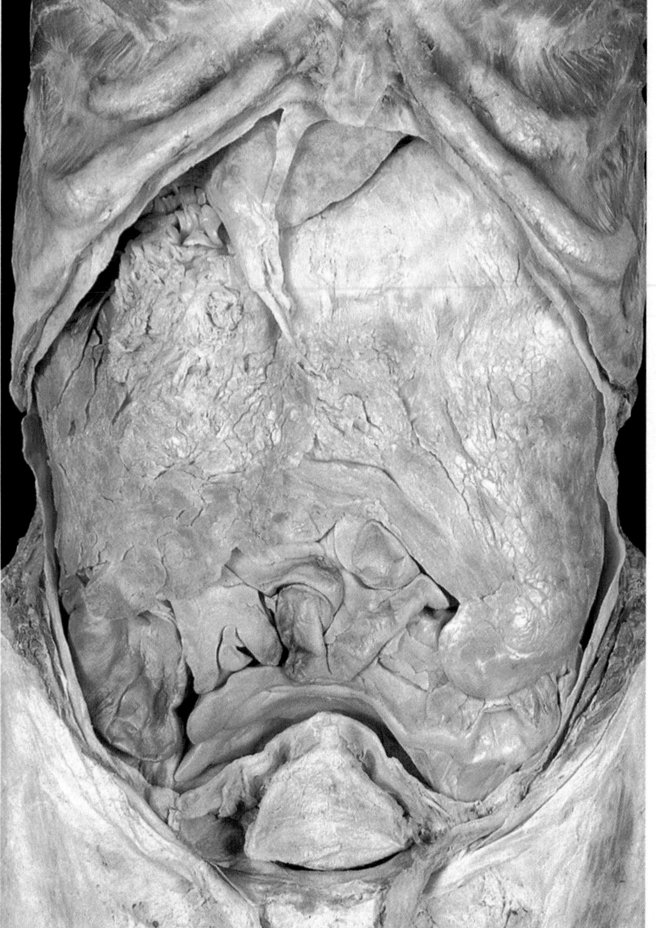

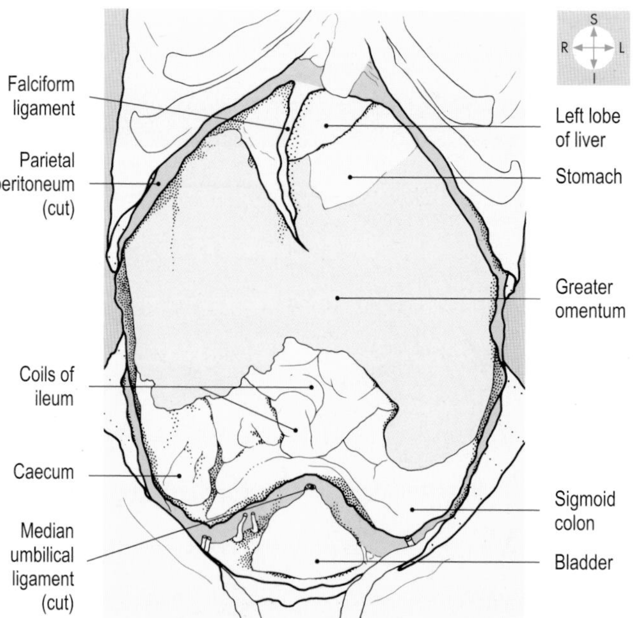

Fig. 4.33 Greater sac after removal of most of the parietal peritoneum. In this specimen the greater omentum is adherent to the right side of the diaphragm, concealing the right lobe of the liver and the gall bladder.

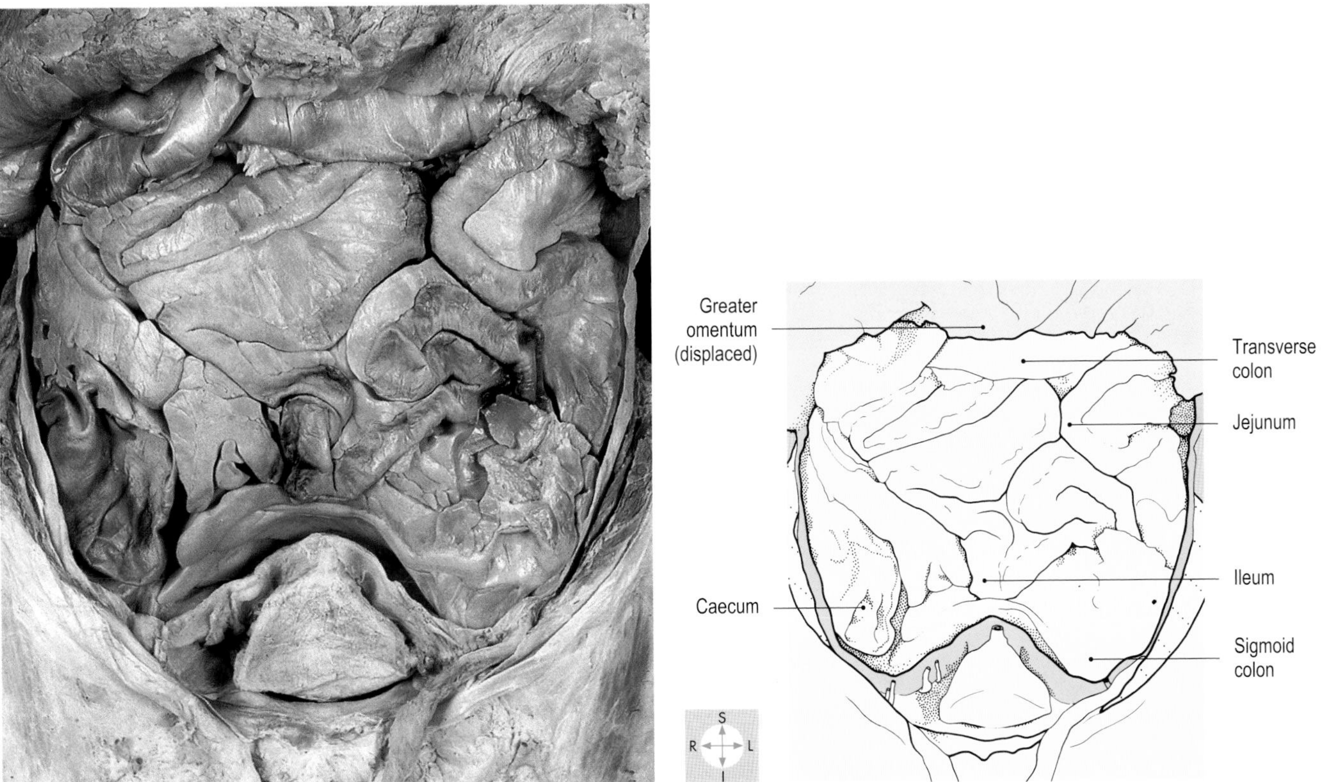

Fig. 4.34 Greater omentum has been turned upwards to display the contents of the infracolic compartment of the greater sac.

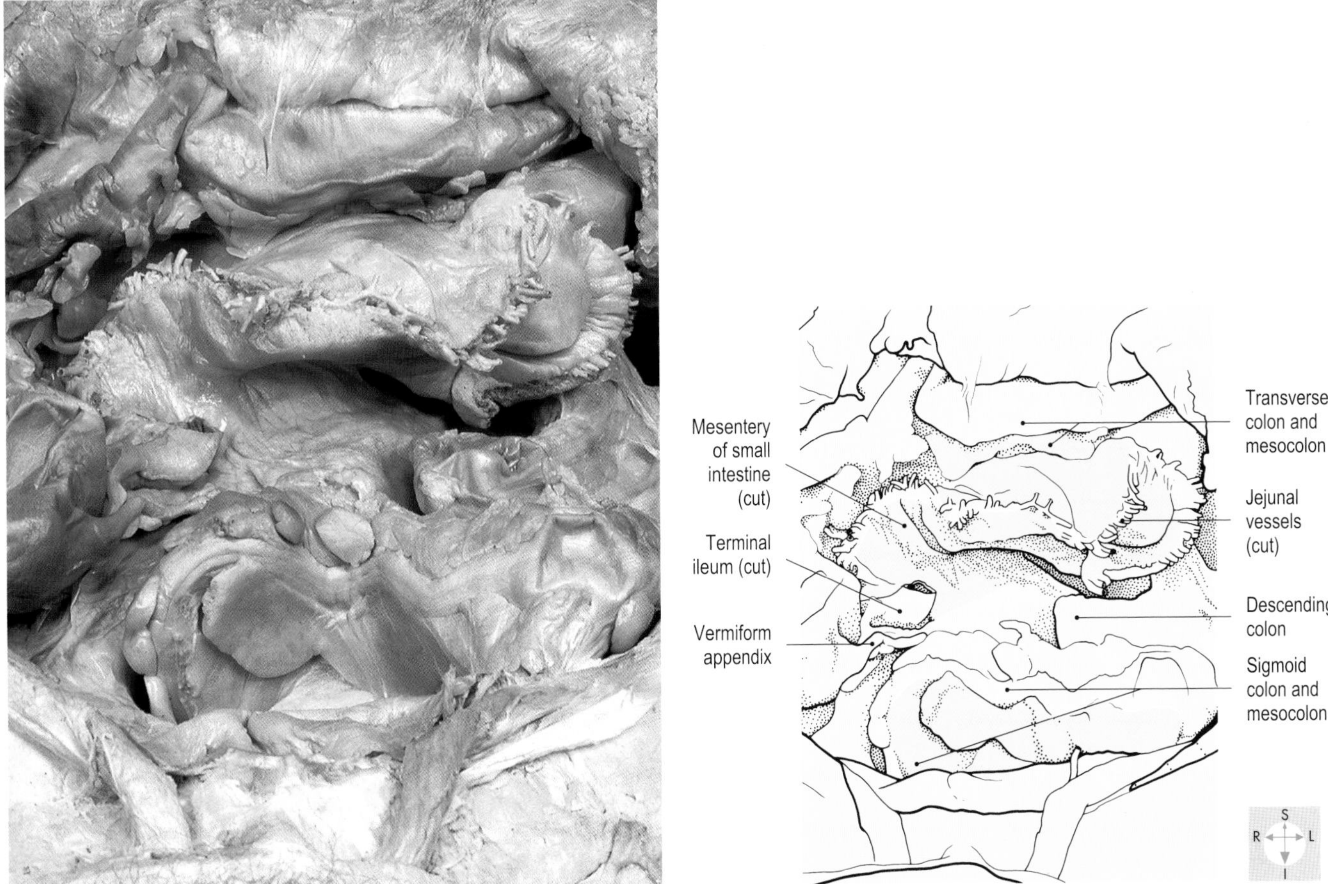

Fig. 4.35 Infracolic compartment of the greater sac. Removal of the jejunum and ileum has revealed their mesenteries. The descending colon is more medially placed than usual.

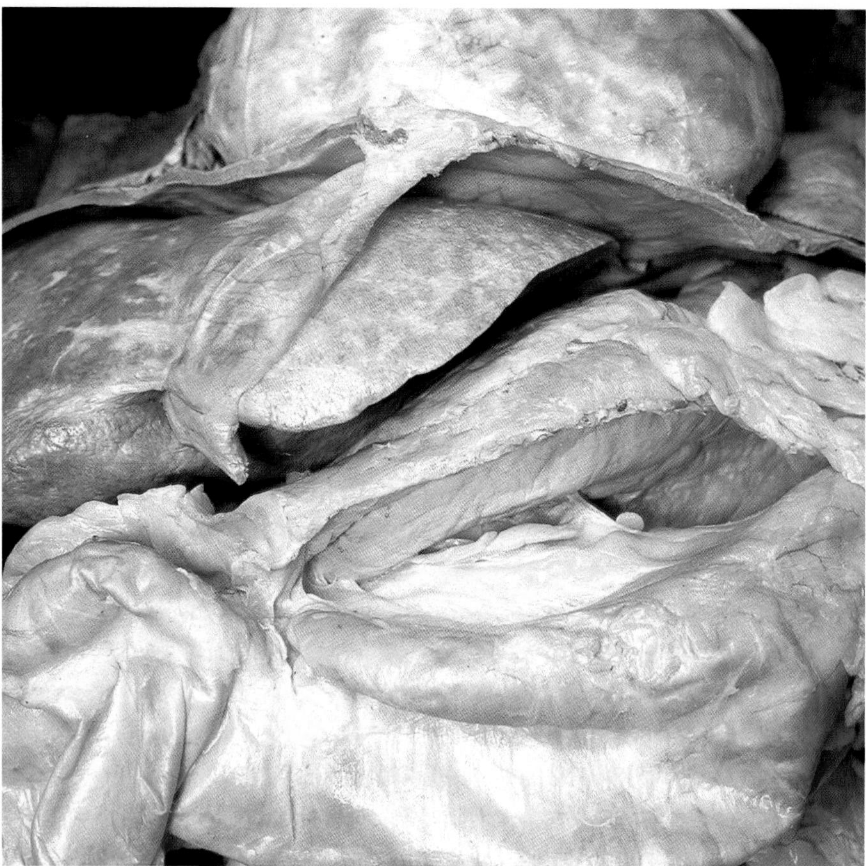

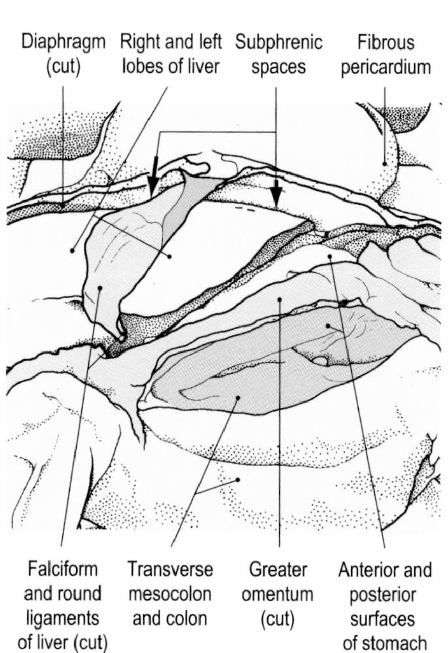

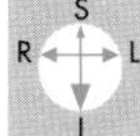

Fig. 4.36 Supracolic compartment of the greater sac. After removal of most of the greater omentum, the greater curvature of the stomach has been displaced upwards to show the position of the omental bursa (pink).

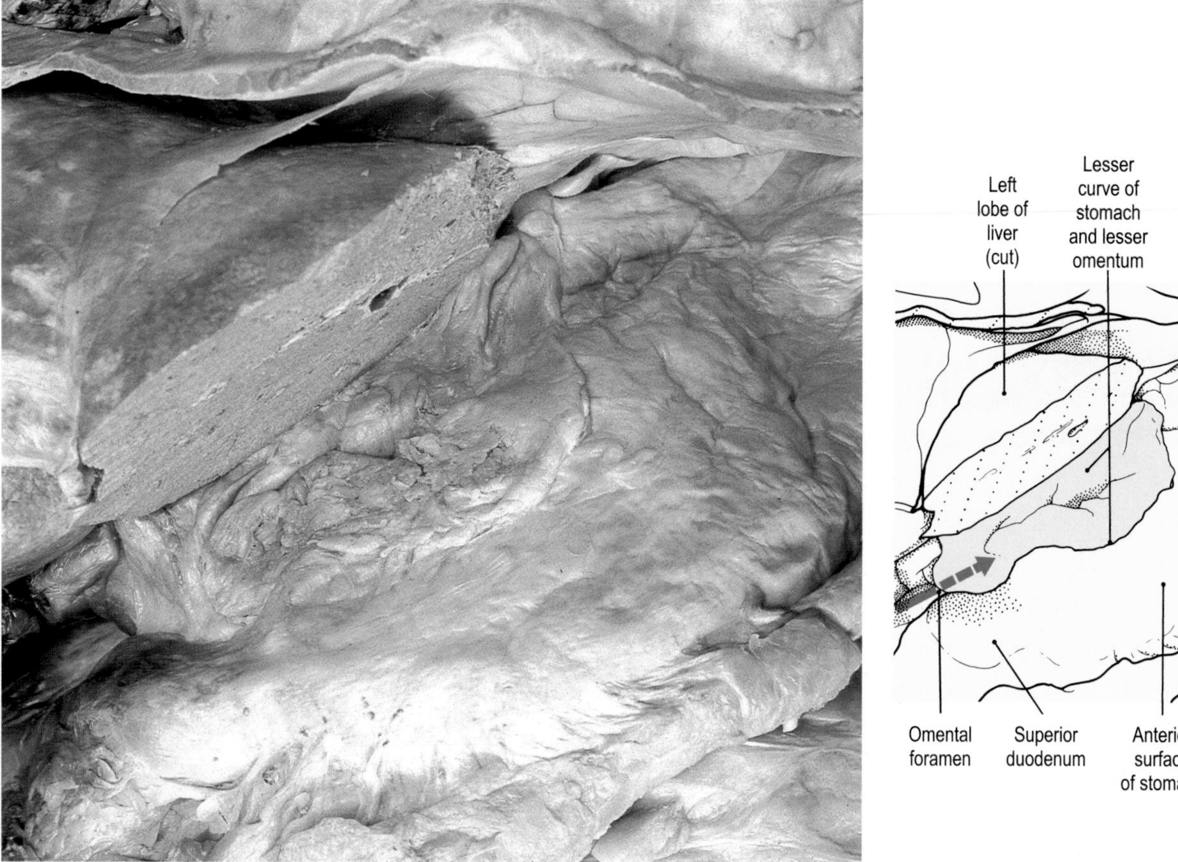

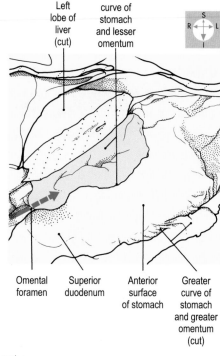

Fig. 4.37 Lesser omentum exposed by removal of part of the left lobe of the liver. The pink arrow traverses the omental foramen into the omental bursa and lies behind the lesser omentum.

Another mesentery, the sigmoid mesocolon, lies in the left lower part of the infracolic compartment. Its root is shaped like an inverted 'V', with its apex overlying the bifurcation of the left common iliac vessels and the left ureter. Behind the sigmoid mesocolon lies the intersigmoid recess, which ends blindly at the apex of the 'V' but is continuous inferiorly with the pelvic cavity.

Small folds of peritoneum may produce additional peritoneal recesses (or fossae) near the ascending duodenum (paraduodenal recesses) and the caecum (retrocaecal and ileocaecal recesses). A loop of bowel can become trapped in a peritoneal recess, producing an 'internal hernia' which may lead to intestinal obstruction.

Nerve supply

The autonomic nerves that supply the abdominal organs also innervate the visceral peritoneum surrounding the organs. Pain conveyed by these nerves tends to be deeply felt and poorly localized.

Supracolic compartment of greater sac

The supracolic compartment lies above and in front of the transverse mesocolon (Fig. 4.36). Its superior part intervenes between the diaphragm and the liver and is divided by the falciform ligament into two subphrenic spaces. The compartment includes the deep recess between the right lobe of the liver and the right kidney (the hepatorenal recess) and extends across the midline below the left lobe of the liver and in front of the stomach. Infection within the abdomen or pelvis can spread through the peritoneal cavity and may accumulate near the liver, producing an abscess. Abscesses between the diaphragm and the liver are termed 'subphrenic' and those below the liver 'subhepatic'.

Omental bursa (lesser sac)

The omental bursa is the small part of the peritoneal cavity behind the stomach (see Figs 4.36 & 4.38). It communicates with the greater sac through a narrow opening, known as the omental or epiploic foramen, which lies between the first part of the duodenum and the visceral surface of the liver (Fig. 4.37).

The omental bursa is isolated from the greater sac by the stomach and several peritoneal folds. One of these folds, the lesser omentum, connects the lesser curvature of the stomach to the posterior surface of the liver (Fig. 4.37). Two further folds, the gastrosplenic and splenorenal (lienorenal) ligaments, attach the spleen to the greater curvature of the stomach and the left kidney respectively (Fig. 4.38).

The omental bursa extends upwards behind the stomach and the caudate lobe of the liver as far as the diaphragm. On the left it continues to the hilum of the spleen, terminating between the gastrosplenic and splenorenal ligaments. Inferiorly the omental bursa usually extends a short distance below the greater curvature of the stomach between the gastric and colic attachments of the greater omentum.

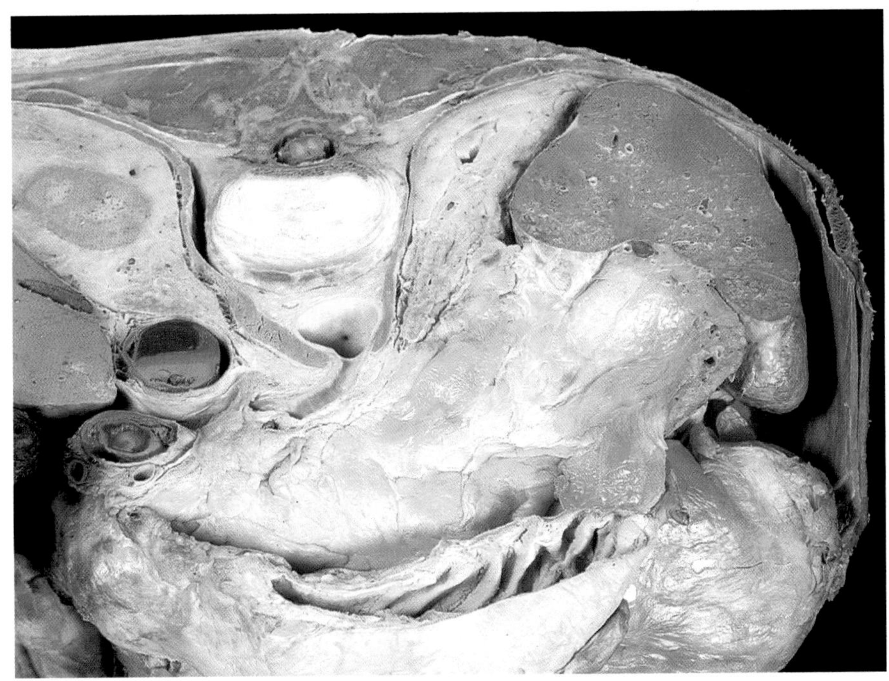

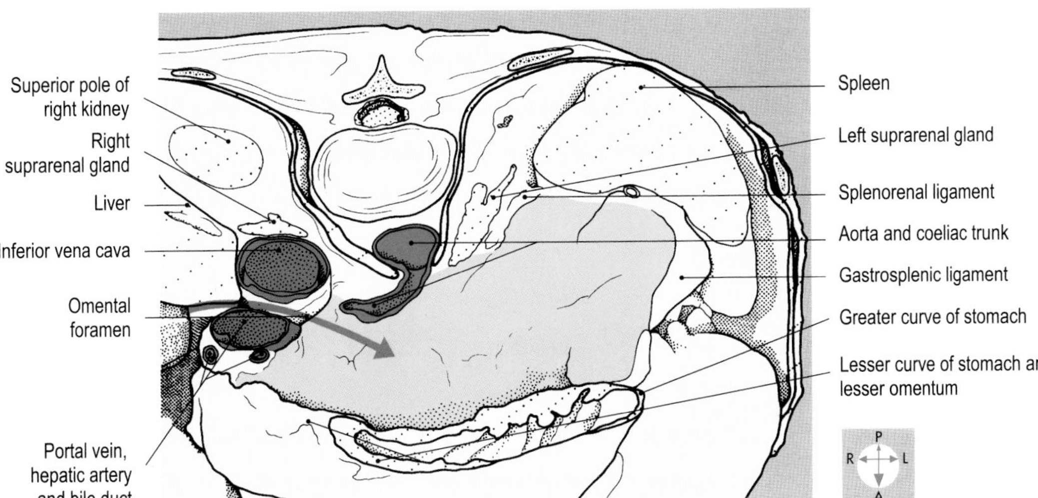

Fig. 4.38 Transverse section at the level of the disc between the twelfth thoracic and first lumbar vertebrae. The pink arrow traverses the omental foramen into the omental bursa (pink area). In this specimen the left kidney lies lower than usual. Superior aspect.

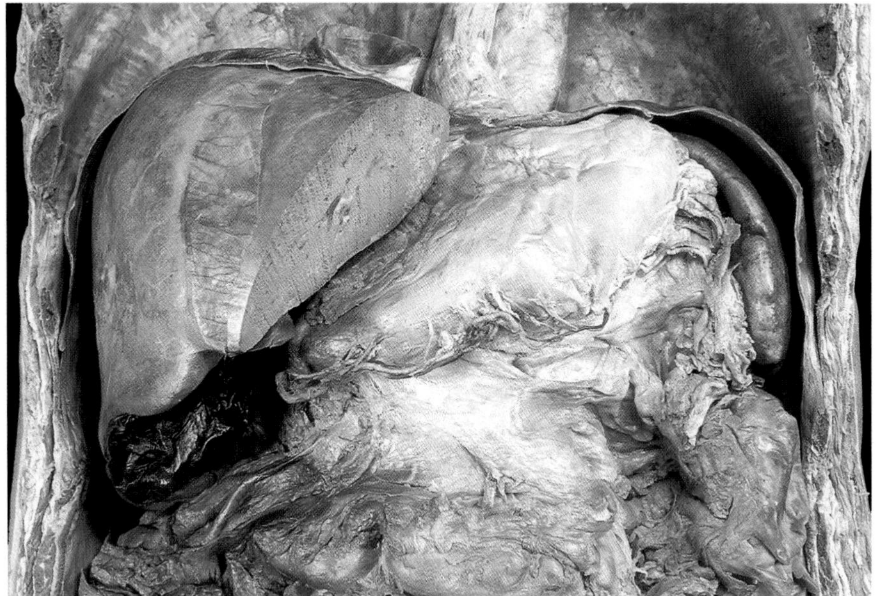

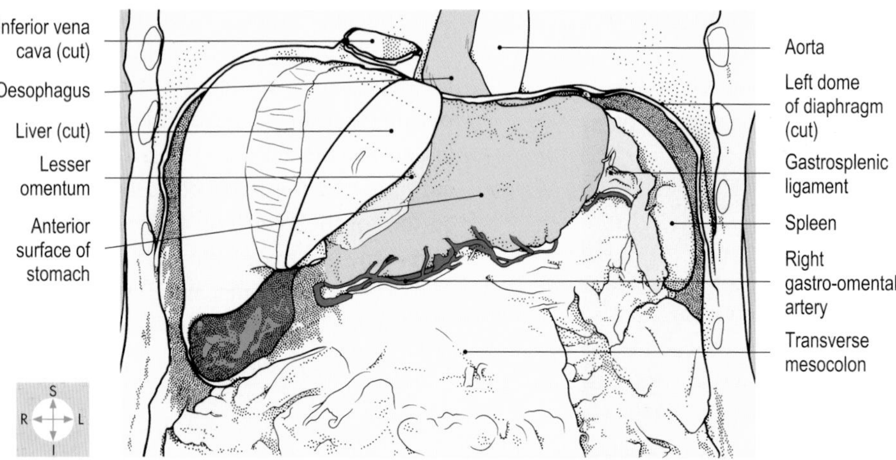

Fig. 4.39 Stomach and some of its relations, seen after removal of the anterior half of the diaphragm and left lobe of the liver and dissection of the greater omentum.

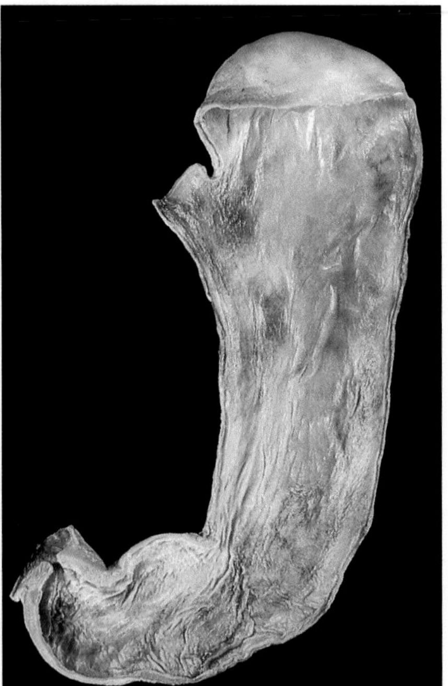

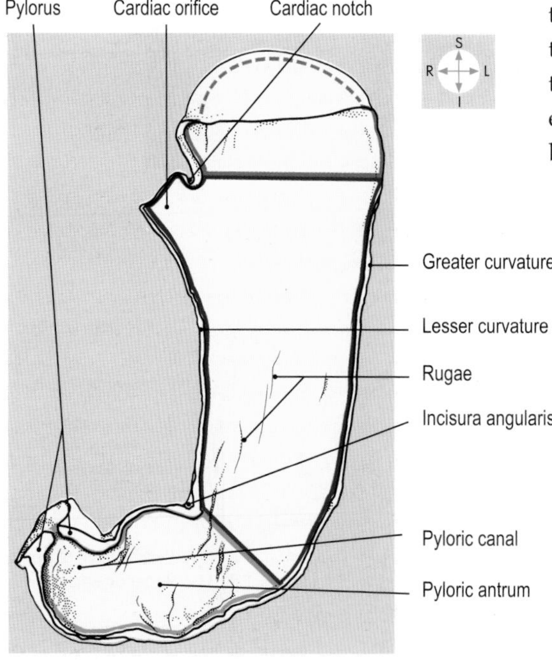

Fig. 4.40 Longitudinal section through the stomach.

Stomach

The stomach is the dilated portion of the gut in which the early stages of digestion take place. It lies in the upper part of the abdomen beneath the left dome of the diaphragm (Fig. 4.39). Proximally, the stomach joins the oesophagus at the cardiac orifice and distally it is continuous with the duodenum at the pylorus. Between these two relatively fixed points, the organ varies considerably in size, shape and location in response to its muscle tone, the quantity and nature of its contents and the position of the individual (Figs 4.41 & 4.42). Usually, the loaded stomach is J-shaped and lies in the left hypochondrium, the epigastrium and umbilical region of the abdomen.

The oesophagus pierces the diaphragm and has a short intra-abdominal course before joining the stomach at the cardiac orifice. This lies a little to the left of the midline at about the level of the eleventh thoracic vertebra (Fig. 4.42). Anatomical and physiological factors produce a sphincteric effect at the gastro-oesophageal junction. If this mechanism fails, gastric contents flow/leak into the oesophagus (gastro-oesophageal reflux), causing inflammation of the oesophageal mucosa.

The stomach has two surfaces, anterior and posterior, which meet at two curved borders, the curvatures (Fig. 4.40). The lesser curvature extends from the cardiac orifice downwards and to the right to reach the upper border of the pylorus. A notch, the incisura angularis, is usually present on the lesser curvature towards its pyloric end. The greater curvature is longer and begins at the cardiac notch on the left side

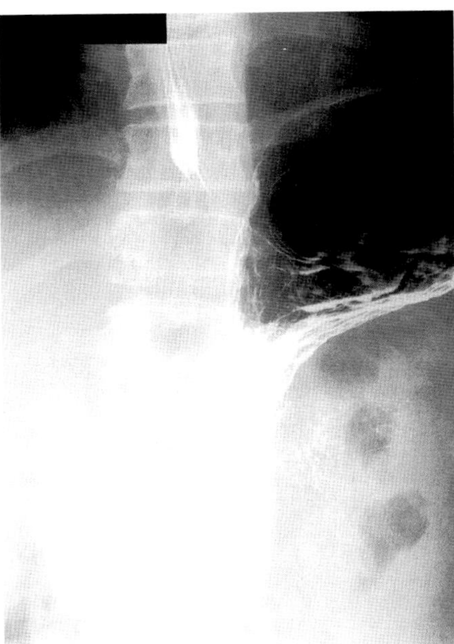

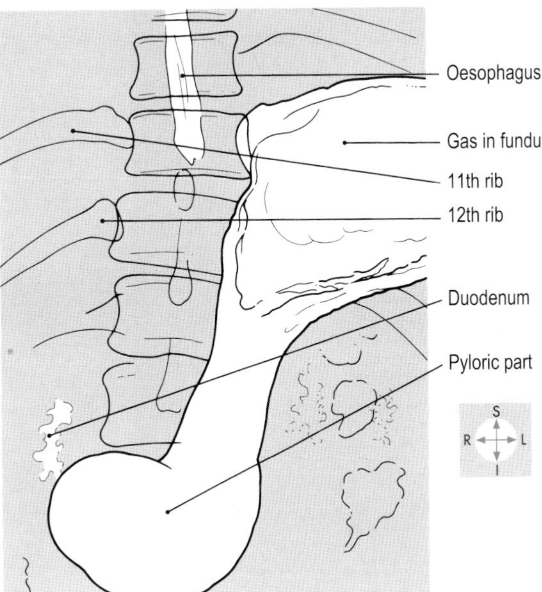

Fig. 4.41 Anteroposterior radiograph following a barium meal. The subject is supine and most of the barium has pooled into the pyloric part of the stomach.

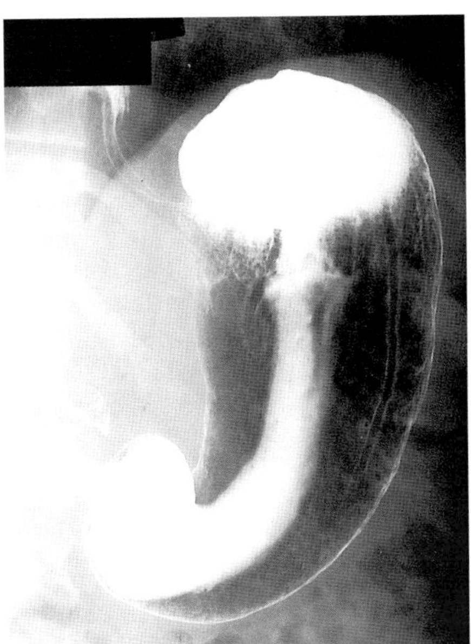

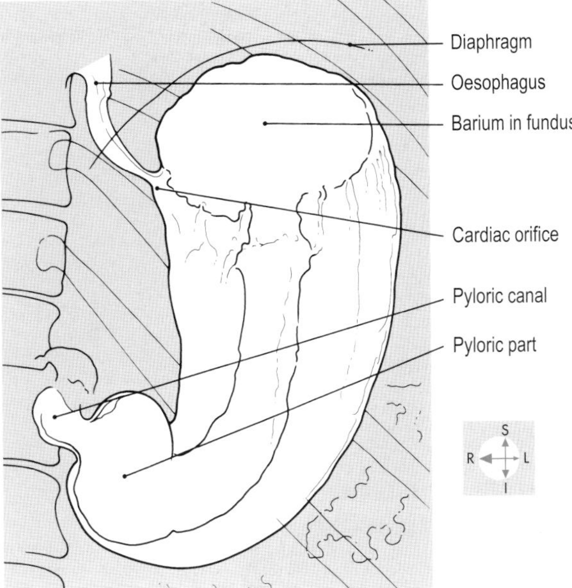

Fig. 4.42 Oblique radiograph of same individual, now lying supine and tilted head down. The barium has flowed into the fundus of the stomach.

of the cardiac orifice. It arches upwards and to the left before descending along the left and inferior aspects of the organ to reach the inferior border of the pylorus.

The pylorus is normally situated just to the right of the midline at the level of the first lumbar vertebra, on the transpyloric plane.

By convention, the stomach is described as having three parts, the fundus, the body and the pyloric part (Fig. 4.40). The fundus lies above an imaginary horizontal plane passing through the cardiac orifice while the antrum lies to the right of the incisura angularis. The body lies between the fundus and the pyloric part and is the largest part of the stomach. In the pyloric part, the cavity of the pyloric antrum tapers to the right into a narrow passage, the pyloric canal.

The mucosal lining presents numerous longitudinal folds or rugae which are most prominent when the stomach is empty (Fig. 4.40). There is a well-developed smooth muscle coat which is thickened around the pyloric canal and pylorus to form the pyloric sphincter.

Relations

The anterior surface of the stomach lies in contact with the diaphragm, the anterior abdominal wall and the left and quadrate lobes of the liver. Posterolateral to the fundus lies the gastric surface of the spleen (Fig. 4.39). The remainder of the stomach's relations are situated posteriorly and collectively form the stomach bed. This includes the diaphragm, left suprarenal gland, upper part of the left kidney, the splenic artery, pancreas, transverse mesocolon and sometimes the transverse colon (see Fig. 4.43). However, these structures are separated from the stomach by the omental bursa (see below). Gastric ulcers can perforate into either the greater sac or the omental bursa. Sometimes, ulceration may involve the pancreas or the splenic artery.

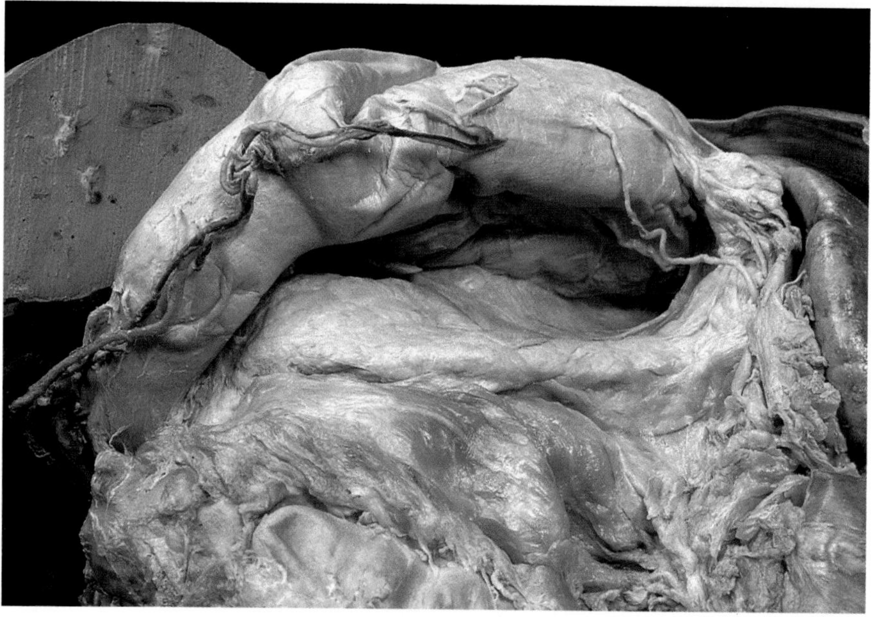

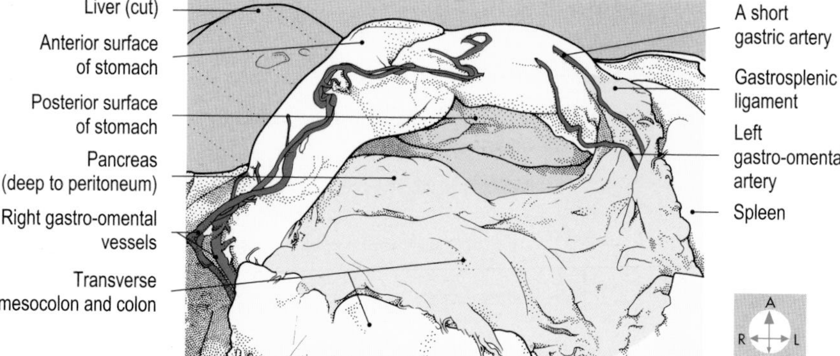

Fig. 4.43 Omental bursa (pink) and stomach bed, seen after removal of the greater omentum and lifting the greater curvature upwards.

Omenta and omental bursa

Peritoneum covers both surfaces of the stomach. Attached to the curvatures are double layers of peritoneum, which form the lesser and greater omenta.

The lesser omentum extends from the liver (see Fig. 4.37) to the lesser curvature of the stomach and also attaches to the abdominal oesophagus and the commencement of the duodenum (see Fig. 4.39). Near the lesser curvature it contains the left and right gastric vessels (Fig. 4.44), accompanied by lymphatics and autonomic nerves, while its free border encloses the portal vein, the bile duct and the proper hepatic artery.

The greater omentum hangs from the distal part of the greater curvature and from the superior duodenum. Near the greater curvature it contains the left and right gastro-omental (gastroepiploic) vessels (Fig. 4.43). To the left the greater omentum is continuous with the gastrosplenic ligament which connects the proximal part of the greater curvature to the hilum of the spleen.

The omental bursa (lesser sac) lies behind the stomach and the lesser omentum (Fig. 4.43). Its opening (the omental foramen) lies above the first part of the duodenum, immediately posterior to the free border of the lesser omentum. From here the omental bursa extends to the left as far as the hilum of the spleen where it is

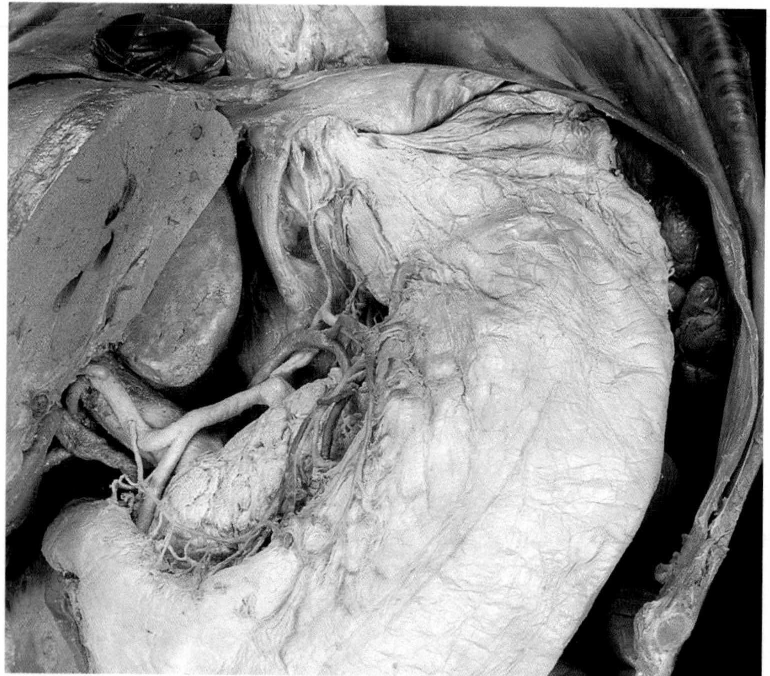

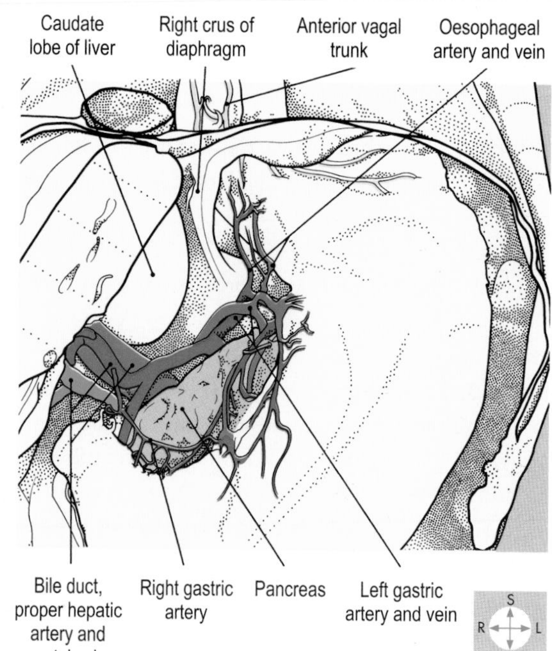

Fig. 4.44 Dissection of the lesser omentum showing structures along the lesser curvature of the stomach.

limited by the gastrosplenic and splenorenal (lienorenal) ligaments. Superiorly it reaches the undersurface of the diaphragm behind the caudate lobe of the liver. Inferiorly the bursa extends a short distance below the greater curvature between the two peritoneal folds that constitute the greater omentum.

Arterial supply

The stomach is supplied by several arteries, which are all derived from branches of the coeliac trunk and which anastomose extensively with each other. The coeliac trunk (Fig. 4.45) is a short, wide vessel arising from the anterior aspect of the aorta just below the diaphragm. It divides into three branches: the left gastric, the common hepatic and the splenic arteries.

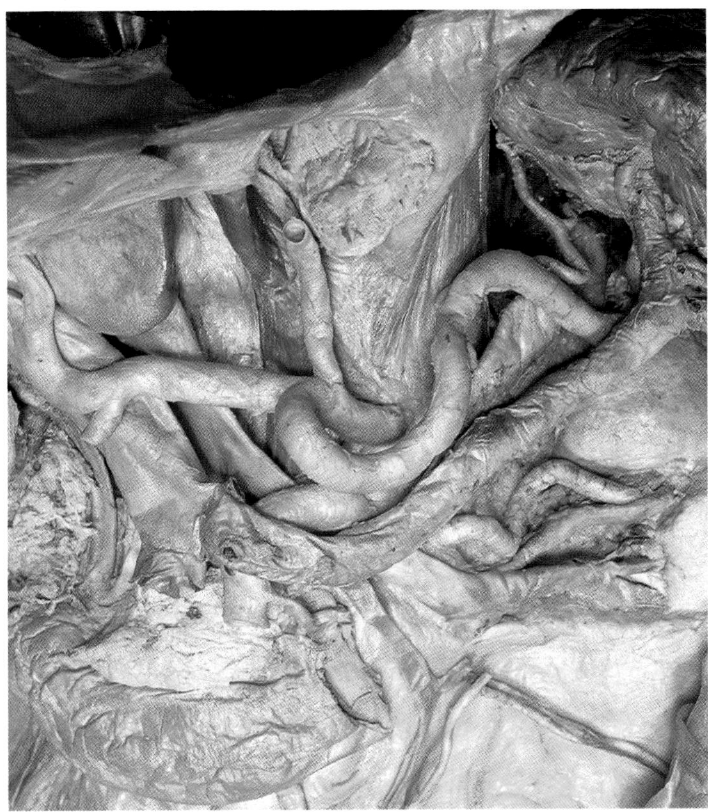

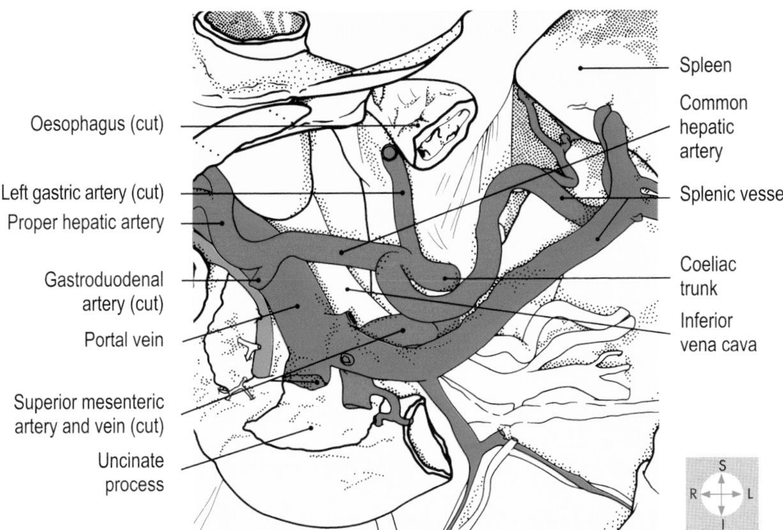

Fig. 4.45 Stomach and most of the pancreas have been removed to reveal the coeliac trunk and its branches.

The left gastric artery is the smallest branch, passing upwards and to the left behind the omental bursa to reach the oesophagus, then descending along the lesser curvature within the lesser omentum (Fig. 4.44). Its branches include two or three to the lower oesophagus which ascend through the oesophageal opening of the diaphragm. Other branches supply the cardia and lesser curvature of the stomach.

The common hepatic artery gives rise to the right gastric and gastroduodenal arteries. The right gastric artery (Fig. 4.44) arises above the superior duodenum and runs to the left within the lesser omentum, supplying the lesser curvature and anastomosing with the left gastric artery. One of the branches of the gastroduodenal artery is the right gastro-omental (gastroepiploic) artery (Fig. 4.43). This vessel runs to the left within the greater omentum, parallel to the greater curvature, giving numerous branches to the pyloric part and body of the stomach.

The splenic artery is the largest branch of the coeliac trunk (Fig. 4.45). It runs a tortuous course to the left along the superior border of the pancreas, initially behind the omental bursa and then within the splenorenal ligament, and terminates near the hilum of the spleen. It provides collateral branches to the pancreas and terminal branches to the spleen and stomach. There are several gastric branches, which pass to the greater curvature by way of the gastrosplenic ligament. Most of these vessels supply the fundus of the stomach and are called short gastric arteries (Fig. 4.43). However, one branch, the left gastro-omental (gastroepiploic) artery, continues downwards and to the right within the greater omentum. It follows the greater curvature, supplies the body of the stomach and may anastomose with the right gastro-omental (gastroepiploic) artery.

Venous drainage

The veins of the stomach accompany the gastric arteries and drain into the portal venous system, the portal vein itself receiving the right and left gastric veins. The splenic vein receives the short gastric and left gastro-omental (gastroepiploic) veins while the right gastro-omental vein usually enters the superior mesenteric vein. The oesophageal tributaries of the left gastric vein (see Fig. 4.44) take part in an important portacaval anastomosis (see p. 185) with tributaries of the azygos venous system within the thorax.

Nerve supply

In the thorax the vagus nerves form a plexus on the surface of the oesophagus. From this plexus emerge two principal nerves, the anterior and posterior vagal trunks, which enter the abdomen on the respective surfaces of the oesophagus. The anterior vagal trunk (Fig. 4.44), derived mostly from the left vagus nerve, gives branches to the anterior surface of the stomach including the pyloric region. Branches from the posterior trunk, whose origin is mainly from the right vagus nerve, pass to the posterior surface of the stomach and also to the coeliac plexus (see pp 197 & 199). The parasympathetic innervation of the stomach by the vagus nerves is important in relation to both secretion and motility of the organ.

Spleen

The spleen is a lymphoid organ lying in the left hypochondrium posterior to the stomach. The fresh spleen is purple in colour and rather variable in size and shape. Since it lies entirely behind the midaxillary line and under cover of the left lower ribs, the normal spleen cannot be palpated in the living subject, even during full inspiration. The spleen is soft and delicate and can be damaged by blunt or penetrating injuries resulting in life-threatening intraperitoneal haemorrhage. The blood may irritate the peritoneum lining the abdominal surface of the diaphragm, producing pain referred to the left shoulder region (see p. 205).

Surface features

The spleen is oval in shape when viewed from its anterior aspect (Fig. 4.46) and its long axis lies parallel to the left tenth rib. The two extremities of the organ are connected by superior and inferior borders. The superior border often possesses one or more notches near its anterior end while the inferior border is usually smooth. The organ has two easily distinguishable surfaces. The diaphragmatic surface faces backwards and laterally and is smoothly convex (Fig. 4.47). The visceral surface faces anteromedially and is characterized by ridges and depressions. The centrally placed hilum is perforated by numerous blood vessels together with lymphatics and nerves. The depressions around the hilum accommodate adjacent organs.

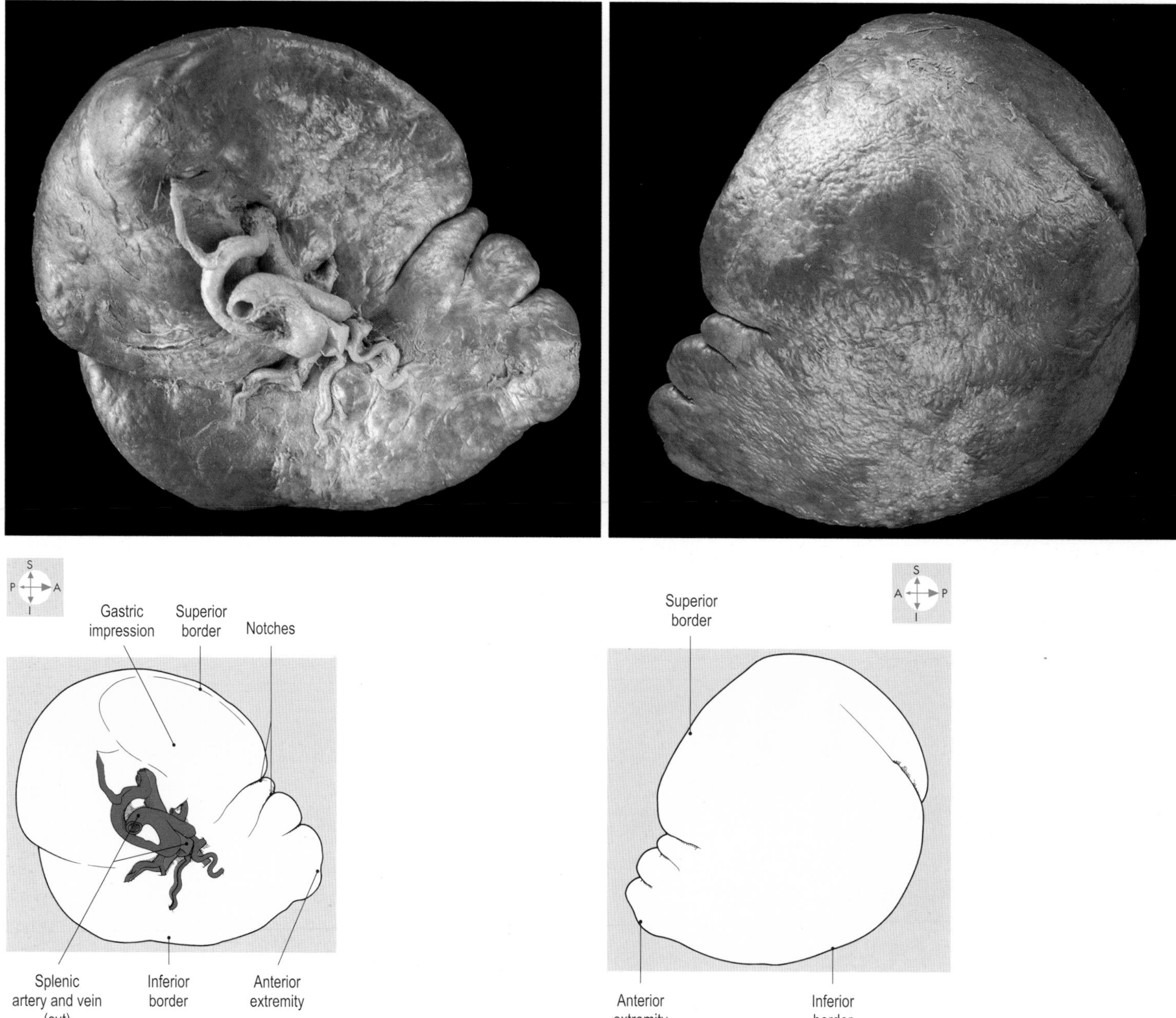

Fig. 4.46 Visceral surface of the spleen.

Fig. 4.47 Diaphragmatic surface of the spleen. This specimen has several well-defined notches on its superior border and a single notch on the inferior border.

Relations

The spleen is an intraperitoneal organ and most of its capsule is covered by peritoneum of the greater sac. However, there is a small bare area near the hilum which gives attachment to two peritoneal folds or ligaments. The splenorenal (lienorenal) ligament runs medially to reach the left kidney while the gastrosplenic ligament connects the spleen to the greater curvature of the stomach. Part of the omental bursa lies between these two ligaments and extends to the left as far as the splenic hilum (see Fig. 4.38).

Arching above the spleen and descending posterior and lateral to it, the left dome of the diaphragm is responsible for movements of the organ during ventilation (Fig. 4.48). The diaphragm separates the spleen from the left lung and pleura, and from the ninth, tenth and eleventh ribs.

On the visceral surface of the spleen, above the hilum, is the gastric impression which accommodates part of the posterior surface of the stomach. Below the medial half of the hilum is the renal impression, which abuts the superior pole of the left kidney.

Near the lateral extremity of its visceral surface the spleen may possess a small colic impression which lies against the left colic flexure. The tail of the pancreas extends laterally into the splenorenal ligament and its tip may reach the splenic hilum (Fig. 4.48).

Blood supply

The splenic artery is a direct branch of the coeliac trunk (see p. 161). It follows a tortuous course along the upper border of the pancreas, giving off several pancreatic branches. The artery traverses the splenorenal ligament and divides into its terminal branches near the hilum of the spleen. Several splenic branches enter the hilum, while the short gastric arteries and the left gastro-omental artery enter the gastrosplenic ligament to supply the fundus and greater curvature of the stomach respectively.

Veins accompany the terminal branches of the splenic artery and unite adjacent to the hilum of the spleen to form the splenic vein. Running to the right, this vein lies posterior to the tail of the pancreas within the splenorenal ligament and continues retroperitoneally posterior to the body of the gland and inferior to the splenic artery. It then crosses the anterior aspects of the left kidney and renal vessels and receives several small tributaries from the pancreas. Posterior to the neck of the pancreas the splenic vein unites with the superior mesenteric vein to form the portal vein and, close to its termination, is usually joined from below by the inferior mesenteric vein. If the pressure rises abnormally in the portal venous system (portal hyper-tension) the spleen may become enlarged (splenomegaly).

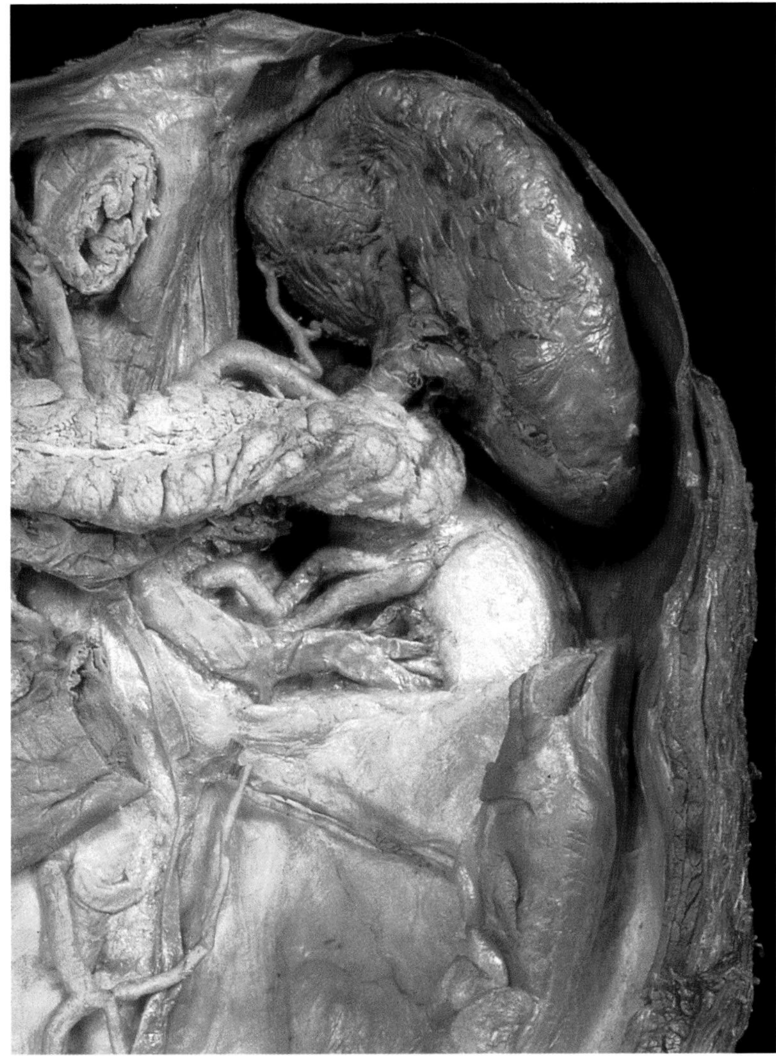

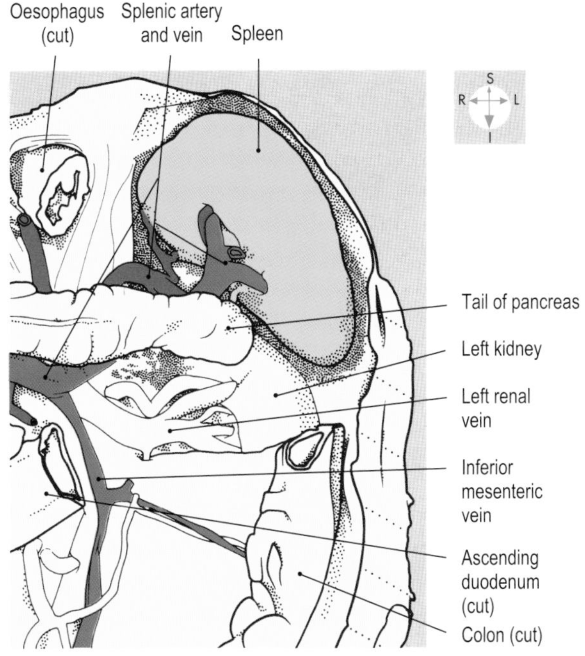

Fig. 4.48 Spleen and its vessels and relationship to the diaphragm, pancreas and left kidney. The stomach and part of the colon and peritoneum have been removed.

Duodenum

The duodenum, the proximal portion of the small intestine, begins at the pylorus and terminates at the duodenojejunal flexure. Deeply placed in the epigastric and umbilical regions of the abdomen, it curves round the head of the pancreas and is shaped like the letter C (Fig. 4.49). Unlike the remainder of the small intestine, the duodenum is mostly retroperitoneal and therefore relatively immobile. The duodenal lumen receives bile and pancreatic secretions via the bile duct and the pancreatic ducts.

Parts and structure

The duodenum is conventionally described as consisting of four parts (Fig. 4.49). The superior (first part of) duodenum begins slightly to the right of the midline at the level of the first lumbar vertebra (on the transpyloric plane) and passes upwards, backwards and to the right. In clinical practice its initial segment is often termed the duodenal bulb or duodenal cap. The descending (second part of) duodenum runs vertically to the level of the third lumbar vertebra. The inferior or horizontal duodenum (third part of) duodenum runs transversely to the left across the midline, arching forwards across the inferior vena cava and aorta. The ascending (fourth part of) duodenum slopes upwards and to the left and terminates at the level of the second lumbar vertebra by turning sharply forwards at the duodenojejunal flexure. Close to the pylorus the duodenal mucosa is smooth but in the second and subsequent parts of the organ it is raised to form numerous circular folds, the plicae circulares (Fig. 4.50).

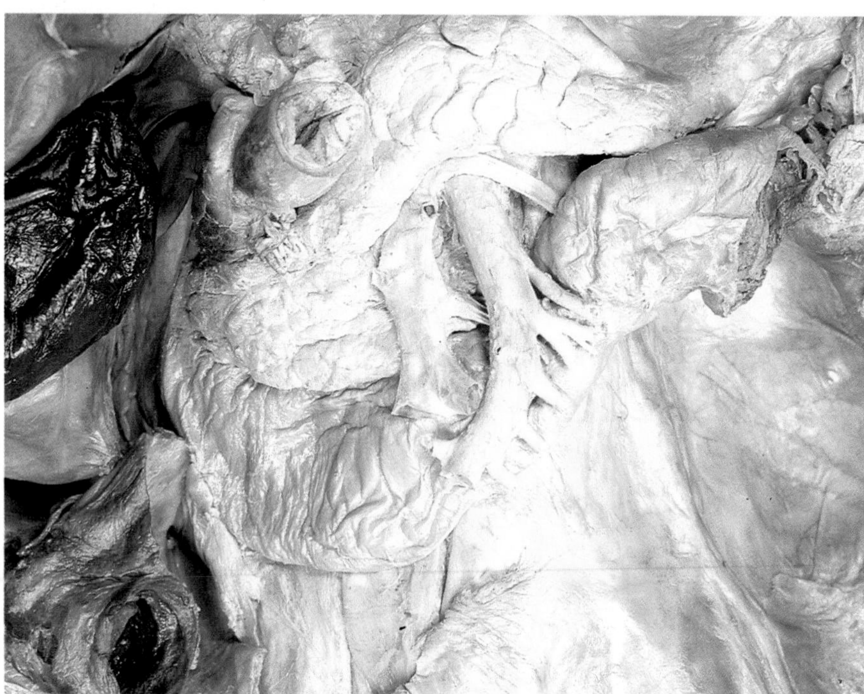

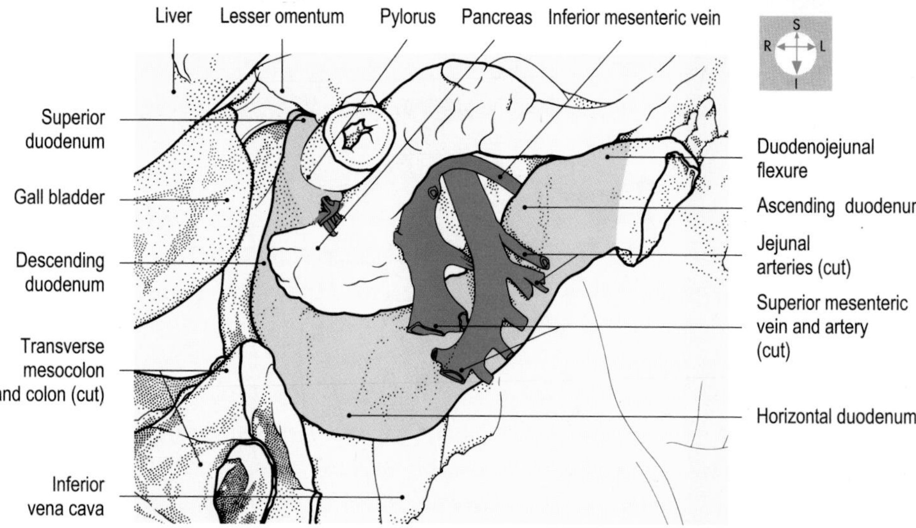

Fig. 4.49 Duodenum and some related structures. The liver and gall bladder have been slightly displaced.

Pancreas

The pancreas is both an exocrine and an endocrine gland. Most of its substance is involved in producing pancreatic juice which is conveyed by a duct system into the descending duodenum. In addition, microscopic clumps of endocrine tissue, the pancreatic islets (islets of Langerhans), are dispersed throughout the gland.

The pancreas is a long and narrow, lobulated organ, deeply located on the posterior abdominal wall. It lies approximately on the transpyloric plane (L1 vertebral level) and slopes slightly upwards from right to left. Its extremities lie in the right and left paravertebral gutters while the intermediate portion is thrust forwards in the midline by the prominence of the vertebral column and aorta.

The gland is divided into four parts, from right to left: the head, neck, body and tail (Fig. 4.53). The head is the broadest part and is surrounded by the loop of the duodenum. Projecting to the left from its lower portion is the uncinate process. The neck is indented posteriorly by the portal and superior mesenteric veins. The body, of fairly uniform width, extends to the left and is continuous with the tail, which tapers as it approaches the hilum of the spleen. The tail is contained within the splenorenal ligament but all other parts are retroperitoneal.

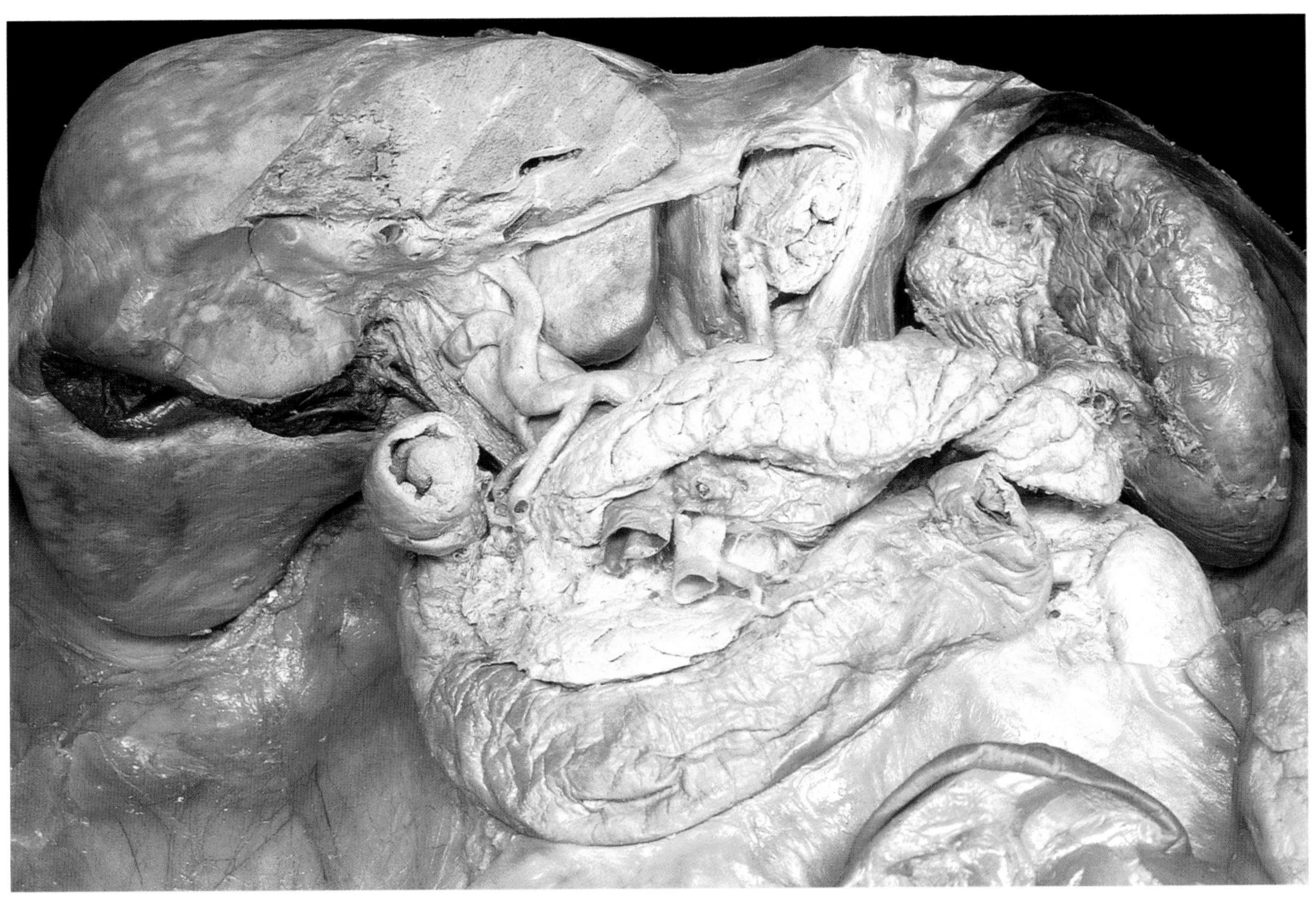

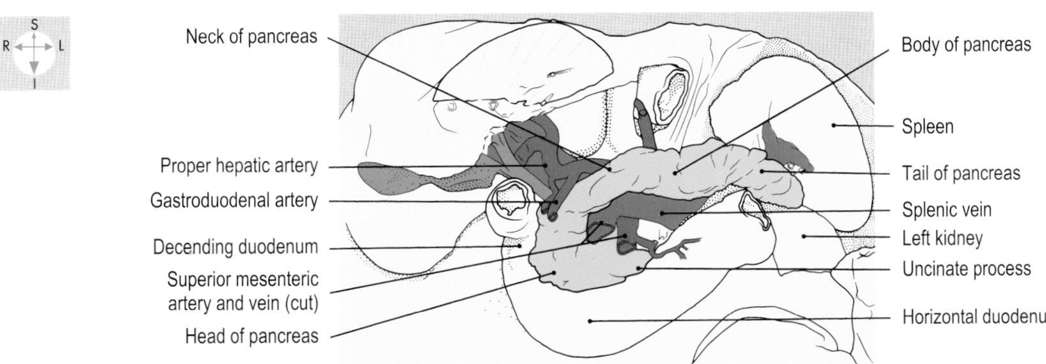

Fig. 4.53 Principal relations and parts of the pancreas.

In cross-section, the pancreas is triangular. It has well-defined superior and inferior borders and a blunt anterior border, to which is attached the transverse mesocolon. The inferior half of the gland is related to the infracolic compartment of the peritoneal cavity while the upper half lies in the floor of the omental bursa and contributes to the stomach bed.

Relations

Surrounded by the loop of the duodenum, the head of the pancreas lies anterior to the inferior vena cava, the right renal vessels and the terminal portion of the bile duct, which is sometimes embedded within the substance of this part of the gland (Fig. 4.54). A tumour in the head of the pancreas can obstruct the bile duct, leading to jaundice. The anterior surface of the head is related to the first part of the duodenum, the transverse colon and the gastroduodenal artery (Fig. 4.53). The uncinate process lies immediately superior to the horizontal duodenum. The superior mesenteric vessels cross the anterior surface of the uncinate process and separate it from the neck of the gland, which lies in front of the superior mesenteric vein and the commencement of the portal vein. The anterior surface of the neck is separated from the pylorus by the omental bursa.

The body of the pancreas crosses the aorta and usually covers the origins of its ventral branches, the coeliac trunk, whose common hepatic and splenic branches are related to the superior border of the gland (Fig. 4.55), and the superior mesenteric artery, which emerges at the lower border (Fig. 4.53). Further to the left the gland covers the left renal vessels and suprarenal gland, and the hilum of the left kidney. Immediately posterior to the body the splenic vein receives a major tributary, the inferior mesenteric vein (Figs 4.54 & 4.55). The inferior border of the body is related to the duodenojejunal flexure, coils of jejunum and the left colic flexure. Overlying the anterior surface of the body are the transverse mesocolon, the stomach and omental bursa, and part of the lesser omentum.

The tail of the gland lies within the splenorenal ligament and is accompanied posteriorly by the splenic vessels (Fig. 4.55). It lies anterior to the visceral surface and hilum of the spleen and posterior to the stomach and omental bursa.

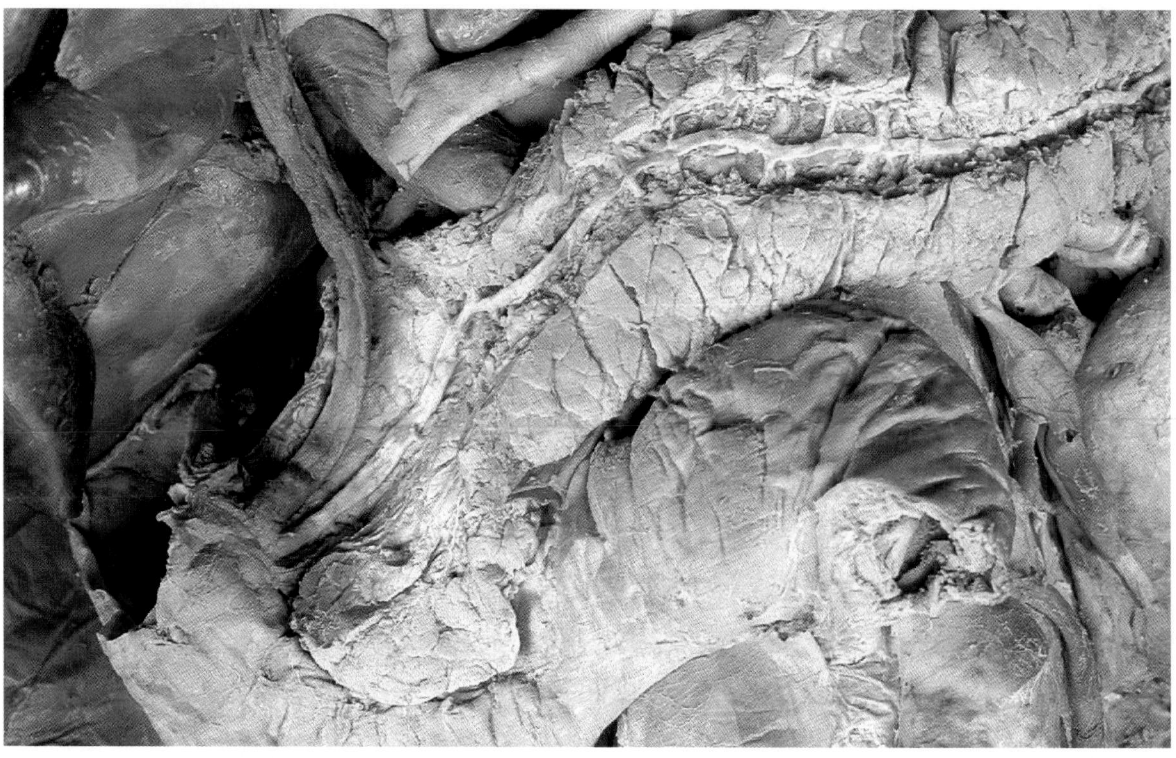

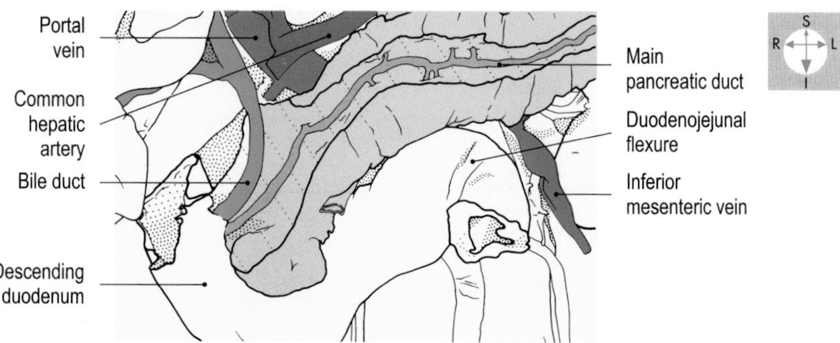

Fig. 4.54 Dissection of the pancreas to expose the terminal portions of the bile and main pancreatic ducts.

Pancreatic ducts

The main pancreatic duct arises in the tail of the gland and traverses the body and neck to reach the head where it curves downwards and to the right to reach the medial wall of the descending duodenum (Fig. 4.54). The duct receives numerous tributaries and gradually increases in calibre from left to right. It pierces the intestinal wall at the greater duodenal papilla (see Fig. 4.51).

The main pancreatic duct and the bile duct usually enter the duodenal wall together and unite to form a common chamber, the hepatopancreatic ampulla (of Vater), in which pancreatic juice and bile may mix before entering the duodenal lumen. There is usually a second and smaller duct, the accessory pancreatic duct, which opens into the duodenum about 2 cm above the main duct, at the minor duodenal papilla.

Blood supply

This is derived from branches of the coeliac and superior mesenteric arteries. The head and uncinate process receive superior pancreaticoduodenal branches from the gastroduodenal artery (a branch of the hepatic artery; Fig. 4.53) and inferior pancreaticoduodenal branches from the superior mesenteric artery (see Fig. 4.52). The remainder of the gland is supplied by branches from the splenic artery (Fig. 4.55). The venous drainage of the pancreas passes into the portal system. Superior and inferior pancreaticoduodenal veins from the head of the gland pass respectively into the portal vein and the superior mesenteric vein. Veins from the remainder of the gland terminate in the splenic vein.

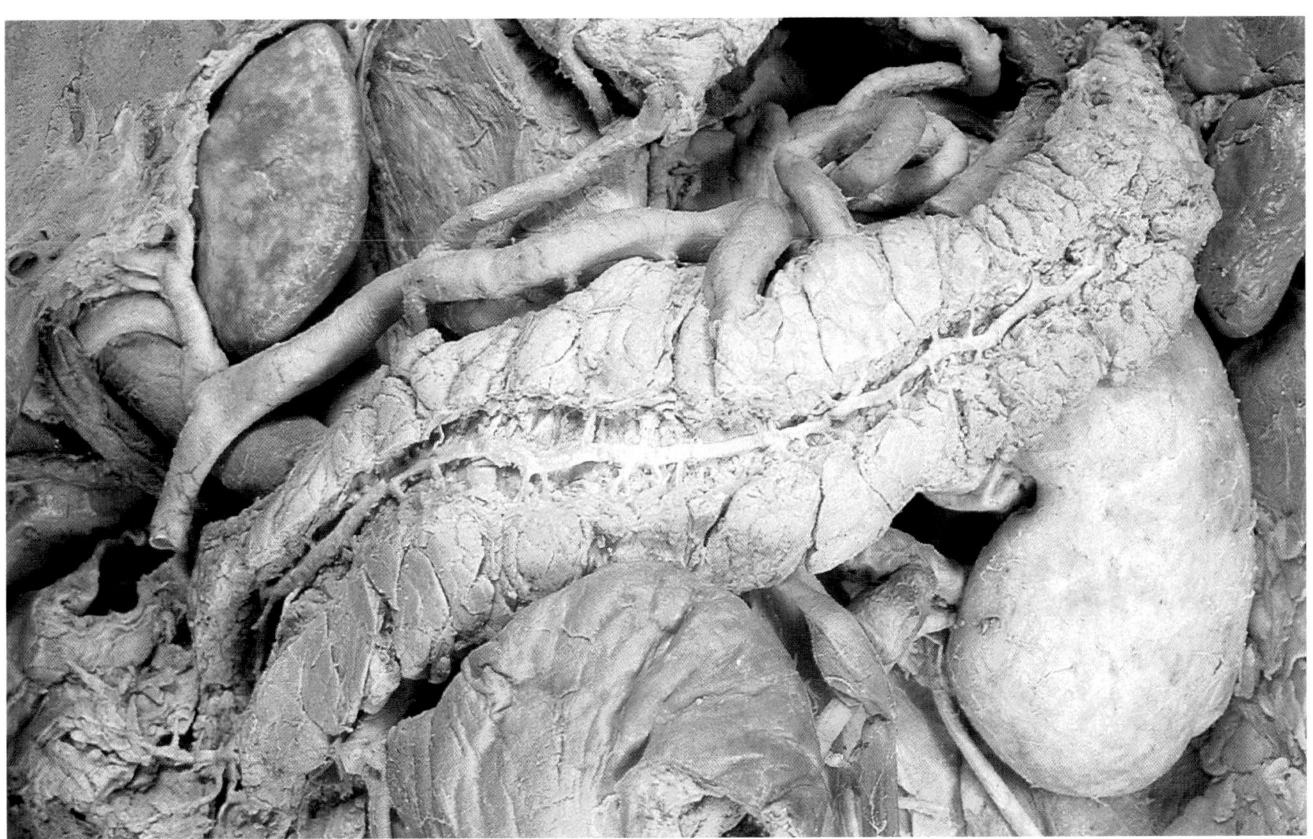

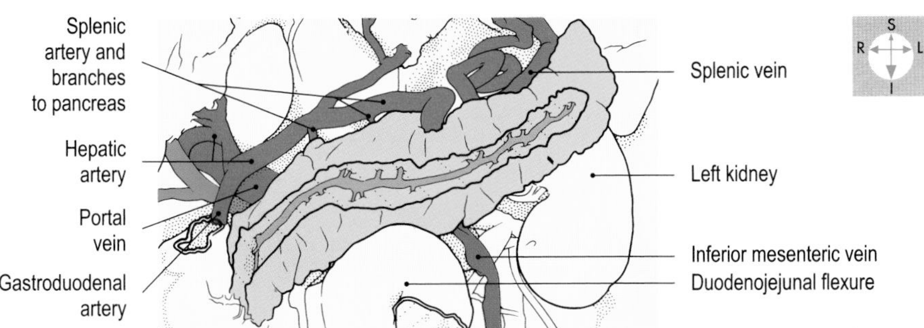

Fig. 4.55 Principal vascular relations of the body and tail of the pancreas.

Liver

The liver is the largest organ in the body and lies in the upper part of the abdominal cavity just beneath the diaphragm and mostly under cover of the ribs. It fills the right hypochondrium and extends across the epigastrium into the left hypochondrium. The living organ is reddish-brown and very soft and delicate.

The surface marking of the inferior margin of the liver coincides with the right costal margin as far anteriorly as the ninth costal cartilage and inclines across the abdomen to the eighth left costal cartilage. The healthy liver is not often palpable in the living subject even during deep inspiration when contraction of the diaphragm pushes the liver inferiorly.

The liver has the shape of a wedge, tapering towards the left (Fig. 4.56). Of its five surfaces, the superior, the anterior and the right lateral merge with no distinct borders intervening. However, a sharp inferior margin separates the anterior from the inferior or visceral surface. The latter faces obliquely downwards, backwards and to the left. The posterior surface blends with the visceral and superior surfaces at indistinct borders. Most of the surface of the liver is clothed in peritoneum.

Surface features and relations

Anterior and lateral surfaces

The anterior and lateral surfaces of the liver are smoothly convex to conform to the diaphragm and the anterior abdominal wall (Fig. 4.57). A two-layered fold of peritoneum, the falciform ligament, connects the anterior surface to the abdominal wall and demarcates the right and left lobes of the organ. In the free lower border of this ligament runs the fibrous remnant of the umbilical vein, the round ligament (ligamentum teres) of the liver, passing from the umbilicus to the visceral surface of the liver.

Superior surface

This surface is gently convex on each side of a shallow depression related to the central tendon of the diaphragm. Above the liver the two layers of the falciform ligament diverge. One layer passes to the right and continues as the superior layer of the coronary ligament (Fig. 4.58); the other extends to the tip of the left lobe where it forms the left triangular ligament. The posterior layer of this ligament, when traced to the right, is continuous with the lesser omentum.

Visceral surface

This surface (Fig. 4.59) is divided into three areas by two vertical features, the gall bladder and the fissure for the round ligament, the upper ends of which are linked by a horizontal cleft. This cleft is the porta hepatis through which pass the branches of the proper hepatic artery and portal vein and the hepatic ducts. The round ligament (ligamentum teres hepatic) ascends along its fissure to reach the portal vein. To the left of the fissure the left lobe of the liver overlies the body of the stomach and lesser omentum. To the right of the fissure is the small rectangular quadrate lobe, which is related to the anterior aspects of the pyloric region of the stomach and the first part of the duodenum. To the right of the

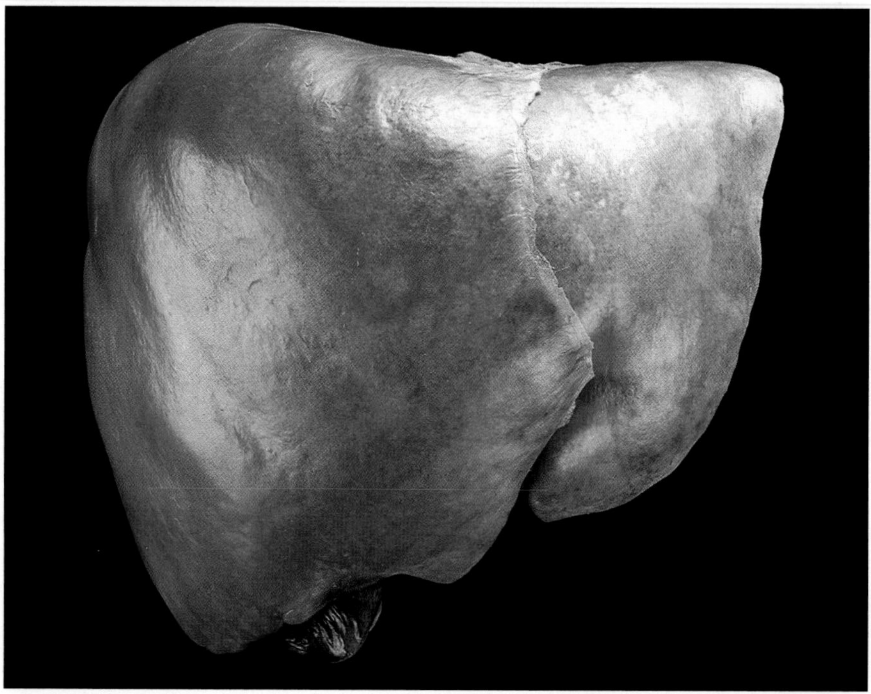

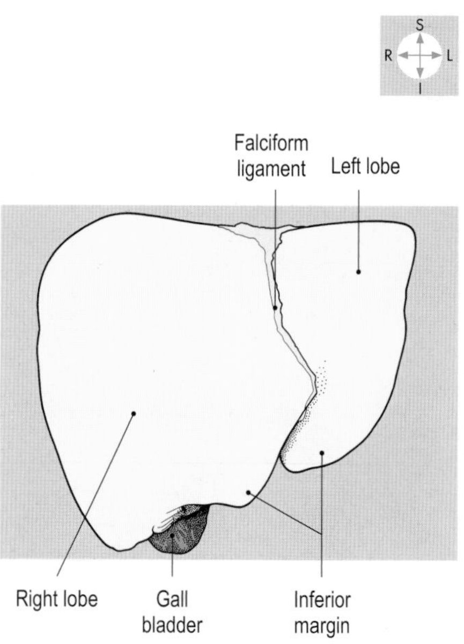

Fig. 4.56 Anterior view of the liver.

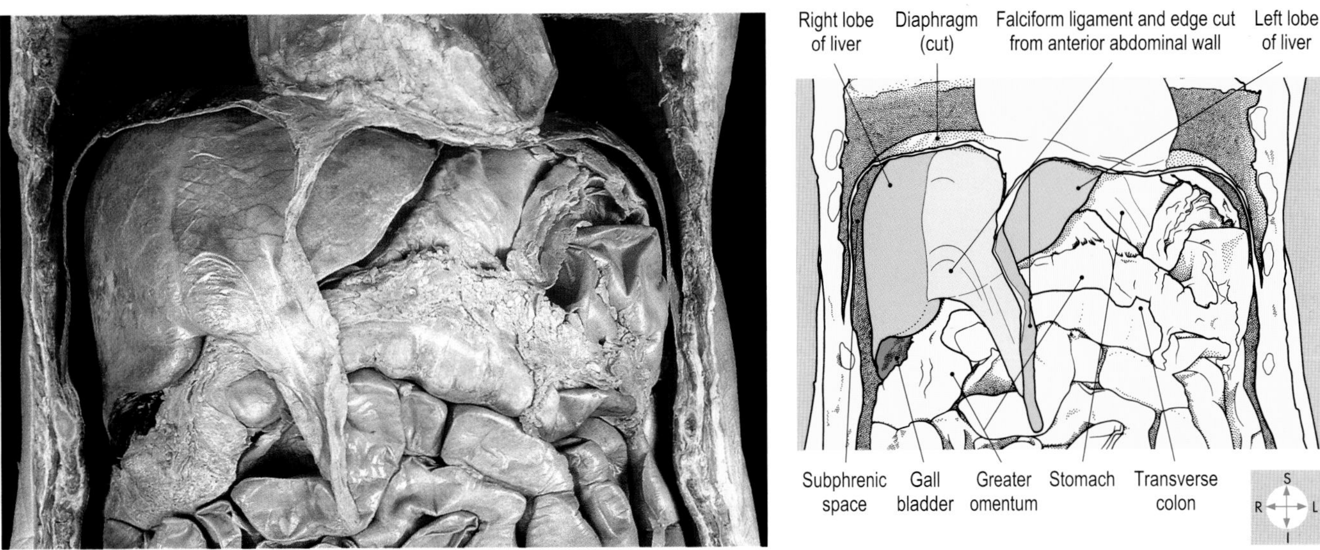

Fig. 4.57 Liver and some of its relations. In this specimen the greater omentum is adherent to the liver and stomach.

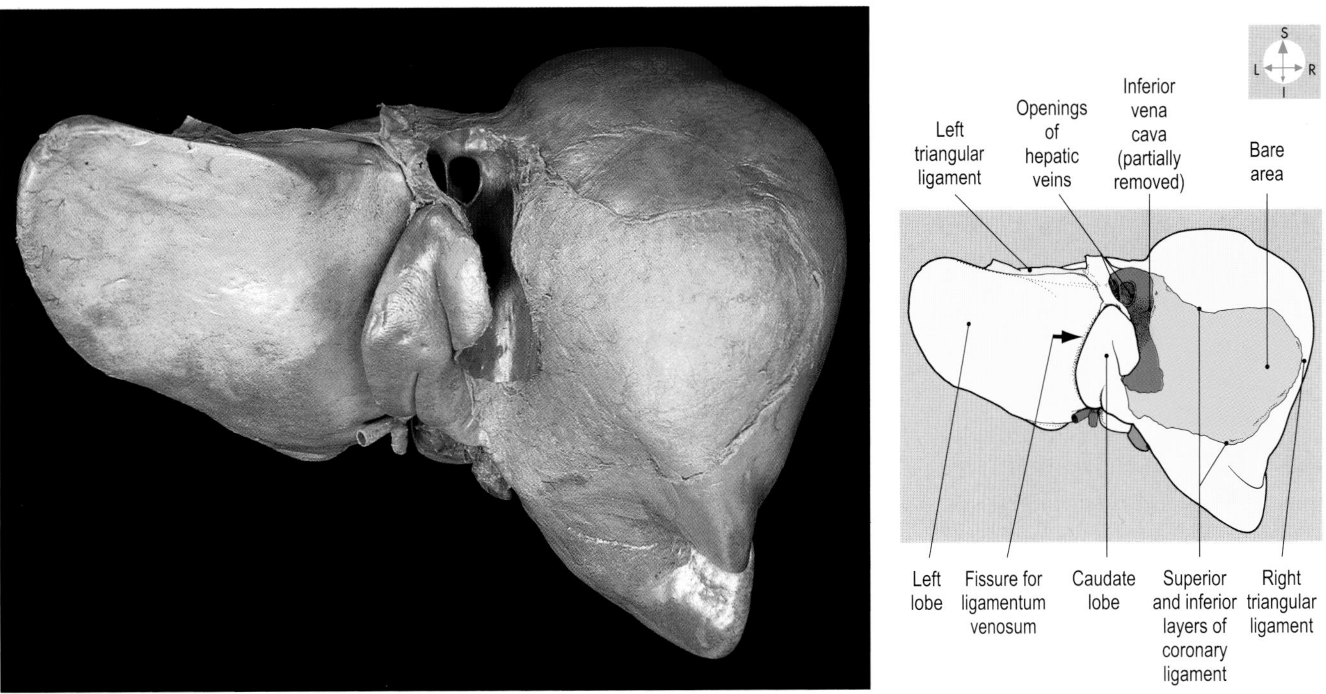

Fig. 4.58 Posterior view of the liver.

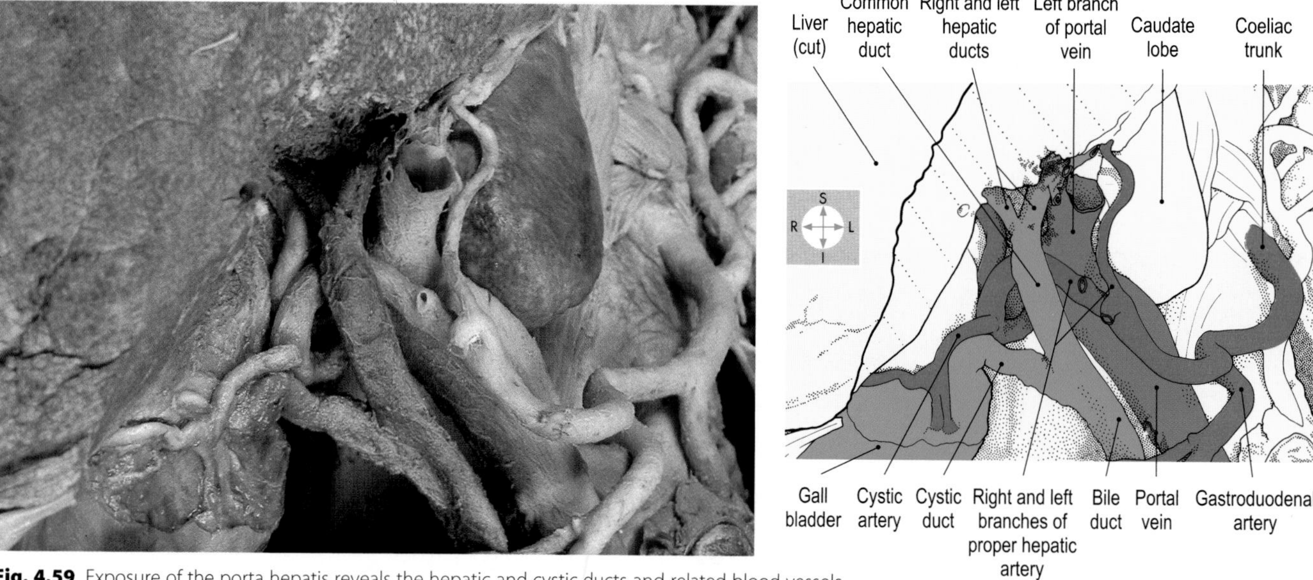

Fig. 4.59 Exposure of the porta hepatis reveals the hepatic and cystic ducts and related blood vessels.

quadrate lobe is the gall bladder, embedded in its fossa. An impression to the right of the gall bladder accommodates the upper pole of the right kidney. This surface of the right lobe is also related to the right colic flexure and the descending duodenum.

Posterior surface

This surface is also divided into three areas (see Fig. 4.58). Extending upwards from the left end of the porta hepatis is the fissure in which lies the ligamentum venosum, the fibrous remnant of the fetal ductus venosus. The lesser omentum attaches to the liver in the depths of this fissure and around the margins of the porta hepatis (Fig. 4.60). The portion of the liver to the left of the fissure covers the front of the abdominal oesophagus and the fundus of the stomach.

To the right of the fissure lies the caudate lobe, facing into the superior recess of the omental bursa. To the right of this lobe lies the inferior vena cava, which usually grooves the liver deeply. Further to the right is the bare area (see Fig. 4.58), where the right lobe of the liver is in direct contact with the diaphragm and the right suprarenal gland with no intervening peritoneum. The bare area is bounded above and below by the two layers of the coronary ligament which converge laterally to form the right triangular ligament.

Subphrenic and subhepatic spaces

The arrangement of the various peritoneal ligaments around the liver produces several clinically important spaces in which fluids may accumulate. Between the liver and the diaphragm are the subphrenic spaces (see Fig. 4.57), separated from each other by the falciform ligament and the superior layer of the coronary ligament. The subhepatic spaces lie below and behind the liver, adjacent to either the stomach or the right kidney.

Biliary apparatus

Ducts

Bile produced by the liver is collected by a system of canaliculi that drain into the right and left hepatic ducts. The two hepatic ducts emerge through the porta hepatis and soon unite to form the common hepatic duct. As this duct descends in the free border of the lesser omentum it is joined from the right by the cystic duct to form the bile duct (Fig. 4.59).

Initially, the bile duct lies in the free edge of the lesser omentum, to the right of the hepatic artery and in front of the portal vein. It then passes behind the first part of the duodenum with the gastroduodenal artery and curves to the right behind the head of the pancreas, sometimes grooving the gland (see Fig. 4.54). The bile duct pierces the wall of the descending duodenum in company with the main pancreatic duct (see Fig. 4.51).

Gall bladder

This is a hollow, pear-shaped organ in which bile from the liver is concentrated and stored (see Fig. 4.61). It lies against the visceral surface of the liver, often partially buried in its substance, and usually projects beyond the inferior margin to end blindly in a rounded fundus. The fundus normally makes contact with the anterior abdominal wall where the lateral edge (linea semilunaris) of the right rectus abdominis muscle crosses the costal margin. The body of the gall bladder is its widest part and tapers superiorly into the neck, which continues as the cystic duct. This duct, through which bile enters and leaves, runs upwards towards the

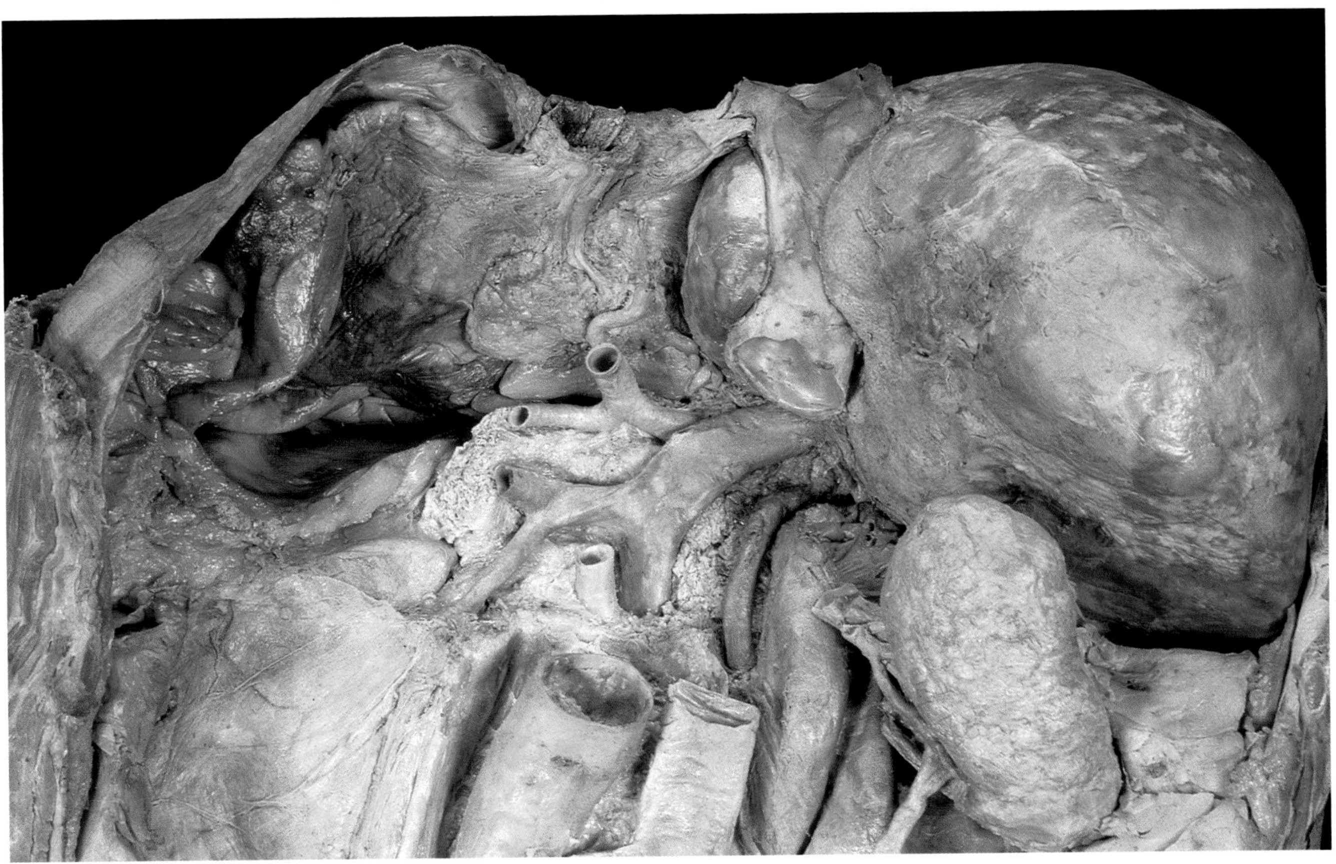

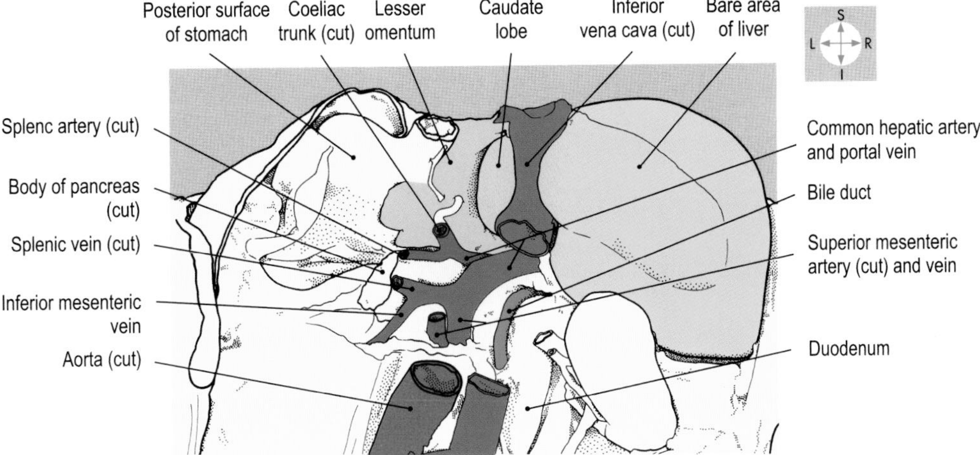

Fig. 4.60 Posterior view of liver, stomach and lesser omentum. The spleen, left kidney, parts of the pancreas, aorta and inferior vena cava have been removed.

porta hepatis and then turns downwards to join the common hepatic duct. The undersurface of the gall bladder is covered by peritoneum continuous with that surrounding the liver. The body is usually related to the proximal part of the duodenum and the fundus often makes contact with the transverse colon. Inflammation associated with gallstones can progress to ulceration, allowing stones to pass from the gall bladder into the duodenum or colon.

The arterial supply to the gall bladder is provided by the cystic artery, which usually springs from the right branch of the proper hepatic artery (Fig. 4.59), though its origin is variable. The cystic vein normally drains into the portal vein or its right branch.

Hepatic blood vessels

Blood is conveyed to the liver by the proper hepatic artery and the portal vein, both of which enter via the porta hepatis. Blood is drained by the hepatic veins embedded in the organ which enter the anterior aspect of the inferior vena cava immediately below the diaphragm (see Fig. 4.58). The common hepatic artery, a branch of the coeliac trunk (Fig. 4.62), runs retroperitoneally downwards and to the right to the superior border of the first part of the duodenum (Fig. 4.59). Here the common hepatic artery gives off the right gastric and gastroduodenal arteries and continues as the proper hepatic artery. The right gastric artery arises

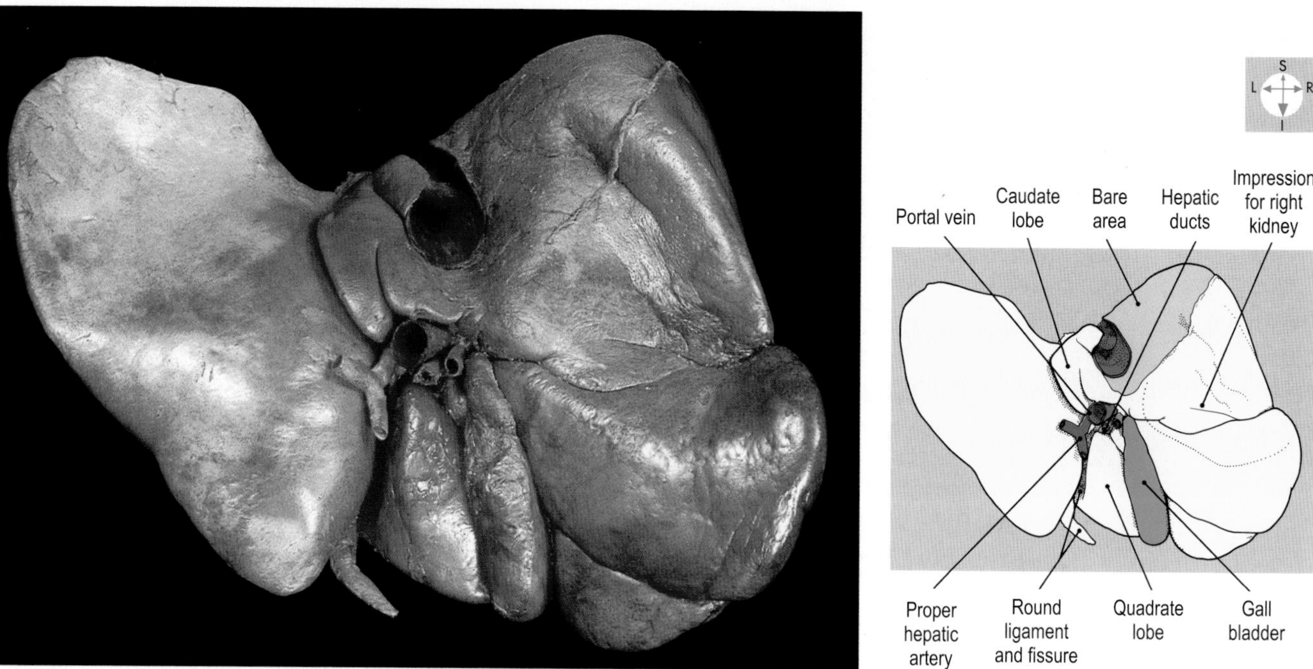

Fig. 4.61 Inferior view of liver and gall bladder showing porta hepatis and visceral surface.

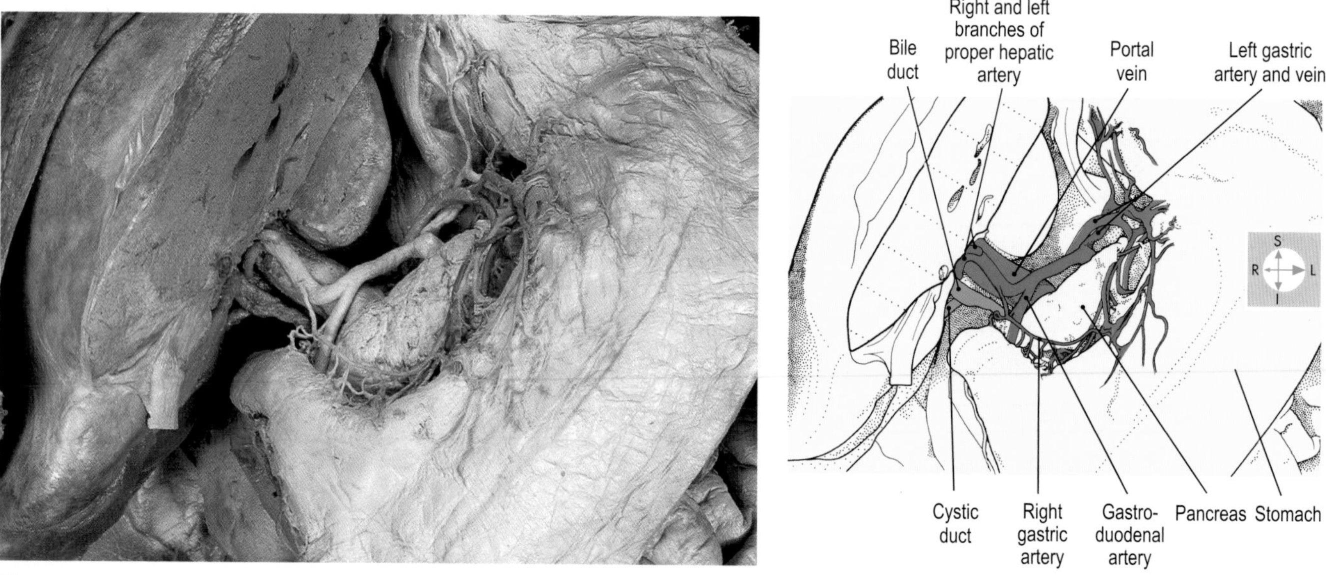

Fig. 4.62 Course and branches of the common hepatic artery. The lesser omentum has been removed.

above the first part of the duodenum and runs to the left within the lesser omentum, supplying the lesser curvature of the stomach. The larger gastroduodenal artery descends behind the first part of the duodenum alongside the bile duct. Its terminal branches are the superior pancreaticoduodenal artery (see Fig. 4.52) and the right gastro-omental artery (see Fig. 4.43). The proper hepatic artery ascends in the free border of the lesser omentum on the left of the bile duct and anterior to the portal vein. Near the porta hepatis it divides into right and left branches to enter the liver with corresponding branches of the portal vein. The left branches of the artery and vein are distributed to the left, quadrate and most of the caudate lobes. The right branches supply the remainder of the liver. The proper hepatic artery also supplies the gall bladder via the cystic artery (Fig. 4.59).

Jejunum and Ileum

The jejunum and ileum constitute the major part of the small intestine. The jejunum commences at the duodenojejunal flexure and the ileum terminates at the ileocaecal junction. Between these two sites the small intestine is about 5 or 6 metres long and forms numerous loops that fill most of the infracolic compartment of the abdomen (Fig. 4.63). By convention, the proximal two-fifths are called the jejunum and the remainder the ileum. However, no precise anatomical feature marks the junction between the two, there being a gradual morphological transition along the whole length of the small intestine.

As the small intestine is traced distally there is a gradual reduction in the size of the lumen. The terminal ileum is the narrowest region and it is here that foreign bodies may lodge. Mucosal folds (plicae circulares) are numerous in the proximal jejunum (Fig. 4.64) but diminish in both size and number so that in the distal ileum they are often absent. This difference in mucosal structure can be detected by palpation and may also be apparent on radiographs. The distribution of lymphoid tissue in the jejunum is diffuse whereas in the mucosa of the ileum it is arranged in discrete clumps (Peyer's patches).

Ileal diverticulum

Within a metre of the ileocaecal junction the ileum occasionally possesses a diverticulum on its antimesenteric border. This diverticulum (Meckel's diverticulum) is the embryological remnant of the vitellointestinal duct and may be connected to the umbilicus. Inflammation of the diverticulum can give rise to clinical features similar to those of appendicitis.

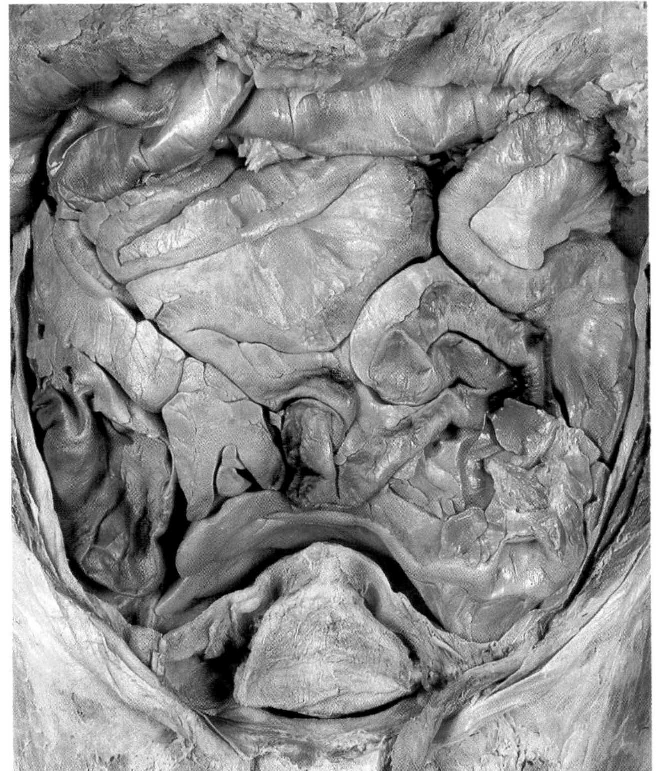

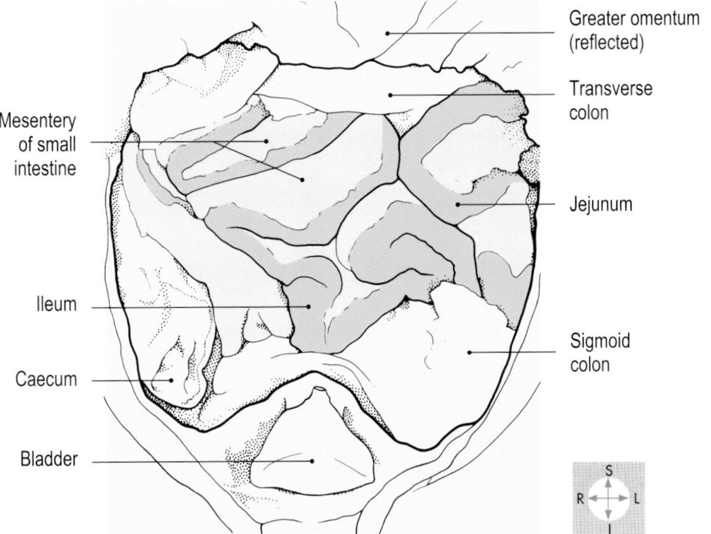

Fig. 4.63 Jejunum and ileum. The greater omentum has been reflected upwards.

Mesentery

The jejunum and ileum are contained within the free border of the mesentery of the small intestine. This fan-shaped structure has a root about 15 cm long attached to the posterior abdominal wall between the duodenojejunal flexure and the ileocaecal junction (Fig. 4.65). The mesentery divides the infracolic compartment of the peritoneal cavity into right and left infracolic spaces. Between its two peritoneal layers the mesentery contains a quantity of fat, which is particularly abundant in the ileal portion. Embedded in this fat are numerous jejunal and ileal blood vessels (see below), lymphatic vessels and nodes, and autonomic nerves.

Location and relations

Because they are suspended from the mesentery, the jejunum and ileum possess considerable mobility and their coils can change position relative to adjacent organs. The jejunum usually occupies the central part of the abdomen, especially the umbilical region, while the ileum lies at a lower level, mostly in the hypogastrium and the pelvic cavity (Fig. 4.63). The terminal ileum usually ascends from the pelvis into the right iliac fossa to reach the medial aspect of the caecum (see Fig. 4.69). The principal anterior relations of the jejunum and ileum are the greater omentum, the transverse colon and its mesocolon, and the anterior abdominal wall. Posteriorly, the coils of small intestine

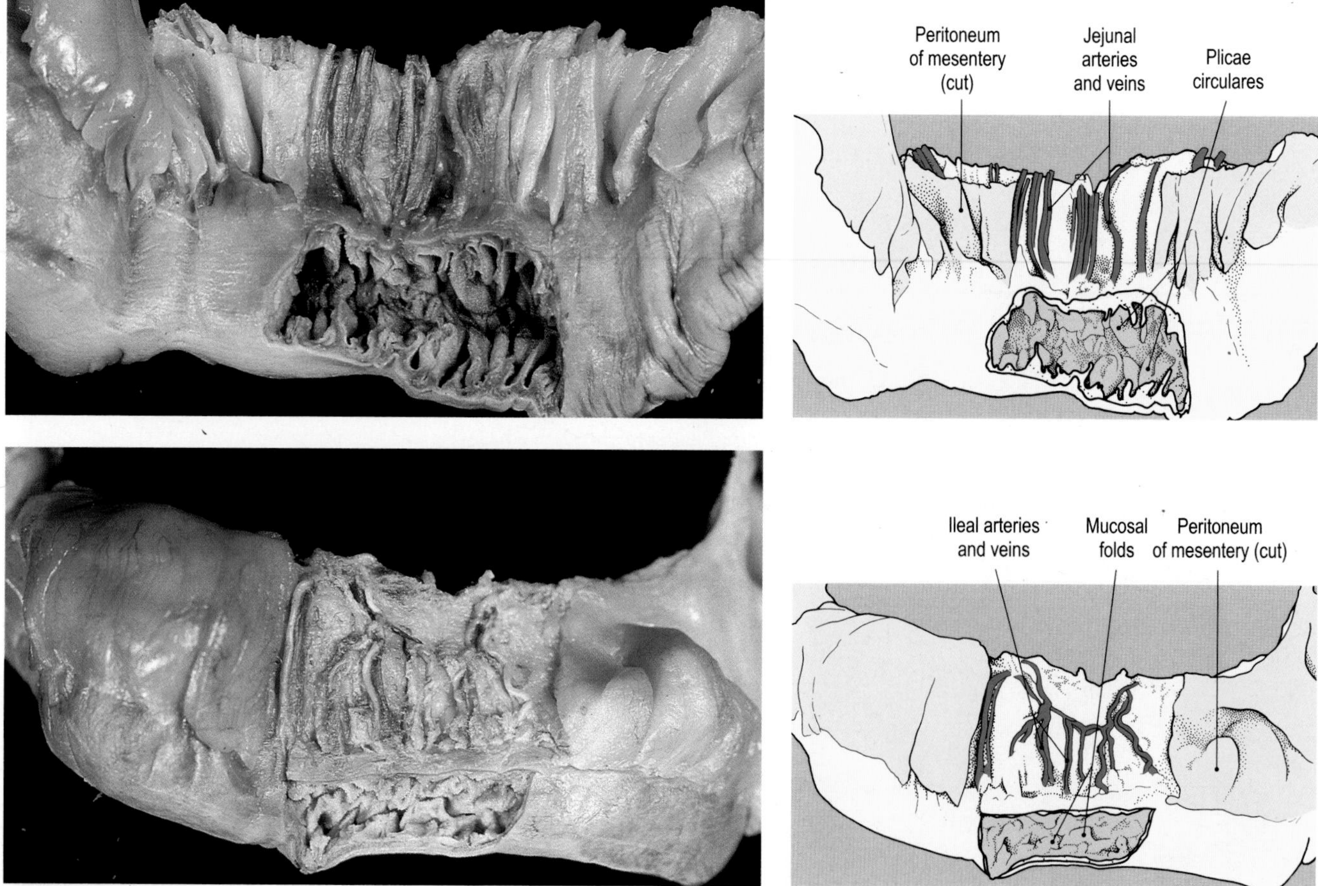

Fig. 4.64 Segments of jejunum (upper) and ileum (lower) opened to show their mucosae. Their mesenteries have been dissected to reveal the blood vessels.

overlie retroperitoneal structures on the posterior wall of the abdomen and pelvis and may also overlap the ascending, descending and sigmoid parts of the colon. Within the pelvis, loops of ileum may lie in contact with pelvic organs such as the rectum and urinary bladder and, in the female, with the uterus and its appendages.

Superior mesenteric vessels

The superior mesenteric artery supplies the intestine from the descending duodenum to the splenic flexure of the colon. The artery is an anterior branch of the abdominal aorta (see Fig. 4.89) at the level of the first lumbar vertebra, just below the coeliac trunk. It descends in front of the left renal vein (see Fig. 4.91) and behind the neck of the pancreas. Inclining to the right, the artery continues downwards in front of the uncinate process of the pancreas and across the horizontal duodenum to enter the root of the mesentery (Fig. 4.66).

The superior mesenteric artery gives rise to middle colic and inferior pancreaticoduodenal branches before gaining the mesentery. As it descends in the root of the mesentery it furnishes the right colic artery, which passes behind the peritoneum to supply the ascending colon. A further branch, also retroperitoneal, is the ileocolic artery, which inclines downwards and to the right towards the caecum. The superior mesenteric artery also gives numerous branches to the jejunum and ileum. Within the mesentery these jejunal and ileal arteries anastomose, producing a series of arterial arcades which are more profuse in the ileal part of

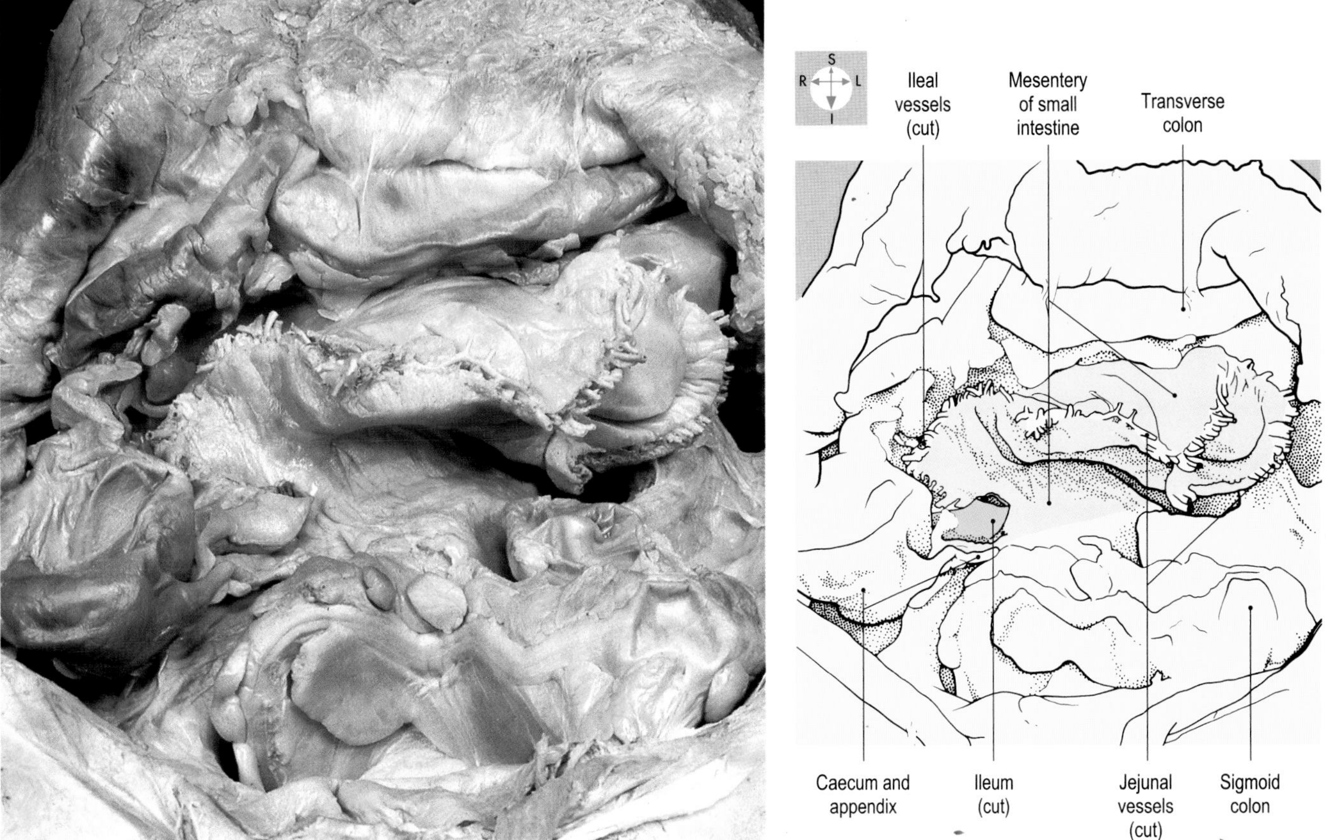

Fig. 4.65 Mesentery of the small intestine. All of the jejunum and most of the ileum have been excised and the cut edge of mesentery trimmed to reveal the jejunal and ileal vessels.

Transverse colon (displaced)
Middle colic artery
Right colic artery
Pancreas
Marginal artery
Ileocolic artery
Ascending colon
Caecal arteries
Ileum (cut)
Caecum
Transverse mesocolon (cut and displaced)
Superior mesenteric vein
Jejunal arteries (cut)
Mesentery of small intestine (cut)
Ileal arteries (cut)
Meso-appendix and appendix
Sigmoid colon
S
R
L
I

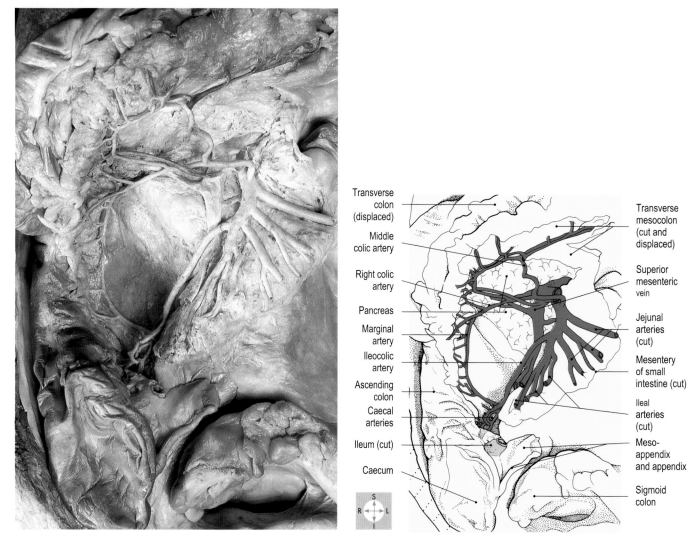

Fig. 4.66 Superior mesenteric artery and its branches. The jejunal and ileal veins have been removed.

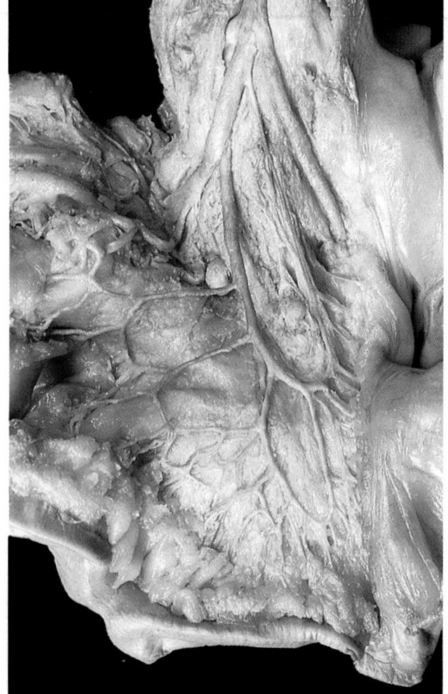

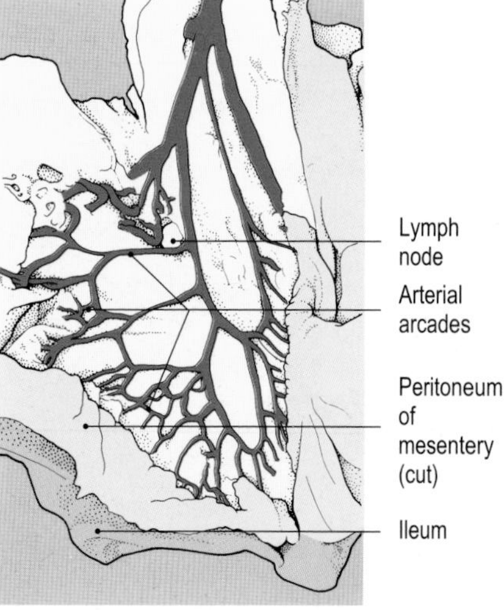

Fig. 4.67 Ileal arteries and their arcades in the mesentery of the ileum.

the mesentery (Fig. 4.67). The superior mesenteric artery terminates at the upper border of the terminal ileum, where it anastomoses with the lower branch of the ileocolic artery and the distal ileal arteries.

The superior mesenteric vein begins above the terminal ileum and ascends in the root of the mesentery. It lies on the right of the superior mesenteric artery and its tributaries correspond to the branches of the artery. The vein terminates behind the neck of the pancreas by joining the splenic vein to form the portal vein. Close to its termination, it may be joined by the inferior mesenteric vein (see Fig. 4.78), but this more commonly enters the splenic vein.

Caecum, Appendix and Colon

The large intestine is approximately 1.5 metres long and comprises the caecum, appendix, colon, rectum and anal canal. The caecum and appendix lie in the right iliac fossa while the colon runs a circuitous course (Figs 4.68, 4.69 & 4.70) before descending into the pelvic cavity to become continuous with the rectum. Descriptions of the rectum and anal canal are given in Section 5.

The lumen of the intestine is relatively wide in the caecum and ascending colon but narrows gradually as the colon is traced towards the rectum.

The outer longitudinal muscle coat of the caecum and colon is thickened to form three longitudinal bands, the taeniae coli (Fig. 4.71). Bulges (haustrations) of the gut wall between the taeniae

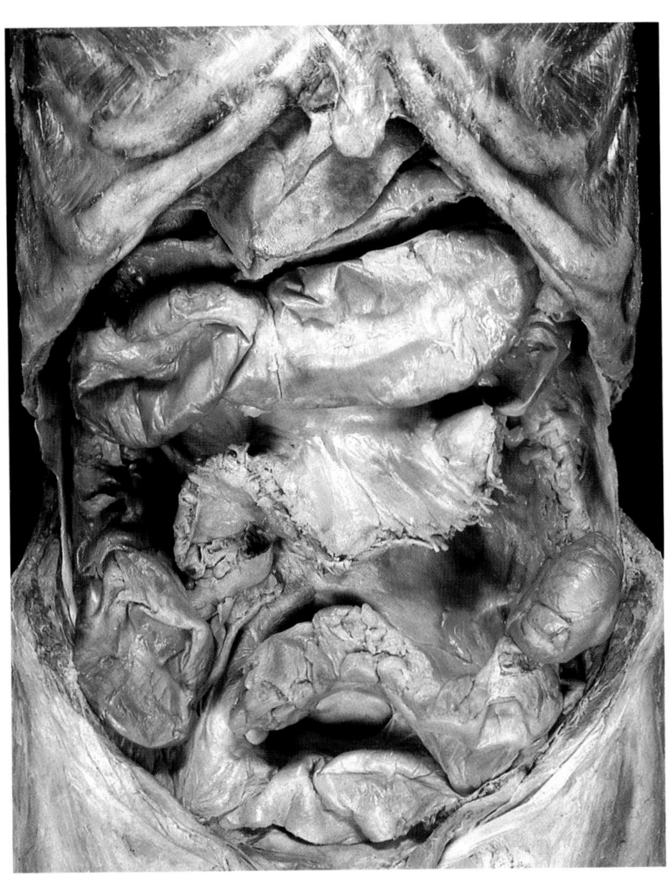

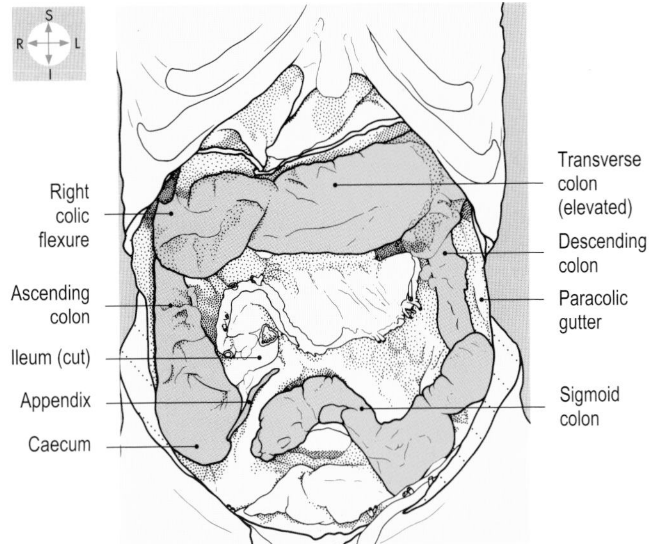

Fig. 4.68 Caecum, appendix and colon after removal of the greater omentum and most of the small intestine. The transverse colon has been raised.

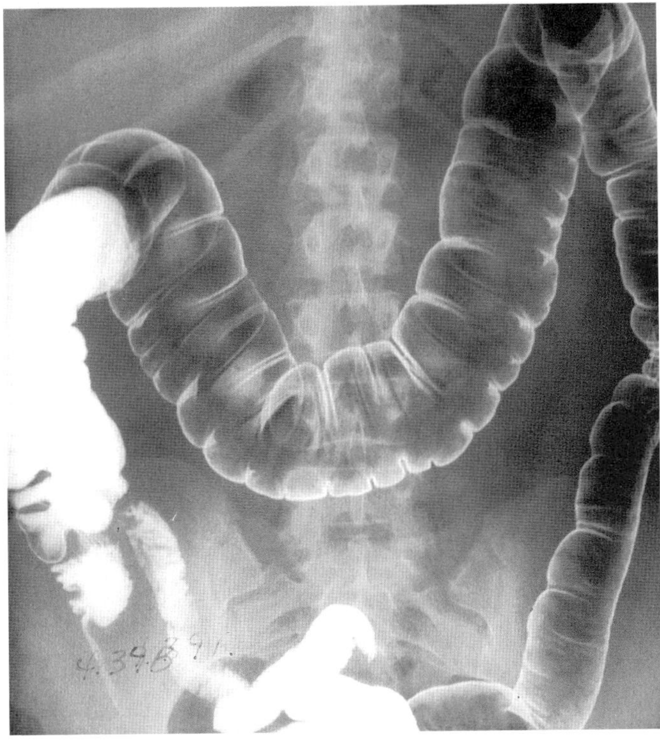

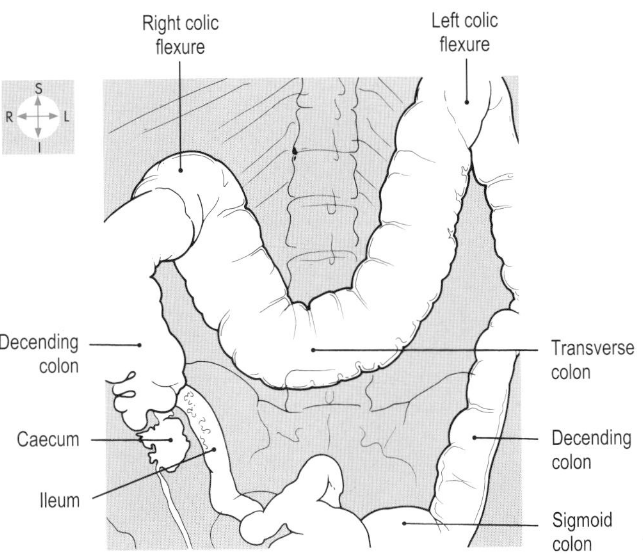

Fig. 4.69 Barium enema radiograph. Most of the colon is gas filled, but barium coats its mucosa and has passed proximally into the ileum.

correspond with sacculations on the mucosal surface. The peritoneal surface of the colon (but not of the appendix or caecum) is characterized by numerous fat-filled tags, the omental appendices (appendices epiploicae).

Caecum

The ileum terminates by opening into the large intestine at a slit-like or oval aperture, the ileal orifice (ileocaecal valve) (Fig. 4.72). The caecum is the blind-ending portion of the large intestine below the level of this orifice. The caecum and ascending colon are in direct continuity and the three taeniae coli descend along the outer surface of the caecum and converge on its posteromedial aspect at the root of the appendix.

The caecum usually lies in the right iliac fossa above the lateral half of the inguinal ligament (Fig. 4.73). Anteriorly, it is related to the abdominal wall, the greater omentum and coils of ileum; the iliacus and psoas muscles lie posteriorly. The caecum may lie

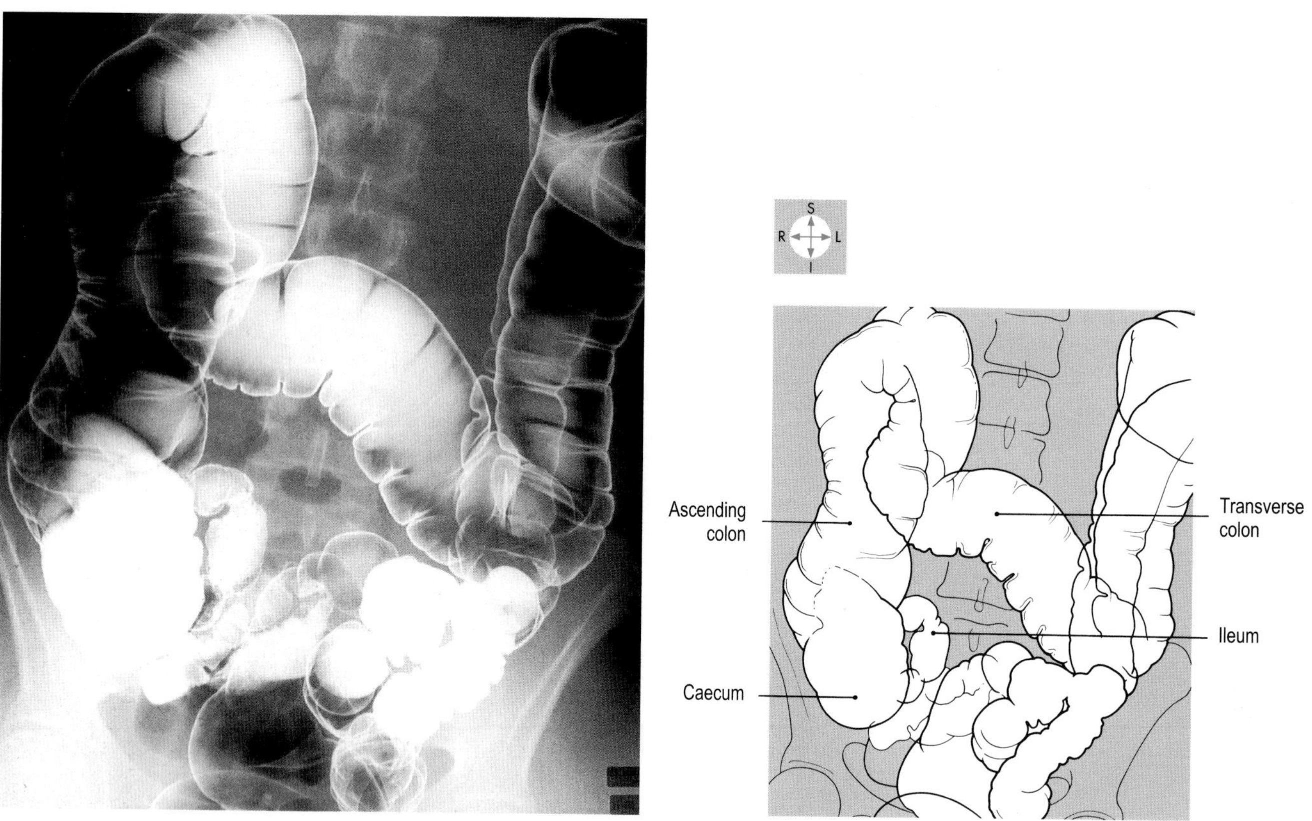

Fig. 4.70 Barium enema radiograph of a different subject from Fig. 4.69, to show variation in bowel anatomy. The transverse colon is more dependent and coils of sigmoid colon overlap each other.

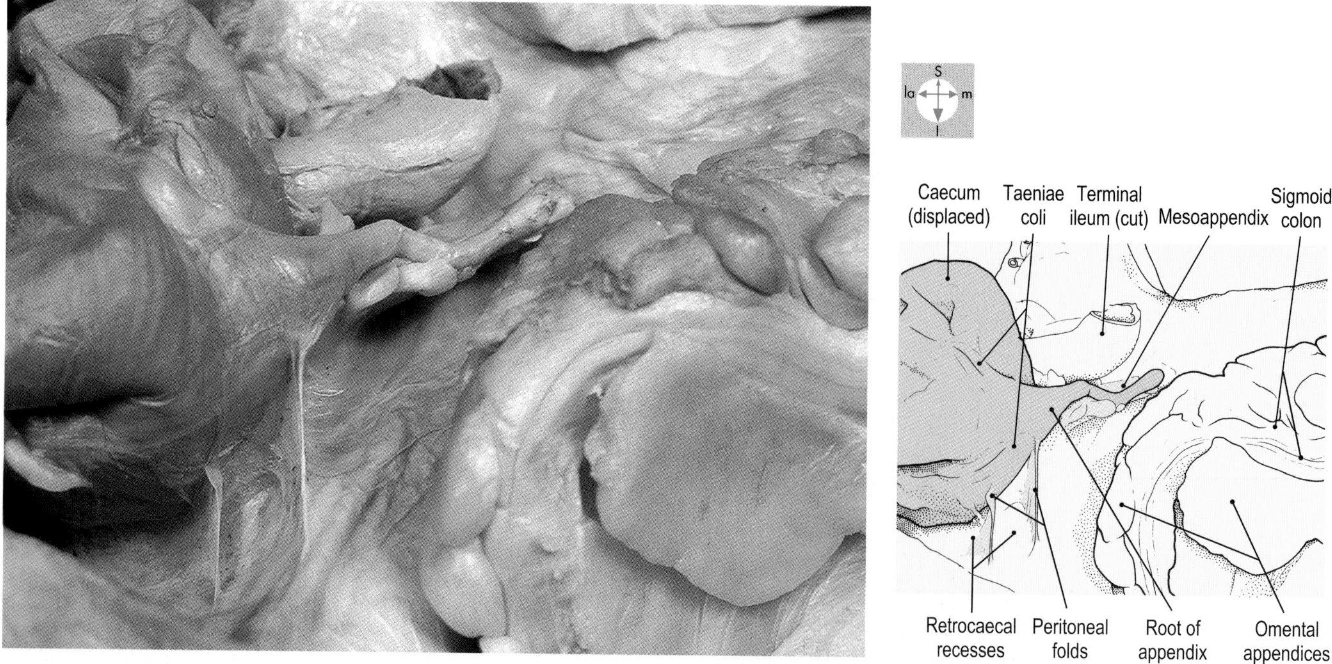

Fig. 4.71 Base of the appendix and retrocaecal folds and recesses revealed by pulling the caecum forwards.

free in the iliac fossa, completely surrounded by peritoneum. Alternatively, it may be attached to the iliac fossa by peritoneal folds forming a retrocaecal fossa (Fig. 4.71). Rarely, the caecum is entirely retroperitoneal. On the medial side of the caecum, adjacent to the terminal ileum, small peritoneal folds may enclose one or more ileocaecal recesses.

Appendix

The worm-like appendix is attached to the posteromedial wall of the caecum where the taeniae coli converge (Fig. 4.71). It is a thick-walled tube with a narrow lumen and, although variable in length, usually measures approximately 10 cm. The surface marking of the root of the appendix is relatively constant, lying one-third of the distance from the anterior superior iliac spine to the umbilicus.

The appendix usually possesses a mesentery, the mesoappendix (Fig. 4.72), which is attached to the mesentery of the ileum and confers upon the appendix a degree of mobility. Although it frequently lies behind the caecum (Fig. 4.74), in front of the iliacus or psoas muscles, it occasionally descends into the pelvis where its tip may lie adjacent to the bladder, the right ureter and, in the female, the ovary or uterine tube (Fig. 4.73). Rarely, the appendix lies anterior or posterior to the terminal ileum. It is a common site of infection (appendicitis) which may spread to adjacent structures. Usually, the pain of appendicitis arises initially from the gut wall and is periumbilical. When the inflammation spreads to the parietal peritoneum the pain become localized to the right iliac region.

Colon

The colon consists of ascending, transverse, descending and sigmoid parts (see Fig. 4.68). The ascending and descending parts are usually retroperitoneal while the transverse and sigmoid parts are suspended by mesenteries. The colon possesses two acute

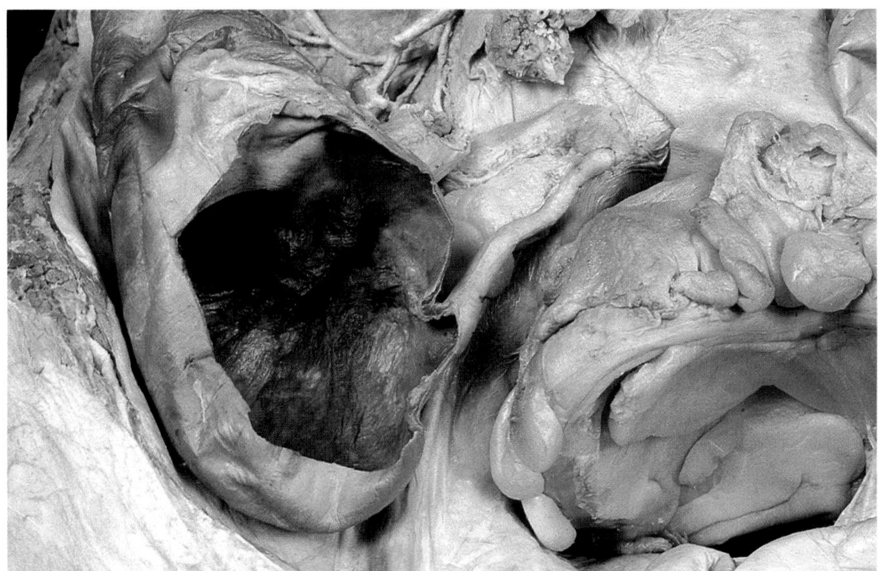

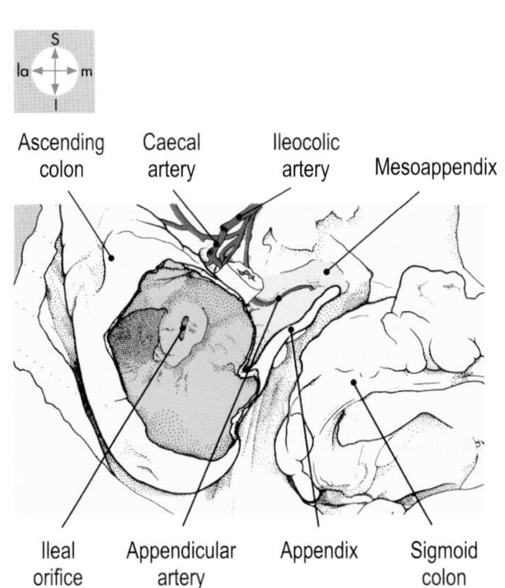

Fig. 4.72 Ileal orifice revealed by removal of the anterior wall of the caecum. The mesoappendix has been dissected to show the appendicular artery.

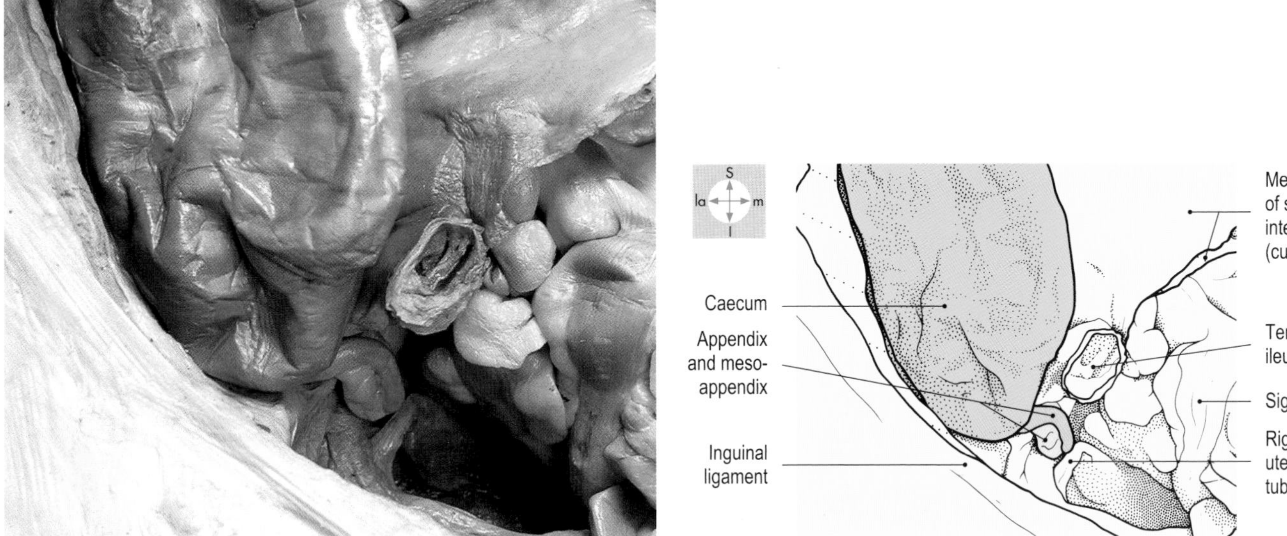

Fig. 4.73 After removal of most of the small intestine, this appendix can be seen descending over the pelvic brim.

angulations, the right (hepatic) and left (splenic) flexures (see Fig. 4.69).

The ascending colon begins at the level of the ileal orifice and runs vertically upwards. At the right colic flexure under the right lobe of the liver, it becomes continuous with the transverse colon. Anterior to the ascending colon lie the abdominal wall, loops of ileum and often the greater omentum. Its posterior relations include the iliacus, transversus abdominis, quadratus lumborum and the right kidney.

The transverse colon extends from the right to the left colic flexure and is suspended by the transverse mesocolon. Typically, its middle portion hangs downwards and crosses the umbilical region (see Figs 4.69 & 4.70). At the left colic flexure just below the splenic hilum, it turns inferiorly to become the descending colon. From right to left, the superior relations of the transverse colon include the liver and gall bladder and the greater curvature of the stomach. Posteriorly lie the descending duodenum, the pancreas, loops of small intestine and the spleen. Anteriorly lie the greater omentum and the abdominal wall. The greater omentum attaches to both the transverse colon and the greater curvature of the stomach (see p. 160).

The descending colon runs from the left flexure to the left iliac fossa and turns medially at the pelvic brim to continue as the sigmoid colon (see Figs 4.68 & 4.76). The upper part of the descending colon is covered anteriorly by coils of jejunum while the lower part usually makes contact with the abdominal wall, through which it is often palpable. Its posterior relations include the left kidney and the psoas, quadratus lumborum and iliacus muscles.

The sigmoid (pelvic) colon begins at the pelvic brim and terminates in front of the third sacral vertebra by joining the rectum. The sigmoid colon varies in length and is mobile on its mesentery, the sigmoid mesocolon. Its proximal portion usually runs to the right across the lower abdomen (see Fig. 4.68) and is related superiorly to loops of small intestine. The remainder of the sigmoid colon lies in the pelvic cavity in contact with the upper surfaces of the pelvic organs.

Blood supply

The blood supply of the caecum, appendix, ascending colon and most of the transverse colon is provided by the superior mesenteric vessels. The remainder of the colon is supplied by the inferior mesenteric vessels.

Branches of superior mesenteric vessels

The origin and course of the superior mesenteric artery are described on page 177. Its branches to the large intestine vary considerably but usually include the middle colic, right colic and ileocolic arteries (Fig. 4.75).

The middle colic artery enters the transverse mesocolon and divides into right and left branches, which supply the proximal two-thirds of the transverse colon. The right colic artery reaches the ascending colon and divides into ascending and descending branches, which supply the organ. The ileocolic artery has anterior and posterior caecal branches and also supplies the ascending colon and terminal ileum. The appendicular branch (see Fig. 4.72) descends behind the terminal ileum, enters the mesoappendix and runs near its free border to the tip of the appendix. The arteries supplying the caecum and colon anastomose, often forming a continuous marginal artery (Fig. 4.75).

Veins corresponding to the branches of the superior mesenteric artery drain into the superior mesenteric vein (Fig. 4.75; see Fig. 4.78).

Inferior mesenteric vessels

The inferior mesenteric artery arises from the anterior aspect of the abdominal aorta 3 cm or 4 cm above the bifurcation, often overlapped by the horizontal duodenum (Fig. 4.76). The artery runs retroperitoneally downwards and to the left to reach the pelvic brim. Here it crosses the common iliac vessels and continues into the pelvis as the superior rectal artery (see p. 218).

The first branch of the inferior mesenteric artery, the left colic artery, runs to the left and gives rise to ascending and descending branches. The former supplies the distal third of the transverse colon and the left colic flexure. The descending branch supplies the descending colon and the commencement of the sigmoid colon. The inferior mesenteric artery gives rise to several sigmoid arteries which reach the sigmoid colon via the mesocolon.

The branches of the inferior mesenteric artery are accompanied by tributaries of the inferior mesenteric vein (Fig. 4.76). The course and termination of this vessel are described with the portal venous system.

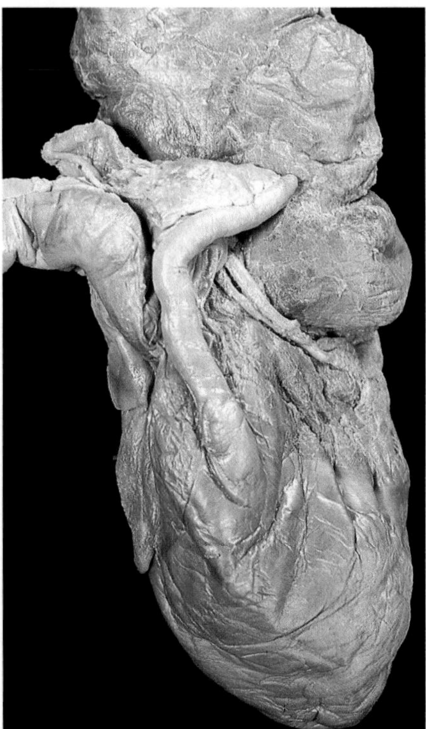

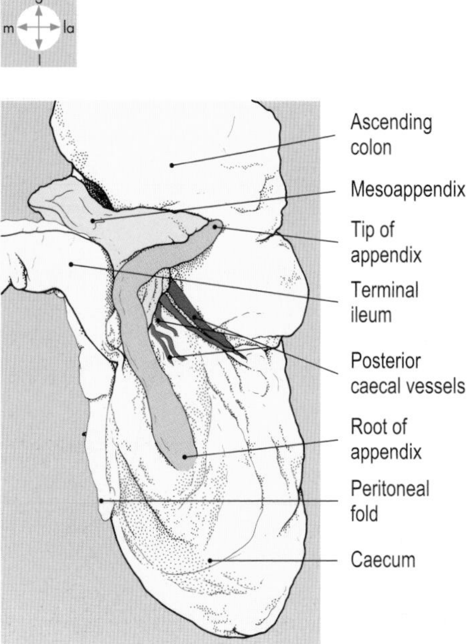

Fig. 4.74 Posterior aspect of the caecum to show a retrocaecal appendix.

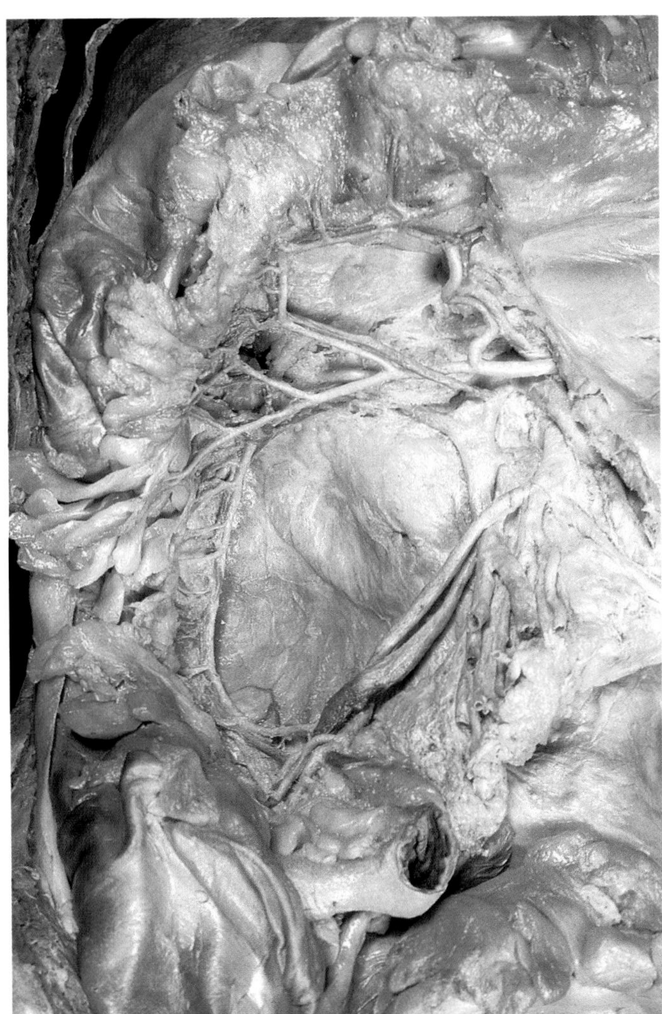

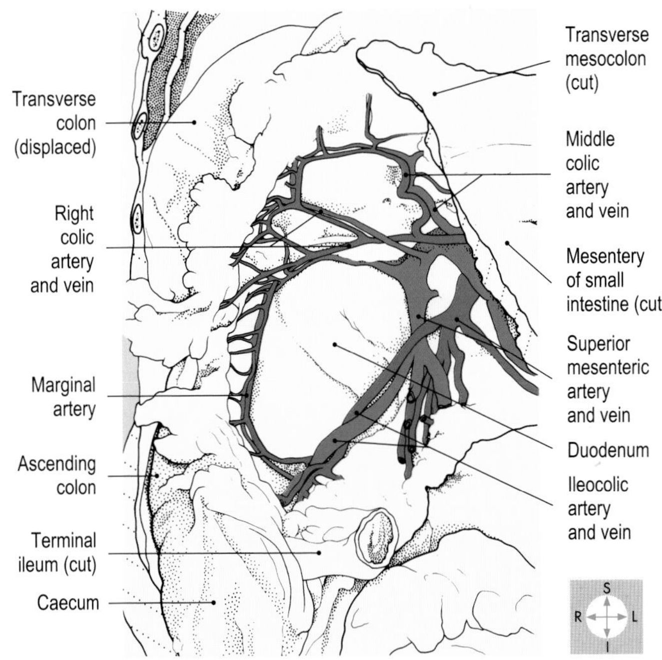

Fig. 4.75 Blood supply to the caecum, ascending and transverse colon. The transverse mesocolon and the mesentery of the small intestine have been dissected to reveal the ileocolic, right colic and middle colic vessels.

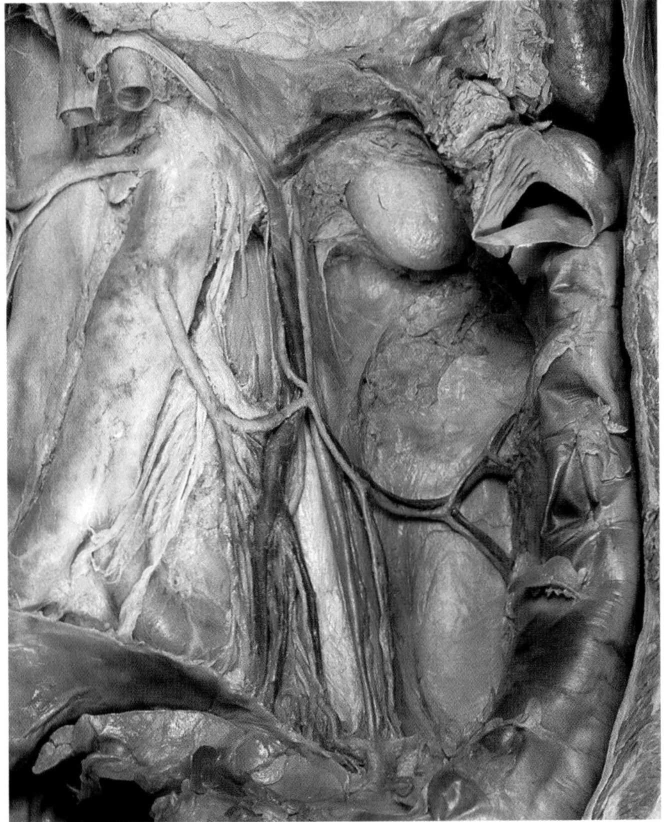

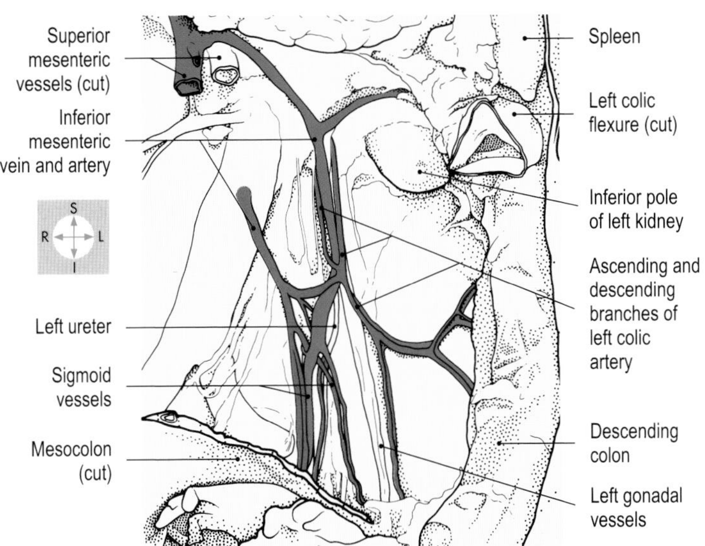

Fig. 4.76 Blood supply to the left colic flexure, descending colon and sigmoid colon. Removal of peritoneum from the posterior abdominal wall to the left of the aorta displays the inferior mesenteric vessels.

Portal Venous System

The hepatic portal venous system drains blood from most of the alimentary tract (including the abdominal oesophagus, stomach, small and large intestines), pancreas, and spleen. Blood from these organs is drained by the superior mesenteric and splenic veins which unite to form the portal vein (Fig. 4.77). This large vein approaches the porta hepatis with the proper hepatic artery, and branches of both vessels enter the liver and further subdivide. The liver is a common site of secondary infection or cancer because blood is conveyed to it from so many other organs. After traversing the liver, blood from both sources is drained by the hepatic veins, which enter the inferior vena cava.

Tributaries

The superior mesenteric vein (Fig. 4.78) receives blood from most of the small intestine and the proximal half of the large intestine. It drains the duodenum distal to the major papilla, the jejunum and ileum, the caecum and appendix, and the ascending and most of the trans-verse colon. The vein accompanies the superior mesenteric artery within the root of the mesentery and its tributaries generally correspond to the branches of the artery.

The splenic vein (Fig. 4.78) drains the spleen and parts of the pancreas and stomach. It arises at the hilum of the spleen and runs to the right in the splenorenal ligament behind the tail of the pancreas. The vein continues behind the body of the pancreas and usually

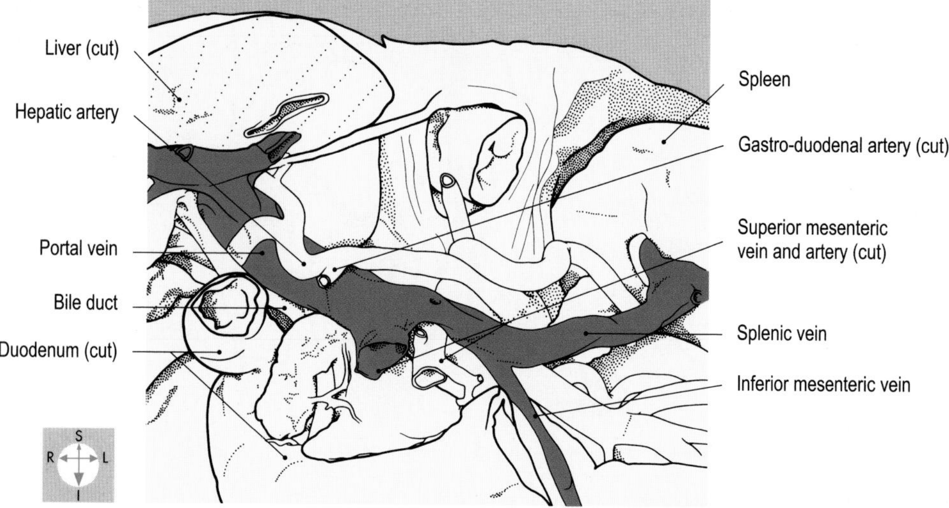

Fig. 4.77 Portal and splenic veins. Most of the pancreas has been removed and the superior duodenum turned aside.

receives the inferior mesenteric vein and other tributaries corresponding to the branches of the splenic artery.

The inferior mesenteric vein drains the upper part of the anal canal, the rectum, the sigmoid and descending parts of the colon and the distal part of the transverse colon. The vein initially accompanies the corresponding artery but in the latter part of its course it ascends the posterior abdominal wall independently, passing to the left of the duodenojejunal junction. The vessel usually terminates by joining the splenic vein behind the body of the pancreas (Fig. 4.77), but it may enter the superior mesenteric vein (Fig. 4.78).

Portal vein

The portal vein is formed behind the neck of the pancreas by the union of the superior mesenteric and splenic veins (Fig. 4.77). It runs upwards and to the right behind the gastroduodenal artery and the first part of the duodenum. The vein then enters the free border of the lesser omentum accompanied anteriorly by the bile duct and the proper hepatic artery (see Fig. 4.44). Near the porta hepatis the vein divides into left and right branches, which enter the liver. Several small veins enter the portal vein directly, including the left and right gastric veins and the cystic vein.

Portacaval anastomoses

There are numerous anastomoses between the tributaries of the portal venous system and those of the systemic venous system. In health, these portacaval anastomoses are microscopic; but if there is obstruction of blood flow through the portal vein or liver they may dilate and give rise to characteristic clinical features. For example, in the wall of the lowest part of the oesophagus, veins draining into the left gastric vein communicate with tributaries of the azygos venous system. Portal vein obstruction can cause gross swelling of these oesophageal veins (oesophageal varices), which may bleed profusely.

Similarly, paraumbilical veins accompanying the round ligament of the liver communicate with the portal vein at the porta hepatis and with veins of the anterior abdominal wall around the umbilicus. Portal vein obstruction, therefore, may result in dilatation of the subcutaneous veins of the abdominal wall. Other sites of portacaval anastomoses include the anal canal and retroperitoneal parts of the intestine.

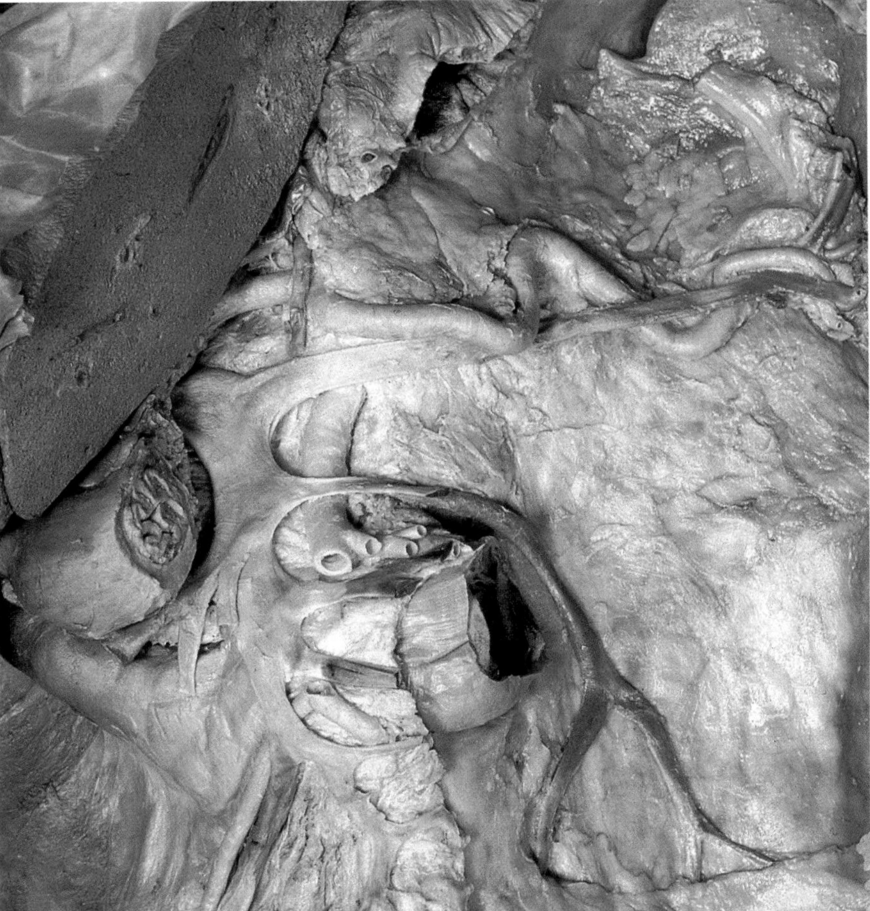

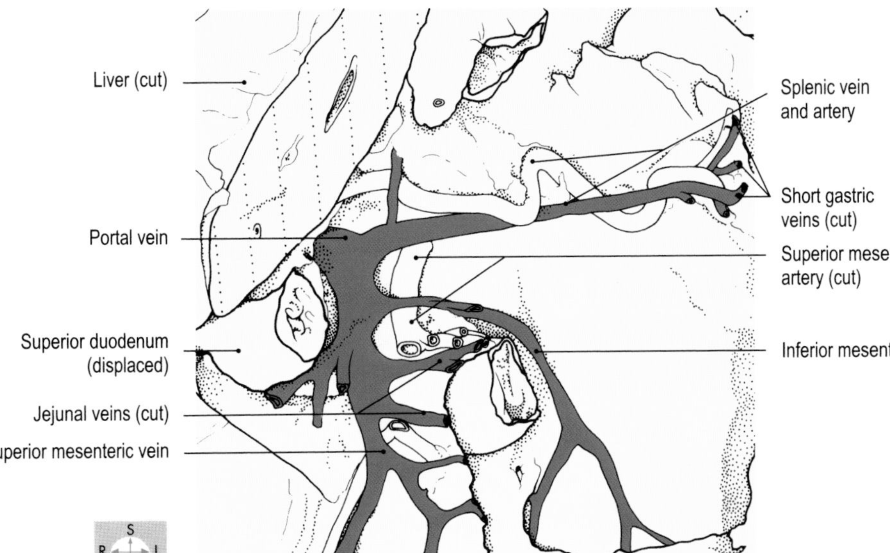

Fig. 4.78 Tributaries of the portal vein. In this specimen the inferior mesenteric vein joins the superior mesenteric vein.

Kidneys and Suprarenal Glands

Kidneys

The two kidneys lie behind the peritoneum on either side of the upper lumbar vertebrae (Fig. 4.79). They are embedded in fat in the paravertebral gutters of the posterior abdominal wall and are placed obliquely, with their anterior surfaces directed slightly laterally (Fig. 4.80). The left kidney usually lies at a higher level than the right.

Each kidney is bean-shaped, flattened anteroposteriorly and approximately 11 cm long. The anterior and posterior surfaces are gently convex and the superior and inferior poles are rounded. The lateral border is convex while the indented medial border bears an aperture, the hilum (Figs 4.81 & 4.82), which is traversed by the renal pelvis or ureter, the renal vessels,

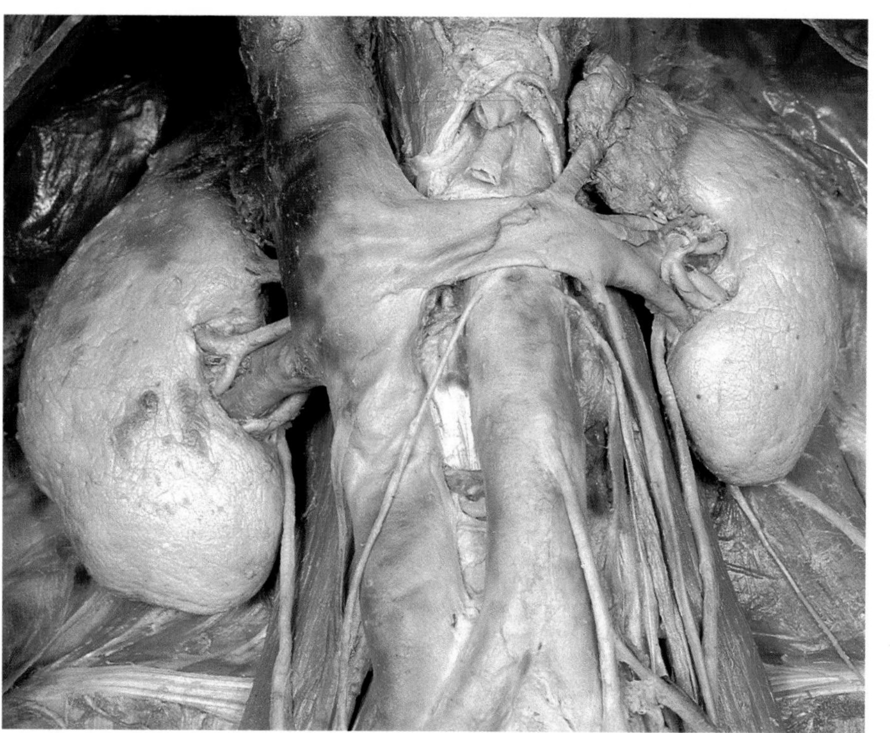

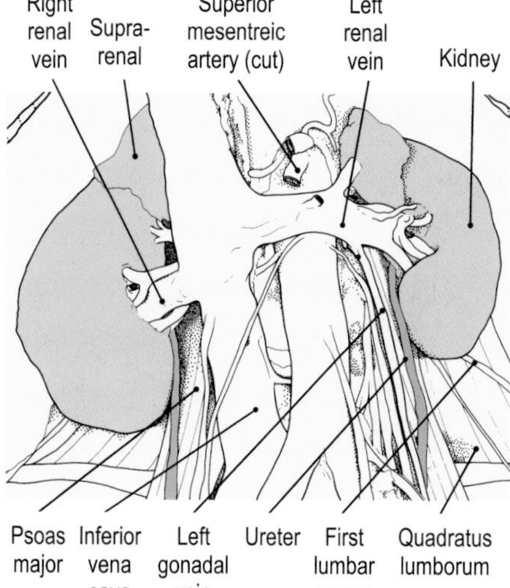

Fig. 4.79 Kidneys, suprarenal glands and some of the vessels associated with them.

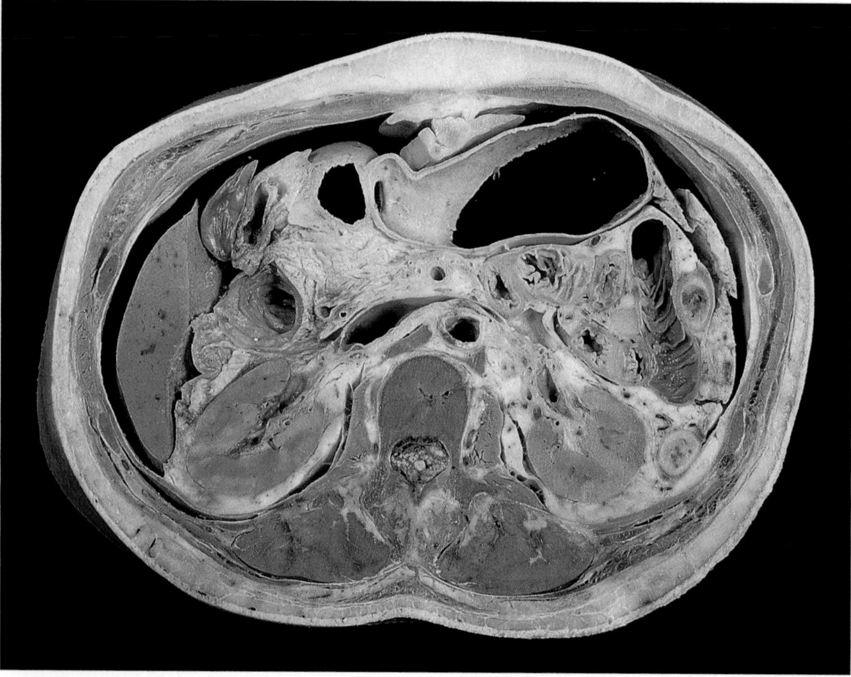

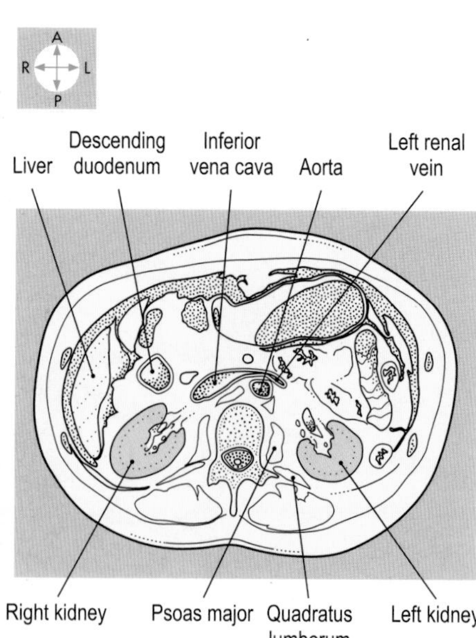

Fig. 4.80 Transverse section at the level of the first lumbar vertebra showing some relations of the kidneys. The spleen is not evident in this specimen. Inferior aspect. Compare Fig. 4.109.

lymphatics and autonomic nerves. The hilum leads into a cavity within the kidney, the renal sinus, which is occupied by the calices and renal pelvis (Fig. 4.83), the renal blood vessels and a quantity of fat.

Covered by a thin capsule, the kidney comprises an outer cortex and an inner medulla. The medulla contains numerous pyramids whose apices project into the renal sinus as the renal papillae. Urine discharged from the papillae is collected by about ten trumpet-shaped chambers, the minor calices (Fig. 4.83), which unite to form two or three major calices. These fuse into the single, funnel-shaped renal pelvis, which lies posterior to most of the vessels and is continuous with the ureter.

Perirenal tissues

Each kidney is surrounded by a layer of perinephric (perirenal) fat enveloped in a thin sheet of connective tissue, the renal fascia (Fig. 4.84). This fascia also encloses the suprarenal gland and the proximal part of the ureter. From the inferior pole of the kidney, the renal fascia tapers downwards into the iliac fossa. Around the fascia is a further layer of fat (paranephric or pararenal fat) lying against the posterior abdominal muscles and covered anteriorly by the peritoneum.

Relations of kidneys

The right and left kidneys have similar posterior relations (see Fig. 4.80). The superior poles lie against the diaphragm and the twelfth

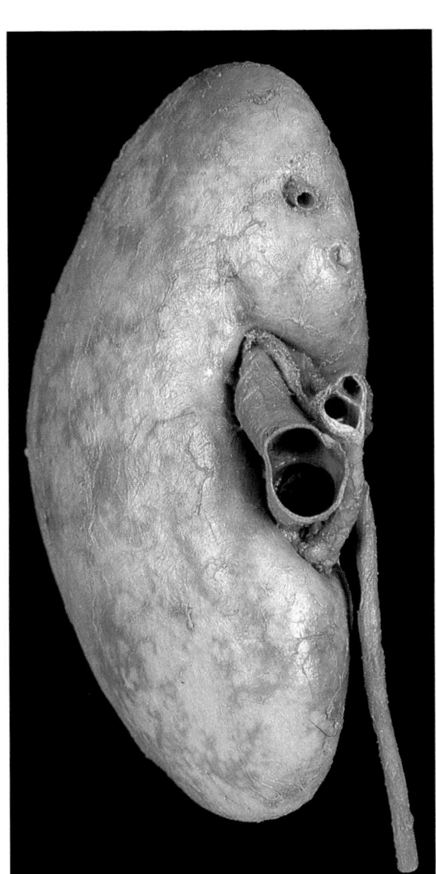

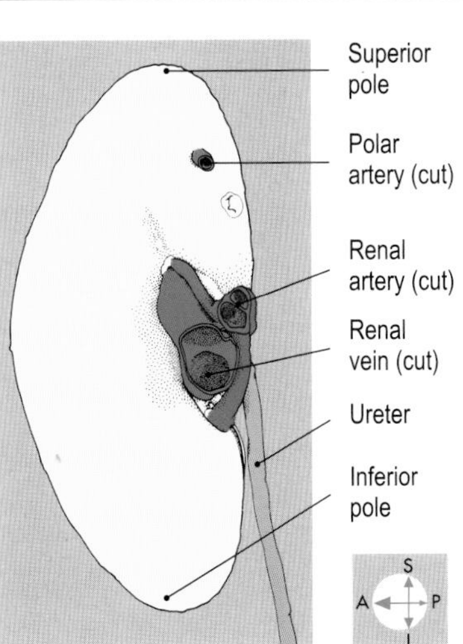

Fig. 4.81 Medial aspect of the right kidney showing the renal vessels passing through the hilum.

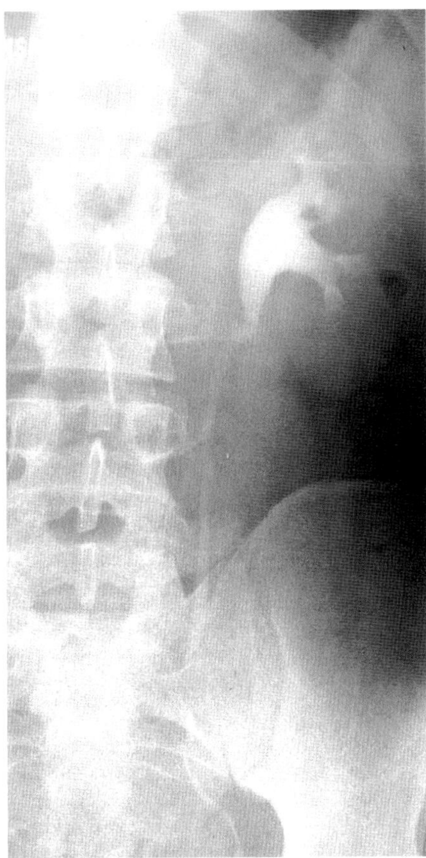

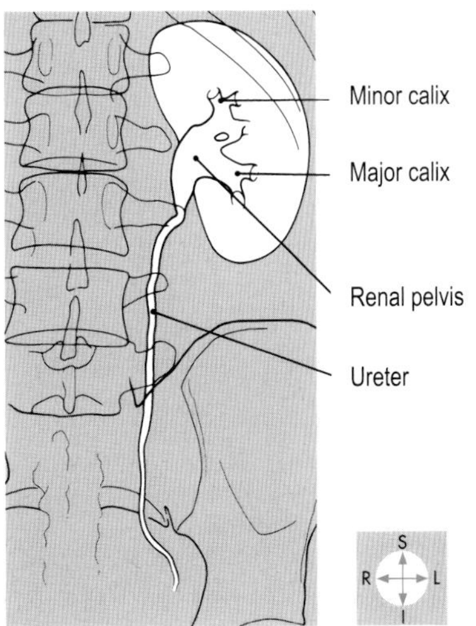

Fig. 4.82 Intravenous urogram showing detail of the pelvicaliceal system.

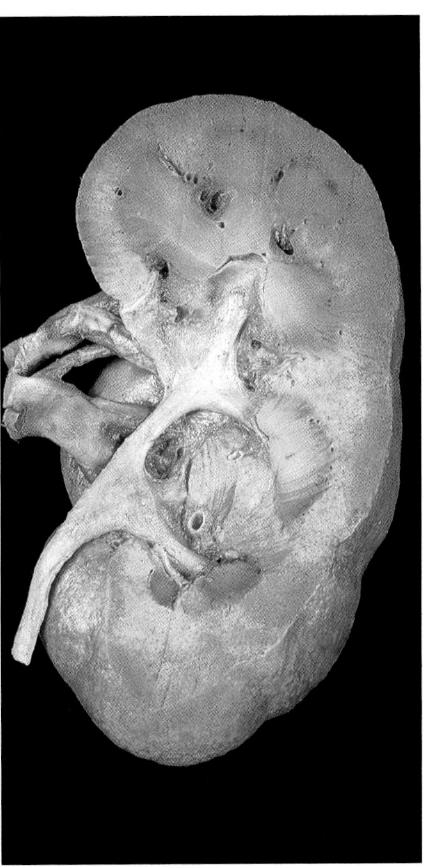

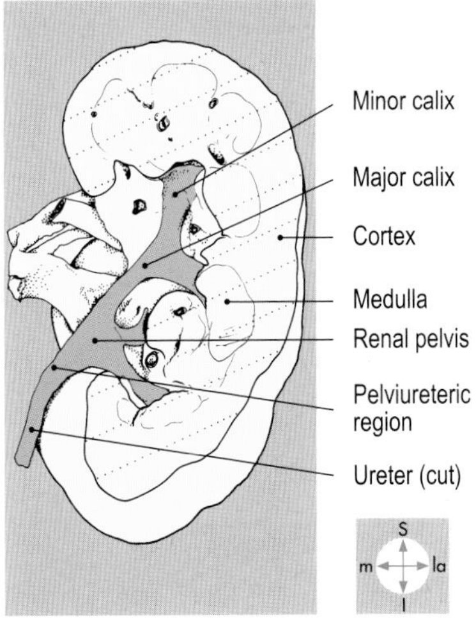

Fig. 4.83 Right kidney dissected from behind to show the renal pelvis and calices.

ribs, below which run the subcostal nerves and vessels. On the left the upper pole is also related, through the diaphragm, to the pleura and eleventh rib. The medial border of each kidney overlaps psoas major (see Fig. 4.79) while the inferolateral portion is related to quadratus lumborum and transversus abdominis, and to the first lumbar nerve.

The anterior relations of the kidneys are asymmetric. On the right, from above downwards, they include the bare area of the liver, the second part of the duodenum (see Fig. 4.80), the right flexure of the colon and coils of jejunum. The medial border of the right kidney is related to the inferior vena cava, the renal vessels and the upper part of the ureter (Fig. 4.84).

On the left, from above downwards, the anterior relations include the stomach and spleen, the splenic vessels, the tail of the pancreas, the left colic flexure and coils of jejunum. The medial border relates to the suprarenal gland, the renal and suprarenal vessels, the left gonadal vein and the proximal part of the ureter (Fig. 4.87).

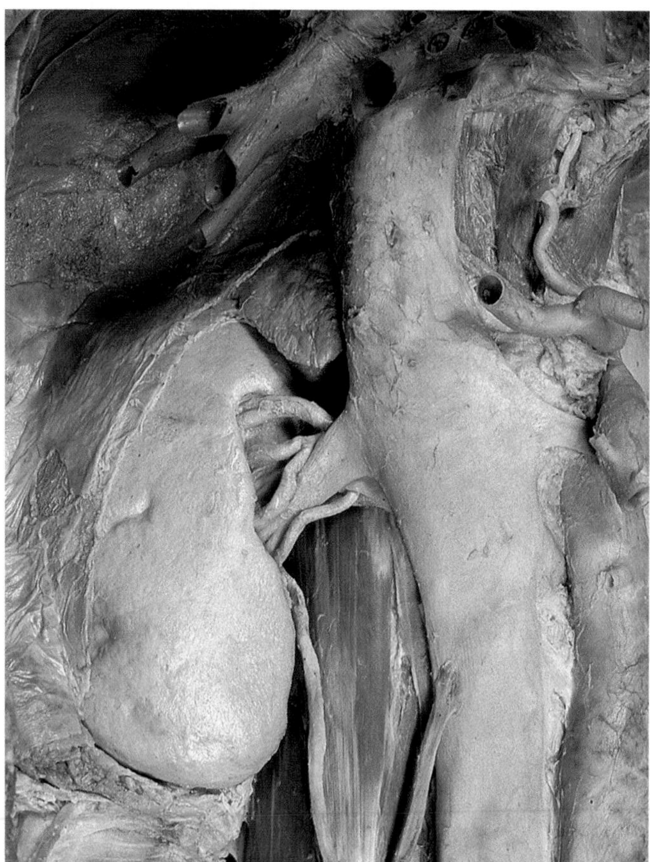

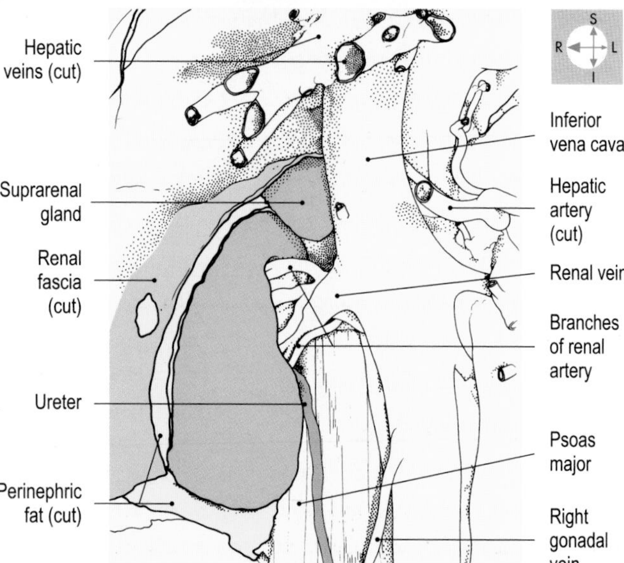

Fig. 4.84 Right kidney and suprarenal gland seen within the renal fascia and perinephric fat, part of which has been removed.

Renal vessels

At the level of the first lumbar vertebra the aorta usually supplies one renal artery to each kidney (Fig. 4.85). Each artery lies behind the corresponding vein, and the artery on the right crosses behind the inferior vena cava. However, there are often supernumerary (anomalous, aberrant or accessory) renal arteries arising from the aorta above or below the typical vessel. Regardless of its origin, each renal artery divides as it approaches the kidney and all the branches usually traverse the hilum. However, a polar artery may occasionally be found entering the medial border of the organ above or below the hilum (see Figs 4.81 & 4.87).

Several veins unite near the renal hilum, anterior to the arteries, forming the renal vein. On the right the vein runs a short course to terminate in the inferior vena cava. The left renal vein is longer and usually receives the suprarenal and gonadal veins before passing in front of the aorta to reach the inferior vena cava (see Fig. 4.79). Because of its termination, the left gonadal vein may become dilated if the renal vein is obstructed. In the male this can lead to swelling of the pampiniform plexus within the scrotum (varicocele).

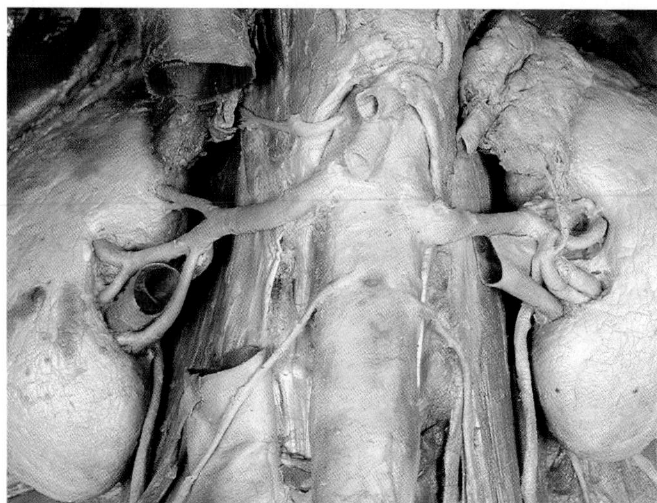

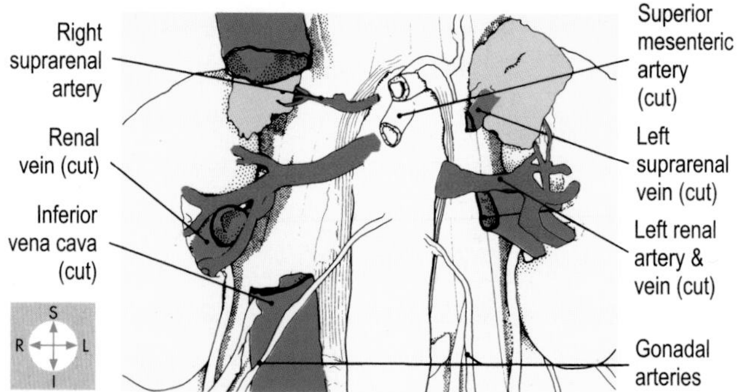

Fig. 4.85 Renal arteries exposed by removal of the renal veins and a portion of the inferior vena cava.

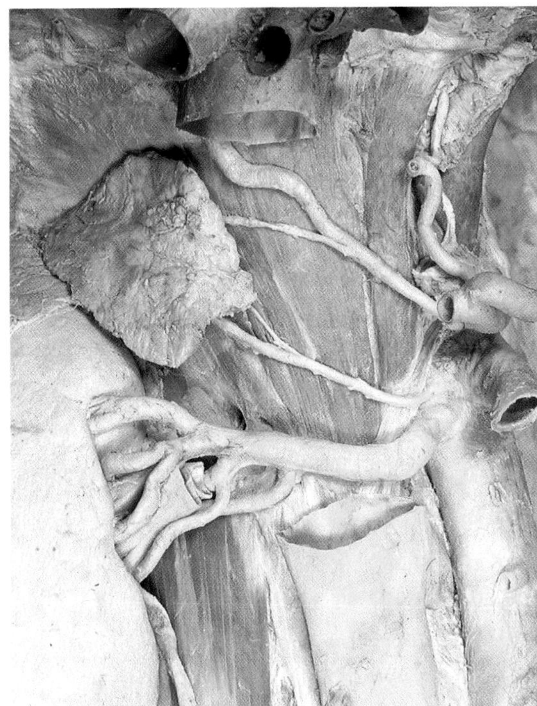

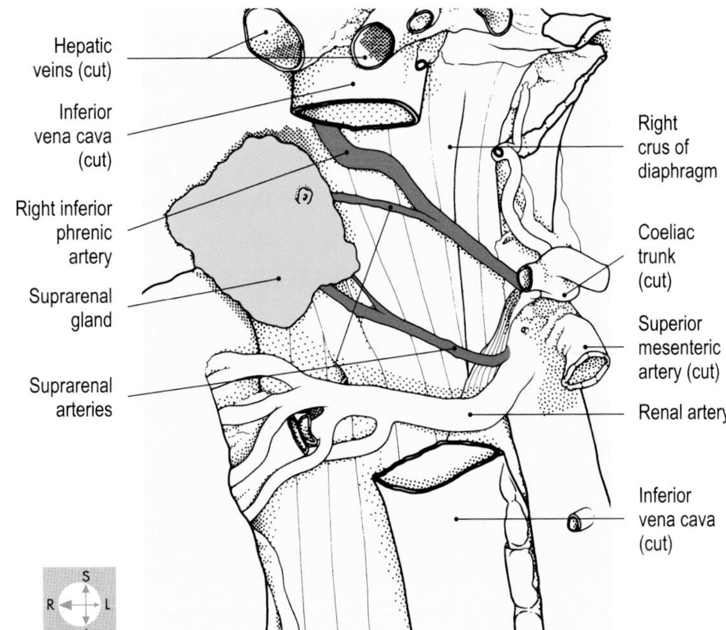

Fig. 4.86 Right suprarenal gland and its arteries exposed by removal of the renal vein and a portion of the inferior vena cava.

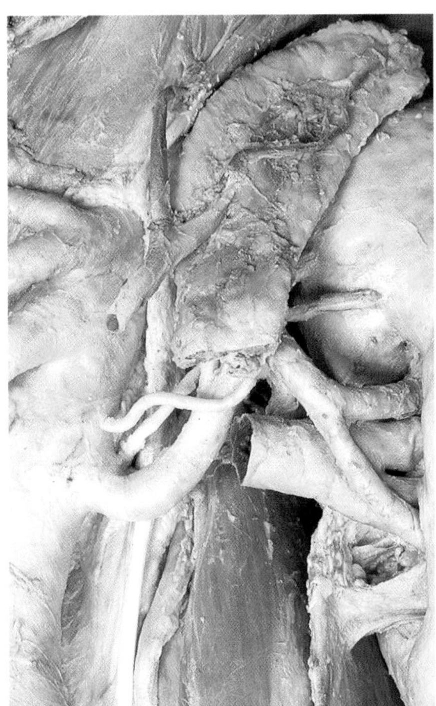

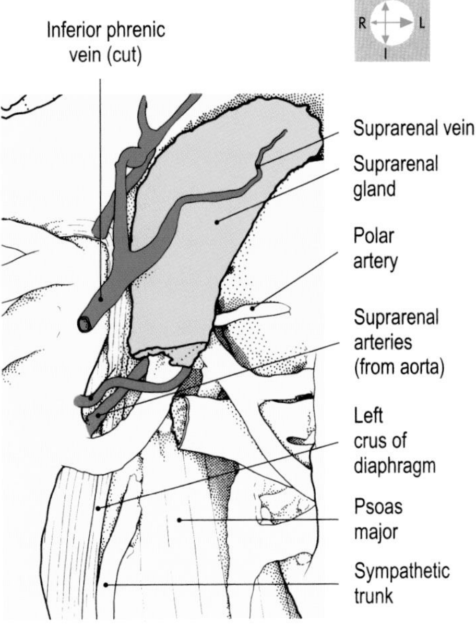

Fig. 4.87 Left suprarenal gland and its vessels. The renal vein and inferior tip of the gland have been excised to reveal the suprarenal arteries.

Suprarenal glands

The suprarenal glands lie adjacent to the superior poles of the kidneys, embedded in the perinephric fat. On the right the gland is tetrahedral and occupies the angle between the superior pole of the kidney and the inferior vena cava (Fig. 4.86). The left gland is crescentic and is applied to the medial border of the kidney above the hilum (Fig. 4.87).

The blood supply to the suprarenal glands is provided by branches of the renal and inferior phrenic arteries and the aorta. The right suprarenal vein is very short and enters the inferior vena cava directly while that on the left descends to enter the left renal vein.

The medulla of each suprarenal gland is richly innervated by preganglionic sympathetic nerves from the adjacent part of the sympathetic trunk.

The blood supply to the abdominal part of the ureter is derived from branches of the renal artery, supplemented by minute peritoneal vessels.

Abdominal parts of ureters

From the pelviureteric region each ureter descends through the retroperitoneal tissues of the posterior abdominal wall as far as the pelvic brim. Here it crosses in front of the external iliac vessels and continues down the lateral wall of the pelvis (see p. 222). Within the abdomen the ureter lies on psoas major (Fig. 4.84), behind which are the lumbar transverse processes (see Fig. 4.82).

The right ureter commences behind the descending duodenum and is crossed by the root of the mesentery, the gonadal vessels and branches of the superior mesenteric artery and accompanying veins. This ureter is also related to coils of small intestine, and sometimes to the caecum and appendix. The left ureter is covered initially by the pancreas and is subsequently crossed by the gonadal vessels, branches of the inferior mesenteric artery and vein (see Fig. 4.76) and coils of small intestine and sigmoid colon. At the pelvic brim, it passes behind the root of the sigmoid mesocolon.

Abdominal Aorta

The aorta enters the abdomen behind the median arcuate ligament of the diaphragm at the level of the twelfth thoracic vertebra. It descends behind the peritoneum, inclining slightly to the left of the midline to its bifurcation in front of the fourth lumbar vertebra (Fig. 4.89). Throughout its course the abdominal aorta is accompanied by lymph vessels and nodes and is surrounded by a plexus of autonomic nerves (see pp 196–199).

Posterior to the aorta lie the left lumbar veins, the anterior longitudinal ligament and the lumbar vertebral bodies. Anterior relations, from above downwards, include the body of the pancreas, the splenic and left renal veins, the horizontal duodenum, the root of the mesentery and coils of small intestine.

To the right of the aorta lie the right crus of the diaphragm and the inferior vena cava (Fig. 4.89). On the left are the left diaphragmatic crus, suprarenal gland and kidney.

Visceral branches

Three arteries arise from the anterior aspect of the aorta to supply the alimentary organs while three pairs of lateral branches pass to the suprarenals, kidneys and gonads respectively.

The coeliac and superior mesenteric arteries arise at the levels of the twelfth thoracic and first lumbar vertebrae respectively whilst the smaller inferior mesenteric artery takes origin at the level of the third lumbar vertebra (Fig. 4.89).

For details of the course and distribution of each of these arteries see pages 161, 177 and 182.

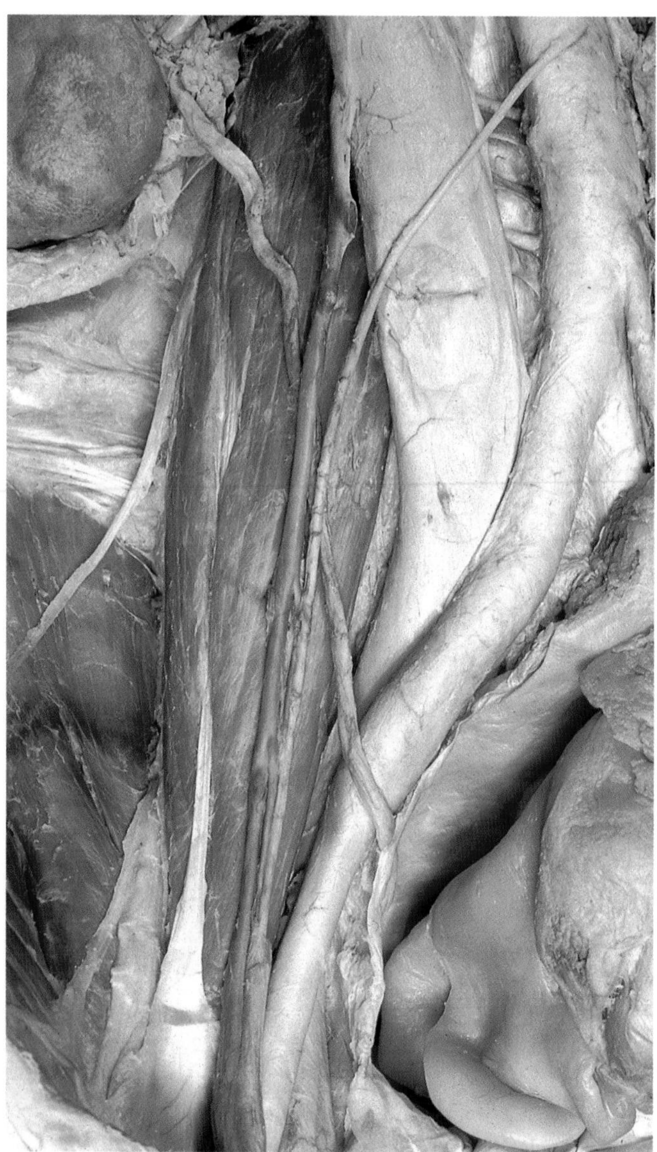

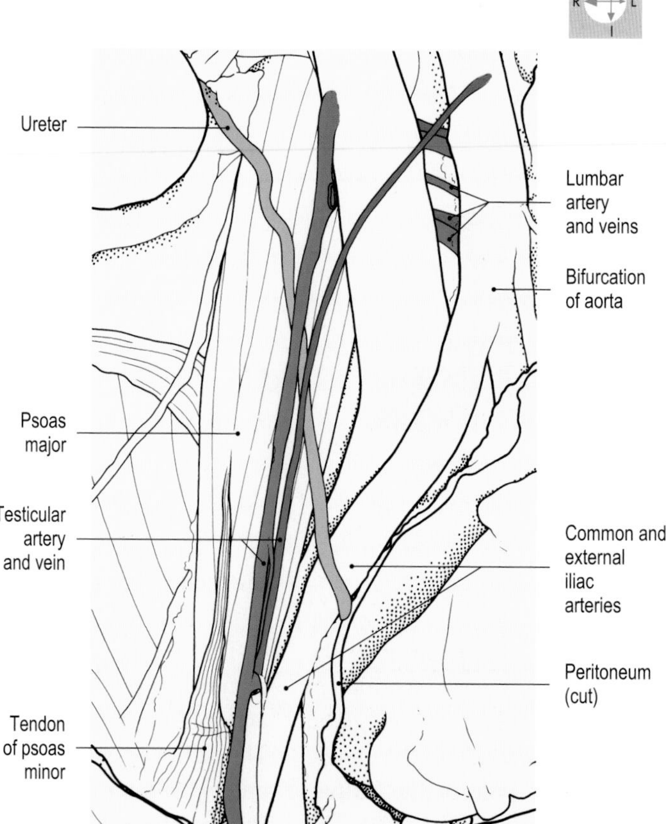

Fig. 4.88 Right testicular vessels within the abdomen. Several lumbar vessels are also seen.

The suprarenal branches of the aorta (Fig. 4.89) are small and variable and are often supplemented by branches from the inferior phrenic and renal arteries (see Fig. 4.86; see also Fig. 4.92). The renal arteries usually arise at the level of the first lumbar vertebra but variations are common (see p. 188).

The long and slender gonadal (testicular or ovarian) arteries usually arise from the aorta just below the renal arteries (Fig. 4.89). The gonadal artery on the right crosses in front of the inferior vena cava, and the arteries of both sides incline downwards and laterally through the retroperitoneal tissues on the psoas major muscles (Fig. 4.88). Each artery is accompanied by one or more gonadal veins and crosses anterior to the ureters but posterior to blood vessels supplying the intestines. Inferiorly the testicular artery follows the psoas major round the pelvic brim and enters the deep inguinal ring (see Fig. 4.23). The ovarian artery crosses the external iliac vessels and pelvic brim to reach the ovary within the pelvis (see p. 221).

Parietal branches

These vessels supply the diaphragm and the posterior walls of the abdomen and pelvis. The paired inferior phrenic arteries are the first branches of the aorta within the abdomen (Fig. 4.89; see Fig. 4.92) and often furnish small branches to the suprarenal glands before arching upwards and laterally on the abdominal surface of the diaphragm.

Four pairs of lumbar arteries usually arise from the posterolateral aspect of the aorta and supply the posterior abdominal wall (Figs 4.88, 4.90 & 4.103). The arteries on the right cross behind the inferior vena cava to curve round the side of the corresponding vertebral body deep to psoas major.

A single small vessel, the median sacral artery, arises from the back of the aortic bifurcation and descends behind the left common iliac vein to reach the anterior surface of the sacrum (Fig. 4.90).

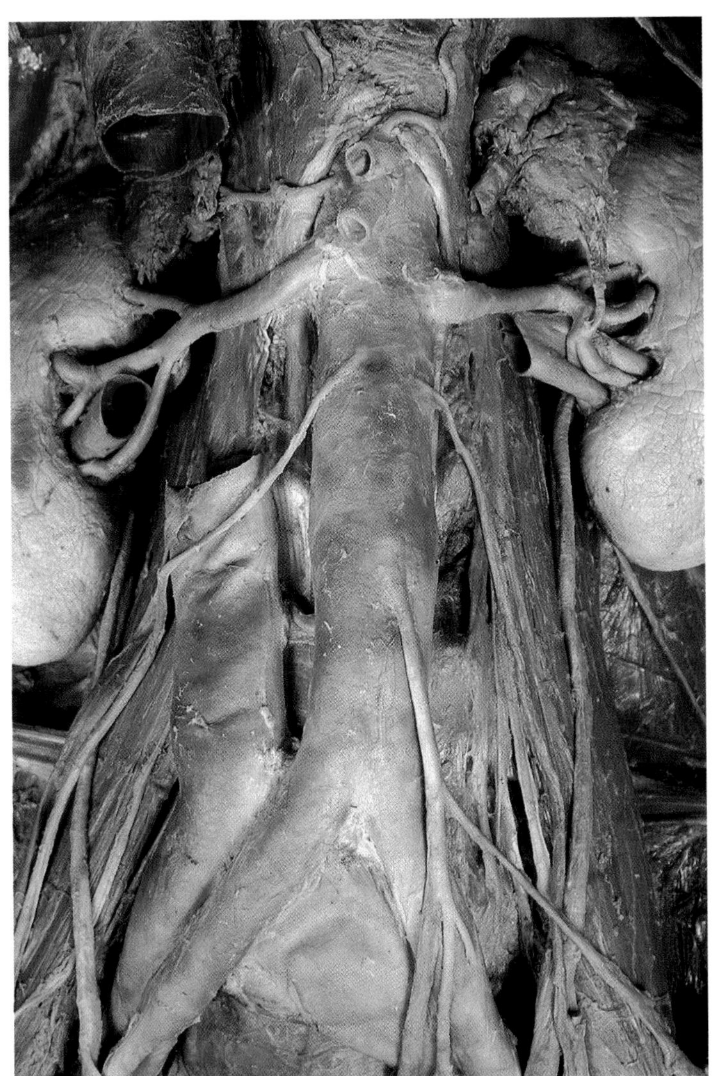

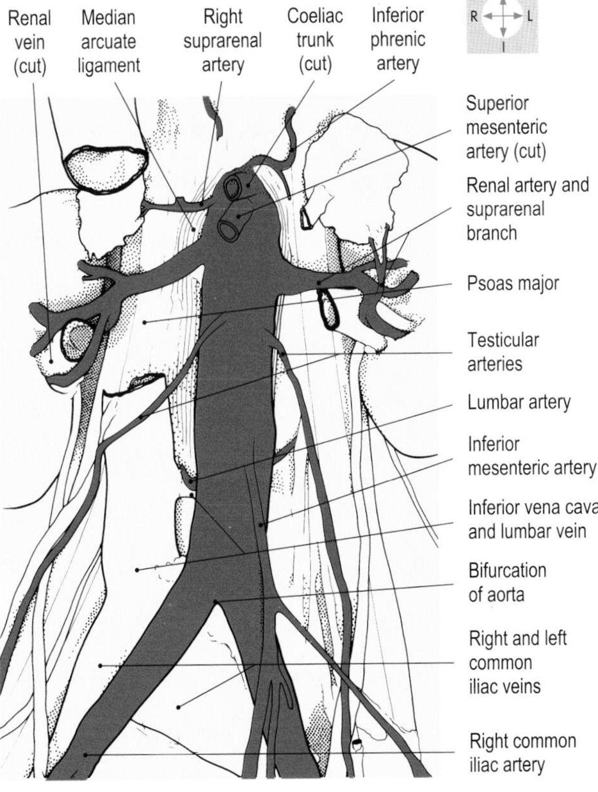

Fig. 4.89 Abdominal aorta and its branches, seen after removal of the renal veins and part of the inferior vena cava.

Iliac Vessels

Common and external iliac vessels

The aortic bifurcation gives rise to the two common iliac arteries, which incline downwards and laterally on the medial aspects of psoas major (Fig. 4.90). The vessels terminate in front of the sacroiliac joints by dividing into internal and external iliac arteries. The right common iliac artery crosses in front of the left common iliac vein, while that on the left is crossed by the inferior mesenteric vessels. The ureter crosses either the lower end of the common iliac artery or the commencement of its external branch (Fig. 4.90). The internal iliac artery begins at the bifurcation of the common iliac artery and descends on the lateral wall of the pelvis (see p. 238).

The external iliac artery curves round the pelvic brim (Fig. 4.90) and, passing behind the inguinal ligament, enters the thigh as the femoral artery (see Fig. 6.19). The external iliac artery is accompanied on its medial side by the corresponding vein and posterolaterally by psoas major. The external iliac vessels are crossed by the ovarian vessels in the female and by the ductus deferens in the male. Near the inguinal ligament the artery gives off the inferior epigastric artery, which runs upwards and medially, medial to the deep inguinal ring (see Figs 4.18 & 4.23).

Each external iliac vein begins behind the inguinal ligament as the continuation of the femoral vein (Fig. 4.90). It receives the inferior epigastric vein, ascends on the medial side of the corresponding artery and joins the internal iliac vein (see p. 239) to form the common iliac vein. The two common iliac veins continue upwards and medially, passing behind the right common iliac artery, by which they may be compressed, before uniting to form the inferior vena cava.

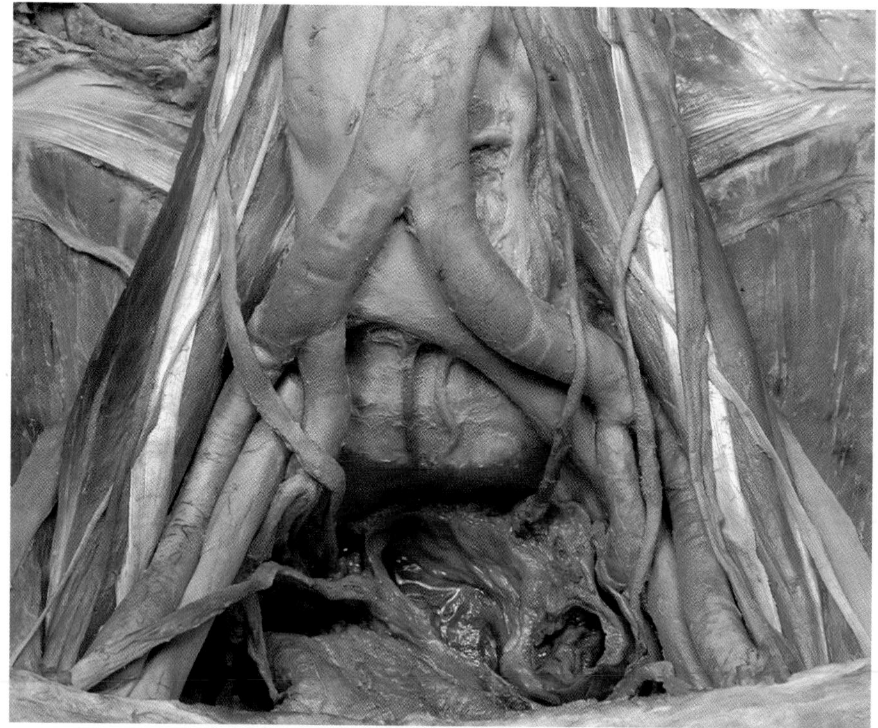

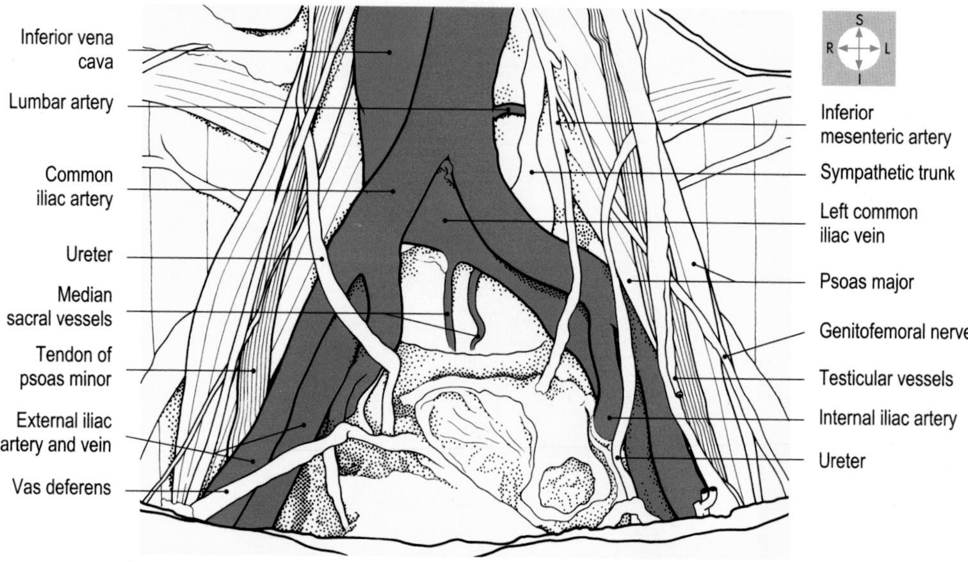

Fig. 4.90 Male pelvis and lower abdomen showing the common and external iliac vessels and some of their relations.

Inferior Vena Cava

The inferior vena cava is formed at the level of the fifth lumbar vertebra, a little to the right of the midline (Fig. 4.91). It ascends the posterior abdominal wall and pierces the central tendon of the diaphragm to enter the thorax at the level of the eighth thoracic vertebra (see Fig. 2.61).

Behind the inferior vena cava lie the lumbar vertebral bodies, the anterior longitudinal ligament, the right sympathetic chain and right psoas major muscle. In addition, the right renal and right lumbar arteries cross behind the vena cava (see Figs 4.88, 4.89) and most of the right suprarenal gland lies posterior to the vessel (Fig. 4.92).

Near its commencement, the inferior vena cava is covered anteriorly by peritoneum and coils of small intestine. Superiorly it is crossed by the root of the mesentery, the right gonadal artery (see Fig. 4.88) and the third part of the duodenum (see Fig. 4.52). It continues behind the omental foramen (see Fig. 4.38) and then grooves the posterior surface of the liver (see Fig. 4.58) before piercing the diaphragm.

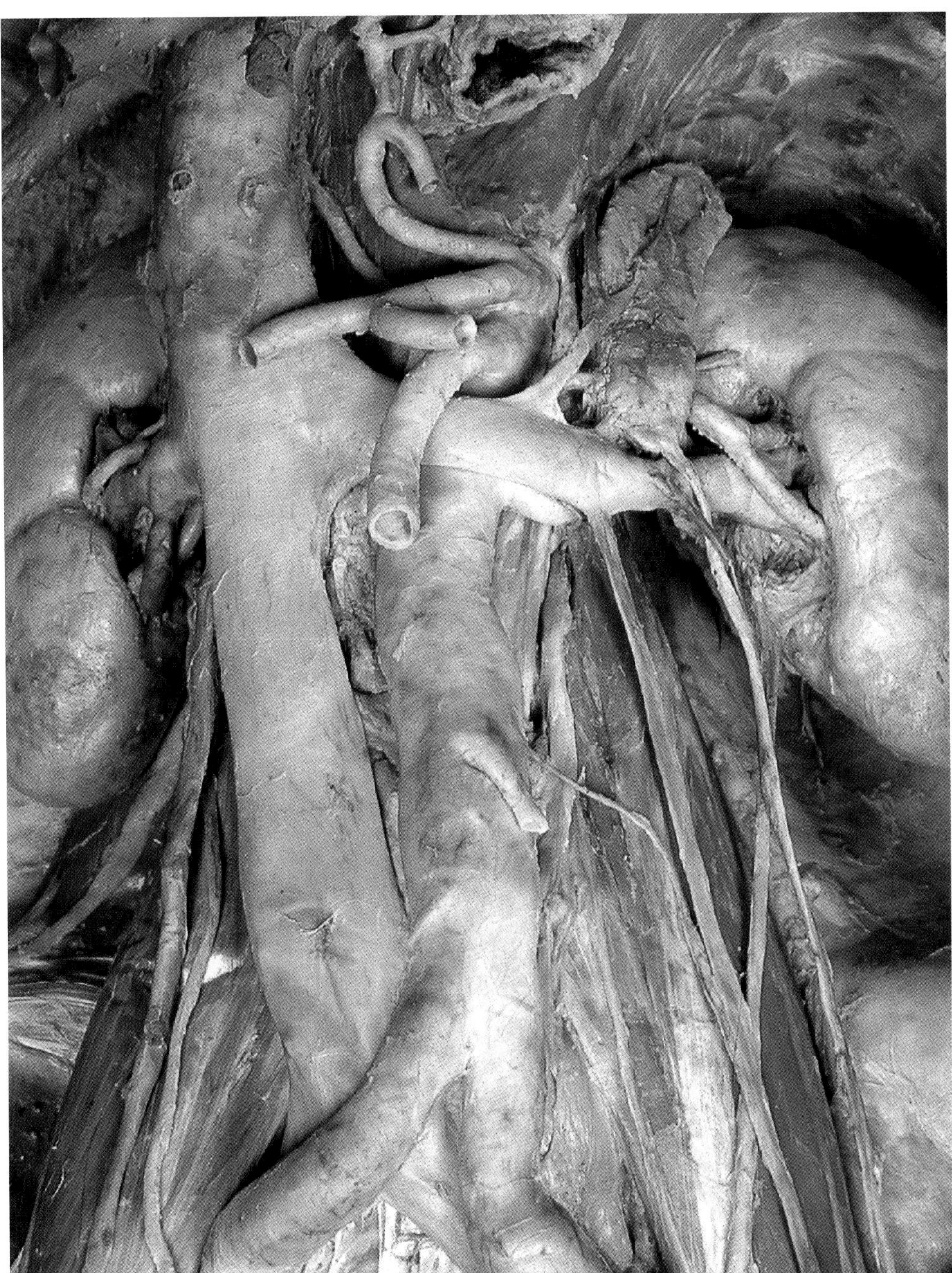

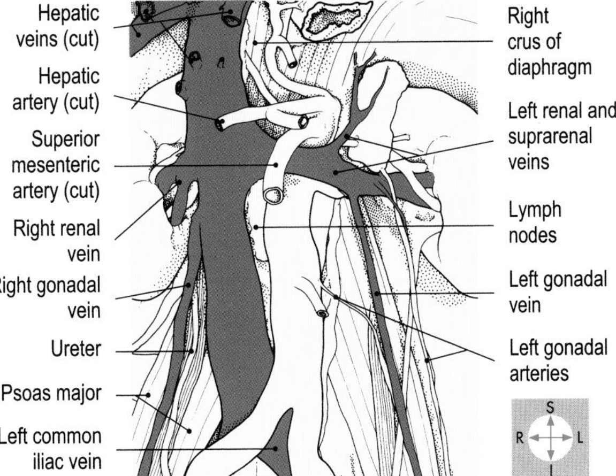

Fig. 4.91 Course and principal tributaries of the inferior vena cava.

To the right of the vena cava lie the gonadal vessels, the ureter, the kidney and renal vessels (Fig. 4.91) and the right lobe of the liver. To the left lie the aorta with its associated lymph nodes, the right crus of the diaphragm and the caudate lobe of the liver.

Tributaries

The venous drainage of the suprarenal glands, the kidneys and the gonads is asymmetric. On the right each of these organs is drained by a vein that passes directly into the inferior vena cava (Figs 4.91 & 4.92) but on the left the renal vein receives the suprarenal and gonadal veins before crossing in front of the aorta to reach the vena cava. Immediately before its passage through the diaphragm the inferior vena cava receives several large hepatic veins (Fig. 4.92).

The parietal tributaries of the inferior vena cava drain the diaphragm and the posterior pelvic and abdominal walls. The lumbar and median sacral veins (see Figs 4.88 & 4.90) accompany the corresponding arteries, the upper lumbar veins often communicating with the renal, suprarenal, azygos and hemiazygos veins. Two or more inferior phrenic veins drain the undersurface of the diaphragm (Fig. 4.92).

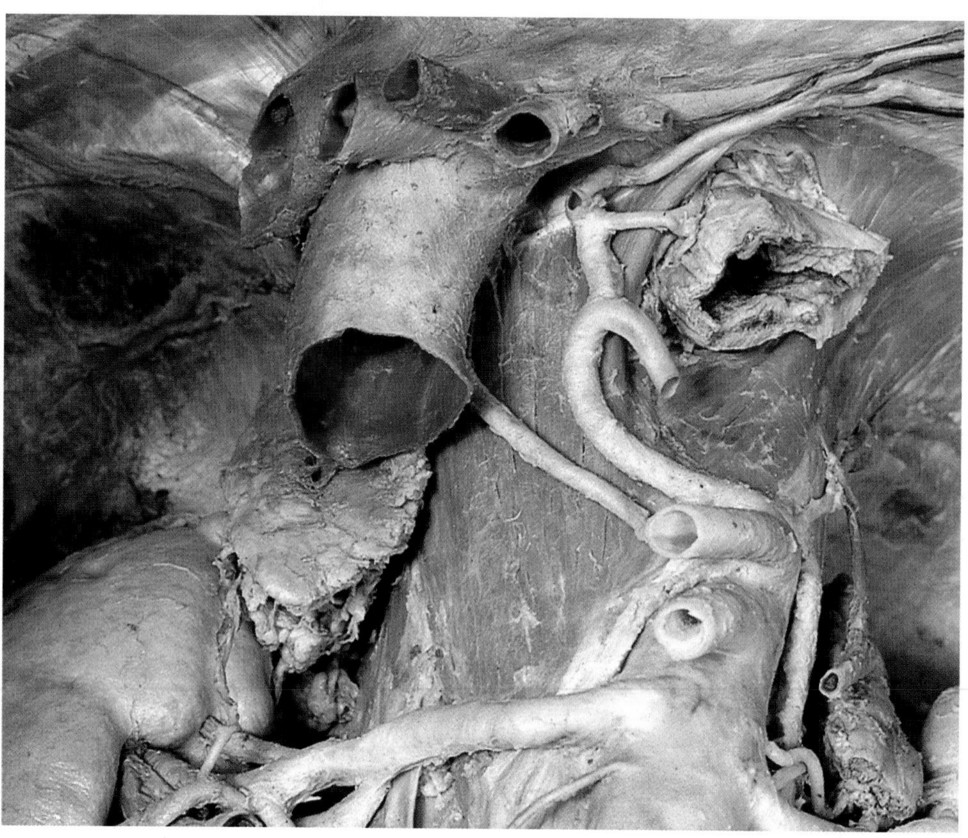

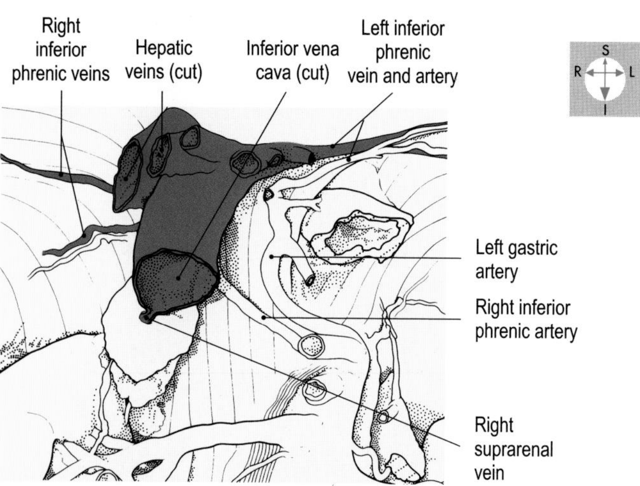

Fig. 4.92 Upper part of inferior vena cava showing its tributaries. In this specimen the left inferior phrenic artery arises from the left gastric artery.

Lymphatics of Abdomen

The lymphatic vessels and nodes of the abdomen drain the abdominal and pelvic organs as well as the pelvic walls and the lower part of the abdominal wall. (The upper part of the abdominal wall is drained by the internal thoracic and axillary nodes; see p. 145.) In addition, the abdominal lymphatics receive lymph from the lower limb, the gonads and the perineum.

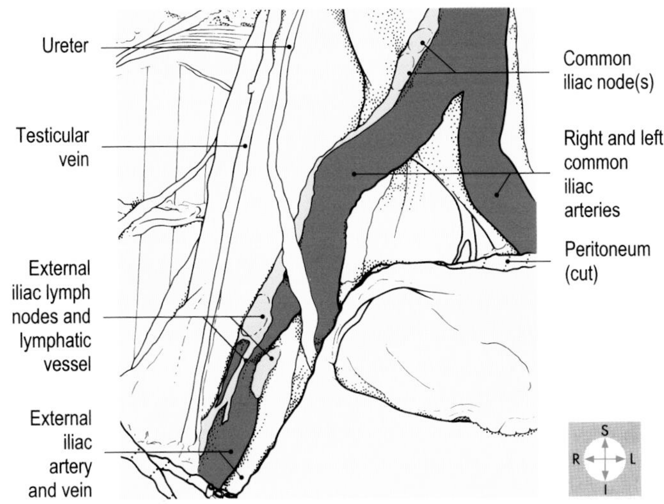

Fig. 4.93 The common and external iliac arteries are accompanied by a chain of lymphatic vessels and nodes.

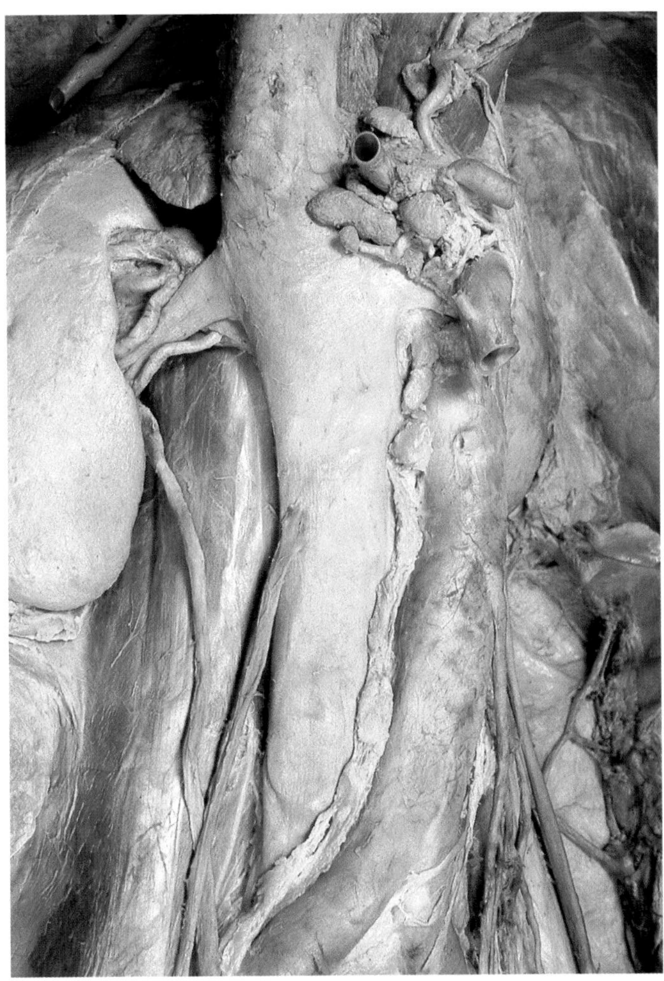

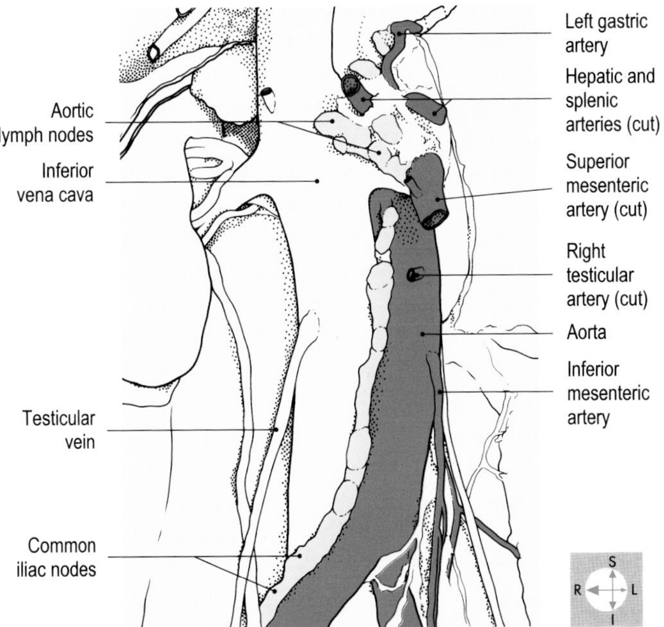

Fig. 4.94 Removal of the autonomic nerves and retroperitoneal connective tissues reveals the lymphatic vessels and nodes lying on the right side of the aorta.

Some lymph nodes are situated adjacent to the organs they drain and include those of the liver and spleen and in the hila of the kidneys. The lymphatic vessels draining most of the abdominal organs accompany blood vessels and pass to nodes grouped around the aorta. Often, lymph passes through intermediate nodes situated along the courses of the arteries. Most of the lymph from the abdominal walls and viscera eventually drains into the thoracic duct.

Because of their deep position, most intra-abdominal lymph nodes are not palpable in the living subject, even when enlarged.

Iliac lymph nodes

The external iliac nodes (Fig. 4.93) receive lymph from the lower limb and perineum via the deep inguinal nodes. In addition, the iliac nodes drain the deeper layers of the abdominal wall below the level of the umbilicus via lymphatic vessels accompanying the inferior epigastric vessels. Lymph from the superficial tissues of the lower abdominal wall reaches the external iliac nodes, having passed first to superficial and then to deep inguinal nodes.

The internal iliac nodes drain the pelvic walls and floor and some of the pelvic organs, including the bladder, lower part of the rectum, prostate and uterus. However, lymph from most of the rectum, sigmoid colon and ovaries drains to the aortic nodes. From the external and internal iliac nodes lymph passes to nodes alongside the common iliac artery (Fig. 4.93) and subsequently to the aortic nodes.

Aortic nodes

The major abdominal lymphatic vessels and their associated nodes are arranged alongside the aorta (Fig. 4.94). The nodes on each side of the aorta receive lymph from the common iliac nodes, posterior abdominal wall, gonads, kidneys and suprarenal glands, while nodes lying immediately anterior to the aorta drain the digestive organs.

Nodes around the origin of the inferior mesenteric artery drain lymph from most of the rectum, and the sigmoid and descending parts of the colon. Nodes lying adjacent to the origins of the superior mesenteric and coeliac arteries drain the spleen, pancreas, liver, stomach, small intestine and the large intestine as far as the splenic flexure.

Cisterna chyli

Efferent lymphatics from the aortic nodes drain into the cisterna chyli (Fig. 4.95). This fusiform sac lies at the level of the upper two lumbar vertebrae, adjacent to the right crus of the diaphragm. It lies behind the right border of the aorta and opens superiorly into the thoracic duct. The duct ascends through the aortic opening of the diaphragm and continues through the thorax to drain into the great veins in the root of the neck (see p. 62).

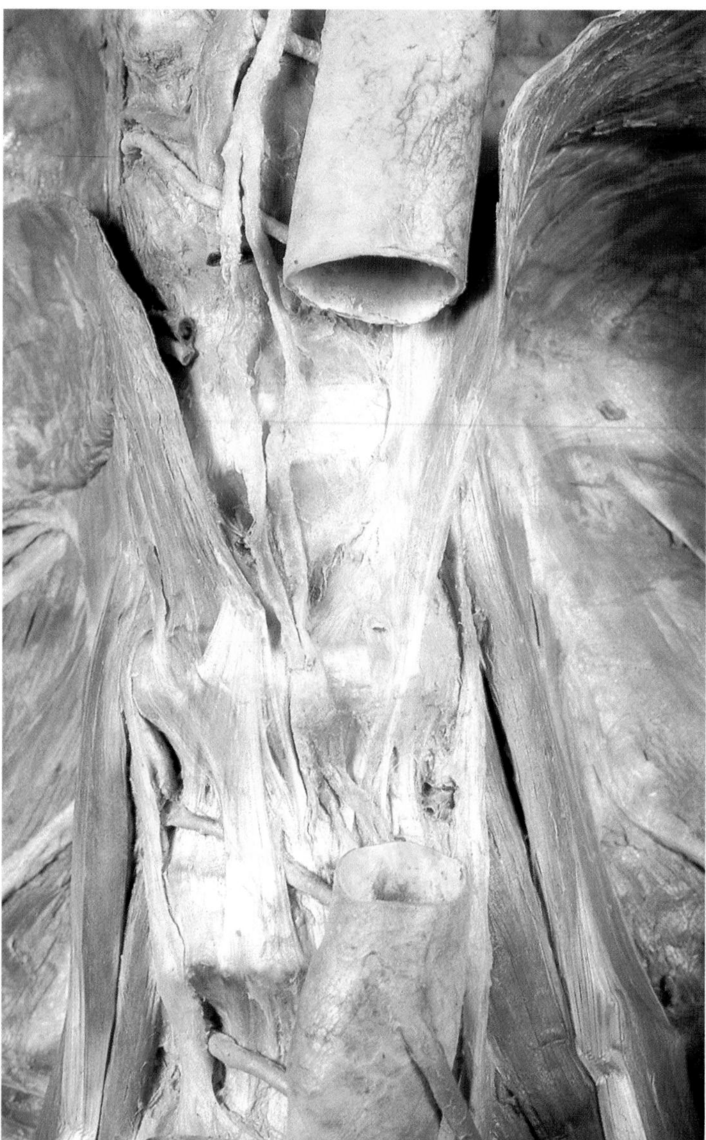

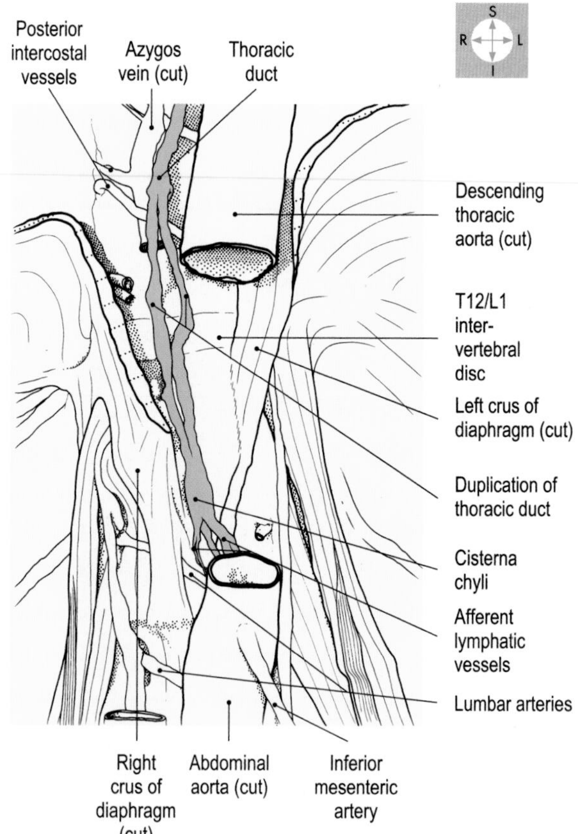

Fig. 4.95 Cisterna chyli, revealed by removal of parts of the crura of the diaphragm and a segment of aorta.

Autonomic Nerves of Abdomen

The autonomic innervation to the abdominal viscera is provided by perivascular plexuses of nerves accompanying the arterial supply to each organ. The plexuses comprise sympathetic and parasympathetic fibres of both motor and sensory type. The autonomic nerves control glandular secretion, smooth muscle activity and vasomotor tone; they are also sensory, mediating the distension of hollow organs and the tension on mesenteries.

Parasympathetic nerves

Most of the parasympathetic supply is provided by the vagus (X cranial) nerves, but there are small contributions to the distal part of the colon from branches of the pelvic splanchnic nerves that arise from the sacral spinal nerves. The vagi and the pelvic splanchnic nerves carry preganglionic parasympathetic fibres which synapse with postganglionic fibres in the walls of the relevant organs.

From the oesophageal plexus (see p. 61) two or more vagal trunks (gastric nerves) emerge and accompany the oesophagus through the diaphragm. The anterior trunk, derived mostly from the left vagus nerve (Fig. 4.96), enters the abdomen in front of the oesophagus and gives branches to the anterior surface of the stomach and to the liver. The posterior trunk, derived mostly from the right vagus, descends behind the oesophagus and supplies the posterior surface of the stomach and the coeliac plexus. From this plexus some vagal fibres pass inferiorly to the root of the superior mesenteric artery. The perivascular plexuses that accompany branches of the coeliac and superior mesenteric arteries convey these vagal fibres to all parts of the digestive system as far distally as the splenic flexure of the colon.

The remainder of the large intestine receives its parasympathetic supply from branches of the pelvic splanchnic nerves (nervi erigentes). These ascend through plexuses in the pelvis (see p. 236) and cross the left common iliac vessels in the root of the sigmoid mesocolon to reach the root of the inferior mesenteric artery. By accompanying branches of this artery, parasympathetic fibres from the sacral segments of the spinal cord supply the descending and sigmoid parts of the colon and the rectum.

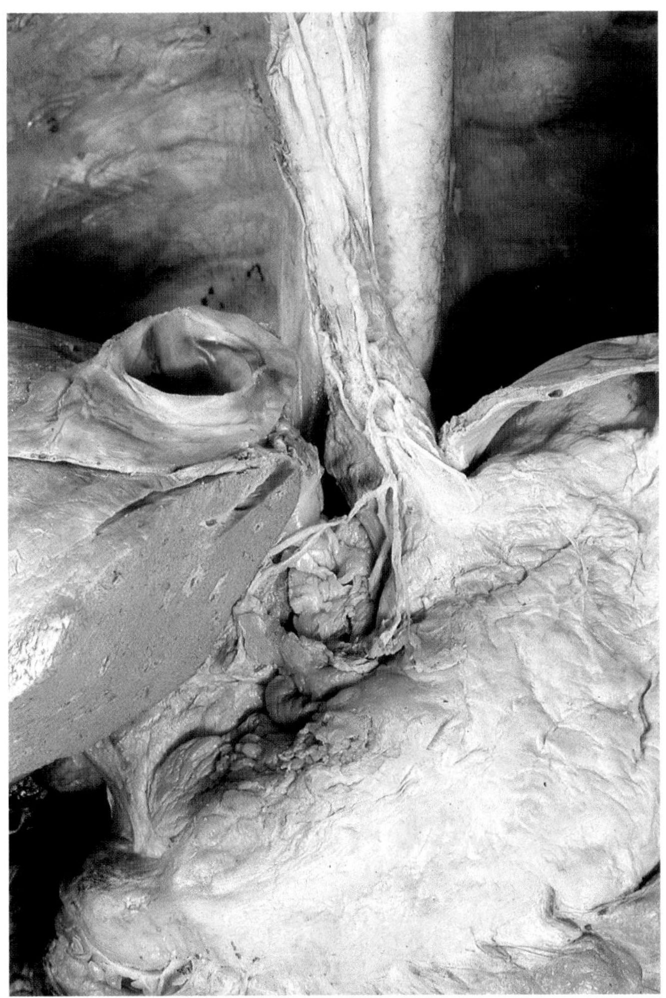

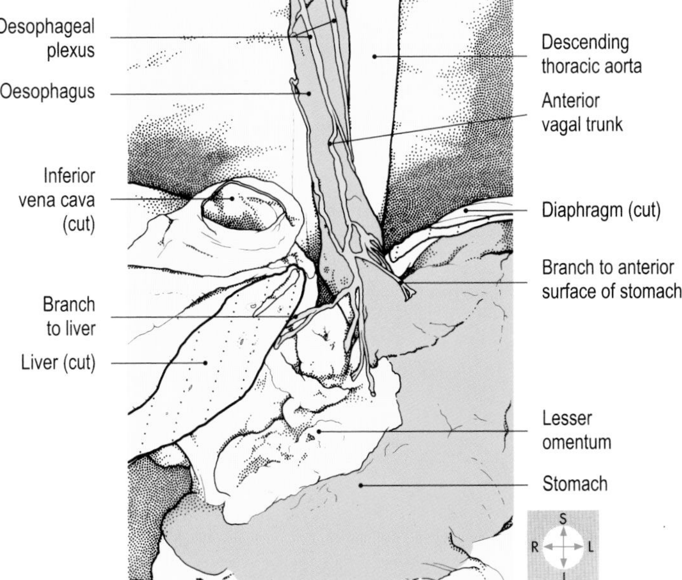

Fig. 4.96 Anterior vagal trunk, revealed by removal of part of the diaphragm and exposure of the lower oesophagus.

Sympathetic nerves

The sympathetic system in the abdomen comprises two ganglionated trunks and a network of nerves (the aortic or prevertebral plexuses) covering the surface of the aorta.

Each sympathetic trunk enters the abdomen behind the medial arcuate ligament of the diaphragm (Fig. 4.97) and descends along the medial border of psoas major, the trunk on the right lying posterior to the inferior vena cava. Each trunk passes behind the common iliac vessels and crosses the pelvic inlet at the ala of the sacrum.

Within the abdomen each trunk bears five lumbar ganglia. Only the upper two ganglia receive fibres from the central nervous system. These preganglionic sympathetic fibres are conveyed in white rami communicantes arising from the first and second lumbar spinal nerves. Some preganglionic fibres synapse in the sympathetic trunk while others pass into branches of the trunk and synapse nearer the target organs.

Each ganglion of the trunk gives a branch, a grey ramus communicans, to the corresponding spinal nerve. The postganglionic sympathetic fibres in the grey rami are distributed to the body wall and the lower limb. In addition, the ganglia supply branches (containing both pre- and postganglionic fibres) to the abdominal and pelvic organs. Branches from the upper ganglia reinforce the aortic plexuses, whilst the lumbar splanchnic nerves descend from the lower ganglia and cross anterior to the common iliac vessels (Fig. 4.98). The lumbar splanchnic nerves from the right and left trunks unite below the bifurcation of the aorta to form the hypogastric plexus from which branches descend to reach the pelvic autonomic plexuses (see p. 236).

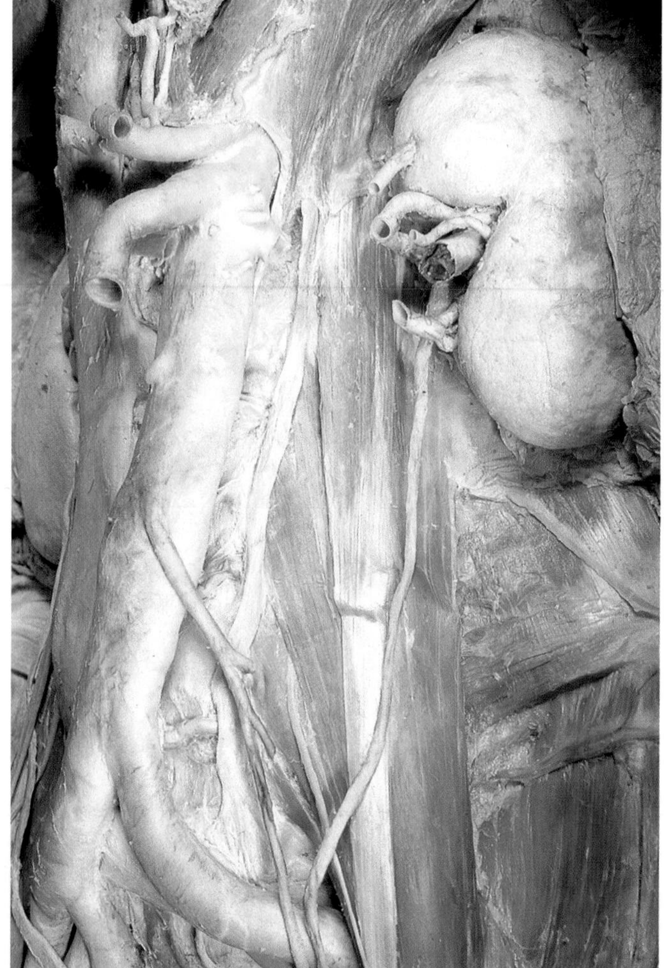

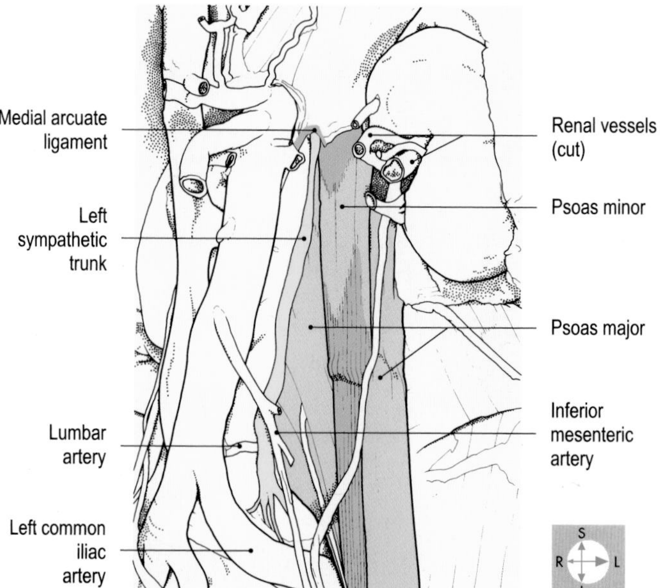

Fig. 4.97 Lumbar portion of the left sympathetic trunk after removal of the aortic plexuses of nerves.

Aortic plexuses

The dense network of autonomic nerves (both parasympathetic and sympathetic) that invests the abdominal aorta (Fig. 4.98) has several component plexuses, which are named according to the larger branches of the aorta. These are the coeliac, aorticorenal, renal, superior mesenteric, intermesenteric and inferior mesenteric plexuses. From these perivascular plexuses nerves are distributed to the abdominal organs.

The parasympathetic fibres in the aortic plexuses are derived mainly from the posterior vagal trunk, which enters the abdomen on the wall of the oesophagus, while the sympathetic fibres are provided principally by the thoracic splanchnic nerves (see p. 63). These branches of the thoracic portions of the sympathetic trunks pierce the crura of the diaphragm to reach the coeliac plexus. Additional sympathetic fibres are provided by the upper ganglia of the lumbar sympathetic chain. Within the aortic plexuses are numerous small ganglia in which the pre- and postganglionic sympathetic fibres synapse.

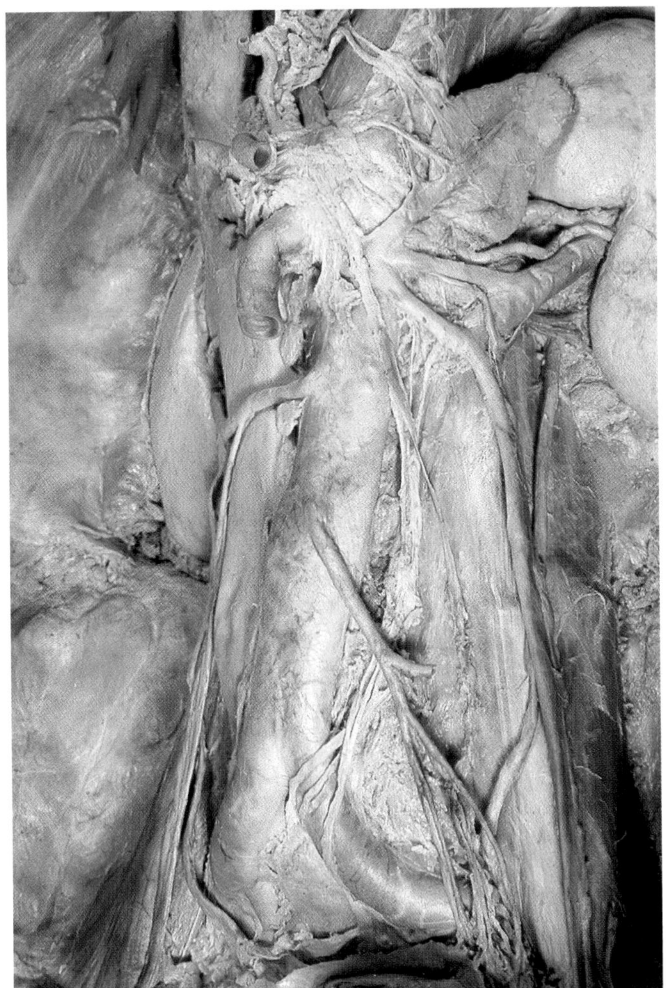

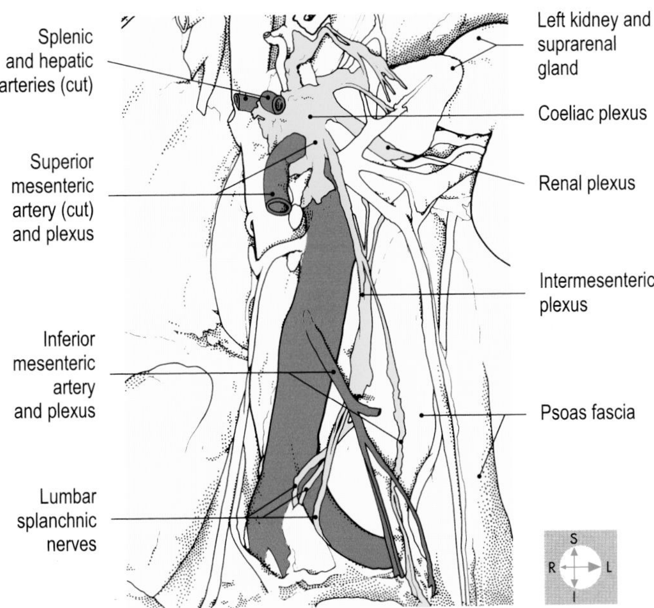

Fig. 4.98 Aortic plexuses of autonomic nerves after removal of aortic nodes and lymph vessels.

Posterior Abdominal Wall

Posterior to the abdominal cavity lie the lumbar spine, the psoas, iliacus and quadratus lumborum muscles, and associated fasciae and nerves (Fig. 4.99). The posterior abdominal wall extends inferiorly to the pelvic brim and superiorly to the attachment of the diaphragm (see p. 203) while laterally it merges with the anterolateral abdominal wall. The lumbar spine and the postvertebral muscles (erector spinae) are considered in Section 8.

Muscles

Psoas major

This long fusiform muscle (Fig. 4.99) attaches to the sides of the last thoracic and all five lumbar vertebral bodies, to the intervening discs and to the fronts of the lumbar transverse processes. At the side of each lumbar vertebral body, psoas major attaches to a fascial tunnel conveying a lumbar artery and vein (see Fig. 4.103).

The muscle inclines downwards, passing behind the inguinal ligament to enter the anterior compartment of the thigh (Fig. 4.100 & 4.101). The psoas major tendon, which also receives most of the fibres of iliacus, passes in front of the hip joint capsule, from which it is separated by a bursa, and attaches to the lesser trochanter of the femur.

Psoas major is innervated by the anterior rami of the upper lumbar nerves and its principal actions are flexion and medial rotation of the hip joint. In addition, the muscle flexes the lumbar spine both anteriorly and laterally. Within the substance of psoas major the anterior rami of the lumbar nerves form the lumbar plexus, whose branches emerge from the lateral, anterior and medial surfaces of the muscle.

Psoas minor

When present, this small muscle lies on the anterior surface of psoas major and gives way to a long narrow tendon (Fig. 4.100), which attaches to the iliopubic eminence of the hip bone.

Iliacus

This fan-shaped muscle attaches to the upper portion of the abdominal surface of the ilium and adjacent part of the sacrum (Fig. 4.100). Most of its fibres attach to the tendon of psoas major although some reach the femur below the lesser trochanter. The muscle is innervated by the femoral nerve (see Fig. 4.103) and assists psoas major in flexing the hip joint.

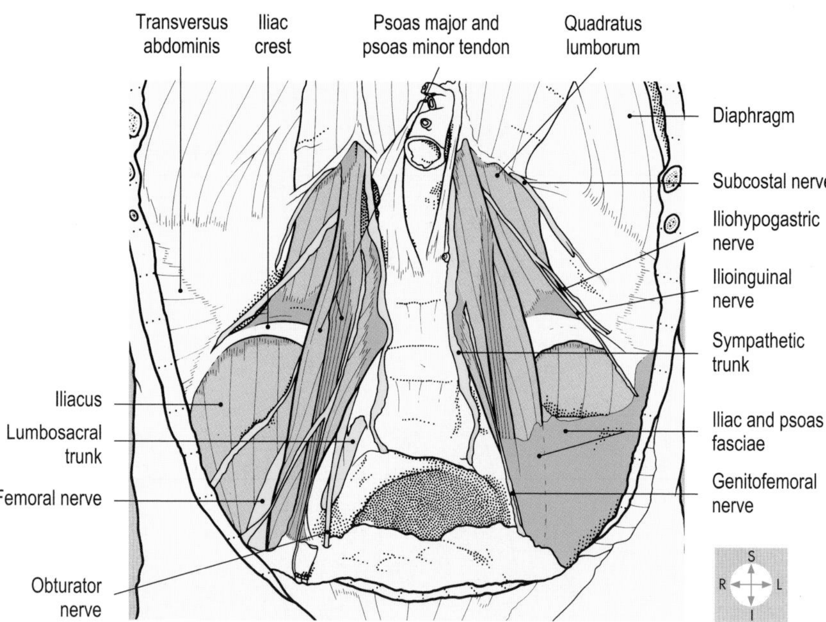

Fig. 4.99 Removal of the abdominal contents reveals the muscles and nerves of the posterior abdominal wall. On one side some iliac and psoas fasciae have been preserved.

Quadratus lumborum

Quadratus lumborum (Fig. 4.99) is anchored inferiorly to the iliolumbar ligament and adjacent part of the iliac crest. Superiorly it reaches the medial part of the lower border of the twelfth rib. There are intermediate attachments to the transverse processes of the upper four lumbar vertebrae. This muscle is innervated by the subcostal nerve and anterior rami of the upper three lumbar nerves, and is a lateral flexor of the lumbar spine. When the diaphragm contracts during inspiration, quadratus lumborum stabilizes the twelfth rib.

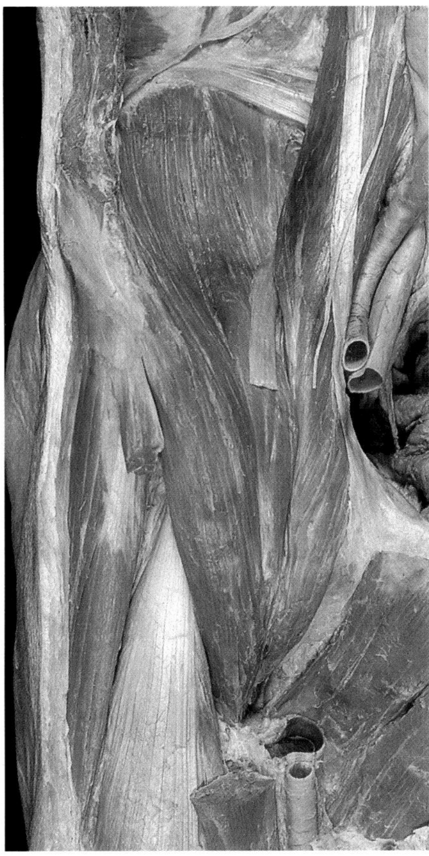

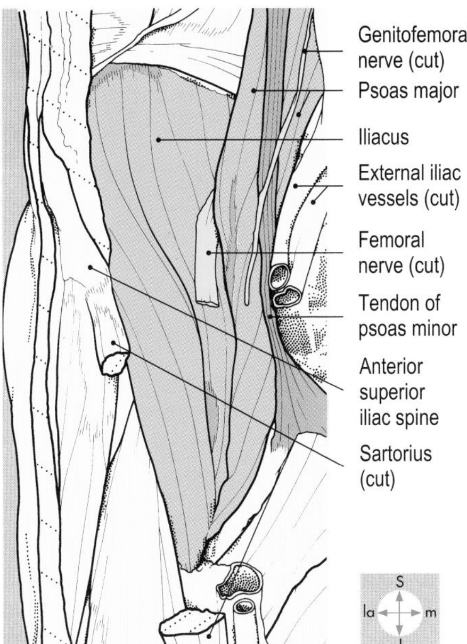

Fig. 4.100 Iliacus and psoas major, seen after removal of the inguinal ligament and part of sartorius, attach to the lesser trochanter of the femur. The psoas minor tendon descends to the iliopubic eminence of the hip bone.

Fasciae

The psoas and iliac fasciae form a continuous layer covering the anterior surfaces of their respective muscles (Fig. 4.99). The psoas fascia fuses superiorly with the diaphragmatic fascia and laterally and inferiorly with the transversalis fascia. Fascial thickenings over the upper parts of psoas major and quadratus lumborum form the medial and lateral arcuate ligaments (lumbocostal arches), which provide attachment for the diaphragm (see Fig. 4.103). Fascial layers covering the anterior and posterior surfaces of quadratus lumborum constitute part of the thoracolumbar fascia. These layers fuse at the lateral border of the muscle and give attachment to transversus abdominis.

Nerves

On each side of the midline the sympathetic trunk enters the abdomen behind the medial arcuate ligament of the diaphragm and descends on the medial border of psoas major (see Fig. 4.97). The anterior rami of the subcostal and lumbar nerves emerge through their respective intervertebral foramina and enter the substance of psoas major. All spinal nerves within psoas receive grey rami communicantes from the sympathetic trunk, but only the last thoracic and upper two lumbar nerves supply white rami to the trunk.

Subcostal (T12) nerve

This nerve follows the lower border of the twelfth rib and enters the abdomen behind the lateral arcuate ligament of the diaphragm. It crosses the anterior surface of quadratus lumborum and continues on the deep surface of transversus abdominis. The nerve pierces transversus to enter the neurovascular plane of the abdominal wall, and its subsequent course is similar to that of the lower intercostal nerves (see p. 145).

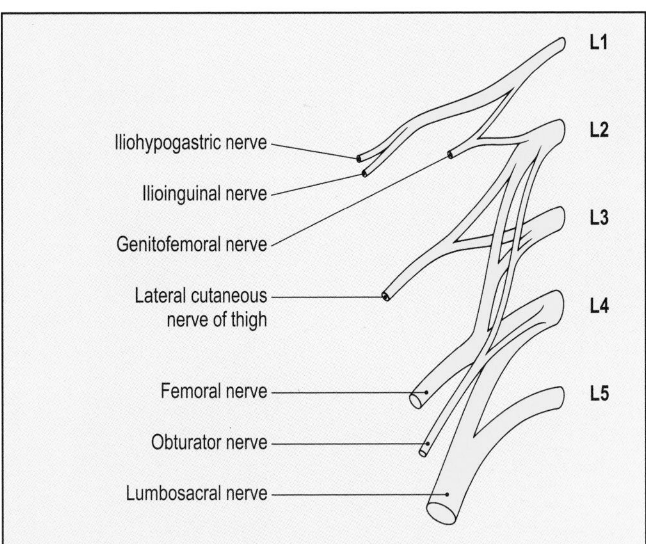

Fig. 4.101 Diagrammatic representation of the lumbar plexus to show the origins of each of its branches.

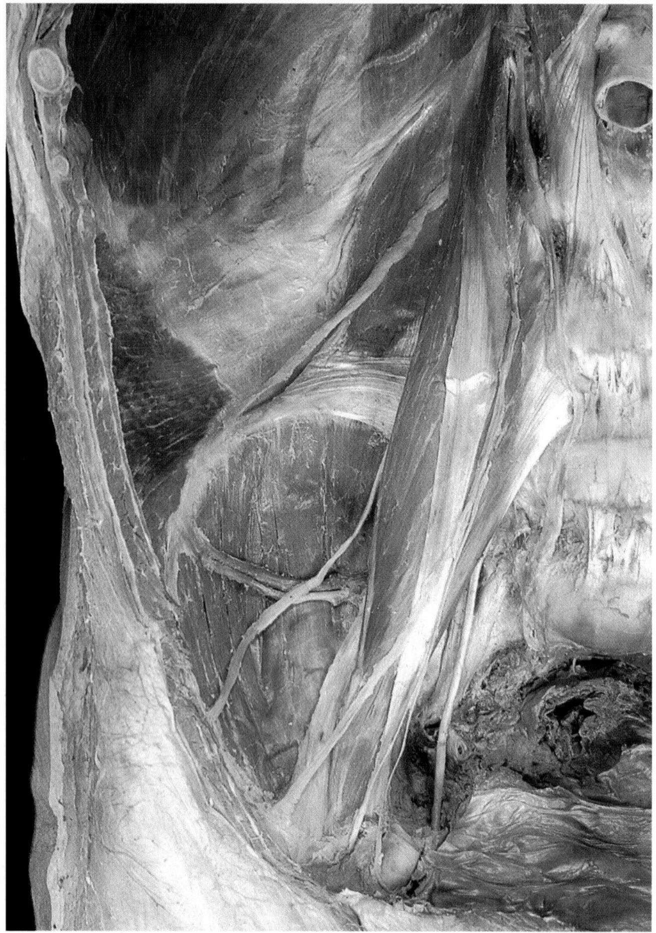

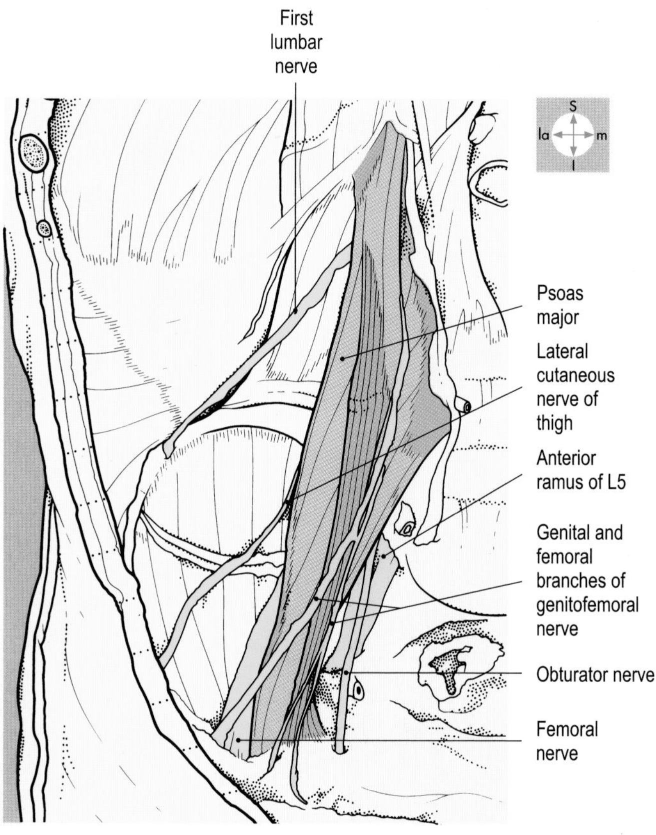

Fig. 4.102 Branches of the lumbar plexus emerge from the substance of psoas major.

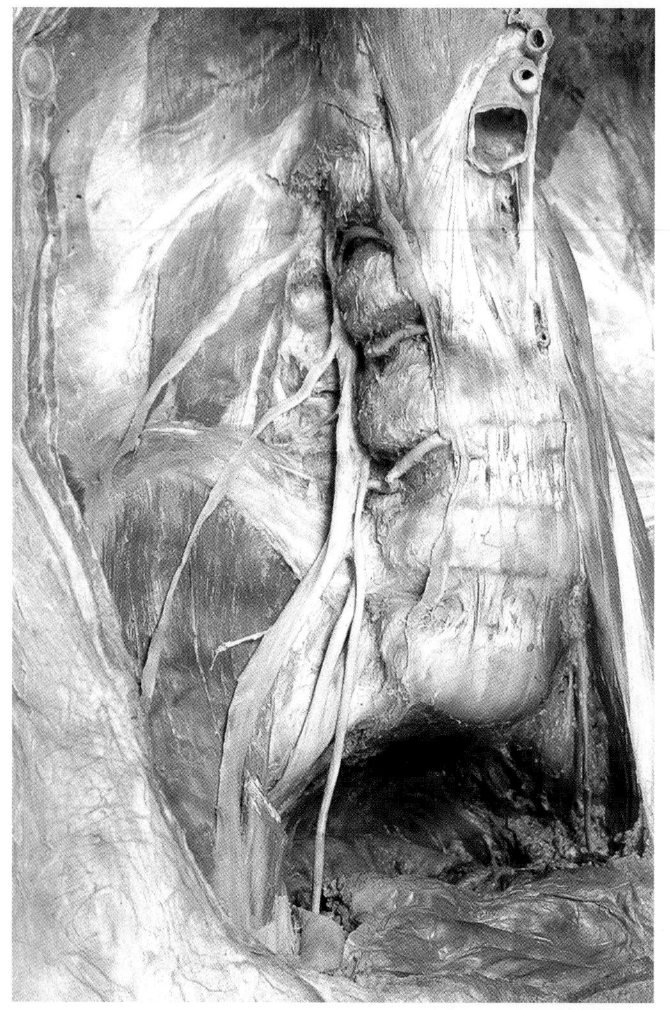

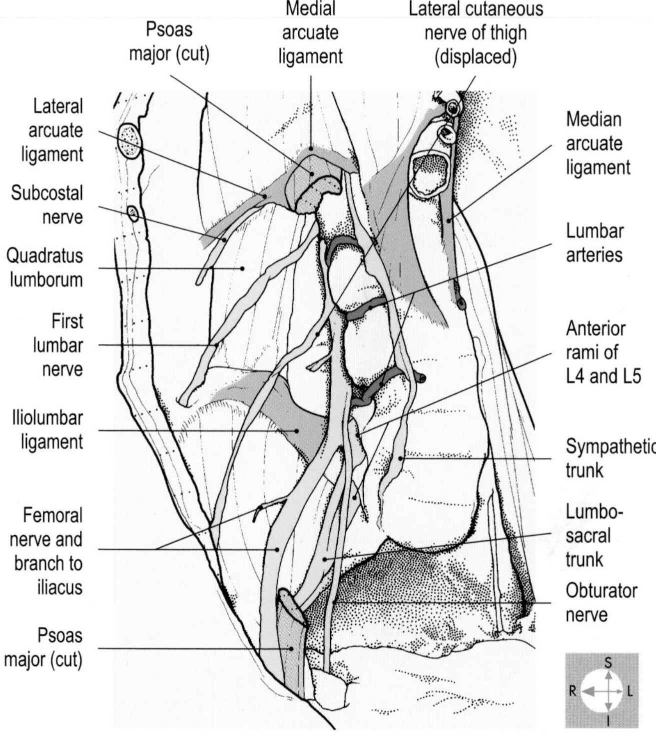

Fig. 4.103 Removal of most of psoas major and the genitofemoral nerve exposes the lumbar plexus.

Lumbar plexus

Within psoas major the anterior rami of the upper four lumbar nerves form the lumbar plexus, whose branches are distributed to the lower part of the abdominal wall, the lower limb and the sacral plexus in the pelvic cavity (see Figs 4.101 & 4.104).

First lumbar nerve

Although a few first lumbar (L1) fibres contribute to the genitofemoral nerve (Fig. 4.101), most form a nerve that emerges from the lateral border of psoas major and crosses the anterior surface of quadratus lumborum (Fig. 4.103).

After a variable distance this nerve divides into iliohypogastric and ilioinguinal branches, which continue into the anterolateral abdominal wall. Their paths and distribution are considered on page 145.

Genitofemoral (L1, L2) nerve

This nerve emerges through the anterior surface of psoas major on which it descends, dividing into two branches (see Fig. 4.101). The genital branch enters the deep inguinal ring and innervates the cremaster muscle, whilst the femoral branch passes behind the inguinal ligament to reach the subcutaneous tissue covering the femoral triangle (see Fig. 6.9).

Lateral cutaneous (L2, L3) nerve of thigh

Emerging from the lateral side of psoas major, this nerve inclines across the anterior surface of iliacus (see Fig. 4.102). It passes behind or through the inguinal ligament close to the anterior superior iliac spine (a site of possible entrapment) and enters the subcutaneous tissue on the anterolateral aspect of the thigh (see Fig. 6.9).

Femoral (L2, L3, L4) nerve

This large nerve appears at the lateral border of psoas major and descends in the gutter between this muscle and iliacus (see Fig. 4.102). It innervates iliacus (Fig. 4.103), passes behind the inguinal ligament lateral to the femoral artery and enters the anterior compartment of the thigh (see Fig. 6.8).

Obturator (L2, L3, L4) nerve

Descending vertically within psoas major, this nerve emerges from the medial border of the muscle near the pelvic brim (Fig. 4.103; see Fig. 4.102). It passes behind the common iliac vessels and runs downwards and forwards on the lateral pelvic wall as far as the obturator canal (see p. 237). Within the canal it divides into anterior and posterior branches, which enter the medial compartment of the thigh (see p. 266).

Lumbosacral trunk

Fibres from the fourth lumbar anterior ramus join those of the fifth to form the lumbosacral trunk (Fig. 4.103). The trunk emerges from the medial side of psoas major and crosses the sacroiliac joint to enter the pelvis where it contributes to the formation of the sacral plexus (see p. 237).

Diaphragm

The diaphragm is a musculotendinous partition separating the thoracic and abdominal cavities. Its periphery consists of skeletal muscle fibres, which merge centrally with an aponeurotic tendon (Fig. 4.104). The diaphragm has a pronounced convexity towards the thorax and has two domes or cupolas, the right usually lying at a higher level than the left (see Figs 4.105 & 4.106).

Musculature

Peripherally, the diaphragmatic muscle is attached to the sternum, the costal margin and the vertebral column. The sternal attachment is by two small slips to the posterior surface of the xiphisternum. The costal attachment is to the inner surfaces of the lower ribs (usually 7–12) and costal cartilages (see Fig. 4.105) by slips that interdigitate with those of transversus abdominis.

The diaphragm attaches to the vertebral column by two crura (pillars), one on each side of the abdominal aorta (Fig. 4.104). Both crura are anchored to the sides of the upper two lumbar vertebral bodies while the longer right crus is also attached to the third lumbar vertebra. The crura are linked in front of the aorta by the median arcuate ligament (Fig. 4.104), the fibres interdigitating as they ascend towards the central tendon. Lateral to each crus the diaphragm attaches to the transverse process of the first lumbar vertebra by the medial arcuate ligament (lumbocostal arch) and to the twelfth rib by the lateral arcuate ligament.

A triangular gap, the lumbocostal triangle (Fig. 4.104), often exists between the fibres attaching to the last rib and those arising from the vertebral column.

Central tendon

The muscle fibres of the diaphragm converge on the margins of the central tendon, a V-shaped area of dense fibrous tissue with its apex directed towards the xiphisternum and its lateral parts running backwards into the domes (Fig. 4.104). The central tendon gives attachment to the fibrous pericardium and is pierced by the inferior vena cava (Figs 4.104 & 4.106).

Structures passing between thorax and abdomen

Apertures in the diaphragm transmit the inferior vena cava and the oesophagus. The opening for the inferior vena cava (caval opening) lies to the right of the midline, and the oesophageal opening (hiatus) is slightly to the left (see Fig. 4.104). During quiet breathing these openings lie at the levels of the eighth and tenth thoracic vertebrae respectively. The caval opening pierces the central tendon and transmits the right phrenic nerve as well as the vena cava. The oesophageal opening, which also transmits the vagal trunks and branches of the left gastric vessels, is surrounded by muscle fibres of the right crus which can constrict the oesophagus (see Fig. 4.104). The left phrenic nerve pierces the left dome adjacent to the apex of the heart while on each side the thoracic splanchnic nerves pass through the crura to reach the coeliac plexus. The left crus may also be pierced by the hemiazygos vein.

The aorta enters the abdomen by descending behind rather than through the diaphragm and is accompanied by the thoracic duct and azygos vein (Fig. 4.107). The three vessels pass behind the median arcuate ligament and in front of the twelfth thoracic vertebral body. The subcostal nerves and vessels enter the abdomen behind the lateral arcuate ligaments anterior to quadratus lumborum while the sympathetic trunks descend behind the medial arcuate ligaments anterior to psoas major (see Fig. 4.104). Close to the xiphisternum, the superior epigastric vessels (branches of the internal thoracic vessels) pass between the sternal and costal slips of the diaphragm to enter the rectus sheath. Around the periphery of the diaphragm, intercostal nerves and vessels pass between the muscular slips to leave the lower intercostal spaces and reach the abdominal wall.

Movements

The diaphragm is an important muscle of inspiration and also assists the muscles of the abdominal walls and pelvic floor in raising the pressure within the abdomen and pelvis. Thus, the diaphragm contracts during acts of lifting and straining (for example, defecation and childbirth).

Its shape and position vary with body position and the phase of ventilation. During full inspiration the central tendon descends to approximately the level of the tenth thoracic vertebra. This descent, which is enhanced by an upright body posture, enlarges the thoracic cavity. When the diaphragm relaxes during expiration, its central tendon is pushed superiorly by intra-abdominal pressure, compressing the thoracic contents. With the body recumbent or head downwards, this upwards displacement is accentuated by the weight of the abdominal organs.

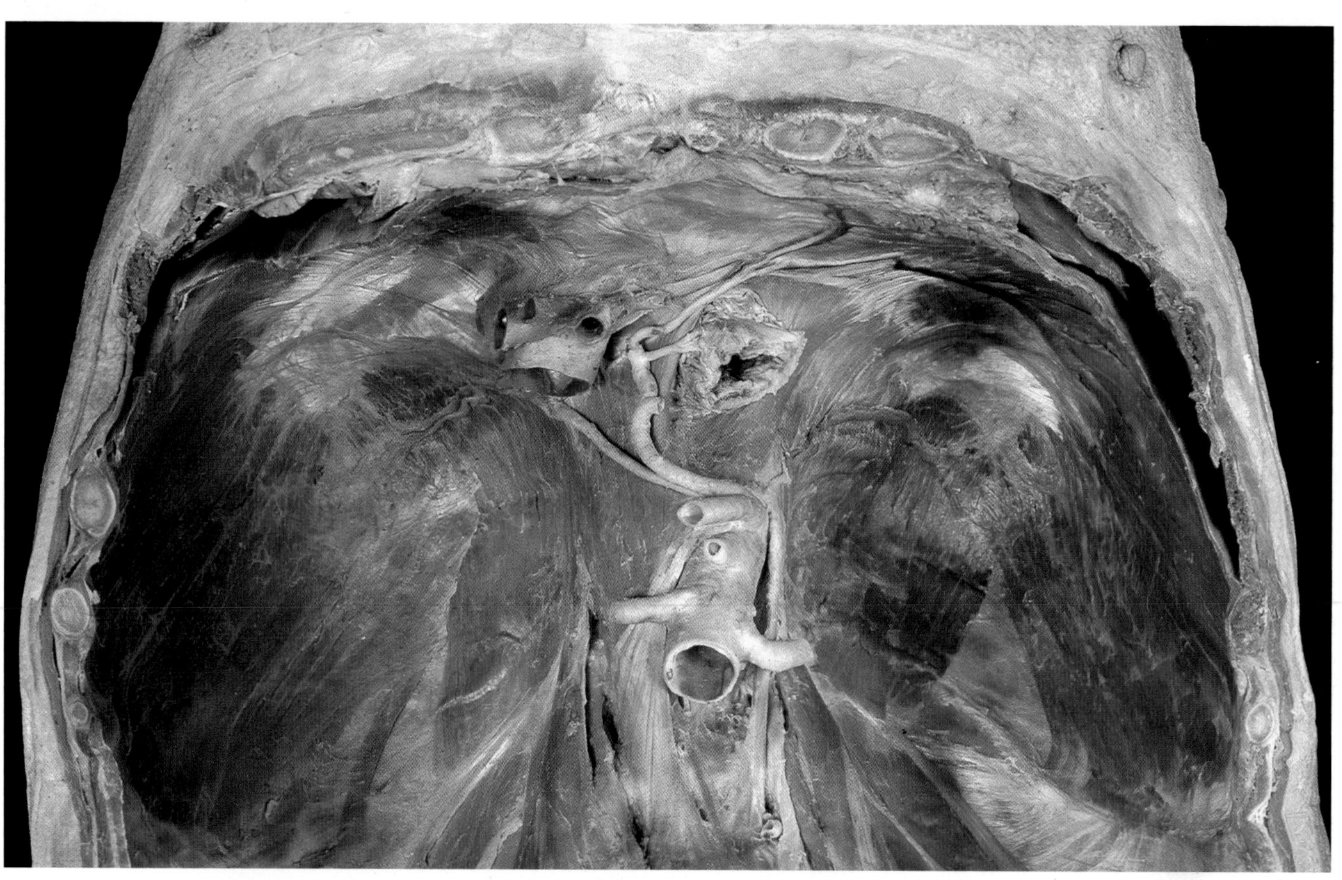

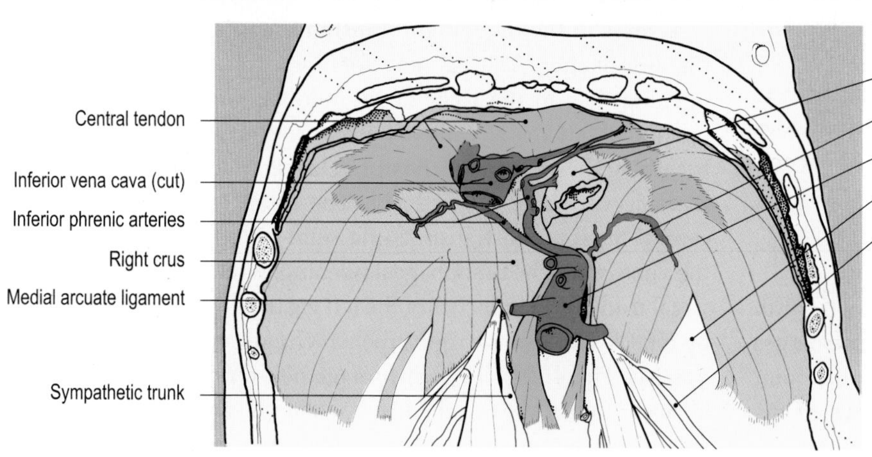

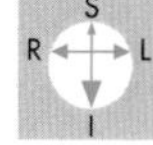

Fig. 4.104 Abdominal surface of the diaphragm after removal of peritoneum. The xiphisternum and anterior costal margin have been excised, including part of the anterior periphery of the diaphragm.

Nerve supply

The right and left phrenic nerves provide the motor and main sensory supply to the diaphragm. The phrenic nerves arise in the neck, from the third, fourth and fifth cervical nerves (see p. 324). Each nerve descends through the thorax (see p. 59) and divides into terminal branches that pierce the diaphragm and innervate it from the abdominal surface.

Each phrenic nerve provides the motor supply to its own half of the diaphragm. In addition, each phrenic nerve carries sensory fibres from the pericardium and from pleura and peritoneum covering the central portion of the diaphragm. Irritation of these sensory fibres may produce pain referred to the shoulder, because the skin covering this area is also supplied by the fourth cervical segment of the spinal cord. Sensory fibres from the peritoneum and pleura covering the periphery of the diaphragm are conveyed by the lower intercostal nerves.

Blood supply

The major blood supply is provided by the inferior phrenic arteries (see Fig. 4.104), which are usually direct branches of the aorta (see Fig. 4.92). The corresponding veins drain into the inferior vena cava. Also, the musculophrenic vessels (terminal branches of the internal thoracic vessels; see Fig. 2.17) supply the periphery of the diaphragm.

Relations

The inferior surface of the diaphragm is in contact with abdominal organs including the liver, kidneys, spleen and stomach. Its thoracic surface is related to the heart and lungs and their associated pericardium and pleura (Figs 4.105 & 4.106). Upward and downward excursions of the diaphragm cause corresponding movements of all the organs related to it. During the later stages of expiration, the periphery of the diaphragm comes into contact with the chest wall as the costodiaphragmatic recesses deepen (Fig. 4.105).

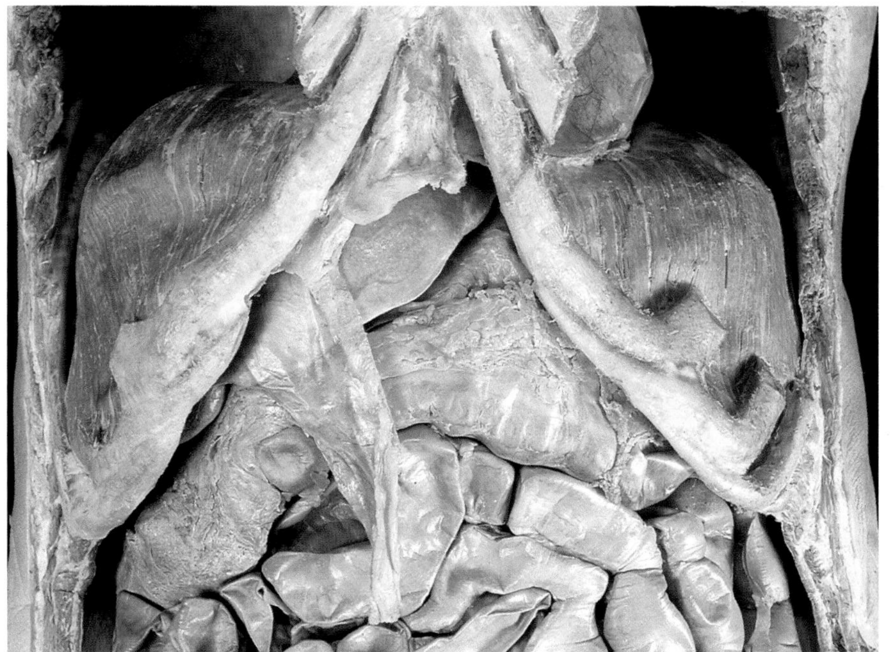

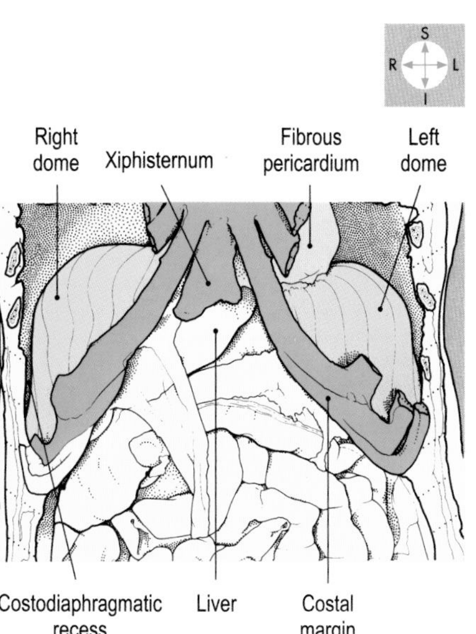

Fig. 4.105 The anterior chest and abdominal walls have been removed (except for the costal margins) to reveal the diaphragm. The abdominal organs are undisturbed but both lungs and the diaphragmatic pleura have been removed.

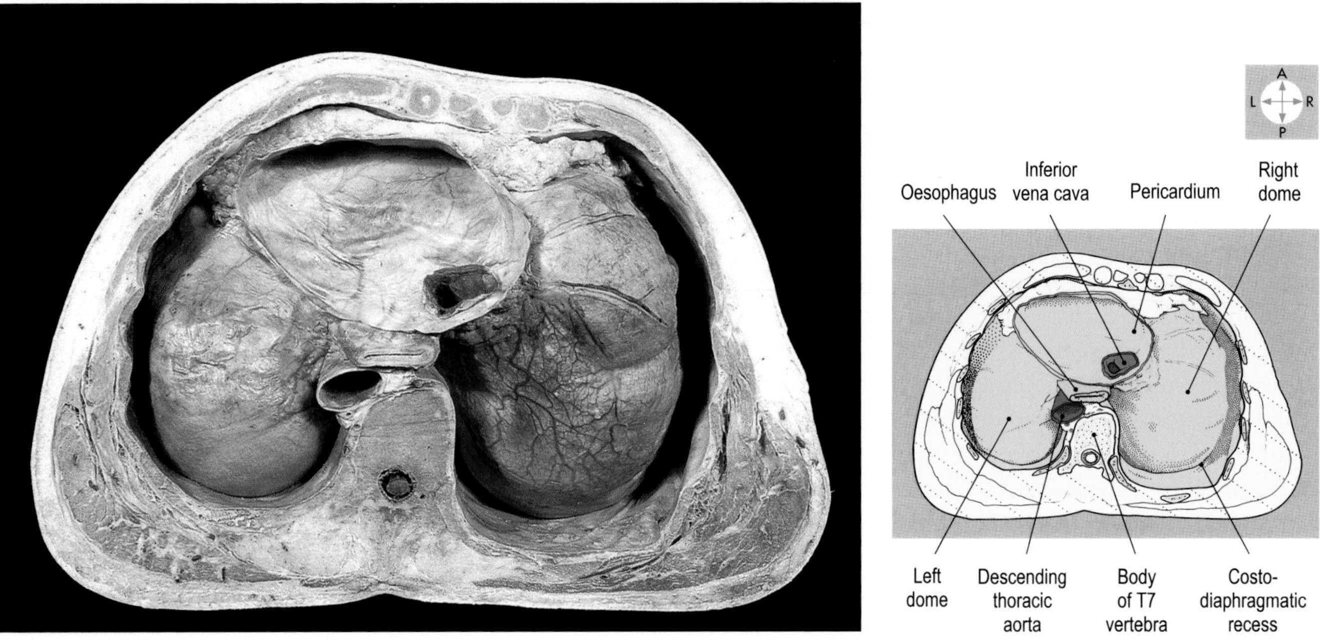

Fig. 4.106 Thoracic surface of the diaphragm. The parietal pleura remains in situ and the base of the fibrous pericardium has been retained.

Pleura (cut)
Posterior intercostal vein and artery
Azygos vein
Thoracic duct
Descending thoracic aorta
Coeliac trunk (cut)
Cisterna chyli
Superior mesenteric artery
Abdominal aorta
S
R
L
I

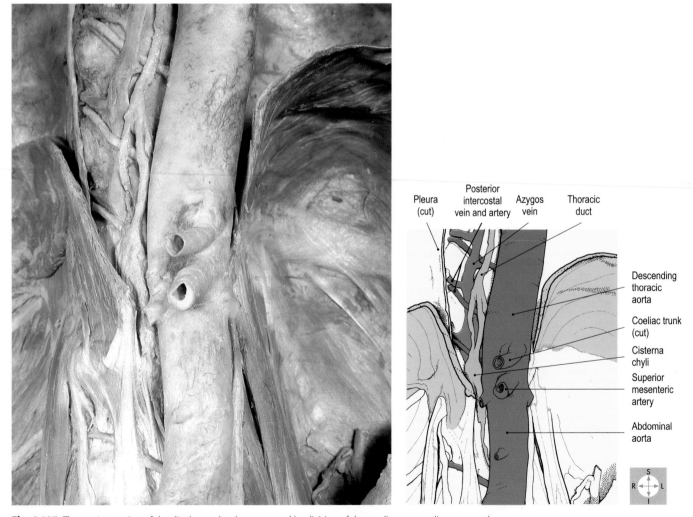

Fig. 4.107 The aortic opening of the diaphragm has been opened by division of the median arcuate ligament and removal of parts of both crura. The aorta is accompanied by the azygos vein and thoracic duct.

Exam Skills

Each of the incomplete statements below is followed by five suggested answers or completions. Decide which are true and which are false. The answers are supplied on page 415.

1. The rectus abdominis muscle:

a) is a powerful flexor of the lumbar spine.
b) is attached to the costal margin.
c) has a lateral border that crosses the ninth costal cartilage.
d) has the inferior epigastric artery as an anterior relation.
e) lies anterior to the inguinal canal.

2. The superior mesenteric artery:

a) arises from the abdominal aorta at the level of the third lumbar vertebra.
b) passes anterior to the horizontal (third part of) duodenum.
c) supplies branches to the head of the pancreas.
d) gives a middle colic branch.
e) supplies branches to the sigmoid colon.

3. The omental bursa (lesser sac):

a) extends superiorly behind the quadrate lobe of the liver.
b) extends to the left as far as the hilum of the spleen.
c) communicates with the greater peritoneal sac via an opening that lies posterior to the portal vein.
d) is closely related to the pancreas.
e) has the gastrosplenic ligament forming part of its posterior wall.

4. The spleen:

a) develops in the dorsal mesogastrium.
b) lies deep to ribs, 9, 10 and 11.
c) may be related at its hilum to the tail of the pancreas.
d) is retroperitoneal.
e) receives its arterial supply from a branch of the superior mesenteric artery.

5. The inferior vena cava:

a) lies anterior to the right sympathetic trunk (chain).
b) passes anterior to the omental foramen.
c) has the right gonadal vein as a direct tributary.
d) pierces the diaphragm at the level of the tenth thoracic vertebra.
e) usually passes anterior to the right renal artery.

6. The diaphragm:

a) contracts during forced expiration.
b) derives part of its motor nerve supply from intercostal nerves.
c) is in direct contact with the liver.
d) derives some arterial supply from the internal thoracic arteries.
e) has an oesophageal opening (hiatus) through which passes the left phrenic nerve.

7. The right kidney:

a) is related posteriorly to the twelfth rib.
b) has a hilum that is directed medially and forwards.
c) is related anteriorly to the head of the pancreas.
d) moves downwards during expiration.
e) is embedded in perirenal fat.

8. Regarding the scrotum:

a) the tunica vaginalis lies posterior to the testis.
b) the epididymis lies medial to the ductus (vas) deferens.
c) the dartos muscle is striated.
d) the ilioinguinal nerve supplies some of the skin.
e) lymph from the subcutaneous tissues drains to inguinal nodes.

9. The body of the pancreas:

a) lies anterior to the splenic vein.
b) has the root of the transverse mesocolon attached to its anterior border.
c) is intraperitoneal.
d) lies at the level of the first lumbar vertebra.
e) receives branches from the splenic artery.

10. The right ureter:

a) lies anterior to the internal iliac artery.
b) is closely related at its commencement to the descending (second part of) duodenum.
c) receives some of its arterial supply from the right renal artery.
d) crosses anterior to the right gonadal vessels.
e) may pass close to the vermiform appendix.

11. The caecum:

a) possesses taeniae coli.
b) usually lies in the right iliac fossa.
c) receives its blood supply from the superior mesenteric artery.
d) usually has the vermiform appendix attached to its lateral side.
e) receives the terminal ileum.

12. Direct relations of the abdominal aorta include:

a) the left renal vein.
b) the descending (second part of) duodenum.
c) the anterior longitudinal ligament.
d) left lumbar veins.
e) the head of the pancreas.

13. Peritoneum related to the liver includes:

a) the falciform ligament, which attaches to the anterior abdominal wall.
b) the left triangular ligament, which attaches to the diaphragm.
c) the lesser omentum, within which lie the gastric vessels.
d) the hepatorenal recess (or pouch) between the liver and the right kidney.
e) the right triangular ligament, which is continuous with the coronary ligaments.

14. The psoas major muscle:

a) attaches to the bodies of all the lumbar vertebrae.
b) laterally flexes the lumbar spine.
c) is innervated by the femoral nerve.
d) has the obturator nerve emerging from its medial surface.
e) extends the hip joint.

15. The liver:

a) usually extends below the costal margin.
b) lies partly in the left hypochondrium.
c) is in direct contact with the left dome of the diaphragm.
d) receives blood from the spleen.
e) has a quadrate lobe which is superior to the porta hepatis.

16. The inguinal canal:

a) has a roof formed by the lowest fibres of the internal oblique and transversus abdominis muscles.
b) has a deep ring that lies lateral to the inferior epigastric vessels.
c) transmits the broad ligament of the uterus.
d) has a superficial ring through which the ilioinguinal nerve emerges.
e) transmits testicular lymphatic vessels to the deep inguinal nodes.

Clinical Skills

The answers are supplied on page 416.

Case Study 1

In the space of two months a boy of two was taken three times to the family doctor because his mother had noticed a swelling in his scrotum. On the first two occasions the doctor had found nothing abnormal but the third time he found a mass and sent the boy into hospital for observation. On arrival in the ward no lump could be found but while having a drink of water the boy spluttered, coughed and began to scream. Now a cylindrical mass was apparent in the lower half of his right groin and extended into the scrotum anterior to the right testis. By the time a surgeon arrived the boy had begun to vomit. The surgeon said an operation was needed.

Questions:

1. What is the diagnosis?
2. Explain how a structure can move from the abdomen into the scrotum.
3. Why did the lump come and go?
4. What anatomical structure does the mass comprise?
5. Why did the boy vomit during the episode in hospital?
6. What will the surgeon do?

Case Study 2

A 20-year-old woman had an accident in her car. While not wearing a seatbelt she collided with a tree. The paramedics found her trapped in the driving seat, partially conscious, pale and sweaty with a weak and rapid pulse. They set up an intravenous drip and took her promptly to hospital. On arrival she was able to tell the doctors about pains in both her abdomen and her left shoulder. The pulse was still rapid and the blood pressure low. Her abdomen was tender, especially on the left side. Preparations were made for a blood transfusion and an abdominal operation. When she recovered from the anaesthetic, she was informed her spleen had been removed.

Questions:

1. The doctors suspected their patient had intra-abdominal bleeding. What was the evidence?
2. The spleen is commonly damaged in victims of blunt trauma to the abdomen. Why is this?
3. Into which part of the peritoneal cavity did the bleeding occur?

Case Study 3

A man in his fifties, who had always been fond of alcohol, especially spirits, visited his family physician with a six-month history of vague ill-health. He had been prompted to seek advice because a few days earlier he had noticed his skin looked yellow.

The physician was confronted by a pale and poorly man with mild jaundice. Examining his patient's abdomen the physician found a tender mass, dull to percussion, in the right hypochondrium which projected 2 cm below the costal margin and descended when a deep breath was taken. The physician gave his patient some stern advice about his diet, which included a ban on any further alcohol intake. He took a blood sample and asked the man to return in a few days.

Questions:

1. What diagnosis did the doctor make?
2. What features led him to this diagnosis?
3. Why did the mass move during inspiration?
   The laboratory reported a raised serum bilirubin concentration and other results consistent with liver failure, but the man did not return and failed to respond to the physician's attempts to get in touch. More than a year later the patient was found dead on the floor of his home in a pool of blood. The post-mortem report mentioned jaundice, ascites, nodularity and hardness of the liver. Varices had been found in the lower oesophagus, one of which had burst. A lot of clotted blood and partially digested food were found in the lungs, pharynx and mouth. The causes of death were asphyxia and shock.
4. How can liver disease produce varices in the oesophagus?
5. Where else might varicose veins be expected in such a patient?

Case Study 4

A man of 45 arrived at an Accident & Emergency department complaining of agonizing pain in the abdomen that had lasted four hours. He had tried unsuccessfully to gain relief by defaecating and emptying his bladder. He was pale, unable to keep still and begging for pain relief. He indicated the current site of the pain in the right iliac fossa but it had started in the small of the back on the right side and radiated into his groin. The physician found mild tenderness in the right iliac fossa, normal bowel sounds and no fever. A rectal examination was normal. A sample of urine looked rather dark to the naked eye, and tested positive for blood.

Questions:

1. What is the anatomical origin of the pain?
2. Why was a rectal examination performed?

   The patient was given an injection of a powerful analgaesic and admitted to a surgical ward. There he was encouraged to drink as much water as possible and all his urine was collected. A plain radiograph was taken of the abdomen and the doctors carefully examined this, along the line of the right ureter, for the shadow of a calculus in the ureter.
3. What is the course of the ureter, as seen on a radiograph?

   An intravenous urogram was performed.
4. What anatomical structures should this investigation depict?

   The patient passed his stone the following day. The pain subsided once the calculus entered the bladder and it travelled easily along the urethra into the collecting vessel.

Observation Skills

Identify the structures indicated. The answers are supplied at the foot of the page.

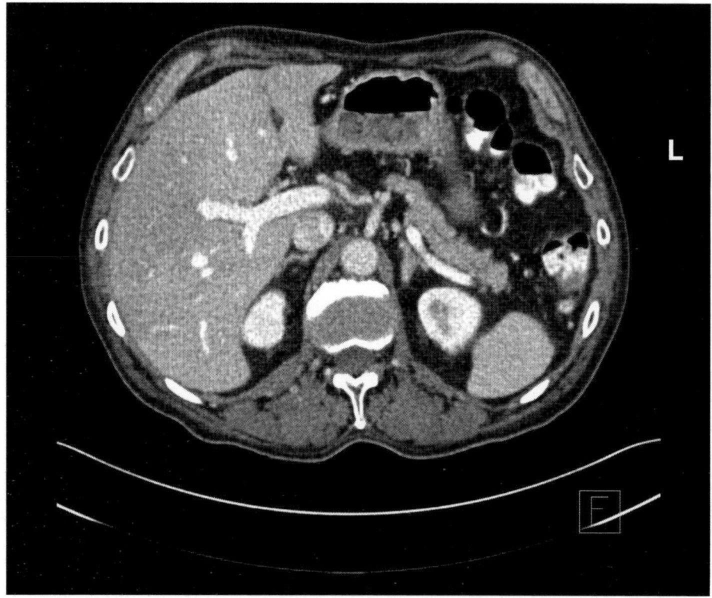

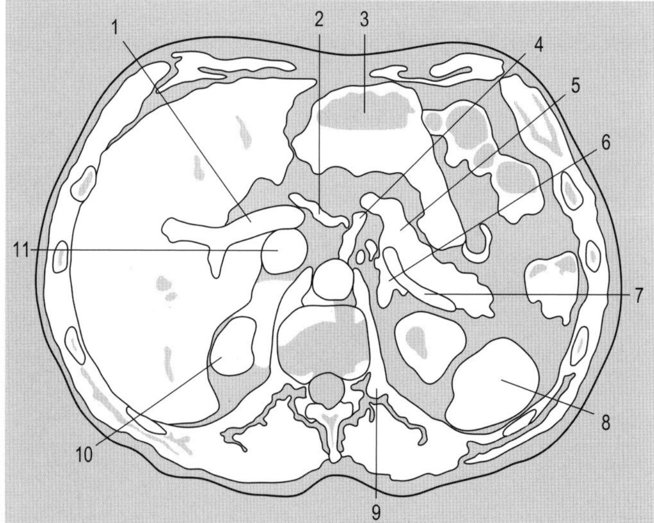

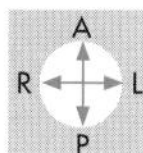

Fig. 4.108 Transverse CT image at the level of the twelfth thoracic vertebra.

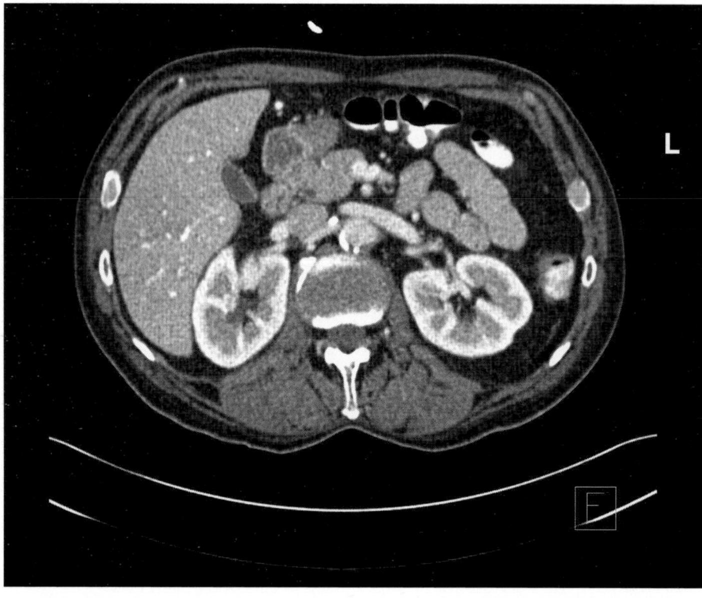

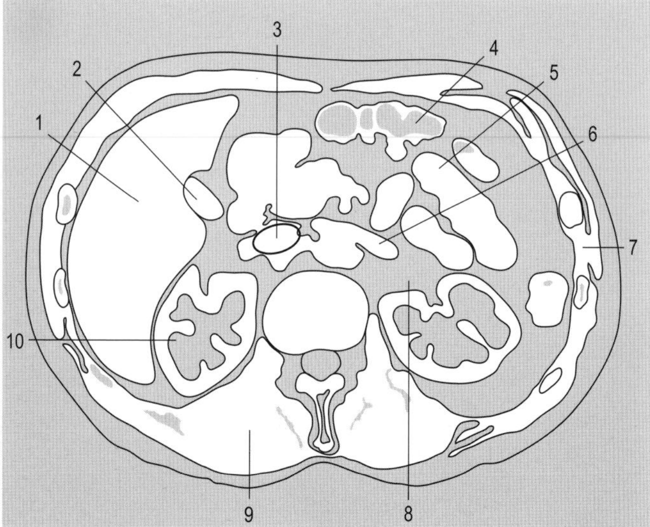

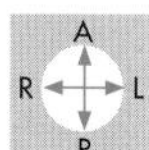

Fig. 4.109 Transverse CT image at the level of the second lumbar vertebra.

Answers

Fig. 4.108 1 = portal vein; 2 = common hepatic artery; 3 = stomach; 4 = coeliac trunk; 5 = body of pancreas; 6 = left suprarenal gland; 7 = splenic vein; 8 = spleen; 9 left crus of diaphragm; 10 = superior pole of right kidney; 11 = inferior vena cava.

Fig. 4.109 1 = liver; 2 = gall bladder; 3 = inferior vena cava; 4 = transverse colon; 5 = small intestine; 6 = left renal vein; 7 = intercostal muscles; 8 = branches of left renal artery; 9 = erector spinae muscle; 10 = right kidney.

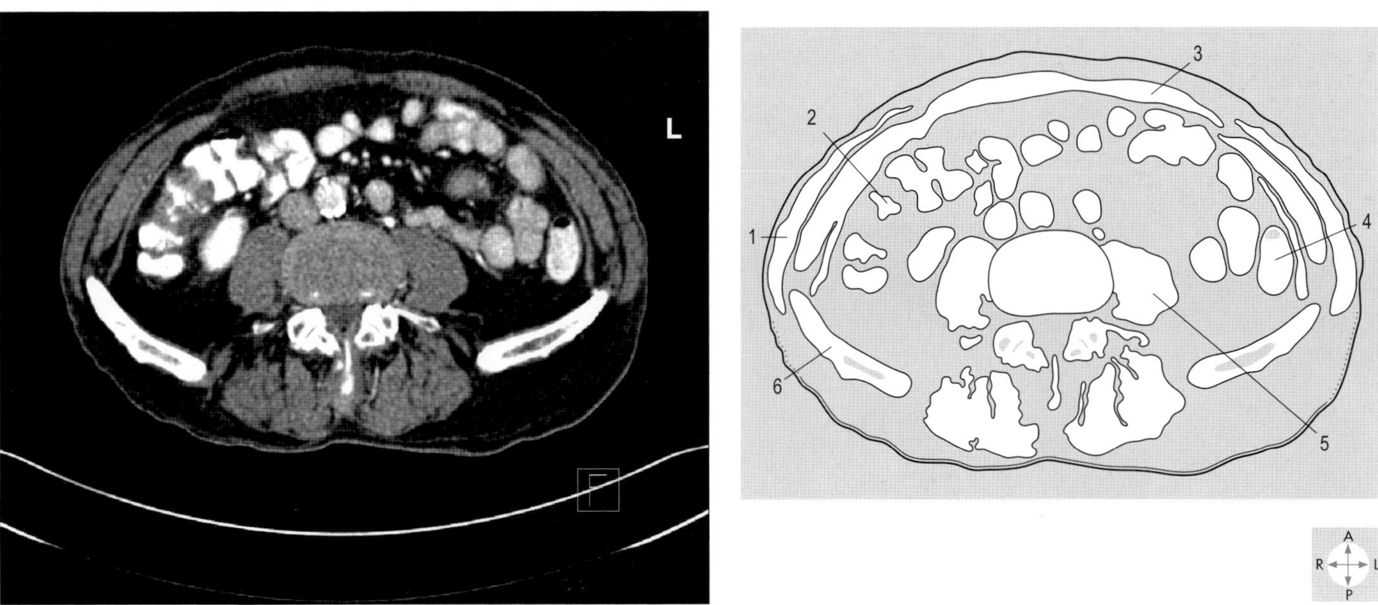

Fig. 4.110 Transverse CT image at the level of the fourth lumbar vertebra. Compare Fig. 4.112.

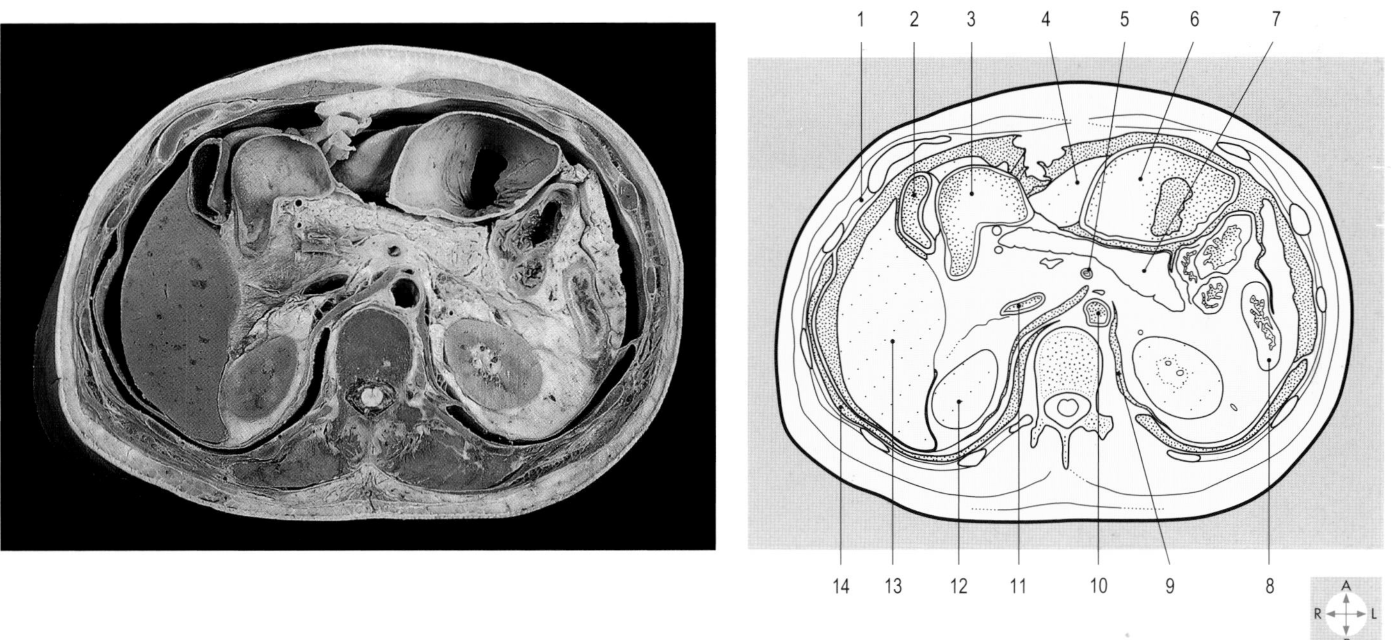

Fig. 4.111 Transverse section at the level of the twelfth thoracic vertebra. Inferior aspect.

Answers

Fig. 4.110 1 = external oblique; 2 = transverse colon; 3 = rectus abdominis; 4 = descending colon; 5 = psoas major; 6 = ilium (*not to be confused with ileum*)

Fig. 4.111 1 = intercostal muscles; 2 = fundus of gall bladder; 3 = descending duodenum; 4 = left lobe of liver; 5 = superior mesenteric artery; 6 = stomach; 7 = pancreas; 8 = descending colon; 9 = left crus of diaphragm; 10 = abdominal aorta; 11 = inferior vena cava; 12 = right kidney; 13 = right lobe of liver; 14 = costodiaphragmatic recess.

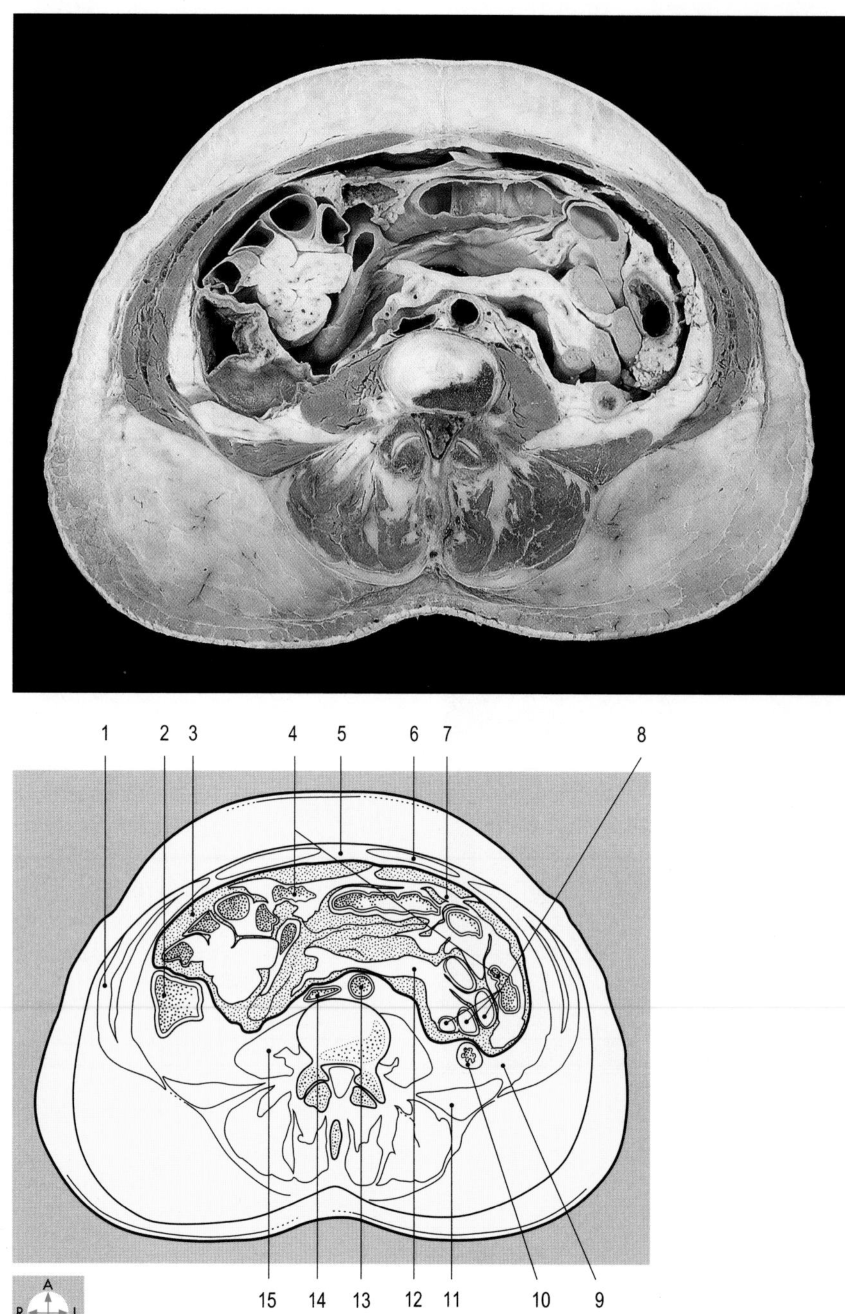

Fig. 4.112 Transverse section at the level of the intervertebral disc between the third and fourth lumbar vertebrae. Inferior aspect. Compare Fig. 4.110.

Answers

Fig. 4.112 1 = external abdominal oblique; 2 = ascending colon; 3 = peritoneal cavity; 4 = transverse colon; 5 = linea alba; 6 = rectus abdominis; 7 = greater omentum; 8 = small intestine; 9 = retroperitoneal fat; 10 = descending colon; 11 = quadratus lumborum; 12 = mesentery of small intestine; 13 = abdominal aorta; 14 = inferior vena cava; 15 = psoas major.

Pelvis and perineum

CHAPTER 5

Introduction

The pelvic cavity is in direct continuity with the abdominal cavity. It extends downwards and backwards within the confines of the bony pelvis as far as the pelvic floor (pelvic diaphragm), inferior to which lies the perineum. Some anatomists and surgeons refer to the 'false pelvis' or 'greater pelvis' (below the iliac crests but above the pelvic inlet) and the 'true pelvis' or 'lesser pelvis' (below the inlet). This chapter deals only with the 'true pelvis' and these other expressions will not be used again.

Pelvis

The pelvic cavity is a basin-shaped region below and behind the pelvic inlet (Fig. 5.1). It is surrounded by the bones of the pelvic girdle supplemented by muscles, ligaments and fascia. The anterior wall, near the pubic symphysis, is shallow while the posterior wall, the sacrum, is deep and concave. Each lateral wall is lined by the obturator internus, a broad muscle covered on its medial surface by fascia. Above this muscle are two apertures providing access for nerves and vessels entering the lower limb. The greater sciatic foramen leads into the gluteal region, the obturator canal into the thigh.

The organs in the pelvis include the bladder and lower ureters, the rectum and possibly coils of small intestine and the sigmoid colon. The male pelvis also contains the prostate (inferior to the bladder) and seminal vesicles (posterior to the bladder) and parts of the ductus deferentes (see Fig. 5.5). In the female, the reproductive organs are interposed between the bladder and rectum, and include the vagina, the uterus, uterine tubes and ovaries (see Fig. 5.6). In the infant, the pelvic cavity is comparatively shallow and therefore parts of the bladder and uterus may lie above the pelvic brim. In the adult, however, the bladder and uterus often lie below the pelvic inlet (brim), though they rise into the abdomen when distended with urine or enlarged by pregnancy.

The peritoneum of the greater sac covers the superior parts of the pelvic organs. In the male it dips into a single pouch between the bladder and rectum while in the female it forms two deeper pouches, anterior and posterior to the uterus. The peritoneum that drapes over each uterine tube is called the broad ligament and the ovary attaches to its posterior aspect (see Fig. 5.8).

The arterial supply to most of the pelvic organs is provided by the internal iliac artery (Fig. 5.2), but the rectum and ovaries are supplied by the inferior mesenteric artery and the ovarian arteries, respectively, from the abdominal aorta. Similarly, most venous blood passes to the internal iliac veins but the rectum drains to the portal venous system via the inferior mesenteric vein, while the ovarian veins enter the inferior vena cava and left renal vein. Much of the lymph from the pelvic organs passes to the internal iliac nodes, but the rectum and ovaries drain to aortic nodes in the abdomen.

Many of the nerves in the pelvis, including the sacral plexuses, are applied to the pelvic walls and are merely in transit to the lower limb. The pelvic organs themselves receive autonomic innervation via the left and right pelvic plexuses which surround the branches of the internal iliac arteries. The parasympathetic contribution to these plexuses comes from the pelvic splanchnic nerves, branches of the second, third and fourth sacral spinal nerves, while the sympathetic innervation is provided by the hypogastric plexus, which descends from around the aortic bifurcation.

The gutter-shaped pelvic floor is formed largely by the left and right levator ani muscles. They arise from the pelvic wall, chiefly from the fascia covering the obturator internus muscles, slope downward and fuse in the midline. There is a narrow midline gap near the pubic symphysis traversed by the urethra and vagina. The central part of the pelvic floor is pierced by the rectum, turning downwards and backwards to become the anal canal.

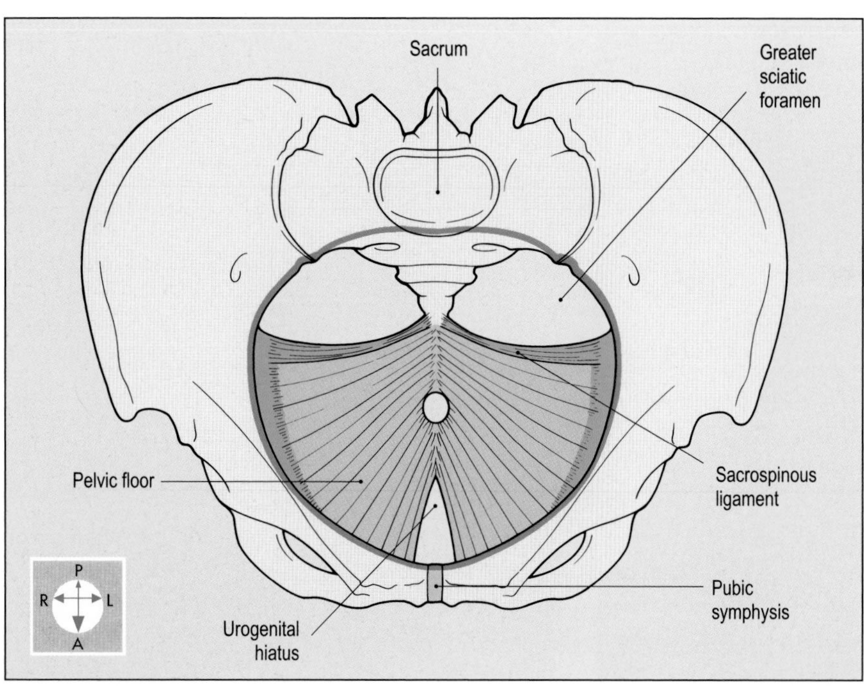

Fig. 5.1 Oblique anterosuperior view of pelvis to show pelvic inlet (pink line) and floor.

Perineum

The perineum is the shallow region that includes the anal canal and the external genitalia. It is bounded by the pelvic outlet: the inferior margins of the bones of the pelvis and their associated ligaments (Fig. 5.3). The region extends forwards to the pubic symphysis, backwards to the coccyx and laterally to the ischial tuberosities. The roof of the perineum is formed by the two levator ani muscles, the floor is the skin and each lateral wall is similar to that of the pelvis: the pubis and ischium covered by the obturator internus muscle.

The posterior half of the perineum, the anal triangle, contains the anal canal, its sphincters and a fat-filled space on each side, the ischioanal (ischiorectal) fossa. Each fossa communicates with the gluteal region via a small aperture, the lesser sciatic foramen. The anterior half of the perineum, the urogenital triangle, includes the external genitalia. In the female, the lower parts of the vagina and urethra are surrounded by the vulva (labia majora and minora and the clitoris), while in the male the distal part of the urethra is enclosed by the penis. Below the root of the penis is the scrotum. Although the scrotum is part of the perineum it is described with the testis and inguinal canal in Chapter 4 (see p. 149).

Most structures in the perineum, including the scrotum but excluding the testes, are supplied by the pudendal nerve and the internal pudendal vessels (Fig. 5.2). The neurovascular bundle arises in the pelvis but does not pierce the levator ani to reach the perineum. Instead, it traverses the greater sciatic foramen, the gluteal region and the lesser sciatic foramen. The nerve and vessels then run forward through the perineum, giving branches to the anal canal, the scrotum or labia and the penis or clitoris. Most of the lymph from these structures passes to the inguinal nodes, which are also the main site of drainage for the lower parts of the vagina and anal canal, but the testes drain to aortic lymph nodes in the abdomen.

The pudendal nerve gives motor branches to many striated muscles in the perineum, including the external anal and urethral sphincters. In addition, it supplies sensory branches to the anal canal, vagina, urethra and most of the perineal skin.

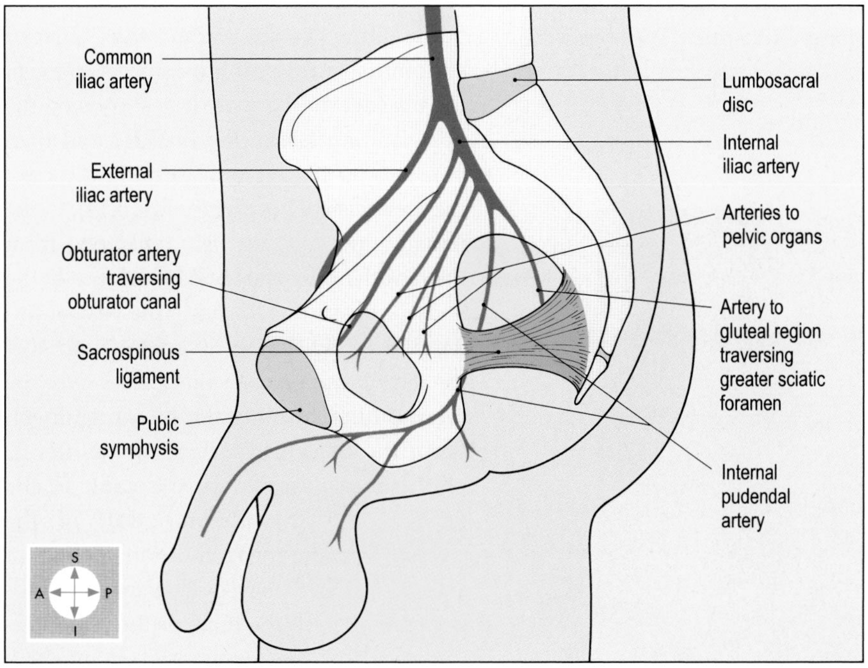

Fig. 5.2 The internal iliac artery and some of its branches to the pelvis, perineum and lower limb.

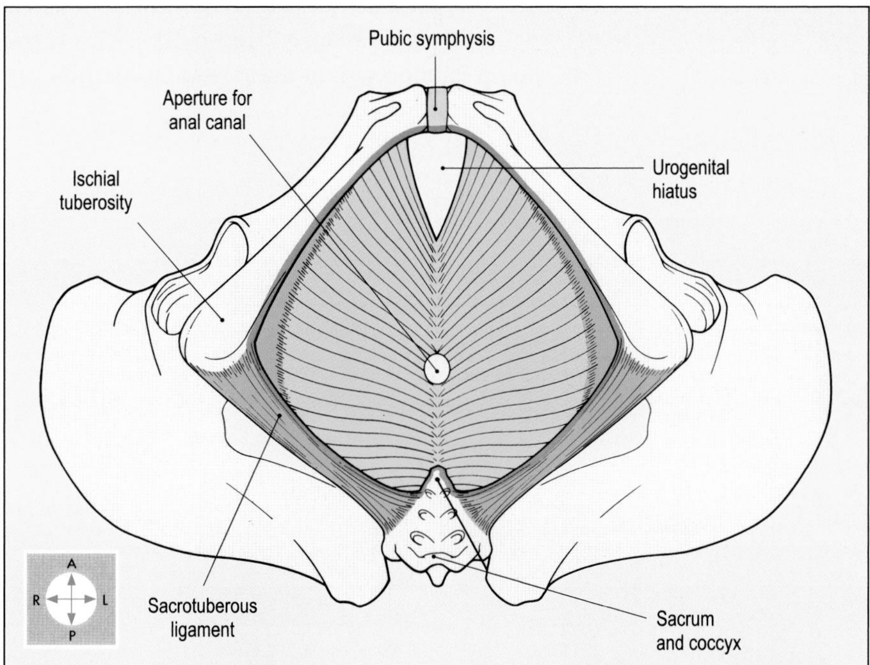

Fig. 5.3 Inferior view of pelvic outlet (pink line) and boundaries of perineum.

Pelvic Cavity

Although the pelvic cavity is in direct continuity with the abdominal cavity the two regions are delineated by the pelvic inlet (pelvic brim). This lies at approximately 45 degrees to the horizontal and comprises the sacral promontory posteriorly, the arcuate and pectineal lines laterally and the pubic crests and upper border of pubic symphysis anteriorly (Fig. 5.4; and see Figs 4.6, 5.26 & 5.27).

The bony walls of the pelvis give attachment to two pairs of muscles. The obturator internus and piriformis muscles arise within the pelvis but their tendons pass out into the gluteal region to reach the femur. The fascia covering the medial surface of obturator internus is dense and provides attachment for the pelvic floor. The piriformis muscles spring from the anterior surface of the sacrum and are partially covered by the large nerves comprising the sacral plexuses (Fig. 5.4).

In both sexes the pelvic cavity contains the rectum and bladder along with the lower parts of the ureters and loops of small or large intestine. The remaining organs differ between the sexes. The male reproductive organs found within the pelvis (Fig. 5.5) are the prostate, seminal vesicles and ductus deferentes. Those of the female (Fig. 5.6) are the ovaries, uterine tubes, uterus and upper part of vagina.

Peritoneum

Peritoneum lines the lateral and posterior pelvic walls and covers most of the pelvic organs (Figs 5.5 & 5.6). In both sexes peritoneum passes from the anterior abdominal wall onto the upper surface of the bladder. In the male it descends on the posterior surface of the bladder and then passes onto the rectum, forming a recess, the rectovesical pouch (see Fig. 5.14). In the female, peritoneum is reflected from the bladder onto the anterior surface of the body of the uterus, forming the vesicouterine pouch (Fig. 5.6). It covers the fundus of the uterus and on each side passes over the uterine tube, forming the broad ligament. From the posterior surface of the uterus, peritoneum passes over the vault of the vagina onto the anterior wall of the rectum, forming the rectouterine pouch (of Douglas). Fluid may collect in the rectovesical pouch of the male or the rectouterine pouch of the female and, if infected, may form a pelvic abscess.

Between the peritoneum and the pelvic organs, and intervening between the organs, lies the extraperitoneal fat or pelvic fascia (see Fig. 5.7 and p. 235). This tissue is important in the spread of infection.

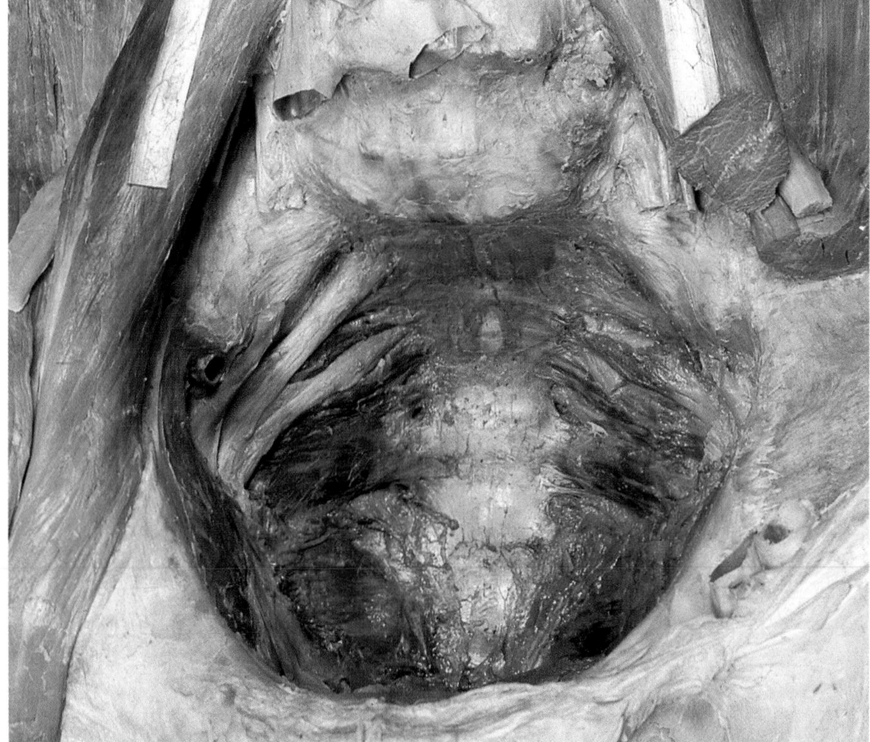

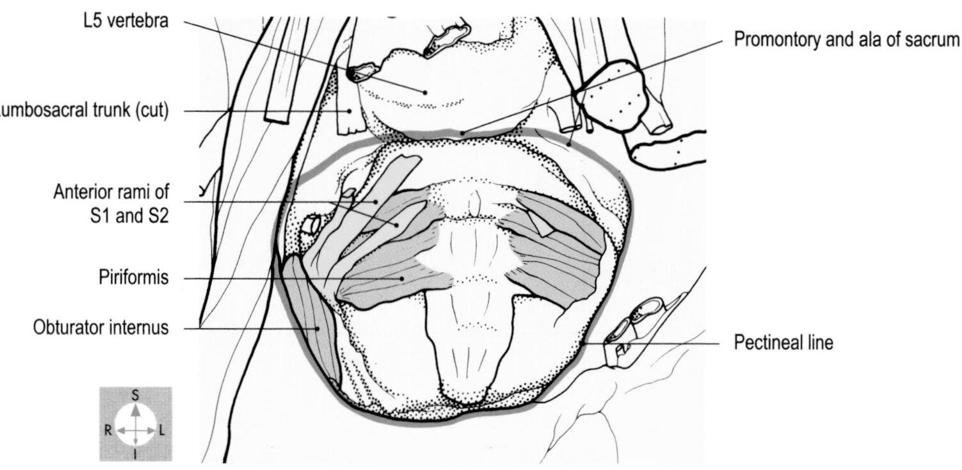

Fig. 5.4 Pelvis and lower abdomen after removal of all the organs and most of the vessels to demonstrate the pelvic inlet (pink line) and cavity.

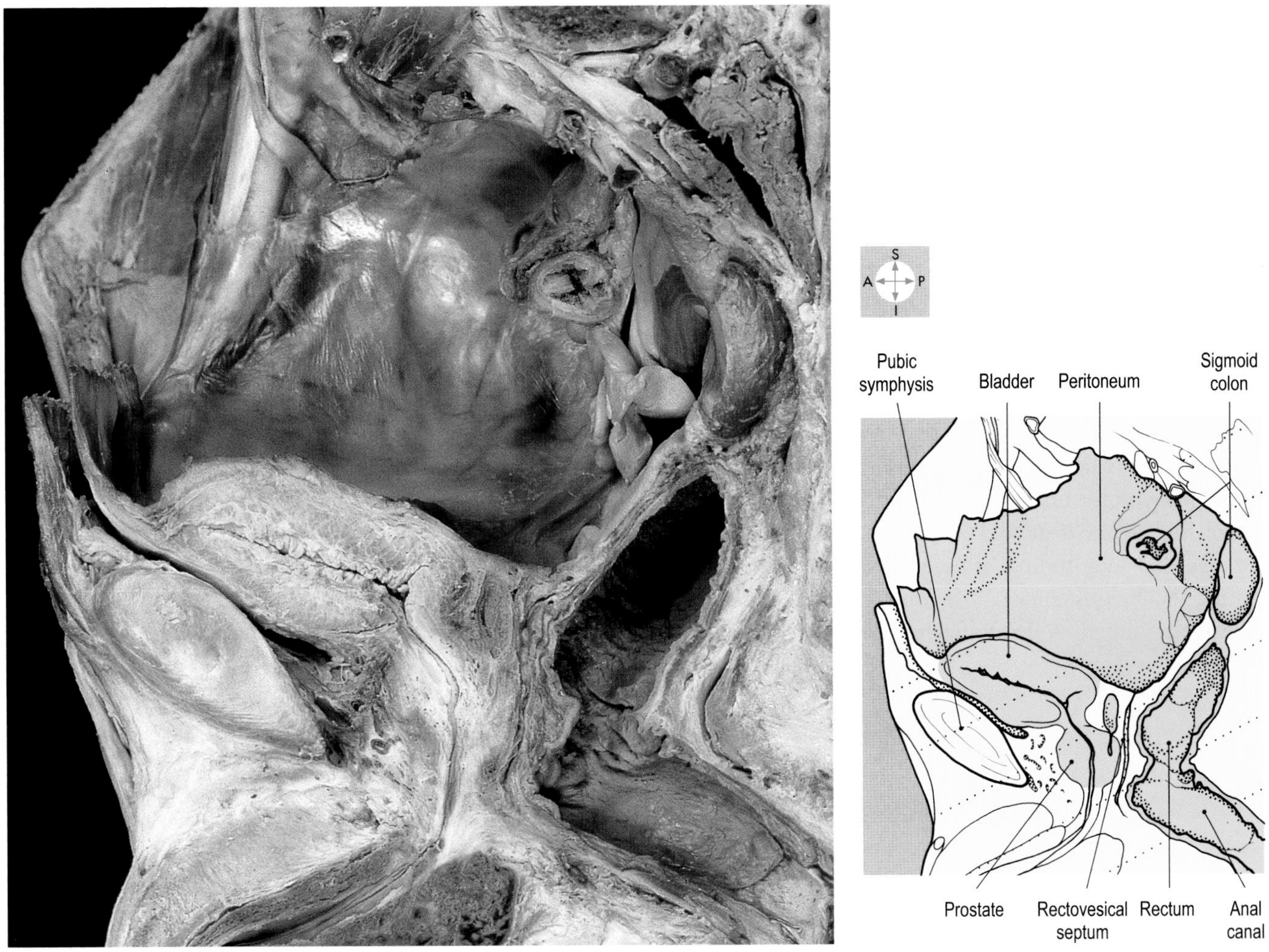

Fig. 5.5 Median sagittal section through the male pelvis to show the peritoneum and the principal pelvic viscera.

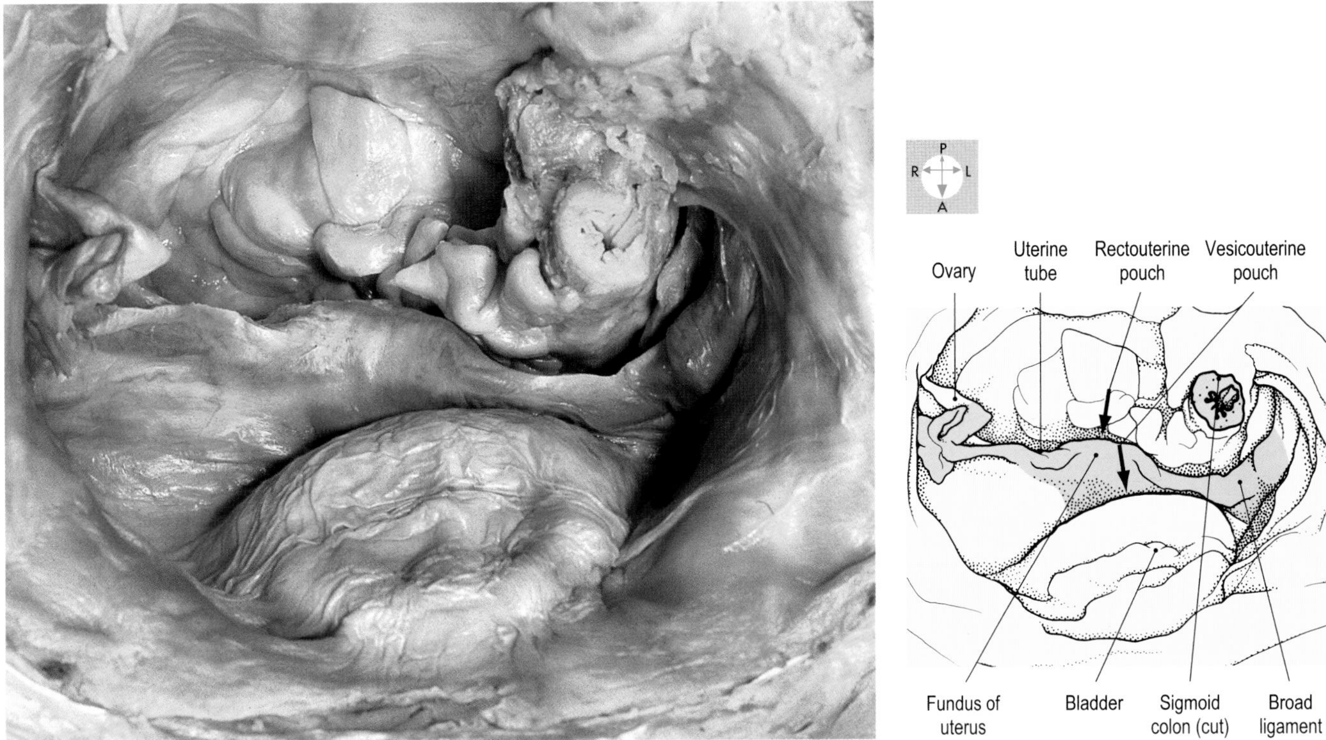

Fig. 5.6 Superior view of peritoneum and organs within the female pelvis. The small intestine and most of the sigmoid colon have been removed.

Rectum

The rectum is the distal portion of the large intestine and lies in the posterior part of the pelvic cavity. It is continuous with the sigmoid colon at the rectosigmoid junction in front of the third piece of the sacrum (Fig. 5.7), where there is often an acute angulation in the intestine which must be navigated with care during colonoscopy. The rectum curves downwards and forwards, lying first on the anterior surface of the sacrum and then on the upper surface of the pelvic floor. It deviates to either side of the midline and these lateral flexures become pronounced when the organ is distended. The lowest part of the rectum, the ampulla, is its most dilatable portion. Turning abruptly downwards and backwards, the rectum pierces the pelvic floor and terminates at the anorectal junction, where it is continuous with the anal canal (see Fig. 5.5).

Unlike the colon, the rectum is devoid of appendices epiploicae and has no taeniae, the longitudinal muscle being distributed uniformly around its circumference. The mucous membrane projects into the rectal lumen as three shelves, which form the horizontal folds.

Relations

The upper two-thirds of the rectum are related to the most inferior portion of the peritoneal cavity. The upper third of the organ is covered anteriorly and on both sides by peritoneum while the middle third, lying behind the rectouterine or rectovesical pouch, has peritoneum only on its anterior surface.

Posterior to the upper part of the rectum are the sacrum, coccyx and the piriformis muscles, while its lower part rests on the levator ani muscles. Descending behind the organ are the superior rectal vessels (Fig. 5.7), the hypogastric plexus of autonomic nerves and, on each side of the midline, the sympathetic trunk and sacral plexus. Lateral to the rectum lie the pelvic plexuses of autonomic nerves and the ureters.

Anterior to the upper portion of the rectum lie those parts of the sigmoid colon and ileum that descend into the pelvic cavity. The anterior relations of the rectal ampulla are of clinical interest because they may be palpated on rectal examination. In the male these are the prostate (see Fig. 5.5), the base of the bladder, the seminal vesicles and ampullae of the ductus. These structures are separated from the rectum by the rectovesical septum. In the female the rectal ampulla lies adjacent to the posterior wall of the vagina; therefore, rectal examination permits palpation of the cervix of the uterus.

Blood supply

The arterial supply to the rectum is derived principally from the superior rectal artery (Fig. 5.7), the continuation of the inferior mesenteric artery (see p. 182). This supply may be supplemented by middle rectal branches from the internal iliac arteries. Venous blood drains into the portal venous system via the superior rectal vein and its continuation, the inferior mesenteric vein. In addition, middle rectal veins drain into the internal iliac veins. As the superior and middle rectal veins interconnect, the wall of the rectum is a site of portacaval anastomosis (see p. 185).

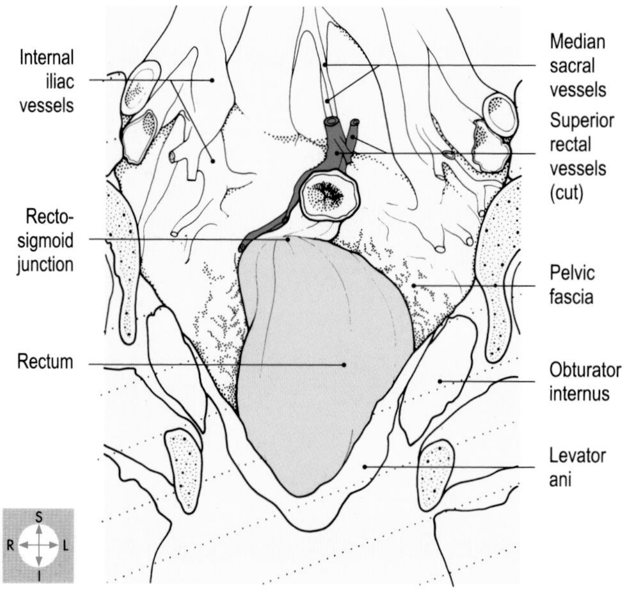

Fig. 5.7 Anterior aspect of rectum seen in a male pelvis sectioned coronally. All peritoneum has been removed.

Female Internal Reproductive Organs

The female internal organs of reproduction include the uterus and vagina and the paired ovaries and uterine (fallopian) tubes. The uterus and ovaries are particularly affected by atrophy (shrinkage) after the menopause.

Uterus

The uterus is a pear-shaped organ approximately 8 cm in length. Its major component is the body (or corpus), which remains somewhat enlarged after pregnancy. Inferiorly the uterus tapers into the cylindrical neck or cervix, which protrudes into the upper part of the vagina (Fig. 5.9).

The uterus is most commonly positioned with its body lying on the superior surface of the bladder (Fig. 5.8). As the bladder fills and empties, the uterine body moves on the relatively immobile cervix. Thus, when the bladder is empty the uterine body is anteflexed (bent forwards on the cervix), but when the bladder is distended the uterus may become retroflexed.

Body

The uterine body possesses anteroinferior and posterosuperior surfaces. The right and left borders give attachment to the broad ligaments and superiorly give origin to the uterine tubes (Figs 5.8 & 5.11). The rounded upper end of the organ between the attachments of the tubes is called the fundus.

On the posterosuperior surface of the uterus lie the sigmoid colon or coils of ileum. Both surfaces are covered with peritoneum, which continues laterally as the broad ligament (Fig. 5.11). Adjacent to the uterus within each broad ligament is the uterine artery and its associated plexus of veins. On each side, the ligament of the ovary and the round ligament of the uterus attach to the uterine body close to the origin of the uterine tube. These ligaments, remnants of the fetal gubernaculum, run laterally within the broad ligament, often raising ridges in the peritoneum. The ligament of the ovary attaches to the medial pole of the ovary while the round ligament of the uterus runs to the lateral pelvic wall and turns forwards in the extraperitoneal tissues. Crossing the external iliac vessels, the round ligament of the uterus enters the deep inguinal ring (see Fig. 5.8), traverses the inguinal canal and terminates in the subcutaneous tissues of the labium majus (see Fig. 4.22).

The wall of the uterine body comprises a thick layer of smooth muscle (myometrium) lined by a vascular mucosa (endometrium), whose thickness varies with the phases of the menstrual cycle. The uterine cavity is narrow in sagittal section but triangular in coronal section, being widest where the uterine tubes enter (Figs 5.10 & 5.11). Tapering inferiorly, the cavity communicates via the internal os with the cervical canal.

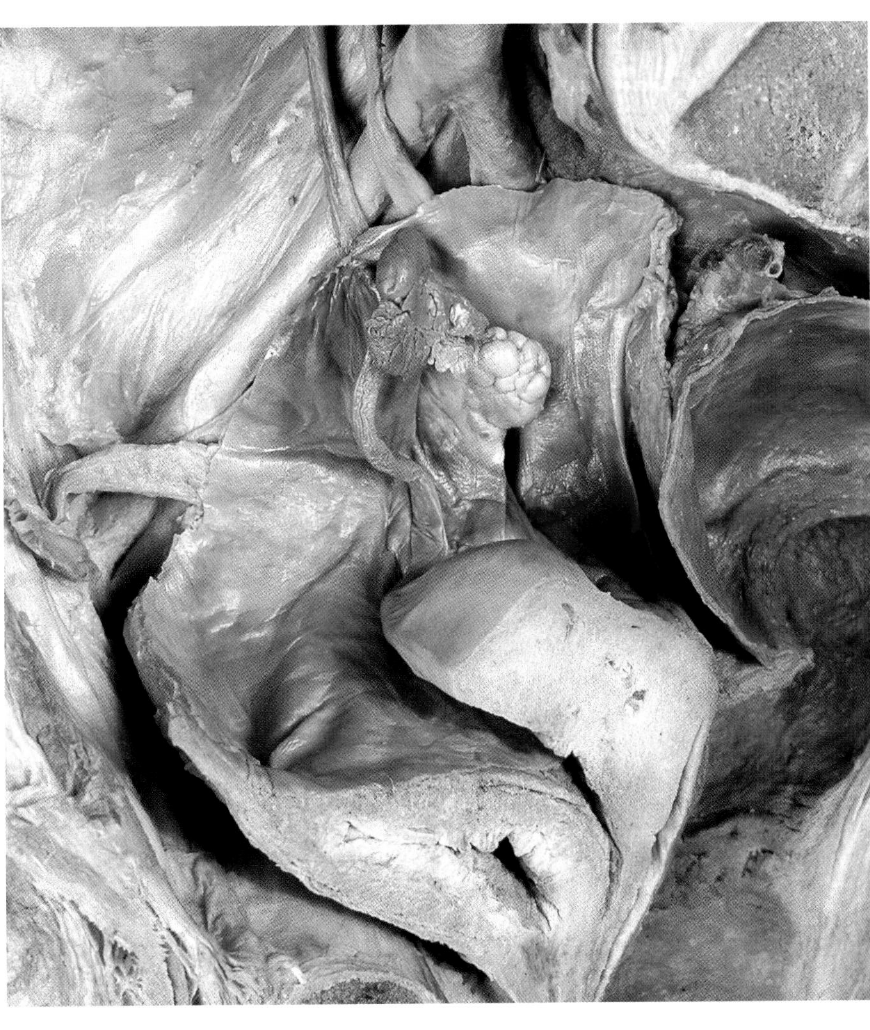

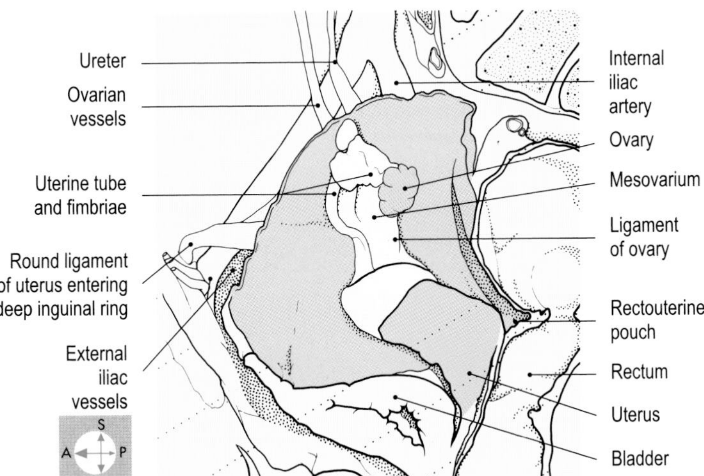

Fig. 5.8 Right ovary and broad ligament.

Cervix

The uterine cervix is thick walled and has a narrow lumen, the cervical canal (Figs 5.9 & 5.11). The canal communicates superiorly with the uterine cavity via the internal os and opens inferiorly into the vagina at the external os. The external os is circular before the first vaginal delivery but thereafter presents an oval aperture. Although approximately in line with the body of the uterus, the cervix lies roughly at right angles to the long axis of the vagina (a position called anteversion). Structures close to the cervix are vulnerable to the local spread of cervical carcinoma. Approximately half of the cervix lies above the vagina (the supravaginal part) and is covered posteriorly by peritoneum passing from the uterine body onto the vault of the vagina. The root of the broad ligament is attached to this part of the cervix and contains the uterine artery (see Fig. 5.13). The vessel runs medially above the ureter then turns upwards at the side of the cervix near the lateral fornix of the vagina. Anteriorly, the supravaginal part of the cervix is related to the posterior surface of the bladder. The lower half of the cervix protrudes through the anterior wall of the vagina, making it accessible for clinical examination.

The uterine body and cervix are supplied by branches of the uterine artery, a branch of the internal iliac artery. Venous blood passes into the uterine venous plexus, which drains into the internal iliac vein (see Fig. 5.13).

Uterine tubes

The paired uterine tubes, each approximately 10 cm long, run in the free upper borders of the broad ligaments (Figs 5.8, 5.10 & 5.11) and convey ova from the ovaries to the uterine cavity. Near the ovary the lumen of each tube communicates with the peritoneal cavity via its pelvic aperture. This opening leads into the funnel-shaped infundibulum, which bears a series of finger-like processes, the fimbriae, one of which attaches to the ovary. The infundibulum leads into the ampulla, which forms the comparatively wide lateral part of the uterine tube. The medial part of the tube, the isthmus, is narrower and continues through the uterine wall as the intramural part of the tube.

The blood supply to the medial part of the uterine tube is provided by terminal branches of the uterine artery. This vessel runs laterally in the upper part of the broad ligament and anastomoses with the ovarian artery, which supplies the lateral portion of the tube. Venous blood drains into veins that accompany the arteries.

Fertilization of ova normally occurs in the uterine tube, usually within its ampulla. Blockage of the tubes is a common cause of infertility.

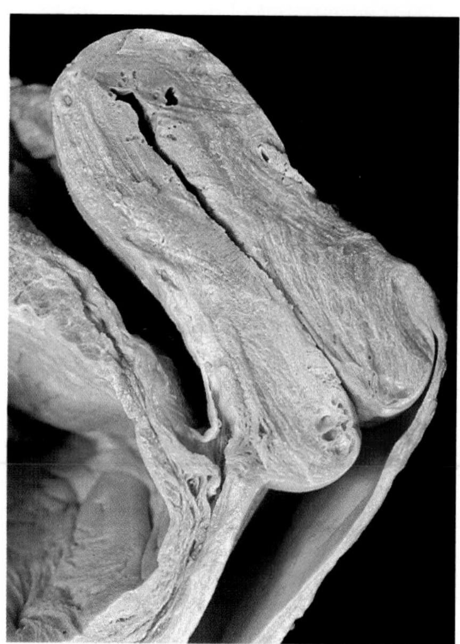

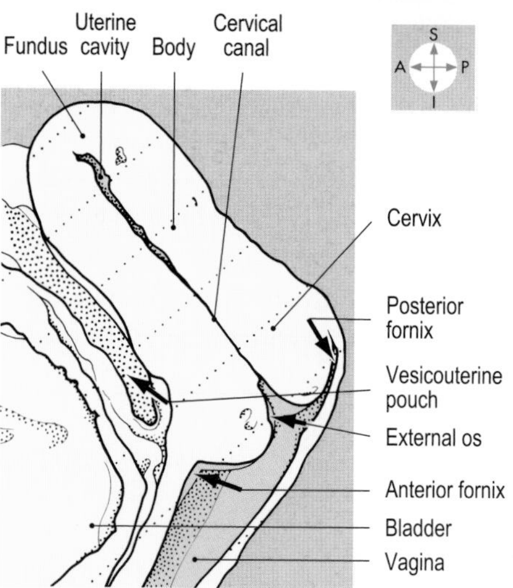

Fig. 5.9 Uterus and vagina in sagittal section.

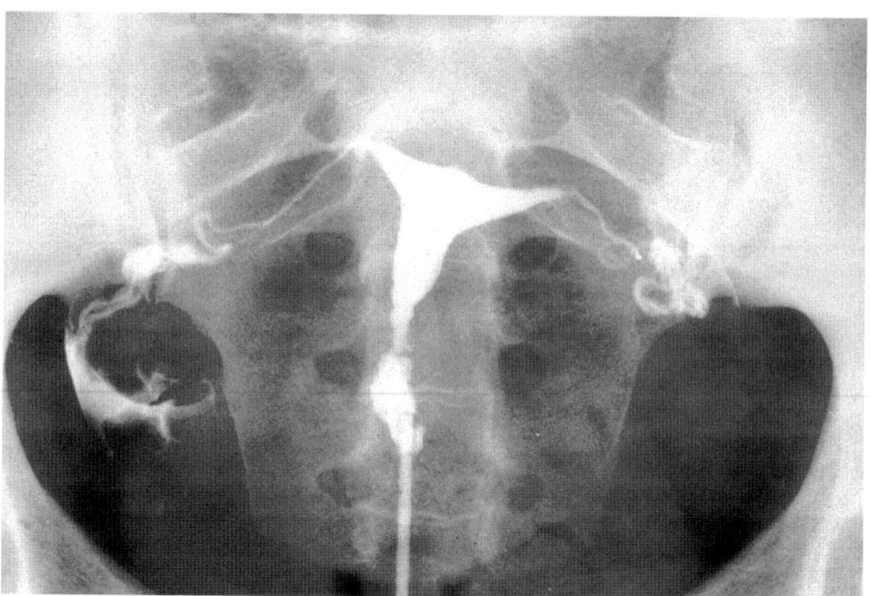

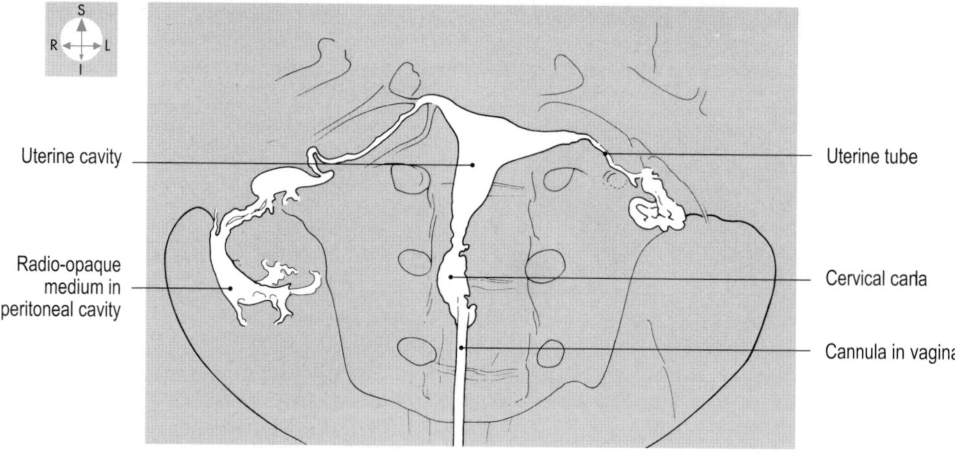

Fig. 5.10 Hysterosalpingogram. Radio-opaque medium has been injected, via a cannula in the vagina, into the uterus and along the uterine tubes.

Ovaries

The ovaries lie close to the lateral pelvic walls, suspended from the posterior surfaces of the broad ligaments (see Fig. 5.8). Each ovary is ovoid, approximately 4 cm long and 2 cm broad, with one pole directed medially towards the uterus and the other laterally towards the fimbriated end of the uterine tube. Each ovary is attached to the broad ligament by a sleeve of peritoneum, the mesovarium, which conveys the ovarian vessels. However, most of the ovarian surface is devoid of peritoneum. The ligament of the ovary attaches to the medial pole of the organ and runs within the broad ligament to reach the side of the uterine body. The ovary often lies in a hollow, the ovarian fossa, on the lateral pelvic wall between the external and internal iliac vessels. The ureter descends in the posterior boundary of the fossa while the obturator nerve and vessels cross its floor (Fig. 5.13; see Fig. 5.16). Therefore, ovarian disease that involves the parietal peritoneum at this site may produce pain referred via the nerve to the medial side of the thigh.

The ovary is supplied by the ovarian artery (Fig. 5.13), a direct branch of the abdominal aorta (see p. 191). After crossing the pelvic brim this vessel traverses the suspensory ligament of the ovary (infundibulopelvic ligament) to enter the broad ligament and divides into terminal branches within the mesovarium. The ovary is drained by numerous veins (the pampiniform plexus), which unite to form the ovarian vein. On the right the ovarian vein terminates in the inferior vena cava while the left ovarian vein usually joins the left renal vein (see p. 194).

Vagina

The vagina is a midline tubular organ approximately 8–10 cm long which slopes downwards and forwards (see Figs 5.8 & 5.9). Its upper two-thirds, including the blind-ending vault, lie in the pelvic cavity. The vagina pierces the pelvic floor and terminates inferiorly by opening into the vestibule between the labia minora (see p. 246). The anterior and posterior vaginal walls lie in mutual contact so that the lumen forms a transverse cleft. The lining possesses numerous transverse ridges (rugae; see Fig. 5.12).

The uterine cervix pierces the upper part of the anterior vaginal wall and an anular groove surrounds the intravaginal part of the cervix. This groove is deepest superiorly where it is termed the posterior fornix (see Fig. 5.9). On either side are the lateral fornices, whilst below the cervix is the comparatively shallow anterior fornix (see Fig. 5.12).

Anteriorly, the vagina is closely applied to the posterior wall of the bladder and urethra. Posteriorly lie the rectouterine pouch of peritoneum and the ampulla of the rectum (Fig. 5.13). Lateral to its inferior third are the medial borders of the levator ani muscles, which provide important support to the vagina and uterus. Weakness of the pelvic floor musculature may lead to prolapse (descent of the uterus into the vagina).

The blood supply to the vagina is provided by branches of the uterine arteries and occasionally by vessels arising directly from the internal iliac arteries (see Fig. 5.32). Venous blood passes into an exten-sive venous plexus surrounding the upper vagina and eventually reaches the internal iliac veins.

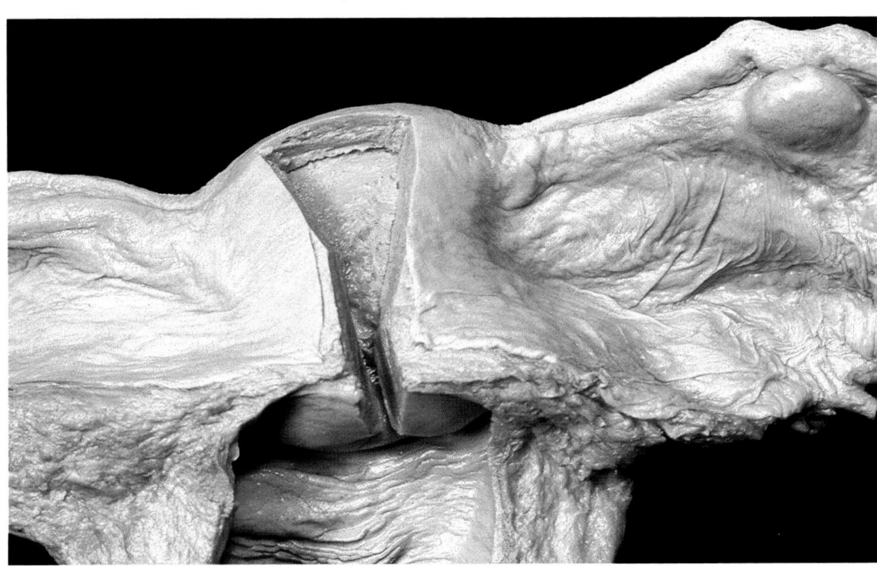

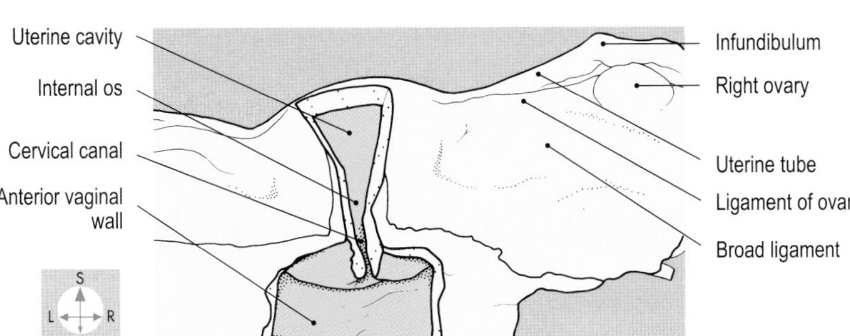

Fig. 5.11 Posterior aspect of uterus and broad ligaments. The uterine cavity, cervical canal and vagina have been exposed by removal of parts of their posterior walls.

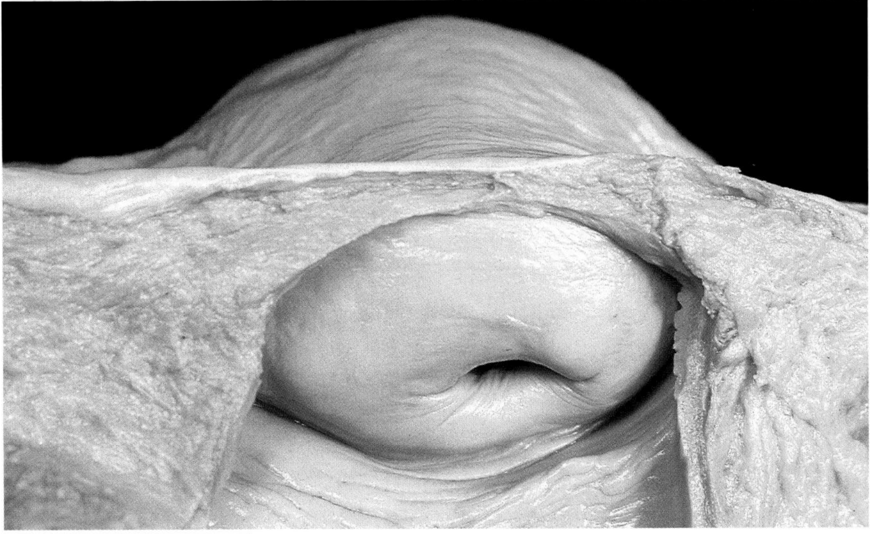

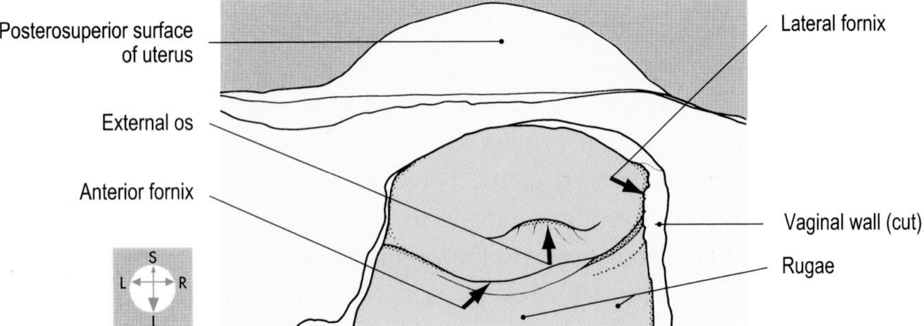

Fig. 5.12 Intravaginal part of the cervix revealed by removal of the posterior wall of the vagina.

Pelvic Ureters

Each ureter enters the pelvis by crossing in front of the common iliac vessels or the commencement of the external iliac vessels (Fig. 5.14). The ureter passes downwards and backwards before curving forwards to reach the posterior surface of the bladder. The ureter crosses the medial aspect of the obturator nerve and vessels and the superior vesical vessels before running forwards along the levator ani muscle. The pelvic peritoneum covers the medial aspect of the ureter and separates it from the rectum, sigmoid colon or coils of ileum.

In the male the ureter passes under the ductus deferens and terminates near the seminal vesicle (Fig. 5.15). In the female the ureter descends close to the posterior aspect of the ovary (Fig. 5.13) and is covered with peritoneum as far as the root of the broad ligament. Here the ureter crosses under the uterine artery and is closely related to the lateral aspect of the uterine cervix.

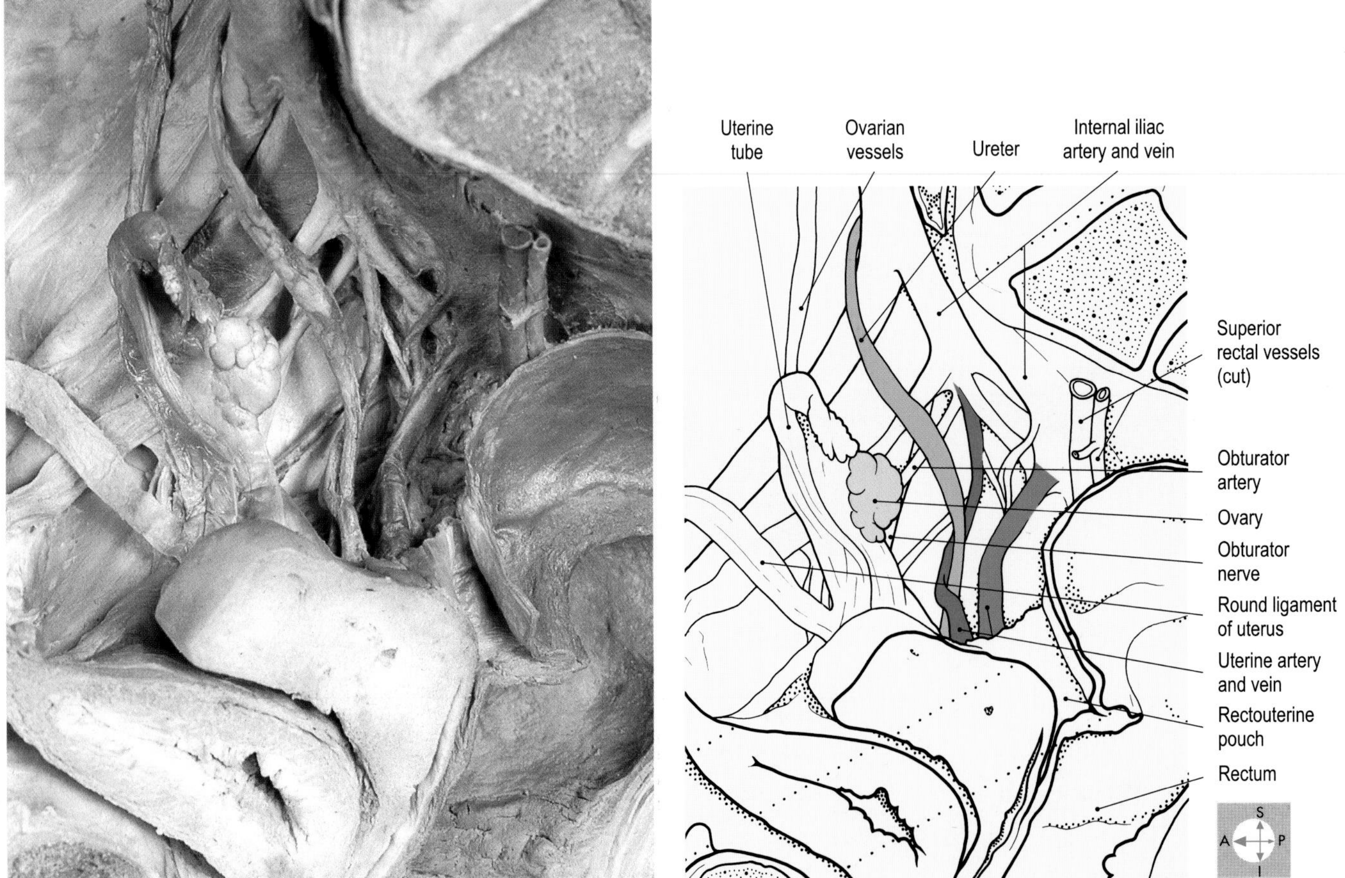

Fig. 5.13 Uterine vessels and the ureter after removal of peritoneum from the lateral pelvic wall.

Bladder

The urinary bladder lies in the anterior part of the pelvic cavity. When distended, the organ has an approximately spherical shape but when empty it assumes the form of a tetrahedron with four angles and four surfaces. The two posterolateral angles receive the ureters while the inferior angle, the bladder neck, is continuous with the urethra. The anterior angle gives attachment to a fibrous cord, the median umbilical ligament (Fig. 5.17). This remnant of the fetal allantois ascends in the extraperitoneal tissues of the anterior abdominal wall to the umbilicus.

The superior surface and the two inferolateral surfaces expand considerably as urine accumulates but the comparatively small posterior surface or base remains relatively fixed. This surface lies between the entrances of the ureters and the bladder neck.

The wall of the bladder consists of smooth muscle (detrusor) whose thickness gradually decreases as the organ fills. Although the interior of the distended bladder is smooth, the mucosa becomes rugose when the organ empties (Fig. 5.17), except in the region of the trigone. This is the triangular area between the ureteric orifices and the internal urethral meatus (see Fig. 5.14). The ureters pierce the musculature of the bladder wall obliquely and open at slit-like orifices.

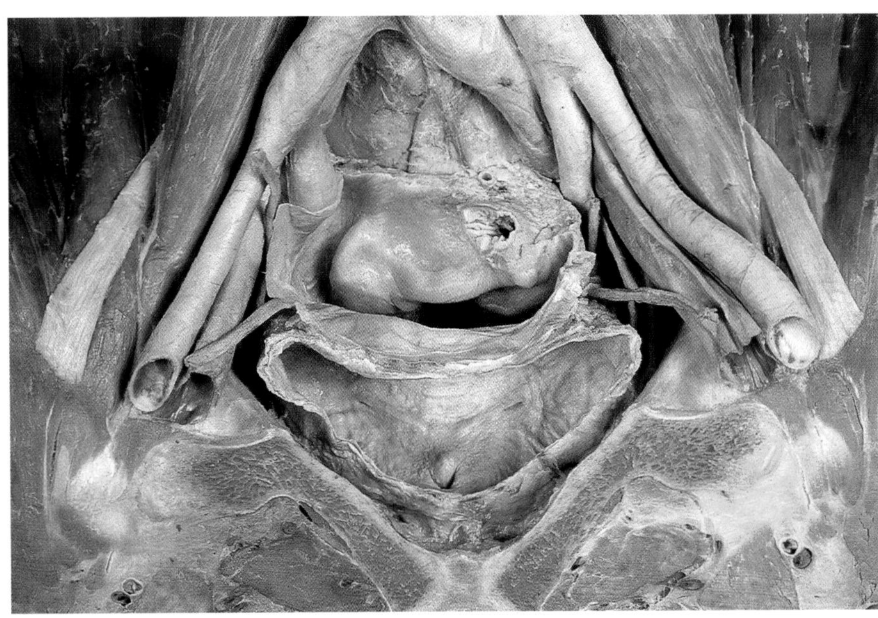

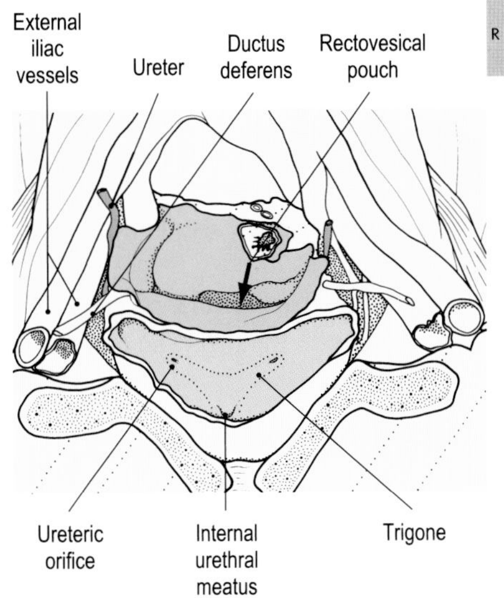

Fig. 5.14 Coronal section through the male pelvis to show the interior of the bladder and some of its relations.

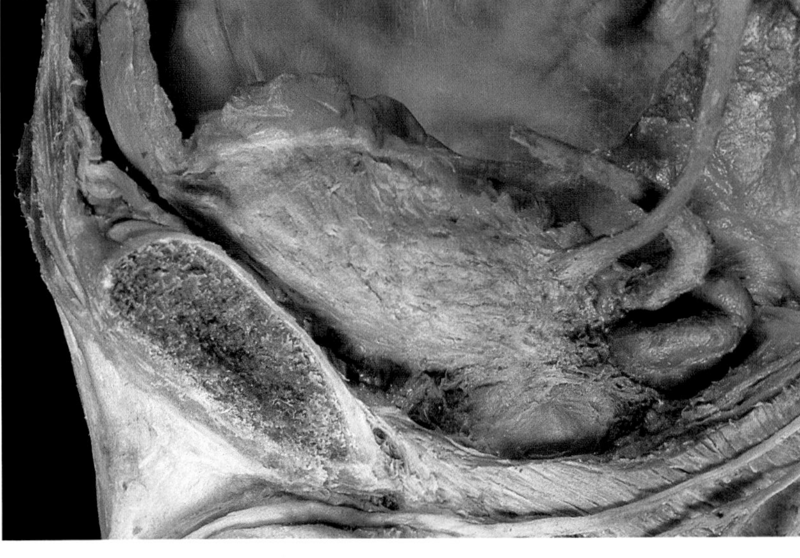

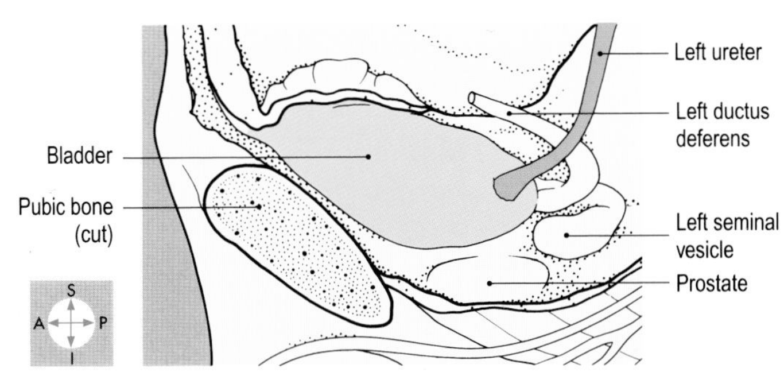

Fig. 5.15 Lateral view of the male bladder after removal of the left pelvic wall.

Relations

The superior surface of the bladder is covered with peritoneum (Fig. 5.17) on which rest coils of ileum and sigmoid colon. In both sexes the inferolateral surfaces lie against the obturator internus and levator ani muscles and their associated fascial coverings. Between the bladder and these muscles run the obturator nerve and vessels and the superior vesical vessels (Fig. 5.16). Anterior to the bladder is the retropubic space, filled with adipose tissue and veins (Fig. 5.17). The empty bladder lies behind the pubic bones but as it fills it rises above the level of the pubic crests and comes into contact with the lower part of the anterior abdominal wall. The distended bladder intervenes between the parietal peritoneum and the abdominal wall (see Fig. 4.29); surgical access to the organ can be made through an abdominal incision without opening the peritoneum.

In the male the seminal vesicle and the ampulla of the ductus deferens are applied to each side of the posterior surface. Peritoneum descends a short distance on this surface before being reflected onto the anterior surface of the rectum to form the rectovesical pouch (see Fig. 5.14). Below the level of this pouch the bladder is related to the rectovesical septum and the ampulla of the rectum. Inferior to the male bladder lie the prostate and the prostatic plexus of veins.

In the female the posterior part of the superior surface of the bladder is related to the body of the uterus (Fig. 5.17). Peritoneum passes from the superior surface of the bladder onto the uterine body, forming the vesicouterine pouch. Against the posterior surface of the female bladder lie the cervix of the uterus and the anterior wall of the vagina. The inferior angle of the bladder in the female lies at a lower level than in the male and is closely related to the two levator ani muscles.

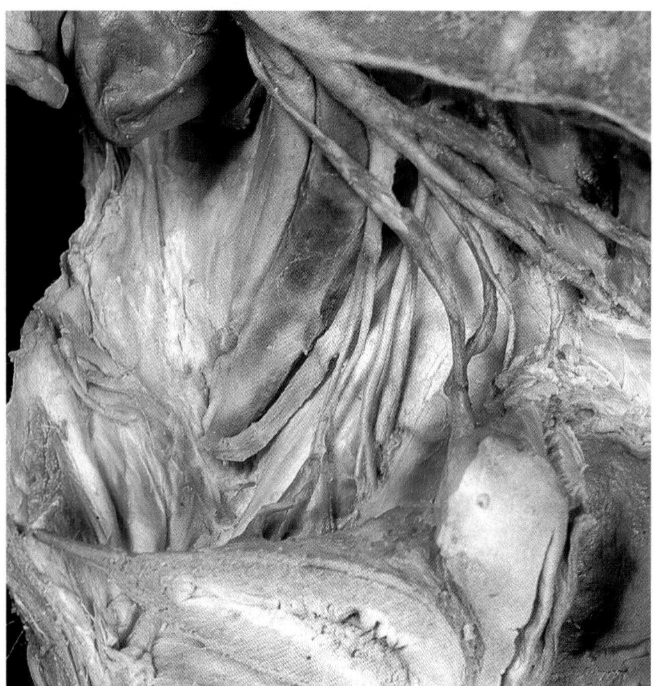

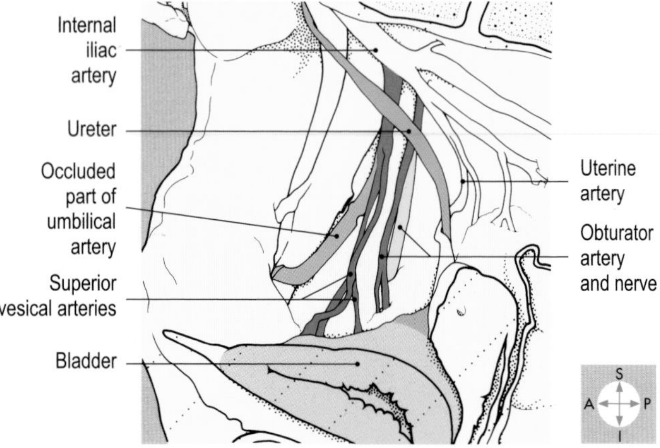

Fig. 5.16 Arterial supply and relations of the bladder in a female pelvis.

Blood supply

The bladder is supplied by branches of the internal iliac arteries. On each side, the patent part of the umbilical artery gives off one or more superior vesical arteries (Fig. 5.16). The bladder receives additional supply from the inferior vesical and obturator arteries. In the female the uterine and vaginal arteries also contribute to the vascular supply of the bladder.

Venous blood passes into an extensive network of veins, the vesical plexus, which communicates with the prostatic or vaginal plexus and drains into the internal iliac veins.

Nerve supply

The motor innervation to the detrusor muscle is by parasympathetic nerves conveyed in the pelvic splanchnic nerves and the pelvic plexus of autonomic nerves (see Fig. 5.30). In the male the smooth muscle surrounding the bladder neck (preprostatic sphincter) is innervated by sympathetic nerves derived from the hypogastric plexus. The parasympathetic motor innervation stimulates contraction of the bladder at the time of micturition, while the sympathetic supply to the male bladder neck prevents reflux ejaculation.

Female Urethra

The female urethra is a fibromuscular tube 3–4 cm long and begins at the internal urethral meatus of the bladder. Embedded in the anterior wall of the vagina, it inclines downwards and forwards through the pelvic floor (Fig. 5.18) and terminates in the vestibule at the external meatus between the clitoris and the vaginal opening.

The urethra passes close to the posterior aspect of the pubic symphysis (Fig. 5.17), to which it is attached by the pubourethral ligaments. The middle third of the urethra is encircled by striated muscle fibres of the external urethral sphincter, whose tone is the principal factor in maintaining continence of urine. Occlusive force on the urethra is also provided by contractions of the levator ani muscles (Fig. 5.18). Micturition occurs when bladder pressure is higher than urethral pressure and is produced by contraction of the detrusor muscle of the bladder wall accompanied by relaxation of the external urethral sphincter.

The arterial supply to the urethra is provided by the inferior vesical arteries, and venous drainage is to the vesical plexus of veins. The mucosa receives its sensory nerve supply from the pudendal nerve, derived from the second, third and fourth sacral segments, which also innervate the external urethral sphincter.

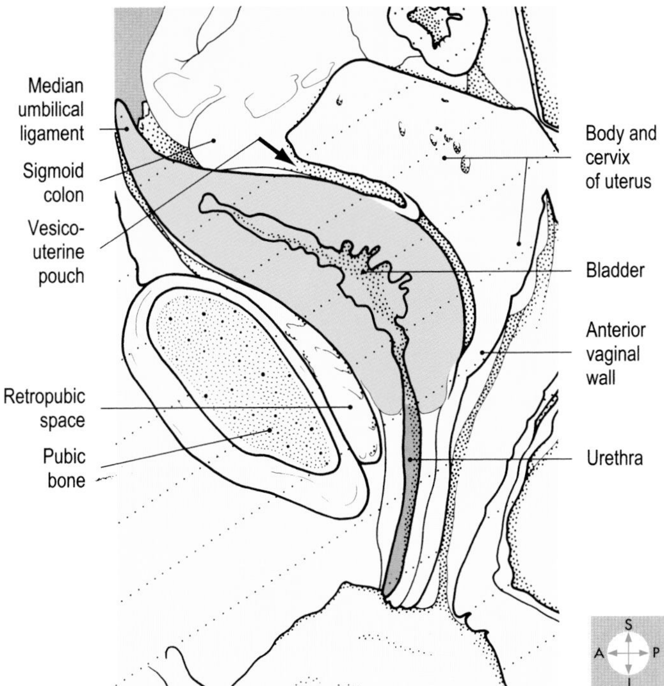

Fig. 5.17 Median sagittal section through the female pelvis to show the bladder and some of its relations.

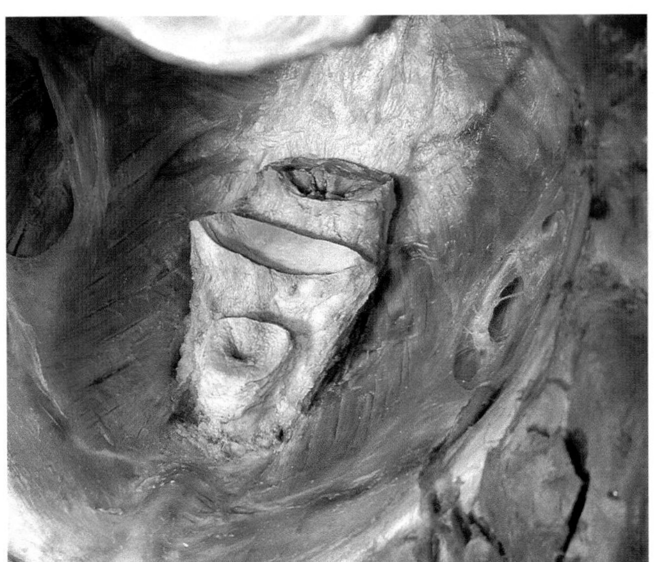

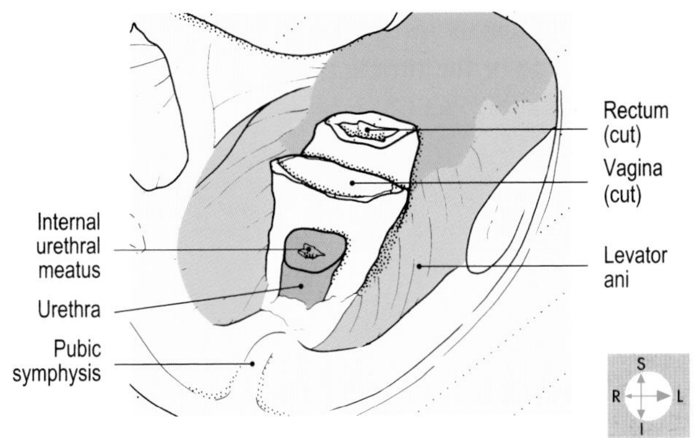

Fig. 5.18 Female urethra and its relationship to the vagina and the levator ani muscles.

Male Urethra

The male urethra is a fibromuscular tube approximately 20 cm long. Beginning at the internal urethral meatus of the bladder, it descends through the prostate and the pelvic floor and enters the bulb of the penis (Fig. 5.19). It then traverses the corpus spongiosum and glans of the penis and terminates at the external urethral meatus. In the male the urethra not only drains urine from the bladder but also receives secretions from the prostatic ducts, the ejaculatory ducts and the ducts of the bulbourethral glands.

The male urethra is described in three parts: prostatic, intermediate (membranous) and spongy. The prostatic and intermediate parts pass downwards while the spongy part turns forwards in the bulb of the penis (Fig. 5.19). This abrupt angulation is of considerable importance when catheters or cystoscopes are being introduced. Furthermore, although the spongy and prostatic parts can be readily dilated, the external meatus and the intermediate urethra are comparatively narrow.

Prostatic urethra

Passing downwards through the prostate, the prostatic urethra is approximately 3 cm long. A midline ridge, the urethral crest, projects from the posterior wall, producing bilateral grooves, the prostatic sinuses (Fig. 5.20). Opening into each sinus are numerous prostatic ducts. The urethral crest is most prominent near its midpoint, where it presents a rounded elevation, the seminal colliculus. A midline orifice on the colliculus leads into a blind-ending sac, the prostatic utricle, which is a remnant of the ducts that give rise to the uterus in the female embryo. On each side of the utricle is the opening of the ejaculatory duct.

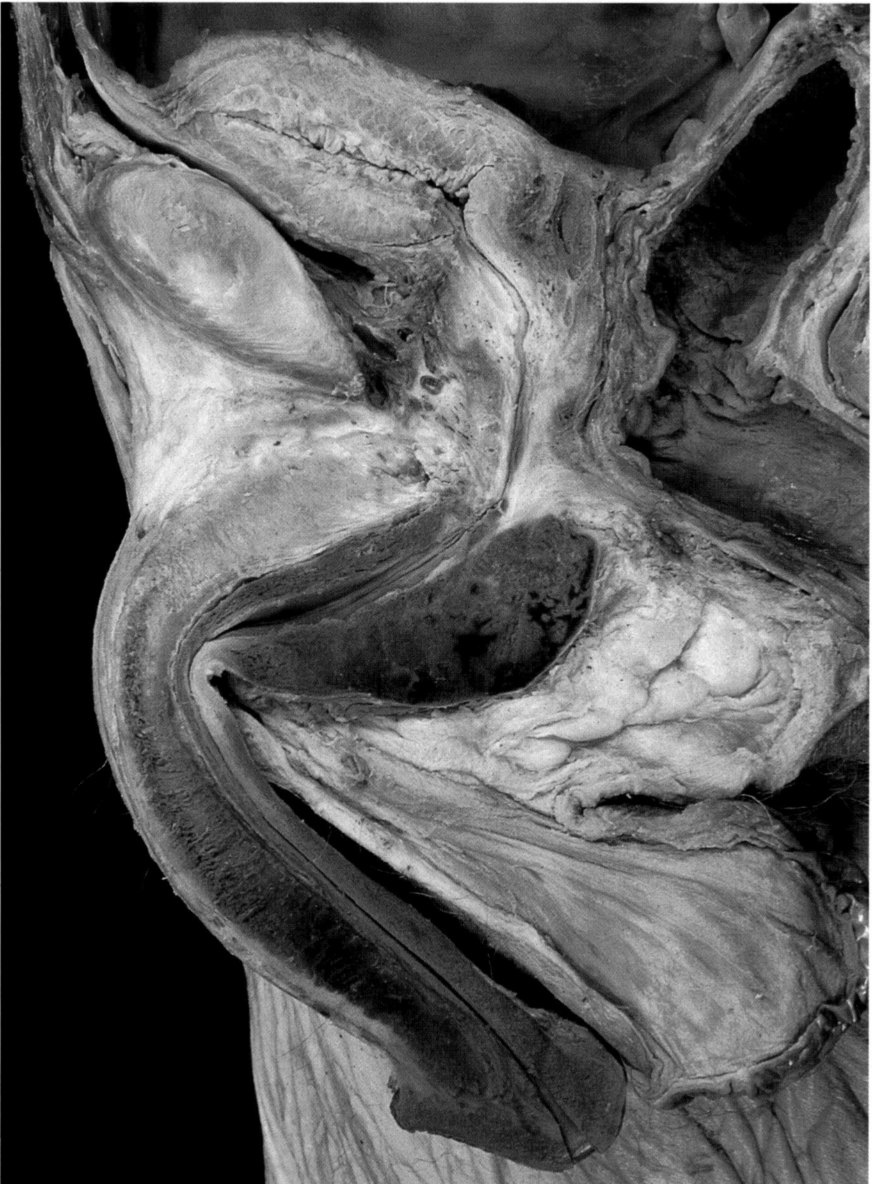

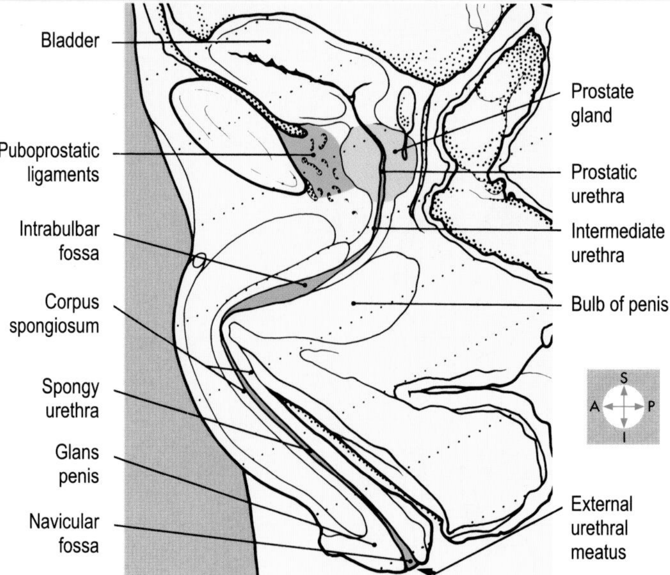

Fig. 5.19 Male urethra in sagittal section.

Intermediate (membranous) urethra

Emerging from the anterior aspect of the apex of the prostate, the intermediate urethra descends through the pelvic floor and pierces the perineal membrane. It is approximately 2 cm long and its mucosa is folded, giving the lumen a stellate appearance on cross-section. Encircling the intermediate urethra is the striated muscle of the external urethral sphincter (Fig. 5.21), the main structure responsible for urinary continence. Lateral to the sphincter are the medial borders of the levatores ani.

Posterolateral to the intermediate urethra are the paired bulbourethral glands, each about 1 cm in diameter (Fig. 5.21). Their ducts pierce the perineal membrane and open into the spongy urethra. An additional posterior relation of the intermediate urethra is the ampulla of the rectum, while anteriorly lies the lower border of the pubic symphysis, to which the urethra is anchored by the pubourethral ligaments.

Spongy (penile) urethra

The spongy urethra is approximately 15 cm in length, commencing in the bulb of the penis and traversing the erectile tissue of the corpus spongiosum and glans (Fig. 5.19). The mucosa presents numerous small recesses or lacunae and most of its lumen forms a transverse slit. Within the bulb the urethra is wider, forming the intrabulbar fossa. The lumen is also expanded within the glans to form the navicular fossa, which opens at the surface as a vertical slit, the external meatus.

Blood supply

The prostatic and intermediate parts of the urethra receive blood from the inferior vesical arteries. The spongy part is supplied by the internal pudendal artery via the dorsal arteries of the penis and the arteries to the bulb. Venous blood passes into the prostatic venous plexus and the internal pudendal veins.

Nerve supply

The principal sensory innervation of the mucosa is provided by the pudendal (S2, S3 & S4) nerve, a branch of the sacral plexus. The same spinal cord segments innervate the external sphincter.

Male Internal Organs of Reproduction

The organs of reproduction in the male comprise the paired testes, epididymides, ductus (vasa) deferentia, seminal vesicles, ejaculatory ducts and bulbourethral glands as well as the prostate and penis. The superficial organs (the external genitalia) include the penis (see p. 245), and the testes and epididymides within the scrotum (see pp 149, 151).

The reproductive organs described here are those that lie within the pelvis, namely the prostate, the seminal vesicles, the intrapelvic parts of the ductus deferentia (Fig. 5.22) and the ejaculatory ducts.

Prostate

The prostate is an approximately spherical organ lying immediately below the bladder (Fig. 5.23). The flattened superior surface (base) is applied to the neck of the bladder and is pierced by the urethra, which descends through the gland and emerges near the blunt apex. The part of the prostate behind the urethra and above and between the ejaculatory ducts (see below) is sometimes described as the median lobe (Fig. 5.24).

Anteriorly, the prostate is anchored by the puboprostatic ligaments (see Fig. 5.19) to the inferior border of the pubic symphysis. Inferior to the organ lies the intermediate urethra (Fig. 5.23) surrounded by the external urethral sphincter, and posteriorly are the rectovesical septum and the ampulla of the rectum. On each side of the prostate is the medial border of levator ani.

With advancing age the gland often enlarges (benign prostatic hypertrophy) and may obstruct the prostatic part of the urethra, thus interfering with micturition.

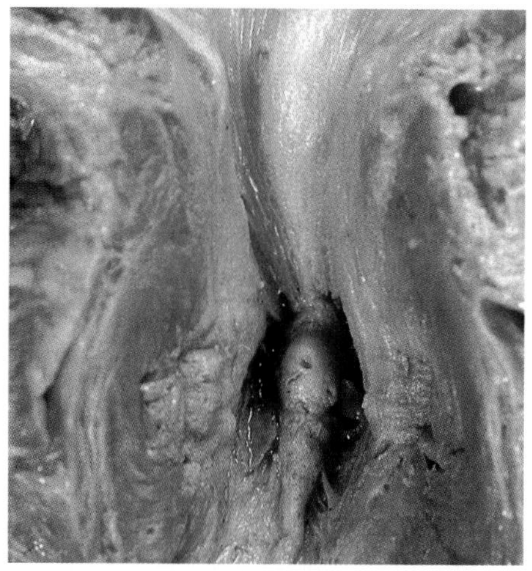

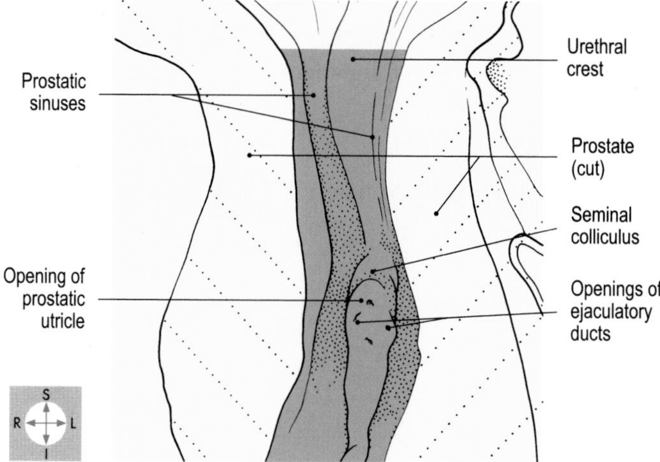

Fig. 5.20 Prostatic urethra opened through its anterior wall to show the urethral crest and seminal colliculus.

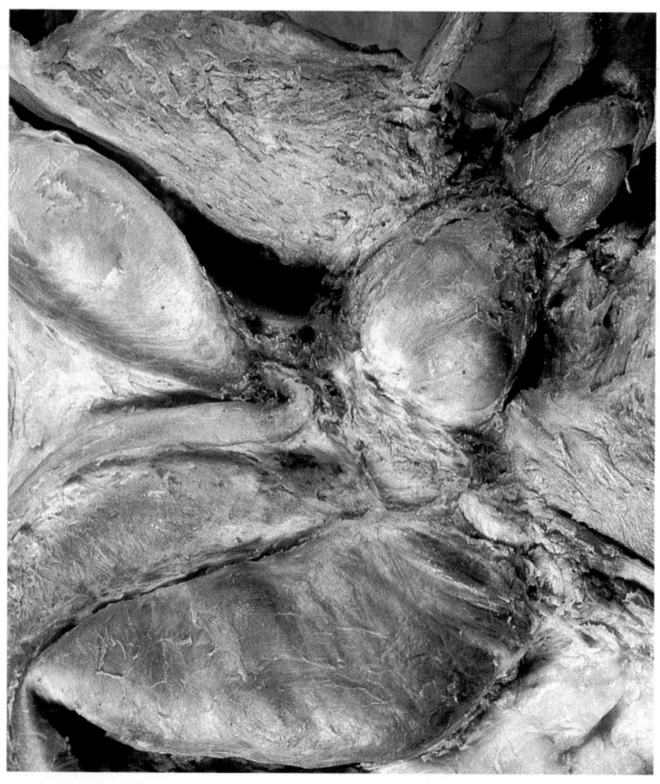

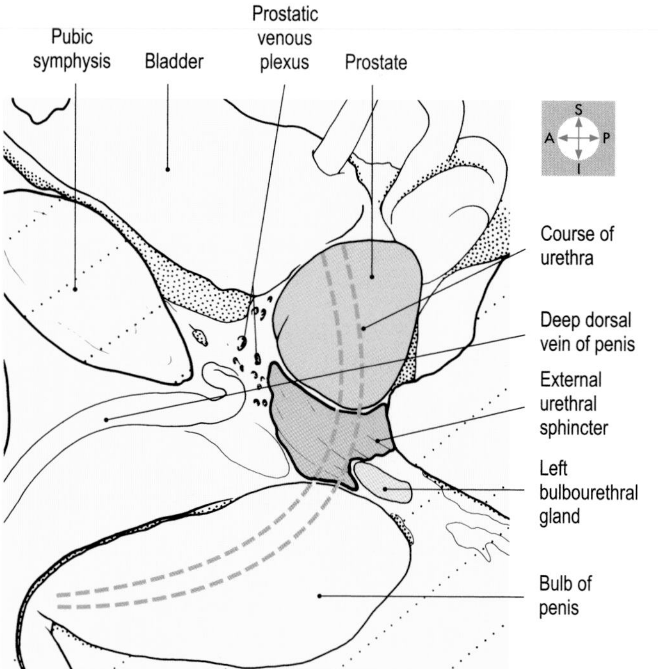

Fig. 5.21 The left pelvic wall and levator ani have been removed to show the prostate gland, external urethral sphincter, left bulbourethral gland and bulb of the penis.

Seminal vesicle

Each seminal vesicle is a sacculated gland approximately 3 cm long, lying lateral to the ampulla of the ductus deferens (Figs 5.24 & 5.25). The seminal vesicles lie in front of the rectum and rectovesical pouch of peritoneum (Fig. 5.23) and extend up the posterior wall of the bladder as far as the terminal parts of the ureters (Fig. 5.25).

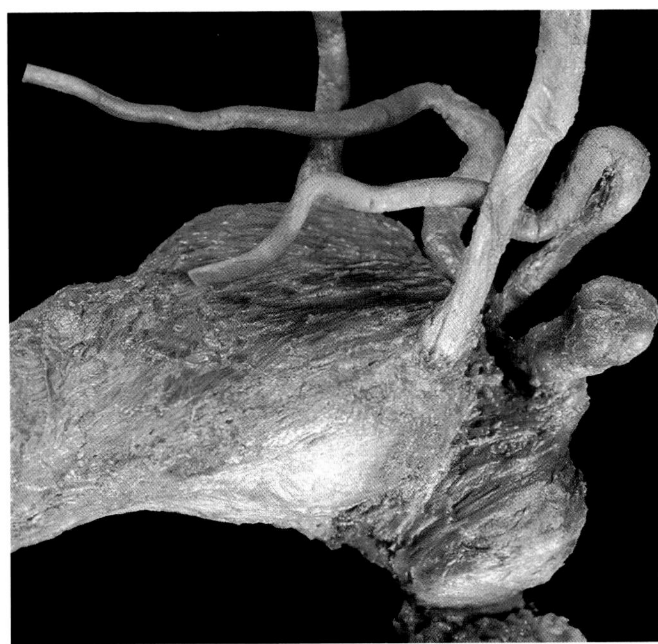

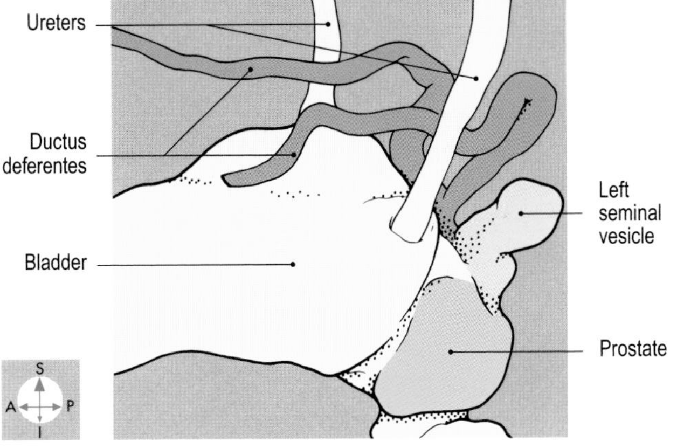

Fig. 5.22 Lateral view of the prostate, left seminal vesicle and both ductus deferentes.

Ductus (vas) deferens

Each ductus (vas) deferens begins at the tail of the epididymis in the scrotum, ascends within the spermatic cord and traverses the inguinal canal (see pp 146–151). After emerging from the deep inguinal ring, the ductus runs along the lateral pelvic wall, covered by peritoneum, and passes medial to the superior vesical vessels and obturator nerve and vessels. The ductus then crosses above the ureter (Fig. 5.25) and turns downwards and medially, posterior to the bladder (Fig. 5.23). The terminal part of the ductus is dilated to form the ampulla, which lies medial to the seminal vesicle. The ampulla is related posteriorly to the peritoneum of the rectovesical pouch and to the rectovesical septum and rectum.

Bulbourethral gland

The bulbourethral glands lie adjacent to the intermediate urethra and are described on page 227.

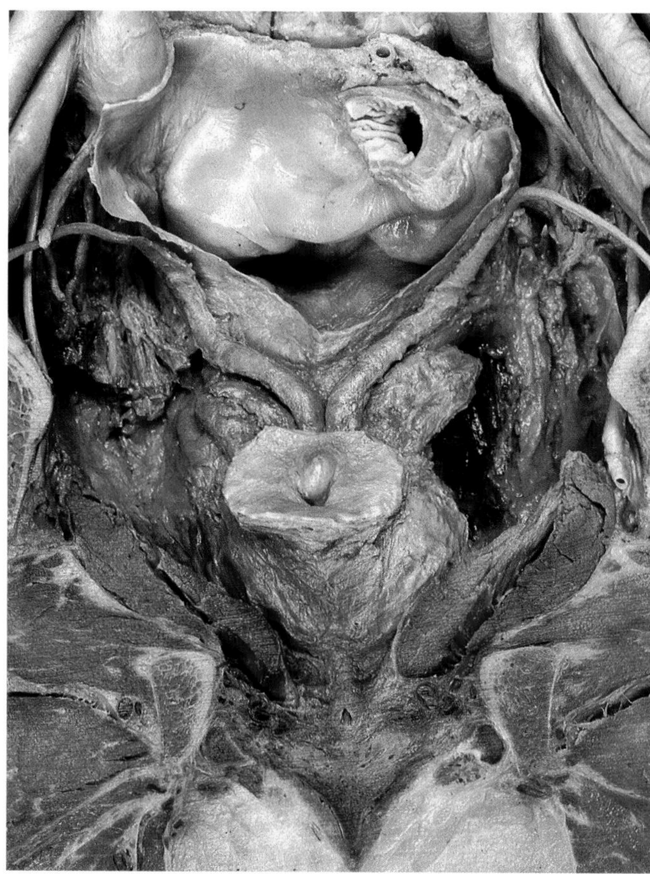

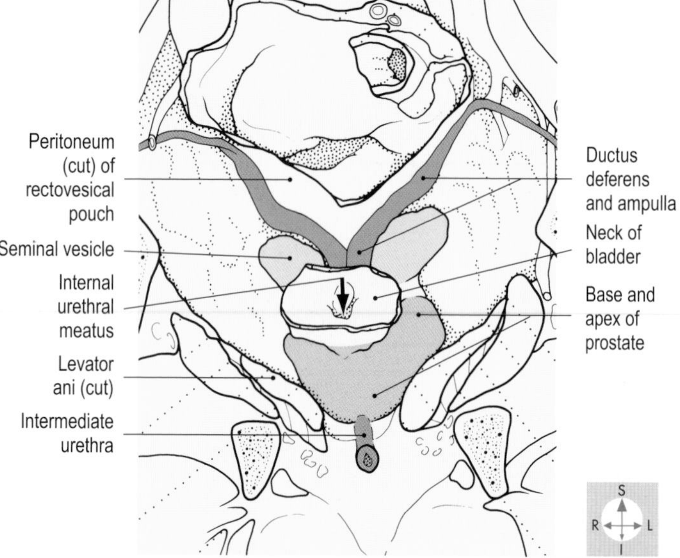

Fig. 5.23 Coronal section of the pelvic walls and floor. Most of the bladder has been removed to reveal the prostate, the seminal vesicles and both ductus deferentes.

Ejaculatory duct

The duct of each seminal vesicle joins the ampulla of the corresponding ductus deferens to form the ejaculatory duct (Fig. 5.24). The right and left ducts pierce the prostate and run downwards, forwards and medially through its substance to open into the prostatic urethra at slit-like orifices on the summit of the seminal colliculus.

Blood supply

The artery to the ductus deferens is usually a small vessel which arises from the superior vesical artery and accompanies the ductus as far as the epididymis. The ampulla of the ductus, the seminal vesicle and prostate are supplied by the inferior vesical artery. From the internal reproductive organs, blood passes into the venous plexus (see Fig. 5.21) surrounding the prostate to drain into the internal iliac veins.

Ejaculation

Semen contains spermatozoa from the testes and secretions from the ampullae of the ductus, the seminal vesicles and prostate. Under the control of the sympathetic nervous system, contraction of smooth muscle in the ductus, seminal vesicles and prostate propels secretions into the prostatic urethra. Semen is then expelled from the urethra by contractions of the bulbospongiosus muscles, which compress the bulb of the penis (see p. 245). Reflux of semen into the bladder is prevented by contraction of the smooth muscle in the wall of the bladder neck, the 'preprostatic sphincter'.

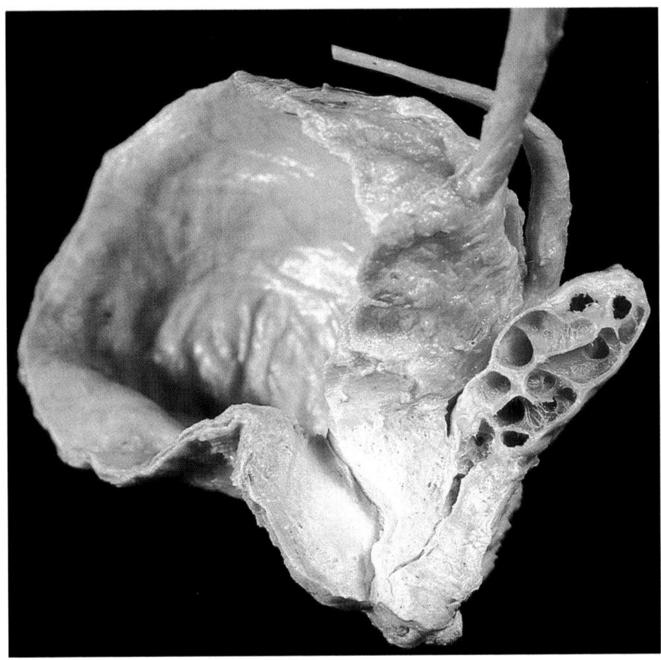

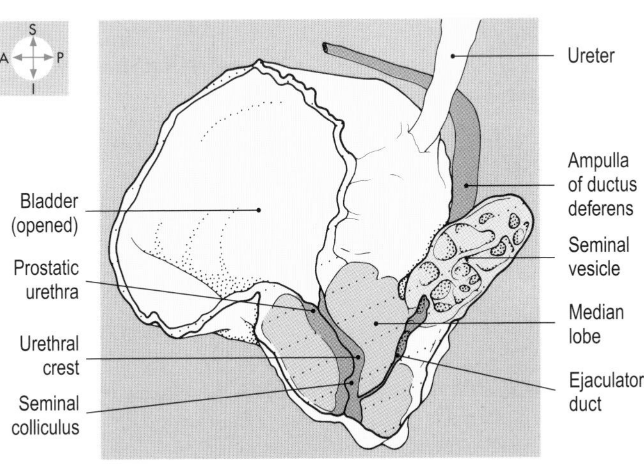

Fig. 5.24 Dissection of prostate and left seminal vesicle.

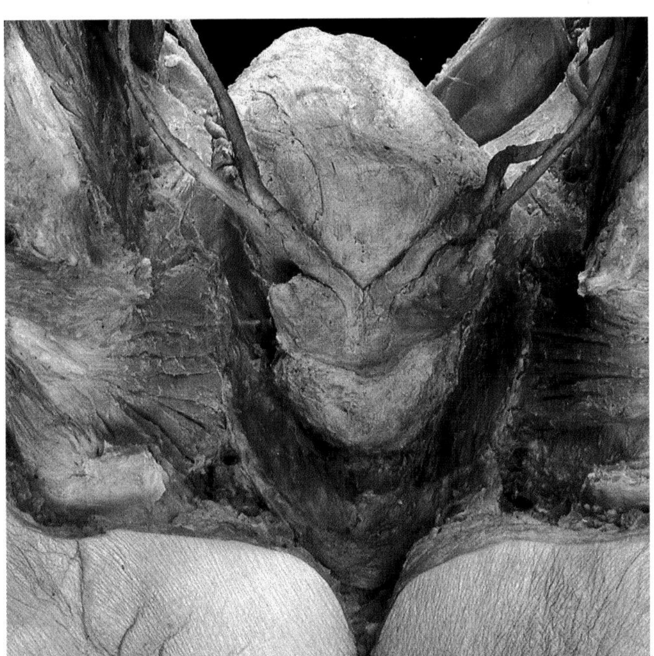

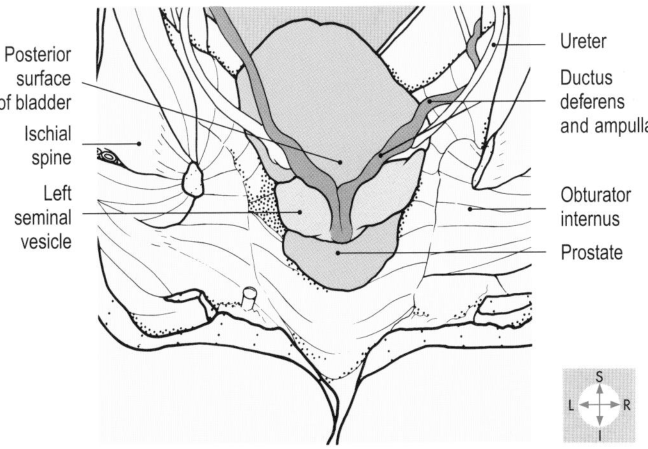

Fig. 5.25 Removal of the rectum and the posterior wall of the pelvis exposes the bladder, prostate, seminal vesicles and ductus deferentes.

Pelvic Wall and Floor

The pelvic wall is formed by the bones of the pelvic girdle and their associated ligaments, muscles and fascia. The bony component comprises the right and left hip bones anterolaterally and the sacrum and coccyx posteriorly. The pelvic cavity is usually wider and shallower in females because of the differences in the shapes of the surrounding bones.

Hip bone

Only the medial or pelvic surface of the hip bone is considered here; the external surface is described on page 269. Each hip bone is formed by the fusion of three components: ilium, ischium and pubis (Figs 5.26 & 5.27). The anterosuperior part of the ilium contributes to the abdominal wall and gives attachment to iliacus. The lower portion of the ilium extends below the pelvic inlet and contributes to the lateral wall of the pelvis. On the posterior part of the bone is the auricular surface, which articulates with the corresponding surface of the sacrum at the sacroiliac joint.

The ischium has a rounded tuberosity inferiorly, which bears body weight in the sitting position. Posteriorly is the pointed spine, which separates the greater and lesser sciatic notches, while anteriorly the ramus of the ischium ascends to fuse with the inferior pubic ramus.

The pubic bone has an iliopubic ramus that merges with the ilium near the iliopubic eminence, and an inferior ramus which is continuous below the obturator foramen with the ramus of the ischium. The bodies of the right and left pubic bones articulate at the pubic symphysis.

The obturator foramen is a large aperture which is almost completely occluded by the obturator membrane (Fig. 5.27). Superiorly the membrane leaves a small gap, the obturator canal, which provides access between the pelvis and the medial compartment of the thigh.

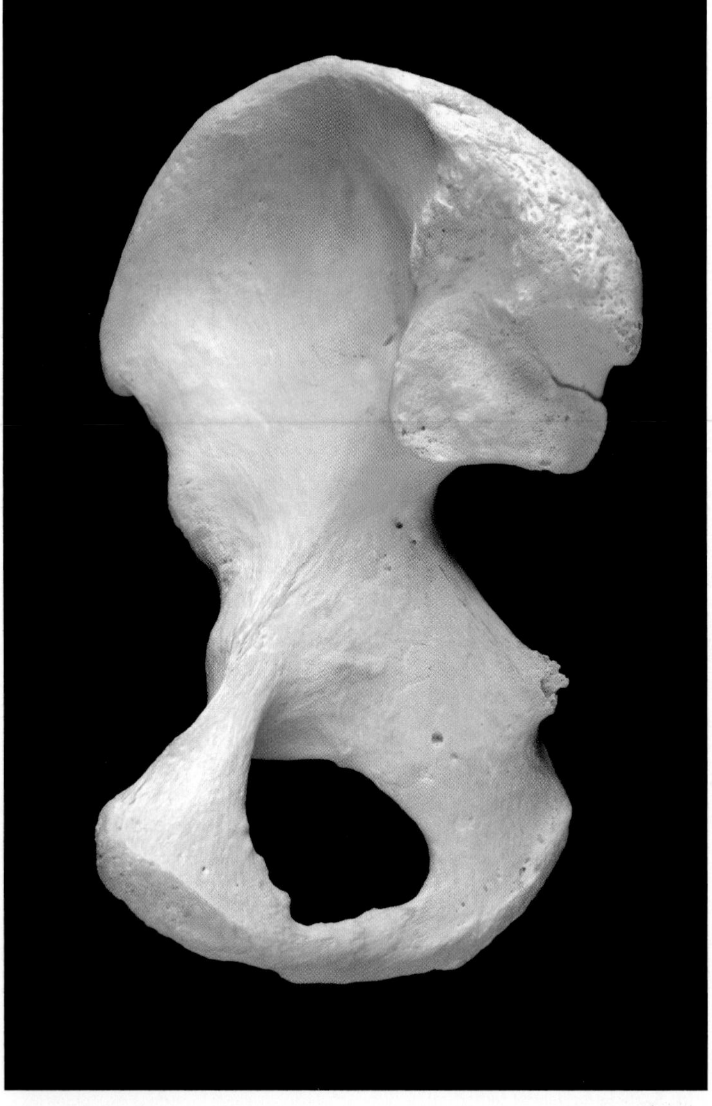

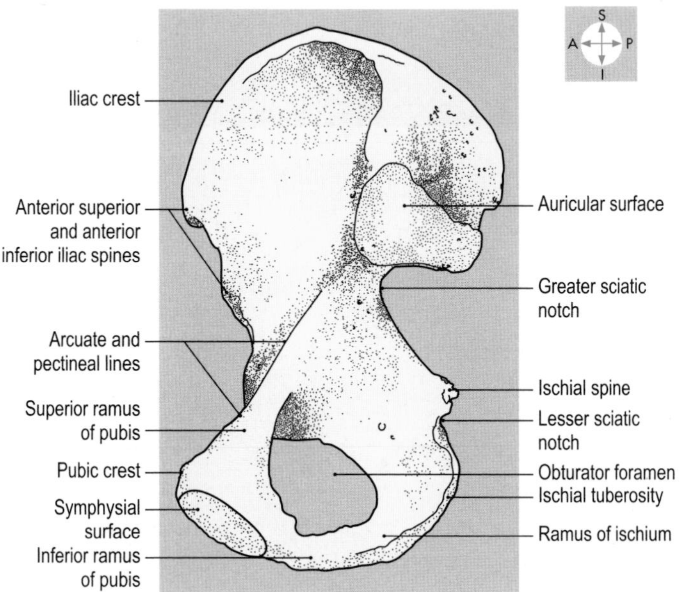

Fig. 5.26 Medial surface of right hip bone.

Pelvic floor

The pelvic floor (or diaphragm) is a muscular partition separating the cavity of the pelvis above from the perineum below. It slopes downwards towards the midline, forming a trough that inclines downwards and forwards (Figs 5.28 & 5.29). In the midline anteriorly, a narrow triangular gap, the urogenital hiatus, between the muscle fibres transmits the urethra in both sexes and the vagina in the female (see Figs 5.1 & 5.18). Posteriorly, the pelvic floor is pierced by the anal canal.

The pelvic floor is formed principally by the right and left levator ani muscles, which are supplemented posteriorly by the coccygeus muscles (Fig. 5.29). The coccygeus muscle is applied to the medial surface of the sacrospinous ligament. Medially, it attaches to the lateral border of the sacrum and coccyx, and laterally to the ischial spine.

Each levator ani muscle has a linear attachment to the pelvic wall. The attachment commences anteriorly on the pelvic surface of the body of the pubis and continues backwards as the tendinous arch along the obturator fascia as far as the ischial spine (Fig. 5.29). The levator ani muscle has two parts; the anterior part comprises pubococcygeus and the posterior part is iliococcygeus.

Pubococcygeus runs backwards and downwards. Its most anterior fibres lie near the midline and pass close to the urethra. In the male they support the prostate (see Fig. 5.23); in the female they attach to the vagina (see Fig. 5.18). The intermediate fibres of pubococcygeus, puborectalis, reach the anal canal and either attach to its wall or loop behind the anorectal junction. The posterior fibres attach to the coccyx or fuse in the midline with fibres from the other side at the anococcygeal raphe.

The fibres of iliococcygeus pass downwards and medially below those of pubococcygeus and attach to the coccyx and to the anococcygeal raphe.

The levator ani muscles support the pelvic contents, actively maintaining the positions of the pelvic viscera. In particular, the pubococcygeus muscles compress the urethra and vagina and provide support for the bladder and uterus. The levator ani fibres that loop behind the anal canal help to maintain the angulation of the anorectal junction and play an important role in the continence of faeces. During defecation, the fibres attaching to the wall of the anal canal pull the organ upwards. Levator ani and coccygeus are innervated by the fourth sacral nerve. Weakening of these muscles, a common gynaecological problem, may result in the descent (prolapse) of the pelvic organs.

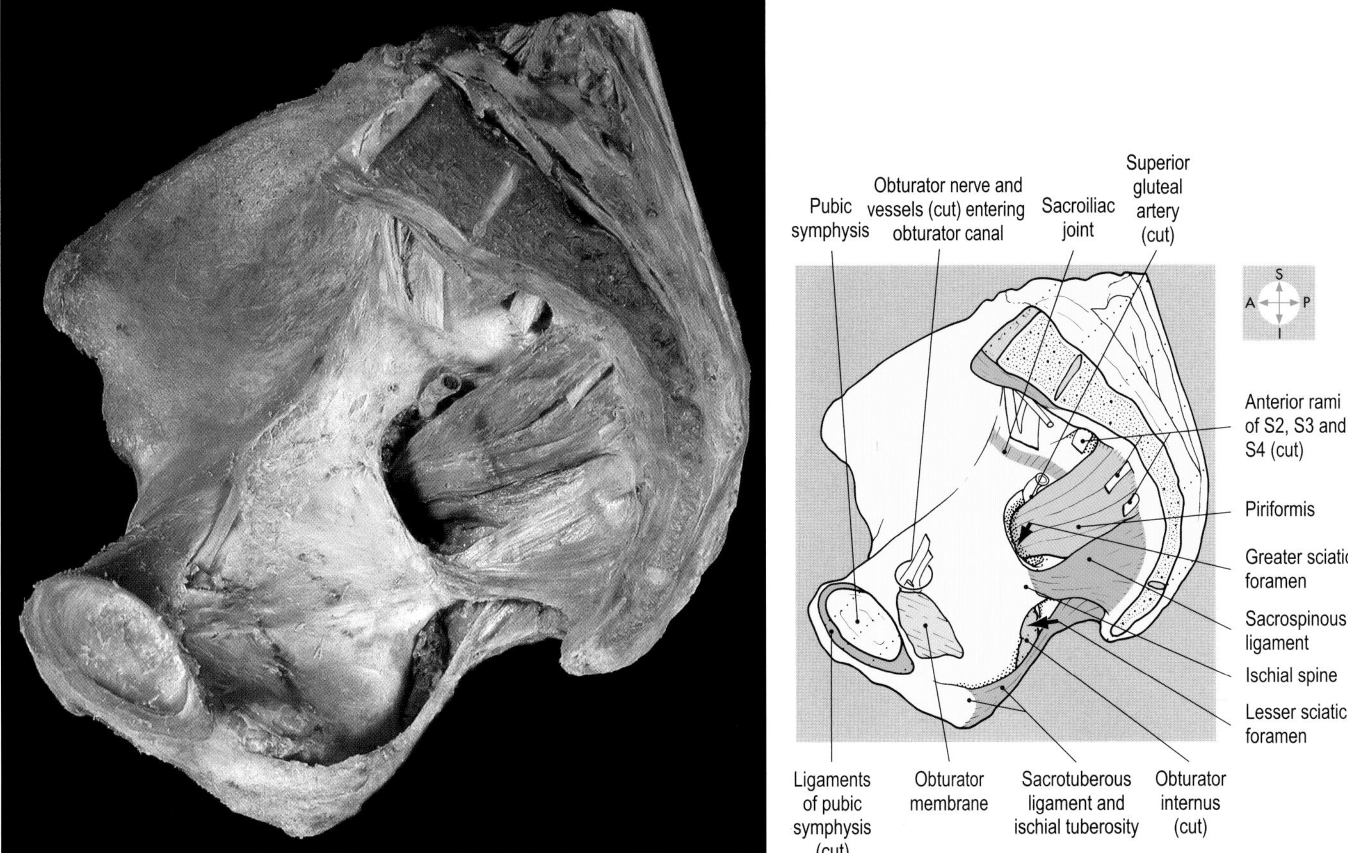

Fig. 5.27 Right hemipelvis showing the pubic symphysis, the obturator membrane, the ligaments and the foramina.

Joints

The pelvic girdle forms a stable ring because its constituent bones are bound together at the two sacroiliac joints and the pubic symphysis.

The symphysis is a secondary cartilaginous joint containing a pad of fibrocartilage, the interpubic disc (Fig. 5.28), that separates the bodies of the right and left pubic bones. The joint is stabilized by ligaments attached around the articular margins.

The sacroiliac joints allow very little movement because the articulating surfaces of their synovial cavities are irregular and behind each cavity is the thick posterior interosseous ligament. Each joint is further supported by the anterior and posterior sacroiliac ligaments and iliolumbar, sacrospinous and sacrotuberous ligaments. Body weight acting downwards through the lumbosacral disc tends to rotate the sacrum, tipping its lower part backwards, a movement prevented by the sacrospinous and sacrotuberous ligaments (Fig. 5.27).

The iliolumbar ligament attaches medially to the transverse process of the fifth lumbar vertebra and laterally to the iliac crest and front of the sacroiliac joint. The sacrospinous ligament passes from the lateral margins of the sacrum and coccyx to the ischial spine. The larger sacrotuberous ligament passes from the side and dorsum of the sacrum and the posterior surface of the ilium to the ischial tuberosity. These two ligaments convert the greater and lesser sciatic notches into the greater and lesser sciatic foramina (Fig. 5.27).

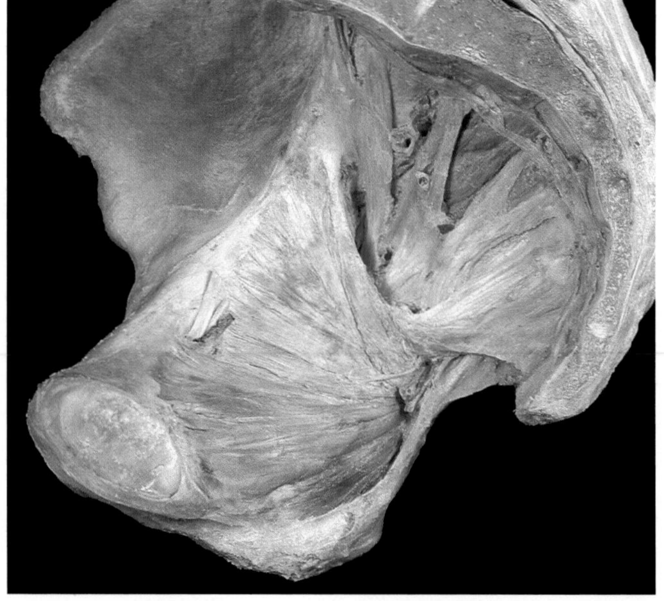

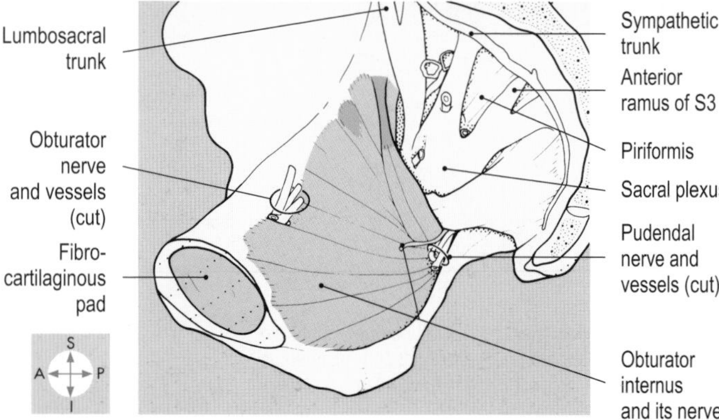

Fig. 5.28 Right hemipelvis showing the pelvic attachment of obturator internus.

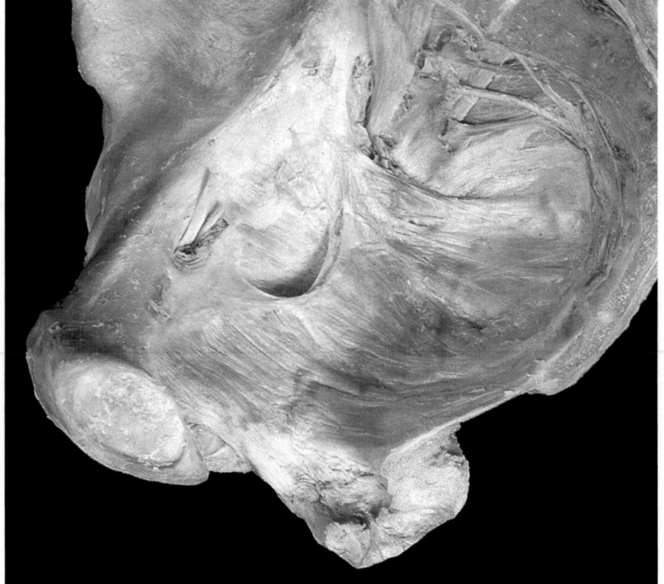

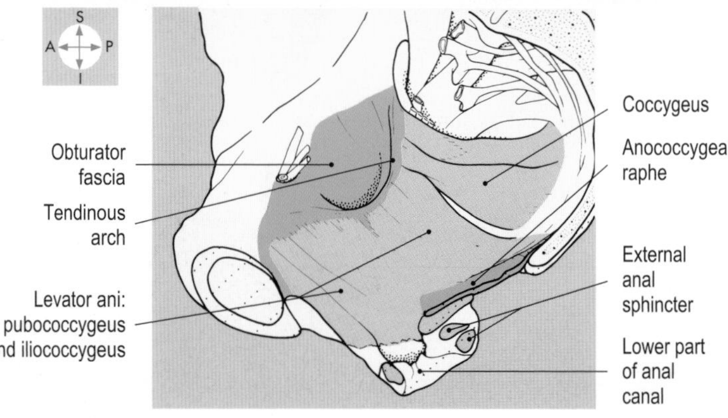

Fig. 5.29 Right levator ani and part of the anal canal, seen in a median sagittal section of the pelvis.

Muscles

Piriformis is a flat muscle attached to the pelvic surfaces of the second, third and fourth pieces of the sacrum (Fig. 5.27). Running laterally through the greater sciatic foramen, it enters the buttock and attaches to the upper part of the greater trochanter of the femur (see p. 271). Piriformis rotates the hip joint laterally and is innervated by the first and second sacral nerves. Numerous vessels and nerves accompany the muscle through the greater sciatic foramen (Fig. 5.28).

Obturator internus is a fan-shaped muscle with an extensive attachment to the margins of the obturator foramen and the pelvic surface of the obturator membrane (Fig. 5.28). The muscle fibres converge on the lesser sciatic foramen to form a tendon, which turns laterally to enter the gluteal region. The tendon is attached to the medial aspect of the greater trochanter (see p. 271). The muscle laterally rotates the hip joint. The nerve to obturator internus (L5, S1 & S2) enters the muscle within the perineum, having traversed the greater and lesser sciatic foramina.

Pelvic fascia

This term includes the fascial lining of the pelvic walls and the extraperitoneal connective tissue surrounding the pelvic viscera (see Fig. 5.7). The pelvic surfaces of obturator internus (Fig. 5.29), piriformis and levator ani are covered by fascia that is continuous superiorly with the transversalis and iliac fasciae. Between the pelvic organs, the pelvic fascia mostly comprises a loose meshwork of connective tissue. However, it is condensed anterior to the rectum to form the rectovesical septum; and some of the arteries to the pelvic organs, notably the uterine and vaginal vessels, are accompanied by thickened bands of fascia termed 'ligaments'. Radiating from the uterine cervix to the pelvic walls are the transverse cervical (lateral sacral) and uterosacral ligaments which provide support to the uterus.

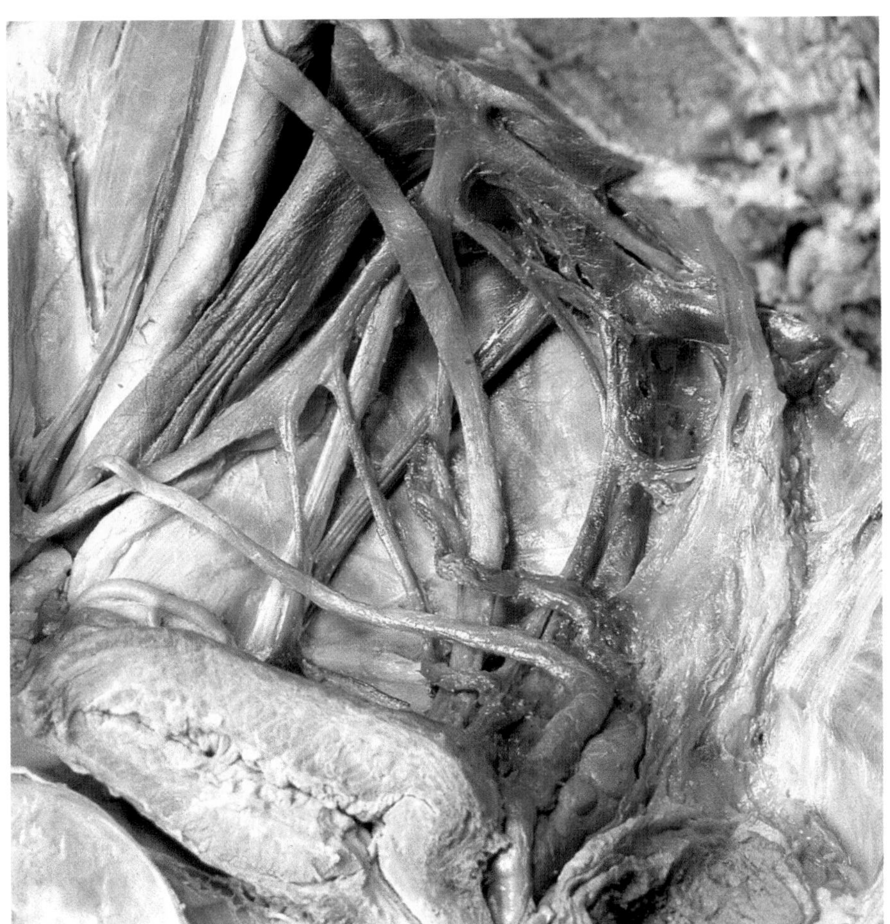

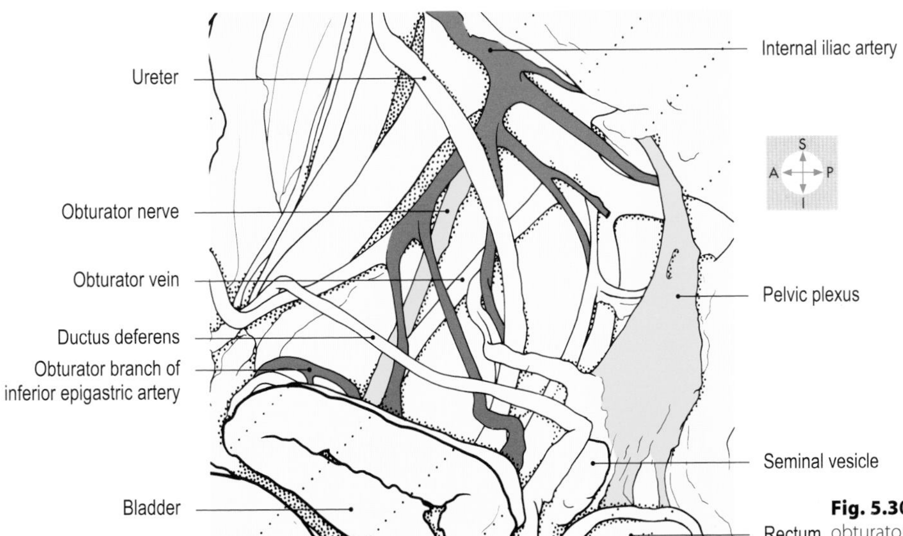

Fig. 5.30 Right pelvic plexus of autonomic nerves. In this specimen the obturator artery is a branch of the inferior epigastric artery rather than the internal iliac artery.

Pelvic Nerves

Autonomic nerves

The pelvic organs receive their autonomic innervation via the right and left pelvic plexuses, which lie adjacent to the internal iliac arteries and their branches (Fig. 5.30). Nerves pass from the plexuses to the bladder, reproductive organs and the rectum by accompanying the arteries to these organs. The plexuses and their branches contain efferent fibres from both the parasympathetic and sympathetic systems, which reach the pelvis from different parts of the spinal cord.

Parasympathetic nerves

The parasympathetic component of the pelvic plexuses is provided by the pelvic splanchnic nerves (nervi erigentes), which leave the spinal cord in the second, third and fourth sacral nerves. The parasympathetic fibres control micturition, dilation of the erectile tissues in both sexes, and defecation. The pelvic plexuses also provide the parasympathetic innervation of the descending and sigmoid parts of the colon. These fibres ascend into the abdomen in the hypogastric plexus and are distributed with the branches of the inferior mesenteric artery.

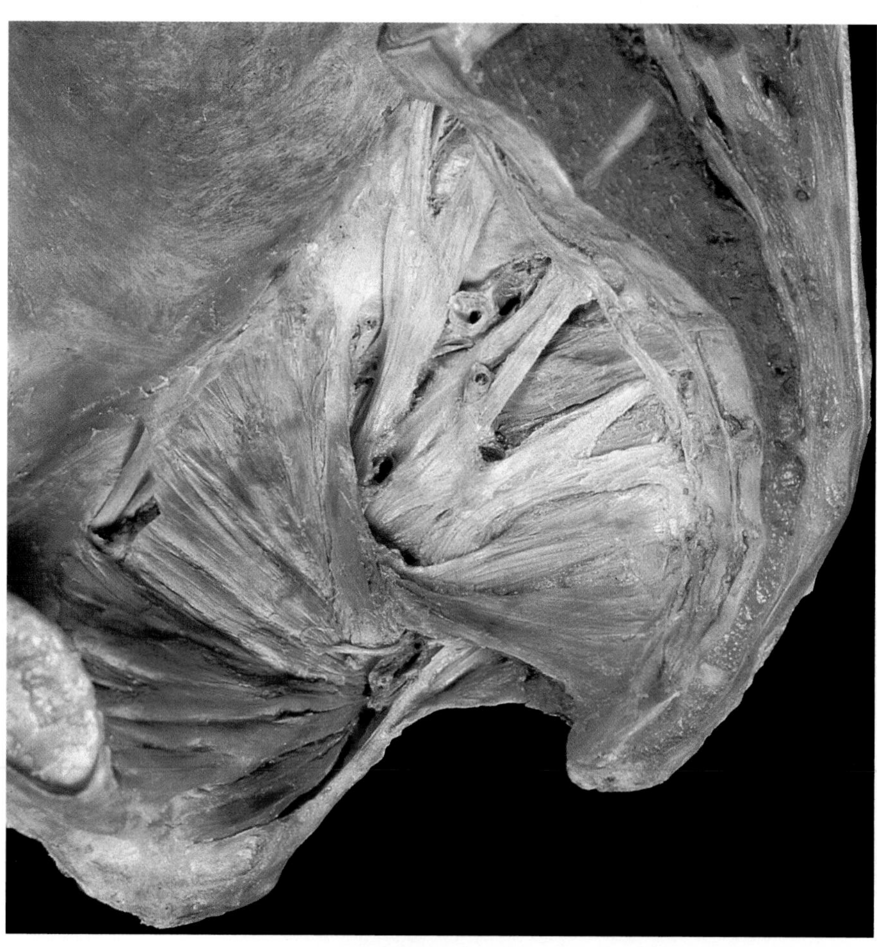

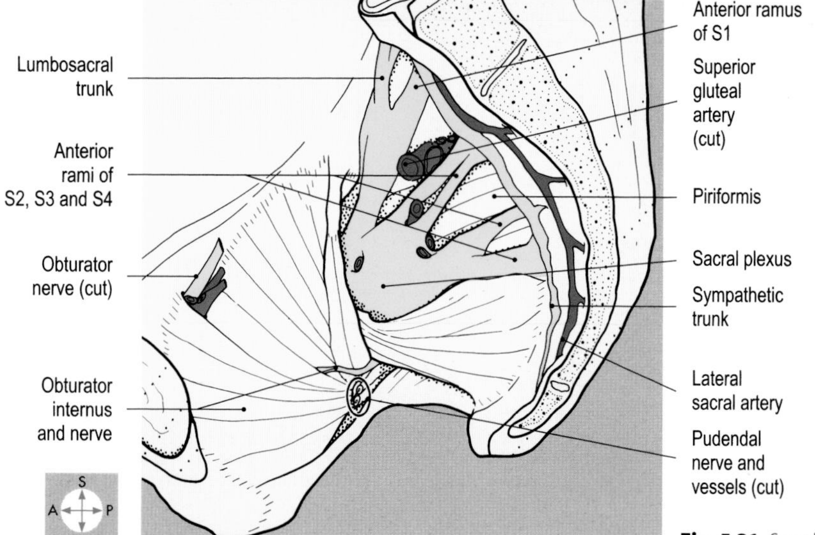

Fig. 5.31 Sacral plexus and pelvic portion of the sympathetic trunk.

Sympathetic nerves

The sympathetic fibres destined for the pelvic autonomic plexuses arise from the lower thoracic and upper lumbar segments of the spinal cord and pass through the lumbar portions of the sympathetic trunks on the posterior abdominal wall. From here they descend in the hypogastric plexus to reach the pelvis. Sympathetic fibres innervate the smooth muscle of the reproductive organs in both sexes, and in the male are responsible for coordinating ejaculation (see p. 231).

The two sympathetic trunks pass from the posterior abdominal wall (see p. 198) into the pelvis by crossing behind the common iliac vessels. Descending in front of the sacrum and piriformis muscles (Fig. 5.31), they incline towards the midline and fuse on the anterior surface of the coccyx. Each trunk bears three or four ganglia and provides grey rami communicantes, consisting of postganglionic fibres, to the sacral nerves. These fibres supply blood vessels and sweat glands in the areas innervated by the appropriate sacral nerves.

Spinal nerves

The lower lumbar and upper sacral spinal nerves are predominantly concerned with the innervation of the lower limb. However, a few fibres derived from these spinal nerves are distributed to the pelvic walls and floor and to the perineum.

Obturator nerve

This branch of the lumbar plexus (see p. 203) emerges from the medial border of psoas major and enters the pelvis by crossing in front of the ala of the sacrum. It descends lateral to the common and internal iliac vessels and the ureter (Fig. 5.30) and reaches the medial surface of obturator internus. The nerve approaches the obturator vessels from above and continues with them through the obturator canal (Fig. 5.31) into the medial compartment of the thigh (see p. 266).

Sacral and coccygeal nerves

The anterior rami of the first four sacral nerves emerge through the anterior sacral foramina and merge to form the sacral plexus (Fig. 5.31). The fifth sacral nerve and the coccygeal nerves are small and do not contribute to the plexus. All the sacral and coccygeal nerves receive grey rami communicantes from the sympathetic trunk.

Sacral plexus

This plexus lies on the posterior pelvic wall in front of piriformis (Fig. 5.31), covered anteriorly by the pelvic fascia. The plexus is formed by the anterior rami of the upper four sacral nerves and is supplemented by the lumbosacral trunk which carries fibres from the fourth and fifth lumbar nerves (see p. 203). The branches of the sacral plexus are distributed to the lower limb, pelvic walls and floor, and perineum.

Those branches that leave the pelvis accompany piriformis through the greater sciatic foramen to enter the buttock (see pp 270 & 271). The nerve to obturator internus and the pudendal nerve then pass forwards through the lesser sciatic foramen to gain the perineum (see Fig. 5.28).

Pelvic Blood Vessels and Lymphatics

The pelvic walls and floor and the pelvic organs receive most of their arterial supply from branches of the internal iliac artery, which also provides branches to the perineum and lower limb. The rectum, however, receives its principal supply from the superior rectal artery (see pp 182 & 218), while the posterior wall of the pelvis is supplied by the median sacral artery (see Fig. 5.31). The ovaries are supplied by the ovarian branches of the abdominal aorta (see p. 221).

Internal iliac artery and branches

The internal iliac artery arises in front of the sacroiliac joint as one of the terminal branches of the common iliac artery (Fig. 5.32). The internal iliac artery runs downwards and backwards on the lateral pelvic wall, giving rise to visceral and parietal branches.

Visceral branches

Before birth, the largest branch of the internal iliac artery is the umbilical artery which conveys blood to the placenta. In the adult, only its proximal part is patent. It runs forward, adjacent to the bladder, giving one or more superior vesical branches (Fig. 5.32) and a slender branch to the ductus deferens. Distally, the vessel becomes a fibrous cord, the occluded part of the umbilical artery or medial umbilical ligament, which continues through the extraperitoneal tissues of the anterior abdominal wall to the umbilicus (see Fig. 4.30). The inferior vesical artery occurs only in the male and supplies the lower part of the bladder, the prostate, the seminal vesicle and the pelvic ureter. The uterine artery runs medially in the root of the broad ligament, crosses above the ureter (see Fig. 5.13) and supplies the vagina and the uterine cervix, body and tube. The artery follows the lateral border of the body of the uterus, then runs laterally in the broad ligament, close to the uterine tube, and terminates by anastomosing with the ovarian artery.

The vagina is supplied by branches of the uterine artery together with one or two small vaginal arteries from the internal iliac artery.

The middle rectal artery (Fig. 5.32) supplies the muscle coat of the rectum and in the male may give additional branches to the prostate and seminal vesicles.

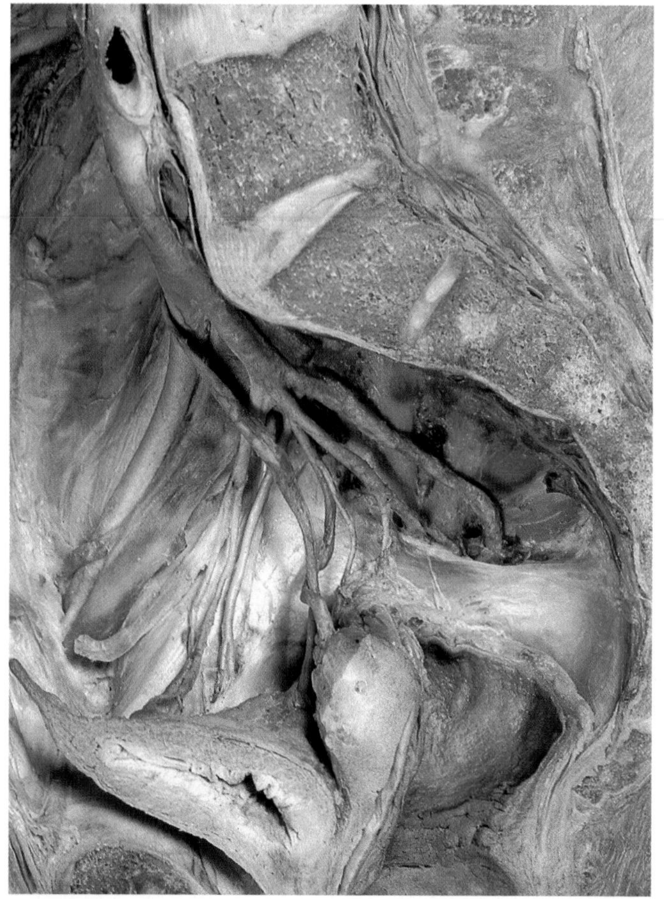

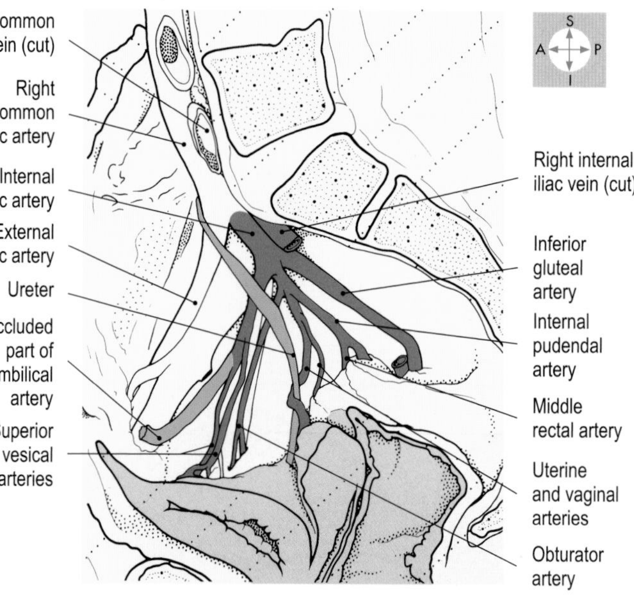

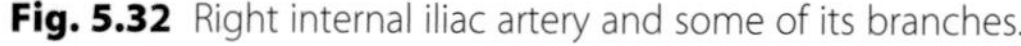
Fig. 5.32 Right internal iliac artery and some of its branches.

Parietal branches

The obturator artery runs downwards and forwards, with the corresponding vein and nerve, to enter the obturator canal. It supplies the proximal part of the medial compartment of the thigh and the hip joint (see p. 266). Occasionally, the obturator artery takes origin from the inferior epigastric artery and descends into the pelvis to reach the obturator canal. Such a vessel, an accessory or 'abnormal' obturator artery (see Fig. 5.30), passes close to the femoral ring and may be damaged during femoral hernia operations.

The superior and inferior gluteal arteries pass through the greater sciatic foramen into the buttock, the superior artery running above piriformis (see Fig. 5.31) and the inferior below (see p. 270).

The internal pudendal artery provides the principal arterial supply to the perineum. The artery passes through the greater sciatic foramen into the gluteal region, curves round the ischial spine and then passes forwards through the lesser sciatic foramen into the perineum (see p. 241).

The iliolumbar artery ascends the posterior abdominal wall to anastomose with the lower lumbar arteries.

The lateral sacral artery (see Fig. 5.31) supplies the posterior wall of the pelvis and anastomoses with the median sacral artery.

Internal iliac vein and tributaries

The branches of the internal iliac artery are accompanied by veins that drain the buttock and perineum, the pelvic walls and most of the pelvic organs. These veins unite to form the internal iliac vein (Fig. 5.33), which ascends on the lateral pelvic wall posterior to the artery. The vein terminates by joining the external iliac vein to form the common iliac vein.

Most of the veins emerging from the pelvic organs anastomose freely, forming extensive venous plexuses (the vesical, prostatic, uterine and vaginal plexuses). While most blood from these plexuses passes into the internal iliac vein, some enters either the superior rectal vein via portacaval anastomoses or the vertebral venous plexus via the anterior sacral foramina. Prostatic carcinoma can spread via these venous plexuses to the sacral and lumbar vertebrae.

Pelvic lymphatics

Lymph from the pelvis is drained by lymphatic vessels that accompany the arteries. Most of the lymph drains into nodes adjacent to the internal iliac artery and then into efferent vessels that pass to the common iliac nodes (see p. 196). However, lymphatic vessels from the ovaries and the rectum pass directly to the aortic nodes, and some vessels from the body of the uterus accompany the round ligament through the inguinal canal to terminate in the superficial inguinal nodes.

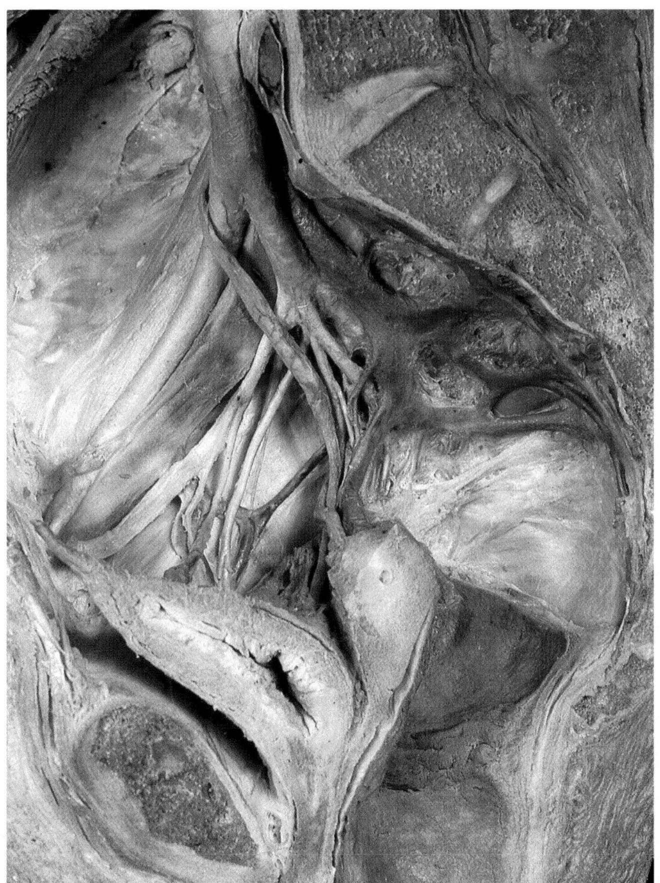

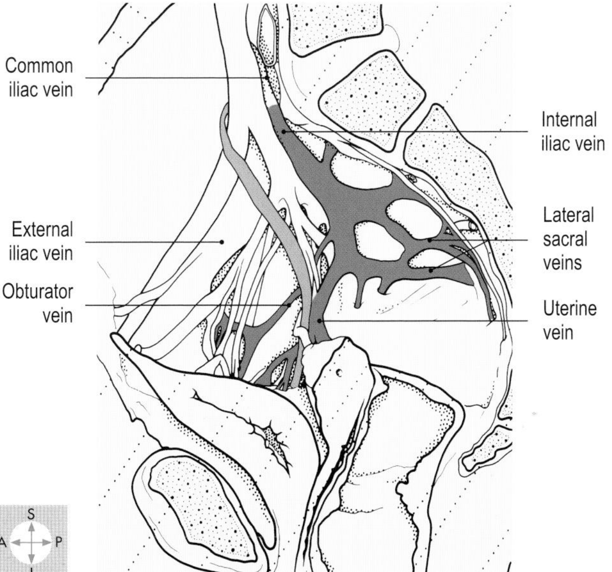

Fig. 5.33 Right internal iliac vein and tributaries.

Perineum

Below the pelvic floor lies the perineum, a superficial region traversed by the anal canal and the lower parts of the genital and urinary tracts. The perineum is diamond-shaped, extending anteriorly to the pubic symphysis, posteriorly to the coccyx and laterally to the ischial tuberosities (Fig. 5.34 see Fig. 5.3). On each side, the region is bounded by the conjoined rami of the ischium and pubis and by the sacrotuberous ligament, which is overlapped by the inferior border of gluteus maximus. Inferiorly the perineum is bounded by skin. By convention, the perineum is divided into two triangular areas by a line joining the ischial tuberosities. Posteriorly is the anal triangle, containing the anal canal and the ischioanal (ischiorectal) fossae, and anteriorly lies the urogenital triangle, containing the external genitalia.

Anal canal

The anal canal is the terminal part of the intestine and is approximately 4 cm long. Beginning at the anorectal junction, it passes downwards and backwards as far as the anus (see Fig. 5.5). Its upper part is lined by mucous membrane bearing several longitudinal ridges, the anal columns; the lower part is lined by skin. The smooth muscle coat of the rectum continues into the wall of the anal canal and thickens to form the internal anal sphincter. Striated fibres from the levator ani muscles (Fig. 5.35) blend with the outer layers of the wall and continue as far as the perianal skin.

In addition, the lower two-thirds of the anal canal are encircled by the external anal sphincter (Fig. 5.36), composed of striated muscle fibres. This sphincter comprises three parts, of which the uppermost, the deep part, blends with the levator ani muscles. Inferior to this lies the superficial part, attached posteriorly to the coccyx and anococcygeal raphe and anteriorly to the posterior border of the perineal membrane. The most inferior component of the sphincter, the subcutaneous part, encircles the anal opening. Continence of faeces is not dependent on the external sphincter alone; the fibres of the levator ani muscles that maintain the anorectal angulation play a major role.

The anal canal is supplied by inferior rectal branches (Fig. 5.36) from the pudendal nerve, which innervate the external sphincter and the cutaneous lining. The internal sphincter and the mucous membrane lining the upper part are innervated, like the rectum, by autonomic nerves (see p. 236). The blood supply is provided by inferior rectal branches of the internal pudendal artery. The anal canal is a site of portacaval anastomosis because venous blood passes not only via inferior rectal veins to the internal iliac veins but also into the superior rectal vein, a tributary of the portal venous system (see p. 185). Lymph drains from the upper part of the canal to the internal iliac nodes, but from the lower part it passes to the superficial inguinal nodes.

The cutaneous lining of the lower part of the anal canal has a rich nerve supply. Tears (fissures) in this skin are painful and produce reflex spasm of the external sphincter.

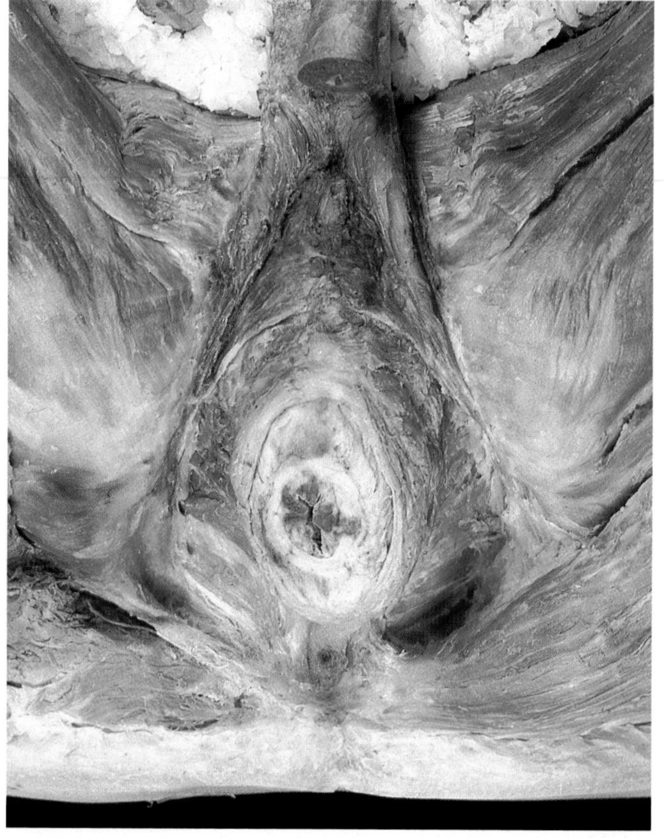

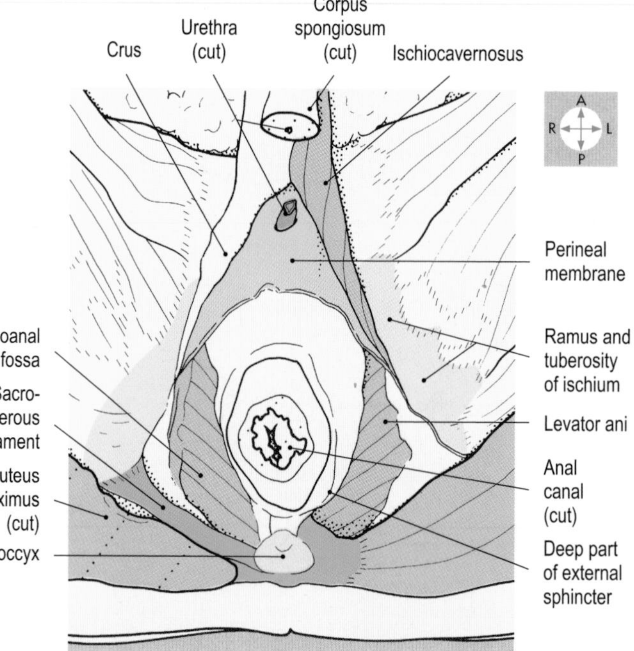

Fig. 5.34 Deep dissection of male perineum. The bulb of the penis has been removed to expose the perineal membrane, and gluteus maximus on one side has been resected to reveal the sacrotuberous ligament.

Ischioanal (ischiorectal) fossa

On each side of the anal canal is a fat-filled space extending laterally as far as obturator internus, upwards to the levator ani muscle and downwards to the perianal skin (see Fig. 5.35). The fossae communicate behind the anal canal. Anteriorly, each fossa tapers and continues above the perineal membrane and external urethral sphincter almost to the pubic symphysis. Entering each fossa from the gluteal region via the lesser sciatic foramen are the nerve to obturator internus, the pudendal nerve (Fig. 5.37) and the internal pudendal artery with its venae comitantes.

The nerve to obturator internus arises from the sacral plexus and supplies the muscle from within the ischioanal fossa (see Fig. 5.28).

The pudendal nerve and the internal pudendal vessels pass along the lateral wall of the fossa in a fascial tunnel, the pudendal canal. Branches from the nerve and artery traverse the upper part of the fossa to supply the anal canal and the posterior part of the scrotum or labium majus (see Fig. 5.36).

Internal pudendal artery

This vessel provides most of the arterial blood to the perineum. Arising from the internal iliac artery within the pelvis (see Fig. 5.32), it enters the buttock through the greater sciatic foramen and then traverses the lesser sciatic foramen to enter the ischioanal fossa. The artery runs forwards along the lateral wall of the fossa in the pudendal canal and gives off inferior rectal branches and posterior scrotal or labial branches. The artery continues above the perineal membrane, where it provides branches to the bulb of the penis or vestibule and crus of the penis or clitoris, and terminates by dividing into deep and dorsal arteries of the penis or clitoris. In the male the dorsal artery passes below the pubic symphysis and continues along the dorsum of the penile shaft (Fig. 5.37), lateral to the deep dorsal vein, and gives branches to the erectile tissue of the corpus cavernosum. The deep artery pierces the perineal membrane and supplies the erectile tissue of the corpus cavernosum. In the female there are comparable but smaller branches to the clitoris. The internal pudendal artery and its branches are accompanied by venae comitantes, which drain into the internal iliac vein.

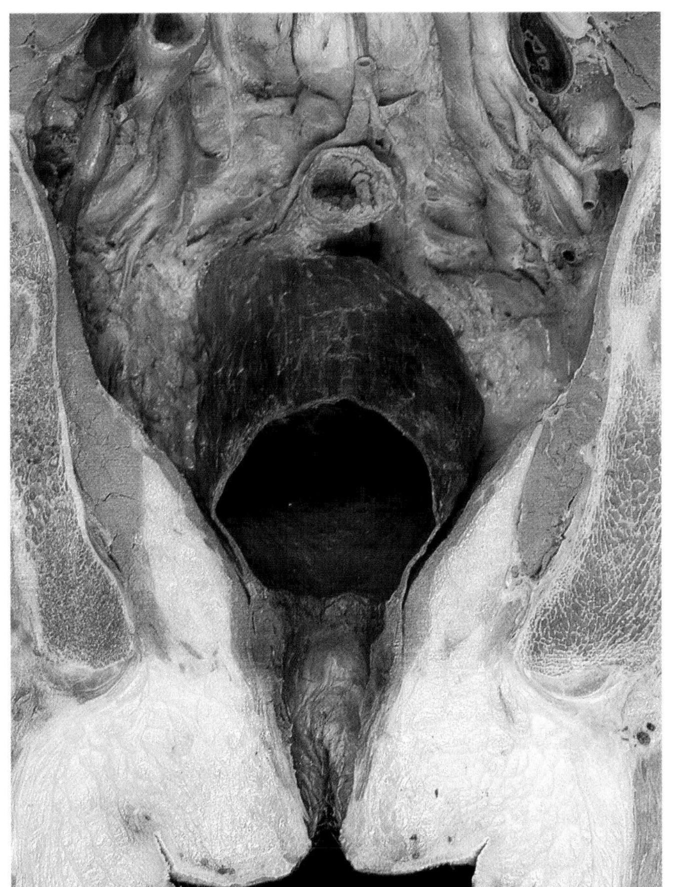

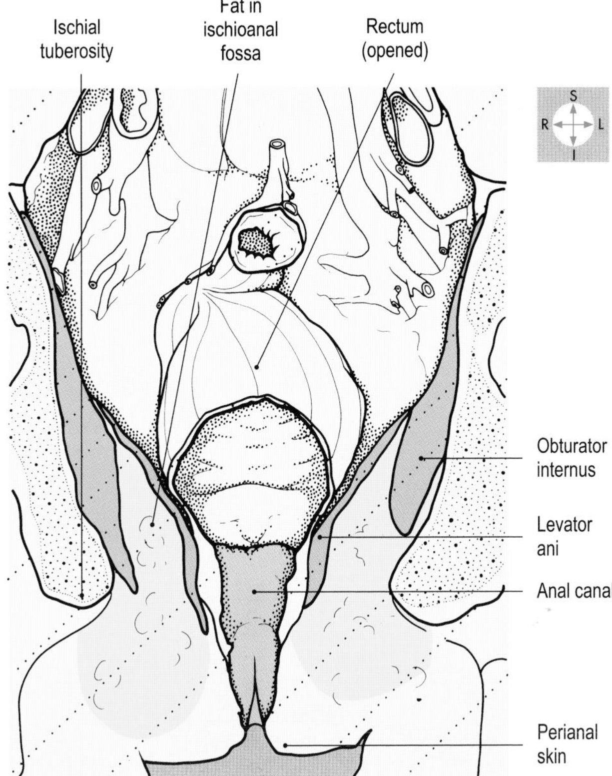

Fig. 5.35 Coronal section through anal canal and ischioanal fossae. Anterior aspect.

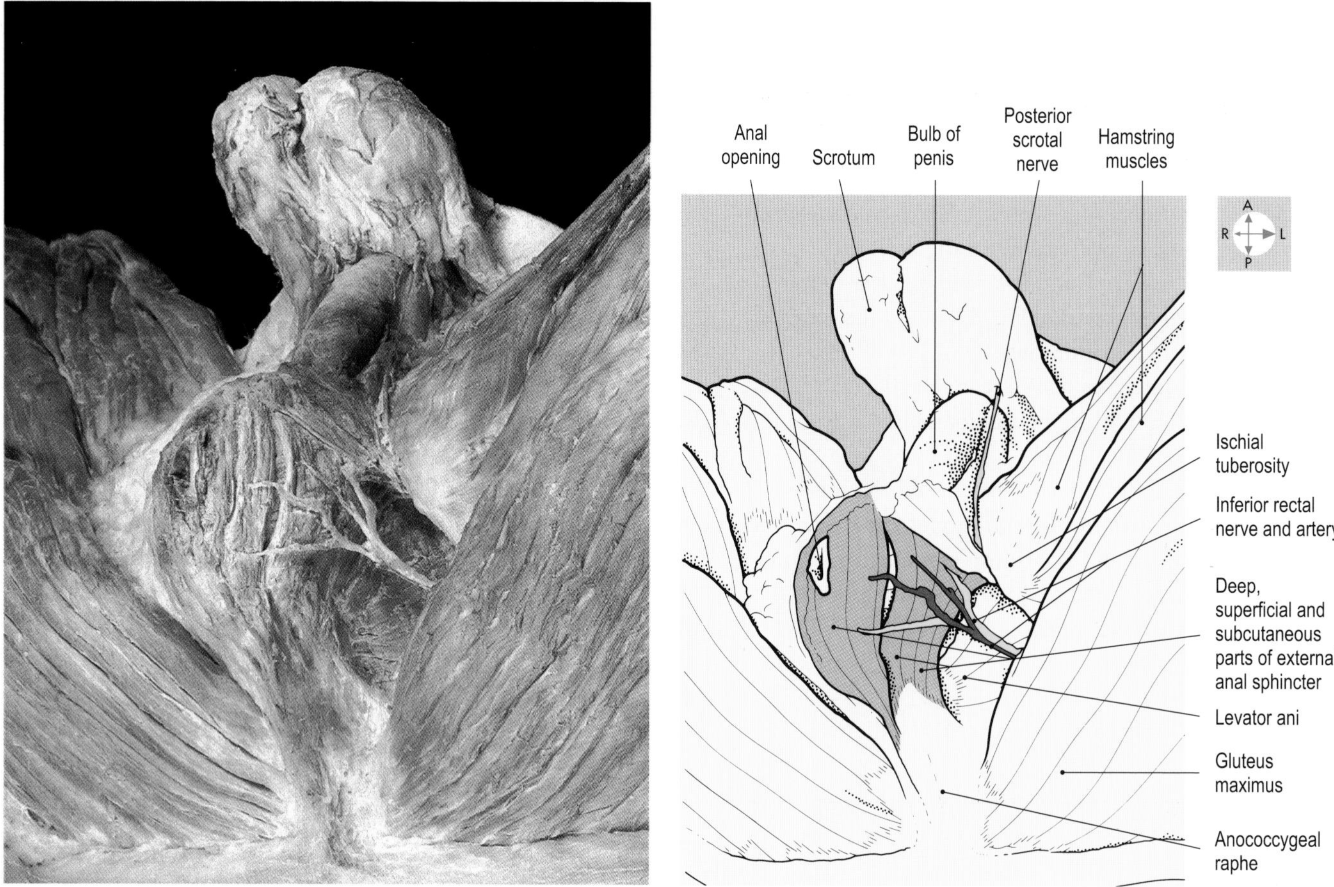

Fig. 5.36 Oblique view of the anal triangle to show the parts of the external anal sphincter and the inferior rectal nerve and artery.

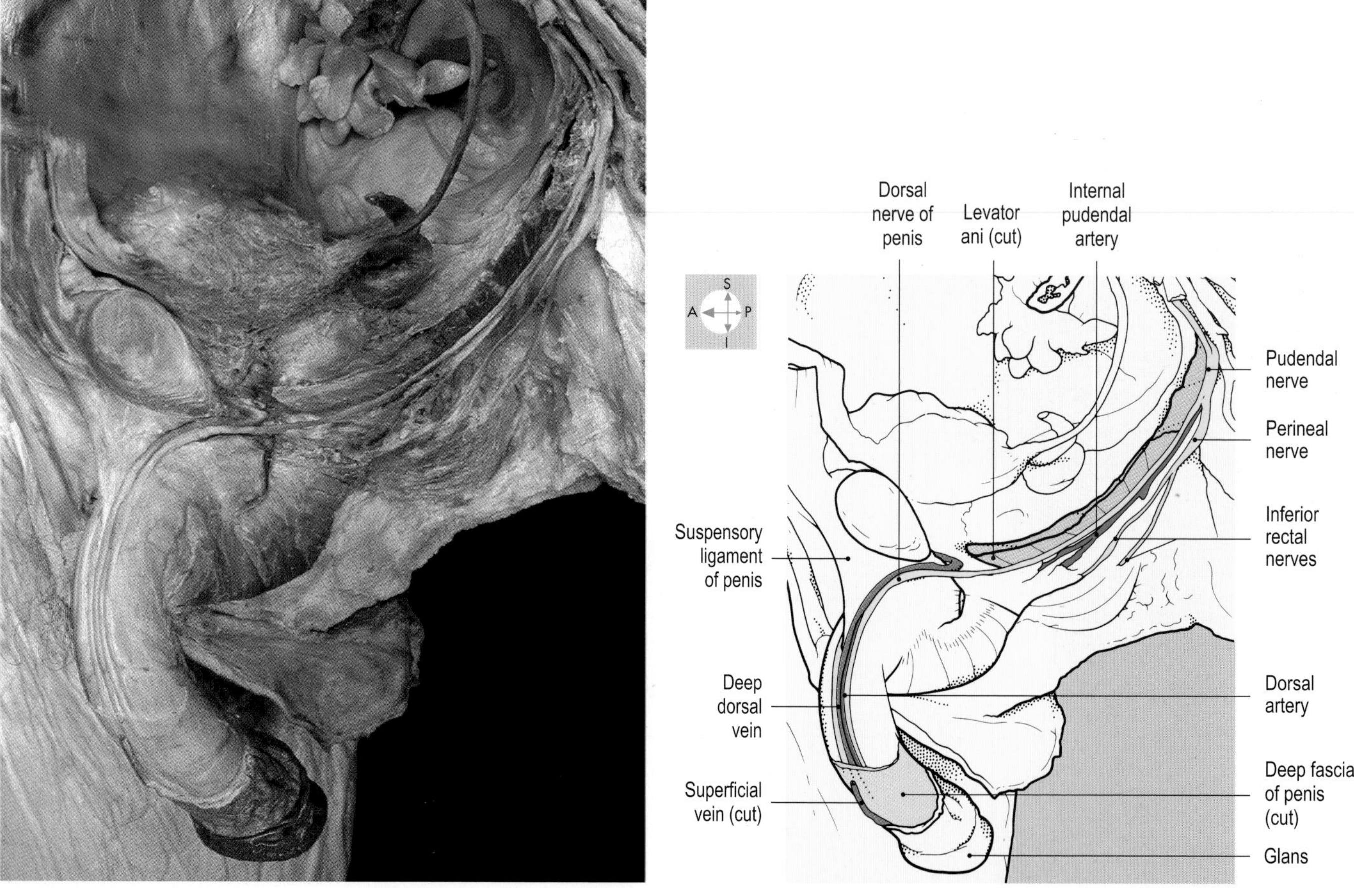

Fig. 5.37 Left pudendal nerve, exposed by removal of the lateral wall of the pelvis.

Pudendal nerve

The pudendal nerve provides the principal innervation to the perineum. It arises from the sacral plexus (S2, S3 & S4) and accompanies the internal pudendal artery into the perineum. In the ischioanal fossa the nerve divides into the dorsal nerve of penis (or clitoris) and the perineal nerve (Fig. 5.37).

The perineal nerve supplies an inferior rectal branch to the anal canal and posterior scrotal or labial branches to the skin of the genitalia (see Fig. 5.36). On reaching the anterior part of the perineum, the perineal nerve gives branches to all muscles in the superficial perineal pouch as well as sensory branches to the urethra.

The dorsal nerve of the penis continues forwards with the internal pudendal artery above the perineal membrane and below the pubic symphysis. It runs along the dorsum of the penis, lateral to the dorsal artery (Fig. 5.39), and innervates the skin of the distal two-thirds of the organ. The dorsal nerve of the clitoris has a similar course and distribution.

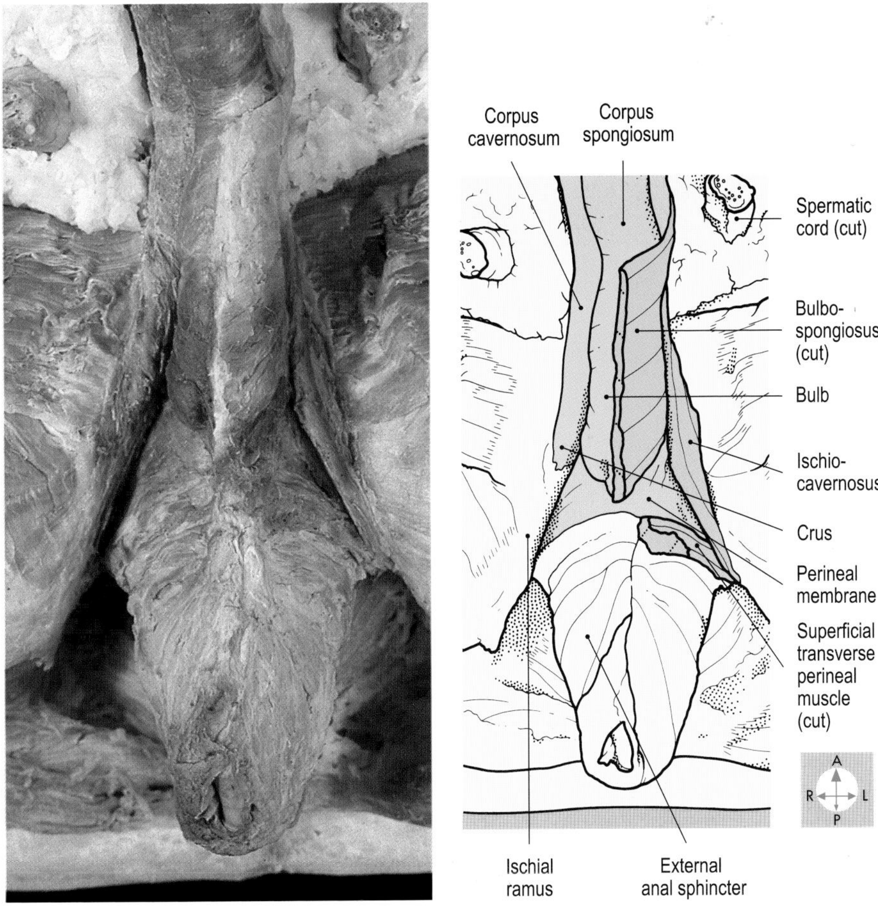

Fig. 5.38 Root of penis. On one side, ischiocavernosus has been excised to reveal the crus and bulbospongiosus removed to expose half of the bulb.

Male External Genitalia

The male external genitalia comprise the scrotum and the penis. An account of the scrotum and its contents is given on pages 149 and 151. The penis consists of a shaft, which is free, and a root, which lies in the superficial perineal pouch, attached to the inferior surface of the perineal membrane.

Perineal membrane and pouches

The perineal membrane is a shelf of dense fascia spanning the triangular interval between the right and left ischial rami and inferior pubic rami (see Fig. 5.34). The membrane has a long free posterior margin and a short anterior margin that is separated from the pubic symphysis by a small gap transmitting the deep dorsal vein of the penis. The central part of the membrane is pierced by the urethra and bulbourethral ducts.

At the root of the penis and around the neck of the scrotum the membranous layer of perineal subcutaneous tissue attaches laterally to the ischial and pubic rami. Posteriorly, the fascia is anchored to the free edge of the perineal membrane. The space contained by the membranous layer of the penis and the scrotum is called the superficial perineal pouch. This pouch communicates with the subcutaneous tissues of the anterior abdominal wall but not with the ischioanal fossae, the thighs or pelvic cavity. If the spongy part of the urethra is ruptured, urine may escape into the superficial pouch (superficial extravasation of urine).

On the pelvic aspect of the perineal membrane lie the external urethral sphincter and bulbourethral glands in a space often called the deep perineal pouch. The term 'urogenital diaphragm' is a misnomer sometimes applied to the deep perineal pouch and its boundaries.

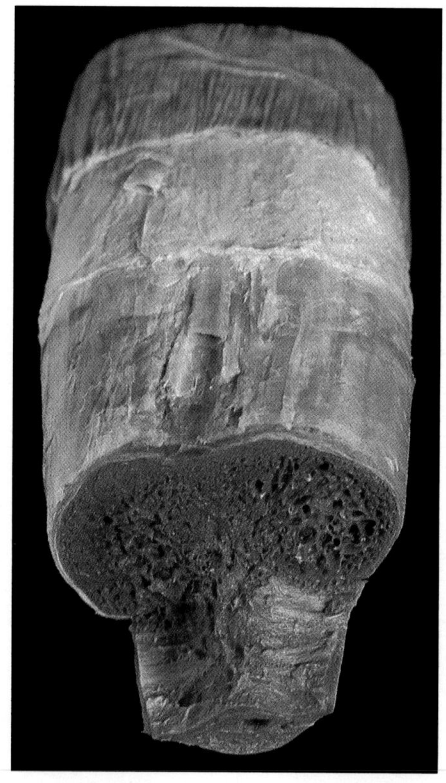

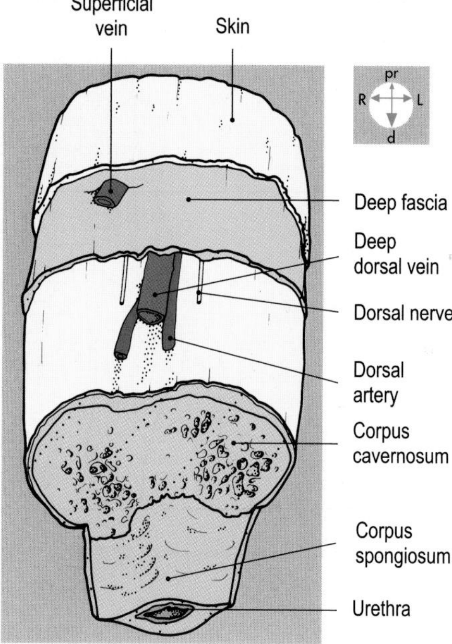

Fig. 5.39 'Step' dissection of the shaft of the penis to show the three corpora and the dorsal vessels.

Penis

The erectile tissue of the shaft of the penis consists of the paired corpora cavernosa, lying in apposition, and the midline corpus spongiosum.

The corpus spongiosum is uniform in diameter except at its extremity, where it expands into the glans (see Fig. 5.19), whose prominent margin forms the corona of the penis. Proximally, the corpus spongiosum continues into the root of the penis to form the bulb, which is attached to the inferior surface of the perineal membrane (Fig. 5.38). The urethra pierces the perineal membrane, enters the bulb from above and curves downwards and forwards. It traverses the corpus spongiosum and glans (see Fig. 5.19) and terminates at the external urethral meatus near the apex of the glans.

Dorsal to the corpus spongiosum are the paired corpora cavernosa (Fig. 5.39), which extend distally as far as the concave proximal surface of the glans. Proximally, the corpora cavernosa continue inferior to the pubic symphysis and diverge as the crura. Each crus tapers posteriorly and is attached to the inferior surface of the perineal membrane and the adjacent rami of the pubis and ischium (Fig. 5.38; see Fig. 5.34).

Fascial layers and skin

The three corpora of the penis are enveloped by a sleeve of deep fascia, which also covers the dorsal vessels and nerves of the organ (see Fig. 5.39). Proximally, the deep fascia is anchored to the front of the pubic symphysis by the suspensory ligament of the penis (see Fig. 5.37), while distally it terminates at the corona by fusing with the corpora. Covering the deep fascia is the superficial fascia.

The subcutaneous tissue of the penis is membranous, devoid of fat and traversed by superficial nerves and vessels (see Fig. 5.39). Proximally, it is continuous with the subcutaneous tissue of the anterior abdominal wall and can be traced around the scrotum, where it contains smooth muscle, the dartos.

The cutaneous covering of the penis is freely mobile except over the glans to which it is adherent. The skin is reflected distally beyond the corona over the glans to form the hood-like prepuce or foreskin. This is attached to the undersurface of the glans by a vascular fold, the frenulum.

Muscles

Surrounding the bulb of the penis are the paired bulbospongiosus muscles (see Fig. 5.38). Their fibres attach to the perineal membrane and pass downwards and backwards to meet at a midline raphe and blend posteriorly with the external anal sphincter. The bulbospongiosus muscles contract during ejaculation and the terminal stages of micturition to compress the urethra and expel its contents.

Covering each crus is the ischiocavernosus muscle (see Fig. 5.38). From the posterior end of each crus a small superficial transverse perineal muscle runs medially to the penile bulb. All the penile muscles are innervated by the perineal branch of the pudendal nerve.

Vessels

The erectile tissues of the penis have a rich blood supply. Each internal pudendal artery (see p. 241) provides branches to the bulb and to the corresponding crus before terminating as the dorsal and deep arteries. The deep artery traverses the length of the corpus cavernosum while the artery to the bulb continues along the corpus spongiosum to reach the glans. The principal venous drainage is via the midline deep dorsal vein, which runs beneath the deep fascia (see Fig. 5.39). This vein is accompanied by the dorsal arteries and passes inferior to the pubic symphysis into the pelvic cavity where it terminates in the prostatic venous plexus (see Fig. 5.21). From this plexus blood drains into either the internal iliac veins or the internal pudendal veins.

Erection of the penis is controlled by parasympathetic nerves (the pelvic splanchnic nerves or nervi erigentes) from the sacral segments of the spinal cord. Stimulation of these nerves causes arterial dilatation and simultaneous venous constriction. This results in engorgement of the erectile tissues leading to enlargement and stiffening of the penis. Diseases affecting these arteries or their autonomic supply may lead to erectile dysfunction.

The skin of the penis and the front of the scrotum are supplied by the external pudendal branches of the femoral arteries. The superficial veins of the penis and the anterior part of the scrotum drain via the external pudendal veins, which are tributaries of the great saphenous vein (see Fig. 6.11). The posterior part of the scrotum is supplied by posterior scrotal branches from the internal pudendal artery, and venous blood passes into the internal pudendal veins.

Cutaneous innervation

The pudendal nerve supplies most of the penis and scrotum via its dorsal and posterior scrotal branches. However, the anterior part of the scrotum and the proximal part of the shaft of the penis are innervated by the ilioinguinal nerve, which descends from the superficial inguinal ring (see p. 145).

Lymphatic drainage

Lymph from the superficial tissues of the penis and scrotum passes to the superficial inguinal nodes while that from the deeper tissues is conveyed via lymphatic vessels accompanying the internal pudendal artery and passes to the internal iliac nodes.

Female External Genitalia

Clitoris and bulbs of vestibule

The perineal membrane is thinner in the female than in the male and is pierced by both the vagina and the urethra. Attached to the inferior surface of the membrane is erectile tissue similar to that in the male, namely the crura of the clitoris and the bulbs of the vestibule covered by the thin ischiocavernosus and bulbospongiosus muscles respectively (Figs 5.40 & 5.41). The right and left crura attach to the medial margins of the ischial and pubic rami. Passing forwards and medially they merge beneath the pubic symphysis to form the shaft of the clitoris. This turns downwards and backwards towards the urethral opening, and its tip is capped by the glans of the clitoris.

The paired bulbs of the vestibule surround the urethral and vaginal openings (Fig. 5.41). Anteriorly they taper and fuse into a midline structure that terminates as the glans of the clitoris. The posterior end of each bulb is expanded and covers the greater vestibular (Bartholin's) gland. This gland is approximately 1 cm in diameter and drains into a minute duct which opens into the vestibule lateral to the vaginal opening. Superficial transverse perineal muscles pass laterally from the bulbs of the vestibule to the ischial tuberosities.

Labia

The most superficial parts of the female external genitalia are the skin folds, the labia majora (Fig. 5.40). These meet anteriorly at the mons pubis. The mons is a pad of fat overlying the pubic symphysis and covering most of the clitoris. Between the labia majora lie the two labia minora, which become more prominent anteriorly. The labia minora fuse in the midline, forming two folds of skin around the glans of the clitoris. The hood-like anterior fold comprises the prepuce of the clitoris and the smaller posterior fold forms the frenulum. Posteriorly, the labia minora are united by a delicate fold, the fourchette, which is usually torn during vaginal delivery.

Vestibule

The labia minora enclose a cleft, the vestibule, into which the vagina and urethra open (Fig. 5.41). The vaginal opening (introitus) is an anteroposterior slit, usually surrounded by a fringe of skin, the hymen. The external urethral meatus lies approximately 1 cm anterior to the vaginal opening.

The term 'vulva' is used to describe the mons pubis, the labia majora and minora, the clitoris and vestibule.

Cutaneous innervation and blood supply

The mons pubis and the anterior parts of the labia are innervated by the ilioinguinal nerves (see p. 145). The posterior part of the vulva receives cutaneous innervation from the labial branches of the pudendal nerves, supplemented by branches of the posterior cutaneous nerves of the thighs and the perineal branches of the fourth sacral nerves.

The skin and subcutaneous tissues are supplied by the internal pudendal artery (see p. 241) and the superficial and deep external pudendal branches of the femoral artery. Most of the venous blood passes into the venae comitantes of the internal pudendal artery, but anteriorly some blood drains by external pudendal veins into the great saphenous vein. Lymph from the skin and superficial tissues, including the vestibule and lower vagina, passes to the superficial inguinal nodes (see p. 145), while lymphatics from deeper structures follow the course of the arteries to reach the internal iliac nodes.

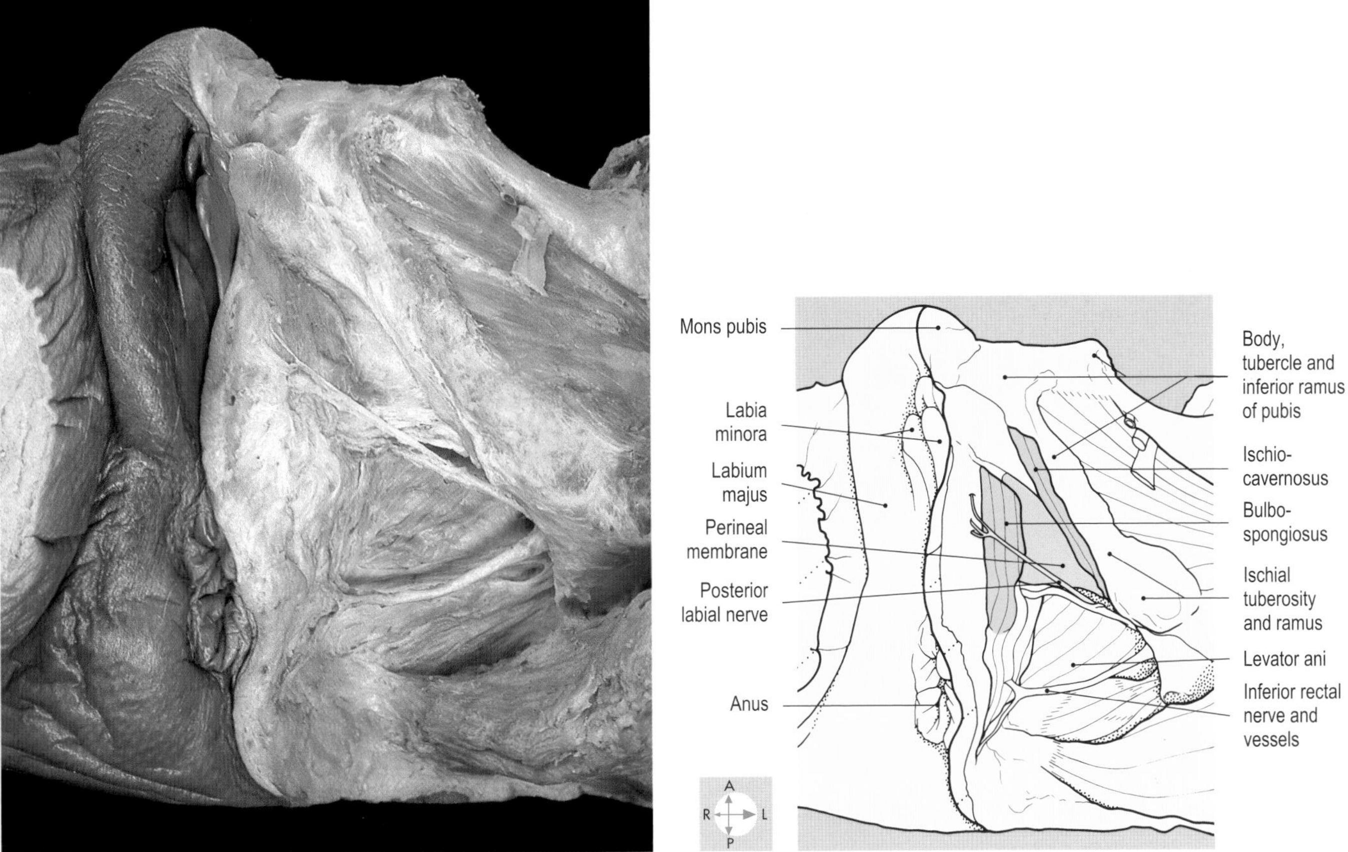

Fig. 5.40 Superficial dissection of one side of the female perineum, showing the muscles and cutaneous nerves.

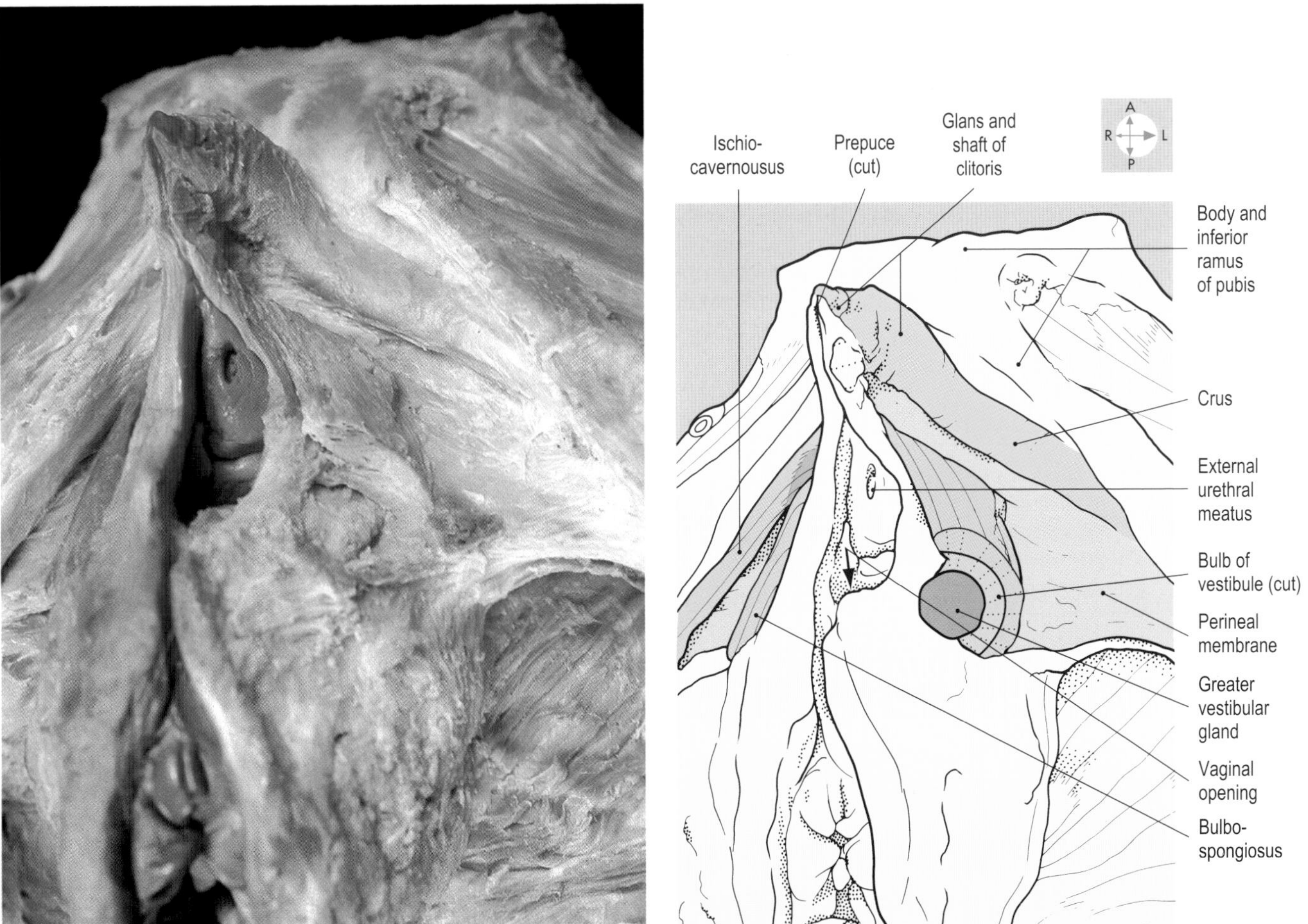

Fig. 5.41 Deeper dissection of the female perineum. The glans, shaft and left crus of the clitoris have been exposed. The left bulb of the vestibule has been cut to reveal the greater vestibular gland.

Exam Skills

Each of the incomplete statements below is followed by five suggested answers or completions. Decide which are true and which are false. The answers are supplied on page 415.

1. The ovary:

a) receives its principal arterial supply from the internal iliac artery.
b) lies in the angle between the internal and external iliac vessels.
c) is attached by the mesovarium to the anterior surface of the broad ligament.
d) may lie in close proximity to the obturator nerve.
e) has a surface which is devoid of peritoneal covering.

2. Peritoneum in the female pelvis:

a) forms the round ligament of the uterus.
b) forms the mesovarium.
c) covers the posterior fornix of the vagina.
d) covers the anterior and lateral surfaces of the whole length of the rectum.
e) is in direct contact with the ureters.

3. The piriformis muscle:

a) attaches to the pelvic surface of the sacrum.
b) passes through the lesser sciatic foramen.
c) attaches to the greater trochanter of the femur.
d) has the pelvic plexus on its anterior surface.
e) is a medial rotator of the hip joint.

4. Concerning the lumbar and sacral plexus:

a) the obturator nerve carries fibres from spinal segments L2, L3 and L4.
b) the femoral nerve emerges from the anterior surface of the psoas major muscle.
c) the pudendal nerve provides the motor supply to the external anal sphincter.
d) sympathetic fibres leave the spinal cord in spinal nerves S2, S3 and S4.
e) the lumbosacral trunk carries fibres from spinal segments L4 and L5.

5. The uterus:

a) is supplied with blood by branches of the internal iliac artery.
b) is supported by the broad ligaments.
c) has most of its lymphatics draining into inguinal nodes.
d) is closely related to the ureters.
e) pierces the anterior wall of the vagina.

6. The obturator internus muscle:

a) attaches to the medial surface of the obturator membrane.
b) has a tendon that enters the gluteal region inferior to the ischial spine.
c) is innervated by the first and second lumbar nerves.
d) contributes to the lateral wall of the ischioanal (ischiorectal) fossa.
e) attaches to the lesser trochanter of the femur.

7. Branches of the internal iliac artery in the female include:

a) the superior gluteal artery.
b) the ovarian artery.
c) the uterine artery.
d) the superior vesical artery.
e) the superior rectal artery.

8. The prostate:

a) is surrounded by a plexus of veins.
b) lies within the deep perineal pouch (space).
c) is pierced by the ejaculatory ducts.
d) lies posteroinferior to the base of the bladder.
e) is innervated by branches from the pudendal nerves.

9. The urinary bladder in the female:

a) has peritoneum on its anterior surface.
b) has the urachus attached to its apex.
c) has a rich parasympathetic nerve supply.
d) is drained by internal iliac lymph nodes.
e) is closely related to the body of the uterus.

10. The bulb of the penis:

a) is attached to the superior surface of the perineal membrane.
b) contains the penile urethra.
c) is compressed by the bulbospongiosus muscle.
d) receives blood from the deep artery of the penis.
e) continues as the corpus cavernosus.

11. The ductus (vas) deferens:

a) begins at the tail of the epididymis.
b) ascends within the spermatic cord.
c) passes above the ureter to reach the posterior aspect of the bladder.
d) terminates as an ampulla, which lies lateral to the seminal vesicle.
e) is innervated by the obturator nerve.

12. Regarding the hip bone:

a) the ischial spine gives attachment to the sacrospinous ligament.
b) the anterior superior iliac spine gives attachment to the inguinal ligament.
c) the obturator foramen is traversed by the nerve to obturator internus.
d) articulates with the sacrum by means of a synovial joint.
e) the lacunar ligament is attached to the pectineal line.

13. The uterine (fallopian) tube:

a) runs within the free border of the broad ligament of the uterus.
b) receives some of its arterial supply from the ovarian artery.
c) has a lumen which is narrowest where it pierces the uterine wall.
d) is closely related to the ureter.
e) opens directly into the peritoneal cavity.

14. The parasympathetic nerves of the pelvis:

a) arise from S2, S3 and S4 spinal cord segments.
b) ascend through the hypogastric plexus to supply the sigmoid colon.
c) are involved in the micturition reflex.
d) carry the nervous impulse responsible for ejaculation.
e) innervate the rectum.

15. The greater vestibular gland:

a) lies in the deep perineal pouch.
b) has a duct which opens into the vestibule of the vagina.
c) is closely related to the bulb of the vestibule.
d) is covered by bulbospongiosus.
e) lies in the labium majus.

16. Rupture of the penile bulbar urethra gives rise to extravasation of urine into:

a) the subcutaneous tissue of the scrotum.
b) the subcutaneous tissue of the penis.
c) the subcutaneous tissue of the thigh.
d) the subcutaneous tissue of the lower anterior abdominal wall.
e) the ischioanal (ischiorectal) fossa.

Clinical Skills

The answers are supplied on page 417.

Case Study 1

A woman of 30 went into labour at the end of her first pregnancy and was admitted to an obstetric unit. For the first few hours she was provided with pain relief by injections of analgesic and the inhalation of an oxygen/nitrous oxide mixture. But after 10 hours of uterine contraction it was decided she was making insufficient progress and the baby should be delivered by forceps. The obstetrician told her he was going to anaesthetize her birth canal by means of two injections and he proceeded to carry out bilateral pudendal blocks. Using a special needle he palpated for features of the patient's bony pelvis from within the vagina in order to place the anaesthetic fluid near the pudendal nerves.

Questions:

1. What cutaneous structures does the pudendal nerve innervate?
2. What bony features did the obstetrician palpate?

Case Study 2

A woman of 25 was brought to her family doctor one morning because she had woken up feeling weak and had fainted soon after getting up. She had had a poor night's sleep because of vague lower abdominal pains. The doctor could find very little when he examined her abdomen apart from suprapubic tenderness on the right side. However, he was worried about her and arranged for admission into hospital. There she was given an intravenous drip and closely observed. A gynaecologist examined her and performed a vaginal examination. He asked her whether she had any pain in her neck or shoulders. Three hours after admission she had an emergency operation. The right uterine tube was found to contain a pregnancy which had ruptured. This was removed as was a large volume of blood and clot in the peritoneal cavity. A blood transfusion was given.

Questions:

1. Explain the abdominal tenderness noted by the family doctor.
2. What might the gynaecologist have noted during the vaginal examination?
3. Why did the gynaecologist ask about pain in the neck and shoulders?

Case Study 3

A woman of 30 with three children, aged six years, three years and four months, complains of incontinence of urine when she laughs. Only a small amount of urine escapes on each occasion but it is distressing her. Questioning reveals she has also passed urine involuntarily when coughing or when lifting the baby. She is worried she might need an operation. After excluding an infection in the bladder her doctor refers her to a nurse who specializes in incontinence to see whether non-operative treatment might be successful. The nurse tells the patient that exercises may solve the problem. She explains how to do the exercises and encourages her to perform them several times a day.

Questions:

1. In terms of physics and anatomy what makes any person of either sex continent of urine?
2. What are the most important structures contributing to urinary continence in women?
3. Why are women rather prone to this complaint?
4. Which nerves stimulate contraction of the smooth muscle of the bladder wall?

Case Study 4

A man of 60 consulted his doctor because he had noticed blood in his stools. The doctor suspected cancer of the colon or rectum and proceeded to examine his neck, chest and abdomen. He did a rectal examination and referred the man to a surgeon for a further opinion. The specialist did a similar examination, carefully percussed the abdomen and ordered a number of investigations including a chest radiograph, blood tests for liver function, sigmoidoscopy and barium enema.

Questions:

1. Why did the doctor examine the man's neck?
2. Why did the surgeon percuss the abdomen?
3. Rectal cancer can invade any structure directly related to the rectum in both sexes. Which structures could become involved in this way?

Observation Skills

Identify the structures indicated. The answers are supplied at the foot of the page.

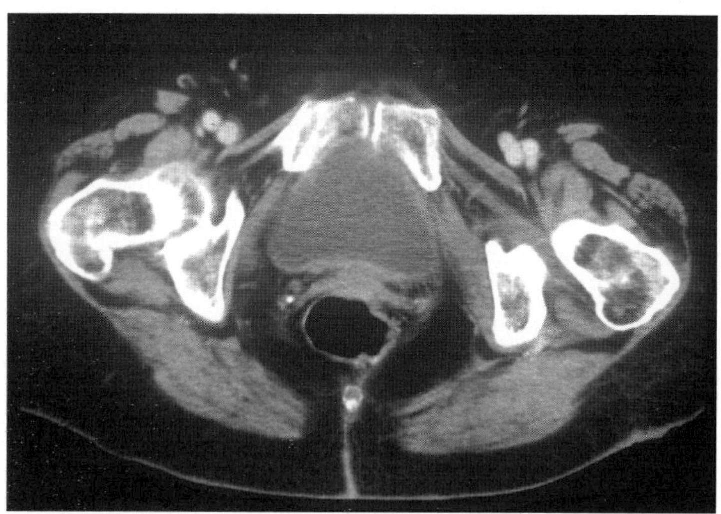

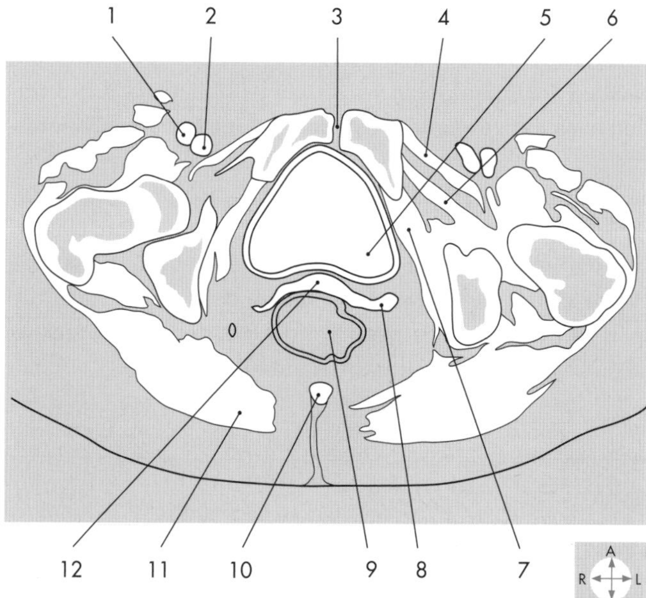

Fig. 5.42 Transverse CT image at the level of the pubic symphysis. Compare Fig. 5.44.

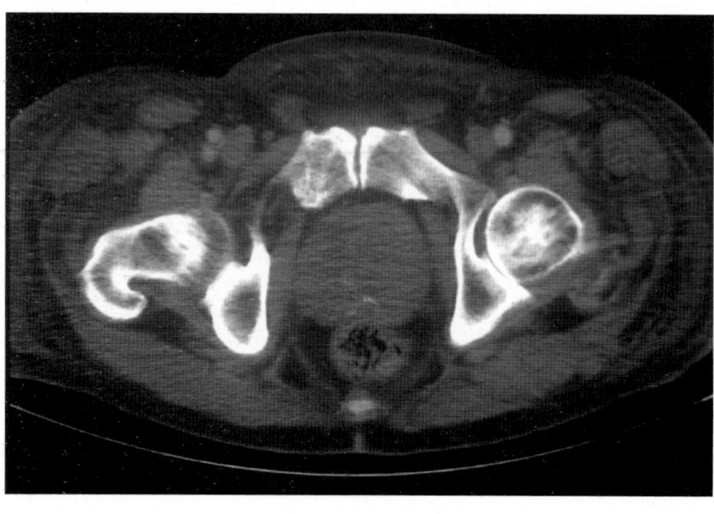

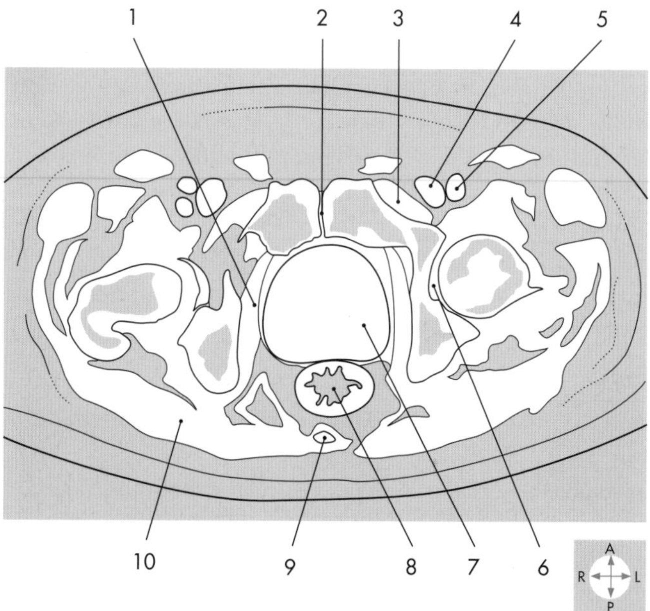

Fig. 5.43 Transverse CT image at the level of the pubic symphysis. Compare Fig. 5.46.

Answers

Fig. 5.42 1 = femoral artery; 2 = femoral vein; 3 = pubic symphysis; 4 = pectineus; 5 = urinary bladder (distended); 6 = obturator externus; 7 = obturator internus; 8 = uterine tube; 9 = rectum (distended); 10 = coccyx; 11 = gluteus maximus; 12 = fundus of uterus.

Answers

Fig. 5.43 1 = obturator internus; 2 = pubic symphysis; 3 = pectineus; 4 = femoral vein; 5 = femoral artery; 6 = acetabular fossa; 7 = prostate (enlarged); 8 = anal canal; 9 = coccyx; 10 = gluteus maximus.

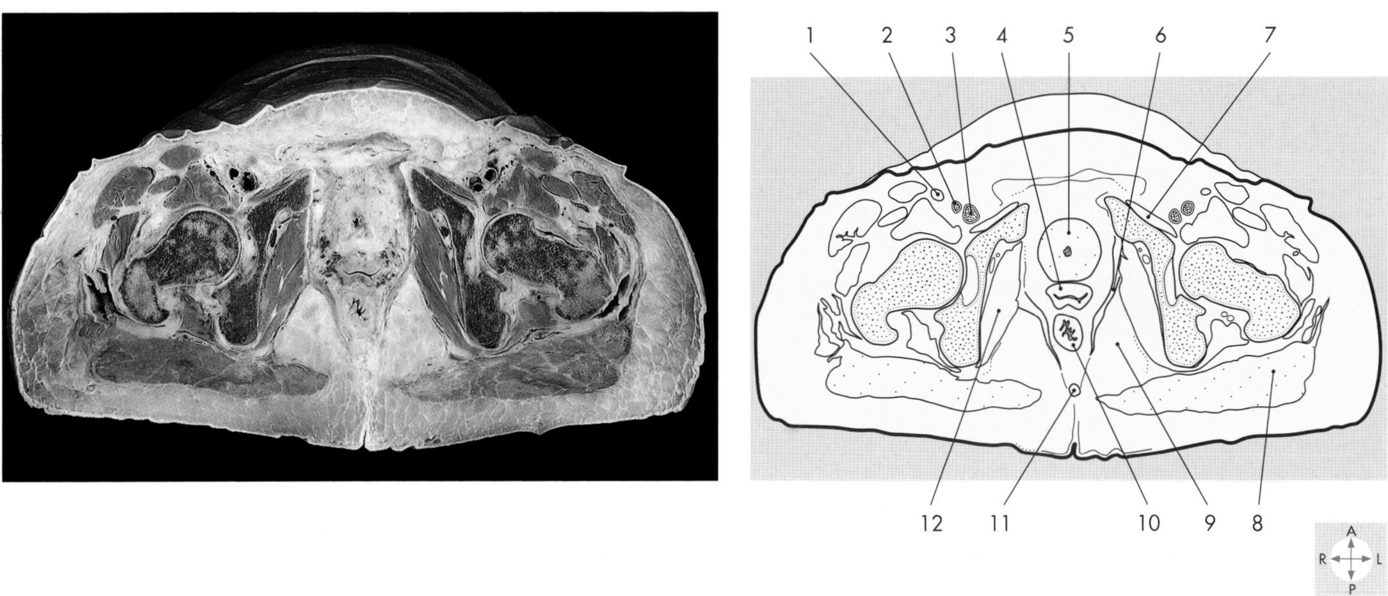

Fig. 5.44 Transverse section just superior to the level of the pubic symphysis. Inferior aspect. Compare Fig. 5.42.

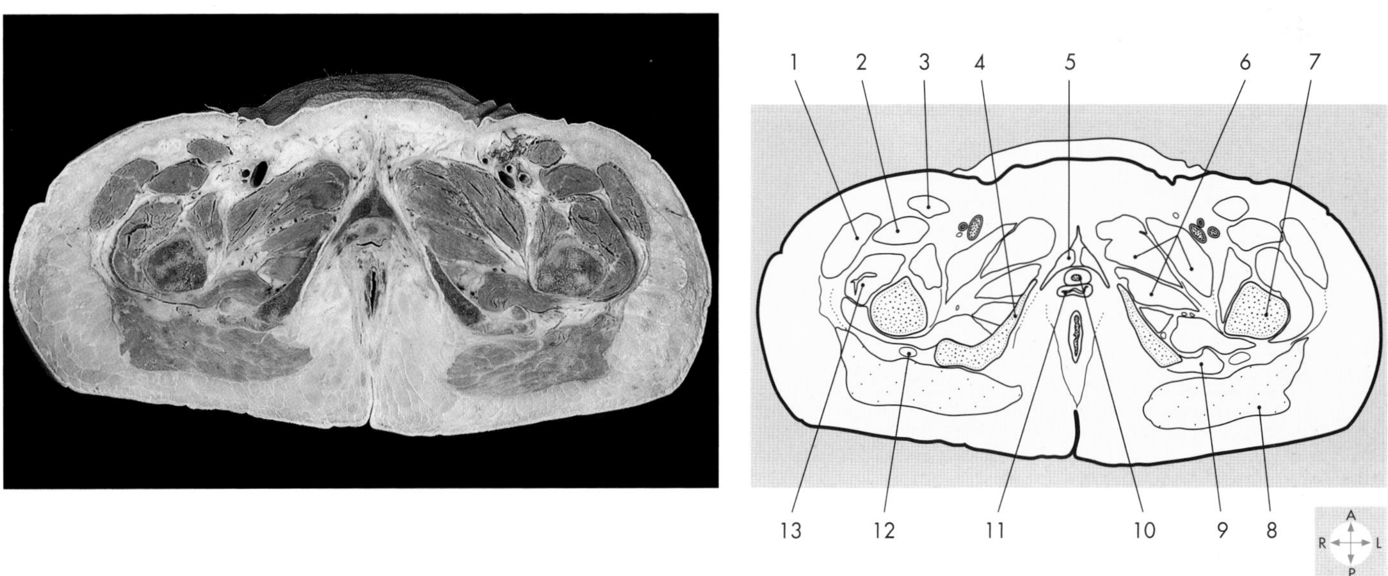

Fig. 5.45 Transverse section at the level of the ischiopubic rami. Inferior aspect.

Answers

Fig. 5.44 1 = femoral nerve; 2 = femoral artery; 3 = femoral vein; 4 = vagina; 5 = neck of bladder; 6 = levator ani; 7 = pectineus; 8 = gluteus maximus; 9 = ischioanal fossa; 10 = anal canal; 11 = coccyx; 12 = obturator internus.

Answers

Fig. 5.45 1 = tensor fasciae latae; 2 = rectus femoris; 3 = sartorius; 4 = ischiopubic ramus; 5 = crus of clitoris; 6 = adductor muscles; 7 = shaft of femur; 8 = gluteus maximus; 9 = tendons of hamstring muscles; 10 = urethra; 11 = vagina; 12 = sciatic nerve; 13 = vastus lateralis.

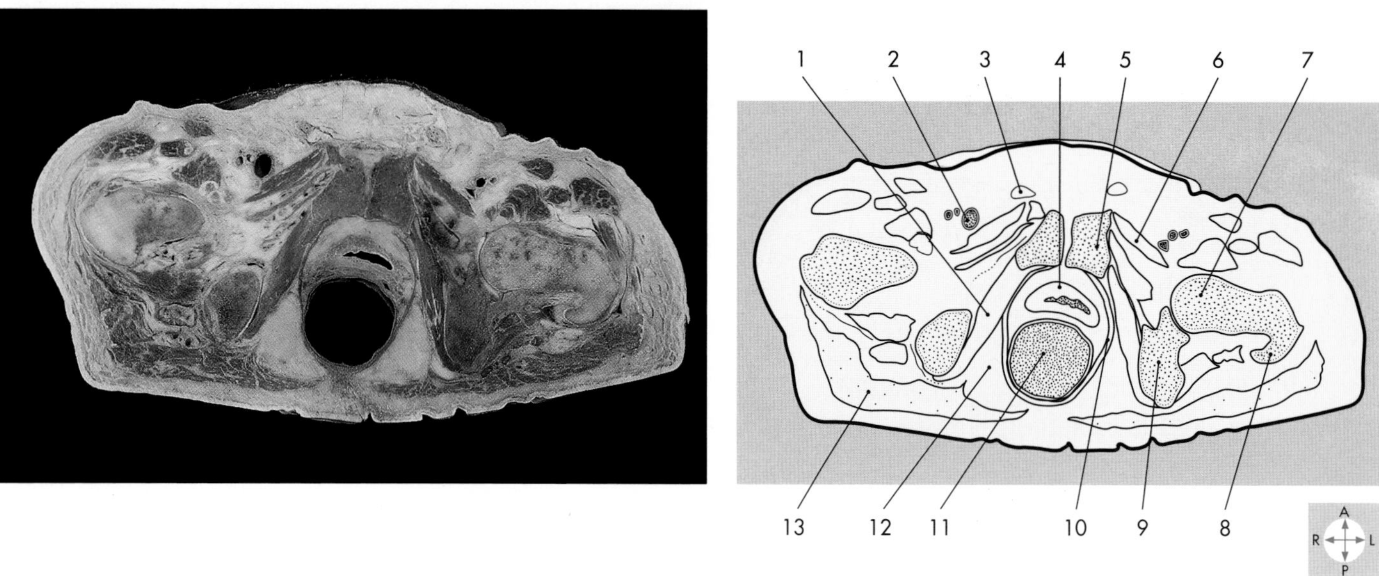

Fig. 5.46 Transverse section at the level of the pubic symphysis. Inferior aspect. Compare Fig. 5.43.

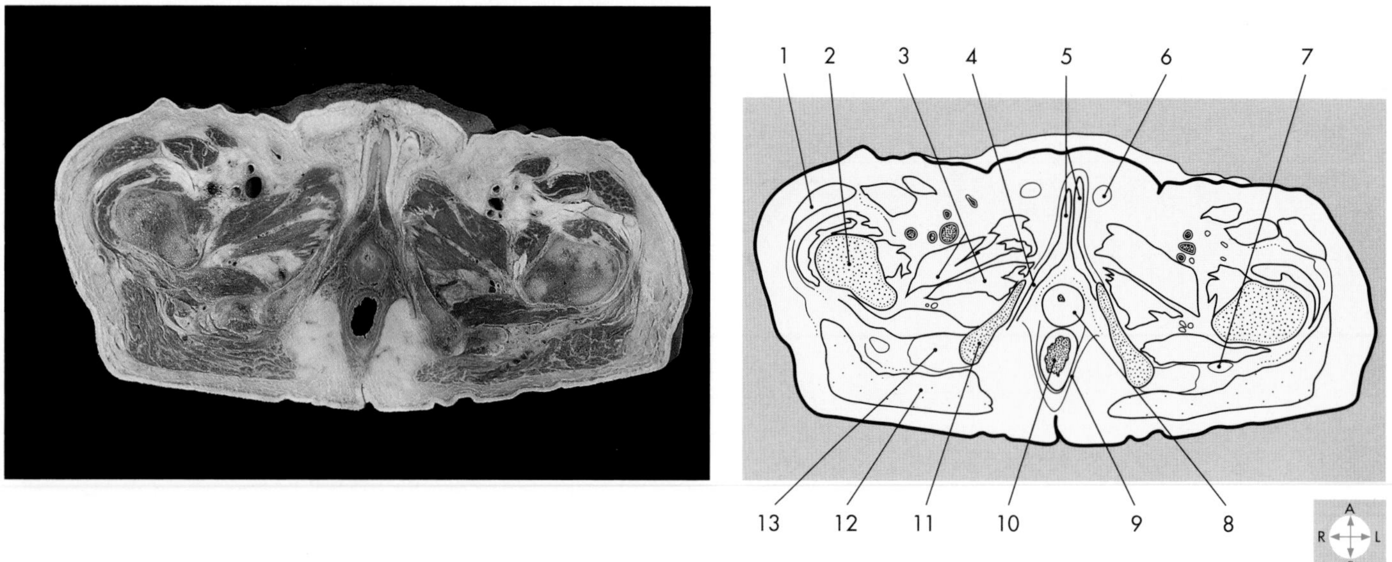

Fig. 5.47 Transverse section at the level of the ischiopubic rami. Inferior aspect.

Answers

Fig. 5.46 1 = obturator internus; 2 = femoral vein; 3 = spermatic cord; 4 = neck of bladder; 5 = pubis; 6 = pectineus; 7 = head of femur; 8 = greater trochanter; 9 = ischial tuberosity; 10 = levator ani; 11 = rectum (distended); 12 = ischioanal fossa; 13 = gluteus maximus.

Answers

Fig. 5.47 1 = tensor fasciae latae; 2 = femur; 3 = adductor muscles; 4 = crus of penis; 5 = corpora cavernosa; 6 = spermatic cord; 7 = sciatic nerve; 8 = bulb of penis; 9 = levator ani; 10 = anal canal; 11 = ischiopubic ramus; 12 = gluteus maximus; 13 = tendons of hamstring muscles.

Lower limb

CHAPTER 6

Introduction

The lower limb supports the body during standing and locomotion. The hip (coxal) bone (Fig. 6.1) provides attachment for muscles of the buttock and thigh, which link the limb to the trunk. The hip joint, between the acetabulum of the hip bone and the head of the femur, is multiaxial and provides versatility of movement.

The femur (Fig. 6.1) is surrounded by the muscles of the thigh and buttock. Its lower end with the patella and upper end of the tibia form the knee joint, a hinge joint. The tibia and fibula, surrounded by the leg muscles, form at their lower ends a socket which articulates with the talus at the ankle joint, also a hinge.

The foot contains three groups of bones: the tarsals posteriorly, the metatarsals more anteriorly and the phalanges within the toes. The skeleton of the foot is adapted for bipedal standing and walking.

The limb is covered by skin, subcutaneous tissue containing vessels and nerves, and by deep fascia. Intermuscular septa separate the muscles into different compartments (Figs 6.2 & 6.3). Each compartment contains muscles with common actions and is supplied by a neurovascular bundle. The thigh has anterior, posterior and medial compartments, whereas the leg has anterior, posterior and lateral compartments. The foot has only two: the dorsum and the sole.

The principal vessels and nerves enter the limb from the abdomen or pelvis by three different routes (Fig. 6.4): posterior to the inguinal ligament from the abdomen to the anterior compartment of the thigh; through the obturator canal between the pelvis and the medial compartment of the thigh; via the greater sciatic foramen, where the pelvis communicates with the gluteal region.

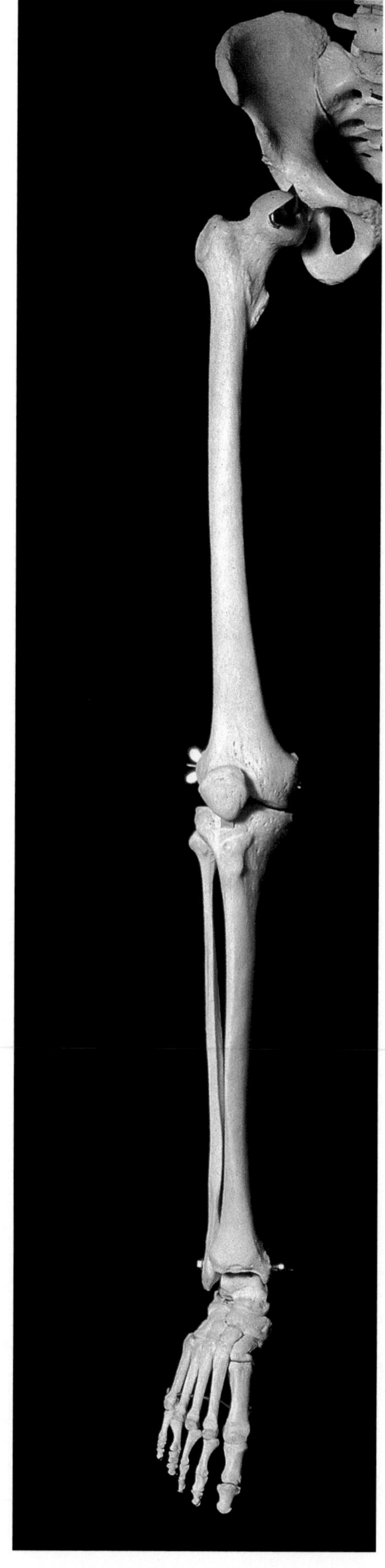

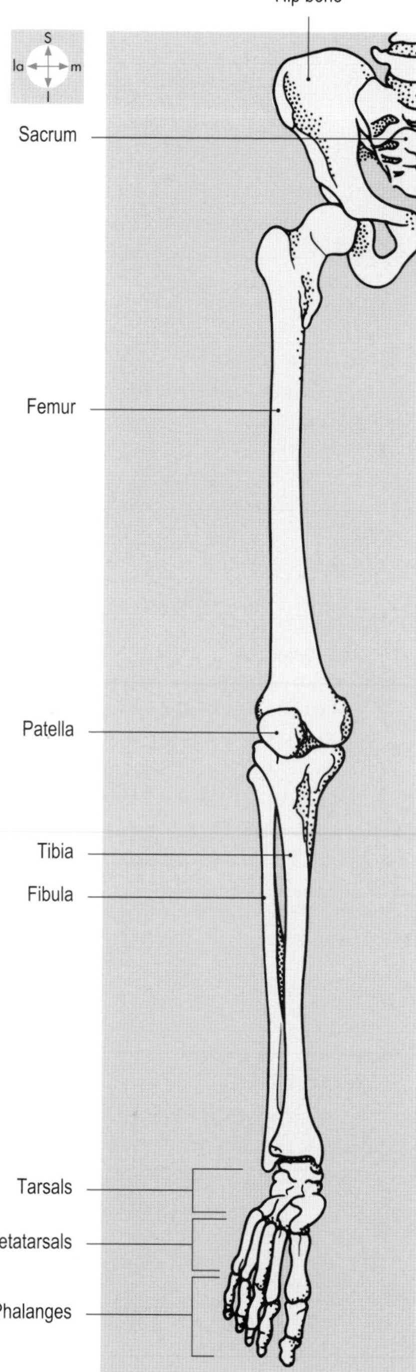

Fig. 6.1 The skeleton of the lower limb.

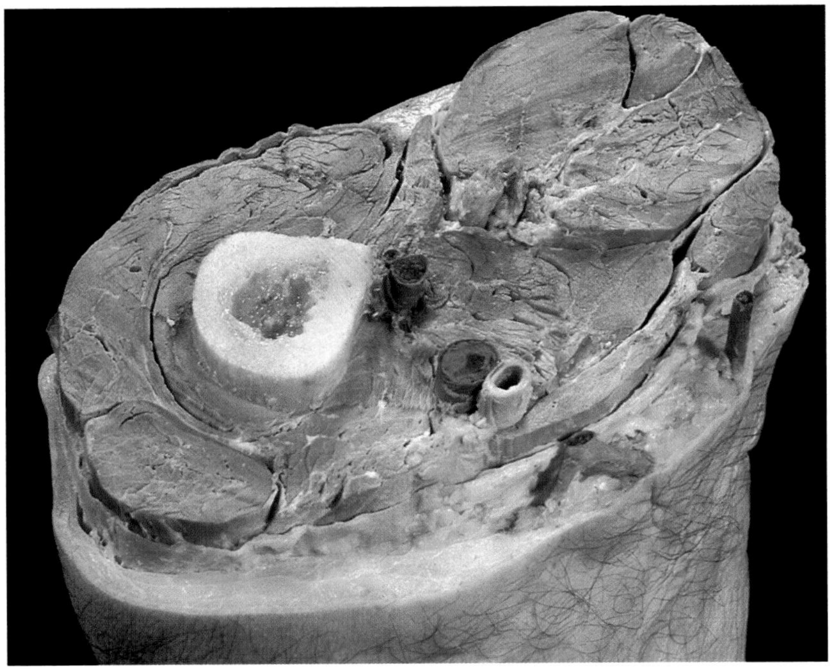

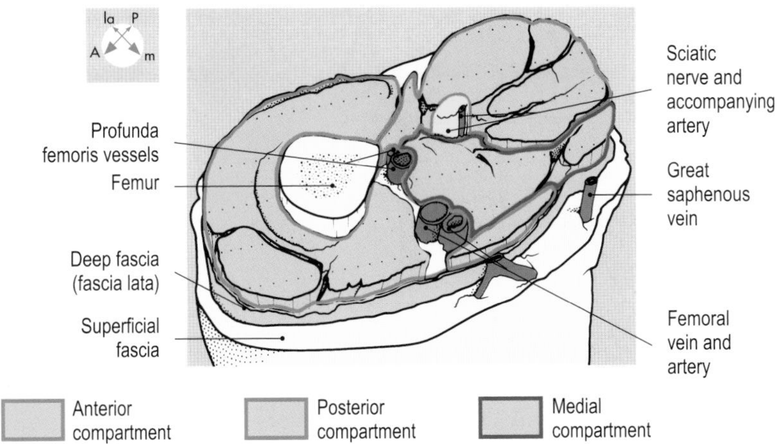

Fig. 6.2 'Step' dissection through the midthigh, showing the relationships of the compartments.

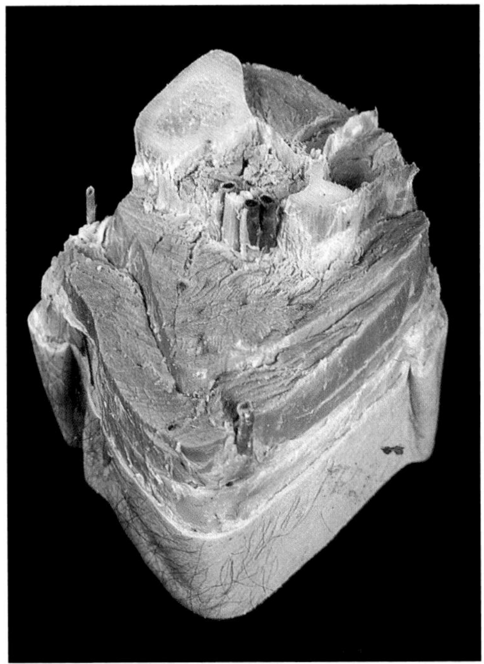

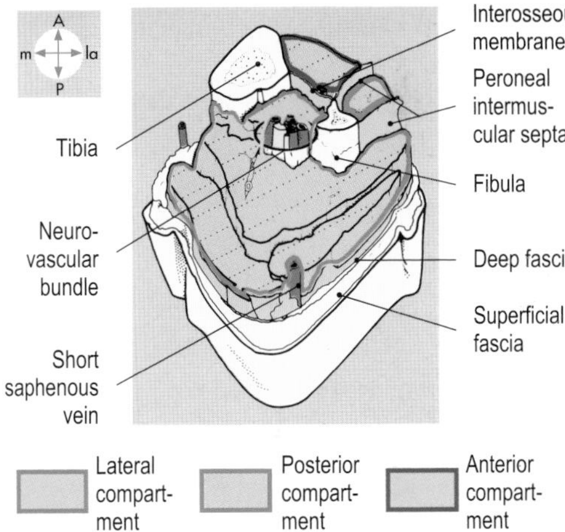

Fig. 6.3 'Step' dissection through the midcalf, showing the relationships of the compartments.

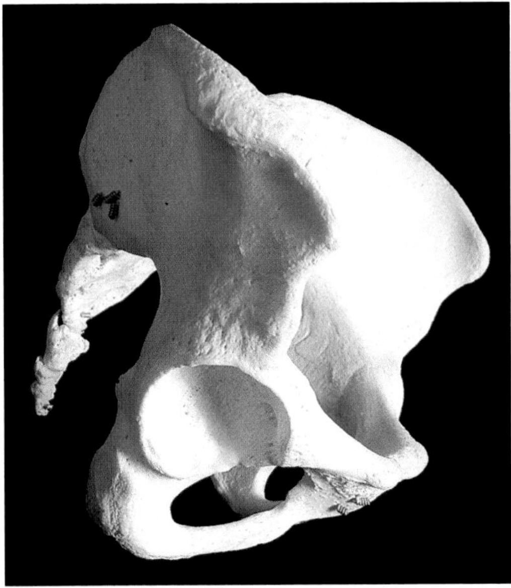

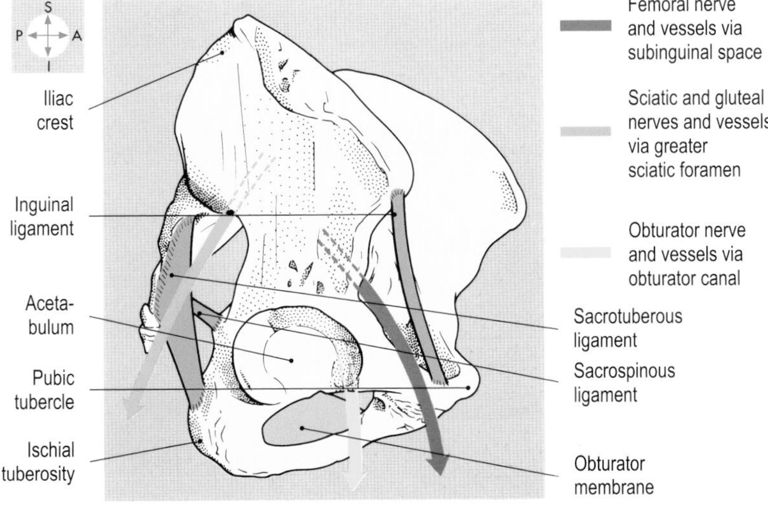

Fig. 6.4 Sites of access of the principal nerves and vessels from the abdomen and pelvis into the root of the lower limb.

Superior and inferior gluteal arteries from the internal iliac artery supply the gluteal region. However, the main supply to the limb is provided by the continuation of the external iliac artery, the femoral artery (Fig. 6.5). This traverses the anterior compartment of the thigh and passes behind the knee to become the popliteal artery, which divides into anterior and posterior tibial branches. The anterior tibial artery passes into the anterior compartment of the leg and continues onto the dorsum of the foot as the dorsalis pedis artery. The posterior tibial artery traverses the posterior compartment of the leg and divides into medial and lateral plantar arteries which supply the sole (plantar compartment) of the foot. Anastomoses occur between arteries in the sole and on the dorsum of the foot.

The superficial and deep veins are linked by communicating (perforating) veins. The superficial veins arise in the foot from the dorsal venous arch (Fig. 6.6). Medially, the great saphenous vein ascends the leg and thigh and drains into the femoral vein just below the inguinal ligament. From the lateral side of the foot the short saphenous vein passes behind the ankle and across the calf to enter the popliteal vein. Deep veins begin distally as venae comitantes, which unite to form the popliteal vein (Fig. 6.6). This becomes the femoral vein in the thigh and continues deep to the

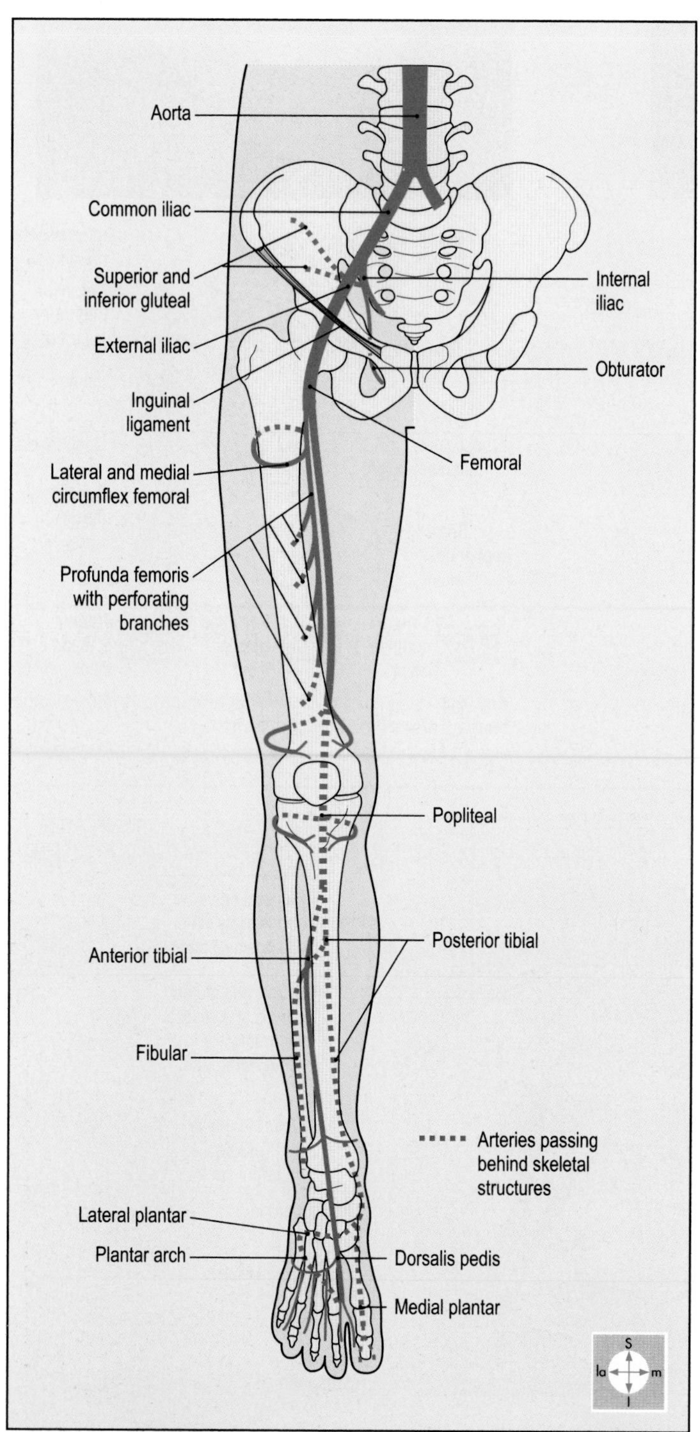

Fig. 6.5 Principal arteries of the lower limb.

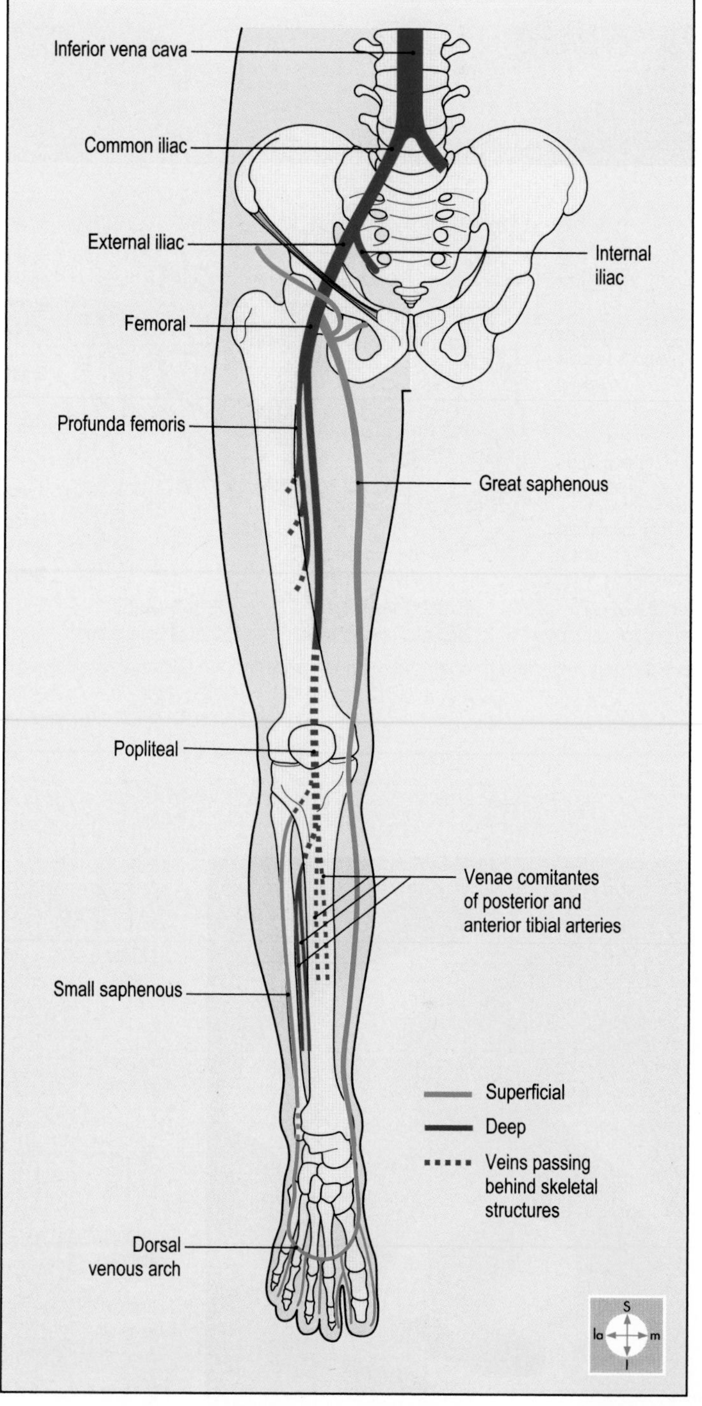

Fig. 6.6 Veins of the lower limb.

inguinal ligament as the external iliac vein. Gluteal veins accompany the corresponding arteries and drain into the internal iliac vein.

There are both superficial and deep lymphatics. The superficial lymphatics accompany the superficial veins. Those with the great saphenous vein terminate in superficial inguinal nodes (Fig. 6.7), which drain into deep inguinal nodes. Lymphatics following the short saphenous vein drain into nodes in the popliteal fossa. The deep lymphatics accompany arteries in the muscle compartments. Those from the leg and foot drain into the popliteal nodes whence lymphatics ascend with the femoral artery to the deep inguinal nodes whose efferents pass to the external iliac group.

The nerves of the lower limb are derived from the lumbar and sacral plexuses. The femoral nerve supplies the anterior compartment of the thigh while the obturator nerve innervates the medial compartment (Fig. 6.8). The sciatic nerve and its branches supply the posterior compartment of the thigh and all compartments of the leg and foot.

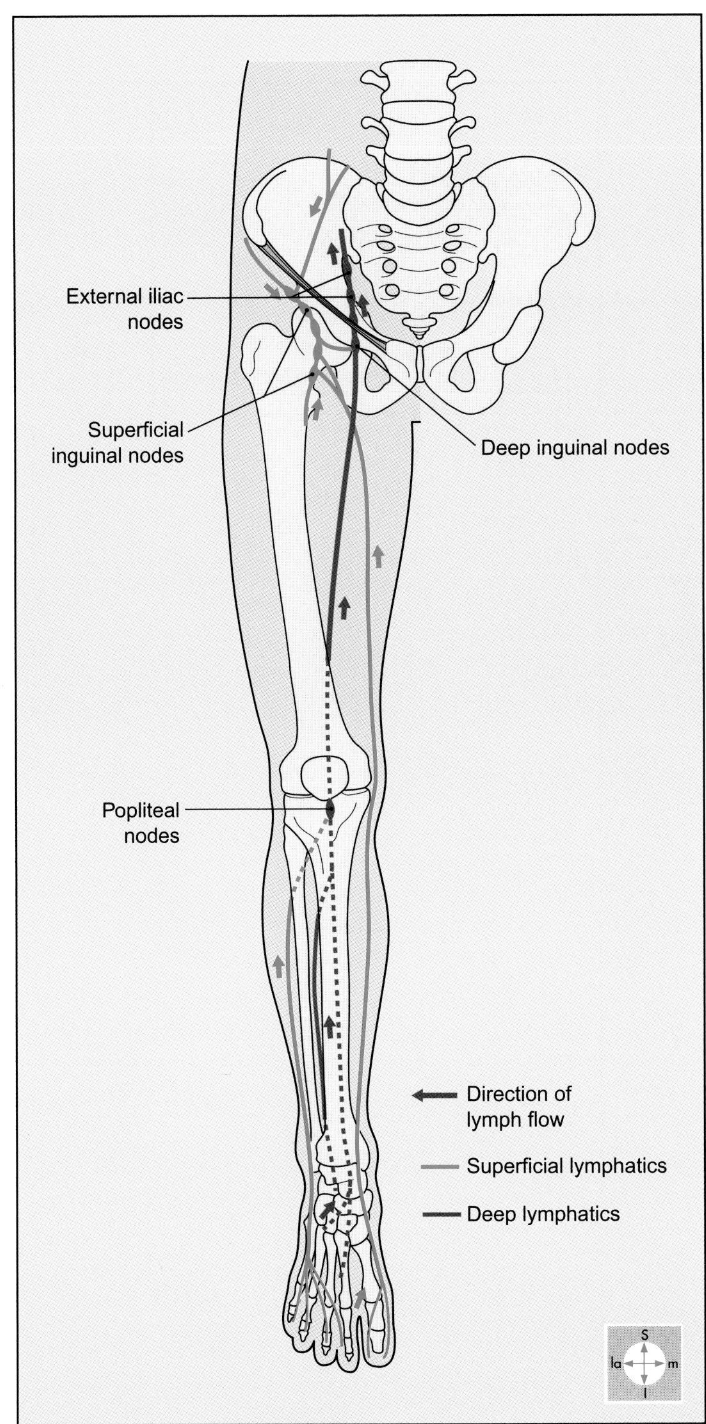

Fig. 6.7 Lymphatics and lymph nodes of the lower limb.

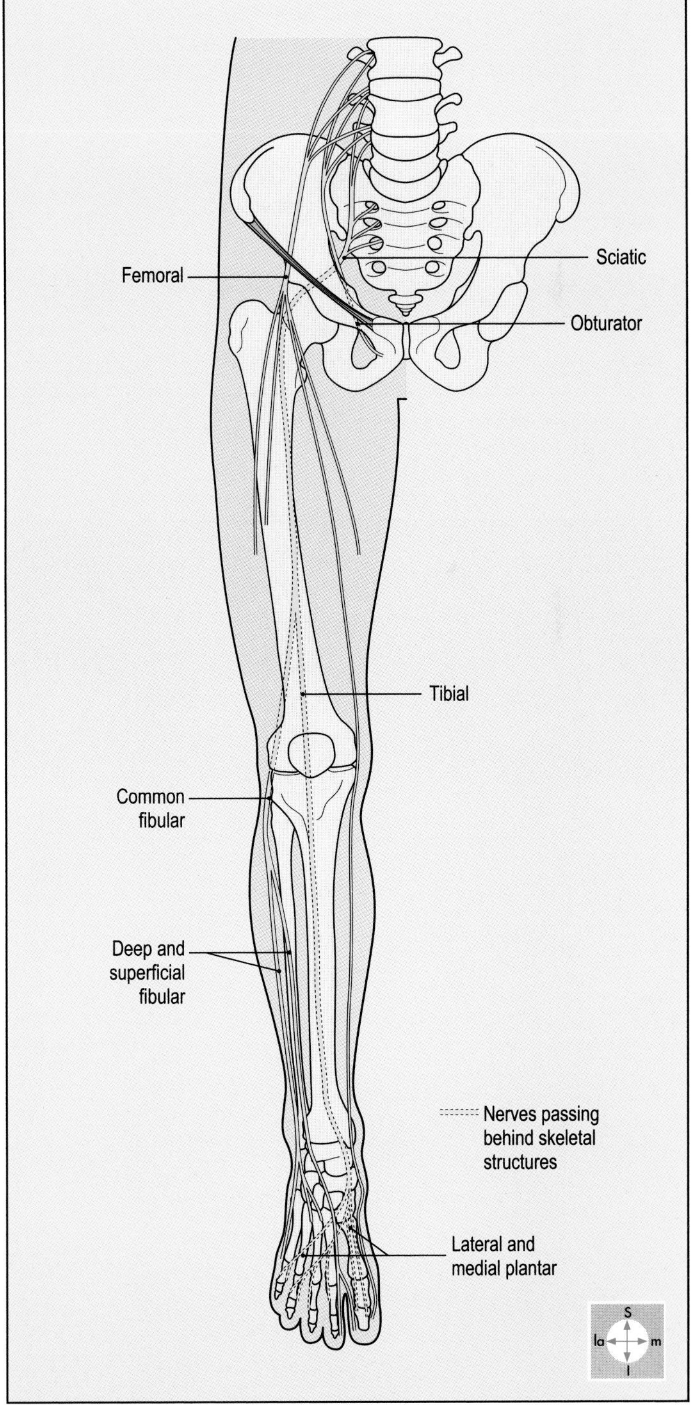

Fig. 6.8 Principal nerves of the lower limb.

Cutaneous nerves (Fig. 6.9) supply areas of skin which vary between individuals. The territories supplied by adjacent nerves overlap and therefore damage to a single nerve usually produces anaesthesia confined to the central part of the area supplied. The dermatome distribution is shown in Figure 6.10. There is some overlap of dermatomes except along the axial lines.

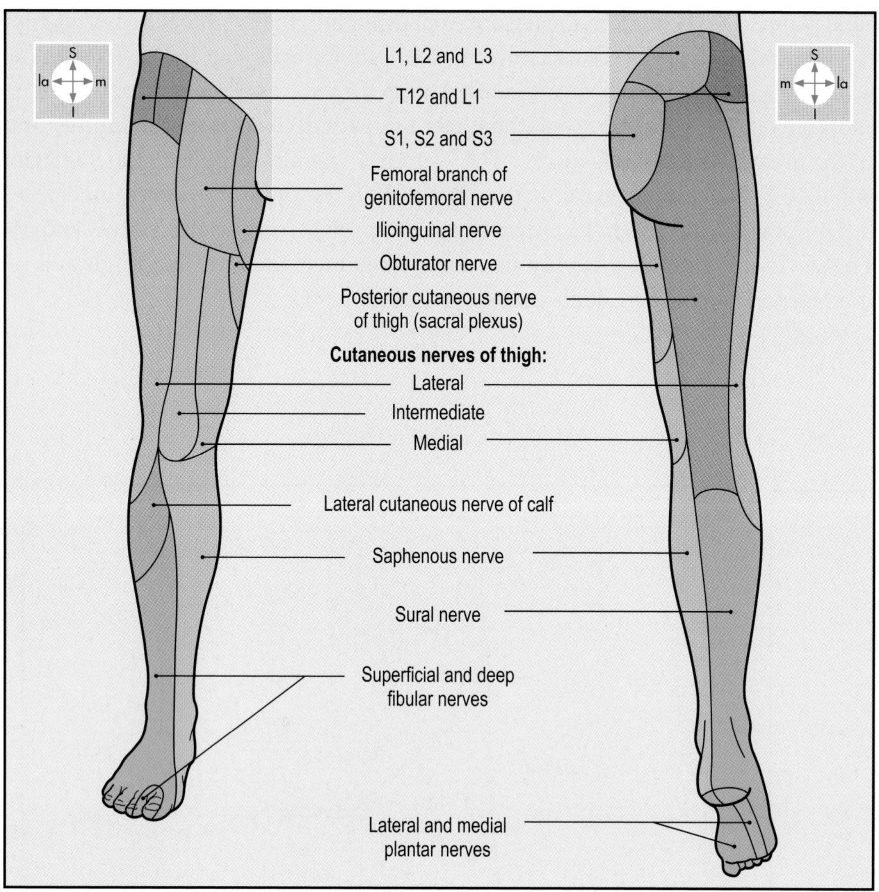

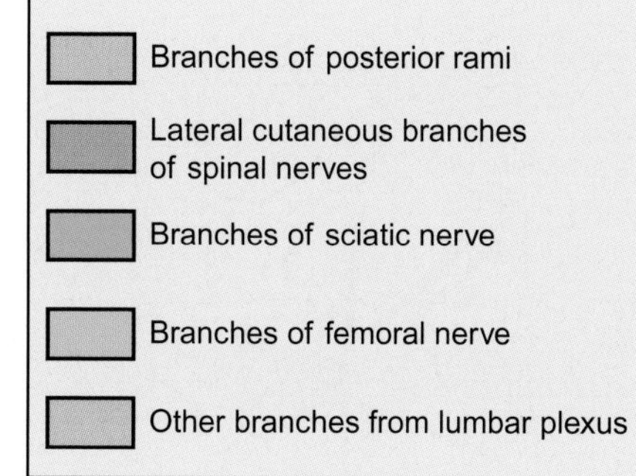

Fig. 6.9 Areas of distribution of cutaneous nerves in the lower limb.

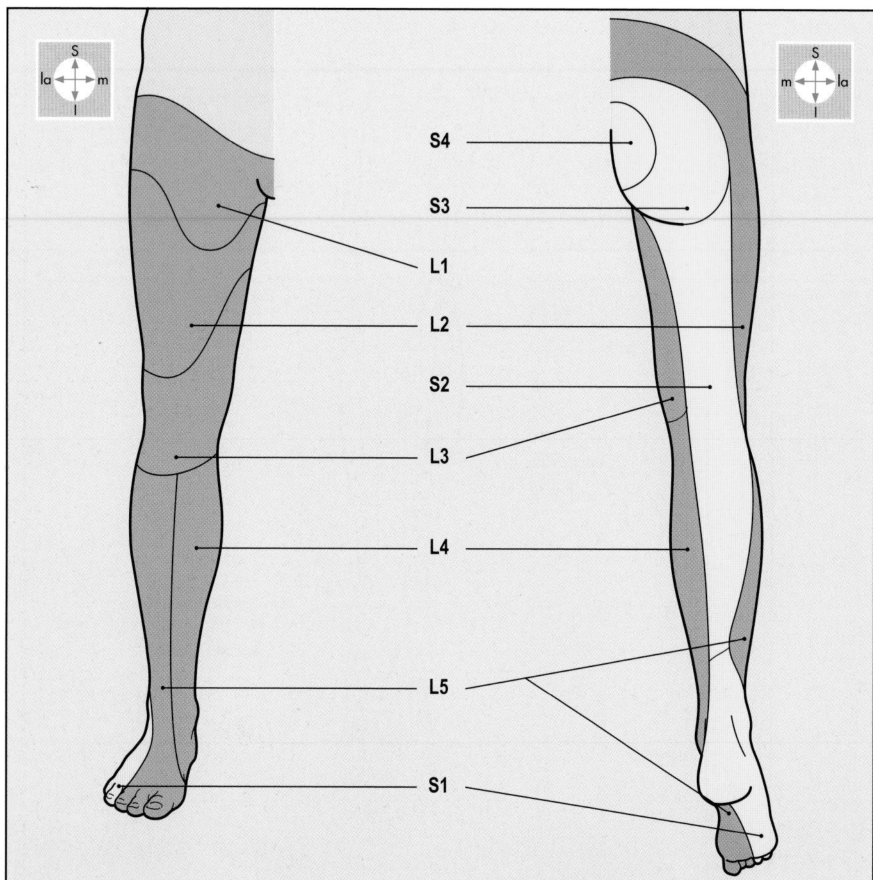

Fig. 6.10 The dermatomes of the lower limb.

Anterior Compartment of Thigh

The anterior compartment is the largest in the thigh, occupying the region between the inguinal ligament and the knee. Lateral and anteromedial intermuscular septa separate the contents from the posterior (hamstring) and medial (adductor) compartments respectively (see Fig. 6.2). The anterior compartment (see Fig. 6.12) contains quadriceps femoris, sartorius and the tendon of iliopsoas, and is innervated by the femoral nerve. The femoral artery and vein, the principal vessels of the lower limb, traverse the compartment and leave via the opening in adductor magnus to gain the popliteal fossa.

Subcutaneous tissue (superficial fascia)

The subcutaneous tissue contains the great (long) saphenous vein and its tributaries with their accompanying arteries, superficial inguinal lymph nodes and cutaneous nerves. The great saphenous vein ascends on the medial side of the thigh (Fig. 6.11) and passes through the saphenous opening in the fascia lata to empty into the femoral vein. The great saphenous vein drains the superficial tissues of the entire limb except the lateral side of the leg and foot. Near its termination the vein receives tributaries which drain the buttock, the perineum and the abdominal wall below the umbilicus. These tributaries are accompanied by corresponding branches of the femoral artery.

The superficial inguinal lymph nodes, often palpable in the living, lie just distal and parallel to the inguinal ligament and adjacent to the termination of the great saphenous vein (Fig. 6.11). These nodes receive lymph from the same superficial tissues as those drained by the great saphenous vein and its tributaries. Efferent lymphatics from the superficial nodes pass through the fascia lata and drain into the

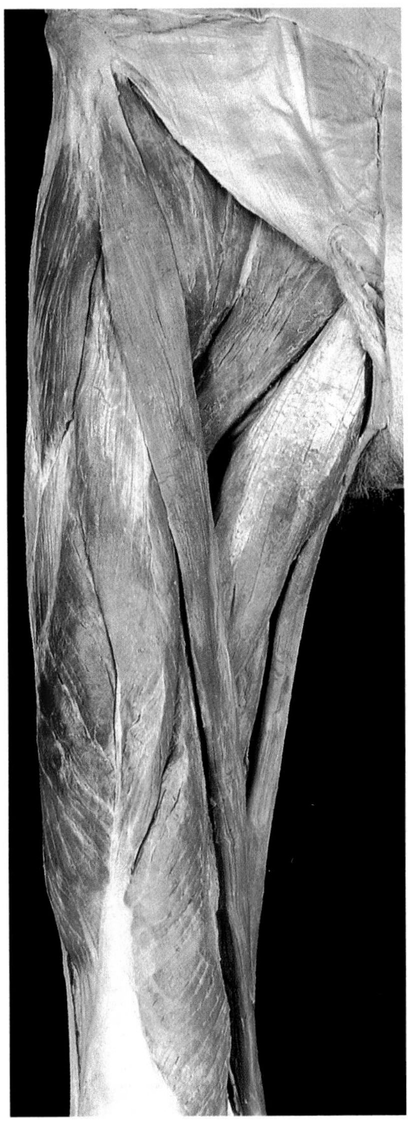

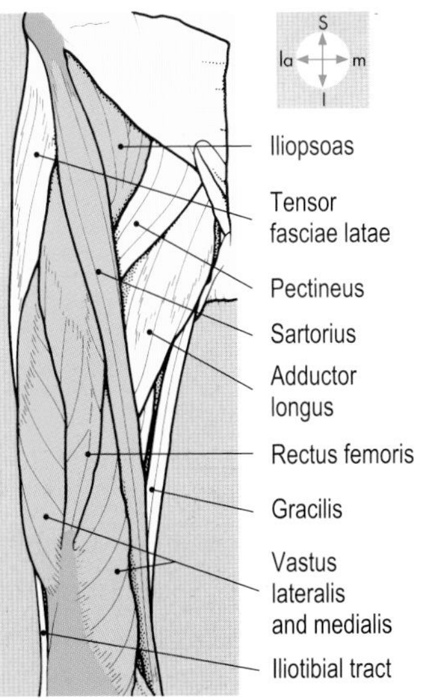

Fig. 6.12 Muscles of the anterior compartment of thigh after removal of the skin and fascia lata.

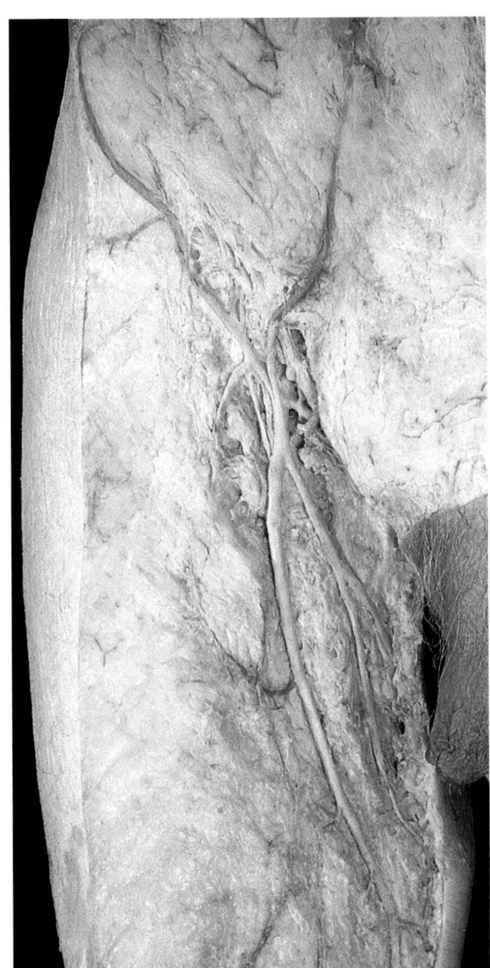

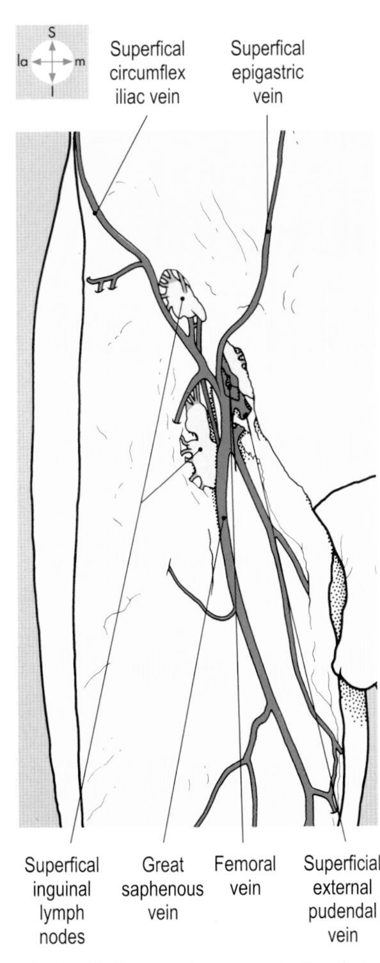

Fig. 6.11 Great saphenous vein, its tributaries and the superficial inguinal lymph nodes lying in subcutaneous tissue.

deep inguinal nodes within the femoral triangle and femoral canal where nodes are a focal point in lymphatic drainage of the lower limb (see p. 257).

The lateral cutaneous nerve of the thigh (L2 & L3) (see Fig. 6.17) pierces the inguinal ligament close to the anterior superior iliac spine where it may become entrapped, causing pain in the thigh. It supplies skin as far as the knee. The intermediate and medial cutaneous nerves of the thigh arise from the femoral nerve and supply the anterior and medial surfaces of the thigh. Usually, the obturator nerve gives a cutaneous supply to the medial side of the thigh. The femoral branch of the genitofemoral nerve (L1 & L2) passes beneath the inguinal ligament to supply skin over the femoral triangle, and the ilioinguinal nerve emerges through the superficial inguinal ring to supply the adjacent medial aspect of the thigh.

Fascia lata

The fascia lata (deep fascia) completely invests the thigh, providing attachment for muscles and associated intermuscular septa in the anterior compartment. It attaches superiorly to the inguinal ligament and iliac crest, and inferiorly is continuous with the deep fascia of the leg. Below and lateral to the pubic tubercle is the saphenous opening, which transmits the terminal part of the long saphenous vein.

Over the lateral aspect of the thigh the fascia lata is particularly thick, forming the iliotibial tract. Gluteus maximus and tensor fasciae latae are attached to its upper part (see Fig. 6.30).

Muscles

Quadriceps femoris

The four parts of quadriceps femoris, namely rectus femoris, vastus lateralis, vastus intermedius and vastus medialis, cover the front and sides of the femur (Figs 6.12, 6.13 & 6.14). Rectus femoris is attached by a straight head to the anterior inferior iliac spine and by a reflected head to the ilium above the acetabulum.

Vastus lateralis attaches to the intertrochanteric line, the lateral lip of the linea aspera and the lateral supracondylar ridge of the femur (Figs 6.15 & 6.16). Vastus intermedius attaches to the upper two-thirds of the anterior and lateral surfaces of the femoral shaft, whilst vastus medialis anchors to the spiral line and medial lip of the linea aspera. Distally, these four muscles form a common tendon which attaches to the upper border (base) of the patella. From the lower border (apex) of the patella the tendon continues as the patellar ligament (see Fig. 6.75) to attach to the tibial tubercle.

Quadriceps femoris is a powerful antigravity muscle, extending the knee joint during standing, walking and running. In addition, rectus femoris flexes the hip. The lower fibres of vastus medialis stabilize the position of the patella (see p. 300). Quadriceps femoris is supplied by branches of the femoral nerve.

Sartorius

This strap-like muscle is attached proximally to the anterior superior iliac spine and descends obliquely across the thigh (see Fig. 6.12), crosses the posteromedial side of the knee and, with gracilis and semitendinosus, attaches to the upper end of the subcutaneous surface of the tibia (see Fig. 6.79). Sartorius flexes and laterally rotates the hip and flexes the knee. It is supplied by the femoral nerve.

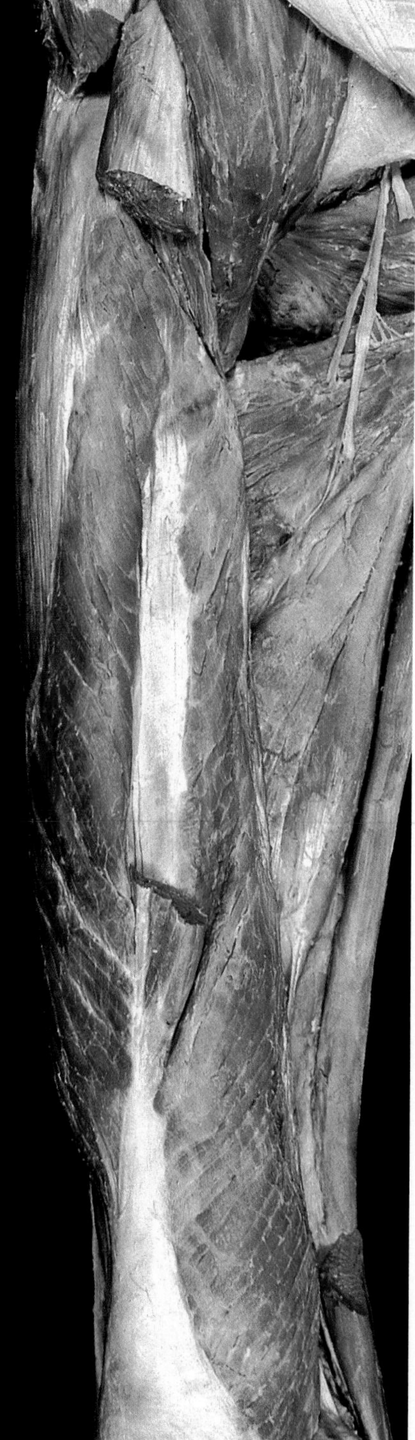

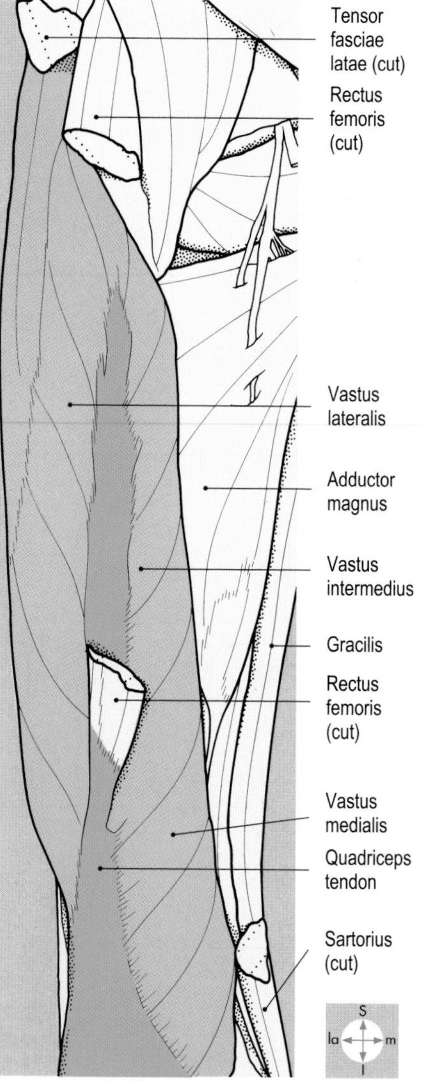

Fig. 6.13 Quadriceps femoris. Vastus intermedius is partially revealed by removal of rectus femoris. Pectineus and adductors longus and brevis have been excised.

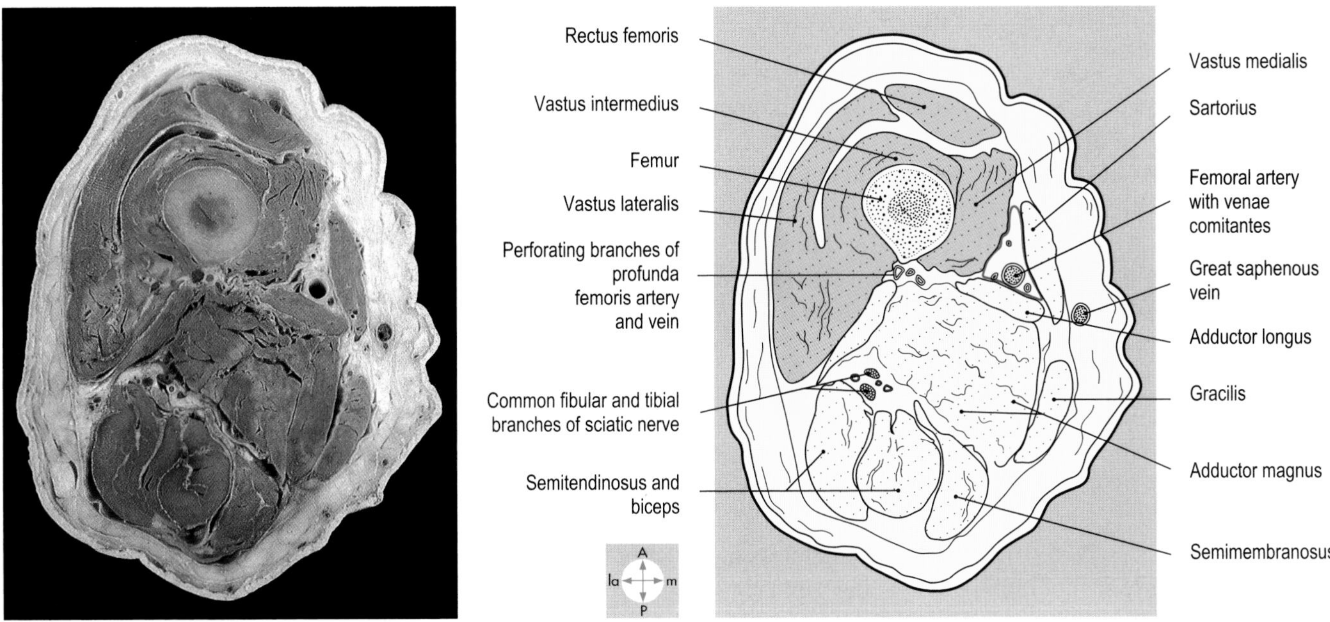

Fig. 6.14 Transverse section through the thigh to show the adductor canal (pink) and components of quadriceps femoris. Inferior aspect.

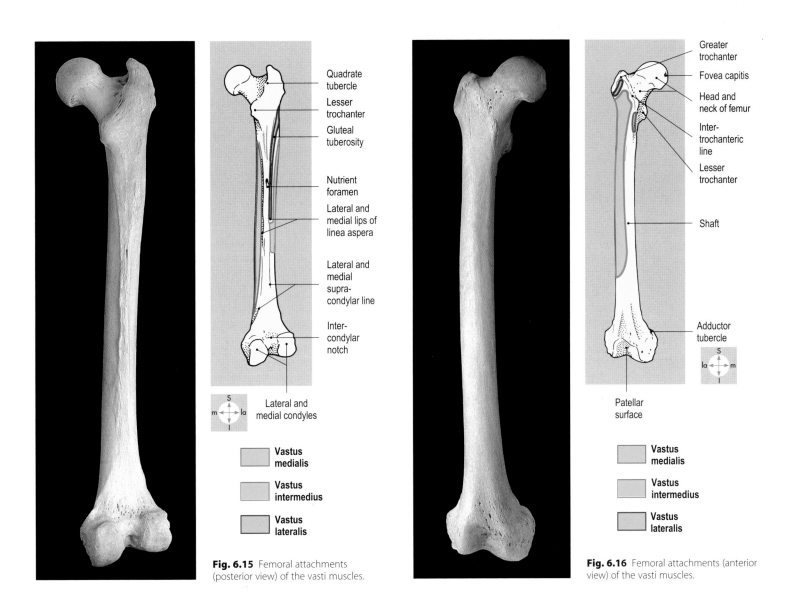

Fig. 6.15 Femoral attachments (posterior view) of the vasti muscles.

Fig. 6.16 Femoral attachments (anterior view) of the vasti muscles.

Femoral triangle

The femoral triangle occupies the upper medial part of the anterior compartment of the thigh. Its upper boundary is the inguinal ligament; its lateral limit is the medial border of sartorius and its medial boundary is the medial border of adductor longus (some authors use the lateral border in their definition). The roof is fascia lata and the floor comprises iliopsoas, pectineus and adductor longus (Fig. 6.17). The triangle contains the femoral vessels and nerve, and the deep inguinal lymph nodes.

Adductor (subsartorial) canal

This canal is an intermuscular space linking the femoral triangle with the popliteal fossa. Triangular in cross-section, it lies beneath sartorius, occupying the groove between vastus medialis and adductor longus, and at its lower end adductor magnus (see Fig. 6.14). Through the canal run the femoral artery and vein, and nerve to vastus medialis and the saphenous nerve (Fig. 6.18).

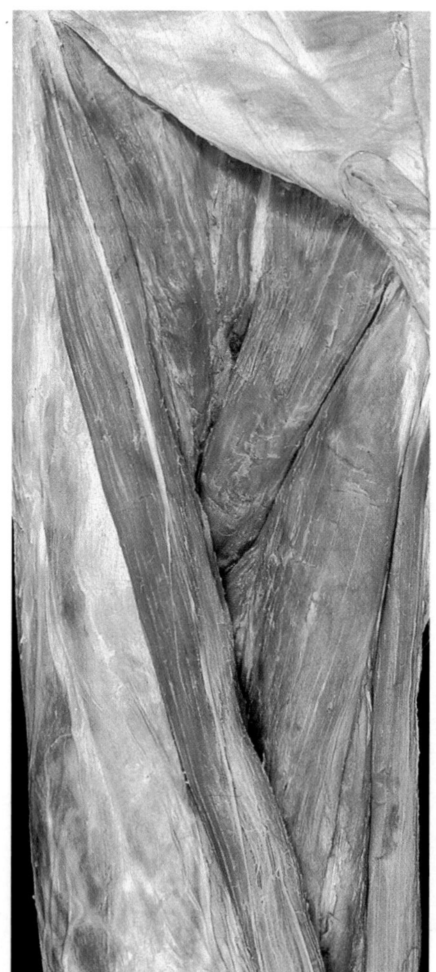

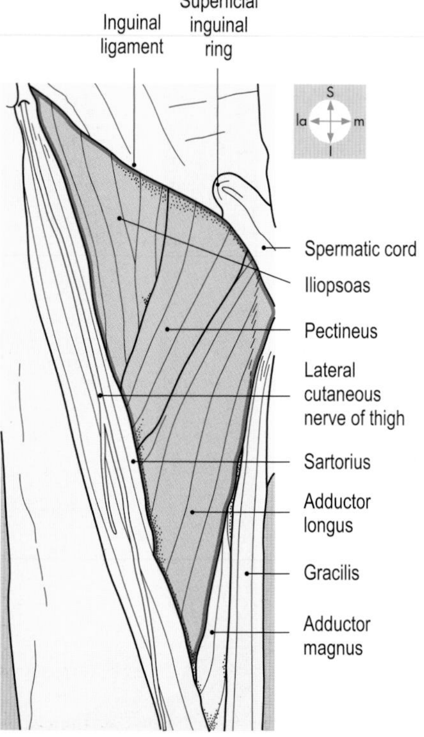

Fig. 6.17 Boundaries and floor of the femoral triangle.

Femoral vessels

The femoral artery, a continuation of the external iliac, is the main artery of the lower limb. It enters the anterior compartment behind the midpoint of the inguinal ligament where it is relatively superficial, easily palpable and accessible for catheterization to perform arteriograms. It is also vulnerable to penetrating or stab wounds. It descends through the femoral triangle (Fig. 6.19) and the adductor canal, and continues through the opening in adductor magnus as the popliteal artery (see p. 275).

The femoral artery or its main branches supply all three compartments of the thigh. Subcutaneous branches of the artery traverse the saphenous opening or pierce the fascia lata to accompany the superficial veins in the groin (see Fig. 6.11). The largest deep branch is the profunda femoris artery (Fig. 6.20), which arises from the posterolateral aspect of the femoral artery about 4 cm below the inguinal ligament and runs distally behind the femoral artery, leaving the triangle by passing between pectineus and adductor longus. The profunda femoris and its perforating branches pass through the adductor muscles and contribute to the anastomosis in the posterior compartment of the thigh. One of the perforating arteries gives a large nutrient branch to the femur. Close to its origin, the profunda femoris artery usually gives medial and lateral circumflex femoral branches (Fig. 6.20). The medial circumflex artery winds round the medial aspect of the femur between iliopsoas and pectineus to join the cruciate anastomosis (see p. 271), and the lateral circumflex artery encircles the femur, passing laterally deep to sartorius and rectus femoris.

The femoral vein is the continuation of the popliteal vein at the opening in adductor magnus. In the adductor canal it lies behind the femoral artery and continues through the femoral triangle, lying medial to the artery (Fig. 6.19). Passing deep to the inguinal ligament the femoral vein becomes the external iliac vein. Tributaries of the femoral vein, except the great saphenous vein, correspond to the branches of the femoral artery.

Femoral sheath

The femoral artery and vein are invested in a thick fascial sleeve, the femoral sheath, derived from the transversalis and iliac fasciae. The sheath passes deep to the inguinal ligament and tapers inferiorly, blending with the adventitia of the vessels about 2.5 cm distal to the ligament.

Two vertical septa divide the sheath into three compartments. The femoral artery lies laterally while the femoral vein occupies the intermediate compartment. The medial compartment is called the femoral canal (Fig. 6.20) and contains fat and lymph nodes. The upper limit of the femoral canal is the femoral ring (see Fig. 4.21), an aperture bounded in front by the inguinal ligament and behind by the superior ramus of the pubis, whilst laterally lies the femoral vein and medially the lacunar ligament. A femoral hernia descends through the femoral ring to enter the femoral canal.

Femoral nerve

The femoral nerve (L2, L3 & L4) enters the thigh beneath the inguinal ligament, lying on iliopsoas lateral to the femoral sheath (Fig. 6.19). After a brief course in the femoral triangle, it divides into several superficial and deep branches. The superficial branches are the intermediate and medial cutaneous nerves of the thigh and the nerves to sartorius and pectineus. The deep branches include the nerves supplying rectus femoris and the vasti, and the saphenous nerve which enters the adductor canal.

Deep inguinal lymph nodes

The deep inguinal lymph nodes lie in the femoral triangle medial to the femoral vein. They receive lymph from the superficial inguinal nodes and from all parts of the limb deep to the investing fascia. They also drain the glans of the penis or clitoris. Efferent vessels pass proximally through the femoral canal to reach the external iliac nodes.

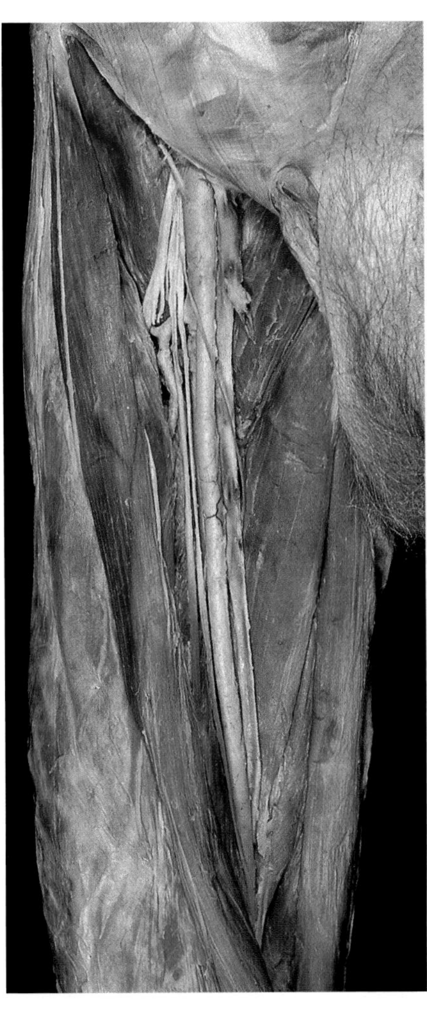

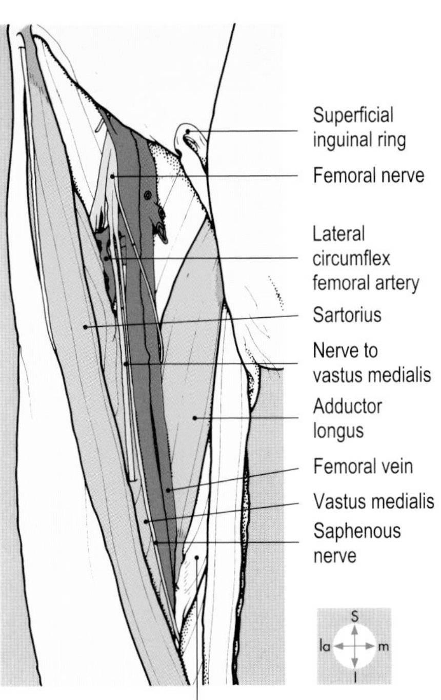

Fig. 6.18 Contents and boundaries of the adductor canal, exposed by displacement of sartorius laterally.

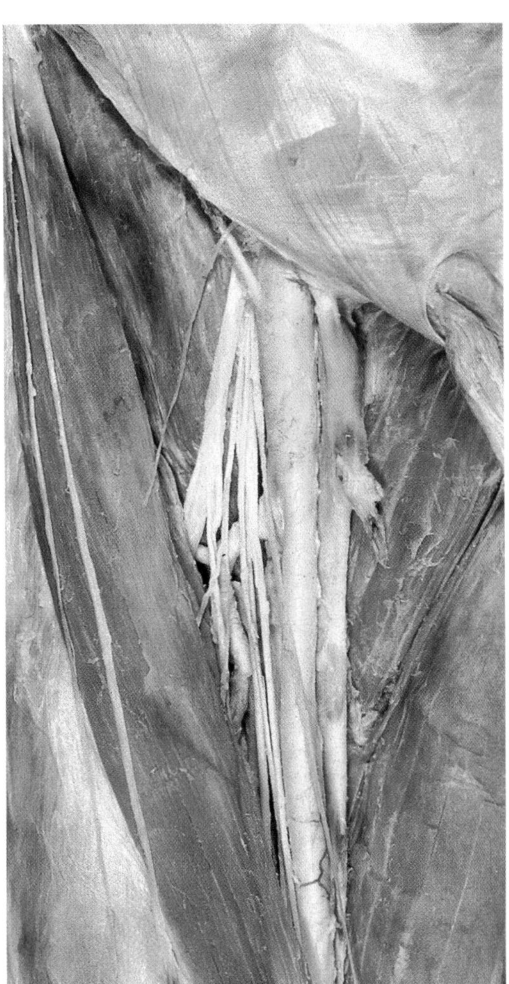

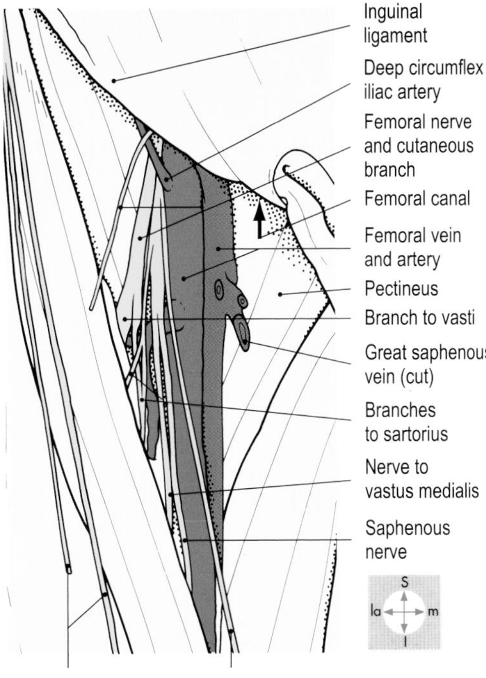

Fig. 6.19 Contents of the femoral triangle exposed by removal of its roof (fascia lata). The deep inguinal lymph nodes lie within the femoral canal.

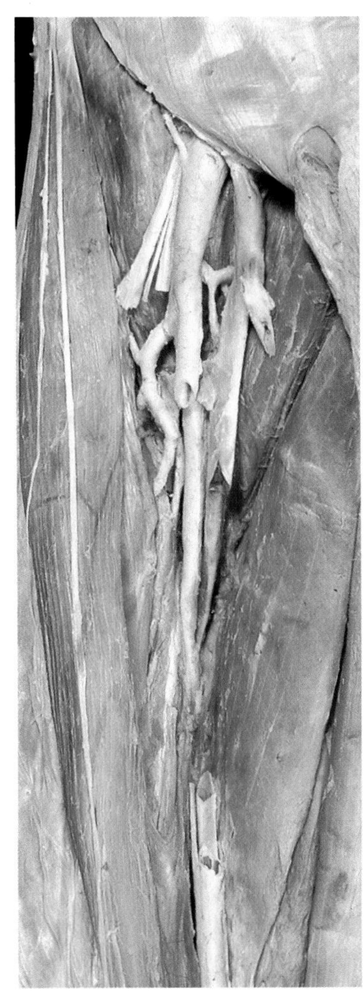

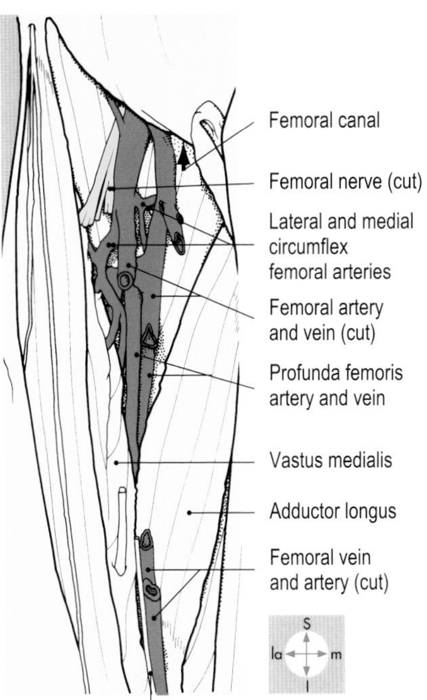

Fig. 6.20 Profunda femoris vessels seen after removal of segments of the femoral artery and vein.

Medial Compartment of Thigh

The medial compartment of the thigh is wedge-shaped and lies between the anterior and posterior compartments. It contains pectineus, adductors longus, brevis and magnus, gracilis and obturator externus. The obturator nerve and vessels and the profunda femoris vessels, together with their perforating branches, supply the compartment.

Muscles

The muscles are arranged in three layers. The anterior layer consists of pectineus, adductor longus and gracilis, from lateral to medial (Fig. 6.21). Deep to these, forming the intermediate layer, is adductor brevis (Figs 6.22, & 6.23). The posterior layer consists of obturator externus and adductor magnus (Figs 6.24 & 6.25). The proximal attachments of these muscles are to the outer surface of the bony pelvis between the superior pubic and ischial rami. In

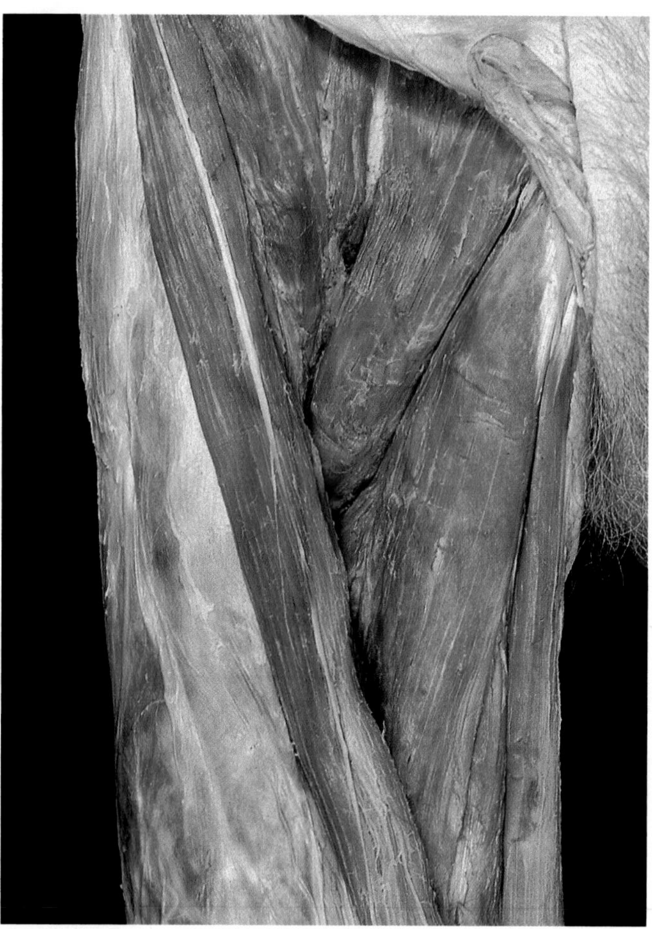

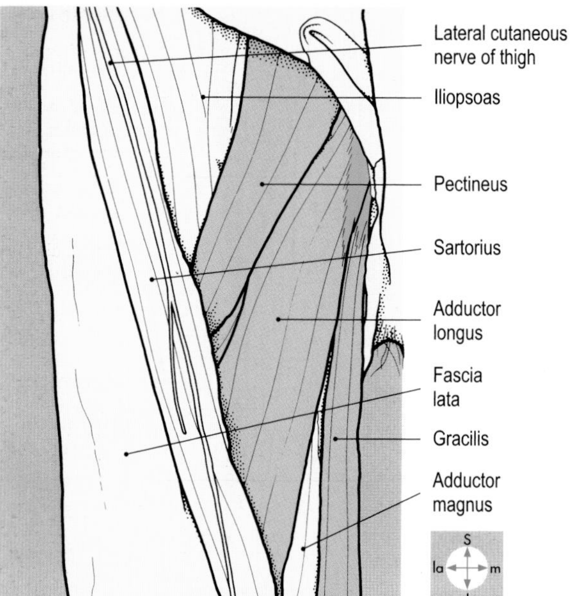

Fig. 6.21 Anterior layer of muscles of the medial compartment of thigh.

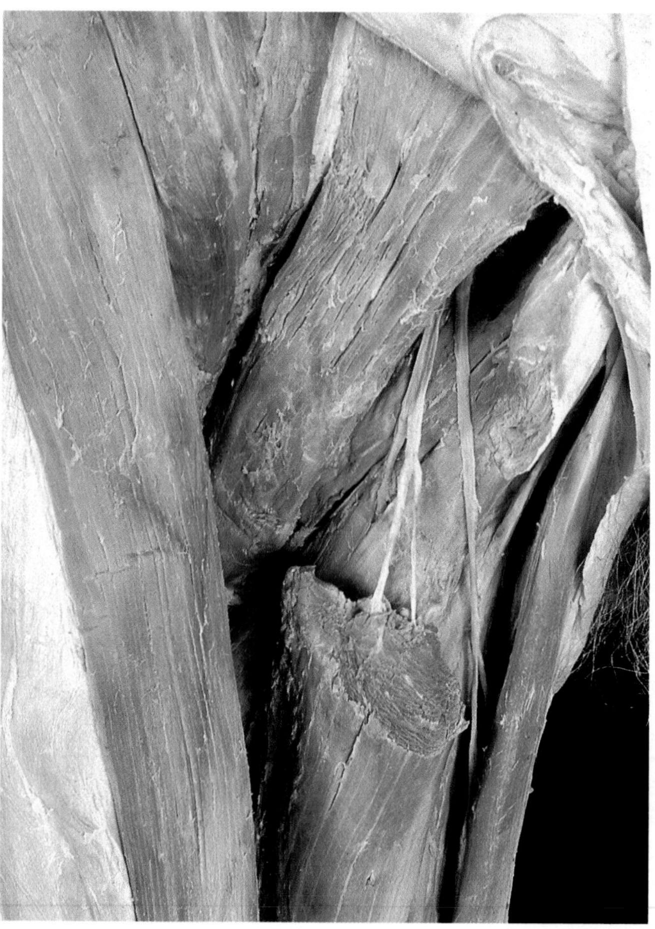

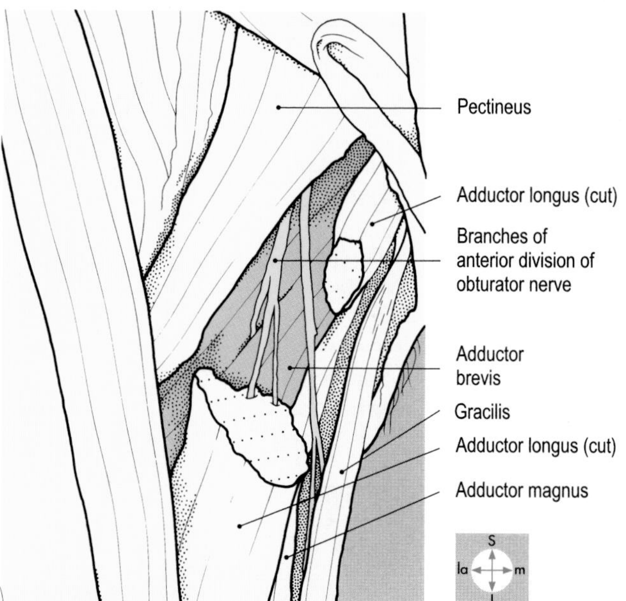

Fig. 6.22 Adductor brevis and branches of the anterior division of the obturator nerve, revealed by removal of part of adductor longus.

addition, obturator externus is attached to the obturator membrane.

The more anterior muscles have higher attachments than those of the deeper layers (Fig. 6.26). Distally, the muscles attach to the femur, except for gracilis (see Fig. 6.79), which descends below the knee to gain the proximal end of the subcutaneous surface of the tibia in company with sartorius and semitendinosus. Obturator externus passes laterally below and behind the capsule of the hip joint (see Figs 6.25 & 6.70) to the trochanteric fossa on the medial aspect of the greater trochanter. Pectineus and adductors longus, brevis and magnus slope downwards and laterally to attach in the region of the linea aspera, the sequence being related to the layer in which the muscle lies (Fig. 6.27). Adductor magnus has the longest attachment, extending from the gluteal tuberosity above to the adductor tubercle below.

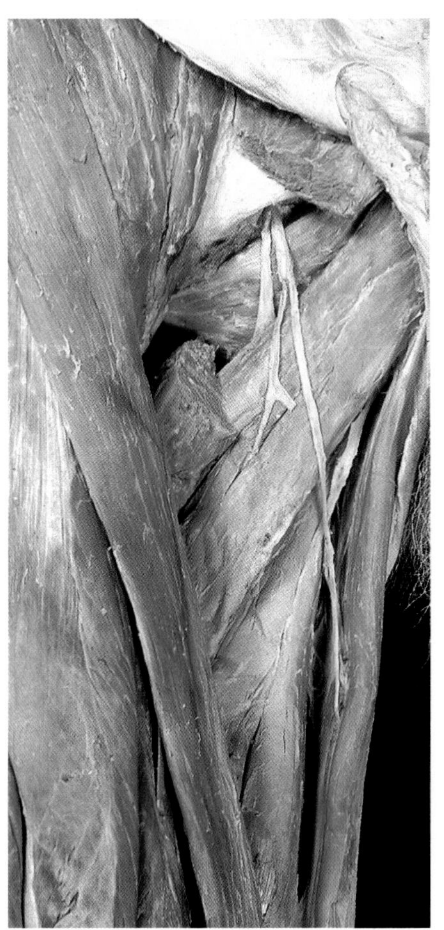

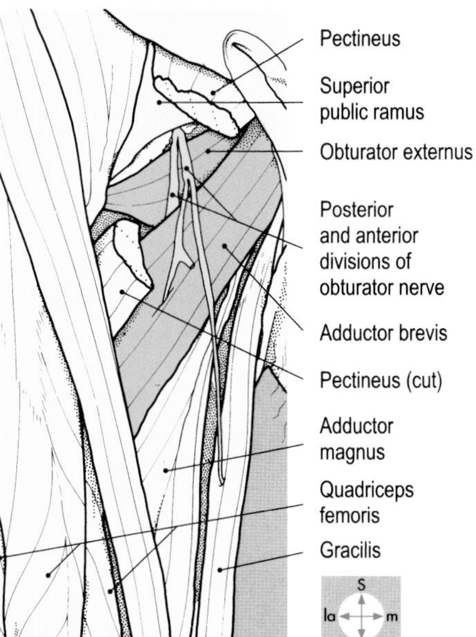

Fig. 6.23 Division of the obturator nerve, revealed by removal of adductor longus and part of pectineus. In this specimen the posterior division lies in front of obturator externus but it usually lies behind or may fan through it.

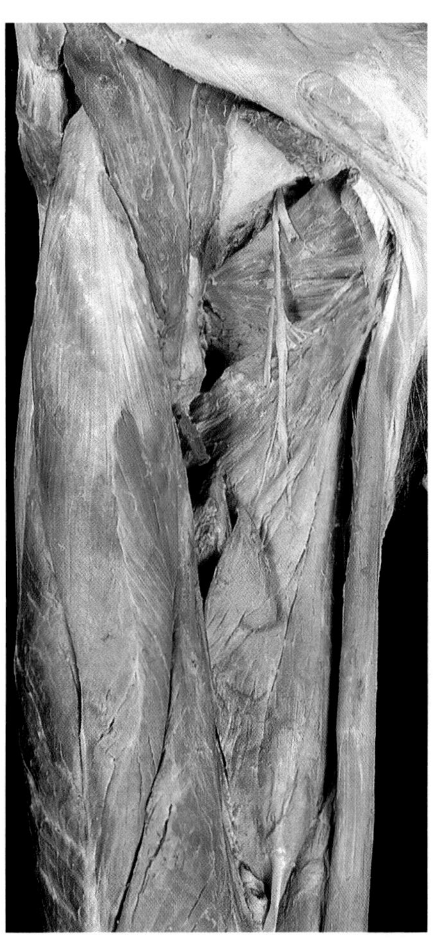

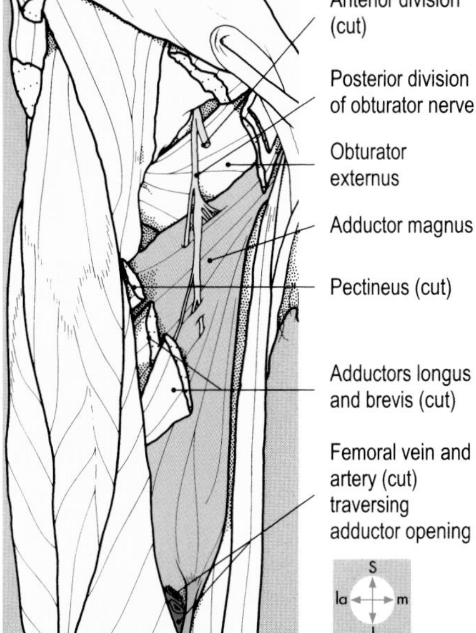

Fig. 6.24 Adductor magnus and the posterior division of the obturator nerve. Adductor brevis has been removed.

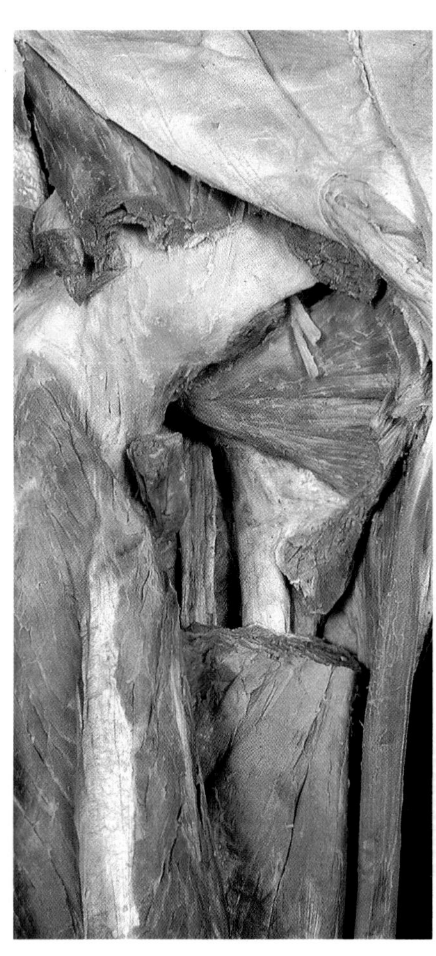

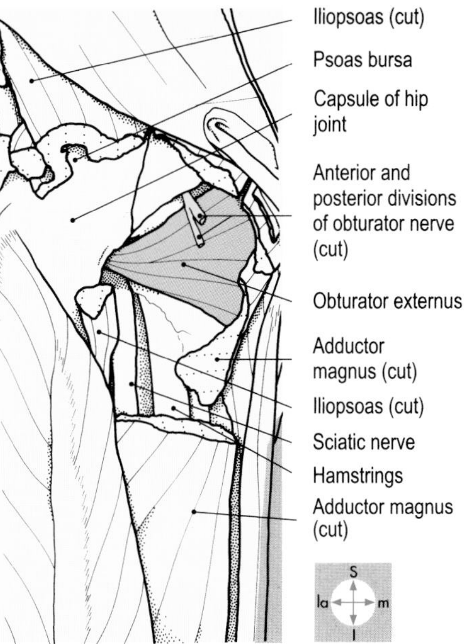

Fig. 6.25 Obturator externus, completely revealed by removal of parts of iliopsoas and adductor magnus.

All the muscles in the compartment except obturator externus adduct the hip joint. During walking they stabilize the femur whilst the abductors of the hip prevent tilting of the pelvis (see p. 270). In addition, pectineus and adductor longus are medial rotators and obturator externus a lateral rotator. Pectineus assists flexion at the hip joint and gracilis flexes and medially rotates the knee joint.

All the muscles in the medial compartment except pectineus are innervated by the obturator nerve. Pectineus usually has a supply from the femoral nerve but may also be supplied by the obturator nerve, and the ischial part of adductor magnus receives fibres from the tibial part of the sciatic nerve.

Obturator nerve

The obturator nerve gains the compartment through the obturator canal and promptly divides into anterior and posterior divisions (see Fig. 6.23). The former passes anterior to obturator externus whilst the posterior division usually pierces and supplies the muscle before emerging onto its surface. The two divisions then descend respectively anterior and posterior to adductor brevis. The anterior division supplies adductors longus and brevis and gracilis (see Fig. 6.22), and gives sensory branches to the hip joint and to skin on the medial side of the thigh. The posterior division lies on and supplies adductor magnus (see Fig. 6.24) and gives sensory branches, which accompany the femoral artery through the opening in adductor magnus to supply the knee joint. Since the obturator nerve innervates the hip and knee joints, disease in one joint may cause referred pain in the other. Pelvic pathology including tumours pressing on the obturator nerve (see p. 222, 234, 237) may also cause referred pain in the hip, knee and medial side of the thigh.

Vessels

The blood supply is derived from the profunda femoris artery and its perforating branches, supplemented by the obturator artery and other branches of the femoral artery. The obturator artery is small and forms an arterial circle around the margins of the obturator membrane, supplying the proximal parts of the muscles. An acetabular branch passes beneath the transverse acetabular ligament and accompanies the round ligament to the head of the femur. Venae comitantes accompanying the arteries in the compartment drain into the profunda femoris or internal iliac veins.

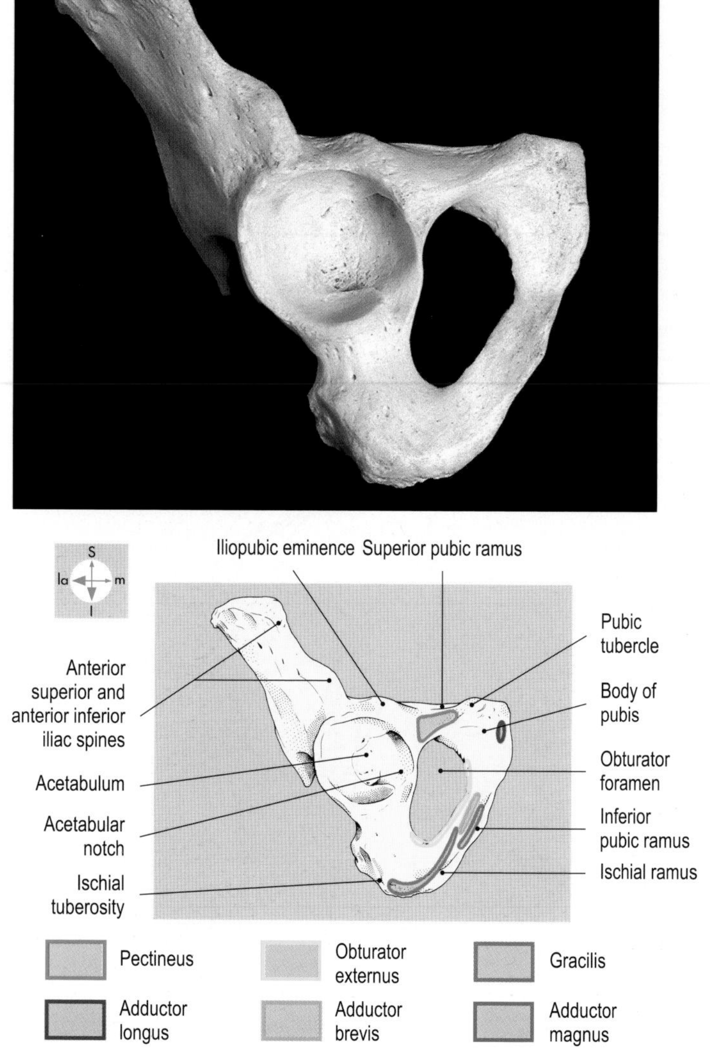

Fig. 6.26 Attachments of the muscles of the medial compartment of the thigh to the hip bone.

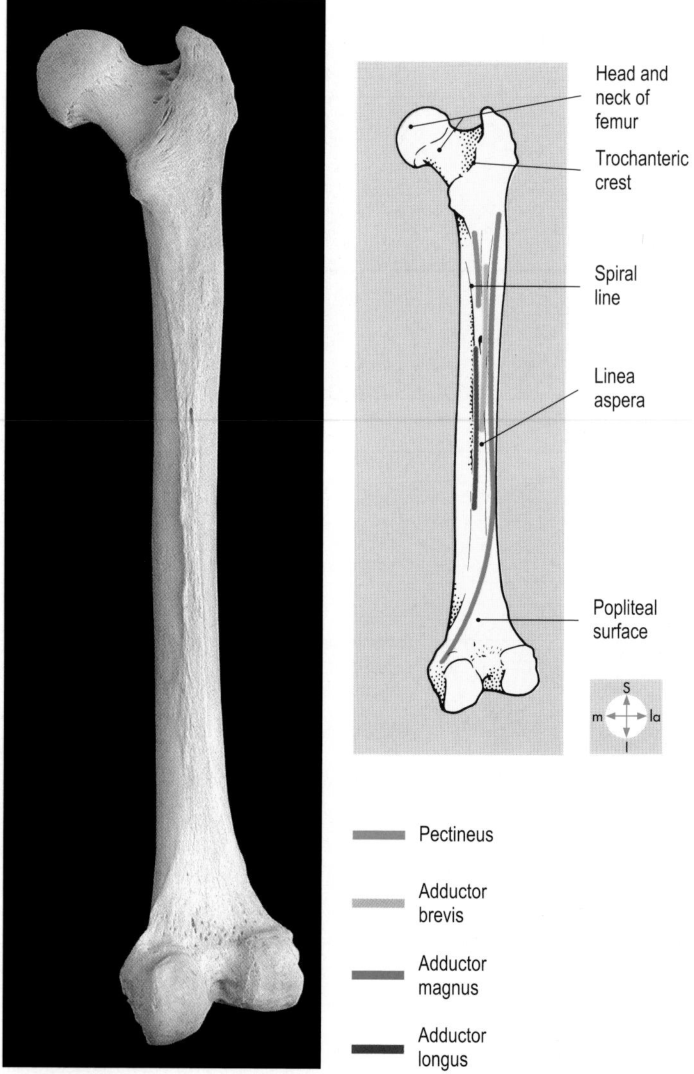

Fig. 6.27 Femoral attachments of the muscles of the medial compartment of the thigh.

Gluteal Compartment

The gluteal region or buttock forms part of the root of the limb. It overlies the dorsum of the ilium, ischium and sacrum and is continuous proximally with the lower trunk and distally with the posterior compartment of the thigh. Three substantial muscles (gluteus maximus, medius and minimus), covered by deep fascia and a thick layer of subcutaneous fat, form the bulk of the buttock and account for its surface contour. The gluteal fold, a prominent surface feature, lies at the junction of the buttock and thigh.

Gluteus maximus

This very large trapezoidal muscle is the most superficial in the buttock. Its fibres slope downwards and laterally (Fig. 6.28) and its lower edge passes obliquely across the gluteal fold. Some of

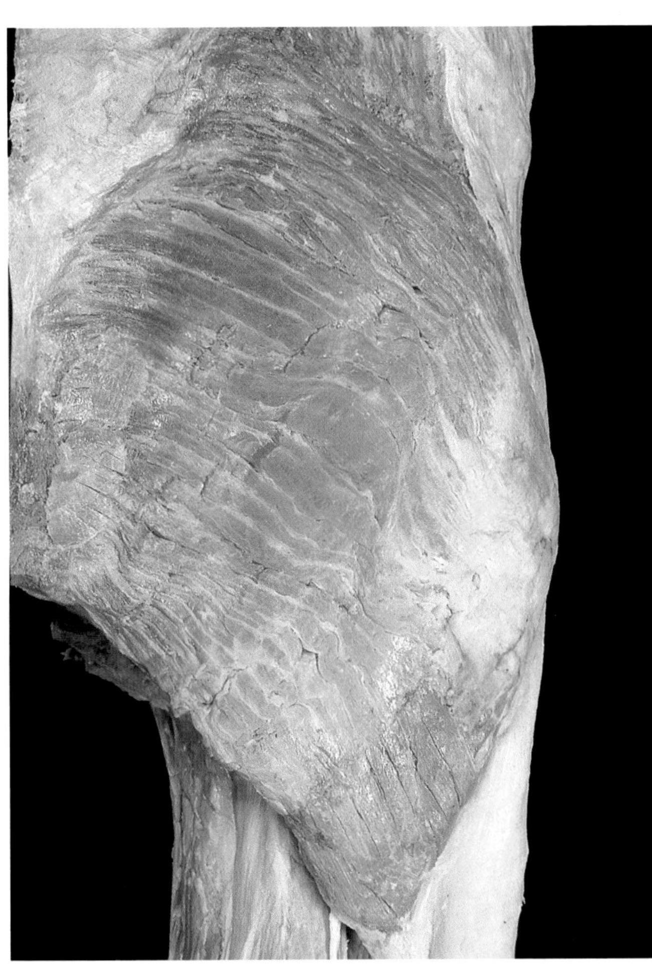

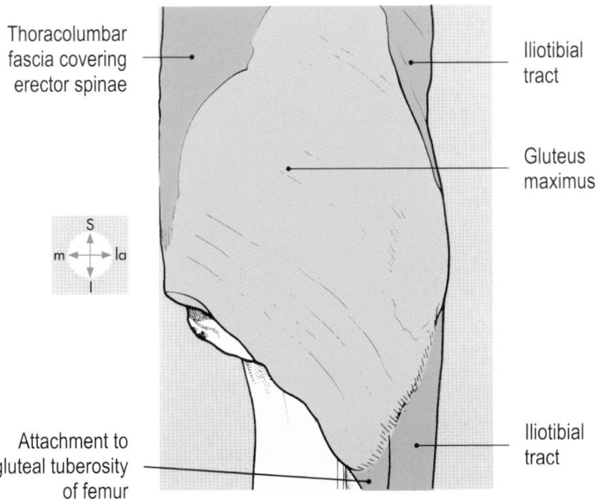

Fig. 6.28 The attachments of gluteus maximus include the thoracolumbar fascia and the iliotibial tract.

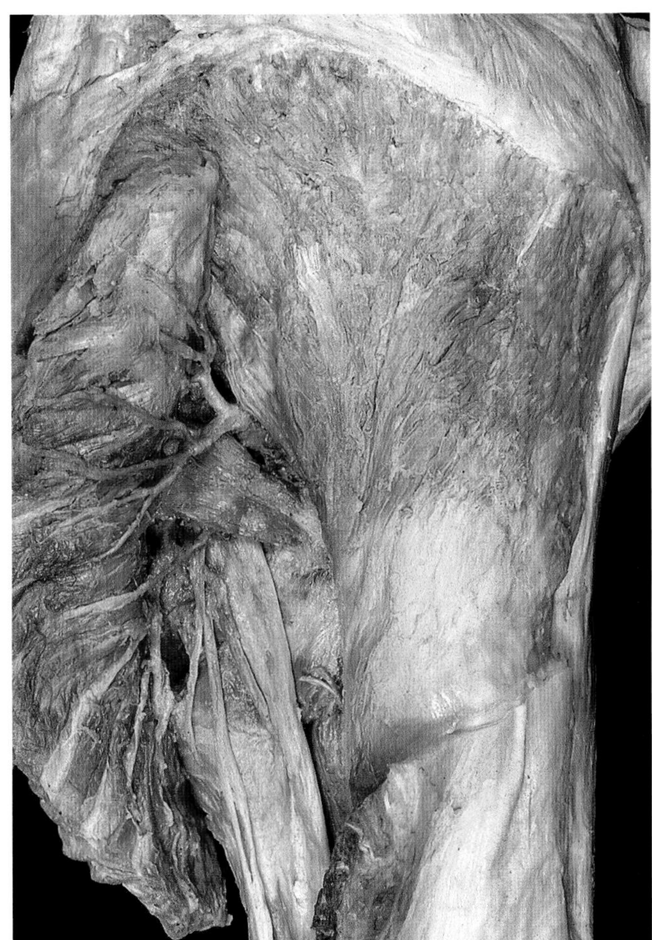

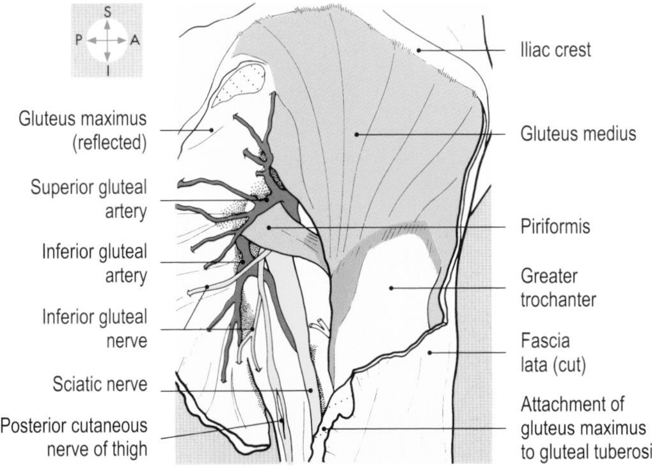

Fig. 6.29 Reflection of gluteus maximus exposes gluteus medius and neurovascular structures.

the sensory nerves to the skin of the buttock penetrate the medial part of the muscle whilst others emerge around its upper and lower borders. Proximally, the muscle has an extensive attachment: to the ilium behind the posterior gluteal line, to the lower part of the sacrum, to the coccyx, to the sacrotuberous ligament and to the thoracolumbar (lumbar) and gluteal fasciae. A synovial bursa is usually present where it crosses the ischial tuberosity. Distally, some of the deeper fibres are attached to the gluteal tuberosity of the femur (Fig. 6.29), but most of the muscle is attached through the iliotibial tract (see Fig. 6.30) to the anterior surface of the lateral tibial condyle. The nerve supply is from the inferior gluteal nerve (L5, S1 & S2).

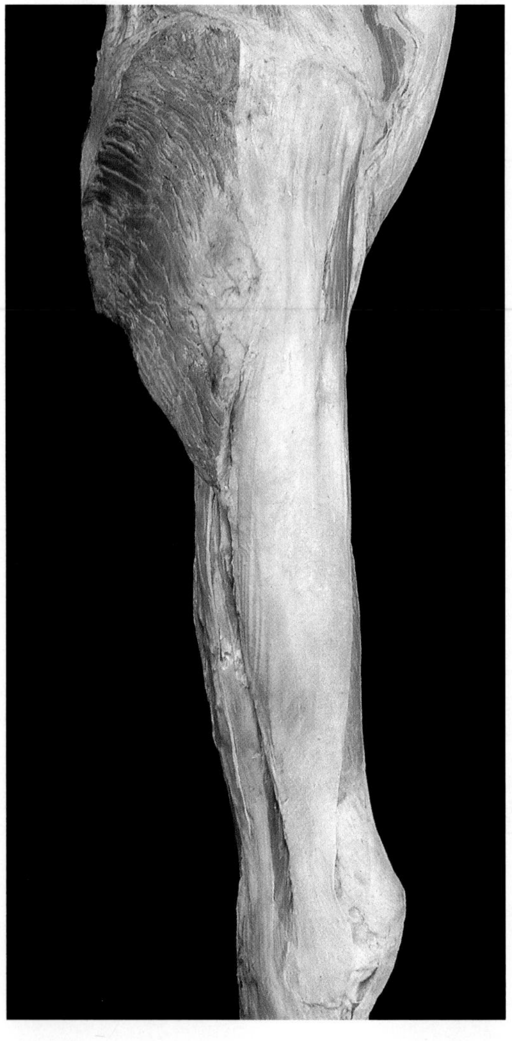

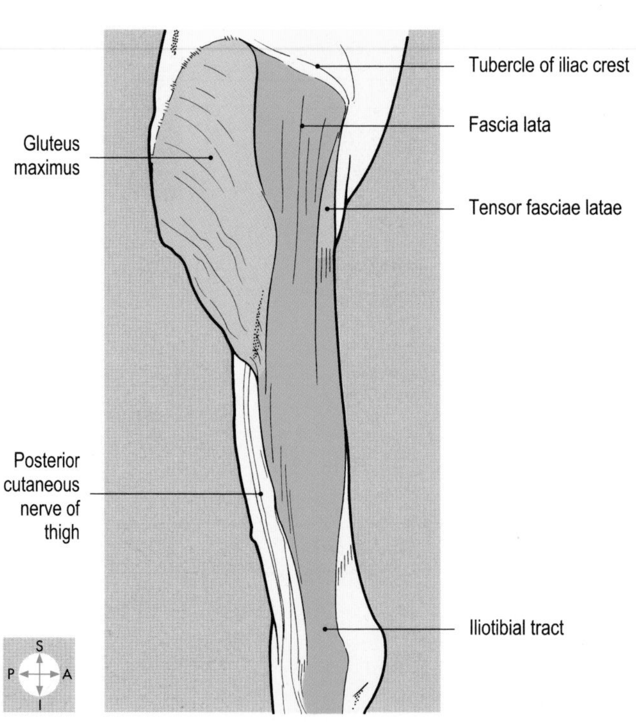

Fig. 6.30 Attachment of gluteus maximus and tensor fasciae latae to the iliotibial tract.

Gluteus maximus is a strong extensor of the thigh, especially during running and climbing, and also produces abduction at the hip joint. As an antigravity muscle it extends the trunk on the hip and through the iliotibial tract it extends and stabilizes the knee joint and the supporting limb during walking and standing.

Tensor fasciae latae

This small muscle is attached proximally to the ilium between the anterior superior iliac spine and iliac tubercle (Fig. 6.31) and distally to the anterior border of the iliotibial tract (Fig. 6.30) which it tenses. It is supplied by the superior gluteal nerve.

Structures deep to gluteus maximus

The arrangement of these structures is clarified by noting whether they enter the buttock above or below the piriformis muscle (see Fig. 6.29), which itself enters via the greater sciatic foramen (see Fig. 6.36).

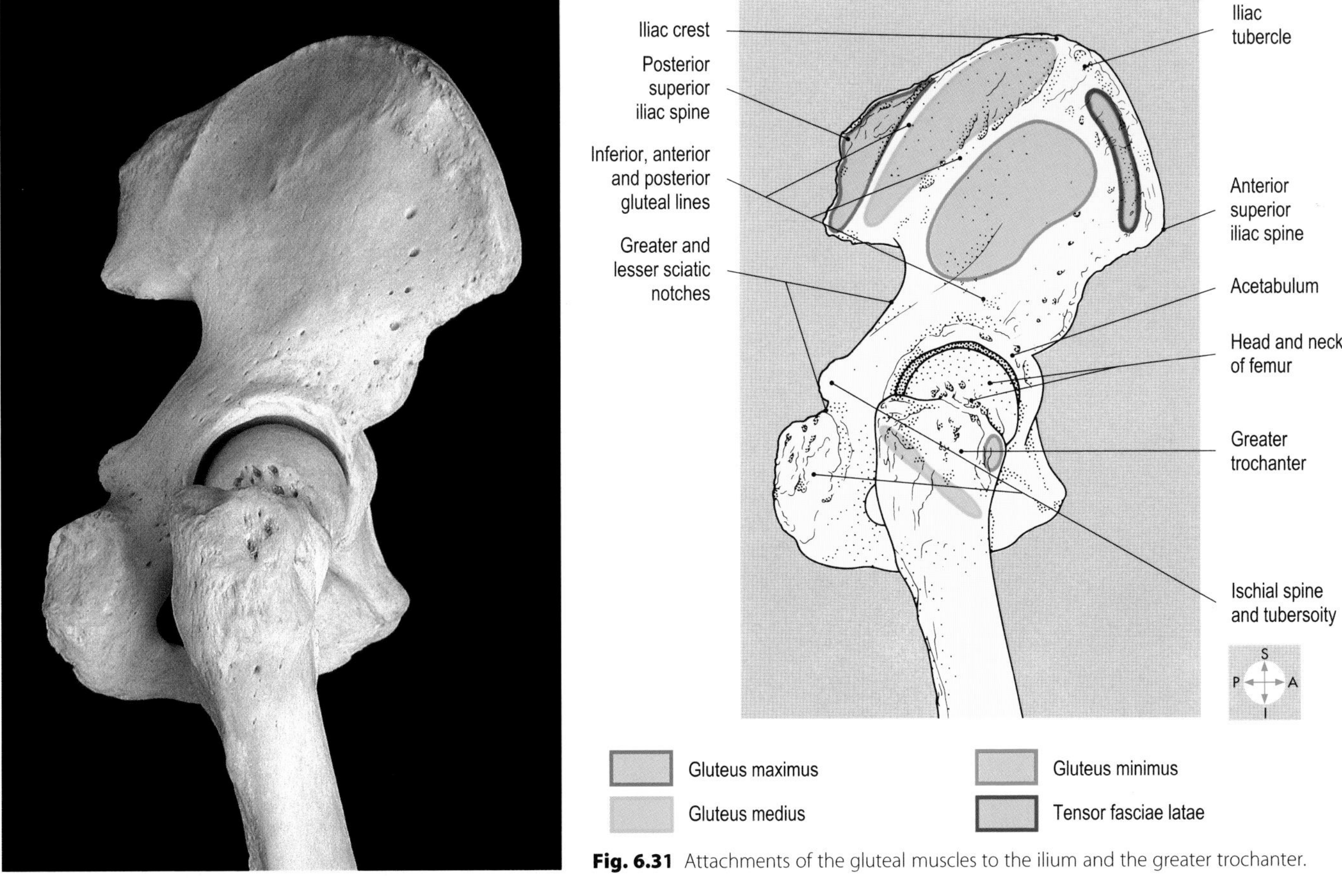

Fig. 6.31 Attachments of the gluteal muscles to the ilium and the greater trochanter.

Structures entering above piriformis

The superior gluteal nerve (L4, L5 & S1) arises within the pelvis from the lumbosacral plexus and enters the buttock through the greater sciatic foramen (see Fig. 6.36), running laterally between gluteus medius and gluteus minimus (Fig. 6.32). It supplies both muscles and terminates in tensor fasciae latae.

The superior gluteal artery arises from the posterior aspect of the internal iliac artery. It enters the buttock accompanying the corresponding nerve and divides into a superficial branch which supplies the overlying gluteus maximus (see Fig. 6.29) and two deep branches, an upper and lower, which supply gluteus medius and minimus (Fig. 6.32). The deep branches also contribute to anastomoses around the greater trochanter and anterior superior iliac spine. The accompanying veins form an extensive plexus between the muscles and drain into the internal iliac vein.

Gluteus medius and minimus

These fan-shaped muscles lie superior to piriformis. Gluteus medius (see Fig. 6.29) is attached proximally to the dorsum of the ilium between the posterior and anterior (middle) gluteal lines and to the gluteal fascia, which separates it from gluteus maximus. Distally, it is attached to the lateral surface of the greater trochanter. Gluteus minimus lies immediately deep to gluteus medius and attaches proximally to the dorsum of the ilium between the anterior and inferior gluteal lines (Fig. 6.31) and distally to the anterior surface of the greater trochanter (Fig. 6.32). Both are supplied by the superior gluteal nerve.

Although both gluteus medius and minimus medially rotate the femur at the hip joint, their importance is in abduction. During walking, gluteus medius and minimus of the supporting limb contract to prevent tilting of the pelvis towards the unsupported side. Failure of this mechanism is the basis of Trendelenburg's sign of hip instability with a dipping gait. It may result from a defective acetabulum (usually congenital), or loss of function in these muscles.

Structures entering below piriformis

These are: three nerves laterally, the sciatic nerve, nerve to quadratus femoris and posterior cutaneous nerve of thigh; medially the internal pudendal artery, pudendal nerve and nerve to obturator internus; and in intermediate position, the inferior gluteal nerve and vessels.

The sciatic nerve (Fig. 6.33), the largest nerve in the lower limb, arises from the spinal nerves L4, L5, S1, S2 & S3 and supplies the entire limb, except for the gluteal structures and the medial and anterior compartments of the thigh. It leaves the greater sciatic foramen about halfway between the posterior superior iliac spine and ischial tuberosity and curves laterally and downwards, crossing the midpoint between the ischial tuberosity and greater trochanter. The nerve is separated from the capsule of the hip joint by obturator internus and the gemelli, quadratus femoris and the upper border of adductor magnus (Fig. 6.33). A branch of the inferior gluteal artery accompanies the nerve.

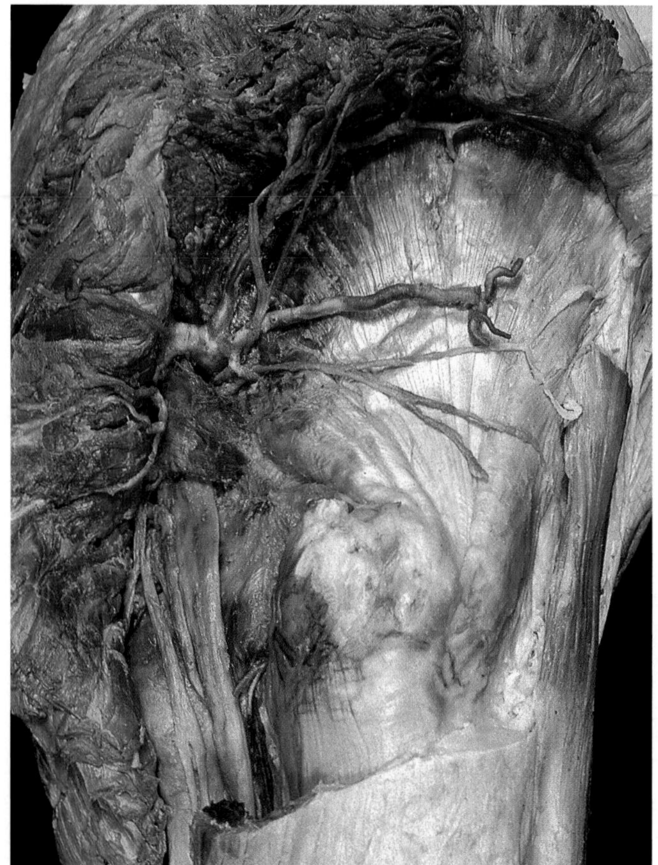

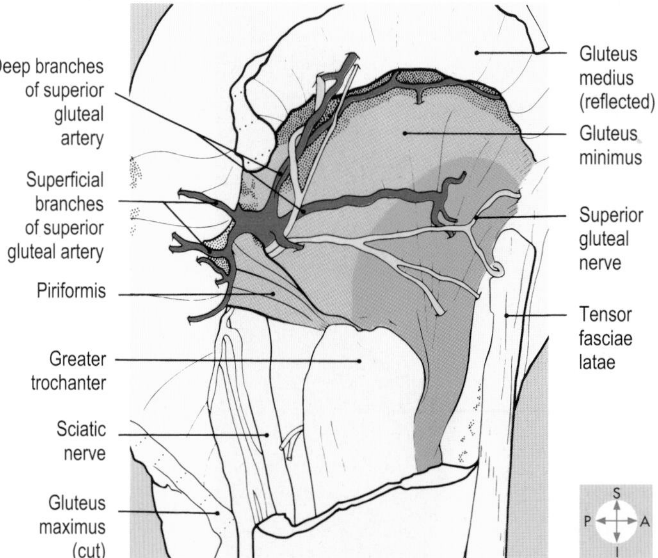

Fig. 6.32 Reflection of gluteus medius reveals gluteus minimus and the superior gluteal artery and nerve entering the buttock above piriformis.

The nerve to quadratus femoris (L4, L5 & S1) lies deep to the sciatic nerve, obturator internus and the gemelli and supplies the inferior gemellus, quadratus femoris and the hip joint.

Superficial and medial to the sciatic nerve is the posterior cutaneous nerve of the thigh (Fig. 6.33), which arises from spinal nerves S1, S2 & S3. Within the buttock its perineal branch runs forwards to supply the skin on the posterior part of the scrotum or labium majus. Other branches curl round the lower border of gluteus maximus to supply the skin over the buttock.

The inferior gluteal nerve and vessels occupy an intermediate position. The nerve turns immediately posteriorly to supply gluteus maximus.

The inferior gluteal artery, a branch of the internal iliac artery, accompanies the nerve and supplies gluteus maximus (see Fig. 6.29) and the short lateral rotators of the hip joint, and contributes to the trochanteric and cruciate anastomoses. Venae comitantes accompany the artery and drain into the internal iliac system.

The pudendal nerve (S2, S3 & S4), internal pudendal vessels, and nerve to obturator internus (L5, S1 & S2), also supplying the superior gemellus, enter beneath the medial part of piriformis (Fig. 6.33). Their course in the buttock is brief before turning forwards into the lesser sciatic foramen, crossing the sacrospinous ligament or ischial spine to enter the pudendal canal (see Fig. 6.36 and p. 243).

Short muscles of buttock

The short muscles of the buttock are, from above downwards, piriformis, obturator internus with the gemelli, and quadratus femoris (Fig. 6.33). Piriformis arises from the ventral surface of the sacrum (see p. 235) and runs laterally through the greater sciatic foramen to converge on the medial border of the greater trochanter. It is innervated within the pelvis by spinal nerves L5, S1 & S2. Obturator internus attaches to the lateral wall of the pelvic cavity (see Fig. 6.72), including the obturator membrane, and runs backwards towards the lesser sciatic foramen where its tendon makes a right-angled turn to run laterally across the buttock to the medial aspect of the greater trochanter above the trochanteric fossa. The superior and inferior gemelli are small muscles arising from the upper and lower margins of the lesser sciatic notch to fuse with the obturator internus tendon.

Quadratus femoris attaches to the lateral margin of the ischial tuberosity and to the quadrate tubercle of the femur and the subjacent shaft. Being behind the hip joint, all the short muscles laterally rotate the hip.

Cruciate arterial anastomosis

The cruciate anastomosis lies at the lower border of quadratus femoris and receives contributions from: above, the inferior gluteal artery; below, the first perforating artery; and on each side, the medial and lateral circumflex femoral arteries.

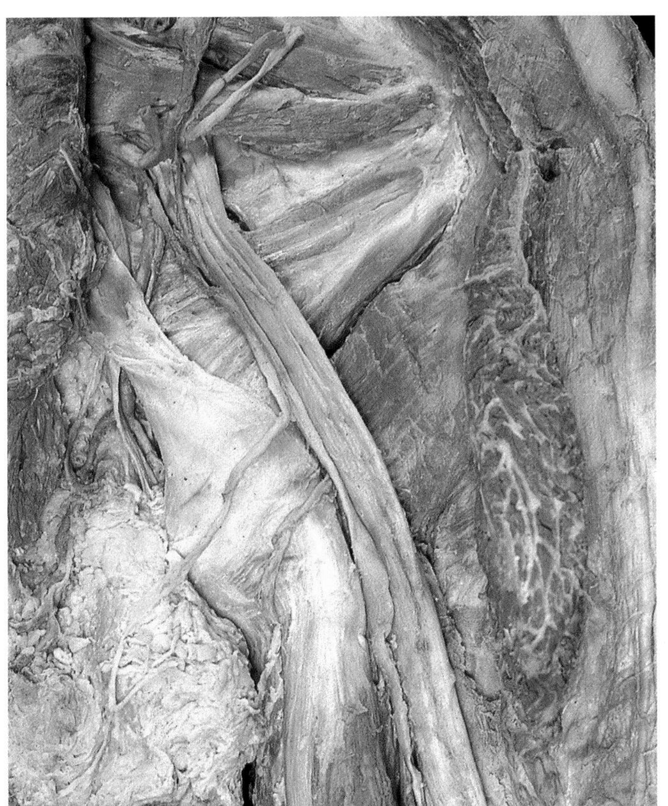

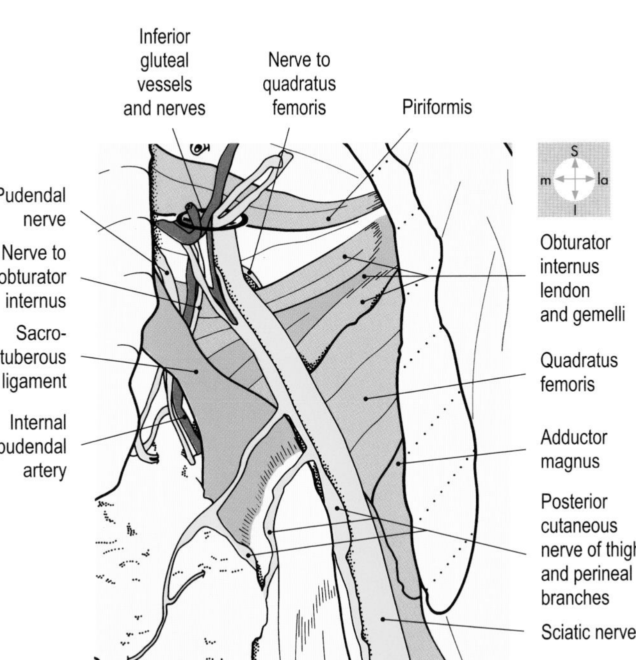

Fig. 6.33 Structures emerging below piriformis and the course and relations of the sciatic nerve.

Posterior Compartment of Thigh

The posterior compartment is enclosed by the fascia lata (Fig. 6.34), and extends from the gluteal region above to the popliteal fossa below. It contains the posterior cutaneous nerve of thigh, 'hamstring' muscles, sciatic nerve and terminal branches of the profunda femoris artery.

'Hamstring' muscles

These three muscles, semimembranosus, semitendinosus and biceps femoris (long head) (Fig. 6.35), attach proximally to the ischial tuberosity (see Fig. 6.36) and distally to the upper end of the tibia or fibula and are innervated by the sciatic nerve. They span the entire length of the femur and act on two joints, the hip for extension and the knee for flexion. After flexion of the trunk, the hamstrings act as antigravity muscles by pulling on the ischial tuberosities, thus extending the trunk into an upright position at the hip. Tears of the hamstrings occur in sports involving jumping, running and kicking.

Semimembranosus

This muscle is attached to the upper and lateral parts of the ischial tuberosity by a wide, flat tendon, which is overlapped by the tendons of biceps and semitendinosus close to the tuberosity, and descends on the medial side of the popliteal fossa to its main

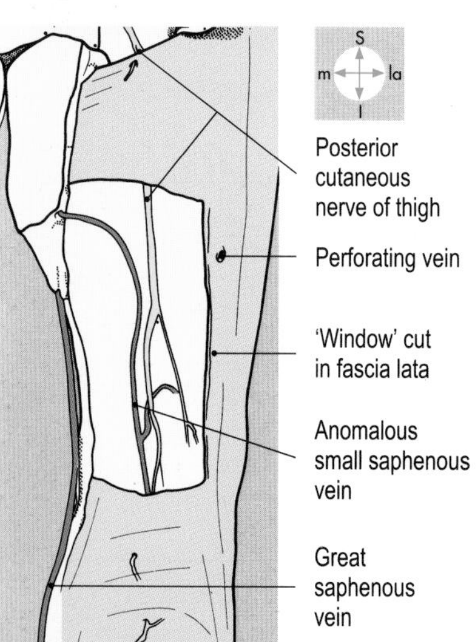

Fig. 6.34 Nerves and veins of the posterior compartment of thigh, seen through a 'window' cut in the fascia lata. This small saphenous vein continues proximally to terminate in the great saphenous vein.

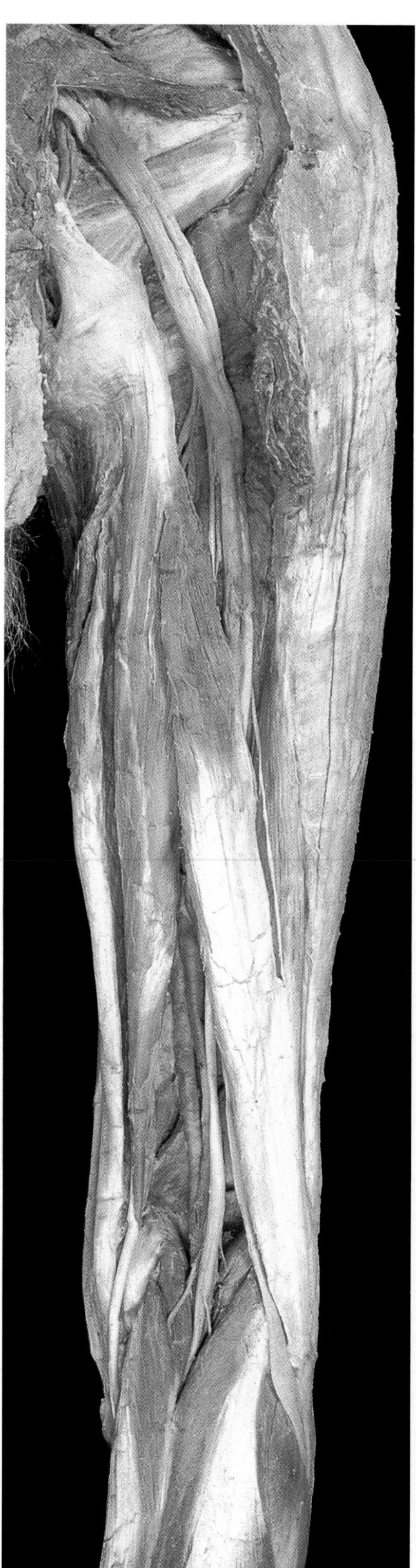

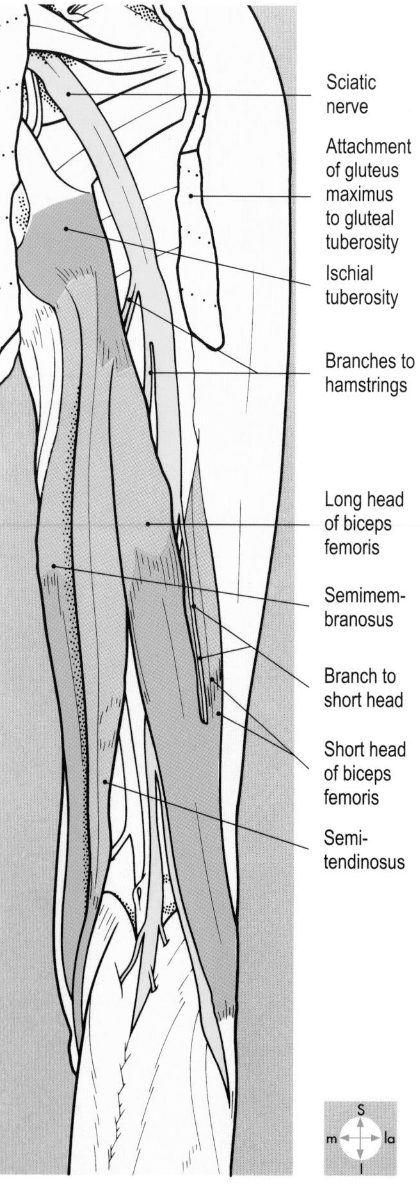

Fig. 6.35 Principal contents of the posterior compartment of thigh, seen after removal of deep fascia.

attachment into a horizontal groove on the posteromedial aspect of the medial tibial condyle. Some of its fibres pass upwards and laterally behind the knee joint to form the oblique posterior ligament; others descend to reinforce the fascia over popliteus (see Fig. 6.39).

Semitendinosus

Proximally, semitendinosus is attached to the medial part of the ischial tuberosity. It descends on the medial side of the popliteal fossa, forming a narrow tendon which overlies semimembranosus, and attaches to the medial surface of the upper end of the tibial shaft close to the attachments of sartorius and gracilis (see Fig. 6.79). Besides contributing to the common actions of the hamstring group, semitendinosus and semimembranosus produce medial rotation of the leg at the knee.

Biceps femoris

This muscle has two heads. Proximally, the long head is attached to the medial part of the ischial tuberosity close to the semitendinosus and descends to the lateral side of the popliteal fossa where it fuses with the short head, which originates from the lateral lip of the linea aspera and lateral supracondylar ridge of femur (see Fig. 6.35). Inferiorly the tendon of biceps is attached to the head of the fibula. In addition to the general actions of the hamstrings, biceps produces lateral rotation of the leg at the knee.

Sciatic nerve

The sciatic nerve emerges at the lower border of gluteus maximus lying just beneath the deep fascia, passes deep to the long head of biceps and descends in the midline of the limb. In the distal third of the thigh it usually divides into two terminal branches, the tibial and common fibular (common peroneal) nerves, which continue into the popliteal fossa (see Fig. 6.40). Division may occur more proximally in the thigh, within the buttock or even the pelvis. In the latter case, the common fibular nerve may pass through the piriformis where it may be compressed. Proximally, fibres from the medial (tibial) part of the sciatic nerve supply the hamstrings (see Fig. 6.35) and the ischial head of adductor magnus. More distally, a branch from the lateral (common fibular) part of the nerve supplies the short head of biceps.

Posterior cutaneous nerve of thigh

The nerve enters the thigh superficial and slightly medial to the sciatic nerve and

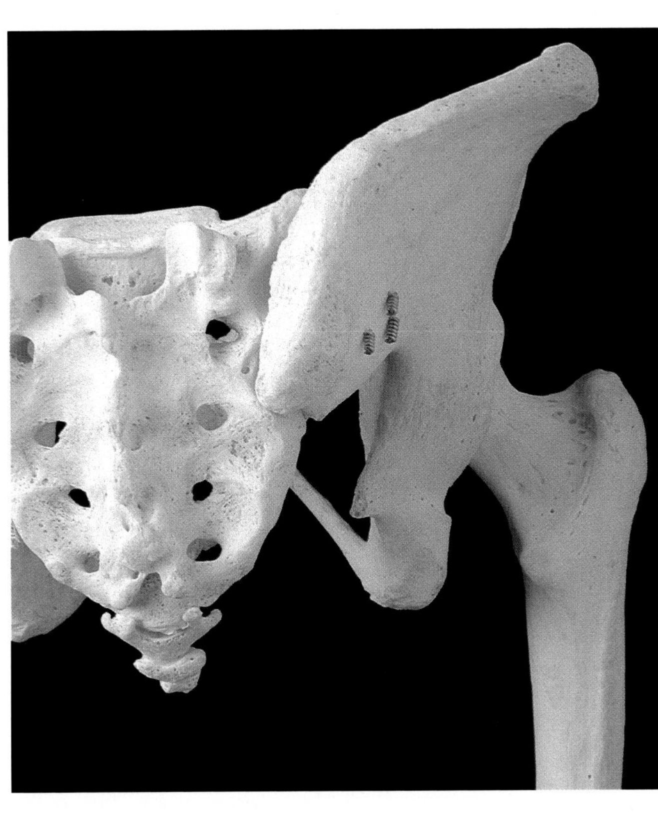

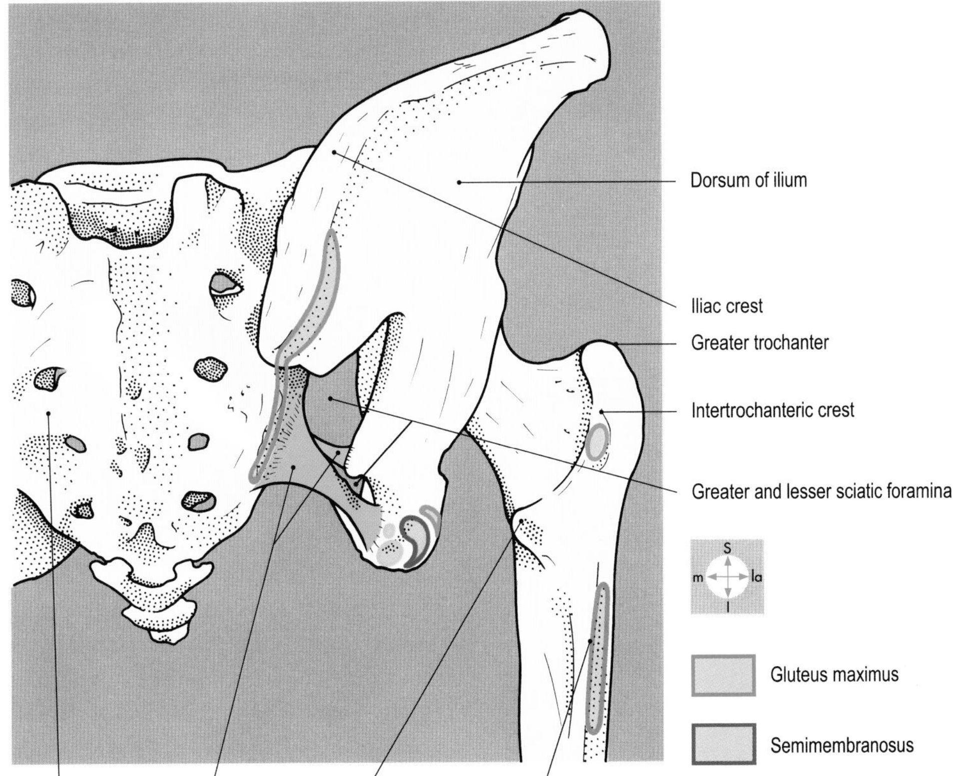

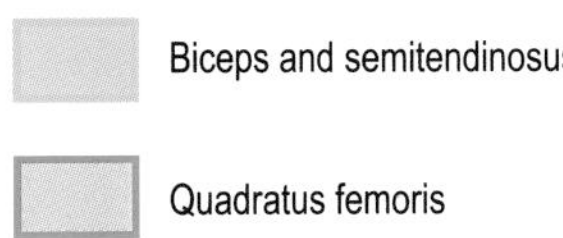

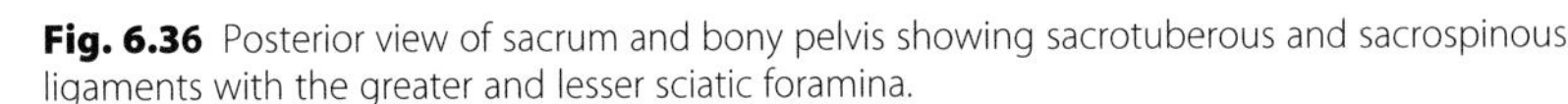

Fig. 6.36 Posterior view of sacrum and bony pelvis showing sacrotuberous and sacrospinous ligaments with the greater and lesser sciatic foramina.

descends beneath the fascia lata to the upper part of the popliteal fossa (Fig. 6.37). Apart from branches arising near the lower border of gluteus maximus, the nerve gives sensory fibres to the skin on the back of the thigh, popliteal fossa and proximal part of leg.

Profunda femoris artery

Perforating branches of the profunda femoris artery penetrate adductor magnus and terminate in the posterior compartment. They anastomose with branches from the inferior gluteal artery above and the popliteal artery below.

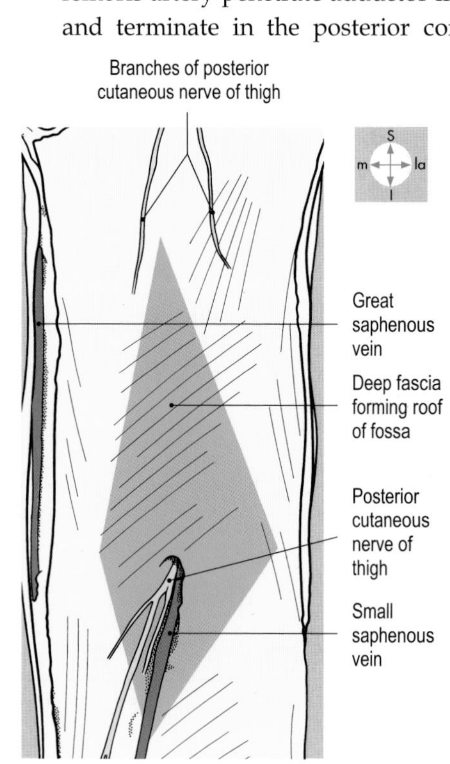

Fig. 6.37 Removal of skin and subcutaneous tissue reveals the cutaneous nerves. The small saphenous vein and accompanying nerve pierce the roof of the popliteal fossa.

Popliteal Fossa

The popliteal fossa is a diamond-shaped space behind the knee joint. It contains the principal blood vessels and nerves passing between the thigh and the leg. It has a roof, four walls and a floor.

Roof

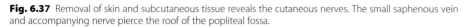

The roof is formed by the investing layer of deep fascia. In the subcutaneous tissue overlying the roof are the posterior cutaneous nerve of the thigh, which continues into the proximal part of the leg, and the small saphenous vein (Fig. 6.37). The vein usually penetrates the roof to drain into the popliteal vein but may drain more proximally into the great saphenou s vein (see Fig. 6.34).

Walls

The walls overhang the fossa. Superiorly they are formed by the diverging tendons of the hamstrings, namely semitendinosus and semimembranosus lying medially and biceps laterally. Inferiorly are the medial and lateral heads of gastrocnemius, which converge at the inferior angle (Fig. 6.38). Adjacent to the lateral head of gastrocnemius is the small plantaris muscle. On each side of the popliteal fossa the hamstring tendons overlap the heads of gastrocnemius, and between the medial head of gastrocnemius and semimembranosus there is frequently a bursa (see Fig. 6.39).

Contents

The principal contents of the fossa are embedded in fat and comprise the popliteal artery and vein together with the two terminal branches of the sciatic nerve, the common fibular and tibial nerves (see Fig. 6.40). These vessels and nerves are responsible for the blood and nerve supply of most of the leg and foot.

The popliteal artery lies deepest and is the continuation of the femoral artery from the thigh. It enters through the opening in adductor magnus and descends vertically on the floor of the fossa to the inferior angle where it leaves beneath the fused heads of gastrocnemius. The artery is so deep that it

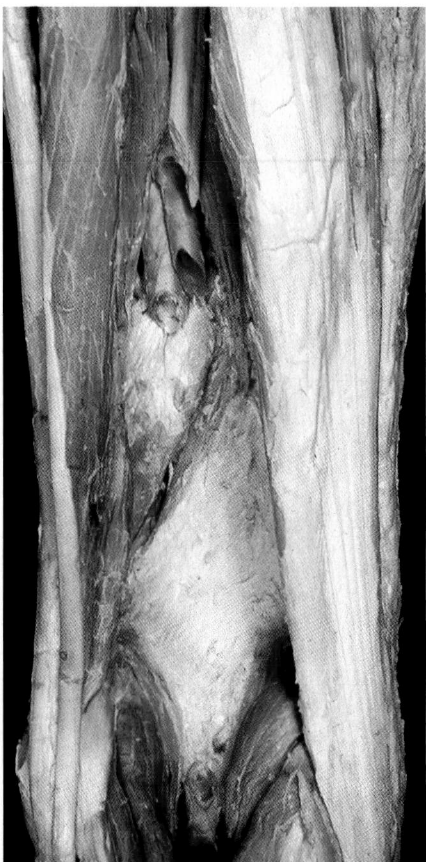

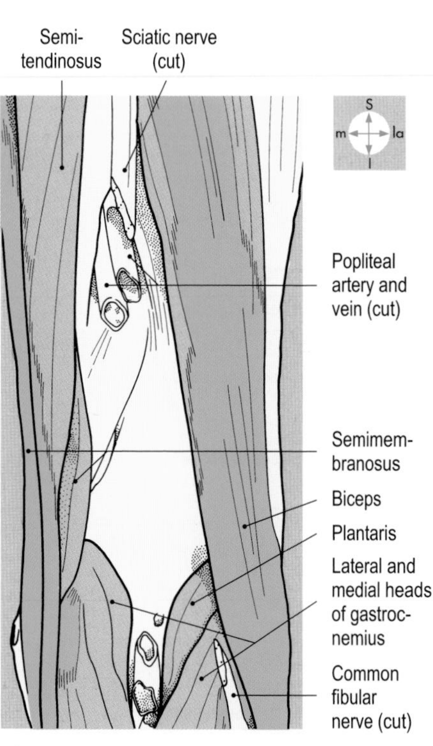

Fig. 6.38 Muscles forming the walls of the popliteal fossa.

is difficult to palpate unless the knee is flexed to relax the boundaries and roof of the fossa. The artery supplies the surrounding muscles and also forms a substantial plexus of articular branches anastomosing symmetrically around the knee joint (see Fig. 1.27).

The popliteal vein lies superficial to the artery and is formed at the inferior angle of the fossa by the union of the venae comitantes that accompany the tibial arteries in the leg. It continues proximally with the artery through the opening in adductor magnus to enter the adductor canal and become the femoral vein.

The tibial and common fibular nerves (Fig. 6.40), entering the fossa from the posterior compartment of the thigh, lie just beneath the roof, superficial to the popliteal vessels. The tibial nerve enters from beneath the hamstrings and descends vertically, bisecting the fossa, and leaves beneath the gastrocnemius at the inferior angle of the fossa, where it enters the posterior compartment of the leg. The tibial nerve is mainly motor in its distribution, supplying gastrocnemius, plantaris, popliteus and soleus. All these branches arise within the fossa. The nerve also gives sensory branches to the knee joint and a large cutaneous branch which passes into the calf to form the sural nerve. The common fibular nerve descends under cover of the tendon of biceps to reach the lateral angle of the fossa, where it enters the lateral (fibular or peroneal) compartment of the leg by winding around the neck of the fibula where it is vulnerable to damage and compression, resulting in foot-drop. It supplies sensory branches to the knee joint and two cutaneous nerves, one to the lateral side of the calf and the other, the lateral sural cutaneous nerve, joining the sural nerve in the calf.

The remaining contents of the popliteal fossa are the deeply placed popliteal lymph nodes which lie close to the popliteal artery. They drain the deep structures of the leg and foot and the knee joint, and receive superficial lymphatics which accompany the short saphenous vein from the lateral side of the foot and leg.

Floor

The floor of the fossa is formed, from above downwards, by the popliteal surface of the femur, the capsule of the knee joint reinforced by the oblique popliteal ligament, and popliteus (Fig. 6.39).

Popliteus

This muscle is attached to a triangular area on the posterior surface of the proximal end of the tibia above the soleal line. The tendon passes upwards and laterally, penetrating the capsule of the knee joint (see Fig. 6.77) to become attached to a pit below the lateral epicondyle of the femur. Its action is to 'unlock' the knee joint by producing lateral rotation of the femur on the tibia during flexion of the joint from the fully extended position. Popliteus is supplied by the tibial nerve.

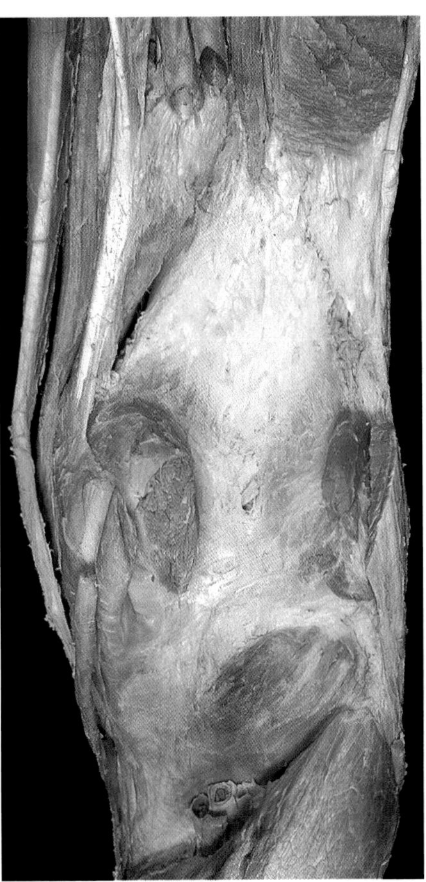

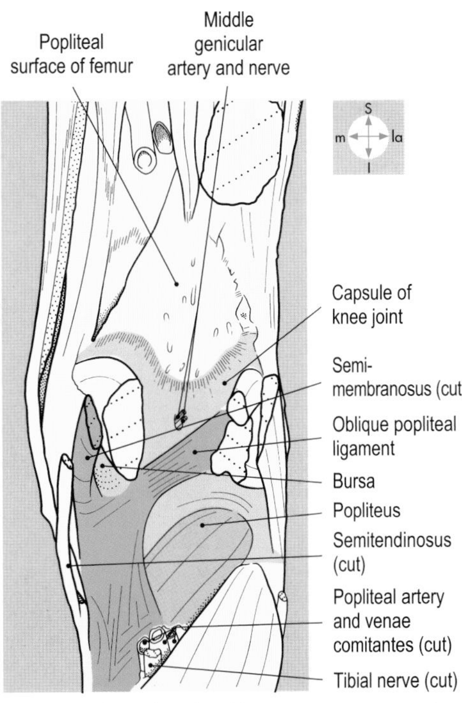

Fig. 6.39 Floor of popliteal fossa, seen after removal of walls and contents of the fossa.

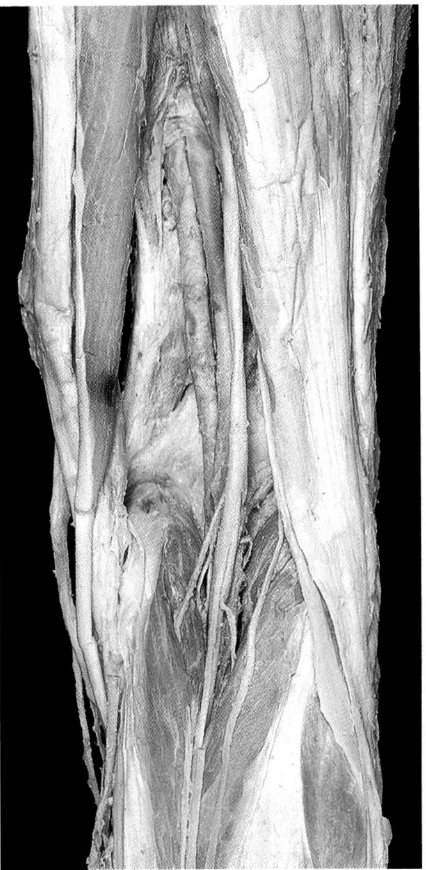

Fig. 6.40 Principal vessels and nerves of the popliteal fossa, revealed by removal of fat.

Posterior Compartment of Leg

The compartment extends from the popliteal fossa above to the ankle below. Gastrocnemius and soleus account for its bulk (Fig. 6.41) and the characteristic contour of the calf. Their common tendon is conspicuous as it passes towards the ankle. Deeper are tibialis posterior and the two long flexors of the toes, flexor hallucis longus and flexor digitorum longus, whose tendons all pass distally into the foot. The posterior tibial artery and its venae comitantes and the tibial nerve pass distally between soleus and the long flexors to enter the foot, where they supply structures in the sole.

Superficial structures and deep fascia

The small (short) saphenous vein begins on the lateral side of the foot as a continuation of the dorsal venous arch. Passing behind the lateral malleolus (Fig. 6.42) it ascends in the midline of the calf and usually terminates by piercing the fascial roof of the popliteal fossa (see Fig. 6.37). The vein has frequent communications with the great saphenous vein and important communicating (perforating) veins which pierce the investing deep fascia to link up with the deep veins of the calf, particularly just above the ankle.

The sural nerve is formed principally from the cutaneous branch of the tibial nerve and descends from the popliteal fossa to pierce the deep fascia in the proximal part of the calf. Here it is joined by the sural communicating branch of the common fibular nerve and continues distally with the small saphenous vein posteroinferior to the lateral malleolus to reach the foot (Fig. 6.42). The nerve supplies skin over the lower two-thirds of the calf and on the lateral side of the ankle and foot.

The deep fascia is continuous proximally with the popliteal fascia, and distally near the heel is thickened in two places. The first forms a thick band stretching between the tibia and fibula over which the tendo calcaneus passes, separated by a bursa. The second thickening, the flexor retinaculum,

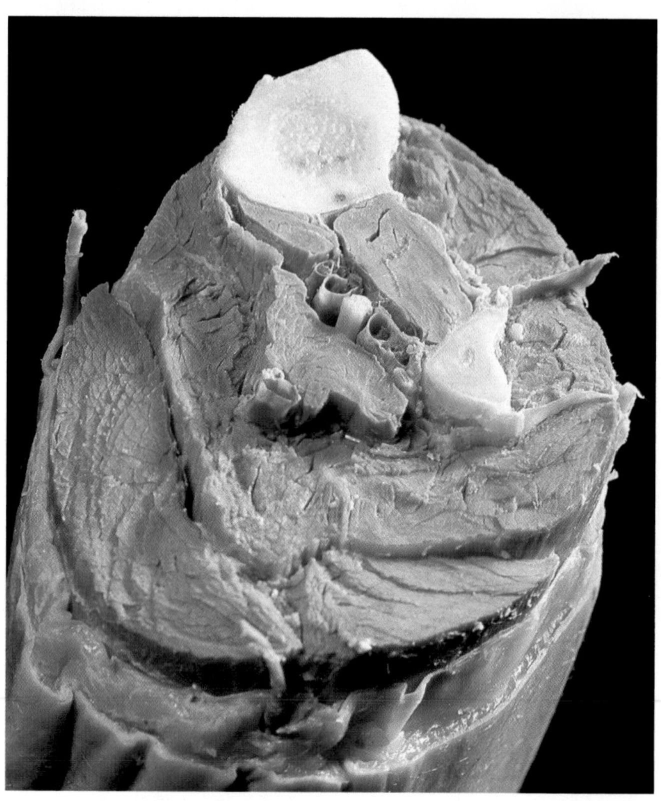

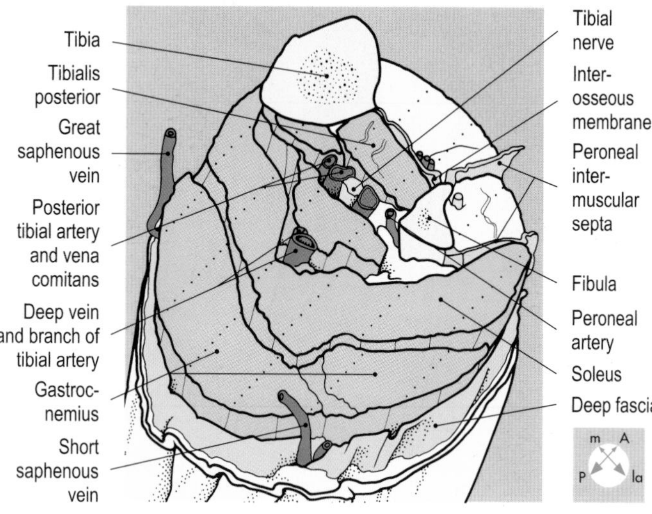

Fig. 6.41 'Step' dissection showing the muscle layers in the upper third of the leg and the location of principal nerves and vessels.

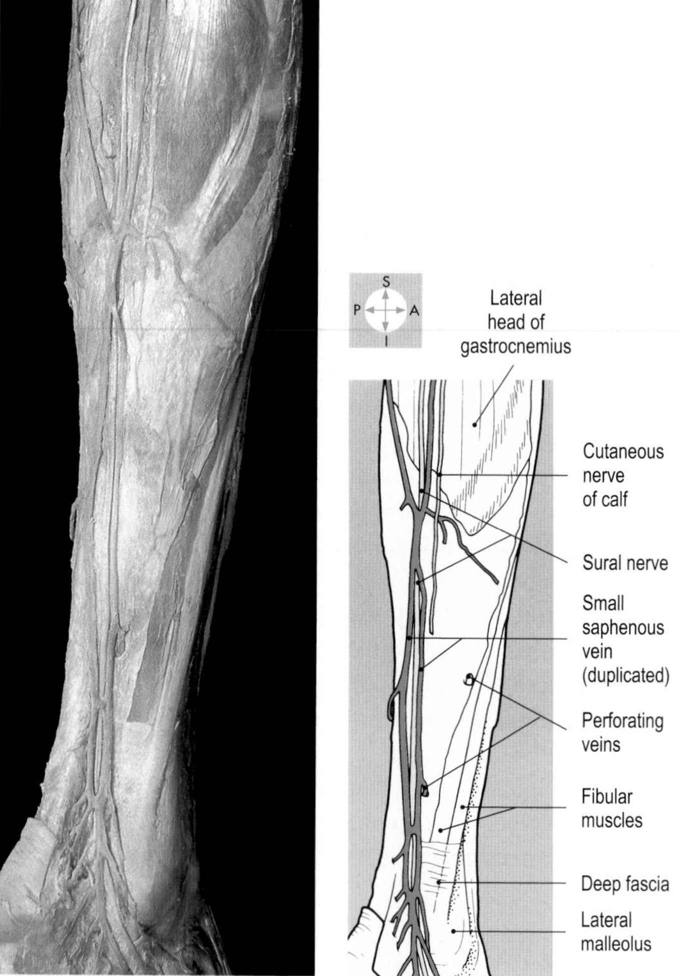

Fig. 6.42 Small saphenous vein and sural nerve. Perforating veins pierce the deep fascia to connect with deep veins in the calf muscles.

bridges the gap between the medial malleolus and the medial surface of the calcaneus, completing a fibro-osseous tunnel similar to the carpal tunnel of the wrist. It is the gateway into the sole of the foot for the tendons of the deep muscles of the compartment and the neurovascular bundle. The tibial nerve may be compressed in the tunnel, causing pain in the heel and foot.

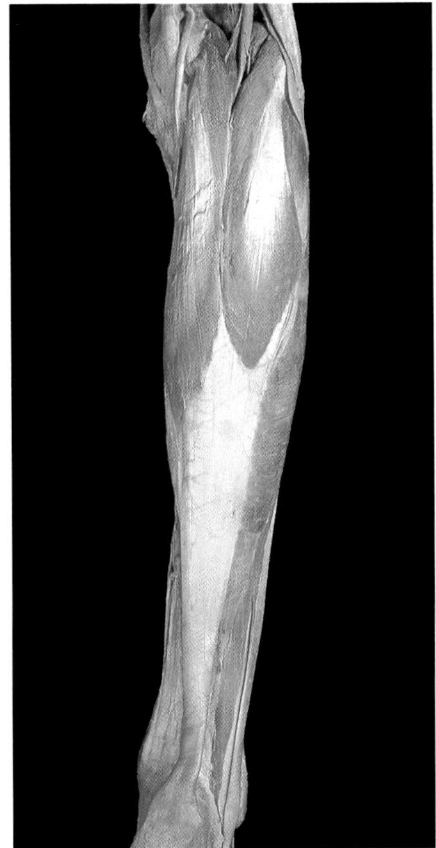

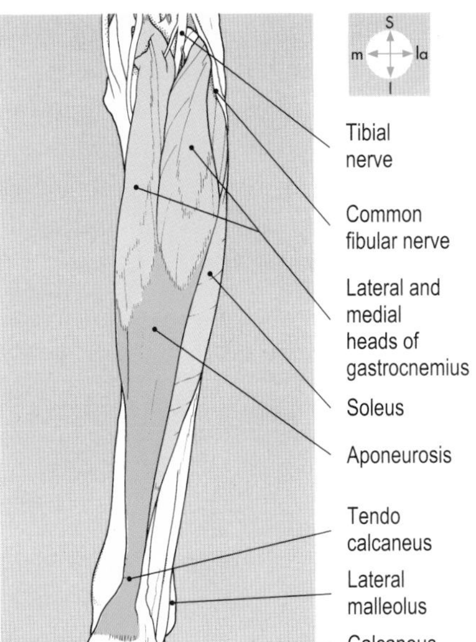

Fig. 6.43 Removal of the deep fascia reveals the superficial flexor muscles, gastrocnemius and soleus.

Superficial muscles

Gastrocnemius

The muscle has medial and lateral heads attached to the respective femoral condyles. The medial head is the larger and its fibres extend more distally. The two heads share a common aponeurosis which overlies that of the subjacent soleus (Fig. 6.43). The long parallel fibres of gastrocnemius provide a large range of movement and are used especially during walking and running. Because of its femoral attachments it is a weak flexor of the knee joint.

Soleus

This muscle attaches to the soleal line on the posterior border of the tibia, from where it arches across to the posterior aspect of the head and upper shaft of the fibula (Figs 6.44 & 6.45). Its short multipennate fibres are continually in action during standing.

The aponeuroses of gastrocnemius and soleus form the tendo calcaneus (Achilles) which attaches to the middle third of the posterior surface of the calcaneus, and via this tendon the two muscles are the principal flexors of the foot at the ankle joint. The tendon, separated from the upper part of the calcaneus, is easily palpable and is used clinically to obtain the stretch (plantar) reflex (S1 & S2).

Plantaris

This muscle attaches to the lower end of the femur close to the lateral head of gastrocnemius. Its long thin tendon passes deep to the medial head of gastrocnemius (Fig. 6.45) between the aponeuroses of gastrocnemius and soleus to insert into the posterior surface of the calcaneus medial to

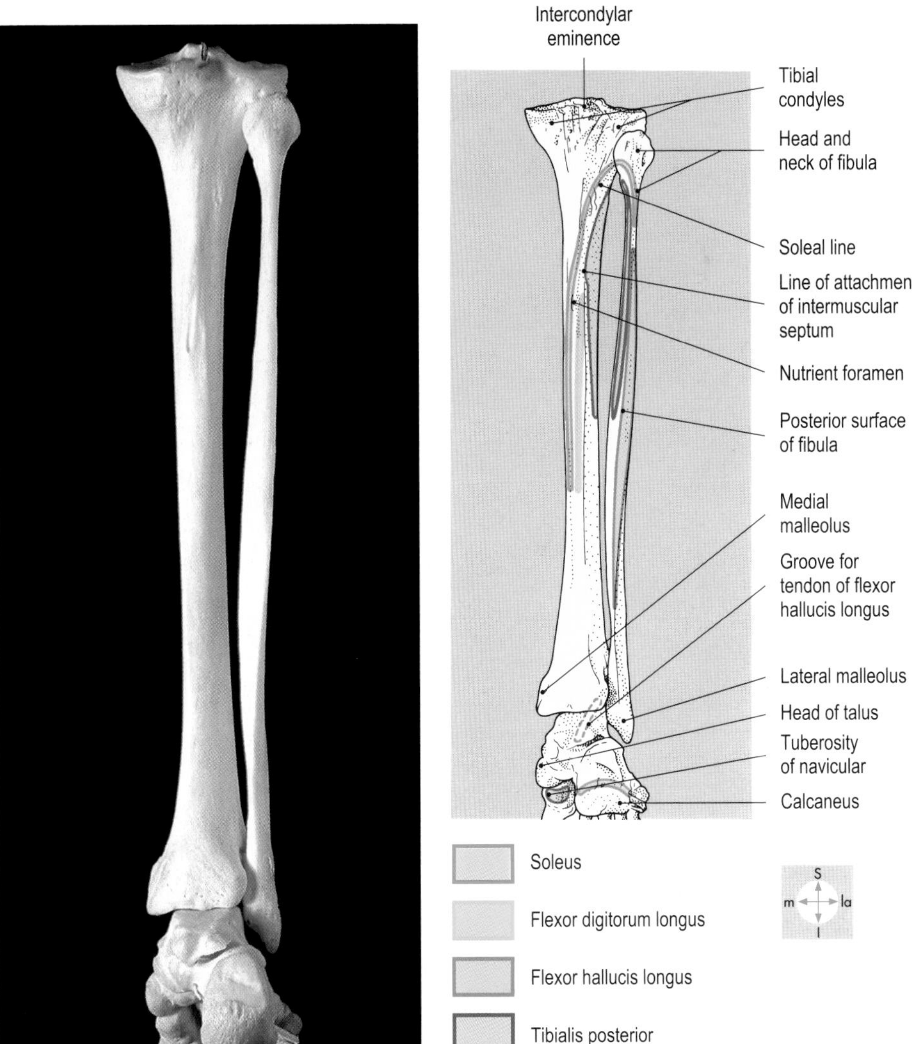

Fig. 6.44 Posterior view of bones of leg and foot. The diagram shows attachments of muscles of posterior compartment.

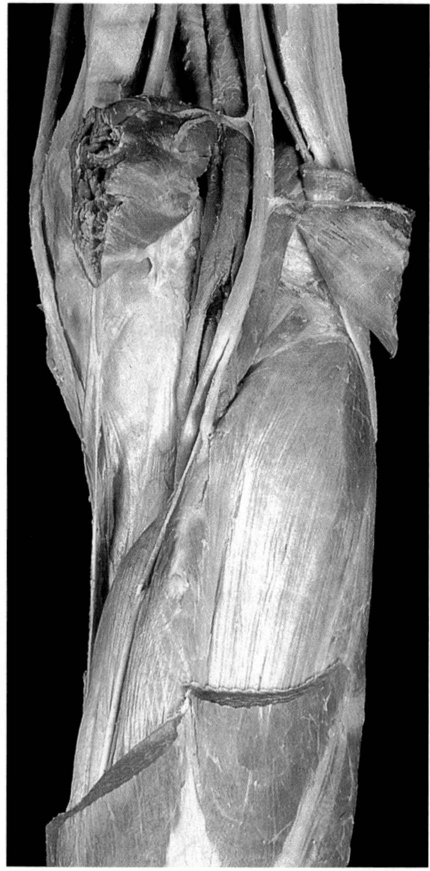

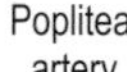

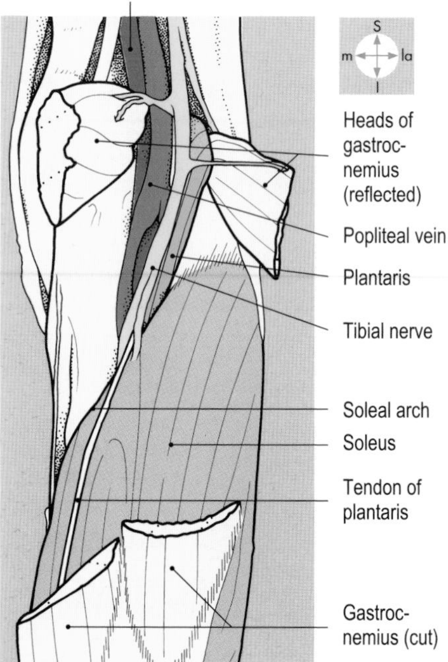

Fig. 6.45 Partial removal of the two heads of gastrocnemius reveals soleus and the neurovascular bundle passing beneath the soleal arch to enter the calf.

the tendo calcaneus. It is a weak flexor of the knee and ankle joints.

Gastrocnemius, soleus and plantaris are supplied by the tibial nerve in the popliteal fossa (see Fig. 6.40). Soleus is further supplied by the tibial nerve as it passes beneath the soleal arch.

Neurovascular structures

Posterior tibial artery

At the lower border of popliteus the popliteal artery divides into two terminal branches, the anterior tibial artery (see p. 290) and the larger posterior tibial artery. The latter, accompanied by its venae comitantes, passes deep to the soleal arch and descends on the fascia of tibialis posterior (see Fig. 6.41) between flexor digitorum longus and flexor hallucis longus. Near the ankle the artery lies on the distal end of the tibia and the capsule of the ankle joint, where its pulsations are easily felt. Passing beneath the flexor retinaculum, it gives calcaneal branches to the superficial tissues of the heel and then divides into medial and lateral plantar arteries. It provides branches to the muscles in the calf and also a large nutrient artery to the tibial shaft.

The most conspicuous branch, the fibular (peroneal) artery, arises just beyond the soleal arch (Fig. 6.46) and passes distally and laterally deep to flexor hallucis longus and upon the fascia of tibialis posterior. It gives muscular branches and a nutrient branch to the fibula. The fibular artery terminates behind the lateral malleolus as lateral calcaneal branches supplying the tissues of the heel. In the lower part of the leg a communicating artery links the fibular and posterior tibial arteries.

A perforating branch of the fibular artery passes forwards through the interosseous membrane into the anterior compartment of the leg. When the anterior tibial artery is small, this perforating artery may substitute for it distally, continuing into the foot as the dorsalis pedis artery.

Tibial nerve

The tibial nerve enters the compartment from the popliteal fossa by passing beneath the soleal arch. Usually, the posterior tibial artery lies medially as it descends through the calf on the fascia of tibialis posterior and on the distal end of the tibia (Fig. 6.46). Like the artery, as it enters the foot it often terminates beneath the flexor retinaculum as two branches, the medial and lateral plantar nerves. It supplies soleus and the deep leg muscles and gives sensory branches to skin over the ball of the heel.

Deep muscles

Lying deep to soleus are flexor digitorum longus, flexor hallucis longus and tibialis posterior (see Figs 6.41 & 6.46). Proximally, their attachments are limited by the origin of soleus from the tibia and fibula. Their tendons enter the foot beneath the flexor retinaculum.

Flexor digitorum longus arises from the posterior surface of the tibia (Fig. 6.44) and from the fascia covering tibialis posterior. In the foot the tendon divides into four slips, which are attached to the bases of the terminal phalanges of the lateral toes. The muscle flexes the toes and assists in plantar flexion of the ankle joint.

Flexor hallucis longus is larger than flexor digitorum longus (Fig 6.46) and has extensive attachments to the posterior surface of the shaft of the fibula (Fig. 6.44), the posterior intermuscular septum and the fascia covering tibialis posterior. Its muscle fibres characteristically extend almost as far as the ankle (Fig. 6.46) and give way to a tendon which passes beneath the flexor retinaculum to insert into the base of the distal phalanx of the great toe. It is a powerful flexor of the hallux, especially in forward propulsion of the foot at the take-off point during walking. Plantar flexion at the ankle joint is also assisted.

Tibialis posterior is the deepest muscle in the compartment and attaches to the posterior surface of the tibia (Fig. 6.44), to the medial surface of the fibula and to the upper two-thirds of the interosseous membrane. Passing under the flexor retinaculum, where it is the most medial structure, the tendon enters the foot to attach principally to the tuberosity of the navicular and by small slips to the other tarsal bones. Together with tibialis anterior its action is to invert the foot. It is also a weak plantar flexor of the ankle joint.

All three deep muscles of the calf are supplied by the tibial nerve. Further details of their tendons in the sole of the foot are given on page 282.

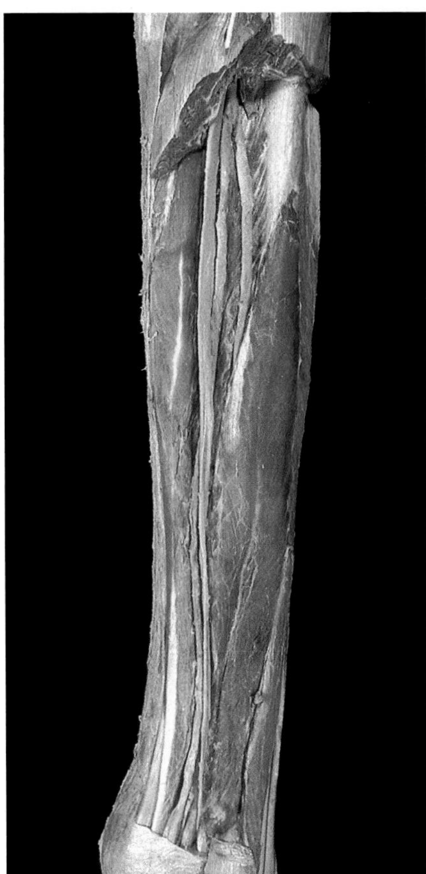

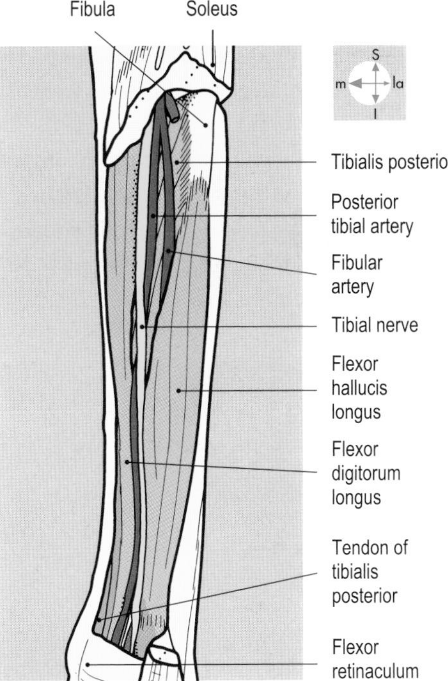

Fig. 6.46 Removal of the superficial flexor group shows the deep muscles of the compartment and the main neurovascular bundle.

Sole of Foot

The sole of the foot contains the plantar aponeurosis, intrinsic muscles, tendons originating from muscles in the leg, and plantar vessels and nerves. The tendons, accompanied by the vessels and nerves, enter the sole deep to the flexor retinaculum (Fig. 6.48) in the tarsal tunnel, between the medial aspect of the calcaneus and the medial malleolus. The skin of the sole is thick and heavily keratinized and is firmly attached to the deep fascia by fibrous septa which traverse and loculate the subcutaneous fat.

Plantar aponeurosis

The plantar aponeurosis, the deep fascia of the sole covering the superficial layer of muscles, is especially thick in its central portion. Posteriorly, the aponeurosis is attached to the medial and lateral calcaneal tubercles. Anteriorly, it widens and diverges into five digital slips (Fig. 6.47), which attach to the fibrous flexor sheaths and plantar metatarsal plates (see Fig. 6.96). These plates give the aponeurosis indirect attachment to the bases of all the proximal phalanges, providing an important support for the longitudinal arches of the foot (see Figs 6.98–6.101). Inflammation of the aponeurosis (plantar fasciitis) is a cause of pain in the foot.

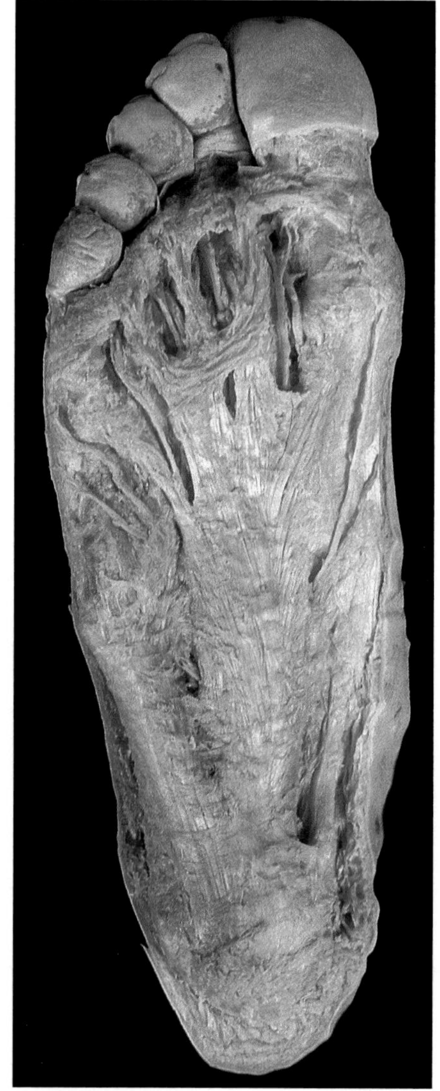

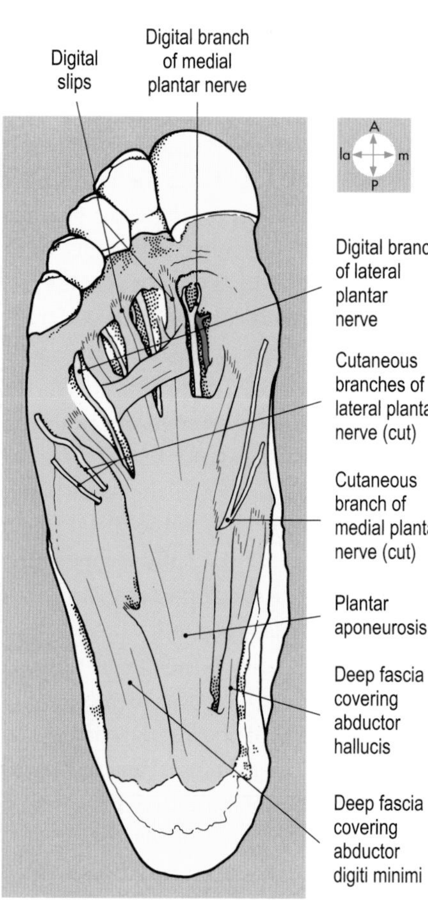

Fig. 6.47 Plantar aponeurosis, deep fascia and cutaneous nerves, revealed by removal of the skin of the sole.

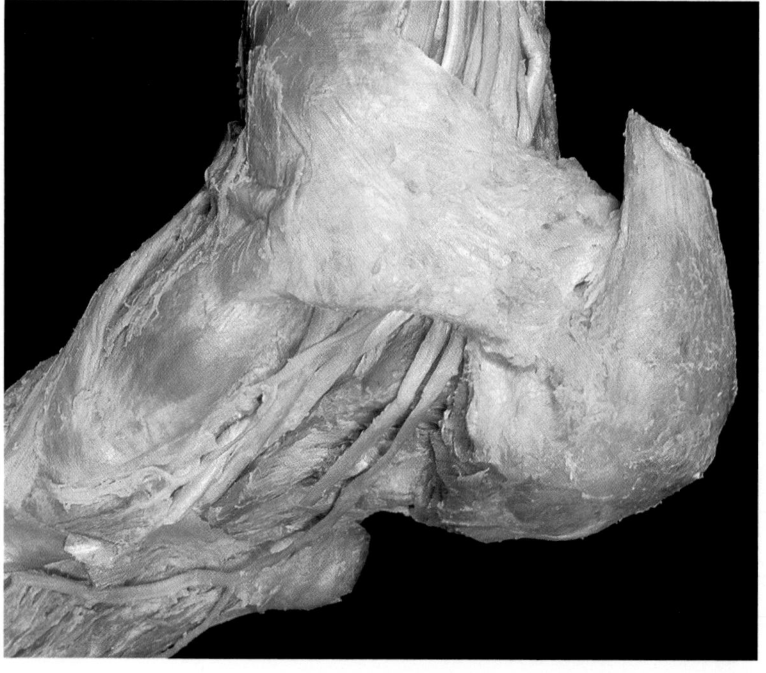

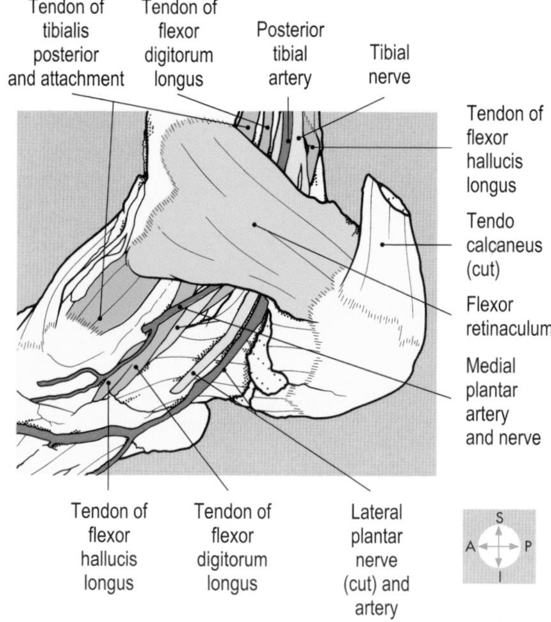

Fig. 6.48 Long tendons and the principal vessels and nerves from the posterior compartment of the leg pass deep to the flexor retinaculum to enter the sole of the foot.

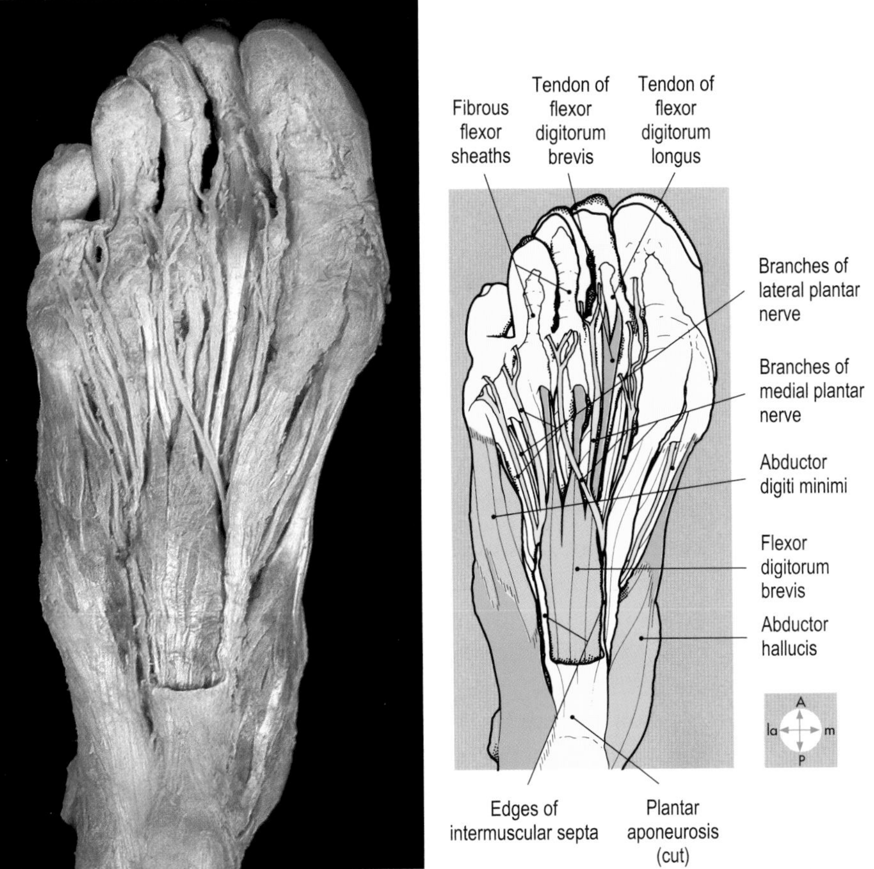

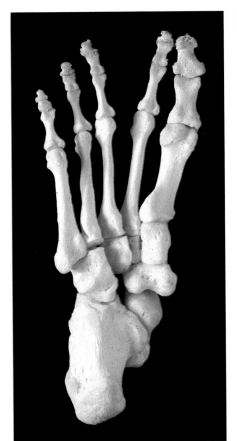

Fig. 6.49 Superficial intrinsic muscles and plantar nerves after removal of deep fascia, part of the plantar aponeurosis and second fibrous tendon sheath. In this specimen, flexor digitorum brevis has only three tendons.

Muscles and tendons

The muscles and tendons in the sole of the foot are arranged in four layers.

Superficial intrinsic muscles

This layer comprises three muscles which span the length of most of the foot and attach to the deep surface of the plantar aponeurosis. Abductor hallucis (Fig. 6.49) lies on the medial side of the foot and arises from the medial calcaneal tubercle and the adjacent flexor retinaculum. Its tendon passes to the great toe with the medial tendon of flexor hallucis brevis and attaches to the medial side of the base of the proximal phalanx. It is supplied by the medial plantar nerve.

Flexor digitorum brevis lies centrally (see Fig. 6.49) and attaches to the medial calcaneal tubercle (Fig. 6.50). It has four tendons which pass forwards to enter the fibrous flexor sheaths of the lateral four toes. Each tendon splits to allow the passage of the long flexor tendon (Figs 6.49 & 6.51), then reunites to attach to the flexor surface of the middle phalanx. Flexor digitorum brevis aids flexion of the proximal parts of the toes and is supplied by the medial plantar nerve.

Abductor digiti minimi traverses the lateral border of the sole (Fig. 6.49) and is attached posteriorly to the medial and lateral calcaneal tubercles. Entering the little toe, its tendon attaches to the lateral side of the proximal phalanx. The muscle is supplied by the lateral plantar nerve.

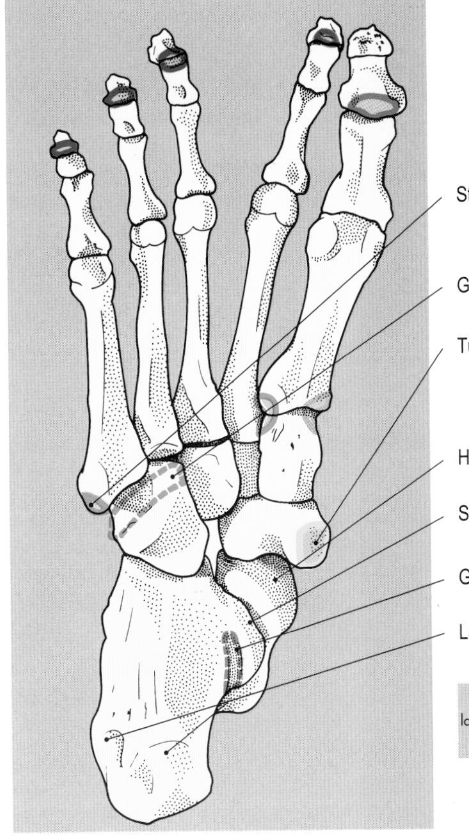

Fig. 6.50 Plantar view of bones of foot showing attachments of some long tendons.

Long flexor tendons and associated intrinsic muscles

This layer includes the tendons of two long flexor muscles which arise in the leg, namely flexor hallucis longus and flexor digitorum longus. Attached to the tendon of flexor digitorum longus (Fig. 6.52) are quadratus plantae (flexor accessorius) and the four lumbricals.

The tendon of flexor hallucis longus grooves the posterior surface of the talus and curves forwards inferior to the sustentaculum tali and the spring (plantar calcaneonavicular) ligament. It passes deep to the tendon of flexor digitorum longus, to which it is usually attached. The tendon of flexor hallucis longus continues forwards inferior to the head of the first metatarsal, where it passes between the sesamoid bones in the two tendons of the flexor hallucis brevis (see below), and enters the fibrous flexor sheath of the great toe to reach its attachment to the base of the distal phalanx (Fig. 6.52). The actions and innervation of flexor hallucis longus are described on page 279.

The tendon of flexor digitorum longus passes forwards medial to the sustentaculum tali and divides into four tendons, one for each of the lateral four toes (see Figs 6.51, 6.52). Each tendon enters its fibrous flexor sheath and passes through the flexor digitorum brevis tendon before attaching to the base of the terminal phalanx. The actions and innervations of flexor digitorum longus are considered on page 279.

Quadratus plantae (flexor accessorius) (Figs 6.51 & 6.52) is quadrangular and is anchored posteriorly to the medial and lateral tubercles of the calcaneus. Anteriorly, the muscle attaches to the tendons of flexor digitorum longus. By pulling on these tendons it can flex the toes irrespective of the position of the ankle. Its nerve supply is from the lateral plantar nerve.

The lumbricals are four small muscles attached proximally to the tendons of flexor digitorum longus (Fig. 6.52). Distally, each slender tendon winds around the medial side of the appropriate digit to attach to the extensor expansion and base of the proximal phalanx. The lumbricals extend the lateral four toes but flex the metatarsophalangeal joints. The first lumbrical is supplied by the medial plantar nerve and the remainder by the lateral plantar nerve.

Deep intrinsic muscles

The three muscles in this layer are located in the anterior part of the foot (Fig. 6.53), adjacent to the metatarsals. Flexor hallucis brevis and adductor hallucis lie medially and are attached to the great toe, whilst flexor digiti minimi brevis lies laterally and acts on the little toe.

Flexor hallucis brevis lies along the medial side of the foot and is attached posteriorly to the cuboid and the three cuneiforms. Passing forwards on either side of the flexor hallucis longus tendon (Fig. 6.52), the muscle gives rise to two short tendons, which lie inferior to the first metatarsophalangeal joint. Each tendon contains a sesamoid bone (see Fig. 6.101) and enters the great toe to attach to the appropriate side of the base of the proximal phalanx. Flexor hallucis brevis flexes the proximal phalanx and is innervated by the medial plantar nerve.

Adductor hallucis (Fig. 6.53) consists of an oblique head which is attached to the bases of the second, third and fourth metatarsals, and a transverse head which lies across the anterior part of the sole, attached to the deep transverse metatarsal ligaments and the lateral three metatarsophalangeal joints. The two heads converge and attach to the lateral tendon and sesamoid of flexor hallucis

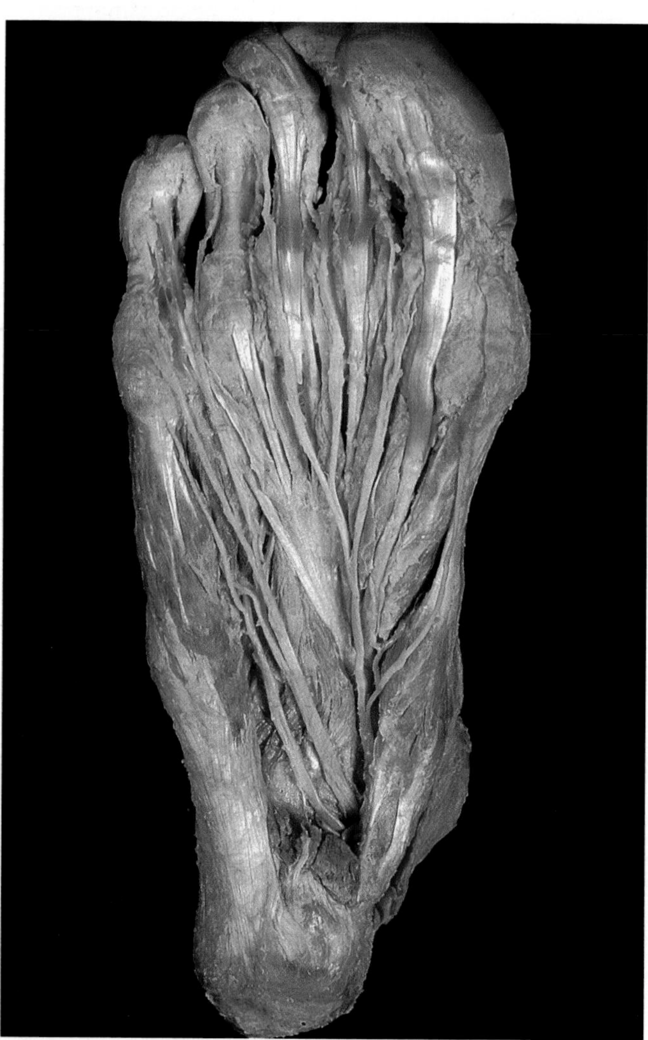

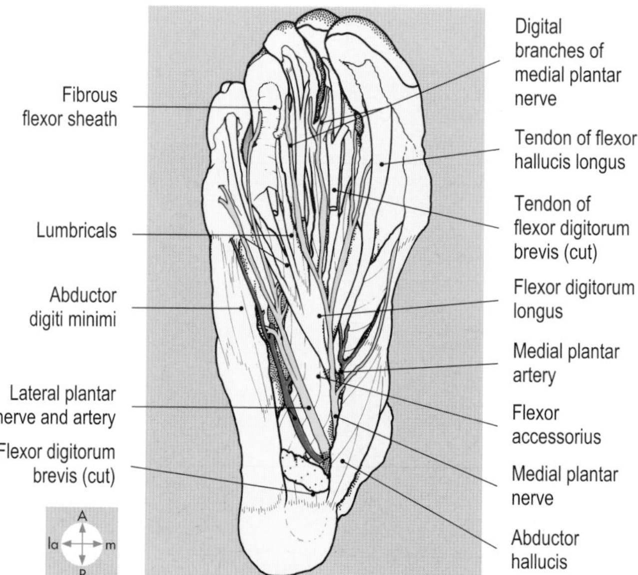

Fig. 6.51 Removal of flexor digitorum brevis has revealed the plantar nerves and arteries, which enter the sole deep to abductor hallucis.

brevis. Adductor hallucis assists flexor hallucis brevis and may help to support the transverse arch of the foot. It is supplied by the lateral plantar nerve.

Flexor digiti minimi brevis lies along the plantar surface of the fifth metatarsal (Fig. 6.53), attaching posteriorly to the base of the bone and anteriorly to the lateral side of the base of the proximal

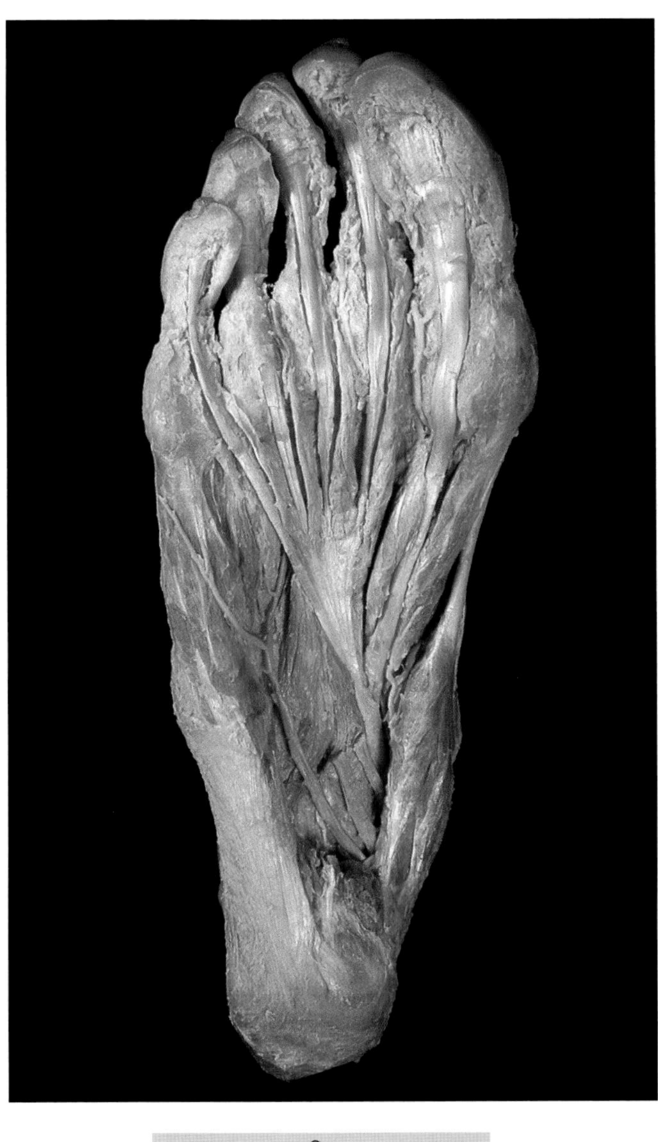

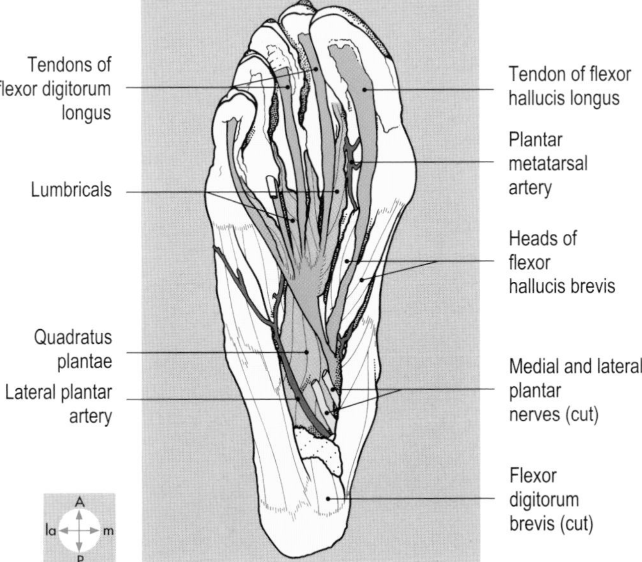

Fig. 6.52 Tendons of flexor digitorum longus, flexor hallucis longus, quadratus plantae and the lumbricals, after removal of medial and lateral plantar nerves and the tendons of flexor digitorum brevis.

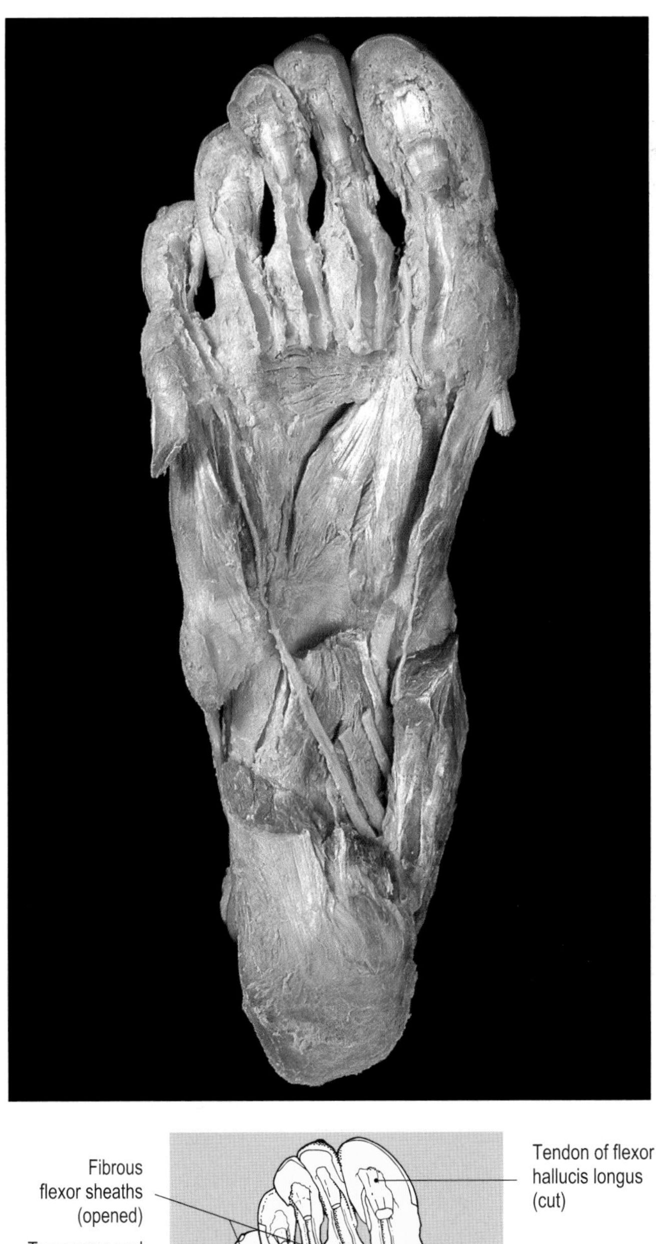

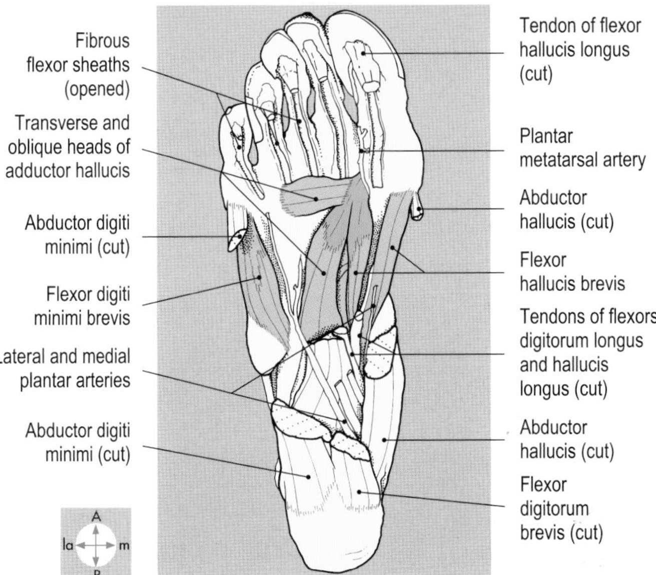

Fig. 6.53 Deep intrinsic muscles, revealed by removal of long flexor tendons and abductors of the great and little toes.

phalanx of the little toe. The muscle flexes the proximal phalanx and is innervated by the lateral plantar nerve.

Interossei and tendons of fibularis (peroneus) longus and tibialis posterior

Lying deeply in the sole, attached to the metatarsals, the three plantar interosseous muscles (Fig. 6.54) attach by single heads to the plantar borders of the third, fourth and fifth metatarsals. The four dorsal interossei (Fig. 6.55) are bicipital and attach to contiguous surfaces of the shafts of the metatarsals. The tendons pass forwards dorsal to the deep transverse metatarsal ligaments and attach to the bases of the proximal phalanges and dorsal extensor expansions. These muscles are supplied by the lateral plantar nerve. They assist extension of the phalanges and flexion of the

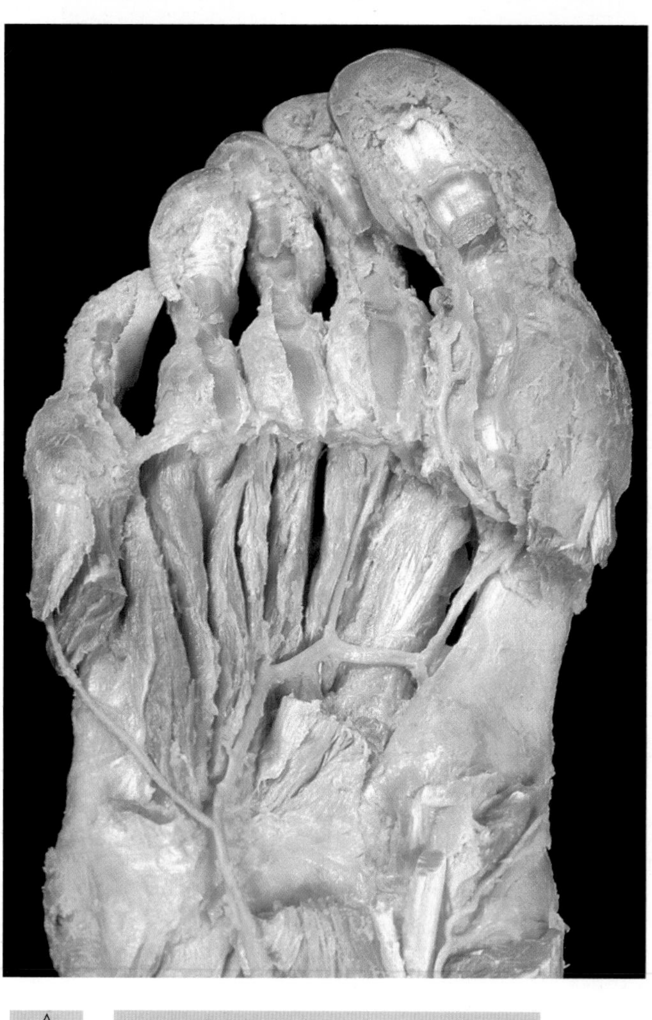

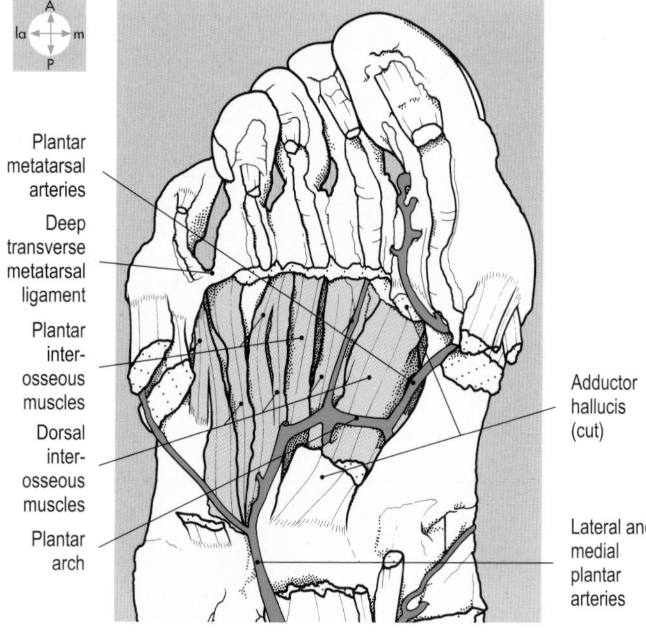

Fig. 6.54 Interosseous muscles and the plantar arterial arch, exposed by removing adductor hallucis.

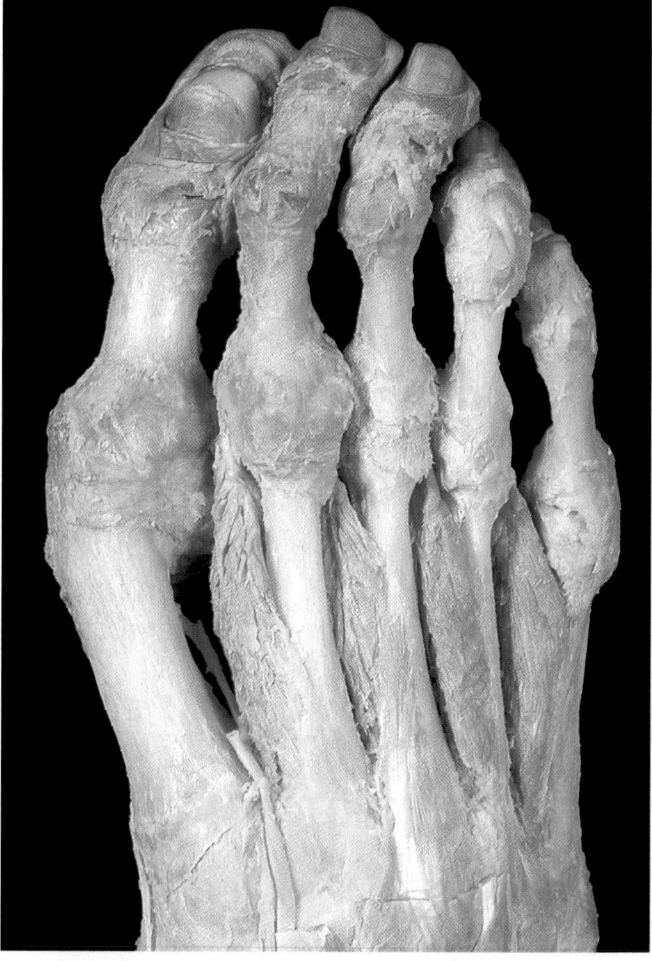

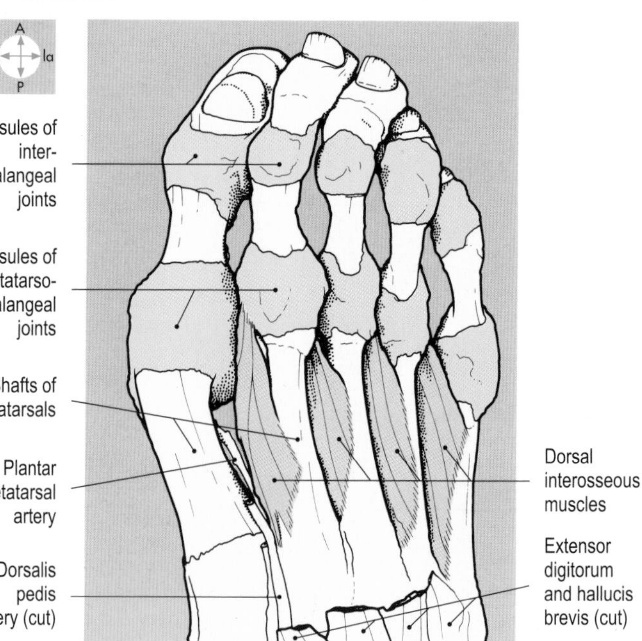

Fig. 6.55 Dorsal aspect of the foot showing the dorsal interosseous muscles after partial removal of extensor digitorum brevis. Extensor expansions have been removed to show joint capsules.

metatarsophalangeal joints. Their attachments indicate that plantar interossei should adduct and dorsal interossei should abduct the toes, but these movements are often poorly developed, especially in the shod foot.

The tendons of fibularis (peroneus) longus and tibialis posterior (Fig. 6.56) pass deeply into the sole to reach their attachments on tarsal and metatarsal bones. The fibularis longus tendon enters the lateral side of the sole and is retained in a groove inferior to the cuboid by the long plantar ligament. The tendon passes forwards and medially to reach the lateral aspect of the base of the first metatarsal and adjacent medial cuneiform (compare with tibialis anterior, p, 288). The tendon of tibialis posterior enters the medial aspect of the foot deep to the flexor retinaculum (Figs 6.48 & 6.56), attaches to the tuberosity of the navicular and sends additional slips to other tarsal bones and the metatarsal bases. These two tendons may help to support the medial longitudinal arch. The other actions of fibularis longus and tibialis posterior and their innervation are considered on pages 279 and 290.

Blood supply

Deep to the flexor retinaculum, the tibial artery divides into medial and lateral plantar branches (see Fig. 6.51). Passing forwards, the medial plantar artery runs deep to the superficial intrinsic muscles, gives off plantar cutaneous branches which pass between abductor hallucis and flexor digitorum brevis, and terminates by supplying digital branches to the medial (and occasionally lateral) side of the great toe. The larger lateral plantar artery passes forwards and laterally (Fig. 6.54) deep to the superficial intrinsic muscles towards the base of the fifth metatarsal. Here the artery inclines medially and deeply to form the plantar arch, lying on the interossei and bases of the metatarsals. A perforating branch between the first and second metatarsals usually links the arch with the dorsalis pedis artery (see p. 290). From the arch, plantar metatarsal arteries (Fig. 6.54) pass distally to the webs of the toes where they divide into digital branches. Venae comitantes accompany medial and lateral plantar arteries and their branches.

Nerve supply

Cutaneous branches of the tibial nerve supply the skin over the heel. Deep to the flexor retinaculum the tibial nerve divides into medial and lateral branches, which supply their respective sides of the sole (see Figs 6.48 & 6.51). The larger medial plantar nerve accompanies the corresponding artery and gives cutaneous branches to the medial three and one-half digits, including the nail beds. The nerve also supplies abductor hallucis, flexor hallucis brevis, flexor digitorum brevis and the first lumbrical.

The lateral plantar nerve accompanies the corresponding artery (see Fig. 6.51) supplying quadratus plantae and abductor digiti minimi and giving cutaneous branches to the sole. Near the base of the fifth metatarsal it divides into superficial and deep branches which supply the remaining muscles of the sole. The deep branch accompanies the plantar arch and terminates in adductor hallucis. In addition to muscular branches, the superficial branch also gives cutaneous branches to the lateral one and one-half toes.

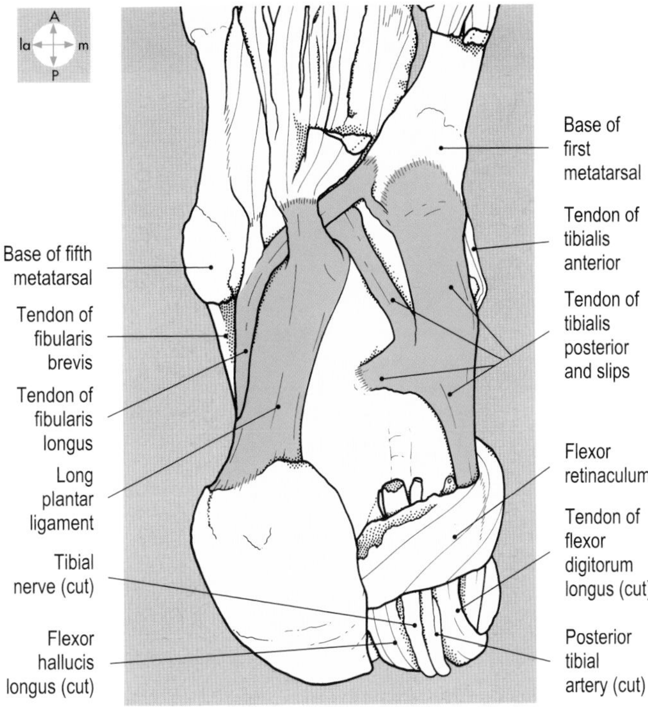

Fig. 6.56 Deep dissection of sole to show long plantar ligament and tendons of fibularis longus and tibialis posterior.

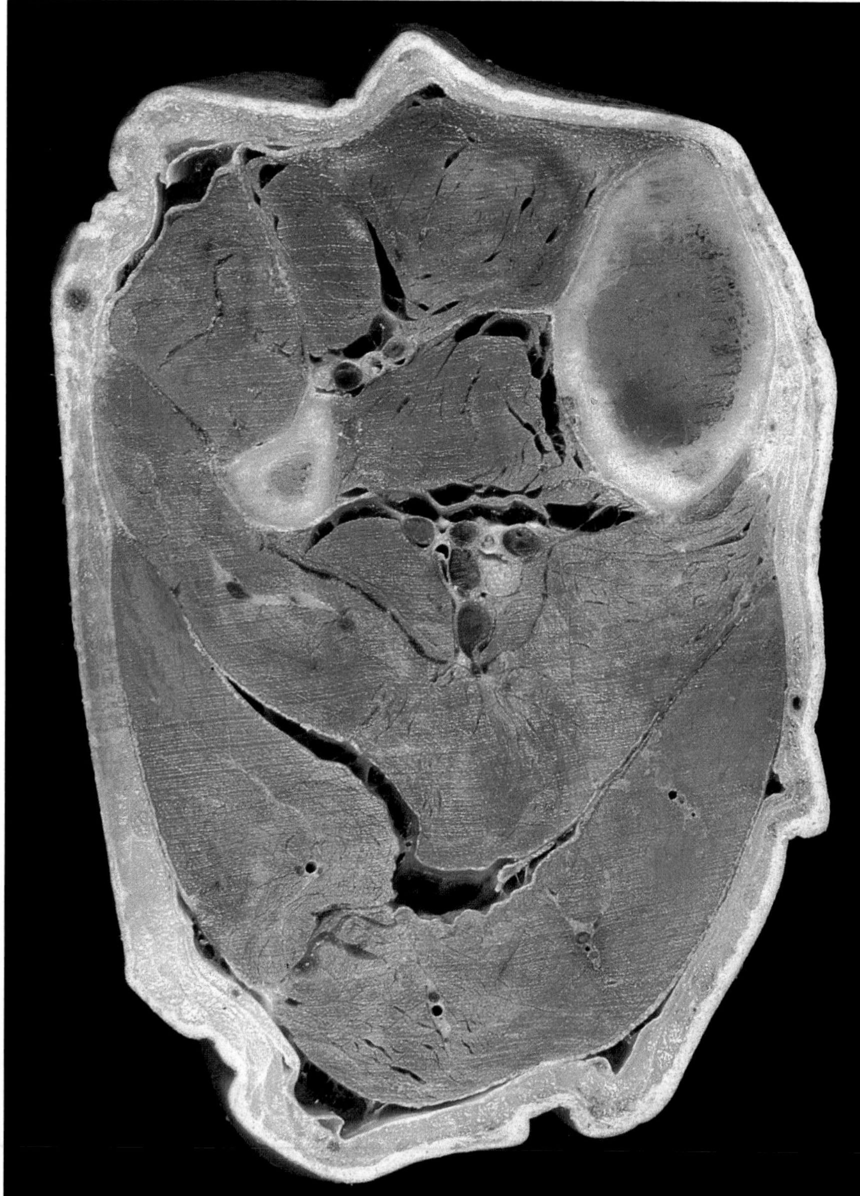

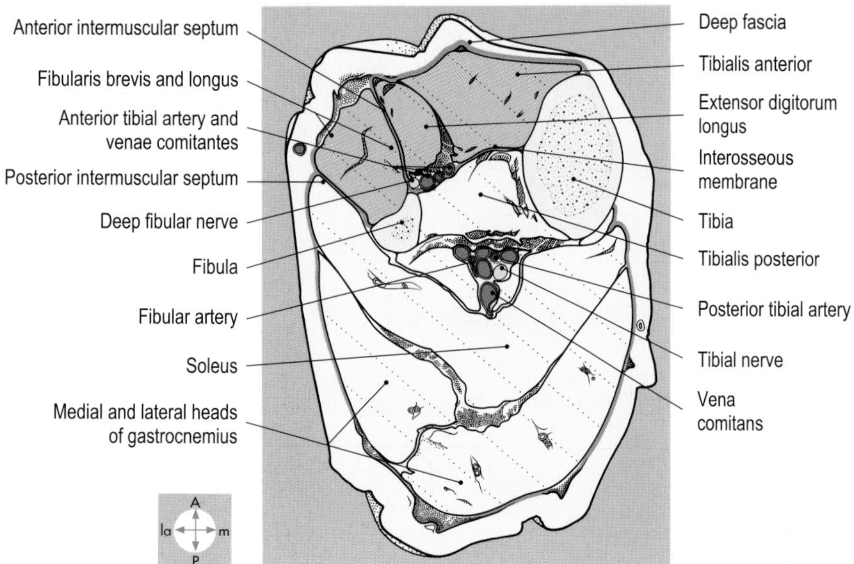

Fig. 6.57 Transverse section through the leg showing anterior and lateral compartments and their contents. Inferior aspect.

Anterior and Lateral Compartments of Leg and Dorsum of Foot

Anterior compartment of leg and dorsum of foot

The anterior compartment of the leg contains muscles that extend the ankle joint and toes and evert and invert the foot. Its neurovascular bundle comprises the anterior tibial artery and its venae comitantes and the deep fibular nerve (Fig. 6.57). The cutaneous branches of the superficial fibular nerve are also present.

On the dorsum of the foot are the long extensor tendons, the dorsalis pedis artery, the dorsal venous arch and, more laterally, the bellies of extensor digitorum brevis and extensor hallucis brevis. The medial and lateral malleoli lie on each side of the ankle.

Superficial structures

The dorsal venous arch (Fig. 6.58) drains blood from the toes and sole of the foot. From its medial end the great saphenous vein passes in front of the medial malleolus where it is palpable and accessible, and then ascends to the posteromedial aspect of the knee. From the lateral side of the arch the small saphenous vein passes behind the lateral malleolus and ascends to the popliteal fossa (see p. 274). The saphenous nerve accompanies the great saphenous vein (Fig. 6.59), supplying skin on the medial side of the leg and medial border of the foot as far as the ball (metatarsophalangeal joint) of the great toe. The sural nerve accompanies the small saphenous vein (Fig. 6.58) and supplies skin along the lateral border of the foot and little toe.

The superficial fibular (superficial peroneal) nerve enters the anterior compartment of the leg from the lateral (fibular or peroneal) compartment at the anterior border of fibularis longus (see Fig. 6.60). Shortly after piercing the deep fascia it divides into medial and lateral branches which supply the skin of the leg and dorsum of the foot (Fig. 6.58). On reaching the toes the medial branch supplies the medial side of the great toe and the contiguous aspects of the second and third toes while the lateral branch innervates the adjacent sides of the third, fourth, and fifth toes. Thus, all of the digital skin is innervated by the superficial fibular nerve except for the cleft between the great and second toes (supplied by the deep fibular [peroneal] nerve) and the lateral aspect of the little toe (supplied by the sural nerve).

The skin and subcutaneous tissues over the anteromedial surface of the tibia are comparatively thin and have a sparse blood supply. As a consequence, lacerations in this region may heal relatively slowly. The subcutaneous tissues of the ankle are a common site for oedema.

Deep fascia

In the region of the ankle and foot there are thickenings of the investing deep fascia forming retinacula (Fig. 6.60) which prevent bowstringing of the long extensor tendons during muscular contraction. As the tendons pass beneath the retinacula to reach the foot they are enveloped in synovial membrane. By convention, superior and inferior extensor retinacula are described (see Fig. 6.64). The superior retinaculum forms a broad band passing between the anterior borders of the tibia

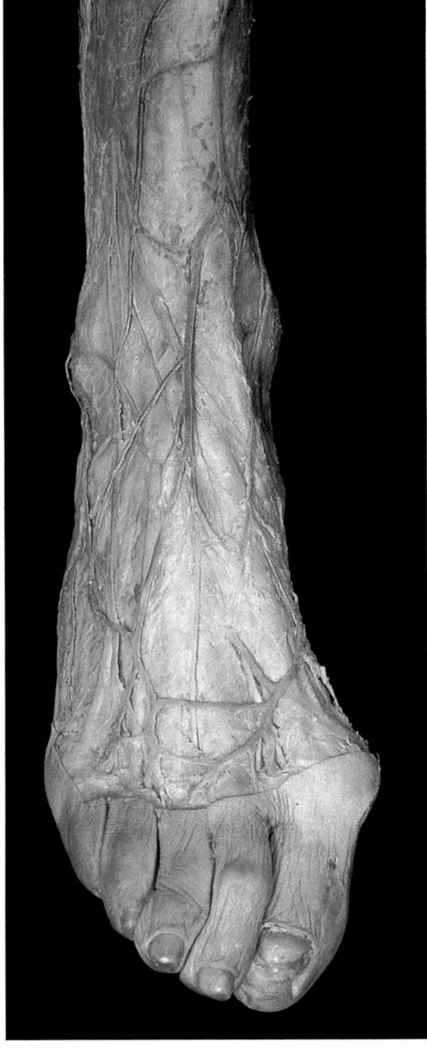

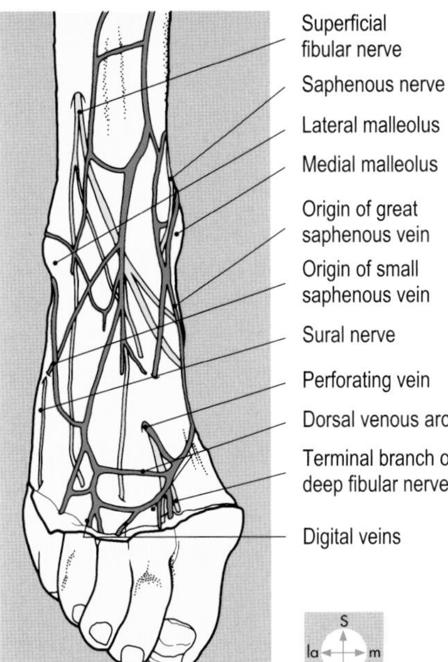

Fig. 6.58 Superficial nerves and veins on the dorsum of the ankle and foot.

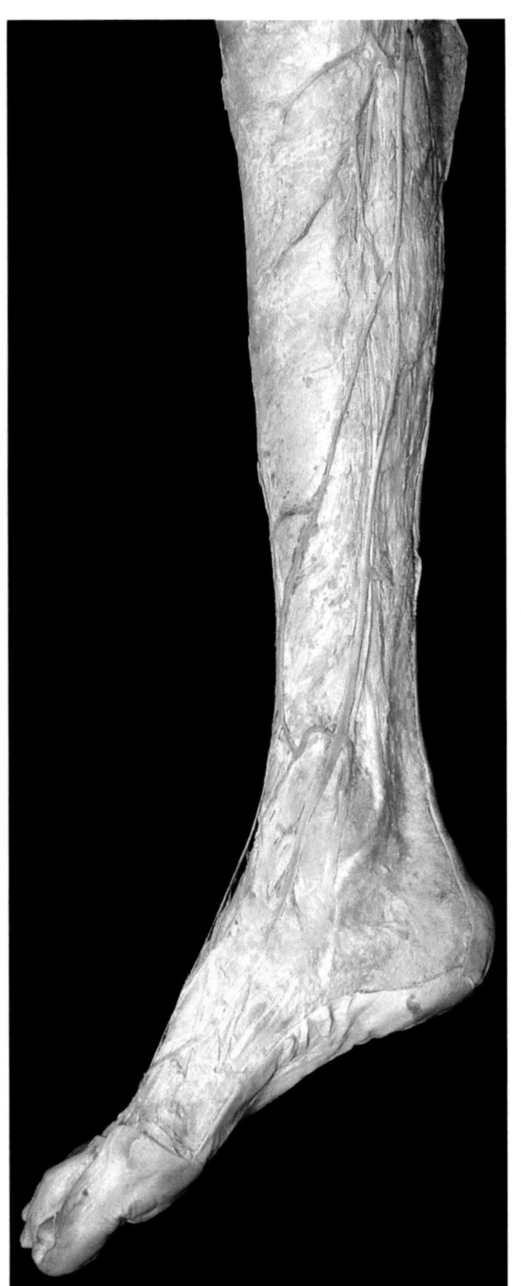

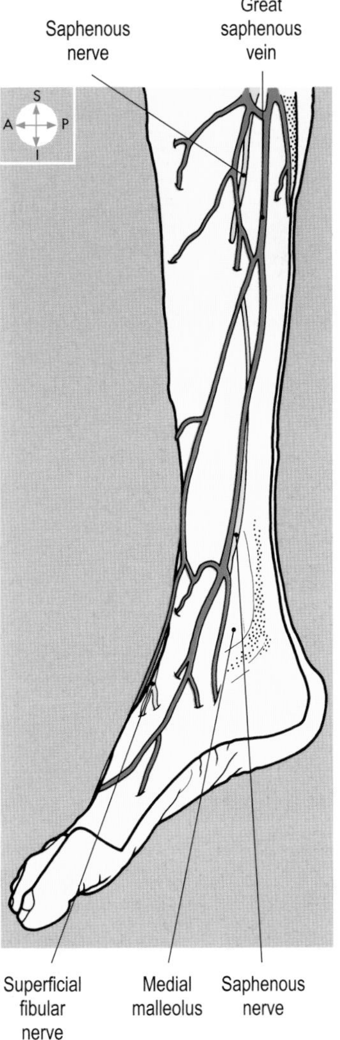

Fig. 6.59 Superficial veins and nerves on the medial surface of the leg and foot.

and fibula. The inferior retinaculum is Y-shaped, with its stem attached to the upper surface of the calcaneus.

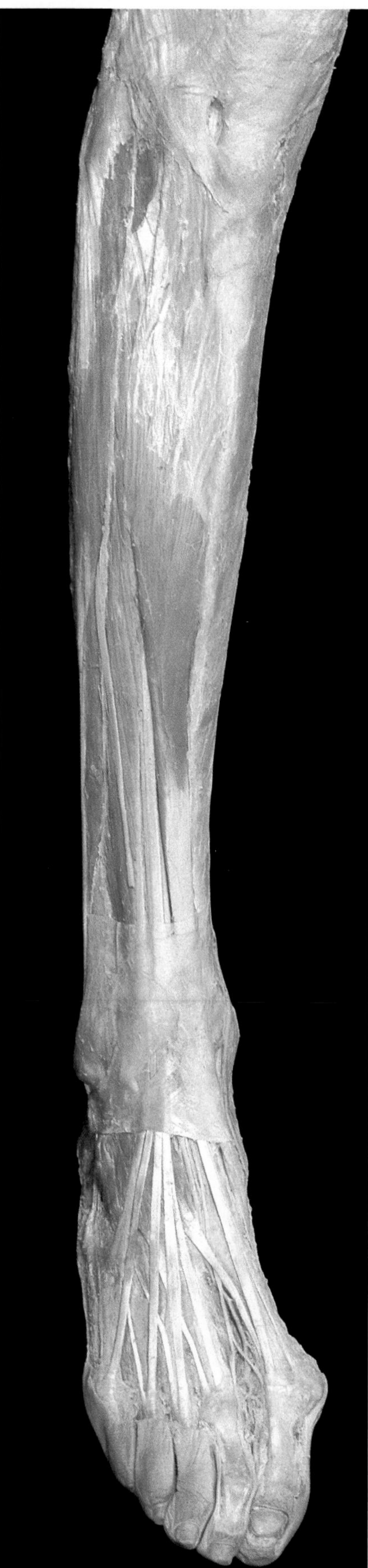

Muscles

The muscles in the anterior compartment are tibialis anterior, extensor hallucis longus, extensor digitorum longus and fibularis (peroneus) tertius. All are supplied by the deep fibular nerve. Tibialis anterior is the most medial (see Figs 6.57 & 6.60), attaching to the lateral condyle and anterolateral surface of the shaft of the tibia, the adjacent interosseous membrane and the deep fascia overlying the muscle. Distally, its tendon crosses the anterior border of the lower end of the tibia and attaches to the base of the first metatarsal and adjacent part of the first cuneiform bone (Fig. 6.61). The muscle inverts the foot and dorsiflexes the ankle joint.

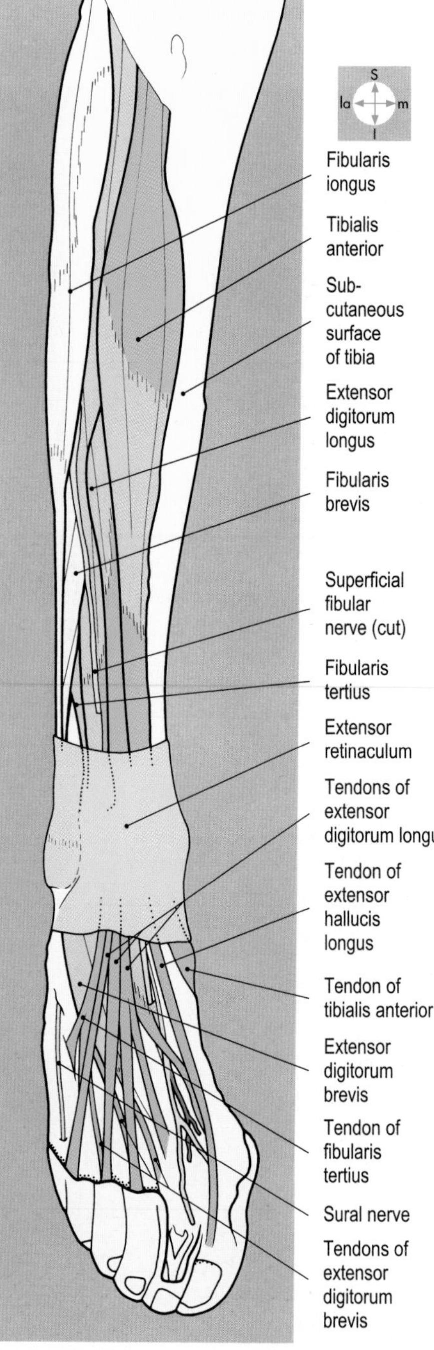

Fig. 6.60 Muscles of the anterior compartment of the leg and tendons on the dorsum of the foot, seen after removal of deep fascia. The extensor retinaculum has been retained.

The other three muscles all attach to the narrow anterior surface of the fibula and adjacent interosseous membrane. Extensor digitorum longus (see Fig. 6.57) is attached to the proximal three-quarters of the bone, fibularis tertius (when present) to the distal quarter, and extensor hallucis longus is overlapped by them medially at midshaft level. In addition, extensor digitorum longus attaches to the anterior intermuscular septum and overlying deep fascia.

The proximal part of extensor hallucis longus is overlapped by adjacent muscles, but in the lower part of the leg its tendon emerges lateral to that of tibialis anterior. As it descends towards the ankle the tendon crosses from the lateral to the medial side of the neurovascular bundle.

In the foot the tendon of extensor hallucis longus runs forwards to the great toe (Fig. 6.62), where it attaches to the base of the distal phalanx. It is a powerful extensor of the toe, dorsiflexor (extensor) of the foot and assists inversion. Lateral to extensor hallucis longus, the muscle belly of extensor digitorum longus gives way distally to four tendons which pass to the dorsal aspects of the lateral four toes. Each tendon forms an extensor expansion that divides into three slips. The central slip attaches to the base of the middle phalanx whilst the two lateral slips combine to insert into the base of the distal phalanx (Fig. 6.62). Extensor digitorum longus extends the lateral four toes and dorsiflexes the foot. Fibularis tertius is a continuation of the belly of extensor digitorum longus. It attaches to the lateral border of the fifth metatarsal (Fig. 6.62) and everts the foot and dorsiflexes the ankle.

The muscles of the anterior compartment of the leg are active during walking in both the supporting and swing phases. In the weight-bearing limb they help to incline the leg forwards while the foot remains stationary on the ground. In the swinging limb the muscles maintain the ankle in dorsiflexion, thereby preventing the foot from dropping.

On the dorsum of the foot, extensor digitorum brevis and extensor hallucis brevis (Fig. 6.62) are attached to the upper surface of the calcaneus and overlying stem of the inferior extensor retinaculum. Extensor digitorum brevis gives rise to three short tendons, which pass deep to the long extensor tendons of the lateral three toes (Fig. 6.62) and attach to the dorsal extensor expansions of the second, third and fourth toes. The tendon of extensor hallucis brevis attaches to the base of the proximal phalanx of the great toe. The muscles assist extension of the toes, particularly when the long extensors are flexing the leg forwards on the foot just before it is lifted from the ground during walking. The nerve supply is the deep fibular nerve.

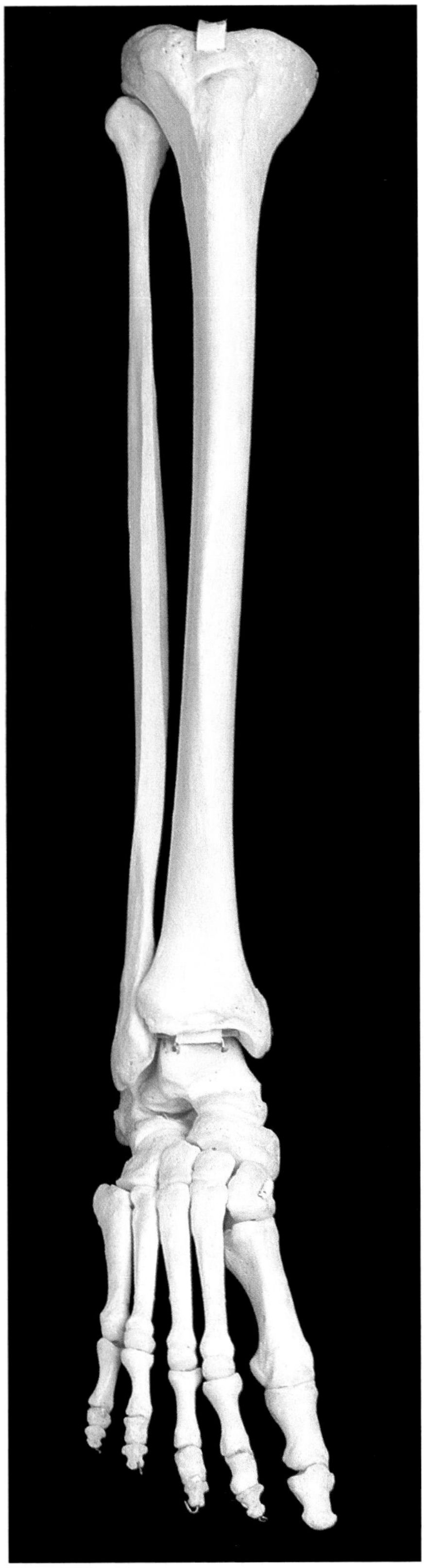

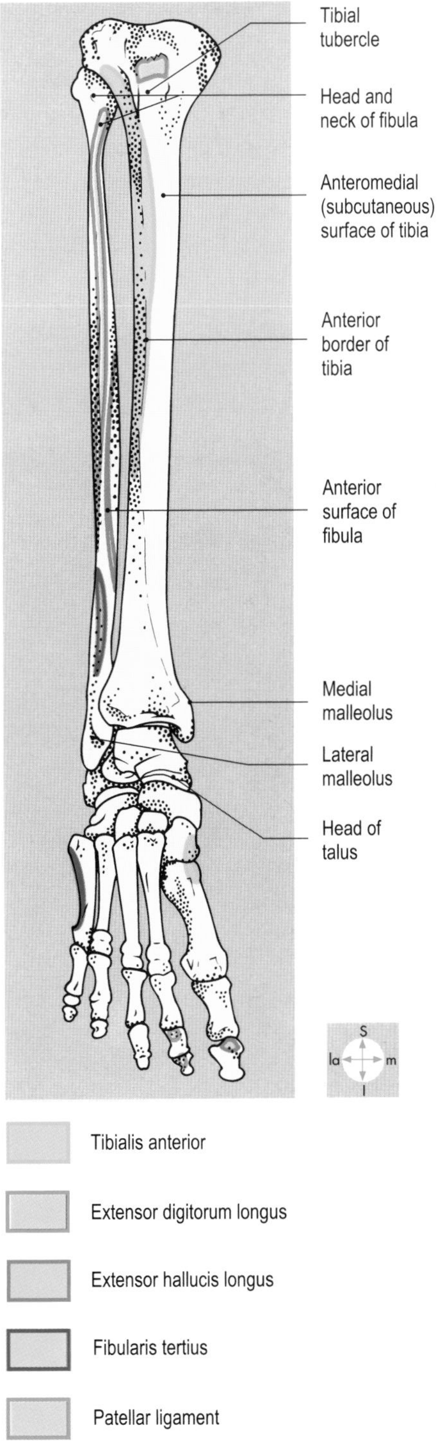

Fig. 6.61 Anterior view of bones of leg and foot showing attachments of muscles of anterior compartment.

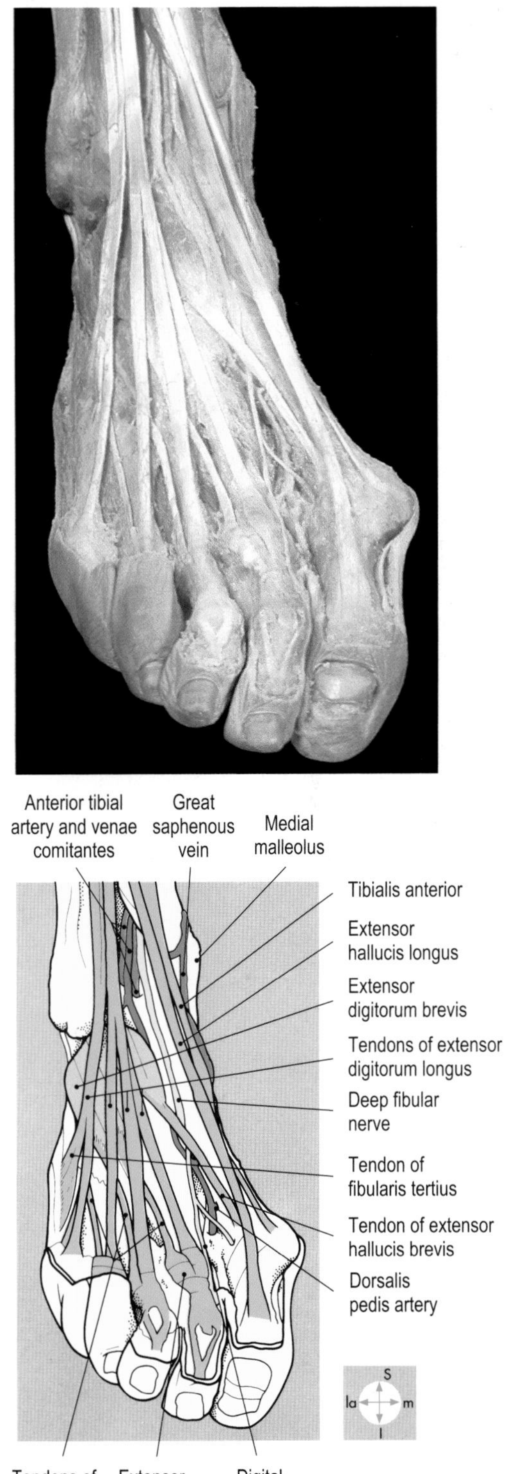

Fig. 6.62 Principal structures on the dorsum of the ankle and foot seen after removal of the extensor retinaculum.

Neurovascular bundle

This comprises the deep fibular nerve and the anterior tibial artery with its venae comitantes (see Fig. 6.57). The artery, a terminal branch of the popliteal artery (see p. 278), reaches the anterior compartment after passing through the interosseous membrane (see Figs 6.76 & 6.83). It then descends on the anterior surface of the membrane (Fig. 6.63) and at the ankle lies midway between the two malleoli. It continues distally as the dorsalis pedis artery on the lateral side of the extensor hallucis longus tendon (see Fig. 6.62), where its pulsations are palpable in the living foot.

At the proximal end of the first intermetatarsal space the dorsalis pedis artery gives a deep branch which passes between the two heads of the first dorsal interosseous muscle to join the plantar arch (see p. 285). This arrangement provides an anastomosis between the anterior and posterior tibial arteries. The dorsalis pedis artery terminates as the first dorsal metatarsal artery, supplying the great toe and adjacent border of the second toe, and the arcuate artery. It turns laterally beneath the extensor tendons across the bases of the metatarsals and gives metatarsal arteries, which divide to supply adjacent borders of the remaining three digits.

The deep fibular (peroneal) nerve, a terminal branch of the common fibular nerve, winds around the neck of the fibula deep to fibularis (peroneus) longus (Fig. 6.63). The nerve accompanies the anterior tibial vessels into the foot and supplies all muscles in the anterior compartment. In the foot the nerve is close to the dorsalis pedis artery, usually lying lateral to the artery but sometimes medial to it (see Fig. 6.62). It gives a branch to extensors digitorum and hallucis brevis and the tarsal joints, and terminates by supplying the skin between the great and second toes (see Fig. 6.62).

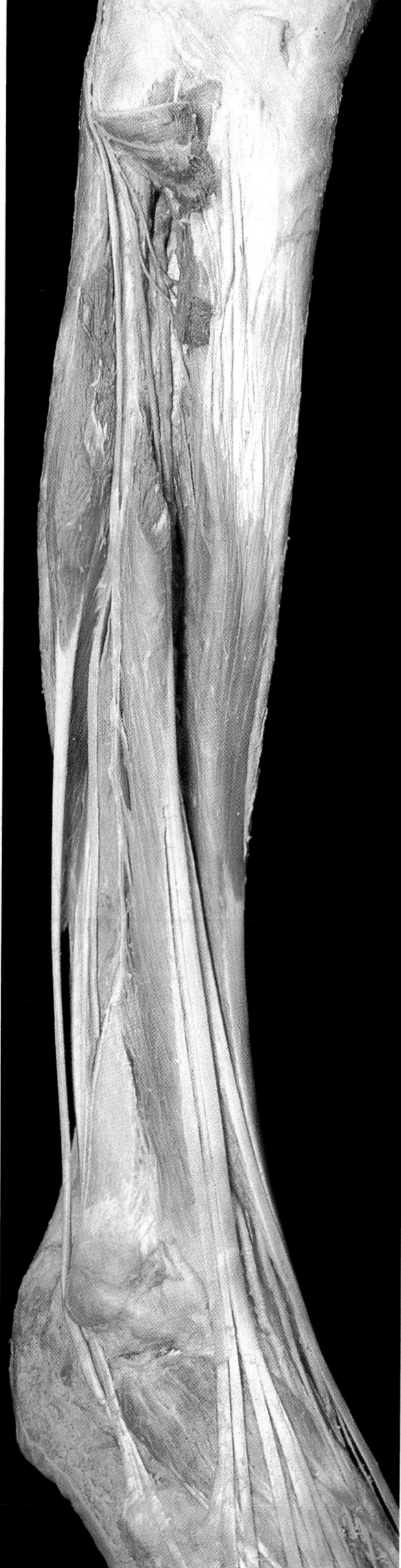

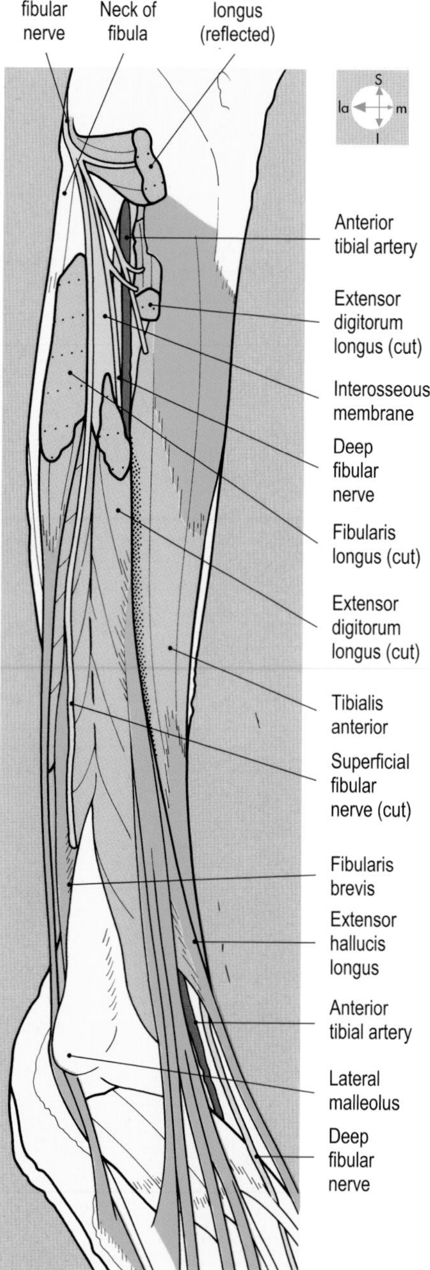

Fig. 6.63 The common fibular nerve and its branches and the anterior tibial artery, seen after deep dissection of both compartments.

Lateral compartment of leg

The lateral (fibular or peroneal) compartment of the leg extends from the head of the fibula above to the lateral malleolus below. Its principal contents are the fibularis longus and brevis muscles (Fig. 6.64). Fibularis (peroneus) longus is attached to the upper two-thirds of the lateral surface of the fibula and fibularis (peroneus) brevis to the lower two-thirds, with brevis being the more anterior. Both muscles are attached to the two crural intermuscular septa and the overlying deep fascia (see Fig. 6.57). On reaching the ankle the tendons pass behind and then below the lateral malleolus, restrained by the superior and inferior fibular retinacula and surrounded by synovial membrane (Fig. 6.64). The tendon of fibularis brevis passes forwards above the fibular trochlea of the calcaneus to attach to the base of the fifth metatarsal. The fibularis longus tendon passes forwards below the fibular trochlea and turns medially into the sole of the foot where it lies in a groove on the cuboid bone (Fig. 6.65). It attaches to the lateral side of the base of the first metatarsal and the adjacent first cuneiform.

Fibularis longus and brevis are evertors of the foot and weak plantar flexors of the ankle joint. Their nerve supply is the superficial fibular nerve, a terminal branch of the common fibular nerve, which enters the lateral compartment by winding around the neck of the fibula where it is palpable and may sometimes be compressed.

Branches of the fibular artery, which arises from the posterior tibial artery (see p. 278) pierce the posterior intermuscular septum to supply fibularis longus and brevis.

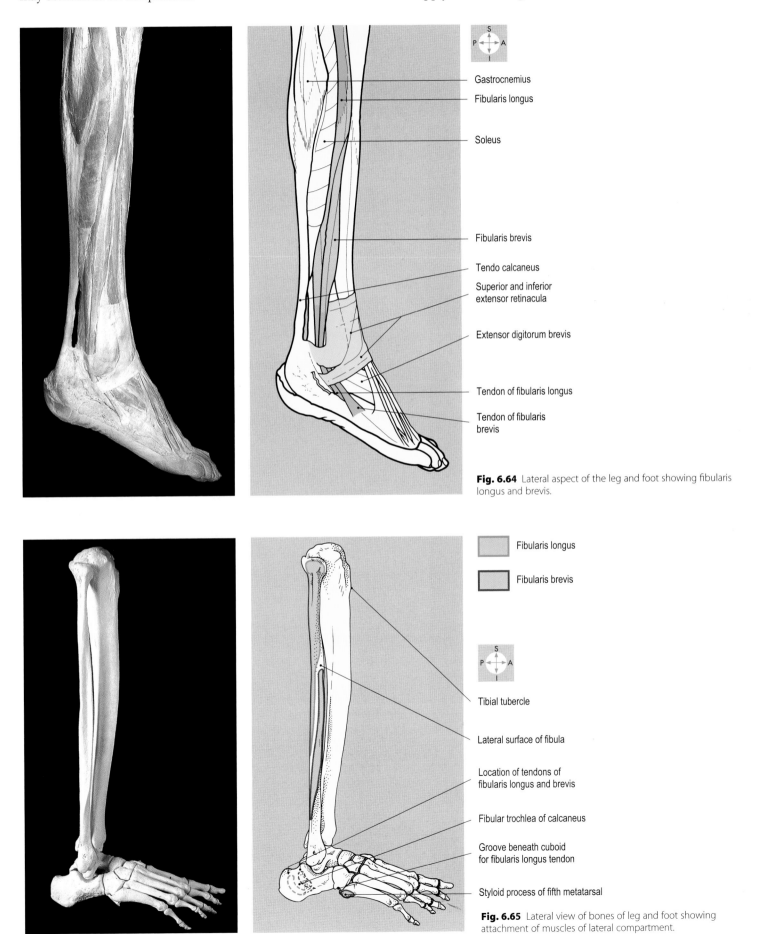

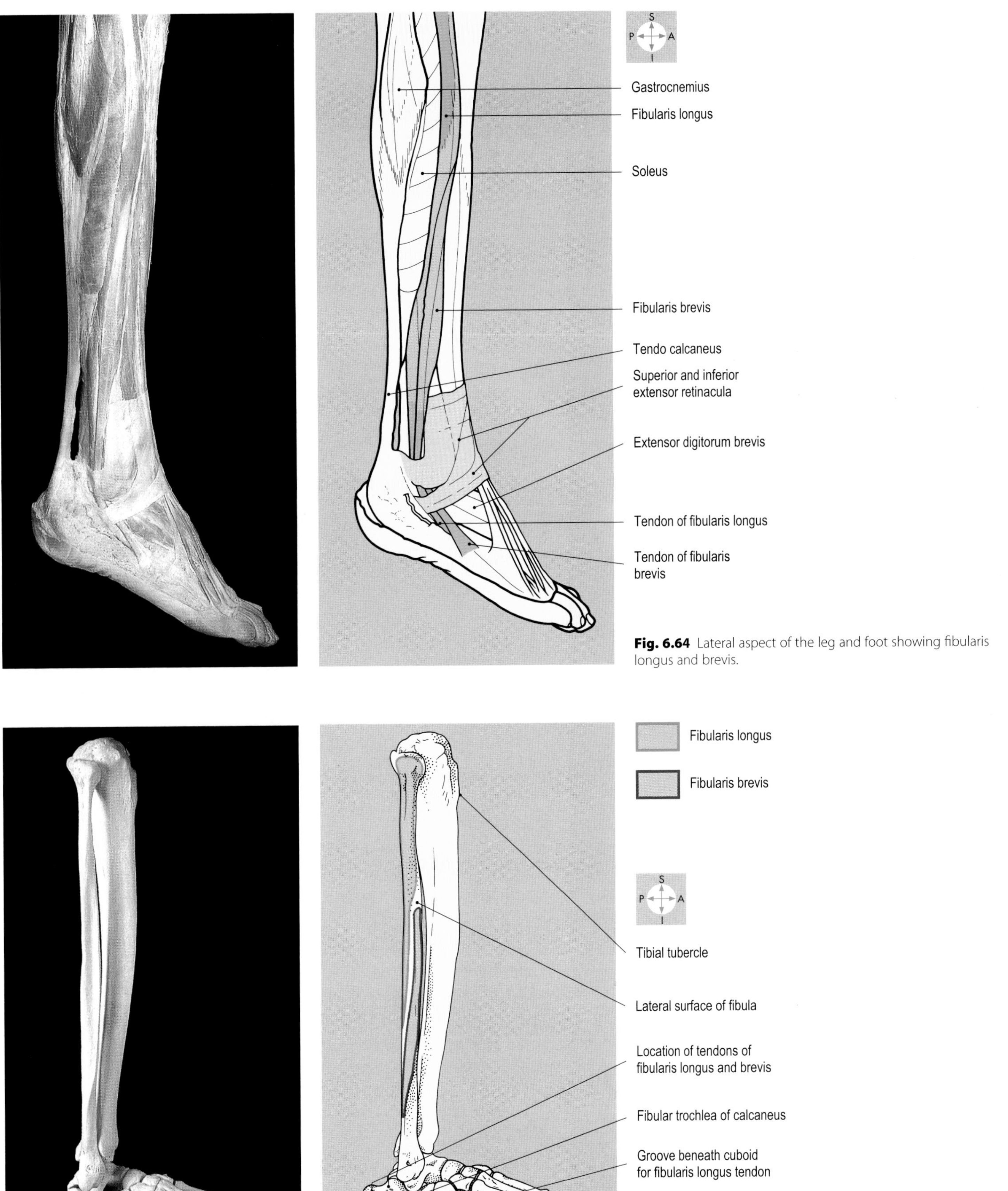

Fig. 6.64 Lateral aspect of the leg and foot showing fibularis longus and brevis.

Fig. 6.65 Lateral view of bones of leg and foot showing attachment of muscles of lateral compartment.

Hip Joint

The hip joint is a synovial ball-and-socket joint between the head of the femur and the acetabulum of the hip bone (Fig. 6.66).

Articular surfaces

The femoral head, covered by hyaline cartilage, forms two-thirds of a sphere and has a central pit (fovea; Fig. 6.66) giving attachment to the round ligament (ligamentum teres). The head surmounts the femoral neck, whose base abuts the medial side of the greater trochanter. The acetabulum is a deep socket with a C-shaped articular area covered with hyaline cartilage and a fat-filled non-articular area (acetabular fossa), whose margins give attachment to the base of the ligamentum teres (Fig. 6.67). The acetabulum is deficient inferiorly at the acetabular notch (Fig. 6.66), where blood vessels, bridged by the transverse acetabular ligament, enter the joint. A fibrocartilaginous labrum, attached to the margins of the acetabulum and the transverse ligament, helps to deepen the socket.

Capsule

Medially, the fibrous capsule is attached to the outer margin of the labrum; laterally the capsule attaches to the intertrochanteric

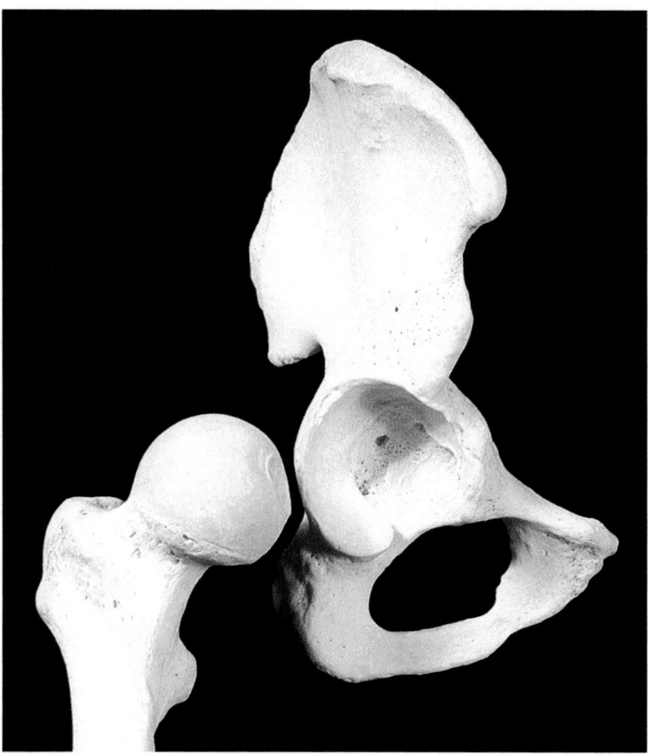

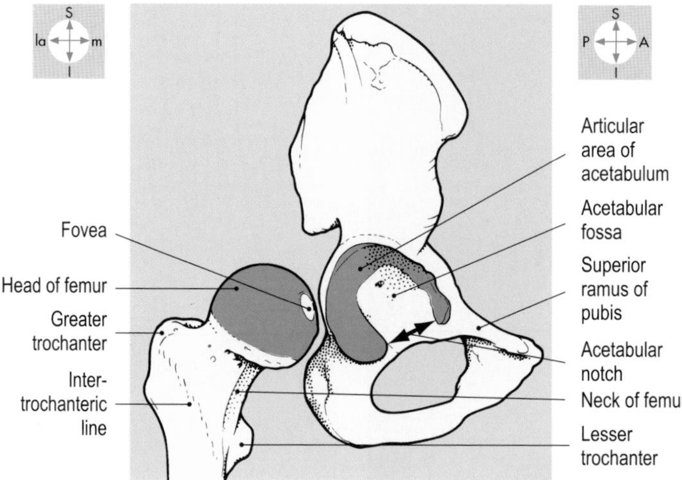

Fig. 6.66 Articular surfaces of the hip joint comprise the acetabulum of the hip bone and the head of the femur.

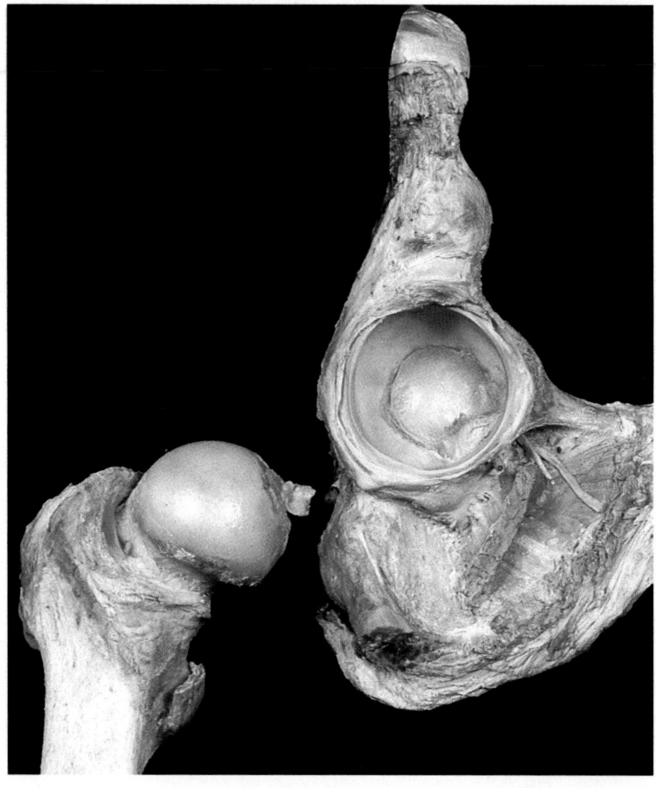

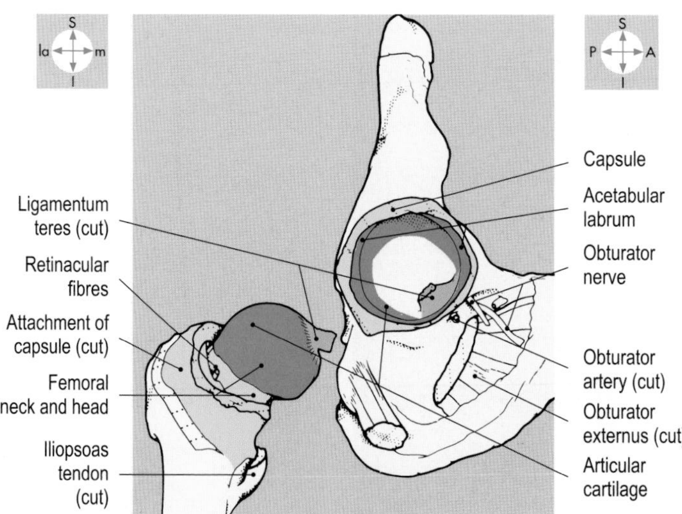

Fig. 6.67 Internal features, revealed by disarticulation of the joint after cutting the ligaments and joint capsule.

line (Figs 6.66 & 6.68) at the root of the femoral neck and to the femoral shaft just above the lesser trochanter. From the femoral attachment of the capsule, retinacular fibres derived from the deep part of the capsule (Fig. 6.67) are reflected medially over the neck to the margins of the head. Posteriorly, the line of attachment of the capsule is such that only the upper (medial) half of the femoral neck lies within the joint.

Ligaments

The iliofemoral, pubofemoral and ischiofemoral ligaments are capsular thickenings that spiral downwards and laterally from the hip bone to the femur. The strong iliofemoral ligament (Fig. 6.68) is an inverted Y shape, the stem attaching to the anterior inferior iliac spine and the limbs to the upper and lower ends of the intertrochanteric line.

The pubofemoral ligament (Fig. 6.68) passes from the iliopubic eminence to the femoral neck just above the lesser trochanter. The ischiofemoral ligament lies posteriorly (see Fig. 6.70) and reaches the root of the greater trochanter.

Within the joint is the ligament of the head of the femur (ligamentum teres femoris) (Figs 6.67 & 6.69), which has the form of a flattened cone, the base attaching to the margins of the acetabular fossa and transverse acetabular ligament and the apex to the fovea on the femoral head.

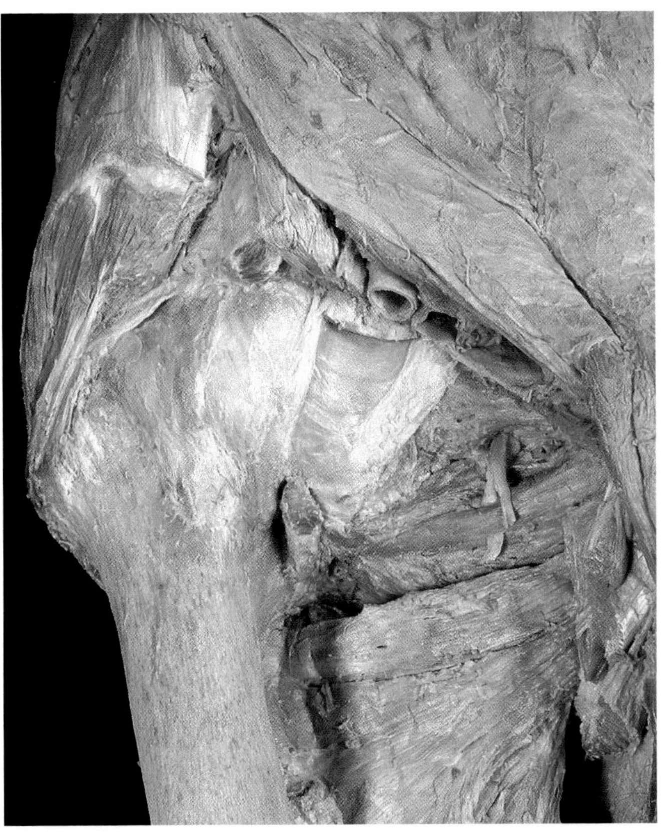

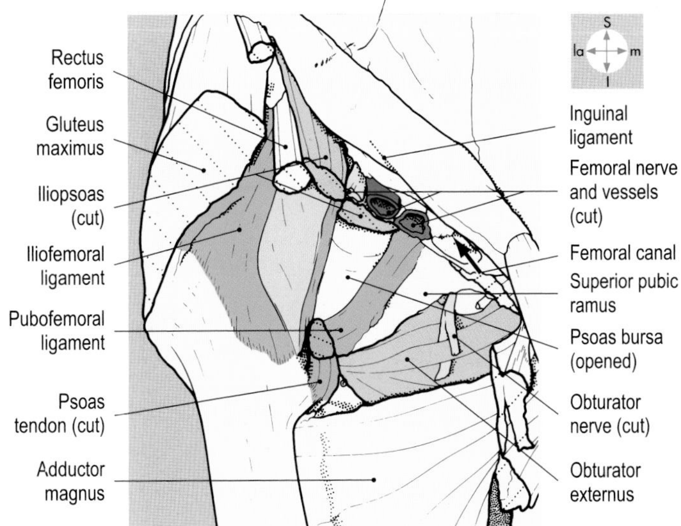

Fig. 6.68 Anterior surface of the joint capsule, its associated ligaments and immediate relations.

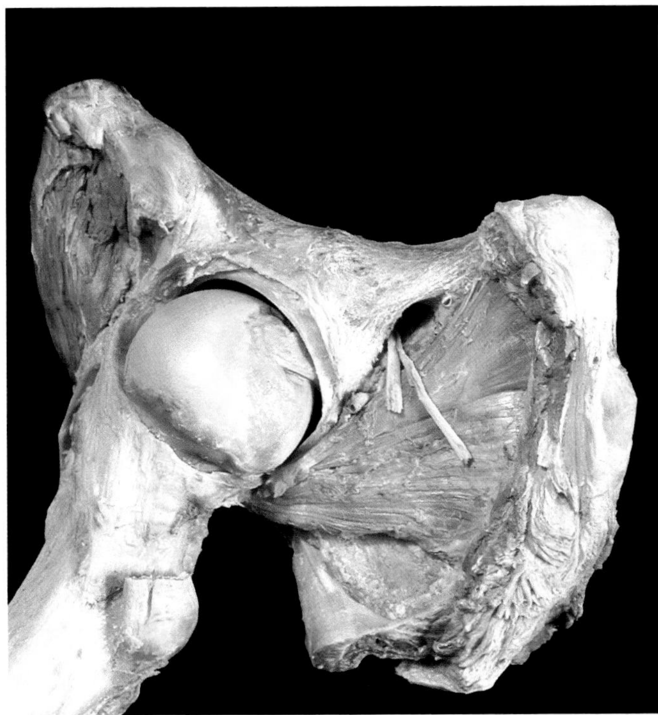

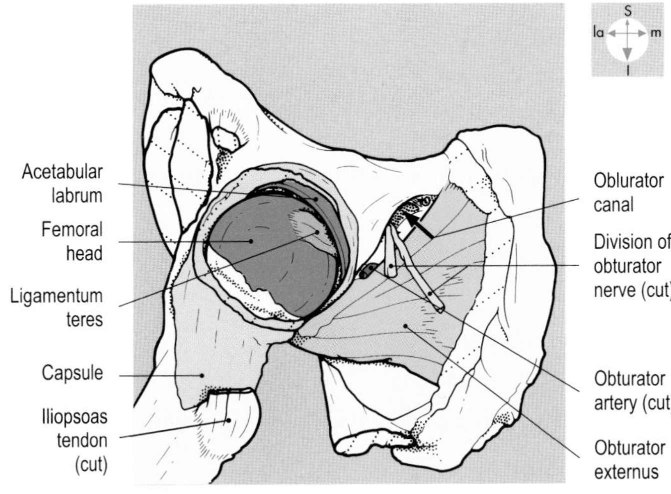

Fig. 6.69 Joint capsule opened anteriorly to show the interior of the joint. The femur has been abducted and externally rotated.

Synovial membrane and bursae

Synovial membrane lines the interior of the capsule and the non-articular surfaces of the joint, clothes the ligament of the head of the femur and is reflected over the retinacular fibres and the femoral neck as far as the head. The iliopsoas tendon and anterior aspect of the capsule are separated by a large bursa (see Fig. 6.68), which often is in communication with the joint cavity.

The tendon of obturator externus is separated from the capsule by a smaller bursa, which may also communicate with the joint.

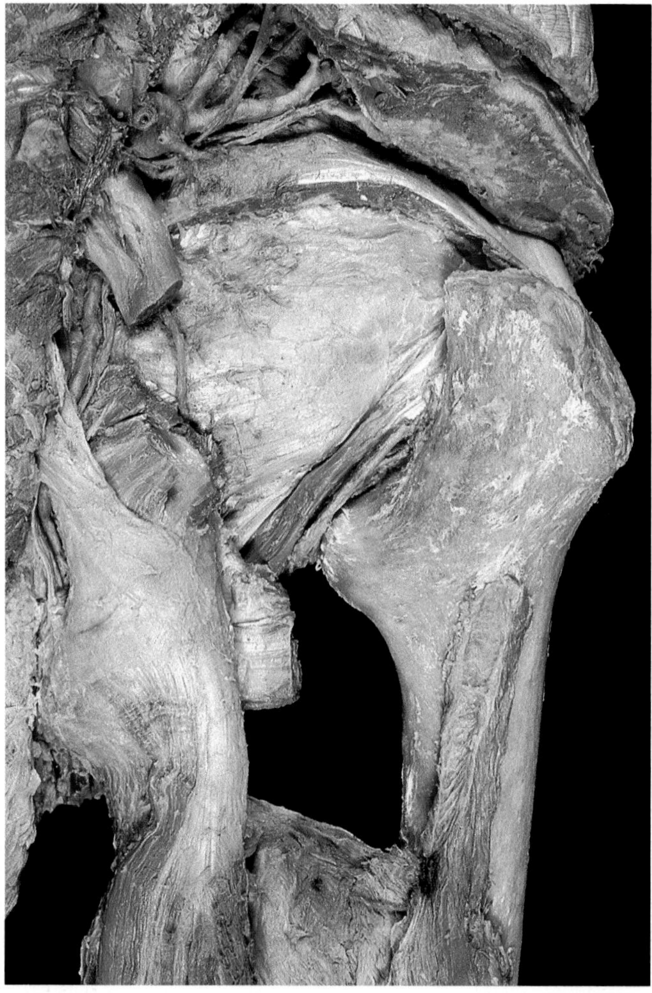

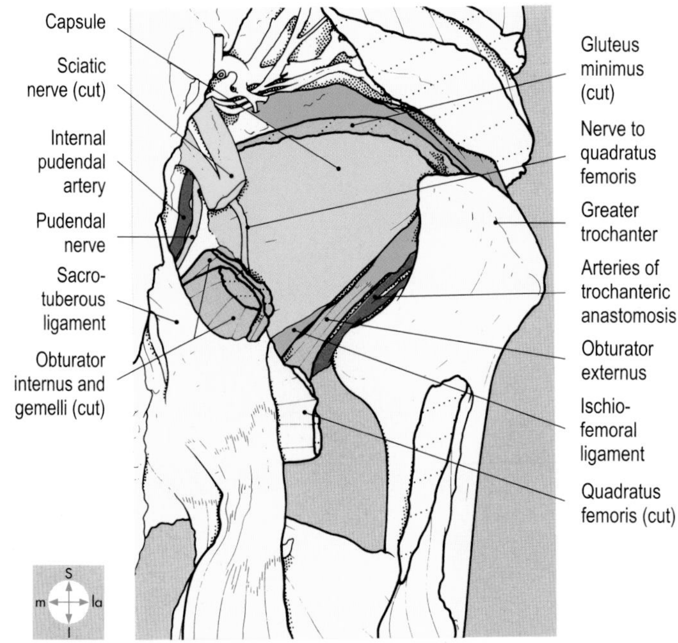

Fig. 6.70 Posterior surface of the joint capsule, the ischiofemoral ligament and close relations.

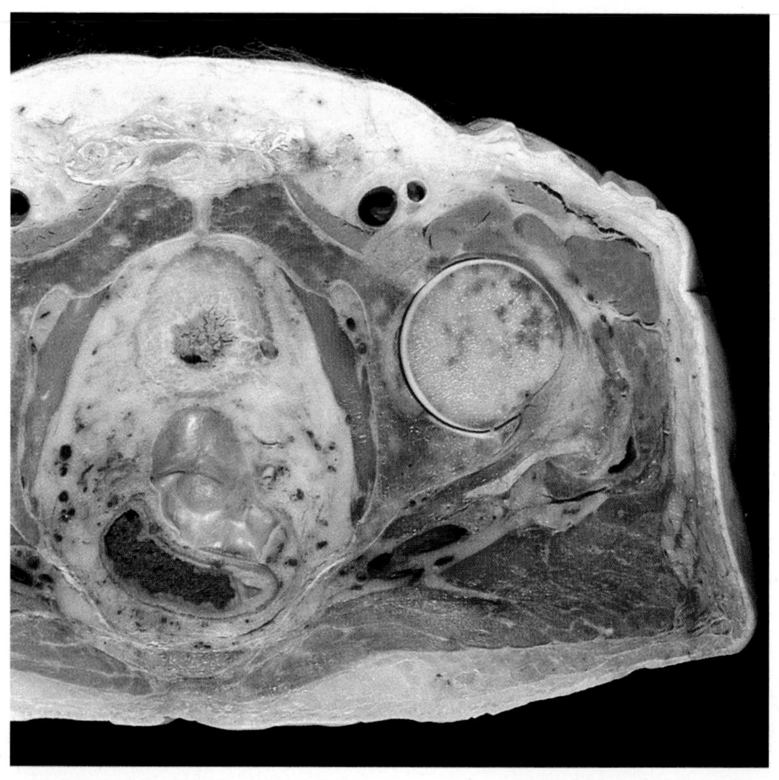

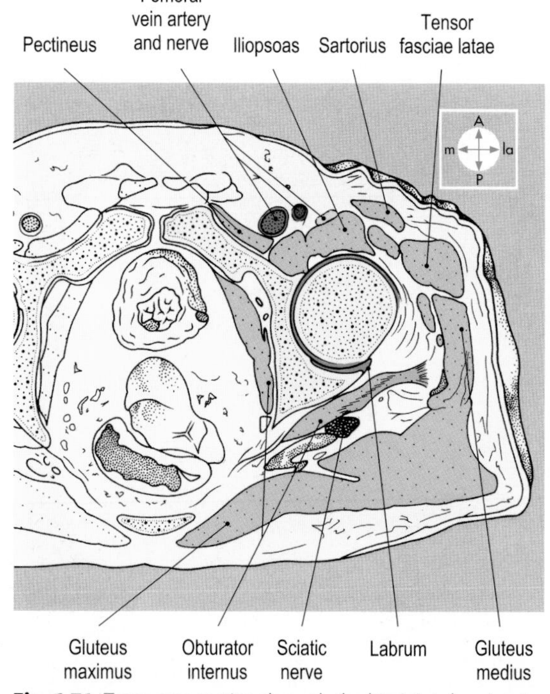

Fig. 6.71 Transverse section through the hip joint showing its relations. Superior aspect. Compare Fig. 5.42.

Movements

The hip joint is multiaxial and permits flexion, extension, abduction, adduction, medial and lateral rotation, and circumduction.

Flexion is produced by iliopsoas, assisted by sartorius, rectus femoris and pectineus. Gluteus maximus and the hamstrings are extensors. Abductors of the hip include gluteus medius and minimus while adduction is produced by adductors longus, brevis and magnus, pectineus and gracilis. Medial rotation is produced by iliopsoas, tensor fasciae latae and the anterior fibres of gluteus minimus and medius. Lateral rotation is produced by piriformis, quadratus femoris, obturator externus and internus and the gemelli.

Stability

The hip joint is very stable, largely because of its bony morphology and the deep fit of the femoral head into the acetabulum. Other important factors include the ligaments and the tone of the muscles crossing the joint. The ilio-, pubo- and ischiofemoral ligaments all limit extension and medial rotation. The iliofemoral ligament, in particular, prevents hyperextension, especially in the upright posture when body weight acts behind the transverse axis of the hip joint and tilts the pelvis backwards. The ligament of the head of the femur limits adduction of the hip.

Relations

The joint is deeply placed behind the midpoint of the inguinal ligament. Laterally, the greater trochanter covers the neck of the femur and is palpable on the lateral side of the thigh. Medially, only the thin bone of the acetabular fossa (Figs 6.71 & 6.72) separates the head of the femur from structures within the pelvis that are vulnerable following acetabular fracture accompanied by medial displacement of the femoral head. Posteriorly lie structures of the gluteal region (Fig. 6.70), including the sciatic nerve, which may be damaged in posterior dislocation. Anteriorly, the joint is covered by the iliopsoas and the femoral vessels and nerve. Obturator externus and the adductor muscles lie inferiorly (Fig. 6.72) whilst superiorly are gluteus medius and minimus.

Blood supply

The arterial supply of the hip joint, especially that of the head and neck of the femur, is of particular clinical importance. The joint receives branches from the obturator artery, superior and inferior gluteal arteries, and medial and lateral circumflex femoral arteries, either directly or from the trochanteric anastomosis they form. From this anastomosis (Fig. 6.70), nutrient arteries travel in the retinacular fibres to enter foramina on the upper part of the femoral neck and terminate in the head. As only the upper half of the neck is covered posteriorly by the joint capsule, fractures at this site may be classified as either intra- or extracapsular. Intracapsular fractures that tear the retinacular fibres may deprive the head of the femur of much of its blood supply. Additional blood supply comes from a branch of the obturator artery conveyed in the ligament of the head of the femur to the femoral head, and from one of the perforating branches of the profunda femoris artery via a nutrient artery that enters the shaft to supply the femoral neck and head.

Nerve supply

Nerves to the joint include the nerve to rectus femoris from the femoral nerve, branches from the anterior division of the obturator nerve, and the nerve to quadratus femoris from the sacral plexus.

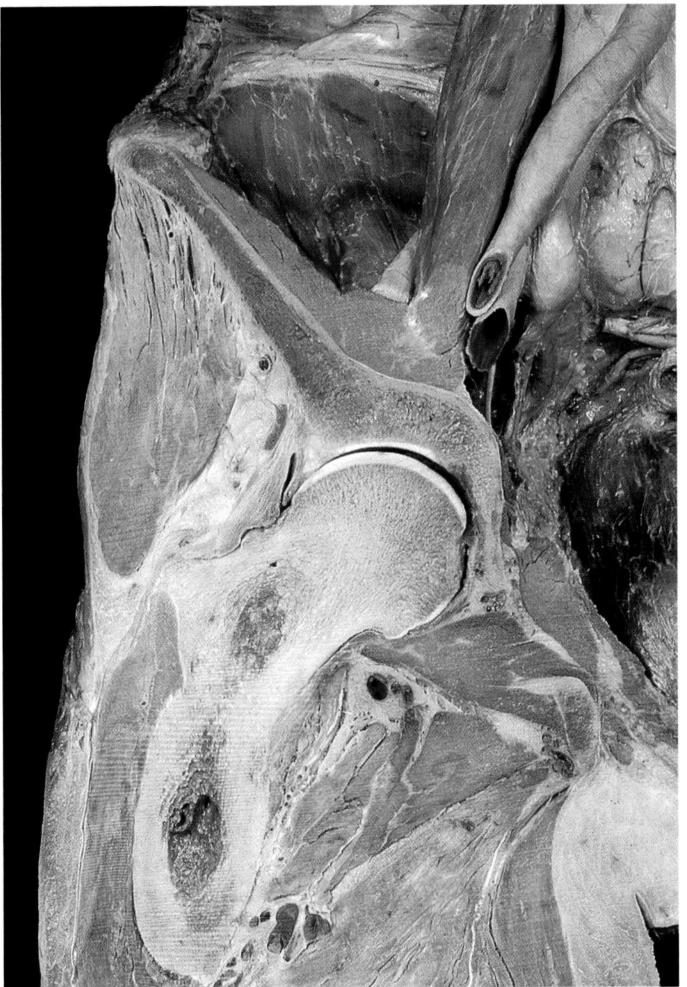

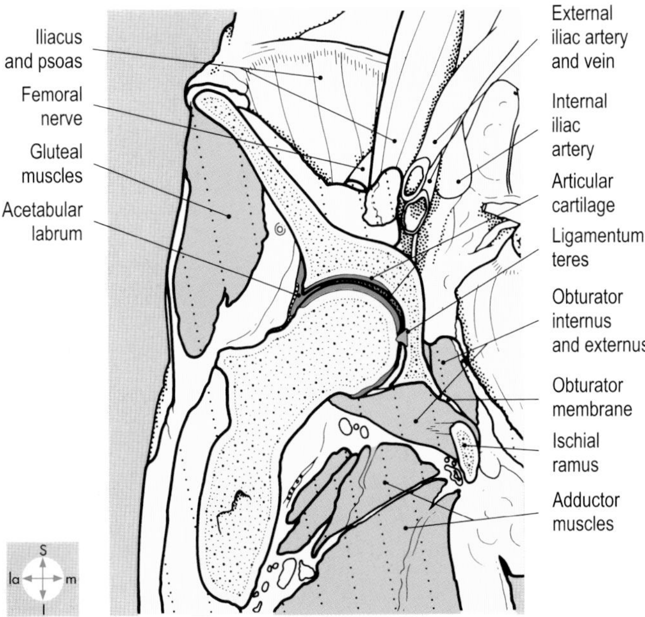

Fig. 6.72 Coronal section through the hip joint showing its relations.

Knee Joint

The knee joint is a synovial joint between the distal end of the femur, proximal end of the tibia and posterior aspect of the patella (Fig. 6.73). It is a hinge joint with a wide range of flexion and extension and limited lateral and medial rotation. The joint is relatively superficial anteriorly, medially and laterally where some of its bony features are palpable but posteriorly is inaccessible, being deeply placed in the floor of the popliteal fossa (Fig. 6.74).

Anteriorly, the patellar ligament (Fig. 6.75) passes from the apex of the patella to the tibial tubercle. It is easily palpable and is used clinically for the stretch reflex (knee jerk, L3 & L4).

Articular surfaces

The medial and lateral condyles of the femur have articular surfaces, covered by hyaline cartilage, which extend over their inferior and posterior aspects and articulate with the respective condyles on the tibia (Fig. 6.73). On the front of the femur lies the patellar articular surface while posteriorly a deep intercondylar fossa separates the two condyles. The articular areas on the tibial condyles are separated by the intercondylar eminence, the lateral articular area being flatter and smaller than the medial area (Fig. 6.73).

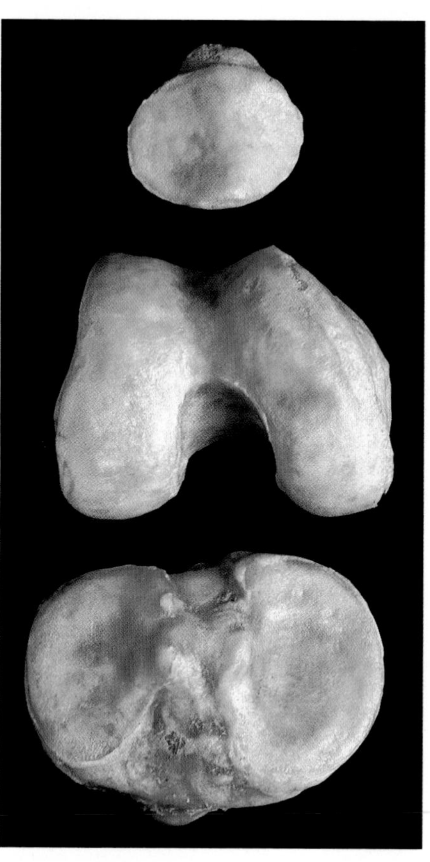

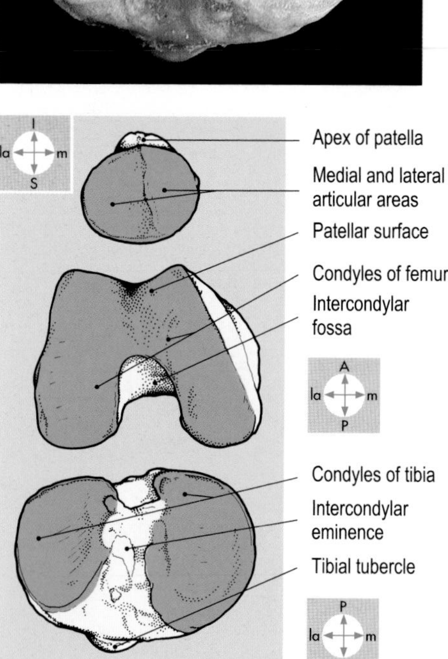

Fig. 6.73 Articular surfaces of the patella, femur and tibia.

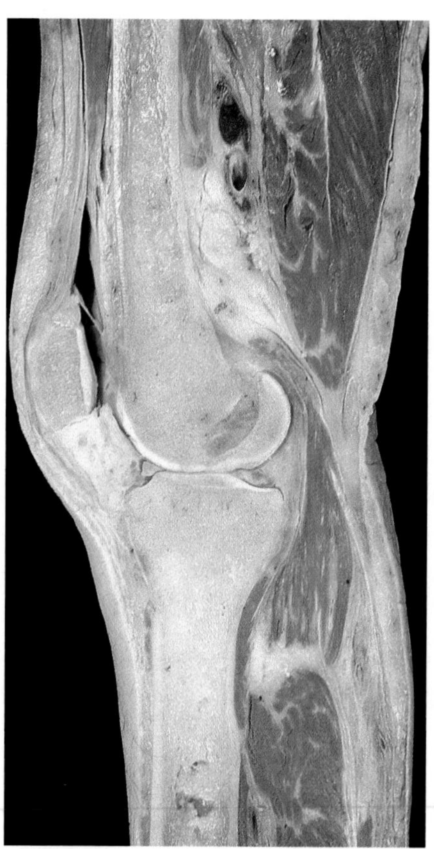

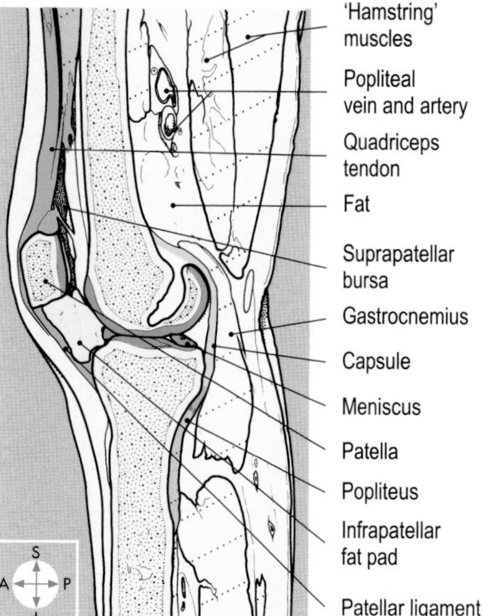

Fig. 6.74 Sagittal section through the knee joint showing the articular surfaces and relations.

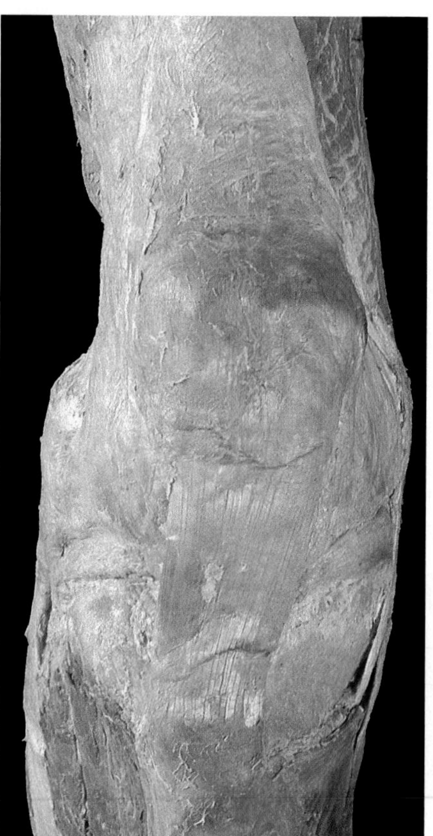

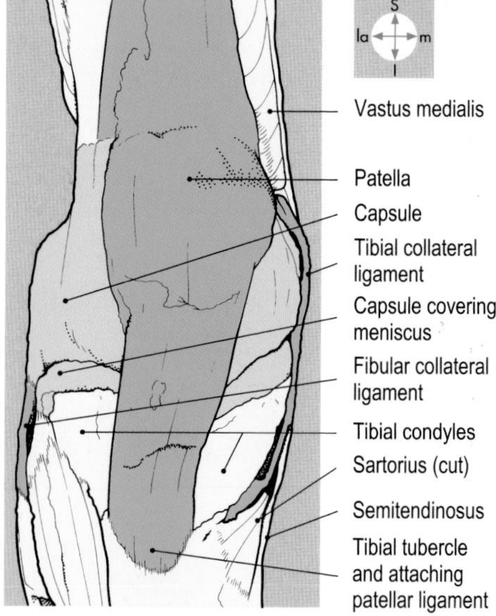

Fig. 6.75 Superficial dissection from the anterior aspect to show patellar ligament, capsule, and collateral ligaments.

Capsule

The capsule is thin anteriorly and posteriorly but is reinforced on each side by strong collateral ligaments. On the sides of the femur the capsule attachment extends up to the epicondyles. Posteriorly, it attaches along the superior margins of the condyles (Figs 6.76 & 6.78) and the intercondylar line whilst anteriorly it extends proximally (Fig. 6.75; see Figs 6.79 & 6.81) to accommodate the synovial membrane that forms the suprapatellar bursa (pouch).

On the sides of the tibia the capsule attaches close to the articular margins. Those parts of the capsule on each side of the joint that loosely anchor the outer borders of the menisci to the tibia are called the coronary ligaments. Posteriorly, the capsular attachment inclines downwards to include the posterior part of the intercondylar area, whilst anteriorly the attachment deviates inferiorly as far as the tibial tubercle. On the patella the capsule is attached close to the articular margins.

Posteriorly, part of the insertion of semimembranosus forms the oblique popliteal ligament, which passes upwards and laterally (Figs 6.76 & 6.77), reinforcing the capsule. Where the posterior part of the capsule is pierced by popliteus, it thickens to form the arcuate ligament (Fig. 6.76).

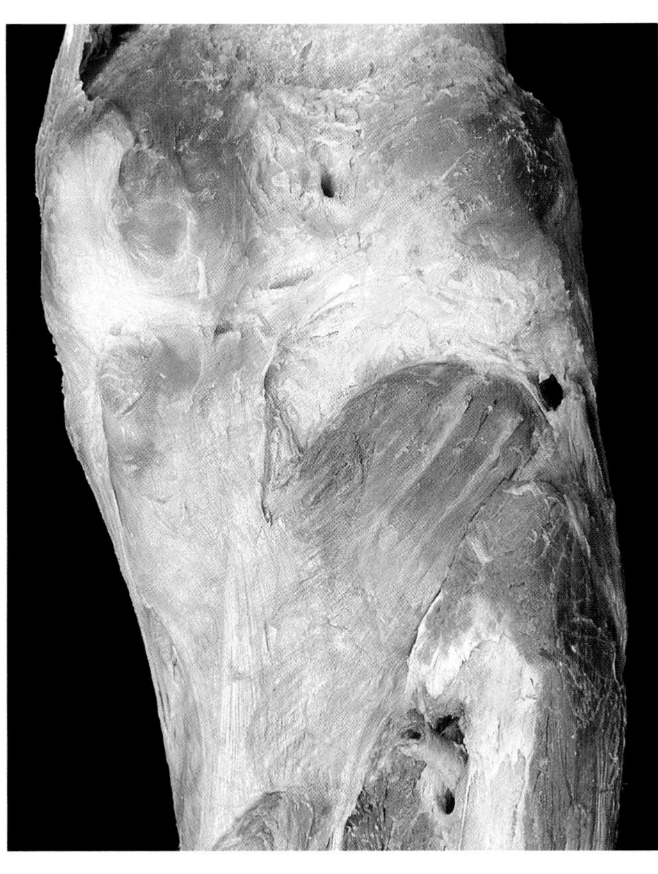

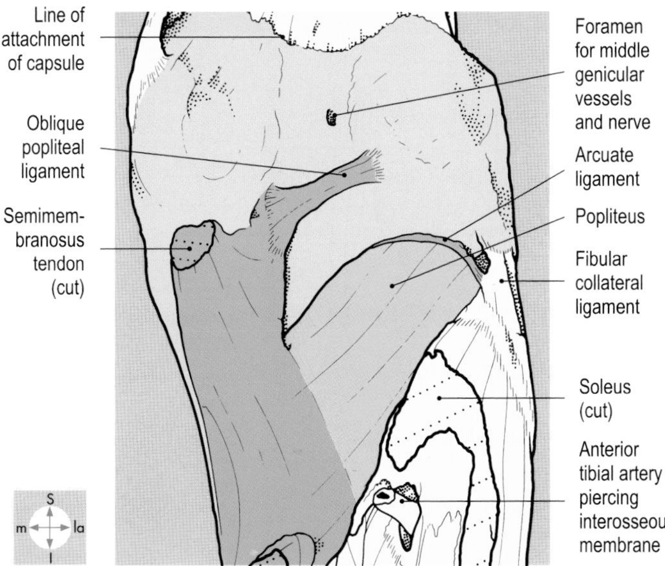

Fig. 6.76 Posterior aspect of joint showing capsule, popliteus and semimembranosus insertion.

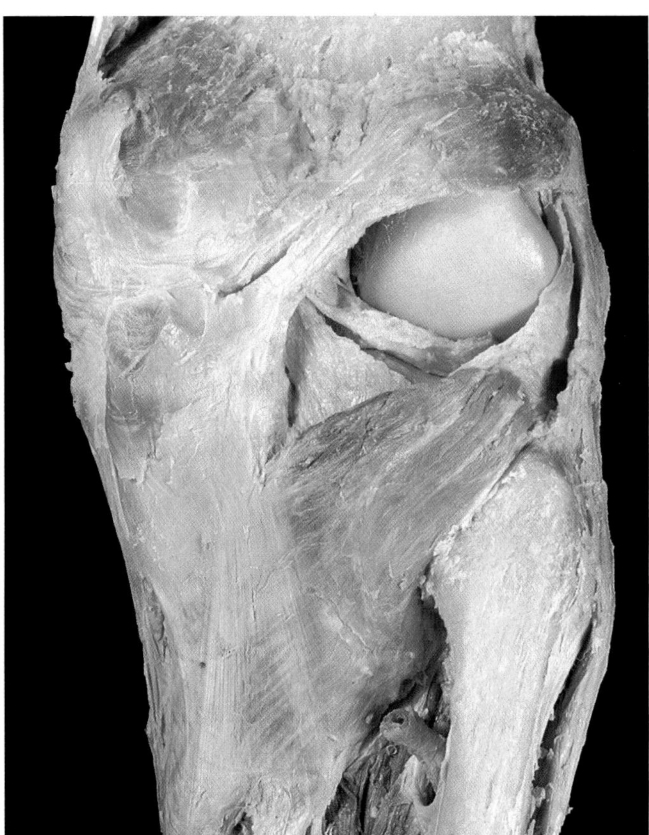

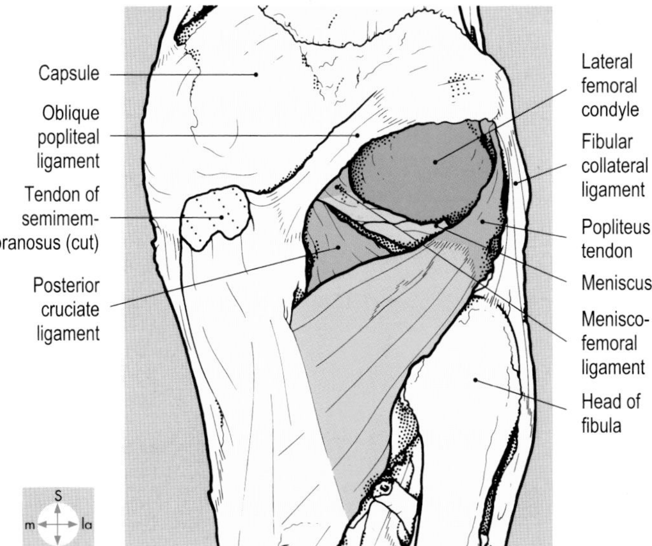

Fig. 6.77 Partial removal of capsule to reveal the meniscofemoral and posterior cruciate ligaments and the tendon of popliteus.

Collateral ligaments

On the medial side of the joint the thick tibial collateral ligament (Fig. 6.79) broadens as it descends from the medial femoral epicondyle to the upper part of the subcutaneous surface of the tibia. Its deep aspect is attached to the outer margin of the medial meniscus (Fig. 6.78), which diminishes mobility of the meniscus, making it more susceptible to tears. On the lateral side the cord-like fibular collateral ligament (Fig. 6.80) descends from the lateral epicondyle of the femur to the styloid process and head of the fibula, separated from the lateral meniscus by the popliteus tendon (Fig. 6.78).

Intracapsular ligaments

The intracapsular ligaments comprise the anterior and posterior cruciate ligaments and the meniscofemoral ligament.

The cruciate ligaments (see Fig. 6.78) are named according to their attachment to the intercondylar eminence of the tibia (see Fig. 6.82). The anterior ligament passes upwards, backwards and laterally to attach to the medial surface of the lateral condyle of the

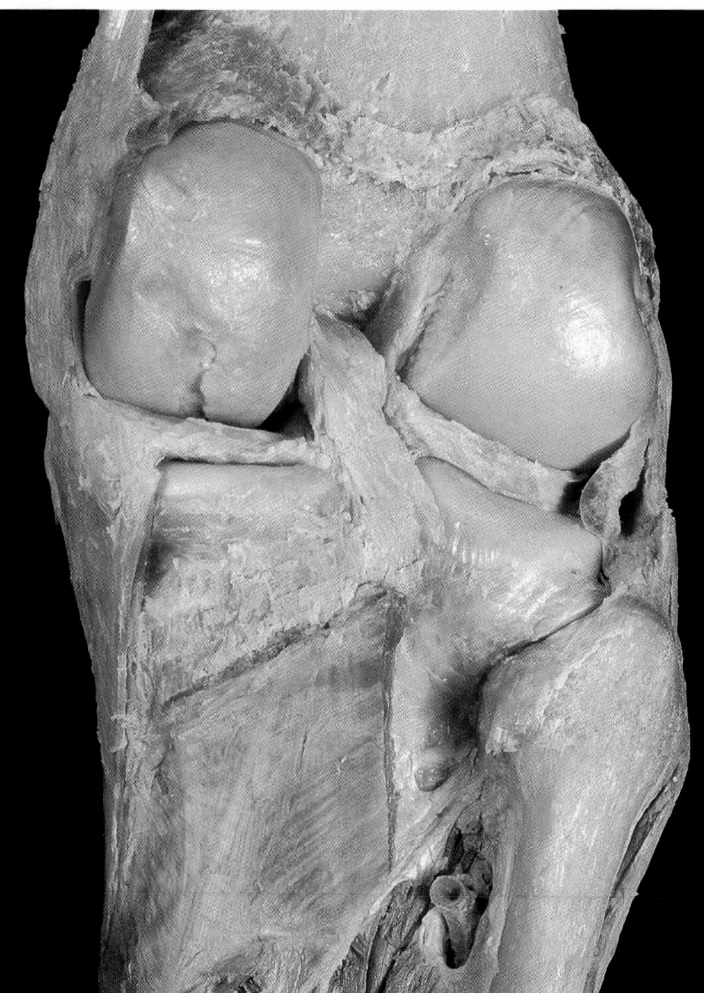

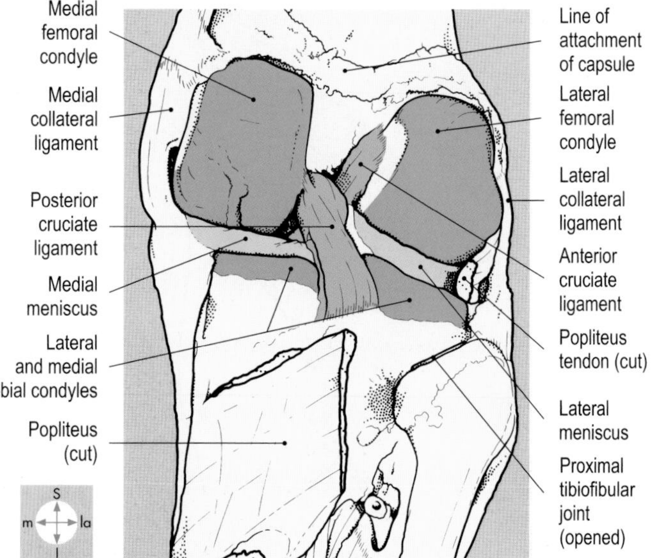

Fig. 6.78 The posterior part of the capsule has been removed to show the cruciate ligaments and menisci.

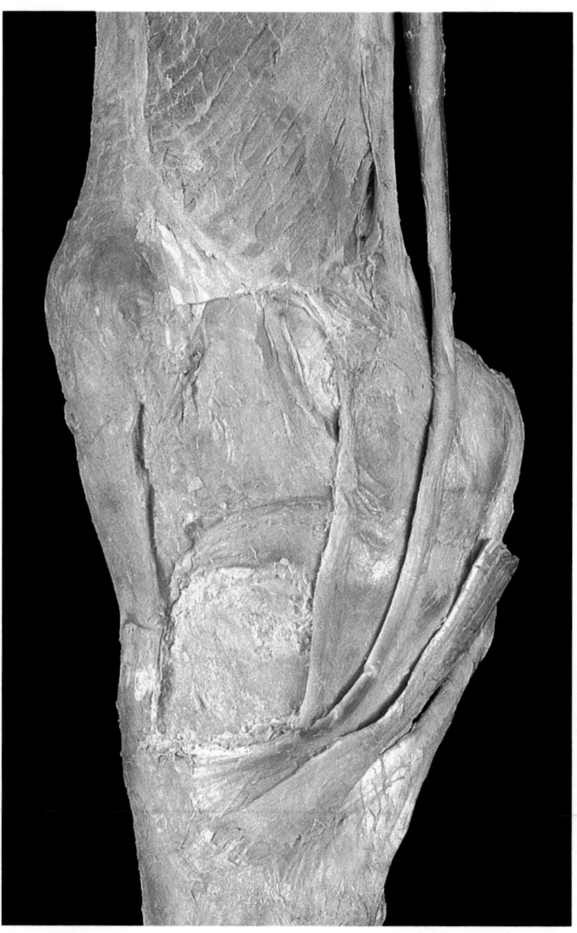

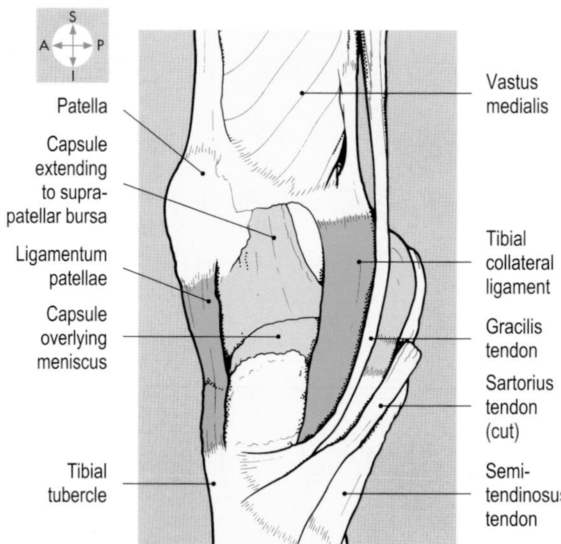

Fig. 6.79 Superficial dissection from the medial aspect showing the tibial collateral ligament, capsule and insertions of sartorius, gracilis and semitendinosus.

femur. The posterior ligament passes upwards, forwards and medially (Fig. 6.78) to attach to the lateral surface of the medial femoral condyle. The meniscofemoral ligament is adjacent to the posterior cruciate ligament (see Fig. 6.77) and attaches the posterior border of the lateral meniscus close to the femoral attachment of the posterior cruciate ligament. It stabilizes the meniscus during rotation of the femur on the tibia. Although within the capsule, the cruciate and meniscofemoral ligaments are covered by reflections of synovial membrane and are therefore not within the synovial cavity.

Menisci

The medial and lateral menisci are C-shaped (Fig. 6.82) with their anterior and posterior horns attached to the intercondylar eminence of the tibia and their outer borders to the joint capsule (coronary ligaments). The menisci differ in size and shape, the medial being narrower though slightly larger so that its horns embrace those of the lateral meniscus. Also, the medial is attached to the medial collateral ligament and in cross-section is deeper than the lateral meniscus. A transverse ligament (see Fig. 6.82) connects the anterior horn of the medial meniscus with the anterior aspect of the lateral meniscus.

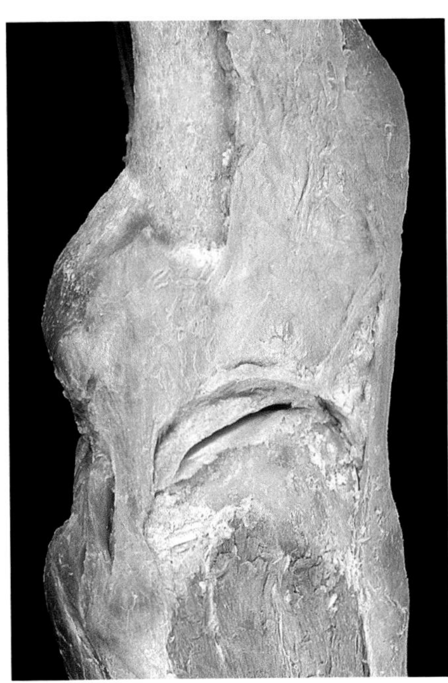

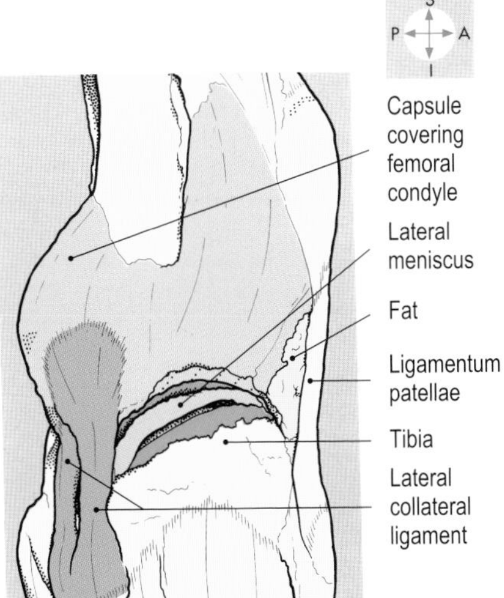

Fig. 6.80 Lateral aspect of joint showing the collateral ligament and the meniscus, revealed by removing part of the capsule.

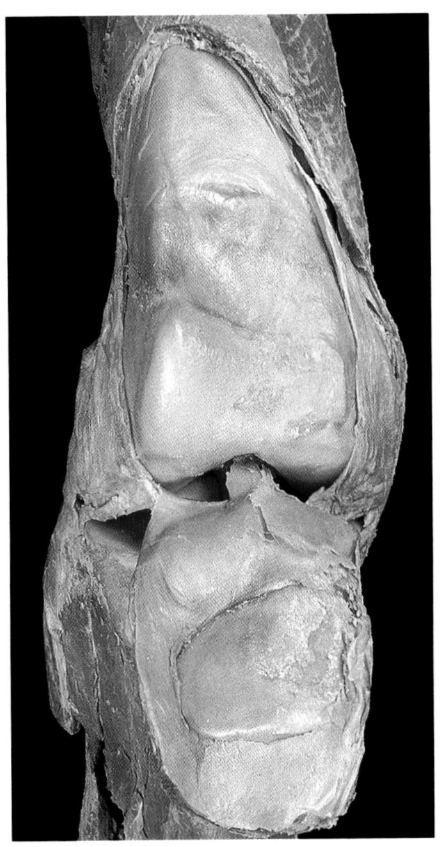

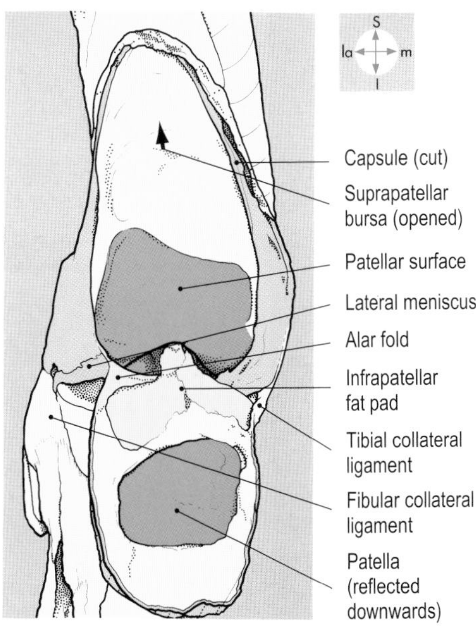

Fig. 6.81 Interior of joint, revealed by opening the capsule anteriorly and reflecting the patella downwards.

Infrapatellar fat pad

Deep to the patellar ligament is a quantity of fat (see Fig. 6.74), which bulges the synovial membrane into the interior of the joint. Folds of synovial membrane, the alar folds (Fig. 6.81), extend on either side from the main pad. Another fold, the ligamentum mucosum, lies in the midline between the anterior part of the intercondylar notch and the lower margin of the patella.

Synovial membrane and bursae

Synovial membrane lines the interior of the capsule but does not cover the menisci. On the femur it is attached to the margins of the intercondylar notch and covers the front and sides of the cruciate ligaments. Synovial membrane also covers the infrapatellar fat pad and the tendon of popliteus.

The suprapatellar bursa (Fig. 6.81; see also Fig. 6.74) is a large pouch of synovial membrane, passing a hand's breadth proximal to the upper border of the patella, deep to quadriceps. Part of vastus intermedius attaches to it. Since the bursa is continuous with the synovial cavity of the joint, it provides a route for injecting fluid into or withdrawing fluid from the joint. After injuries to the joint, fluid accumulates (effusion) in the suprapatellar bursa, causing typical fullness around the knee and the basis for the patellar-tap test. Several other bursae lie near the knee joint and may enlarge, causing swellings. Bursae between the capsule and the two heads of gastrocnemius often communicate with the knee joint while that beneath the medial head may also communicate with the overlying semimembranosus bursa. Other bursae, which do not communicate with the joint, are the pre- and infrapatellar bursae beneath the skin covering the patella and patellar ligament respectively.

Popliteus

From its tibial attachment the popliteus passes upwards and laterally (see Fig. 6.76), penetrating the posterior aspect of the capsule of the knee joint deep to the arcuate ligament. Within the joint its tendon, covered by synovial membrane, attaches to the posterior border of the lateral meniscus and to the femur (see Fig. 6.77) immediately below the lateral epicondyle. Popliteus is supplied by the tibial nerve and its actions are considered below.

Movements

The principal movements of the knee joint are flexion and extension. Flexion is produced mainly by the hamstrings (semimembranosus, semitendinosus and biceps) assisted by the two heads of gastrocnemius. Extension is produced by quadriceps femoris acting through the patellar ligament. Gluteus maximus, acting through the iliotibial tract, maintains stability of the knee in the extended position.

Because of the shape of the articular surfaces, the femur rotates medially during the later stages of extension. The lateral condyle and meniscus (moving in unison because of the meniscofemoral ligament) glide forwards on the lateral tibial condyle whilst the medial condyle completes its movement of extension on the medial meniscus. Full extension is achieved with completion of medial rotation and further movement is prevented by tension in the collateral and oblique posterior ligaments. During the early stages of flexion, lateral rotation of the femur on the tibia is produced by popliteus, which also pulls the lateral meniscus posteriorly. During flexion and extension the patella glides over the patellar surface of the femur.

Slight active rotation of the tibia on the femur can occur when the knee is in a flexed but non-weight-bearing position. Sartorius, gracilis and semitendinosus rotate medially while biceps femoris rotates laterally.

Stability

The knee joint is very stable. The most important factors are muscle tone, especially in quadriceps, and the ligaments. The cruciate ligaments stabilize the femur on the tibia, preventing excessive anteroposterior movement. The collateral ligaments assist medial and lateral stability while the iliotibial tract stabilizes the knee during extension. All of these ligaments, together with the oblique posterior ligament, prevent hyperextension. Cruciate and collateral ligament injuries together with meniscal tears commonly occur in sports, particularly following twisting movements during which the foot is anchored to the ground.

Owing to angulation of the femur relative to the tibia, contraction of quadriceps femoris tends to displace the patella laterally. This displacement is prevented firstly by the lowest fibres of vastus medialis, which insert into the medial patellar border and whose active contraction resists lateral movement of the patella, and secondly by the large size and prominence of the lateral femoral condyle, making lateral patellar movement mechanically difficult. Occasionally, the lateral femoral condyle fails to develop normally, resulting in patellar instability.

Innervation

Branches from the femoral, obturator and sciatic nerves supply the joint, sensory fibres from the femoral nerve travelling with the branches to the vasti and sartorius. Genicular branches from the tibial and common fibular divisions of the sciatic nerve, together with fibres from the posterior division of the obturator nerve, also supply the joint.

Blood supply

The knee joint receives its blood supply from the extensive genicular anastomosis derived mainly from branches of the popliteal, anterior and posterior tibial arteries (see Fig. 1.27).

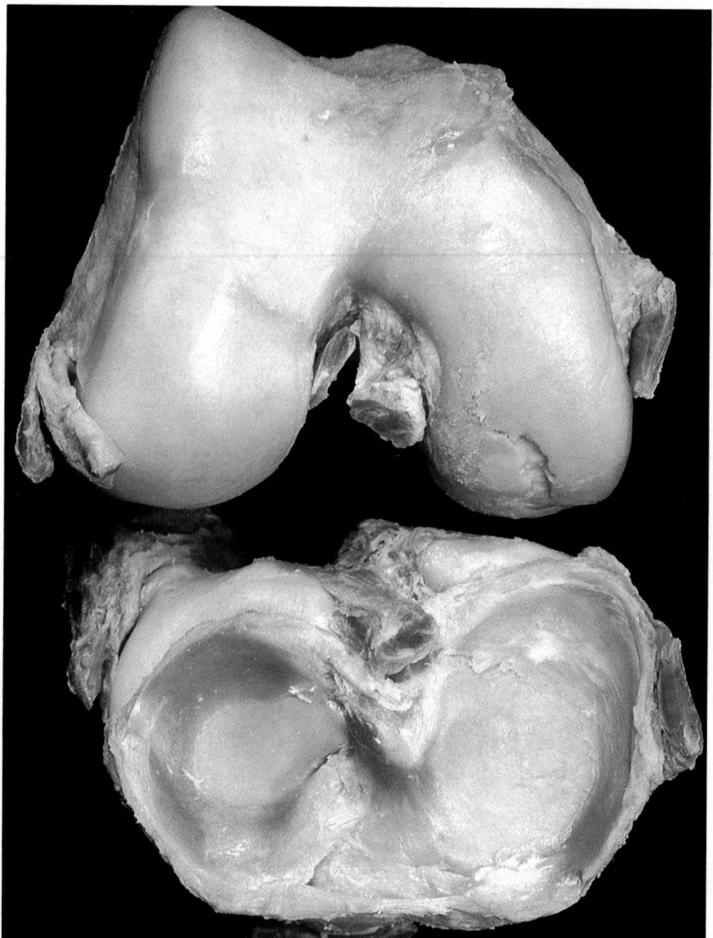

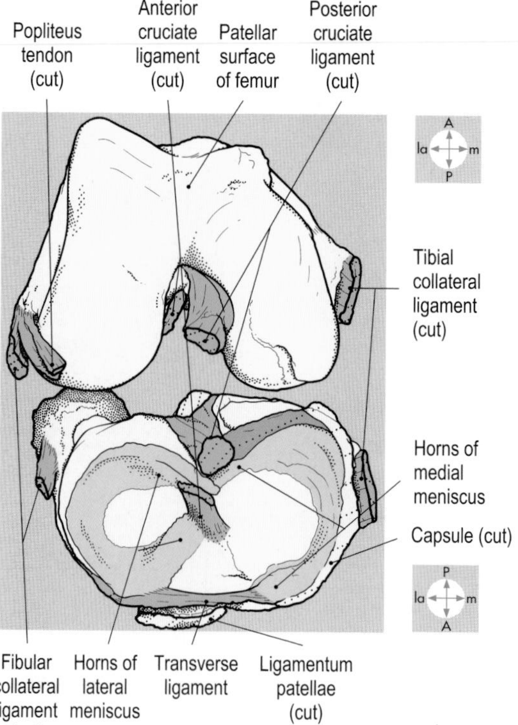

Fig. 6.82 Disarticulation of joint reveals menisci and attachments of cruciate ligaments.

Tibiofibular Joints

The tibia and fibula articulate at proximal and distal tibiofibular joints and are also connected by an interosseous membrane (Fig. 6.83), which unites the interosseous borders of the bones and separates the flexor and extensor compartments of the leg.

The proximal tibiofibular joint is a plane synovial articulation between the lateral condyle of the tibia and head of the fibula, and is supplied by the common fibular nerve. The capsule is reinforced by anterior and posterior ligaments, and the synovial cavity does not communicate with the knee joint.

The opposed triangular surfaces at the lower ends of the tibia and fibula are bound together by an interosseous ligament, forming the fibrous distal tibiofibular joint, which is strengthened by anterior and posterior tibiofibular ligaments. The transverse ligament, an inferior extension of the posterior ligament, contributes to the articular socket of the ankle joint (see Fig. 6.85), whose cavity frequently extends for a short distance between the tibia and fibula. The ankle is stabilized by the ligaments of the distal tibiofibular joint, which prevent separation of the malleoli. Innervation is by the deep fibular and tibial nerves.

Very little movement occurs at the tibiofibular joints, but slight rotation of the fibula may accompany flexion and extension of the ankle.

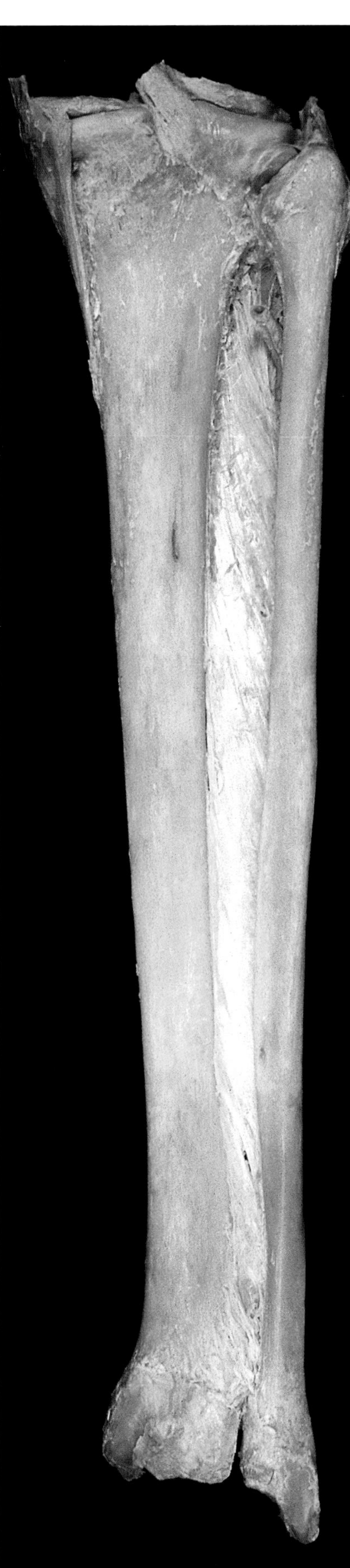

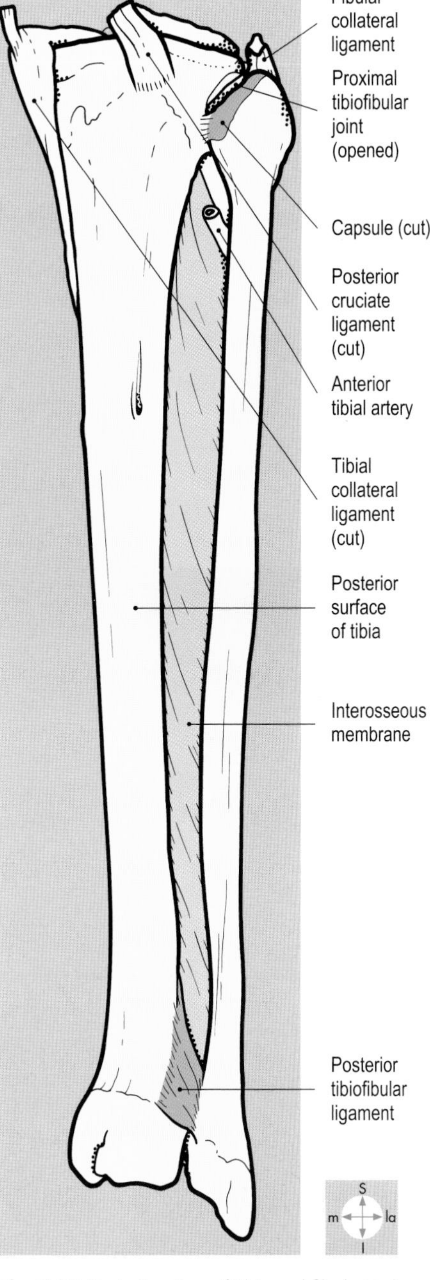

Fig. 6.83 Posterior view of tibia and fibula to show tibiofibular joints and interosseous membrane. The lower part of the tibiofibular ligament has been removed.

Ankle Joint

The ankle joint is a synovial hinge joint between the lower ends of the tibia and fibula and the upper part of the talus (Fig. 6.84), and all the articular surfaces are covered by hyaline cartilage. The proximal articular surface comprises the distal end of the tibia and the medial and lateral malleoli, which together form a deep socket (Fig. 6.85), completed posteriorly by the posterior tibiofibular ligament (see below). The socket is wider anteriorly than posteriorly and is completely congruous with the upper part of the talus, which is reciprocally wedge shaped (Figs 6.84 & 6.86). The articular surface on the lateral side of the talus is more extensive than that on the medial side.

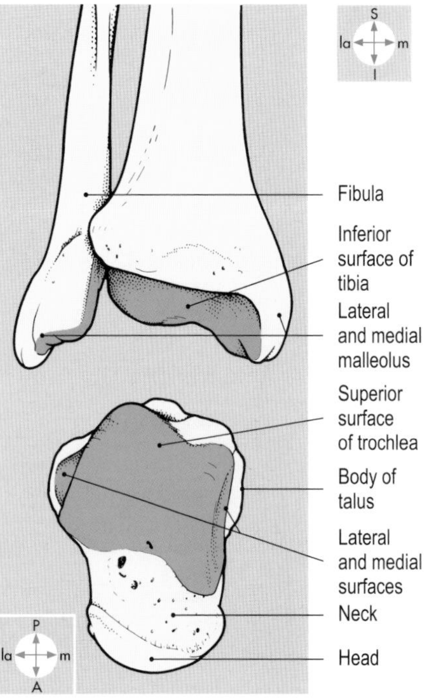

Fig. 6.84 Bones of the ankle joint showing their articular surfaces.

Capsule and synovial membrane

The fibrous capsule attaches to the margins of the articular surfaces, but anteriorly extends forwards onto the neck of the talus (Fig. 6.86). The capsule is thin anteriorly and posteriorly, but is reinforced on each side by ligaments. Synovial membrane lines the capsule internally and covers the intracapsular part of the neck of the talus.

Ligaments

The posterior tibiofibular ligament spans the gap between the distal ends of the tibia and fibula, contributing to the articular socket posteriorly (see Fig. 6.85). There are two collateral ligaments. The medial

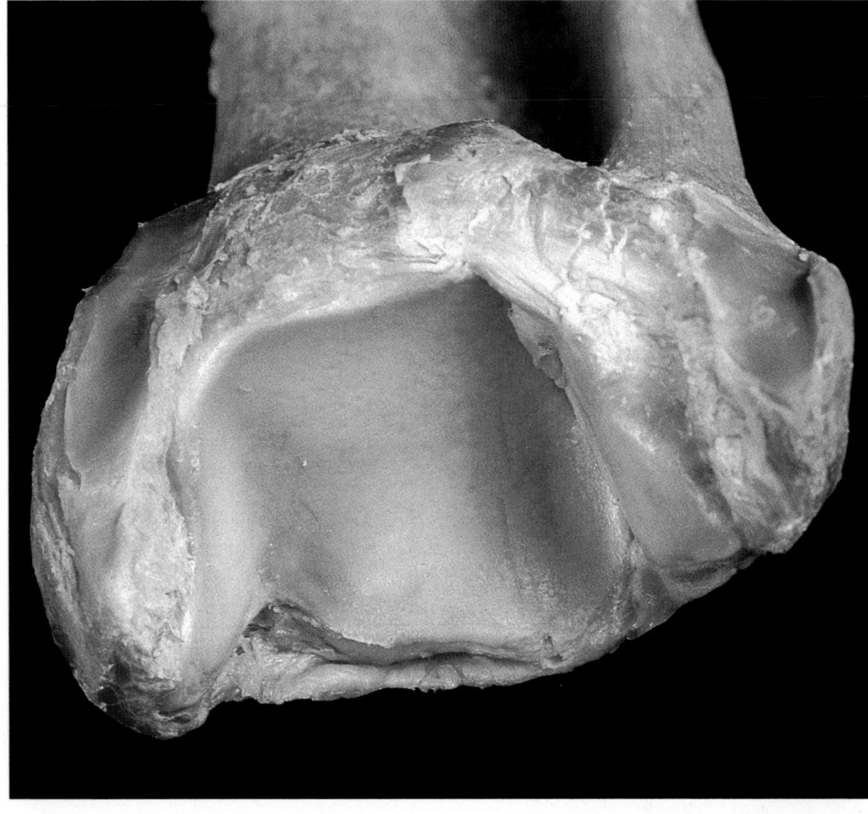

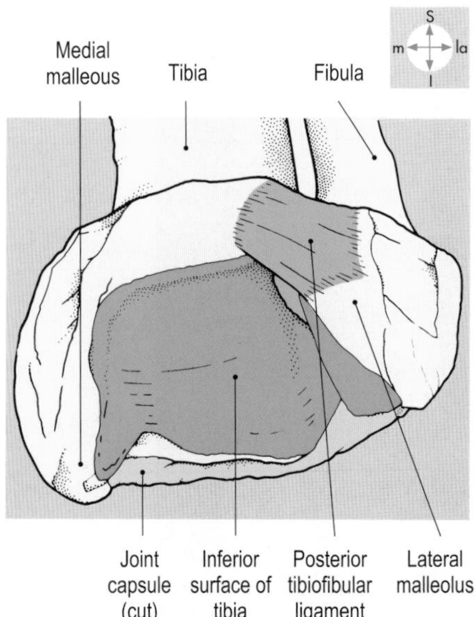

Fig. 6.85 Oblique inferior view of the wedge-shaped articular socket of the ankle joint.

(deltoid) ligament (Fig. 6.89) is attached by its apex to the tip of the medial malleolus. Its deeper fibres descend to the margin of the articular surface on the medial side of the talus and its longer superficial fibres attach to the tuberosity of the navicular, the medial border of the spring (plantar calcaneonavicular) ligament and the sustentaculum tali.

The lateral ligament has three components: the anterior and posterior talofibular and the calcaneofibular ligaments (Figs 6.87 & 6.88). All attach to the lateral malleolus. The anterior talofibular ligament passes forwards to the lateral side of the neck of the talus, the posterior talofibular ligament medially to the posterior tubercle of the talus, and the calcaneofibular downwards and backwards to the side of the calcaneus.

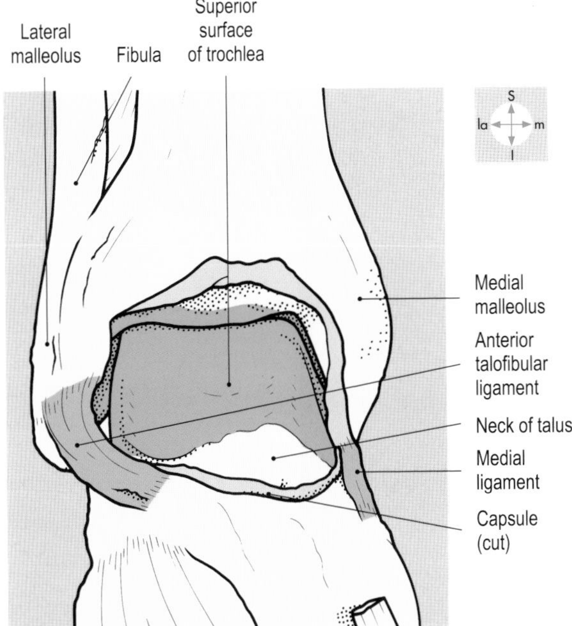

Fig. 6.86 Anterior view of the ankle joint showing articular surfaces, revealed by removal of the capsule.

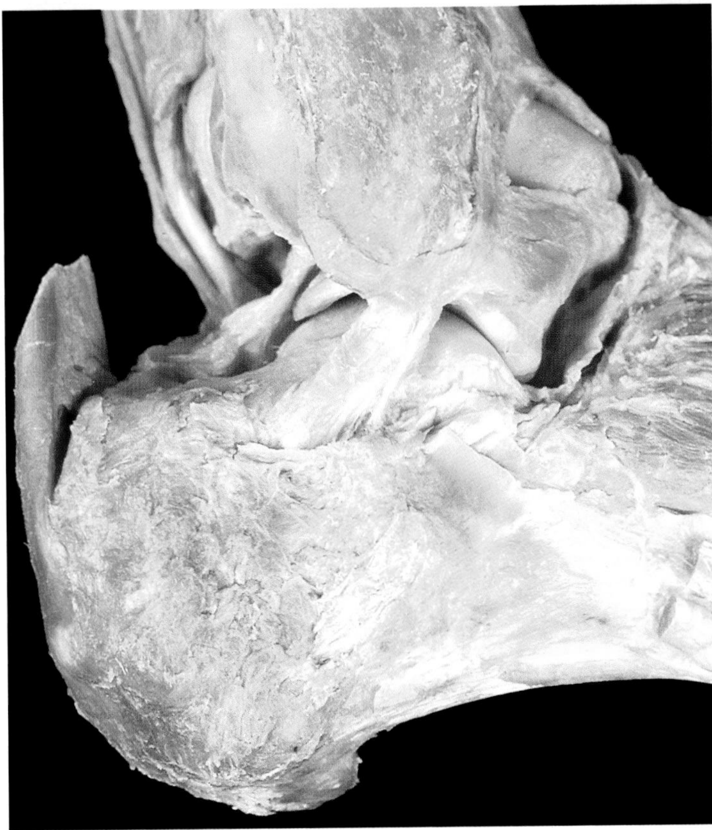

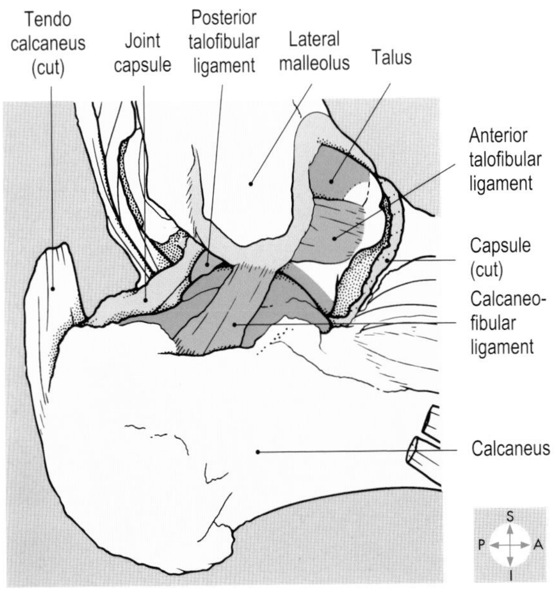

Fig. 6.87 Lateral aspect of joint to show lateral collateral ligament.

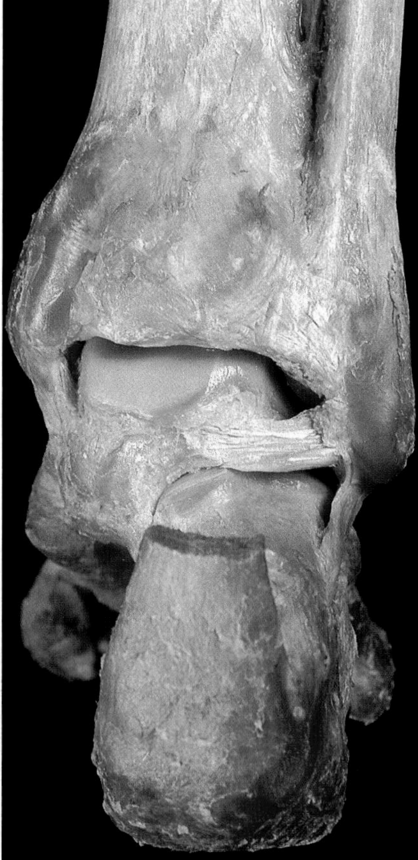

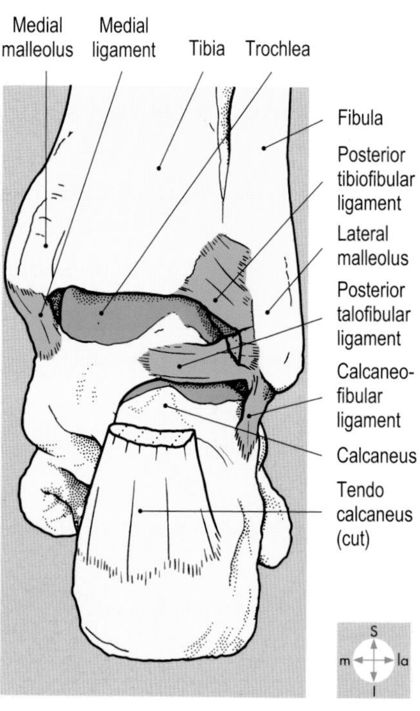

Fig. 6.88 Posterior view of the ankle joint showing the articular surface of talus after removal of the capsule.

Movements

Only extension (dorsiflexion) and flexion (plantar flexion) occur at the ankle joint, around a transverse axis between the malleoli. Plantar flexion is produced by soleus and gastrocnemius, assisted by tibialis posterior, flexors hallucis longus and digitorum longus, and fibularis longus and brevis. Extension (dorsiflexion) is produced by tibialis anterior, extensors hallucis longus and digitorum longus, and fibularis tertius.

Stability

The joint is very stable due to the wedge shape of the articulating surfaces and the strong collateral ligaments. During standing and walking, body weight tends to displace the tibiofibular socket forwards so that it becomes closely packed against the wider anterior part of the talus, which further enhances stability during dorsiflexion. Excessive forward displacement of the tibia and fibula on the talus is prevented by the posterior fibres of the medial (deltoid) ligament and by the calcaneofibular and posterior talofibular ligaments. However, in plantar flexion the narrow part of the talus articulates with the wider anterior part of the socket, allowing some side-to-side movement. In this position, forced inversion of the foot may damage the anterior talofibular ligament, one form of 'sprained ankle'.

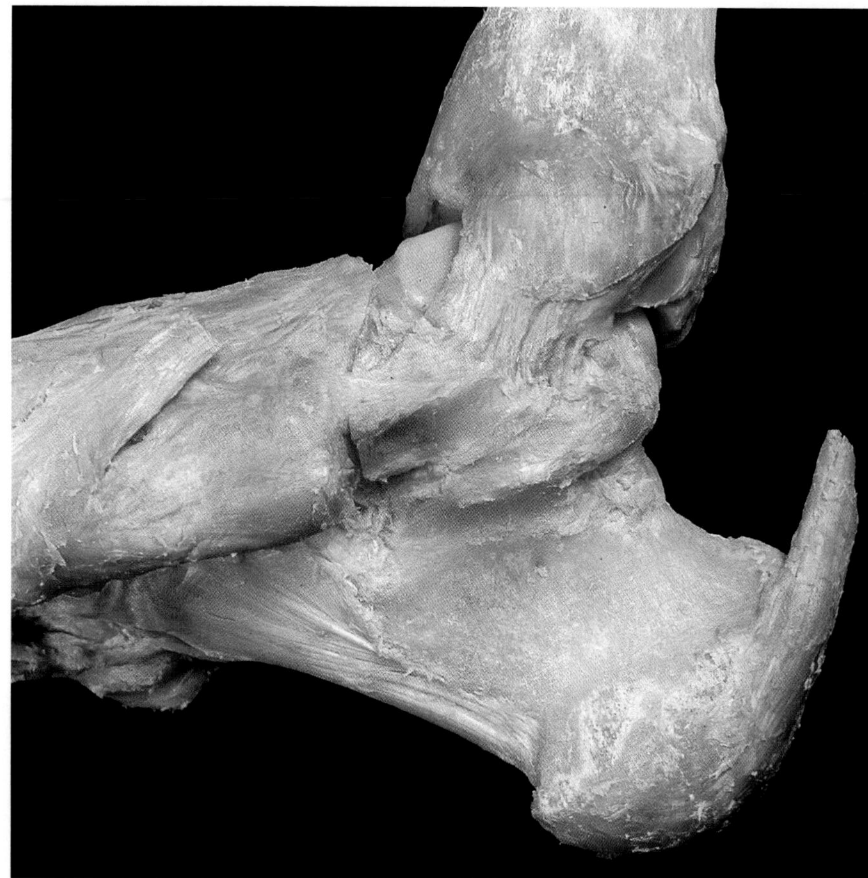

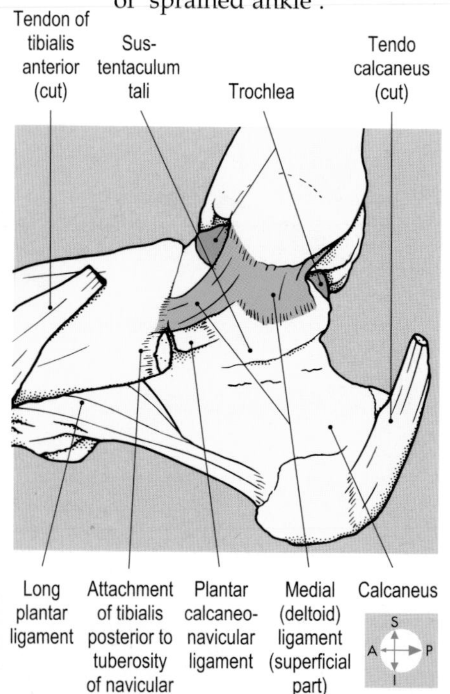

Fig. 6.89 Medial (deltoid) ligament (superficial part) of the ankle joint.

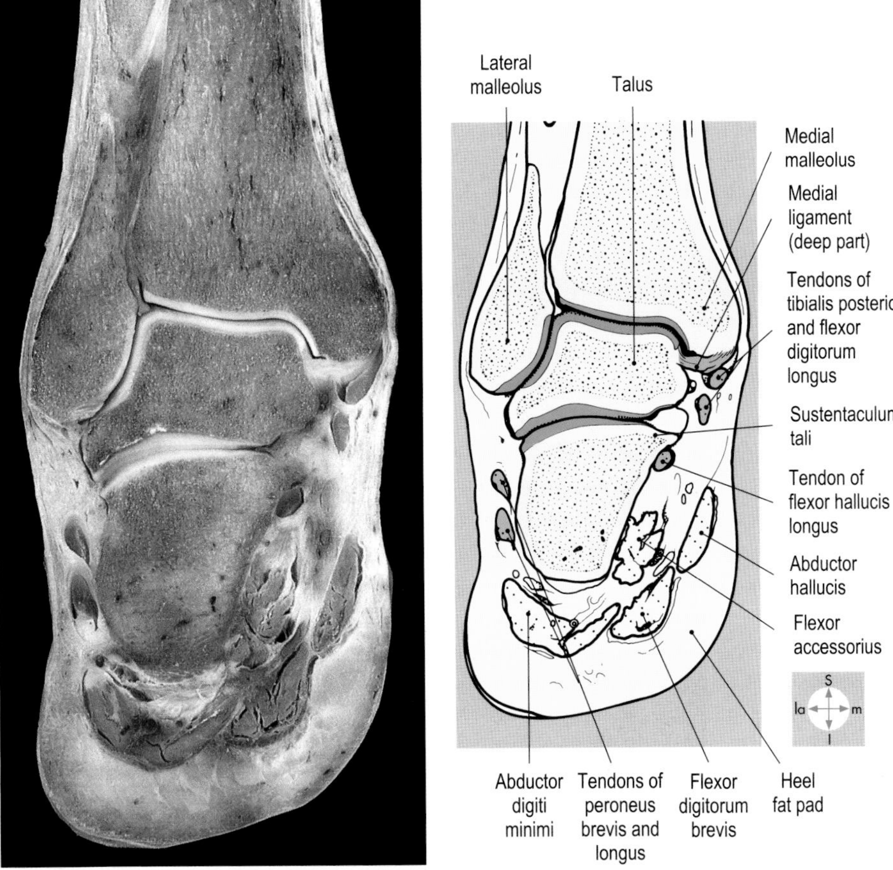

Fig. 6.90 Coronal section through ankle and talocalcaneal joints showing their relations.

Blood and nerve supply

Branches of the anterior and posterior tibial arteries, including the fibular, anastomose at the level of the malleoli and supply the joint. Innervation is from the deep fibular and tibial nerves.

Relations

The sides of the joint, the bony malleoli, are superficial (Fig. 6.90) and easily palpable. Passing subcutaneously in front of the joint are branches of the superficial fibular nerve and, just anterior to the medial malleolus, the saphenous nerve and great saphenous vein. On a deeper plane are the tendons of tibialis anterior and extensor hallucis longus, the dorsalis pedis artery, the deep fibular nerve, and the tendons of extensor digitorum longus and fibularis tertius (Fig. 6.91).

Posteriorly, the tendo calcaneus (Achilles) lies separated from the joint capsule by a bursa and pad of fat. Behind the medial malleolus are the tendons of tibialis posterior, flexor digitorum longus and flexor hallucis longus (Fig. 6.90), accompanied by the tibial nerve and posterior tibial artery (Fig. 6.91). Passing below the medial malleolus, they enter the foot beneath the flexor retinaculum. Passing superficially behind the lateral malleolus are the small saphenous vein and sural nerve and, more deeply, the tendons of fibularis longus and brevis (Fig. 6.91).

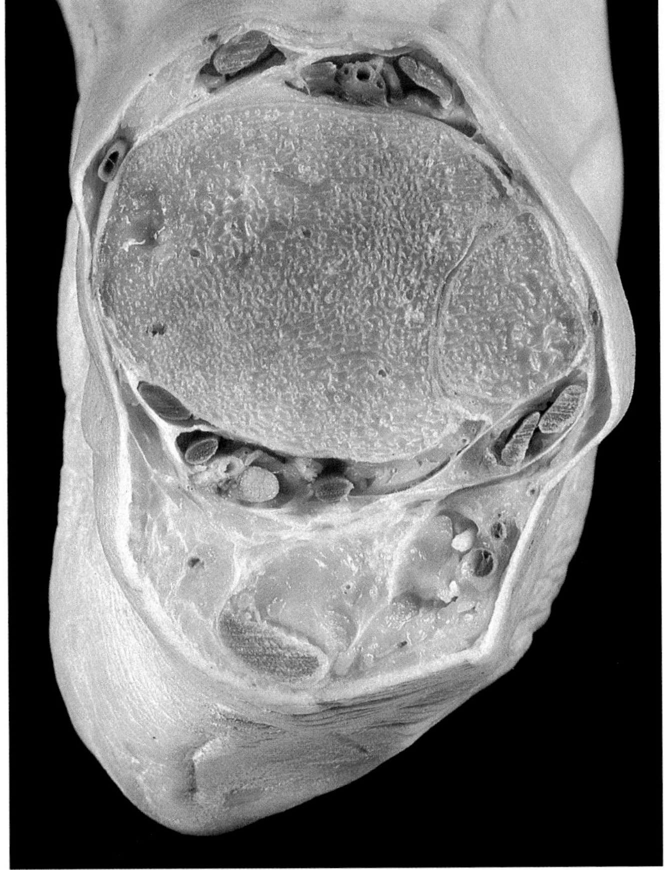

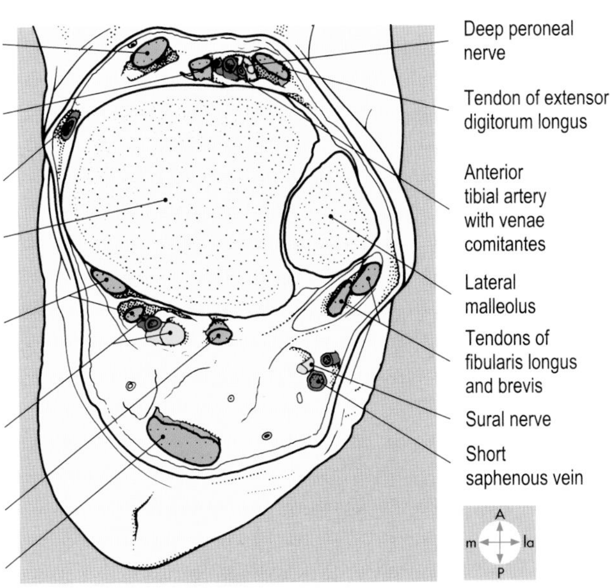

Fig. 6.91 Transverse section immediately above the ankle joint cavity showing relations.

Joints of Foot

These joints include those between the tarsal bones, the metatarsals and the phalanges. They are all synovial and have shapes related to their movements.

Tarsal joints

Although the tarsal joints are articulations between individual bones, they are usually classified into groups according to their locations (Fig. 6.92). The posterior tarsal group involves the talus and calcaneus; the midtarsals are between the talus and navicular on the medial side of the foot and between the calcaneus and cuboid on the lateral side; the anterior tarsals include the navicular, three cuneiforms and cuboid. All these joints are extremely stable.

Talocalcaneal joint

There are two articulations between the talus and calcaneus, each with a separate synovial cavity. Posteriorly is a saddle joint between the convex surface on the middle third of the calcaneus and the reciprocally concave surface on the body of the talus (Fig. 6.93). Anteriorly, two small flat facets on the anterior part of the calcaneus, including the sustentaculum tali, articulate with corresponding facets beneath the head of the talus (Fig. 6.93).

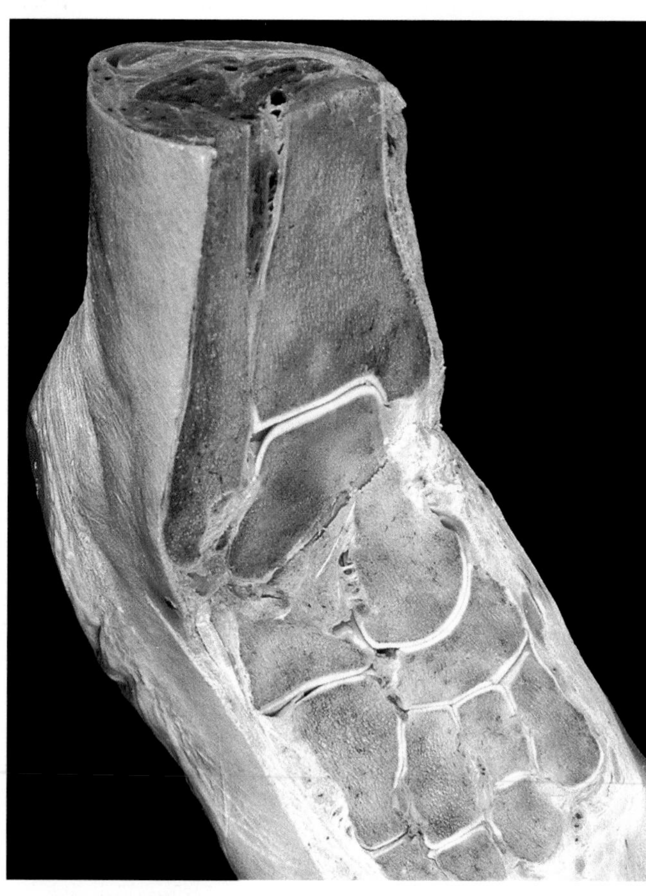

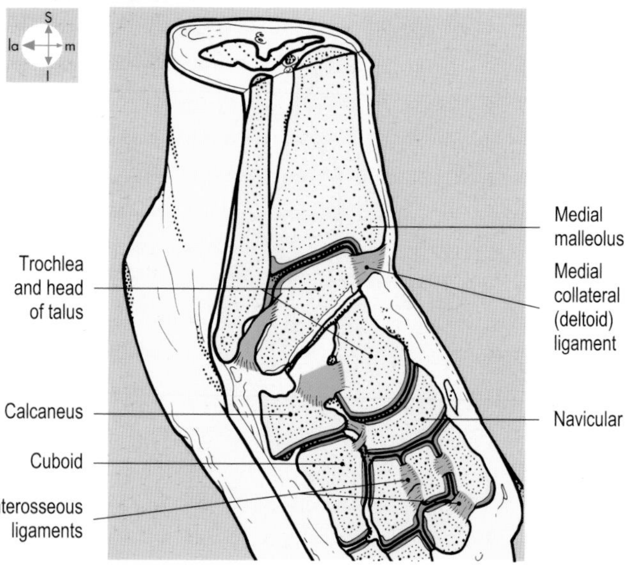

Fig. 6.92 Sections in two different planes through the ankle and foot to show ankle and tarsal joints.

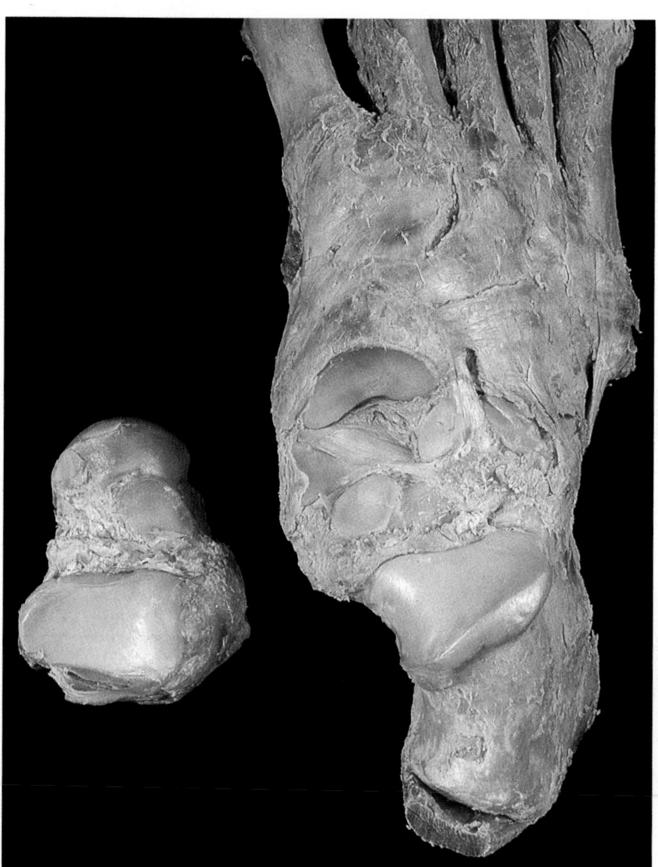

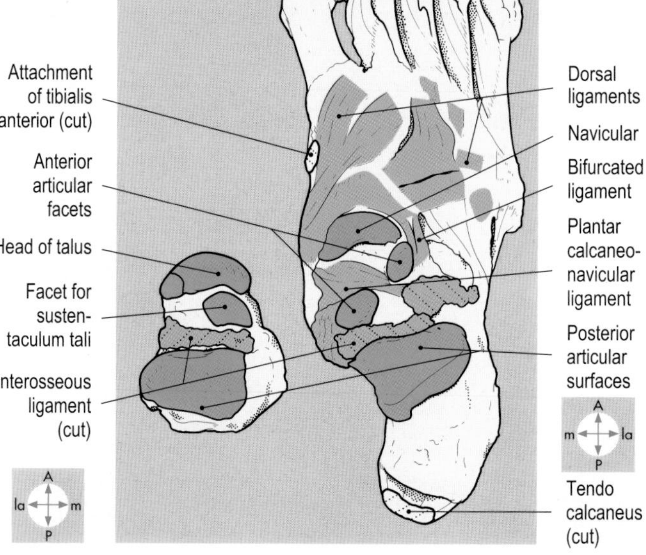

Fig. 6.93 Talocalcaneal and talonavicular joints. The talus has been disarticulated and turned over.

Talonavicular joint

The head of the talus forms a ball-and-socket joint with the posterior surface of the navicular. This joint shares a common synovial cavity with the anterior part of the talocalcaneal articulation. The combined joint, which involves the head of the talus, is termed the talocalcaneonavicular joint. The posterior talocalcaneal and talocalcaneonavicular joints form the subtalar joint.

Calcaneocuboid joint

At this plane joint, the flat anterior surface of the calcaneus articulates with the posterior surface of the cuboid (Fig. 6.92).

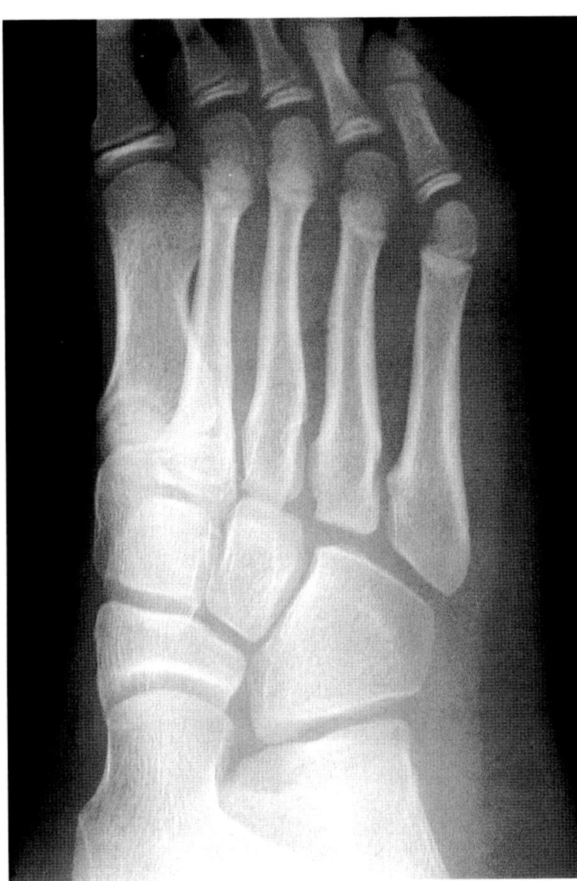

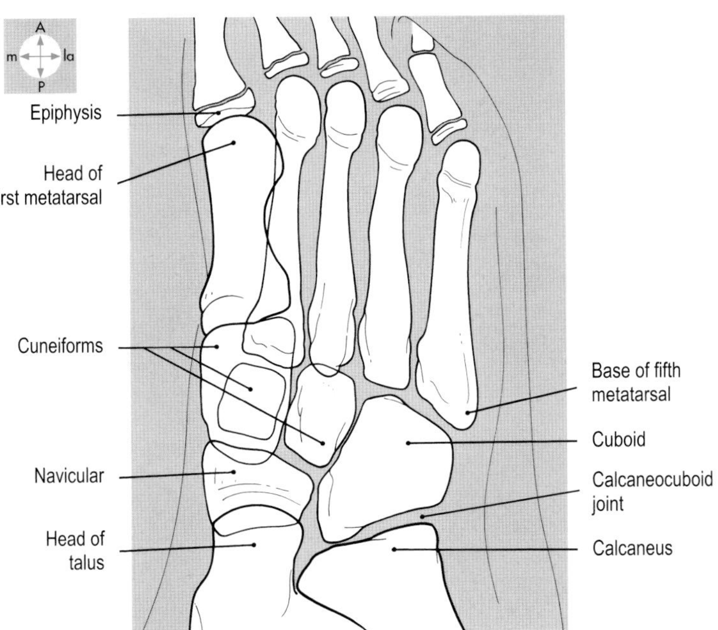

Fig. 6.94 Radiograph of juvenile foot showing tarsal bones and joints.

Other tarsal joints

Plane joints occur between the opposing surfaces of the navicular, the three cuneiforms and the cuboid (Fig. 6.92) and their synovial cavities freely communicate.

Capsules and ligaments

The fibrous capsules are attached around the margins of the articular surfaces. Short ligaments on the dorsum of the joints (Fig. 6.93) reinforce the capsules and, with the interosseous ligaments (Fig. 6.92), keep the articulating surfaces closely opposed. The strong interosseous talocalcaneal ligament (Fig. 6.93) in the sinus tarsi holds the talus and calcaneus together. The stem of the bifurcated ligament attaches to the anterior part of the calcaneus and its limbs to the navicular and cuboid. Beneath the tarsals, the long and short plantar ligaments (see Fig. 6.56) unite the plantar surfaces of the calcaneus and cuboid. The plantar calcaneonavicular (spring) ligament (Fig. 6.93) unites the navicular and sustentaculum tali, supporting the head of the talus and completing the socket by which the head articulates with the navicular and calcaneus.

Movements

The most mobile of the tarsal joints is the talocalcaneonavicular joint. Its ball-and-socket shape permits rotation around an oblique axis which passes upwards, forwards and medially through the neck and head of the talus. This rotation, together with gliding movements at the other tarsal joints, enables the anterior part of the foot to twist in respect to the more posterior part. These twisting movements involve raising either the medial or lateral border of the foot. Raising the medial border is called inversion and is produced by tibialis anterior and posterior, assisted by extensor hallucis longus. Raising the lateral border is called eversion and is brought about by fibularis longus, brevis and tertius.

Because of the oblique axis of the talocalcaneonavicular joint, inversion is always accompanied by plantar flexion and adduction of the foot whilst eversion is accompanied by dorsiflexion and abduction. These additional movements can be compensated by simultaneous movements at other joints. Thus, the plantar flexion accompanying inversion can be offset by slight dorsiflexion at the ankle joint whilst adduction can be offset by lateral rotation of the leg at the knee and hip joints.

Innervation

The tarsal joints are innervated by branches of the medial and lateral plantar nerves and the deep fibular nerve.

Tarsometatarsal and intermetatarsal joints

These are plane joints in which the bases of the fourth and fifth metatarsals articulate with the cuboid whilst the bases of the first, second and third metatarsals articulate with the respective cuneiforms (Fig. 6.94). Dorsal, plantar and interosseous ligaments reinforce the joint capsules. These joints allow gliding movements during alterations in the height of the arches. Innervation is by plantar and deep fibular nerves.

Metatarsophalangeal and interphalangeal joints

In each of the ball-and-socket metatarsophalangeal joints the metatarsal head articulates with the base of the proximal phalanx and the associated fibrocartilaginous plantar plate (Figs 6.95 & 6.96). A capsule enclosing the articular surfaces is reinforced on each side by a collateral ligament and dorsally by the extensor expansion. The principal movements are flexion and extension with only minimal abduction or adduction. The first metatarsophalangeal joint is especially important, bearing body weight during walking. Two sesamoid bones (see Fig. 6.101) are usually present in the plantar plate of this joint, closely associated with the insertions of the intrinsic muscles of the great toe (see p. 282).

The interphalangeal joints (Figs 6.95 & 6.97) are hinge joints, allowing flexion and extension. The muscles moving these joints are described on page 282. The joints of the toes are innervated by digital branches of the medial and lateral plantar nerves.

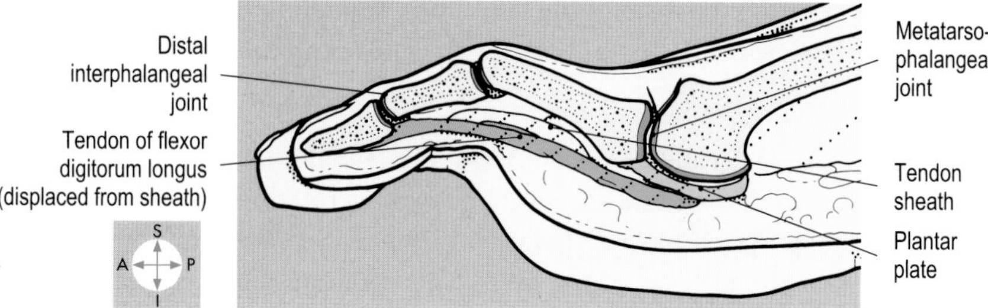

Fig. 6.95 Sagittal section through the third toe showing the metatarsophalangeal and interphalangeal joints.

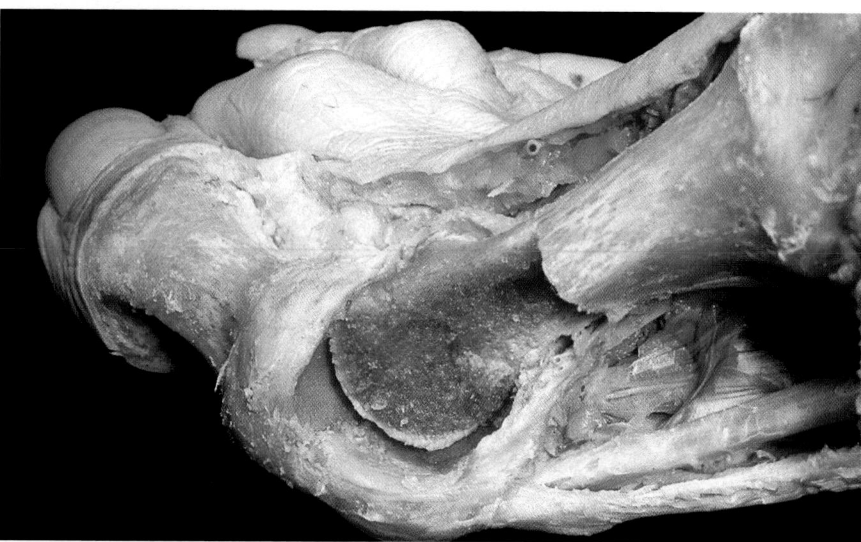

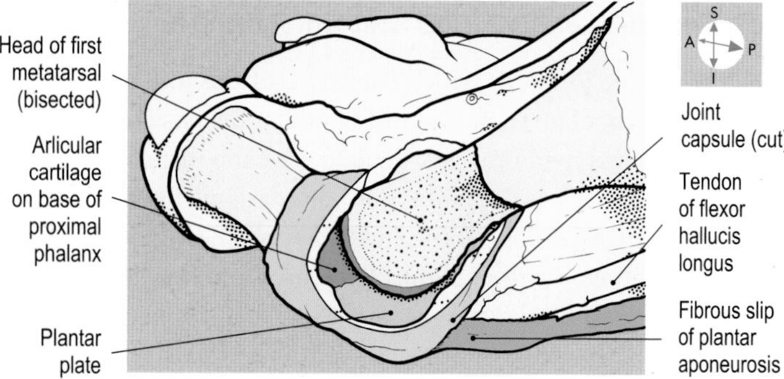

Fig. 6.96 Internal features of the first metatarsophalangeal joint. Part of the capsule and the distal part of the metatarsal bone have been removed.

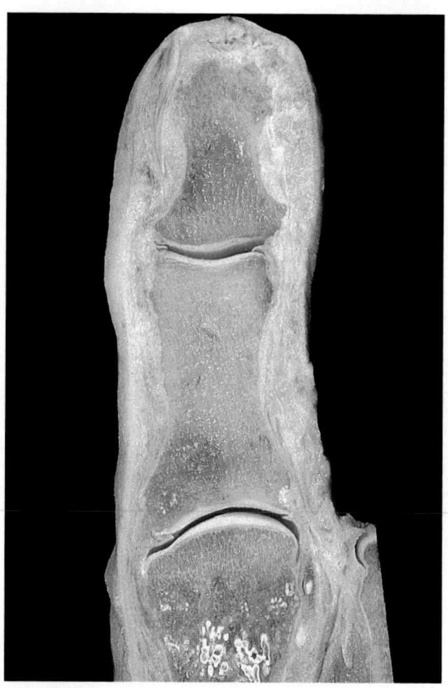

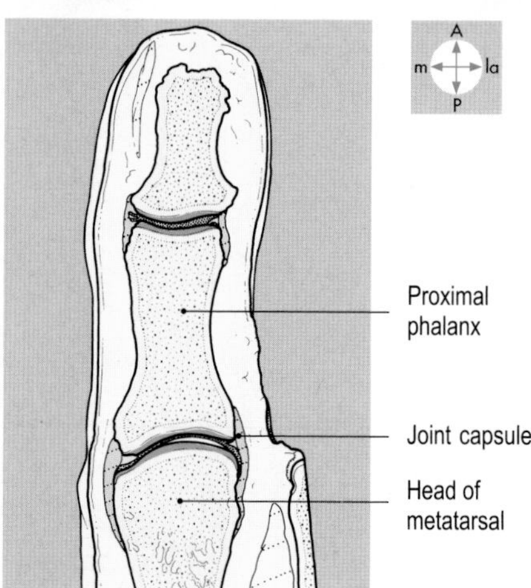

Fig. 6.97 Longitudinal section through the great toe showing its joints.

Arches of Foot

The tarsal and metatarsal bones form two longitudinal arches, medial and lateral. The medial arch is higher, forming the instep of the foot, and consists of the calcaneus, talus, navicular, three cuneiforms, and medial three metatarsals (Figs 6.98, 6.99 & 6.100). The lateral arch comprises the calcaneus, cuboid and lateral two metatarsals (Fig. 6.98). Each arch has an anterior and a posterior pillar, which together transmit body weight to the ground. The posterior pillar of each arch is the same, namely the tubercles on the inferior surface of the calcaneus. However, the anterior pillars are separate, being formed by the heads of the appropriate metatarsals. The arches are important in relation to human bipedalism, as they enhance forward propulsion.

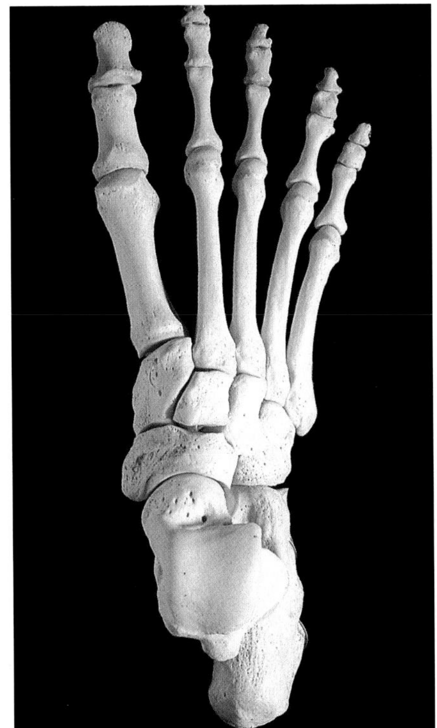

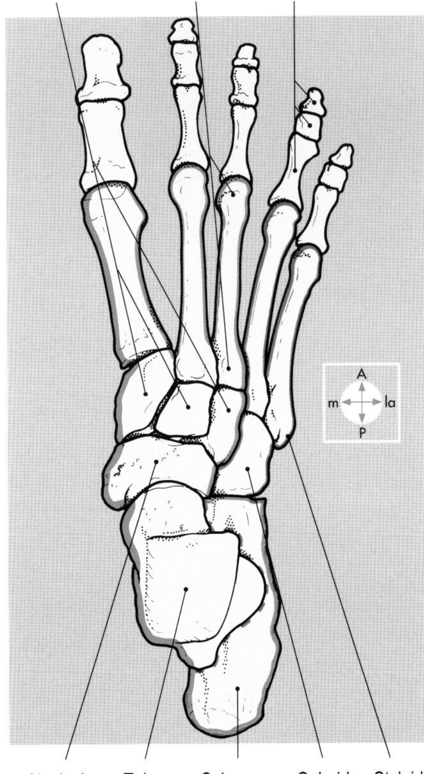

Fig. 6.98 Dorsal aspect of the bones of the foot showing the medial and lateral longitudinal arches.

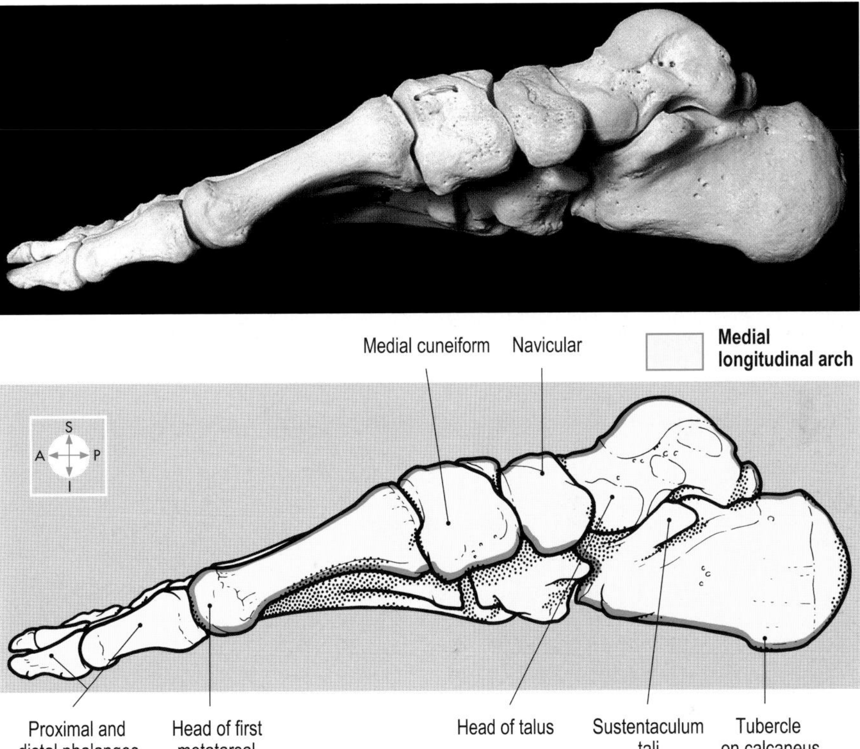

Fig. 6.99 Medial aspect of the bones of the foot to show the medial longitudinal arch.

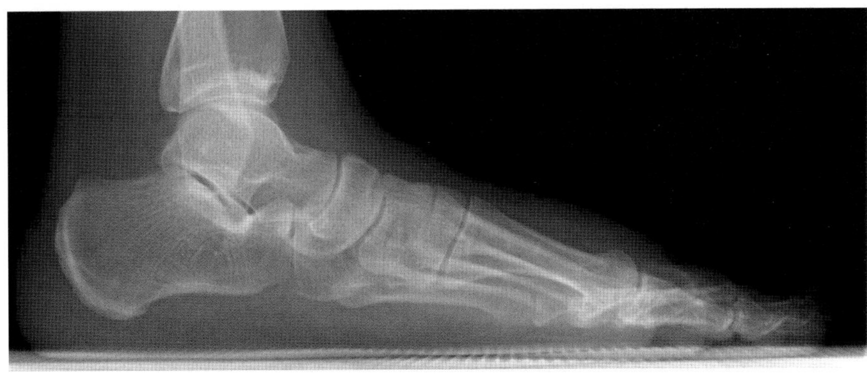

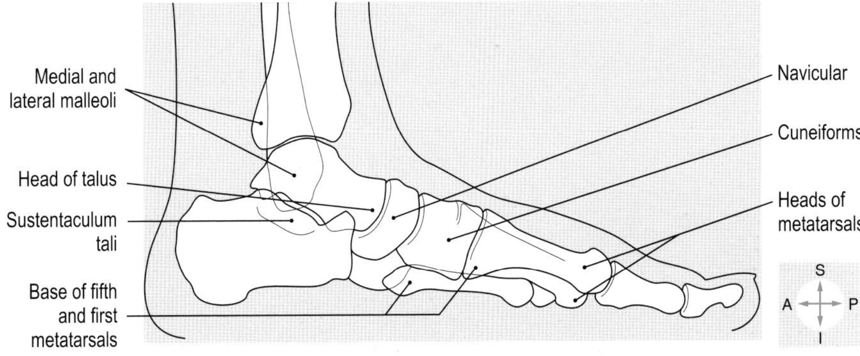

Fig. 6.100 Radiograph of foot showing longitudinal arches.

Stability

Factors in maintaining the arches include skeletal structure, ligaments, the plantar aponeurosis, and tendons and muscles. Skeletal structure is important in the medial arch, where at its highest point the head of the talus articulates in a wedge-like manner with the navicular anteriorly and the sustentaculum tali posteriorly (Fig. 6.101). The head of the talus is supported inferiorly by the plantar calcaneonavicular (spring) ligament (see Figs. 6.93 & 6.101), lying immediately above the tendon of flexor hallucis longus and a slip from the tendon of tibialis posterior, which passes backwards to the sustentaculum tali (see Fig. 6.56). Tibialis anterior, through the attachment of its tendon to the first cuneiform and first metatarsal, may also support the medial arch, which it raises during inversion.

The lateral arch is supported by the long and short plantar ligaments and the tendon of fibularis longus. Both longitudinal arches derive support from the long flexor tendons of the toes and from the plantar aponeurosis, whose digital slips gain indirect attachment to the proximal phalanges (see Fig. 6.96). When the heel rises from the ground the aponeurosis is passively tightened by extension of the toes at the metatarsophalangeal joints, thereby raising the longitudinal arches.

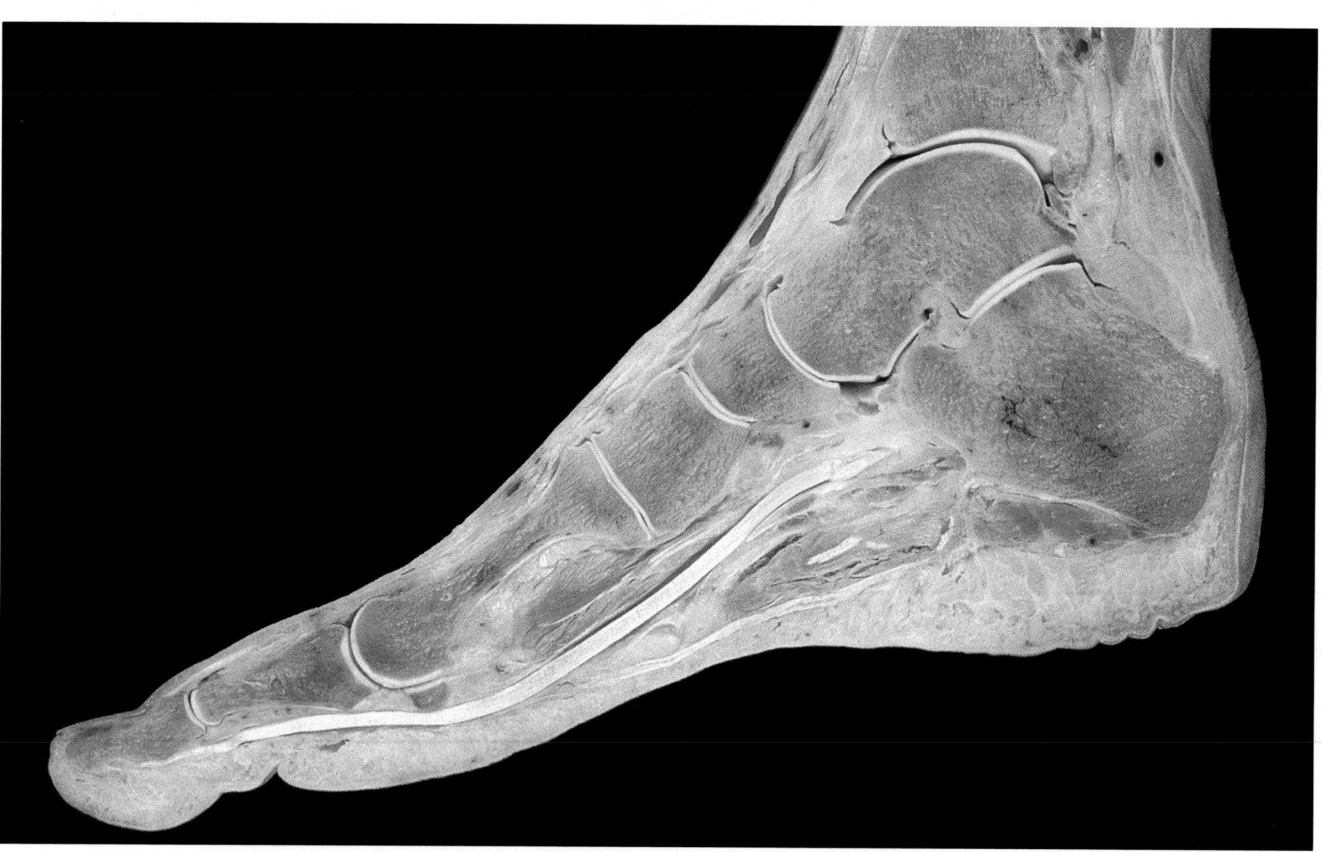

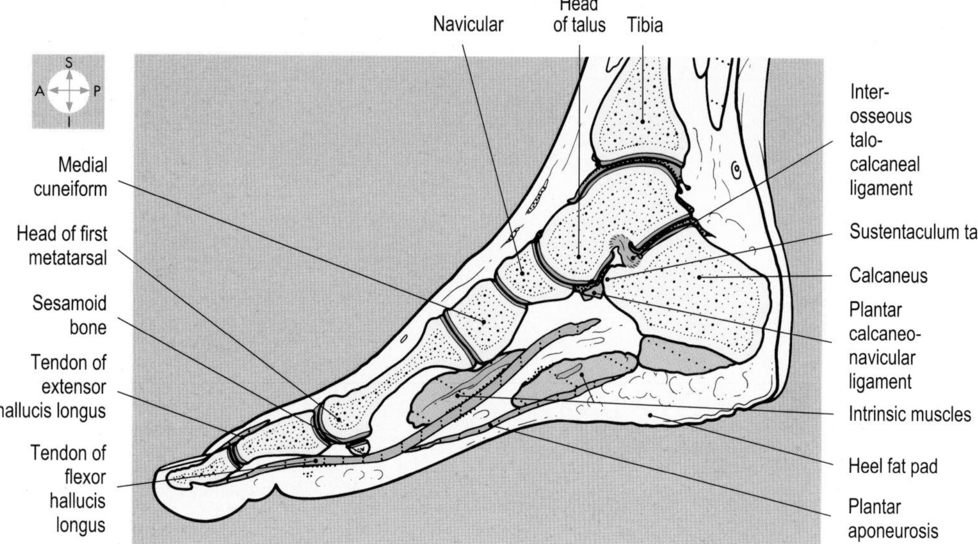

Fig. 6.101 Sagittal section of foot showing the medial longitudinal arch.

Exam Skills

Each of the incomplete statements below is followed by five suggested answers or completions. Decide which are true and which are false. The answers are supplied on page 415.

1. The gluteus maximus muscle:

a) has distal attachment principally to the iliotibial tract.
b) has a bursa separating it from the ischial tuberosity.
c) extends the hip and flexes the knee.
d) is supplied by the inferior gluteal nerve.
e) is attached to the sacrotuberous ligament.

2. Gluteus minimus muscle:

a) attaches to the anterior surface of the greater trochanter.
b) is supplied by the superior gluteal nerve.
c) is covered by the gluteus medius.
d) laterally rotates the hip.
e) during walking contracts in the weight-bearing limb.

3. Concerning nerves in the lower limb:

a) the sciatic nerve passes through the greater sciatic foramen.
b) the obturator nerve innervates the obturator internus.
c) the femoral nerve lies in the femoral sheath.
d) the lateral cutaneous nerve of the thigh passes through the inguinal ligament.
e) the genitofemoral nerve innervates skin on the anterior surface of the thigh.

4. Dermatomes in the lower limbs are located:

a) over the femoral triangle for L1.
b) along the medial border of the foot for L5.
c) over the gluteal region for S3.
d) over the footprint on the sole of the foot for S1.
e) on the lateral side of the leg for L4.

5. Concerning muscles in the thigh:

a) adductor longus separates the femoral from the profunda vessels.
b) vastus medialis forms the lateral wall of the adductor canal.
c) vastus intermedius attaches to the capsule of the knee joint.
d) iliopsoas forms the medial part of floor of the femoral triangle.
e) obturator externus lies below the capsule of the hip joint.

6. The femoral nerve:

a) has root origins from L2, L3 and L4 spinal cord segments.
b) lies lateral to the femoral artery.
c) gives cutaneous branches to the lateral side of the thigh.
d) supplies the sartorius muscle.
e) has a branch passing distally to supply the medial side of the foot.

7. The obturator nerve:

a) supplies obturator externus.
b) innervates the gracilis muscle.
c) has two divisions separated by adductor brevis.
d) supplies skin on the medial side of the thigh.
e) gives branches to the knee and hip joints.

8. Concerning the hip joint:

a) iliopsoas is a powerful flexor and medial rotator.
b) posterior dislocation endangers the sciatic nerve.
c) the surface marking lies just below the midinguinal point.
d) the iliofemoral ligament prevents backward tilting of the pelvis.
e) the neck of the femur lies intracapsular.

9. Concerning the patella:

a) the medial femoral condyle provides stability.
b) when dislocated it displaces laterally.
c) dislocation is more common in the female.
d) vastus medialis is attached to its medial border.
e) the prepatellar bursa is subcutaneous.

10. Concerning arteries in the lower limb:

a) the femoral artery is palpable at the midpoint of the inguinal ligament.
b) the popliteal artery lies close to the capsule of the knee joint.
c) the anterior tibial artery arises in the posterior compartment of the leg.
d) the posterior tibial artery passes behind the lateral malleolus.
e) the dorsalis pedis artery anastomoses with the plantar arch.

11. Concerning venous drainage of the lower limb:

a) communicating (perforating) veins direct blood from superficial to deep veins.
b) the great saphenous vein lies anterior to the medial malleolus.
c) the deep veins below the level of the knee comprise venae comitantes.
d) the small saphenous vein is accompanied by the sural nerve.
e) the superficial epigastric vein drains directly into the femoral vein.

12. Regarding the femoral sheath and its contents:

a) fascia iliaca forms the posterior part of the sheath.
b) the femoral vein lies in the lateral compartment.
c) branches of the ilioinguinal nerve pass anteriorly.
d) the femoral canal and ring are in the medial compartment.
e) pectineus muscle lies posteriorly.

13. Concerning the lymphatic system of the lower limb:

a) the main drainage is to inguinal lymph nodes.
b) skin on the lateral side of the foot drains into popliteal nodes.
c) superficial inguinal nodes drain the lower part of the anal canal.
d) lymph from the lower limb will reach the lumbar lymph trunk.
e) deep parts of the buttock drain into the deep inguinal nodes.

14. Concerning inversion and eversion of the foot:

a) inversion is produced by tibialis anterior.
b) inversion is produced by tibialis posterior.
c) inversion and eversion involve the subtalar joints.
d) inversion is produced by fibularis (peroneus) tertius.
e) eversion is produced by fibularis (peroneus) longus.

15. Concerning the knee joint:

a) the suprapatellar bursa reaches a hand's breadth above the patella.
b) the popliteus muscle attaches to the medial meniscus.
c) the tibial collateral ligament attaches to the medial meniscus.
d) the oblique popliteal ligament is derived from semimembranosus tendon.
e) the collateral ligaments limit extension.

16. Concerning the ankle joint:

a) forced eversion may tear the anterior talofibular ligament.
b) the calcaneofibular ligament prevents forward displacement.
c) the capsule extends onto the neck of the talus.
d) part of the innervation is from the deep fibular (peroneal) nerve.
e) it is less stable when plantar flexed.

Clinical Skills

The answers are supplied on page 417.

Case Study 1

A 24-year-old athletic male soccer player was brought to the Emergency Department with a history of having fallen hard during a game and twisting his knee after being tripped.

On examination he was lying with his left knee partially flexed. It was beginning to swell with fullness visible at the sides and above the patella together with a slight patellar 'tap'. All passive movements were painful. There was localized pain on deep pressure just medial to the patellar ligament over the joint line, and also severe pain over the joint line on the medial border of the knee. It became excruciating with firm medialward pressure applied over the lateral side of the joint at the same time as attempted abduction of the leg at the knee.

A plain frontal radiograph including a film taken whilst manoeuvring the joint as described with attempted abduction of the leg at the knee, showed inequality of the femur/tibia joint line with widening on the medial side.

Questions:

1. What is the anatomical basis for patellar 'tap'?
2. What structure was injured to be the cause of pain on deep pressure medial to the patellar ligament?
3. What structure was injured to explain pain on the medial border of the knee, accentuated by pressure over the lateral side with concomitant abduction of the leg?
4. Which ligaments are extracapsular and which are intracapsular? What are their roles in stabilizing the joint?

Case Study 2

The patient, a 45-year-old female shop assistant, complained of pain and aching in her right leg over a period of several years. The symptoms were particularly bad at the end of the day. Recently a lump had appeared in the left groin, which disappeared when she lay down on her bed, but reappeared on rising in the morning, and it became bigger when she coughed.

The patient was tall and not overweight. On standing, a large tortuous vein appeared beneath the skin, extending from the foot up the medial side of the limb into the groin. There was also a swelling, the size of an egg, just below the medial part of the crease in the groin. It disappeared when the patient was recumbent and especially if the limb was elevated.

The swelling, lying below and lateral to the pubic tubercle, had a smooth surface, was soft and uniform, and could be easily compressed. A direct impulse and thrill could be felt when the patient coughed. A large varicose vein was present along the whole length of the medial side of the limb. Trendelenburg's test was positive.

Questions:

1. Which vein was varicose?
2. What structure was giving rise to the swelling in the groin, and why was there a thrill over it when the patient coughed?
3. What mechanism is important in venous return from the lower limb and at what levels in the limb does it operate?

Case Study 3

The patient, a 60-year-old male, was diabetic. For more than a year he had experienced increasing difficulty in walking due to cramps and pain in the calves of his legs. Although the pain was easier when he rested it was becoming severe even at rest and interfered with his sleep at night. In the last two months he had noticed a black area at the end of his right big toe, which was getting worse.

The skin of both lower limbs, especially below the knee was shiny, thin and hairless. No arterial pulses could be felt in the limb on the right side. The skin over the distal half of the right hallux was shrunken and black, being gangrenous with a sharp line of demarcation separating it from the more proximal part of the toe.

An arteriogram showed severe and widespread narrowing with irregularity of the walls and occlusion of the main artery just above the adductor tubercle. Extensive collaterals were present above and around the knee.

Questions:

1. Where is an arteriogram performed in the lower limb and why?
2. Where are the locations for detecting arterial pulsation in the lower limb?
3. What comprises the genicular anastomosis and which arteries contribute?

Case Study 4

A 20-year-old male presented to the neurology clinic with a five-month history of weakness in the left leg and numbness in the left foot. There was a six-month previous history of a chest infection during an overseas holiday for which he was given two intramuscular injections in the left gluteal region.

The patient walked without any obvious limp although slight foot drop was evident on the left side. There was weakness of plantar flexion, and further weakness on flexing the hallux. Midcalf wasting was evident on the left side. Diminished pain and touch sensation was noted over the left sole of the foot and the ankle-jerk reflex was absent.

Motor nerve conduction studies showed slowing of conduction in the left common fibular (peroneal) nerve compared with the right side, and sensory nerve conduction studies showed slowing in the left sural nerve compared with the right side.

Questions:

1. What nerve supplies the posterior compartments in the lower limb, and which of its branches supplies the muscles of the posterior compartment of the leg?
2. What does wasting of the calf muscles indicate about the level of the lesion?

Observation Skills

Identify the structures indicated. The answers are supplied at the foot of the page.

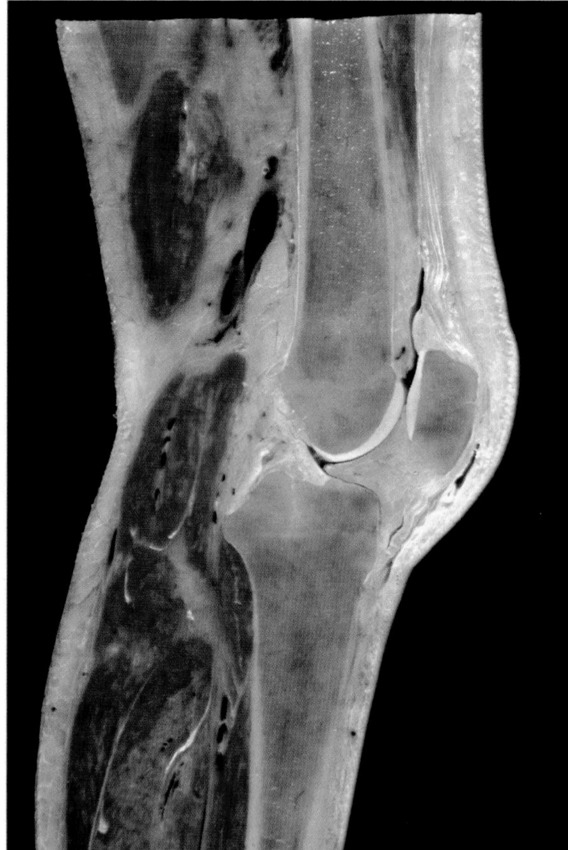

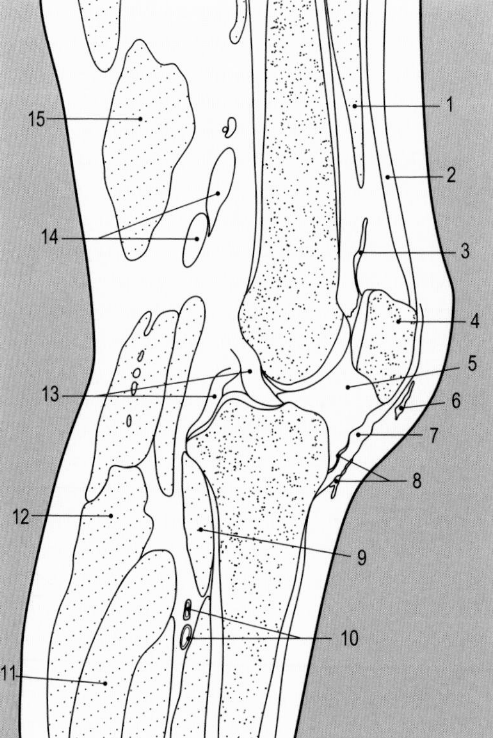

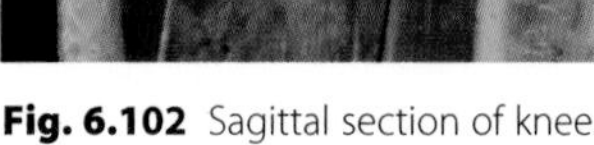

Fig. 6.102 Sagittal section of knee.

Answers

Fig. 6.102 1 = vastus intermedius; 2 = quadriceps tendon; 3 = suprapatellar bursa; 4 = patella; 5 = infrapatellar fatpad; 6 = prepatellar bursa; 7 = patellar ligament; 8 = infra patellar bursae superficial and deep; 9 = popliteus; 10 = popliteal artery and vein; 11 = soleus; 12 = gastrocnemius; 13 = anterior and posterior cruciate ligaments; 14 = popliteal artery and vein; 15 = hamstring

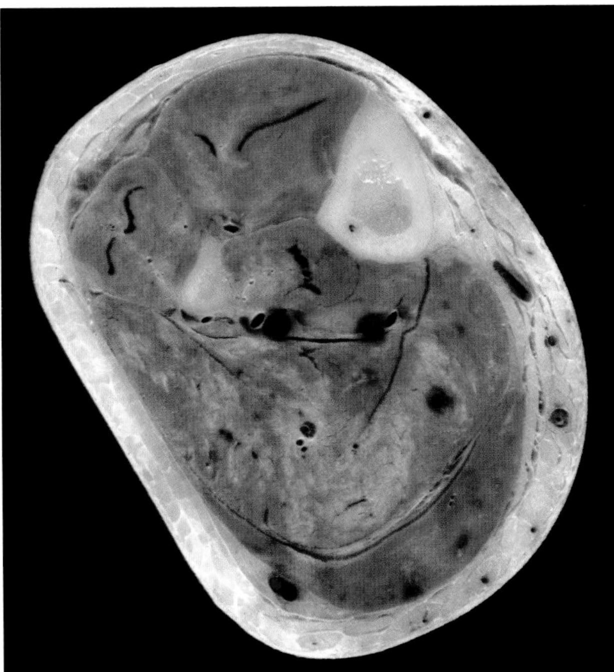

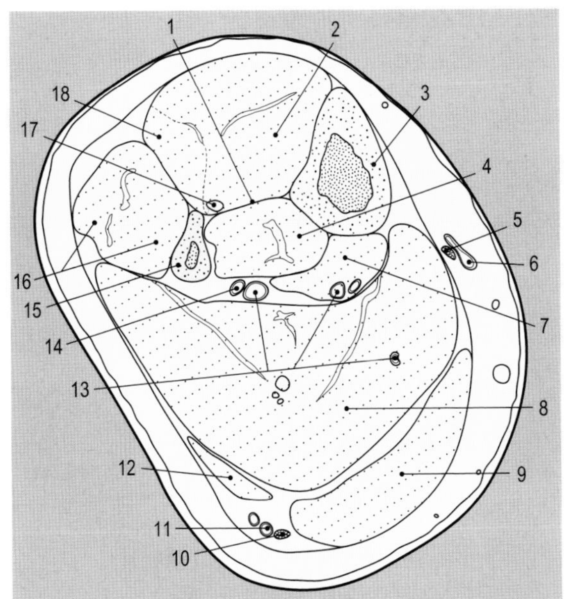

Fig. 6.103 Transverse section of leg.

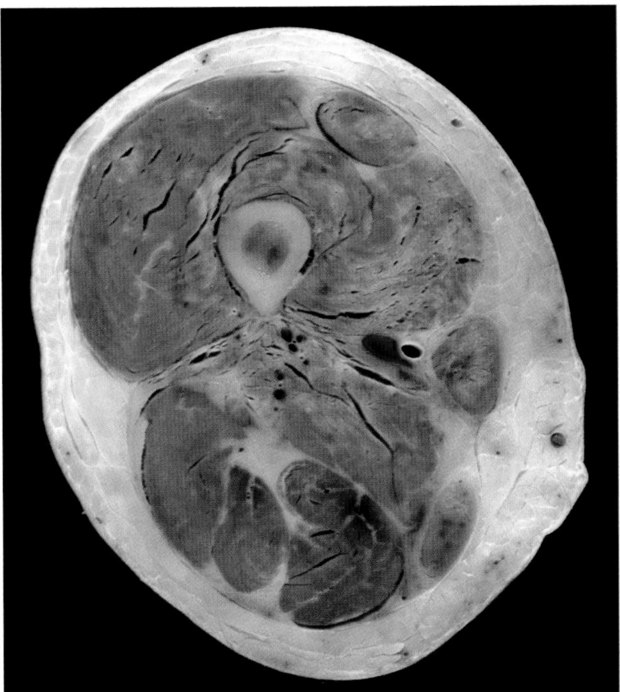

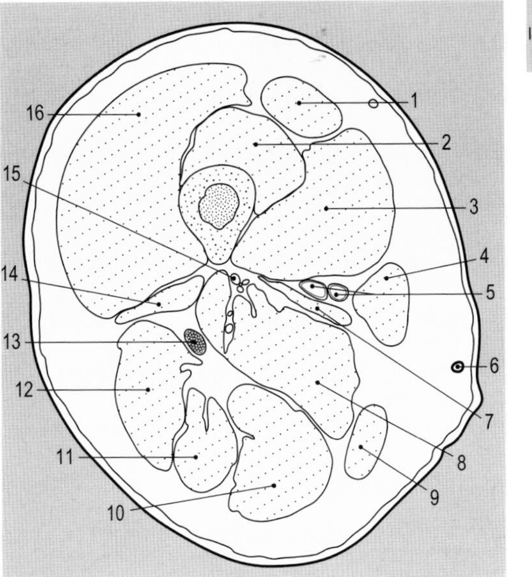

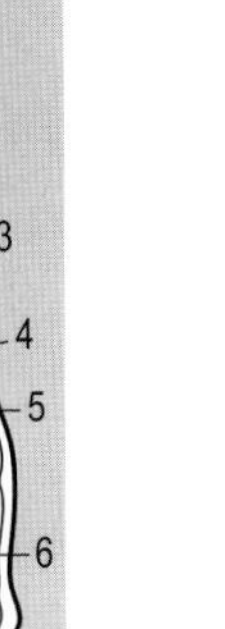

Fig. 6.104 Transverse section of thigh.

Answers

Fig. 6.103 1 = interosseous membrane; 2 = tibialis anterior; 3 = tibia; 4 = tibialis posterior; 5 = saphenous nerve; 6 = great saphenous vein; 7 = flexor digitorum longus; 8 = soleus; 9 = medial head of gastrocnemius; 10 = sural nerve; 11 = small saphenous vein; 12 = lateral head of gastrocnemius; 13 = deep veins; 14 = posterior tibial artery; 15 = fibula; 16 = peroneal muscles; 17 = anterior tibial artery; 18 = extensor digitorum longus

Fig. 6.104 1 = rectus femoris; 2 = vastus intermedius; 3 = vastus medialis; 4 = sartorius; 5 = femoral artery and vein; 6 = great saphenous vein; 7 = adductor longus; 8 = adductor magnus; 9 = gracilis; 10 = semimembranosus; 11 = semitendinosus; 12 = long head of bicepsfemoris; 13 = sciatic nerve; 14 = short head of biceps femoris; 15 = profunda femoris vessels; 16 = vastus lateralis

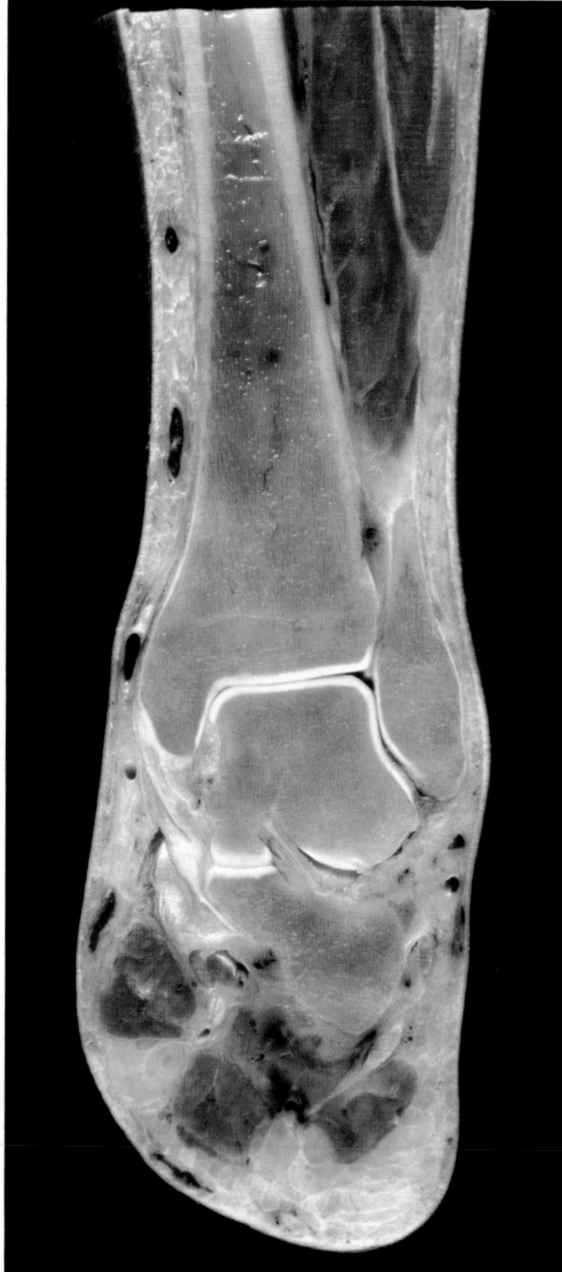

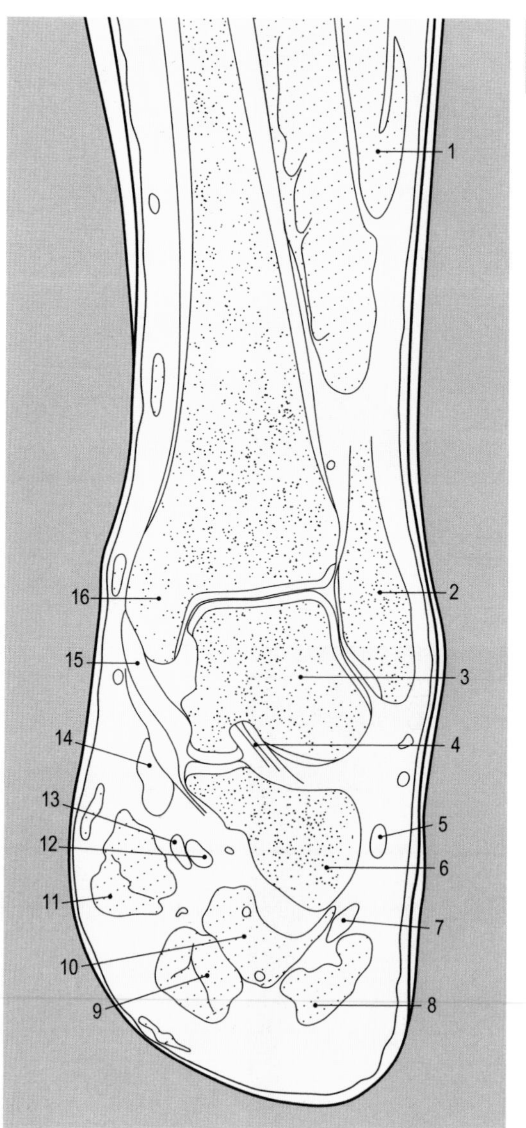

Fig. 6.105 Coronal section of ankle.

Answers

Fig. 6.105 1 = peroneal muscles; 2 = lateral malleolus; 3 = body of talus; 4 = interosseous talocalcaneal ligament; 5 = fibularis brevis tendon; 6 = calcaneum; 7 = fibularis longus tendon; 8 = abductor digiti minimi; 9 = flexor digitorum brevis; 10 = quadratus plantae; 11 = abductor hallucis; 12 = flexor hallucis longus tendon; 13 = flexor digitorum longus tendon; 14 = tibialis posterior tendon; 15 = medial ligament; 16 = medial malleolus

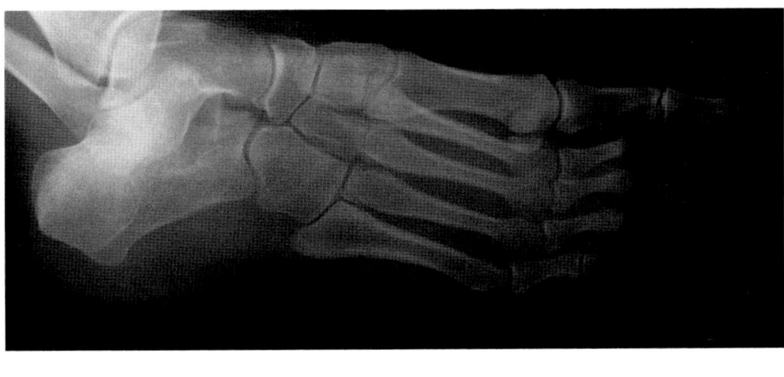

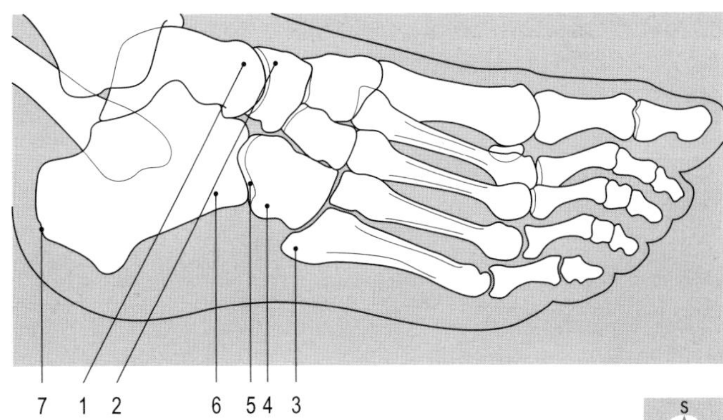

Fig. 6.106 Oblique radiograph of ankle and antero posterior radiograph of foot.

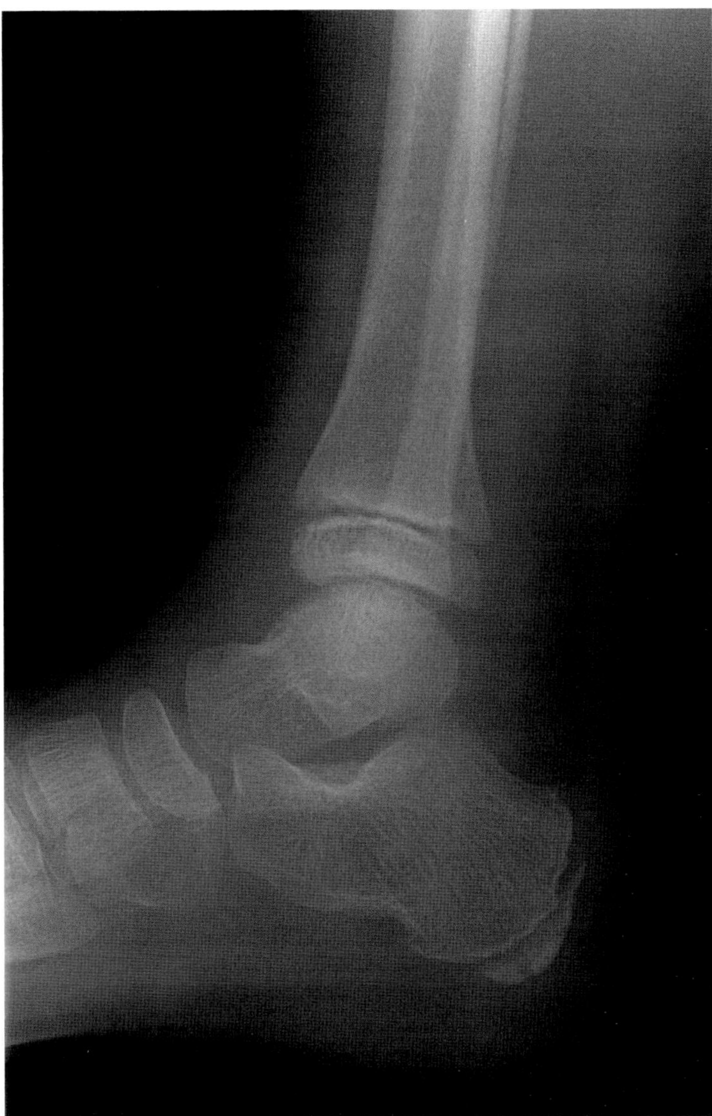

Fig. 6.107 Lateral radiograph of juvenile ankle.

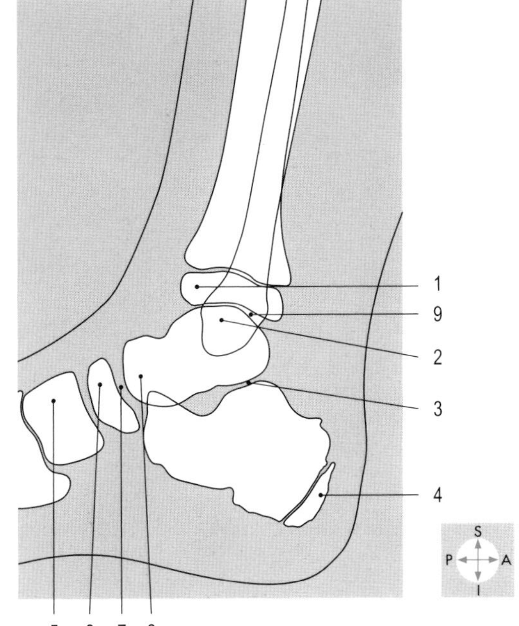

Answers

Fig. 6.106 1 = head of talus; 2 = navicular; 3 = base of fifth metatarsal; 4 = cuboid; 5 = calcaneocuboid joint; 6 = calcaneum; 7 = tubercle for tendo calcaneus

Fig. 6.107 1 = epiphysis on distal end of tibia; 2 = dome of talus; 3 = subtalar joint; 4 = posterior traction epiphysis on calcaneum; 5 = medial cuneiform; 6 = navicular; 7 = talonavicular joint; 8 = head of talus; 9 = ankle joint

Head and neck

CHAPTER 7

Introduction

The bones of the head and neck include the skull, the mandible and the cervical vertebrae (Fig. 7.1). The skull (cranium) comprises the neurocranium, which contains the brain and meninges, and the bones of the face (viscerocranium), attached to the anterior aspect of the neurocranium and clothed by soft tissues. The facial bones enclose the orbits, the nose and paranasal air sinuses, and the mouth and pharynx. The mandible articulates with the neurocranium at the temporomandibular joints.

The neck is the junctional region between the head and the thorax and the upper limbs, and is bounded above by the mandible and the base of the skull and below by the superior thoracic aperture (thoracic inlet) and pectoral girdle. The neck contains the seven cervical vertebrae and associated muscles, parts of the alimentary and respiratory tracts and the thyroid gland. In the midline immediately anterior to the vertebrae is the pharynx, which continues as the cervical oesophagus. Anterior to these are the larynx and upper trachea with the thyroid gland. On each side of the organs major vessels pass between the thorax and the head, accompanied by nerves and lymphatics. The cervical vertebrae support the skull, allowing it to be moved in relation to the trunk.

Within the cervical vertebral column lies the vertebral canal, containing the spinal cord enclosed by meninges. The neck is enclosed by investing fascia, subcutaneous tissue and skin.

Arising from the brainstem are twelve pairs of cranial nerves (Fig. 7.2), which provide innervation for structures in the head and neck. One cranial nerve, the vagus (X), is distributed not only to the head and neck but also to structures in the thorax and abdomen. Eight pairs of segmental spinal nerves arise from the cervical part of the spinal cord. The upper cervical spinal nerves are distributed to the head and neck, whereas the lower ones descend into the upper limbs and thorax. Dermatomes of the head and neck are derived from the trigeminal (V) nerve and from cervical spinal nerves (Fig. 7.3).

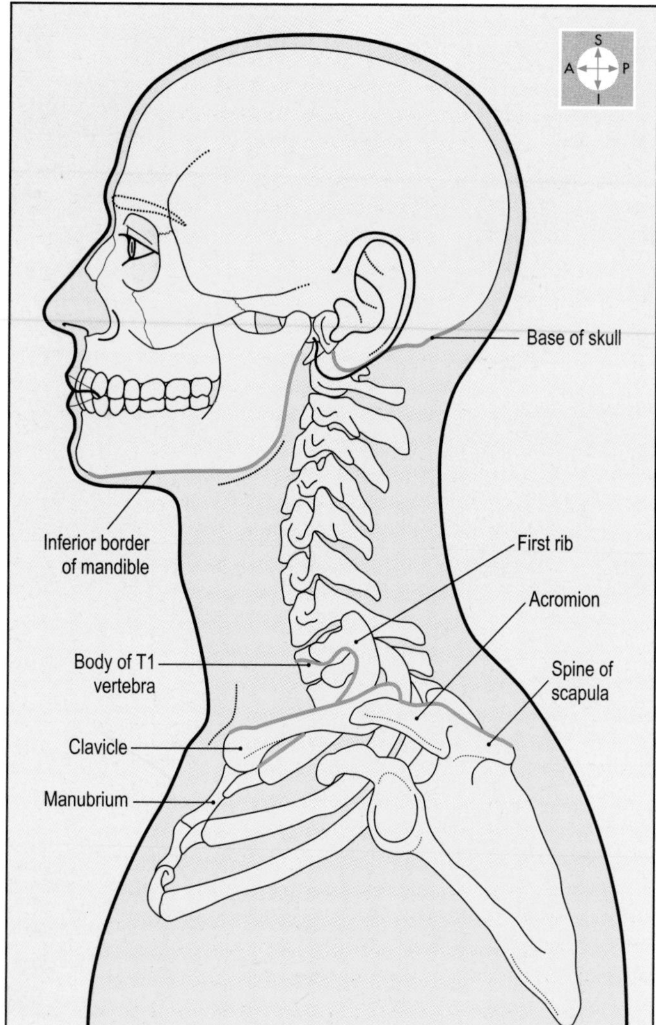

Fig. 7.1 Skeleton of head and neck. Boundary of neck, pink line.

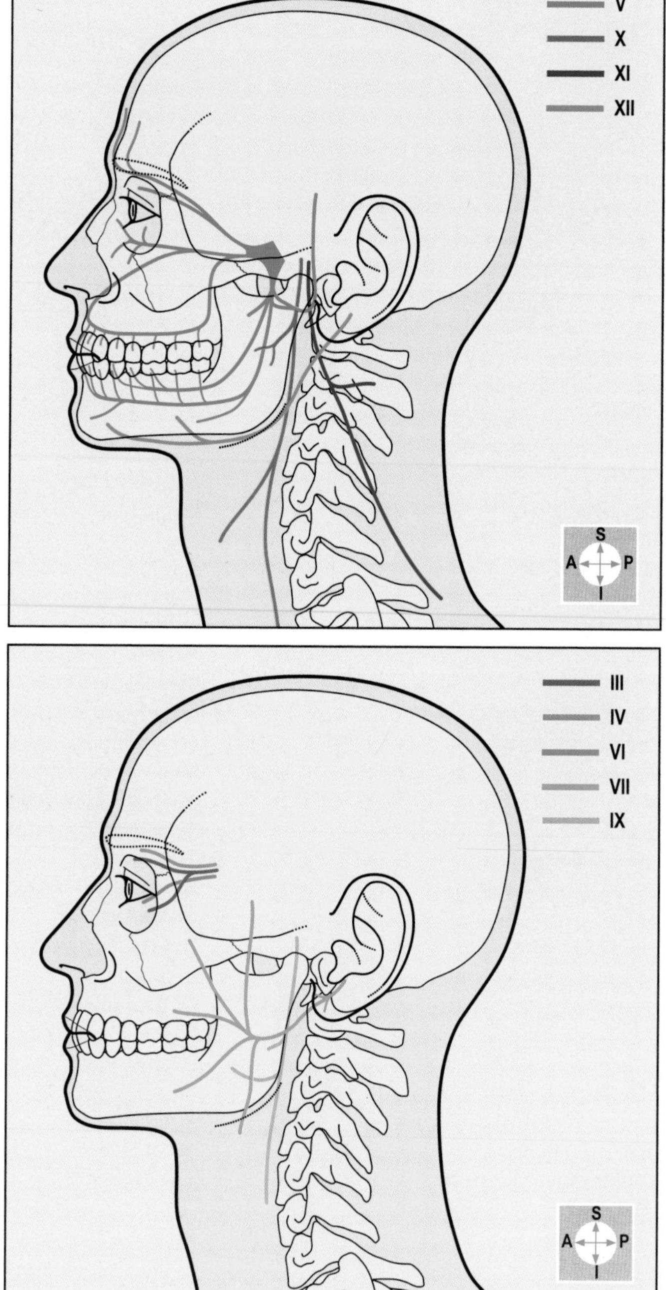

Fig. 7.2 Extracranial parts of cranial nerves III–VII and IX–XII.

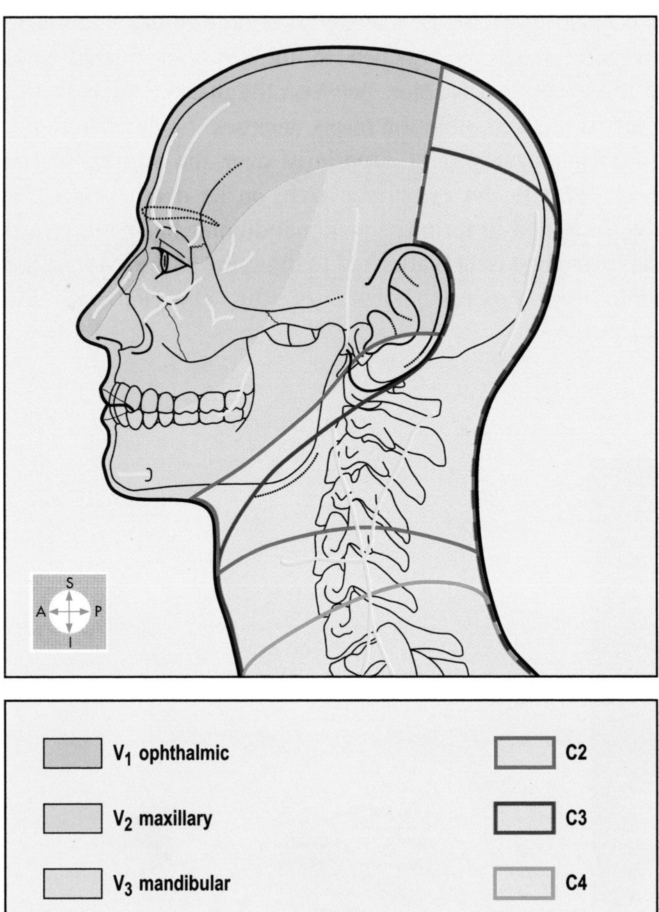

Fig. 7.3 The dermatomes of the head and neck. Cutaneous nerves are shown in yellow.

The arterial supply to the head and neck (Fig. 7.4) is derived from the paired common carotid and vertebral arteries. Each common carotid artery divides to form an internal carotid artery, supplying the contents of the neurocranium and the orbit, and an external carotid artery which supplies the face, most of the scalp and the upper part of the neck. Branches from the subclavian arteries supply structures in the root of the neck. Each vertebral artery ascends through foramina in the transverse processes of the cervical vertebrae and enters the skull via the foramen magnum to assist in the supply to intracranial structures.

Venous drainage (Fig. 7.4) occurs through superficial and deep systems, which communicate in several places. Superficial veins of the face, scalp and neck drain via the external jugular veins into the subclavian veins. Blood from deeper structures of the face and from within the neurocranium drains through the internal jugular veins into the brachiocephalic veins.

Lymph drains through a chain of lymph vessels and nodes lying along the internal jugular vein and is returned to the venous system, usually at the junction of internal jugular and subclavian veins.

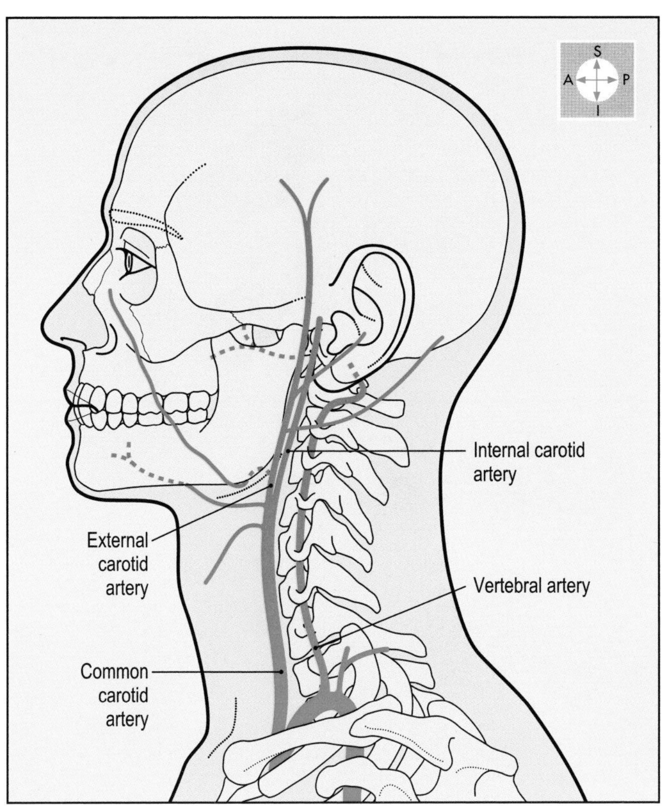

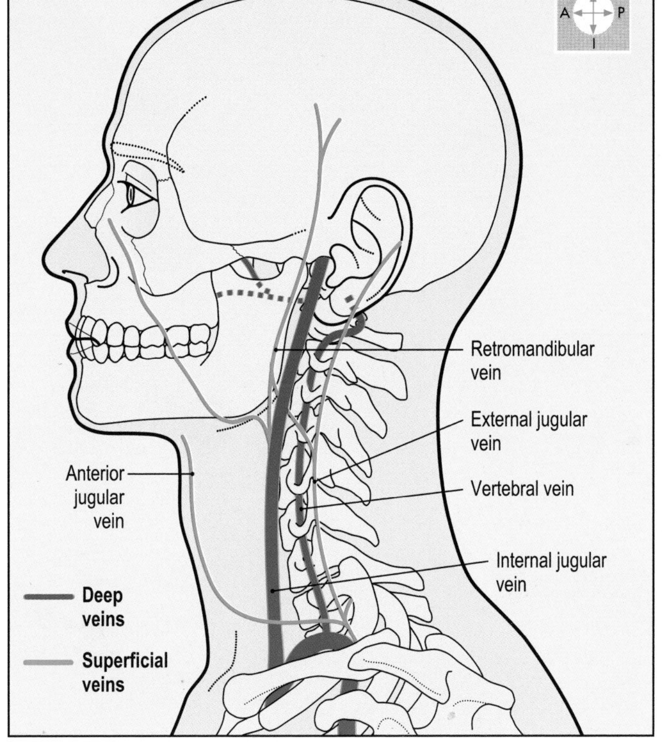

Fig. 7.4 The main arteries and veins of the head and neck.

Neck

Fascial layers

These are complex and are divided into four components: investing fascia, prevertebral fascia, pretracheal fascia and carotid sheaths (Fig. 7.5). The investing fascia is analogous to deep fascia in the limbs. Deep to the skin and superficial tissues, it surrounds the neck, extending from the pectoral girdle below to the base of the skull and mandible above, and splits to enclose trapezius and sternocleidomastoid. Superiorly the investing fascia is attached to the superior nuchal lines and to the mastoid processes. Between the mastoid process and the angle of the mandible the fascia encloses the parotid gland. Its superficial layer passes superiorly over the surface of the gland to attach to the zygomatic arch; on its deep surface the fascia is thickened to form the stylomandibular ligament. Inferiorly the investing fascia is attached to the spine of the scapula, the acromion, the superior border of the clavicle, and the manubrium.

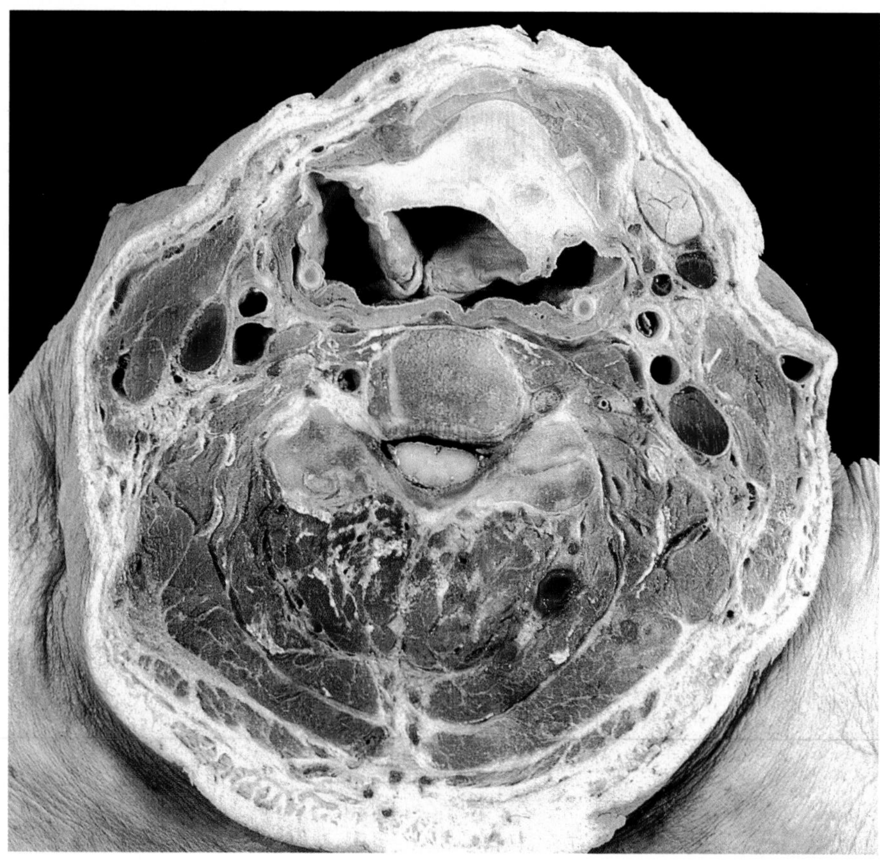

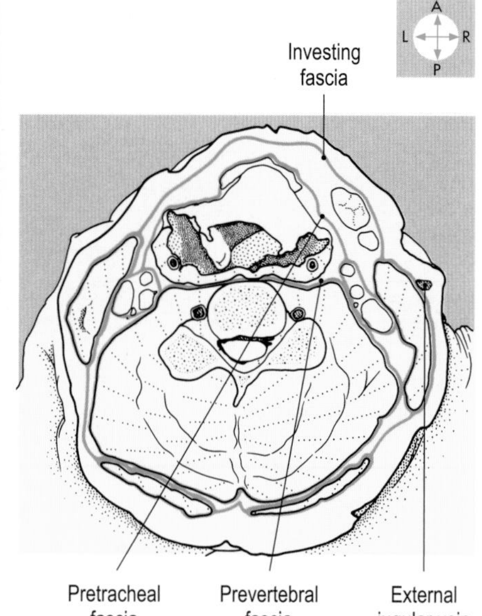

Fig. 7.5 Transverse section at the level of the fourth cervical vertebra showing the layers of cervical fascia (green lines). Superior aspect. Compare Fig 7.95. The layers are shown separately in the diagrams below.

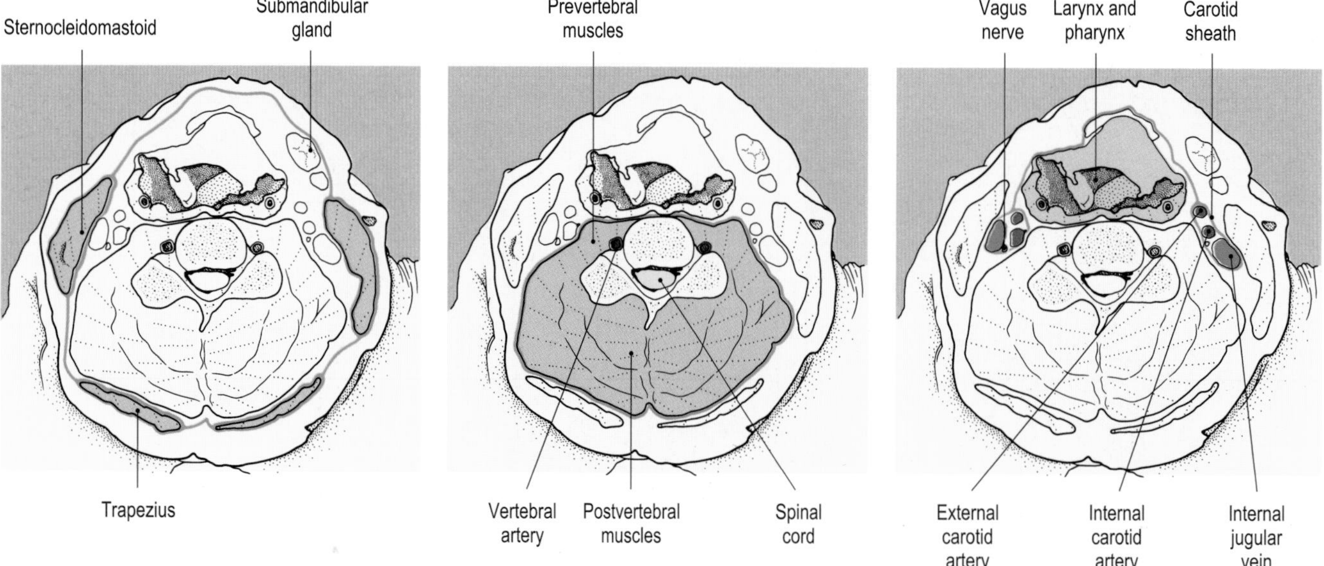

The investing fascia and its enclosures.

The prevertebral fascia and its enclosures.

The pretracheal fascia and carotid sheaths and their enclosures.

The prevertebral fascia encloses the vertebral column, pre- and postvertebral muscles and origins of the cervical and brachial plexuses. Superiorly it attaches to the base of the skull and inferiorly it extends into the superior mediastinum.

The pretracheal fascia covers the anterior and lateral aspects of the trachea and larynx, limited superiorly by the hyoid bone and by the oblique lines on the thyroid cartilage. It splits to enclose the thyroid gland and inferiorly fuses with the adventitia of the aortic arch in the superior mediastinum. Posterolaterally on each side, the pretracheal fascia blends with the carotid sheath.

Each of the two carotid sheaths contains a common, an internal and part of an external carotid artery, a vagus nerve and an internal jugular vein. The sheaths are attached to the base of the skull around the jugular and carotid foramina and pass inferiorly to the aortic arch and brachiocephalic veins to fuse with the adventitia covering these vessels.

For purposes of anatomical description the superficial part of each side of the neck is divided into anterior and posterior triangles separated by sternocleidomastoid.

Sternocleidomastoid (sternomastoid)

This muscle passes obliquely upwards and backwards from the manubrium and the medial end of the clavicle to the mastoid process and superior nuchal line of the skull (Fig. 7.6). One sternocleidomastoid acting alone turns the head towards the opposite shoulder, whereas acting together both muscles protrude the head forwards. Sternocleidomastoid is innervated by the spinal part of the accessory nerve (XI).

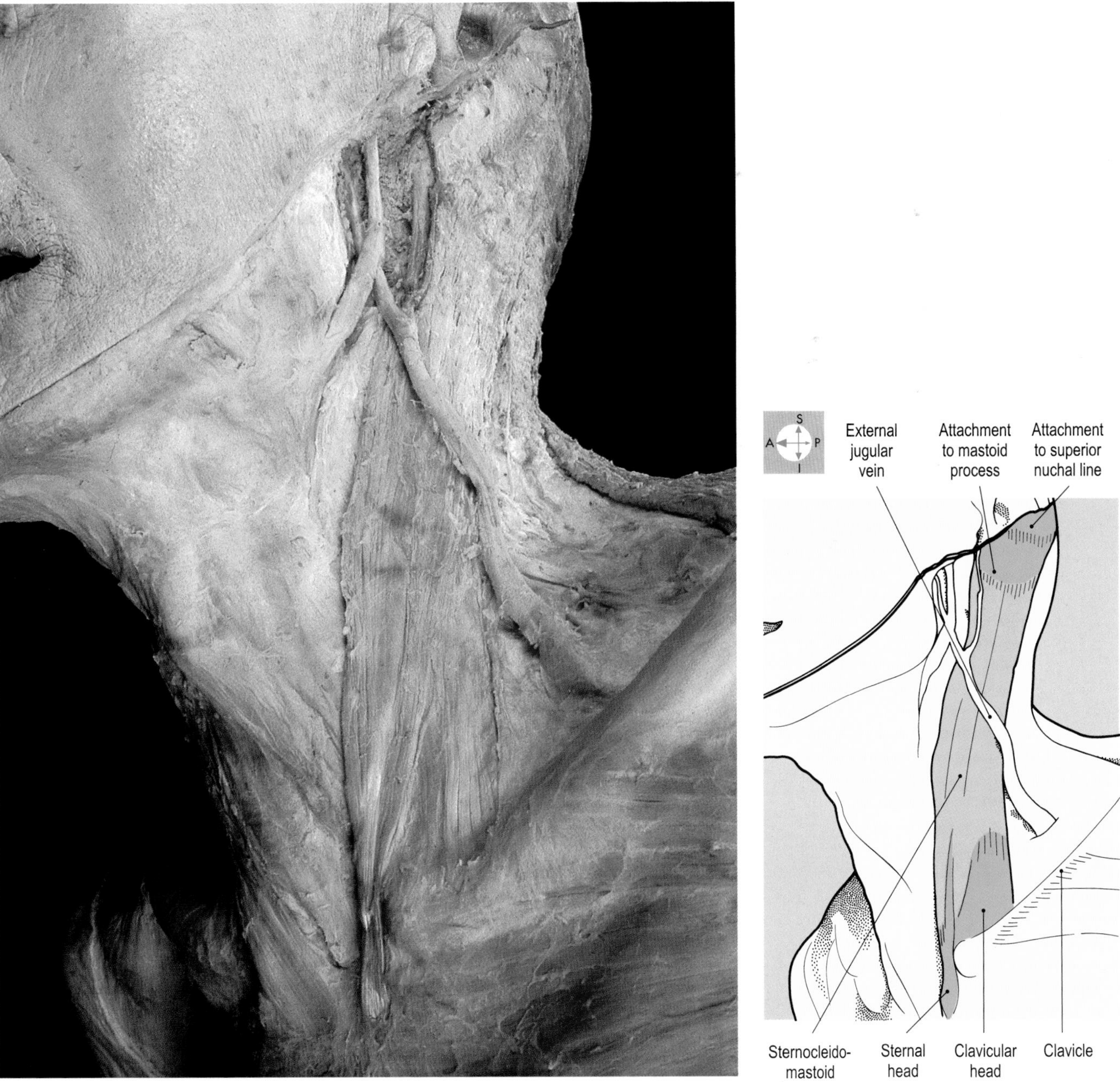

Fig. 7.6 Oblique view of the neck showing sternocleidomastoid after removal of the investing fascia covering sternocleidomastoid and trapezius.

Posterior triangle of neck

This triangle is bounded anteriorly by sternocleidomastoid and posteriorly by trapezius. Inferiorly the upper border of the clavicle forms the base whilst superiorly the attachments of sternocleidomastoid and trapezius converge onto the superior nuchal line to form the apex of the triangle. The posterior triangle does not lie in a flat plane but spirals so that the inferior portion is directed anteriorly, whilst the apex faces posterolaterally.

Roof

The roof of the triangle is formed by the investing fascia which spans the interval between trapezius and sternocleidomastoid. The external jugular vein initially lies vertically over the sternocleidomastoid just beneath the skin and then passes onto the roof of the lower part of the triangle. The vein pierces the roof just above the clavicle to enter the triangle and drain into the subclavian vein. Cutaneous branches of the cervical plexus (see below) also lie superficial to the roof of the triangle (Fig. 7.7).

Floor

The floor of the posterior triangle is formed by the prevertebral fascia covering the paravertebral muscles, which are, from above downwards, splenius capitis, levator scapulae and scalenus posterior, medius and anterior (Fig. 7.8). Deep to the prevertebral fascia are the subclavian artery, the three trunks of the brachial plexus and the cervical plexus. Continuing laterally to reach the axilla, the brachial plexus and the subclavian artery are enclosed in a prolongation of the prevertebral fascia, the axillary sheath. Injection of local anaesthetic inside the axillary sheath blocks sensation from the upper limb. Deep to the scalene muscles, subclavian vessels and brachial plexus are the pleura and apex of the lung.

Contents

Between the floor and the roof of the triangle lie the contents (Fig. 7.9), which include a number of vascular structures, the spinal part of the accessory (XI) nerve, components of the cervical plexus and supraclavicular and occipital lymph nodes. The spinal part of the accessory nerve passes obliquely across the triangle from beneath the posterior border of sternocleidomastoid to leave deep to the anterior border of trapezius. It supplies both of these muscles. In the lower part of the triangle the inferior belly of omohyoid passes towards its scapular attachment. Two branches of the thyrocervical trunk, namely the transverse cervical and suprascapular arteries, also pass laterally across the triangle to the scapula. At the apex of the triangle the occipital artery emerges to supply part of the scalp. The subclavian vein is sometimes visible just above the clavicle.

Cervical plexus

The cervical plexus is formed from the anterior rami of the first four cervical spinal nerves and supplies the paravertebral muscles with segmental branches. It provides a branch from C1 to the hypoglossal nerve and branches from C2 and C3, which all contribute to the ansa cervicalis. The phrenic nerve, the principal innervation of the diaphragm, is formed from C3, C4 and C5 and runs vertically downwards on the anterior surface of scalenus anterior, behind the prevertebral fascia.

Sensory branches from the cervical plexus (Fig. 7.7) pass through the triangle and emerge by piercing the roof near the

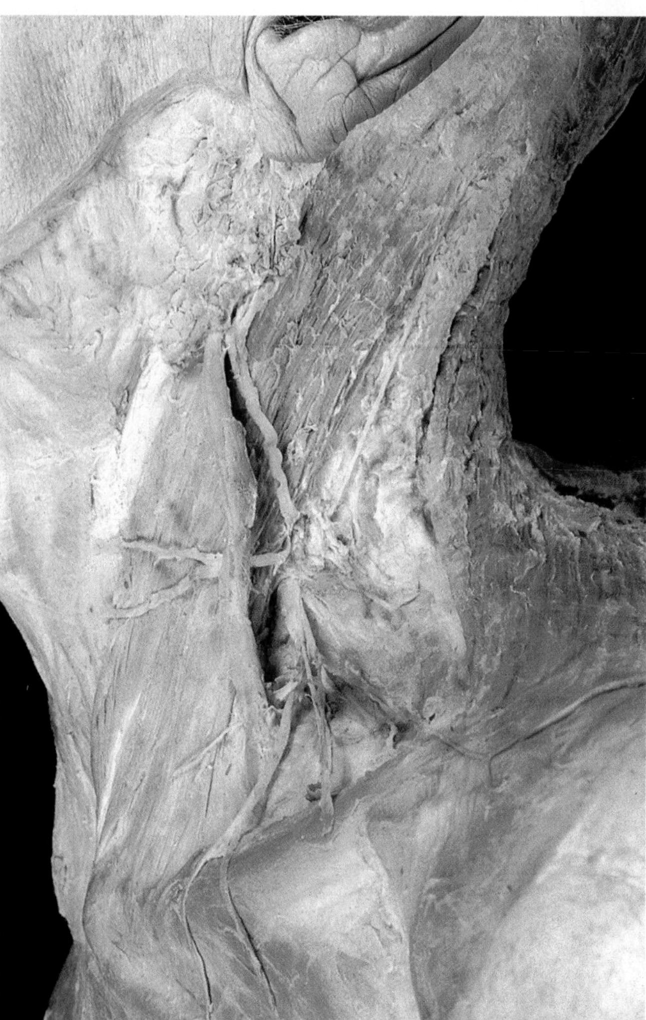

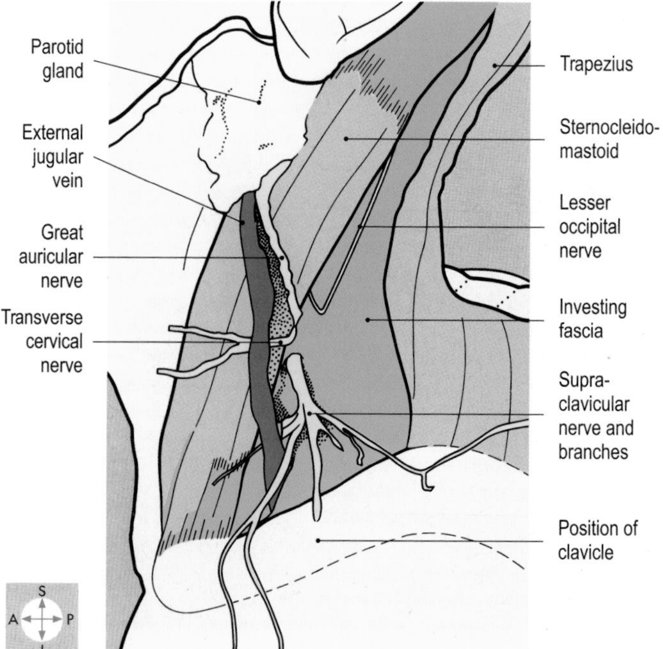

Fig. 7.7 Boundaries and roof of the posterior triangle of the neck. The external jugular vein and cutaneous branches of the cervical plexus, lying superficial to the roof, are also present.

midpoint of the posterior border of sternocleidomastoid. These convey sensation from the neck, the lower part of the face and pinna, the side of the scalp and the upper part of the thoracic wall. The lesser occipital nerve (C2) ascends along the posterior border of sternocleidomastoid and supplies the side of the occipital region of the scalp. The great auricular nerve (C2 & C3) runs vertically upwards across sternocleidomastoid and conveys sensation from the lower part of the pinna and the skin over the parotid gland. The transverse cervical nerve (C2 & C3) passes horizontally, supplying the skin over sternocleidomastoid and the anterior triangle. Finally, the supraclavicular nerves (C3 & C4) radiate downwards to convey sensation from skin over the upper part of the anterior thoracic wall and the shoulder region.

Anterior triangle of neck

By convention, the two anterior triangles of the neck extend medially to the midline. Posterolaterally each triangle is bounded by the anterior border of sternocleidomastoid and superiorly by the inferior border of the mandible. That part of the triangle above the hyoid bone will be described with the mylohyoid and related structures.

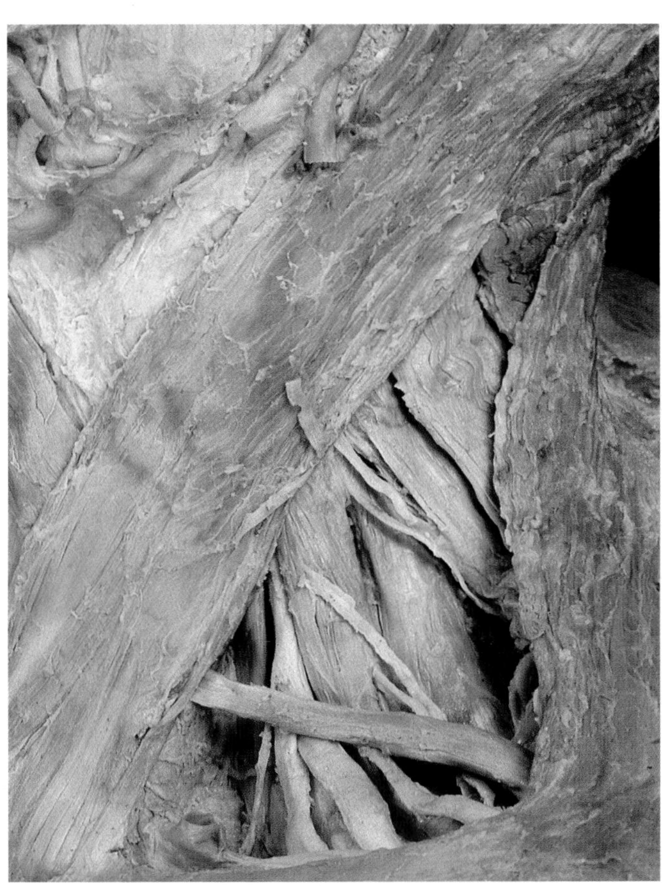

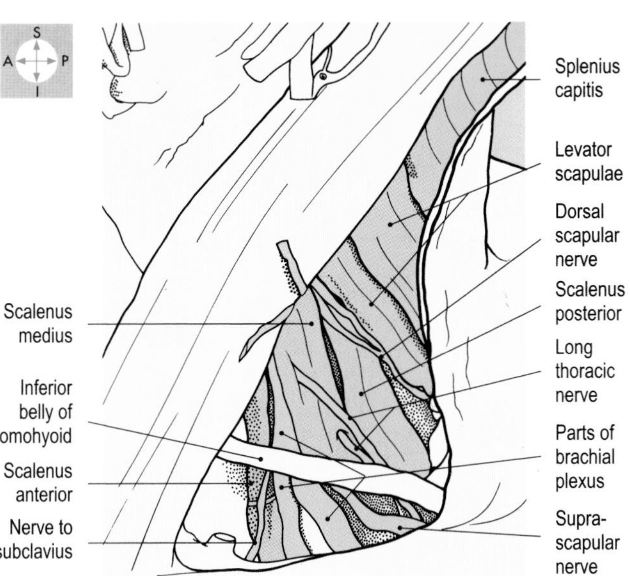

Fig. 7.8 Floor of the posterior triangle from which the prevertebral fascia has been removed. The inferior belly of the omohyoid muscle, one of the contents of the triangle, is still present.

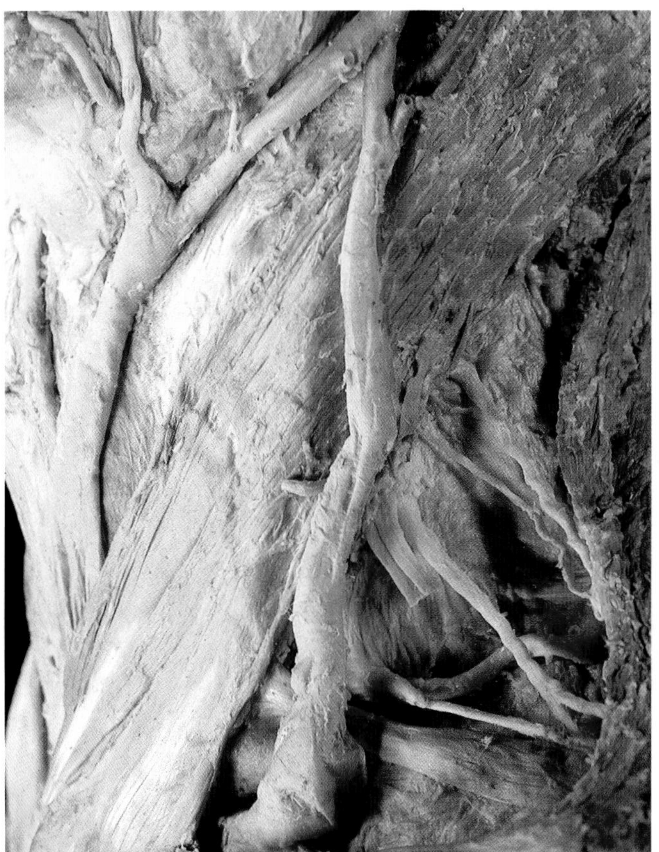

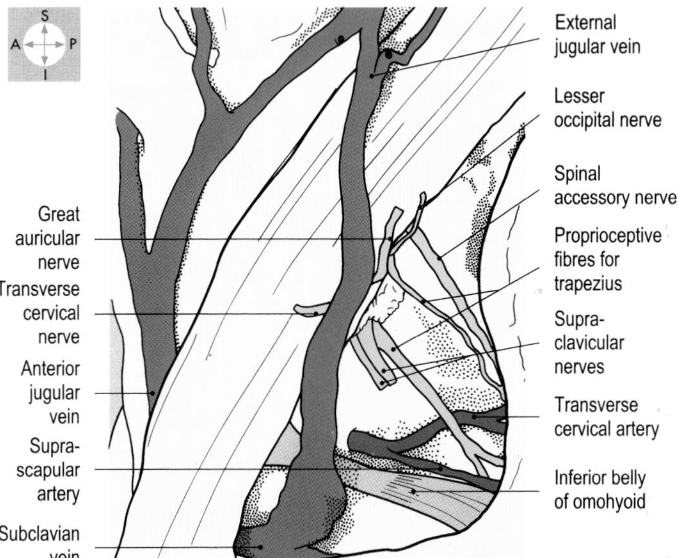

Fig. 7.9 Contents of the posterior triangle. The external jugular vein is in continuity with the anterior jugular system.

Roof

The roof of the anterior triangle (Fig. 7.10) is formed by the investing fascia of the neck. Superficial to the fascia are platysma (see p. 334) and the anterior jugular vein. This vessel pierces the roof and passes deep to sternocleidomastoid to drain into the external jugular vein just before its termination in the subclavian vein. The cutaneous innervation of the skin over the triangle has already been described (see p. 325).

Floor

The floor of the anterior triangle is composed of the pretracheal fascia and posterolaterally the carotid sheath. The thyroid gland (Fig. 7.13) is enclosed by the pretracheal fascia whilst the larynx and trachea lie deep to it. Laterally, the carotid arteries, internal jugular vein and vagus (X) nerve all lie within the carotid sheath.

Contents

The contents of the anterior triangle (Fig. 7.11) comprise infrahyoid or strap muscles (sternohyoid, sternothyroid, thyrohyoid and omohyoid) and their immediate nerve supply. The most superficial muscle, sternohyoid, is attached inferiorly to the deep surface of the manubrium and superiorly to the lower border of the body of the hyoid bone. Deep to sternohyoid are both sternothyroid and thyrohyoid. Sternothyroid extends from the manubrium to the oblique line on the lamina of the thyroid cartilage. In the same plane, thyrohyoid runs from the thyroid cartilage to the inferior edge of the body of the hyoid bone. Omohyoid consists of two bellies linked by an intermediate tendon. The inferior belly is attached to the suprascapular ligament and the adjacent part of the scapula. It crosses the posterior triangle and ends deep to sternocleidomastoid in the intermediate tendon is anchored to the clavicle by a loop of investing fascia. The superior belly continues upwards to its attachment on the lower border of the hyoid bone lateral to the other muscles.

All four muscles are supplied segmentally by branches from the first three cervical spinal nerves. Thyrohyoid is supplied by fibres from C1 that have travelled with the hypoglossal (XII) nerve; the remaining muscles are supplied via the ansa cervicalis. The infrahyoid muscles depress the hyoid bone and the larynx.

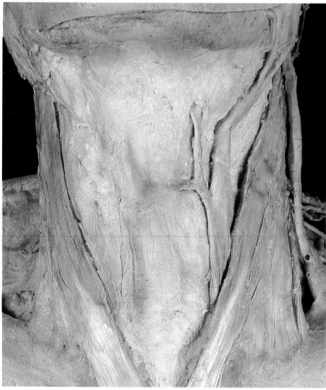

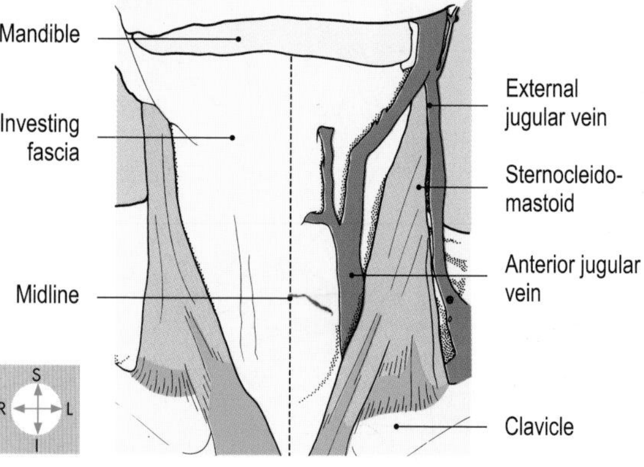

Fig. 7.10 Boundaries and roofs of both anterior triangles of the neck. The midline is the division between the two triangles.

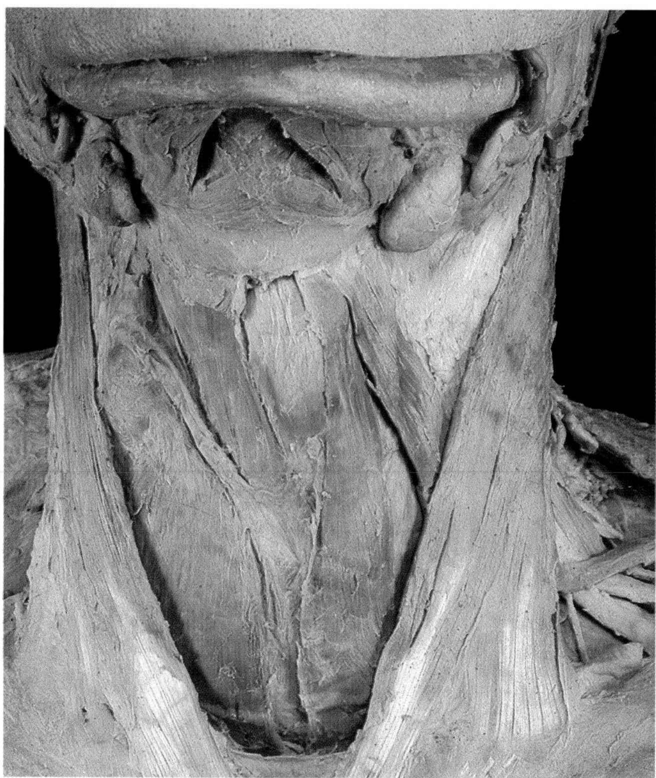

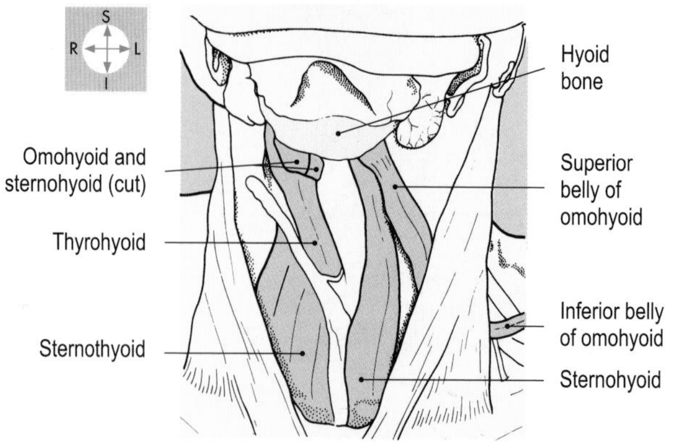

Fig. 7.11 Contents of the anterior triangle. The right omohyoid and sternohyoid muscles have been removed to show the deeper thyrohyoid and sternothyroid muscles.

Ansa cervicalis

Under cover of sternocleidomastoid two nerves, the roots of the ansa, unite to form a loop, the ansa cervicalis (Fig. 7.12), which provides the motor supply to the strap muscles. The superior root (descending limb) from the hypoglossal nerve consists solely of C1 fibres and descends to join the inferior root, C2 and C3 fibres from the cervical plexus, to form the ansa.

Thyroid gland

The thyroid gland (Fig. 7.13) is a vascular endocrine gland enclosed by the pretracheal fascia and closely applied to the anterior and lateral surfaces of the trachea. The fascia links the gland to the larynx so that during swallowing both structures are elevated simultaneously. The two lateral lobes of the gland are joined across the midline by a narrow isthmus at the level of the third tracheal ring. A single pyramidal lobe is often present and projects upwards from the isthmus. Each lateral lobe is pear-shaped with its superior extremity reaching the oblique line on the thyroid cartilage whilst its lower pole lies at the level of the fifth tracheal ring.

Lying anterior to the isthmus of the gland are the sternothyroid muscles and the anterior jugular veins. The lateral lobes are covered anterolaterally by the other infrahyoid muscles and the anterior borders of the sternocleidomastoid muscles. Posterolaterally lie the carotid sheaths whilst posteromedially are the trachea, larynx and oesophagus. In the interval between the oesophagus and trachea the recurrent laryngeal nerves course upwards towards the larynx where they are vulnerable during thyroid or parathyroid surgery. A superior and an inferior parathyroid gland are embedded in the posterior surface of each lateral lobe.

The thyroid gland is a highly vascular organ and is supplied on each side by superior and inferior thyroid arteries. The superior thyroid artery, from the external carotid artery, descends to the upper pole of the gland. The inferior thyroid artery, from the thyrocervical trunk of the subclavian artery, ascends to enter the posterolateral aspect of the gland from behind the carotid sheath. A venous plexus on the surface of the gland drains via superior and middle thyroid veins into the internal jugular veins and via inferior thyroid veins to the left brachiocephalic vein. Lymph drains from the gland into the jugular chain of nodes.

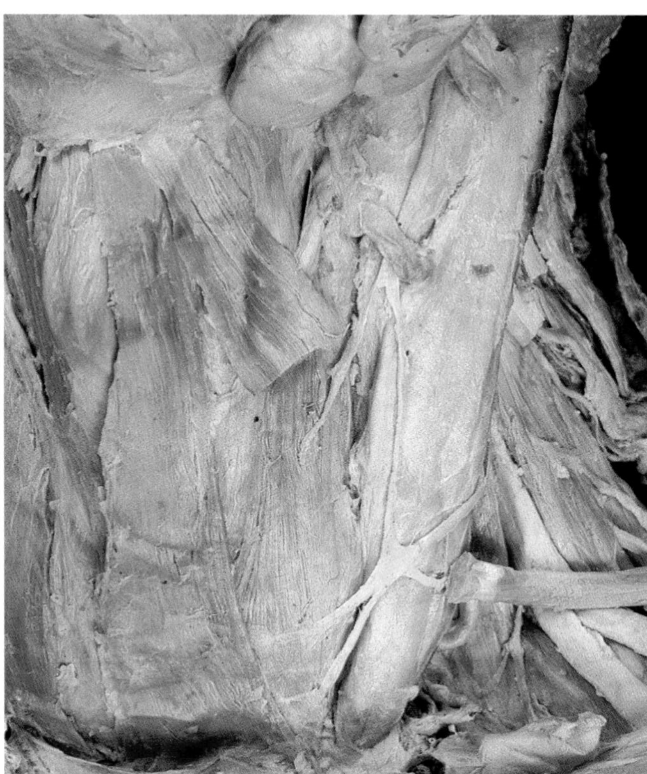

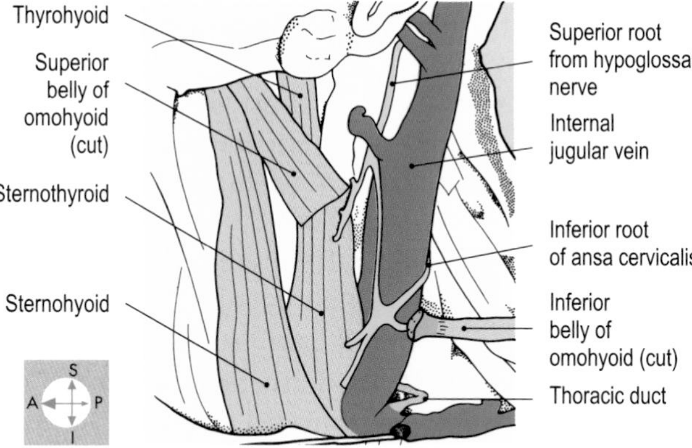

Fig. 7.12 Ansa cervicalis, lying on the internal jugular vein, and its branches to the strap muscles.

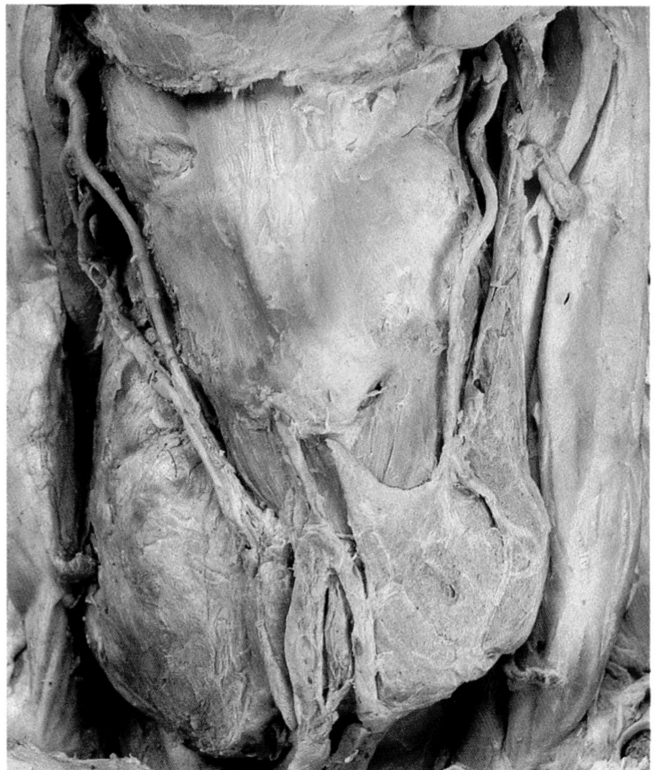

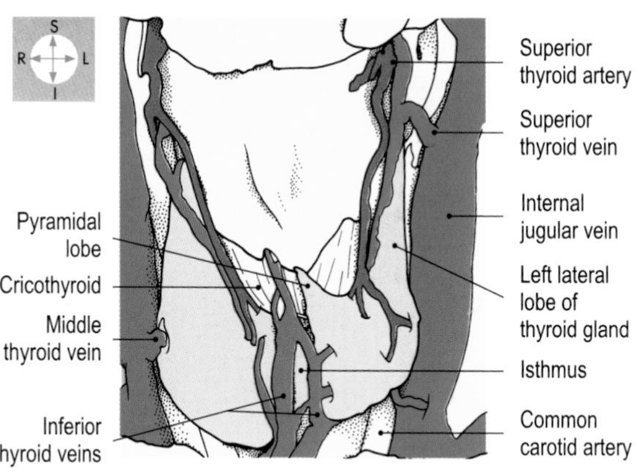

Fig. 7.13 Thyroid gland and its immediate blood supply, revealed by removal of the pretracheal fascia.

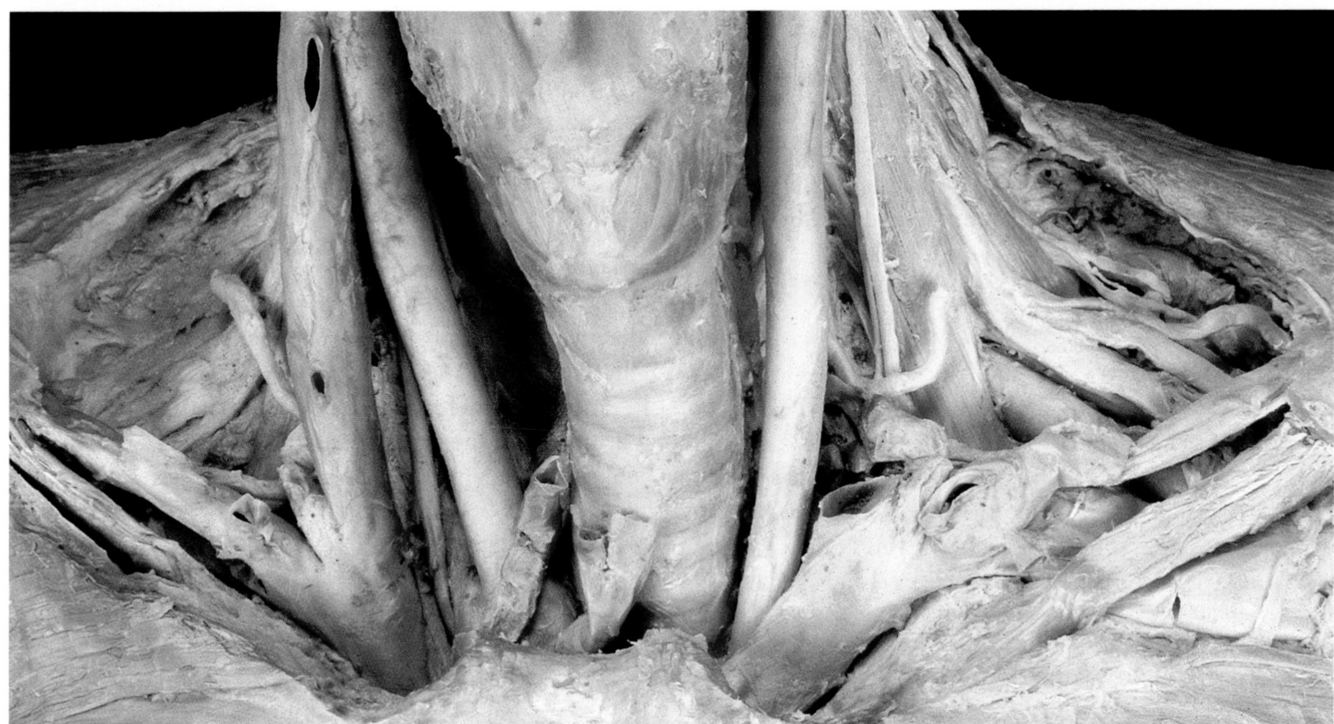

Root of neck

The root of the neck is the region immediately above the superior thoracic aperture (see p. 320). In the midline are the trachea and oesophagus, descending into the superior mediastinum (Fig. 7.14) between the apices of the lungs which are covered with pleura and suprapleural membrane (Fig. 7.15). The other major structures in the root of the neck are vessels and nerves, which will be described in relation to scalenus anterior and its attachment to the scalene tubercle of the first rib (see p. 28).

Veins

Each subclavian vein (Fig. 7.14) begins at the outer border of the first rib as the continuation of the axillary vein (see p. 80). The vessel passes over the rib in front of the attachment of scalenus anterior and receives the external jugular vein from above. The subclavian and internal jugular veins unite at the medial border of scalenus anterior to form the brachiocephalic vein, which enters the thorax anteriorly alongside the trachea. On each side of the neck a major lymphatic trunk terminates by drainage into the angle where the subclavian and internal jugular veins unite. On the left, this lymphatic vessel is the thoracic duct, which arches laterally over the apex of the lung from its position alongside the oesophagus. The duct passes between the carotid sheath and the vertebral vessels, crossing in front of the phrenic nerve and the subclavian artery. The thoracic duct is the ultimate drainage channel for lymph from the lower limbs, pelvis, abdomen, left upper limb and the left side of the thorax, head and neck. On the right side of the neck the smaller right lymphatic trunk terminates similarly, draining lymph only from the right upper limb and the right side of the thorax, head and neck. Canulating the thoracic duct allows collection of lymphocytes for immunological investigation and treatment.

Arteries

The left common carotid and left subclavian arteries emerge from the thorax on the left of the trachea and oesophagus (Fig. 7.14).

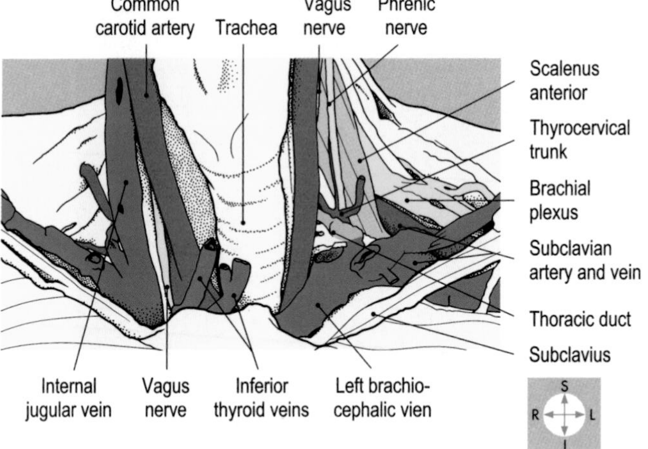

Fig. 7.14 Root of the neck after removal of the clavicles, pretracheal fascia, thyroid gland, carotid sheaths and left internal jugular vein.

On the right, the brachiocephalic trunk divides at the level of the superior thoracic aperture to form the right common carotid and right subclavian arteries (Fig. 7.14). Each common carotid artery ascends into the neck within its sheath and gives no branches before its termination. Each subclavian artery passes laterally over the upper surface of the first rib posterior to scalenus anterior and continues into the axilla as the axillary artery (see p. 79).

Three branches of the subclavian artery, internal thoracic, thyrocervical and vertebral arteries (Figs 7.14 & 7.15), arise medial to scalenus anterior. The internal thoracic artery (see p. 34) descends into the thorax to supply the anterior thoracic and abdominal walls. The thyrocervical trunk is short and divides into three branches, the inferior thyroid (see p. 327), suprascapular and transverse cervical arteries. The latter two vessels cross the posterior triangle of the neck. The suprascapular artery supplies the scapula and related structures and the transverse cervical artery supplies superficial structures in the posterior part of the neck. The vertebral artery (Fig. 7.15) inclines upwards and backwards medial to scalenus anterior and crosses in front of the transverse process of the seventh cervical vertebral, before continuing superiorly through the foramina

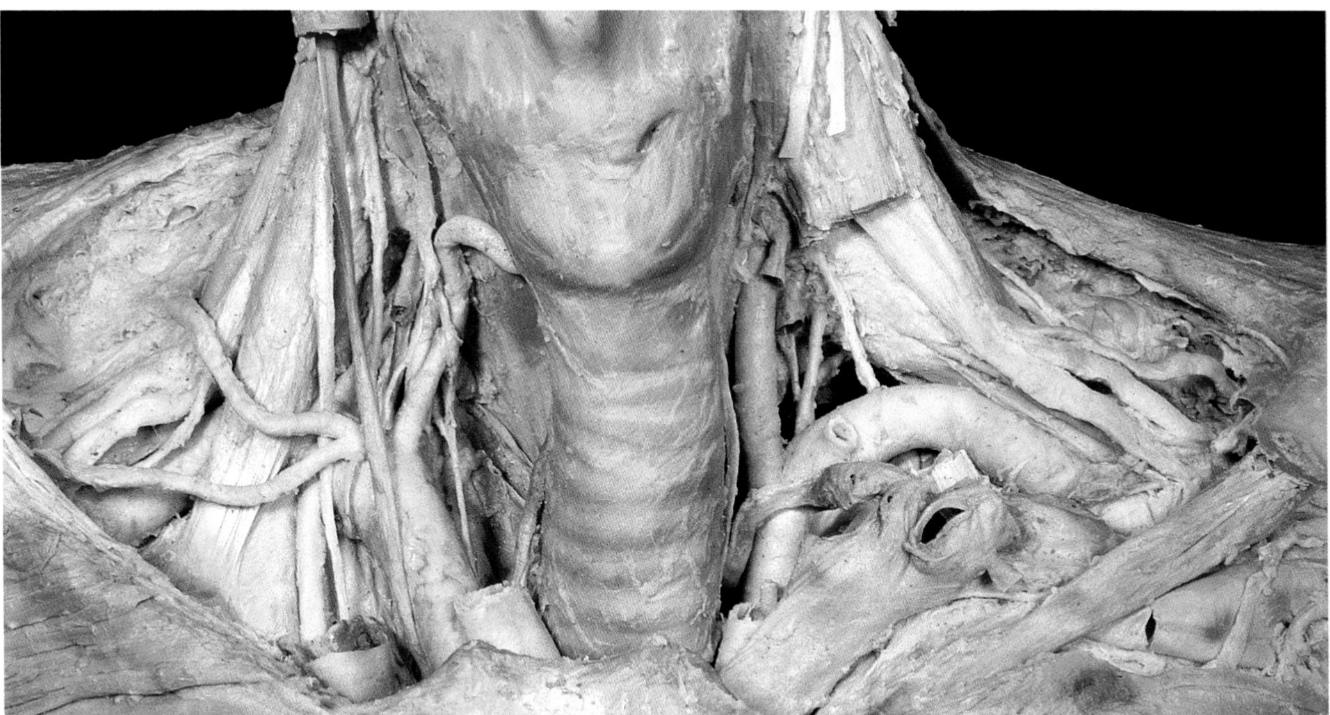

transversaria of the upper six cervical vertebrae, to enter the skull through the foramen magnum (see p. 373).

The costocervical trunk (Fig. 7.15) arises from the subclavian artery behind scalenus anterior and arches backwards over the suprapleural membrane as far as the neck of the first rib, where it divides to form the superior intercostal artery supplying the upper two intercostal spaces (see p. 35) and the deep cervical artery, which supplies the muscles of the back of the neck.

Nerves

The vagus (X) and phrenic nerves, both sympathetic chains and parts of both brachial plexuses all traverse the root of the neck. Each vagus nerve (Fig. 7.14) descends within the carotid sheath and enters the superior mediastinum between the main arterial and venous structures medial to the phrenic nerve. On the right side of the neck the recurrent laryngeal nerve arises from the vagus, hooking under the subclavian artery to ascend in the groove formed by the lateral surfaces of the trachea and oesophagus. On the left, the recurrent laryngeal nerve follows a similar course but arises from the vagus in the thorax (see p. 61).

The phrenic nerve (Fig. 7.15), formed from the anterior rami of the third, fourth and fifth cervical spinal nerves, passes inferiorly on the anterior surface of scalenus anterior beneath the prevertebral fascia. It leaves the medial side of the muscle near its lower end and enters the thorax between the main arterial and venous structures lateral to the vagus nerve.

The sympathetic trunks (Fig. 7.15), covered by the prevertebral fascia, lie alongside the bodies of the cervical vertebrae. In the neck each trunk bears only three sympathetic ganglia, the superior, middle and inferior. The lowest ganglion fuses frequently with the first thoracic ganglion to form the stellate (cervico-thoracic) ganglion. The trunk continues into the thorax in front of the neck of the first rib. The middle and inferior cervical sympathetic ganglia are often linked by a nerve, the ansa subclavia, which curves around the subclavian artery.

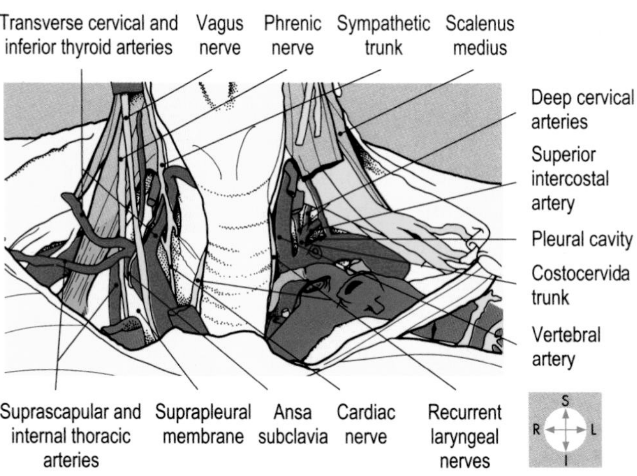

Fig. 7.15 Deeper structures of the root of neck, revealed by removal of most of the left vagus and phrenic nerves, the left scalenus anterior, both common carotid arteries and the large veins.

The brachial plexus (Fig. 7.14) originates from the anterior rami of the lowest four cervical and first thoracic spinal nerves which, partly covered by scalenus anterior, constitute the roots of the plexus. They combine to form the trunks of the plexus, which emerge from behind the lateral border of the muscle. The plexus continues into the upper limb enclosed with the axillary artery in a prolongation of the prevertebral fascia called the axillary sheath. (A detailed account of the brachial plexus is given on page 80.)

Scalene muscles

Scalenus anterior (Fig. 7.15) is attached superiorly to the transverse processes of the third, fourth, fifth and sixth cervical vertebrae. Inferiorly it attaches to the scalene tubercle on the first rib (see p. 28). Behind it lie scalenus medius (Fig. 7.15) and scalenus posterior, which arise from the transverse processes of the lower six cervical vertebrae and attach inferiorly to the upper surfaces of the first and second ribs respectively. These muscles are supplied segmentally by cervical spinal nerves. They elevate the first and second ribs and laterally flex the neck.

Contents of Carotid Sheath

The carotid sheaths form part of the fascial layers of the neck (see pp 322 & 323) and extend from the base of the skull into the superior mediastinum. Each sheath contains the common, the internal and part of the external carotid arteries, the internal jugular vein and parts of the glossopharyngeal (IX), vagus (X) and accessory (XI) nerves.

Carotid arteries

The common carotid artery arises on the left from the aortic arch and on the right from the brachiocephalic artery, then ascends within its sheath into the neck. At the upper border of the thyroid cartilage it divides into internal and external carotid arteries (Fig. 7.17). At its origin the internal carotid artery is dilated to form the carotid sinus. The vessel ascends within the carotid sheath without branching and, in company with its sympathetic nerve plexus, enters the carotid canal. In the cranial cavity the internal carotid artery terminates as the anterior and middle cerebral arteries (see p. 374), having given rise to the ophthalmic artery, which supplies the contents of the orbit.

The external carotid artery leaves the carotid sheath, inclines superolaterally and enters the deepest part of the parotid gland, where it divides into terminal branches at the level of the neck of the mandible. Separating the external and internal carotid arteries are the styloid process, stylopharyngeus, the glossopharyngeal (IX) nerve and the pharyngeal branch of the vagus (X) nerve.

The external carotid artery usually has eight branches (Fig. 7.17), supplying much of the extracranial portion of the head and upper part of the neck. The ascending pharyngeal artery arises on the medial aspect of the external carotid artery and ascends on the lateral surface of the pharynx. The next branch, the superior thyroid artery, inclines downwards and forwards from the anterior surface of the external carotid to supply the thyroid gland and the larynx. The lingual artery passes forwards from the anterior surface of the external carotid artery into the base of the tongue (see p. 349). The facial artery, another anterior branch, supplies the tonsil and descends under the body of the

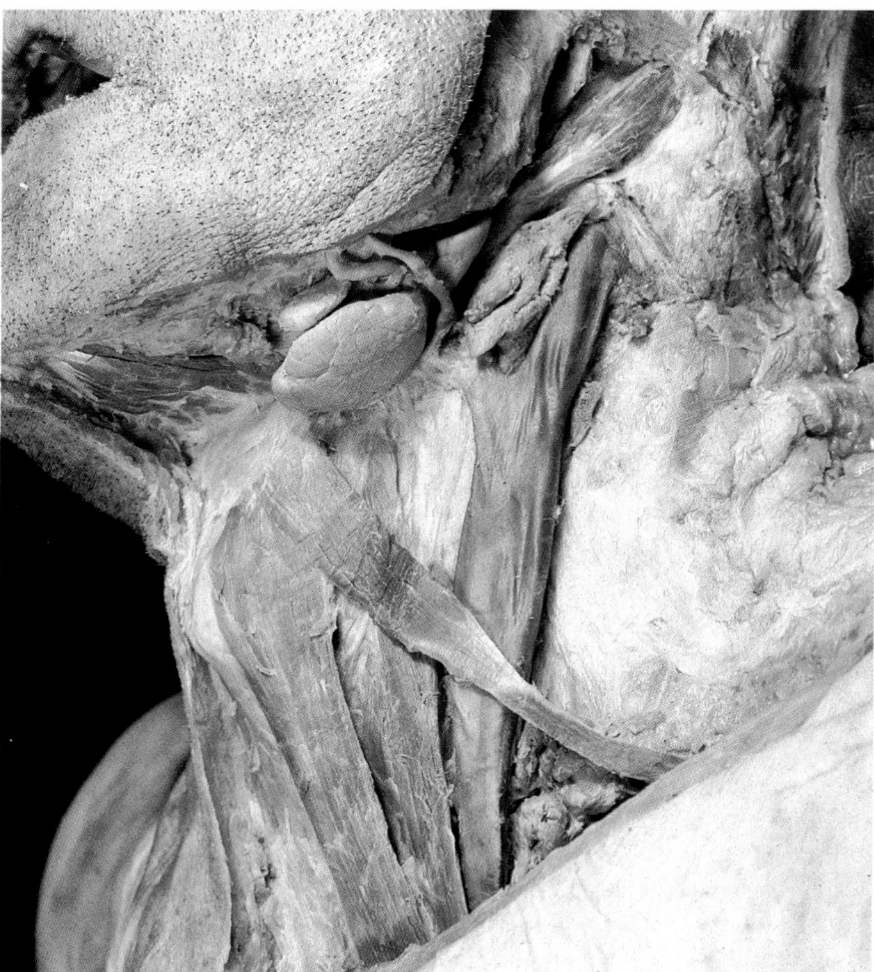

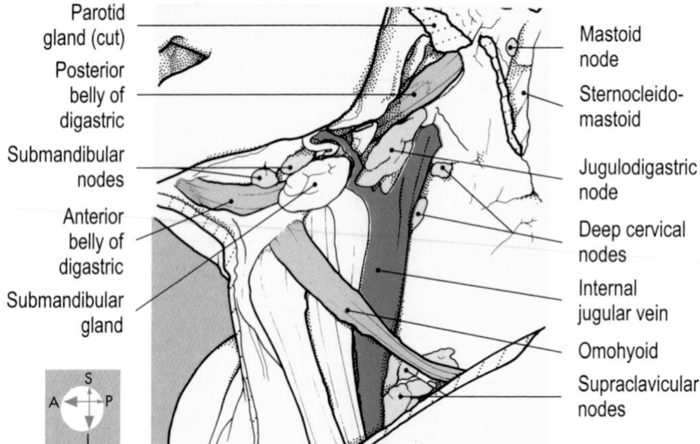

Fig. 7.16 Internal jugular vein and some cervical lymph nodes, revealed after removal of sternocleidomastoid and part of the parotid gland.

mandible, grooving the submandibular gland and emerging from beneath the mandible at the anterior border of masseter to supply the face (see Fig. 7.35).

Arising from the posterior surface of the external carotid artery, the occipital artery passes upwards and backwards deep to sternocleidomastoid (Fig. 7.17; see Fig. 7.24). The vessel crosses the apex of the posterior triangle of the neck to supply the posterior part of the scalp. The posterior auricular artery arises below the pinna and passes upwards and backwards to supply the pinna and the scalp.

The terminal branches of the external carotid artery, the superficial temporal and maxillary arteries, arise within the parotid gland. The former supplies the lateral part of the scalp while the maxillary artery supplies the infratemporal fossa, pterygopalatine fossa and lateral wall of the nose. Postganglionic sympathetic nerve fibres accompany the external carotid artery and its branches.

Internal jugular vein

The internal jugular vein (Figs 7.16 & 7.17) is formed within the jugular foramen by the union of the sigmoid and inferior petrosal dural venous sinuses. The vein descends through the neck within the carotid sheath and receives the facial, lingual, pharyngeal, and superior and middle thyroid veins. The internal jugular vein also communicates with the external jugular system via the anterior branch of the retromandibular vein. It terminates by uniting with the subclavian vein to form the brachiocephalic vein.

Nerves

Within the carotid sheath lie the glossopharyngeal (IX), vagus (X) and accessory (XI) nerves, which leave the skull via the jugular foramen. The glossopharyngeal nerve passes inferiorly, leaves the sheath and winds around the posterolateral surface of stylopharyngeus to enter the posterior third of the tongue. The nerve supplies stylopharyngeus and gives a sensory branch which innervates the carotid sinus (see p. 350).

The vagus (X) nerve (Fig. 7.17) bears two sensory ganglia, one in the jugular foramen and one below the base of the skull, between which the nerve receives the cranial part of

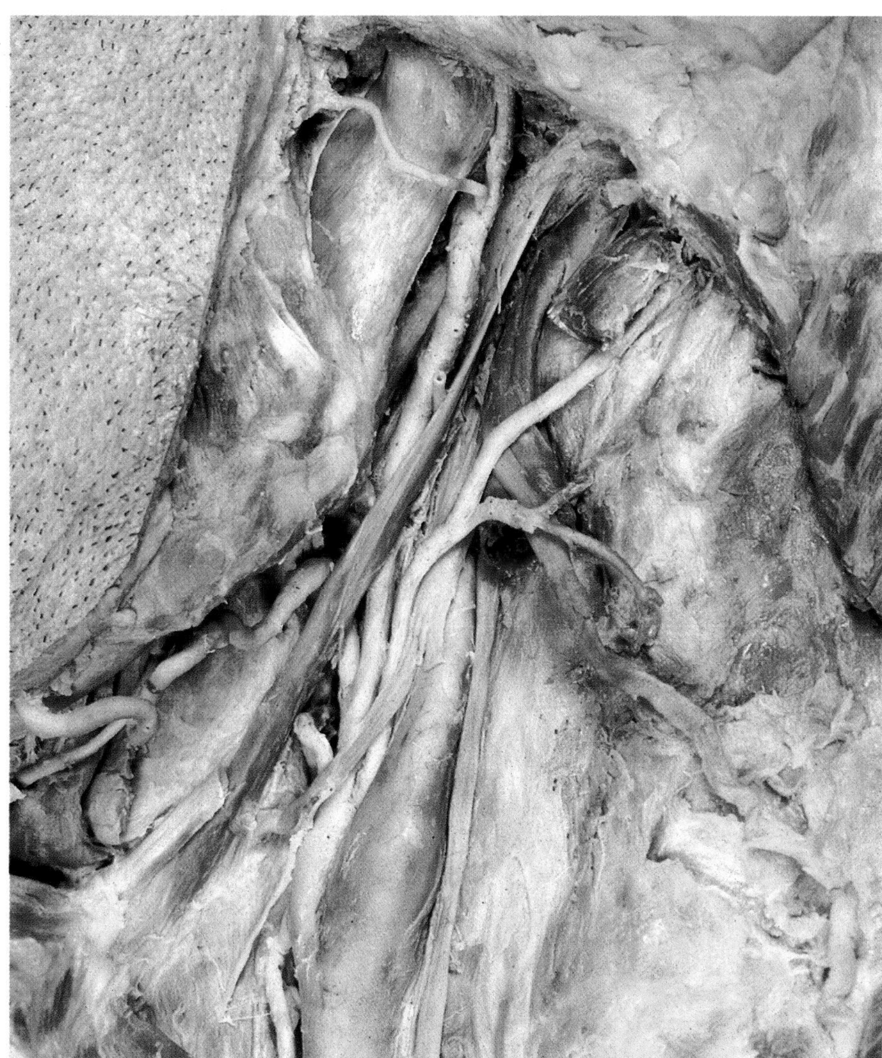

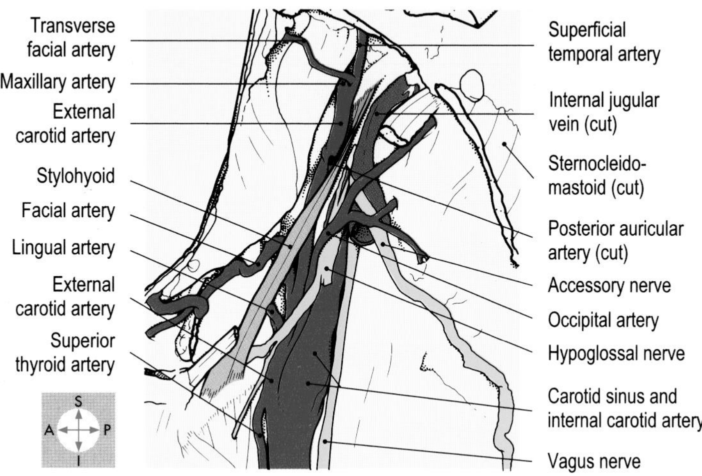

Fig. 7.17 Branches of the external carotid artery and the vagus, accessory and hypoglossal nerves, after removal of part of the internal jugular vein, carotid sheath and posterior belly of digastric.

the accessory nerve. The vagus nerve descends in the posterior part of the carotid sheath between the carotid artery and internal jugular vein and gives rise to pharyngeal, superior laryngeal and cardiac branches before traversing the superior thoracic aperture. The pharyngeal branch passes forwards between the internal and external carotid arteries to the outer surface of the pharynx, contributing to the pharyngeal plexus. The superior laryngeal nerve accompanies the superior thyroid artery and vein supplying the larynx. The cardiac branches of the vagus join those from the sympathetic trunk and descend into the thorax. The right vagus gives a recurrent laryngeal branch in the neck which curves around the right subclavian artery and passes superiorly to reach the larynx (see p. 329). The left recurrent laryngeal nerve arises from the left vagus nerve in the thorax and passes around the aortic arch before ascending into the neck.

The accessory (XI) nerve (see Fig. 7.17) is formed by the fusion of cranial and spinal roots in the posterior cranial fossa. In the jugular foramen the nerve divides into a cranial part joining the vagus nerve and a spinal part which supplies sternocleidomastoid and trapezius.

Lymphatics

Lymphatic vessels from structures in the head and neck accompany the vascular supply and drain into superficial or deep groups of lymph nodes.

Superficial lymph nodes

Several groups of superficial nodes form an incomplete ring around the lower part of the head. The submental nodes lie between the anterior bellies of the two digastric muscles, draining lymph from the tip of the tongue and the mental region. The submandibular group (see Fig. 7.16) lies on the superficial surface of the submandibular gland and receives lymph from the submental nodes, from the remainder of the anterior two-thirds of the tongue, from the floor of the mouth (including the gums and teeth), and from the nose, face and anterior part of the scalp. The parotid nodes lie on or within the parotid gland, the mastoid group (see Fig. 7.16) on the lateral surface of the mastoid process, and the occipital lymph nodes at the apex of the posterior triangle of the neck. These three groups drain the remainder of the face and scalp, including the external ear. Lymph from all the superficial nodes drains into the deep cervical nodes.

Deep cervical lymph nodes

The deep cervical or jugular lymph nodes (see Fig. 7.16) form a chain in and around the carotid sheath. Two of the deep cervical nodes are of particular clinical significance. The jugulodigastric node receives lymph mainly from the tongue and tonsil and the jugulo-omohyoid node drains the tongue. From the deep cervical nodes lymph drains inferiorly, via the jugular lymphatic trunk, usually into the thoracic duct on the left and into the right lymphatic duct on the right.

Superficial Structures of Face and Scalp

The subcutaneous tissue of the face and scalp is highly vascular and is traversed by several nerves. Most of the nerves are sensory to skin and include branches of the trigeminal (V) and upper cervical spinal nerves. In addition, there are branches that are motor from the facial (VII) nerve to a group of muscles in the subcutaneous tissues of the face, scalp and front of the neck, known as the muscles of facial expression.

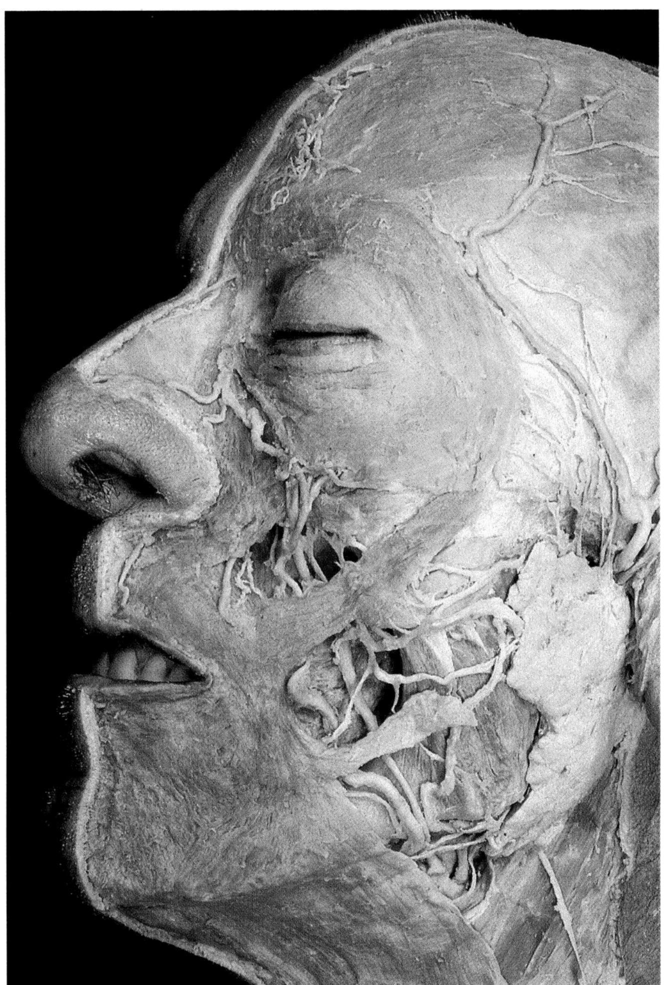

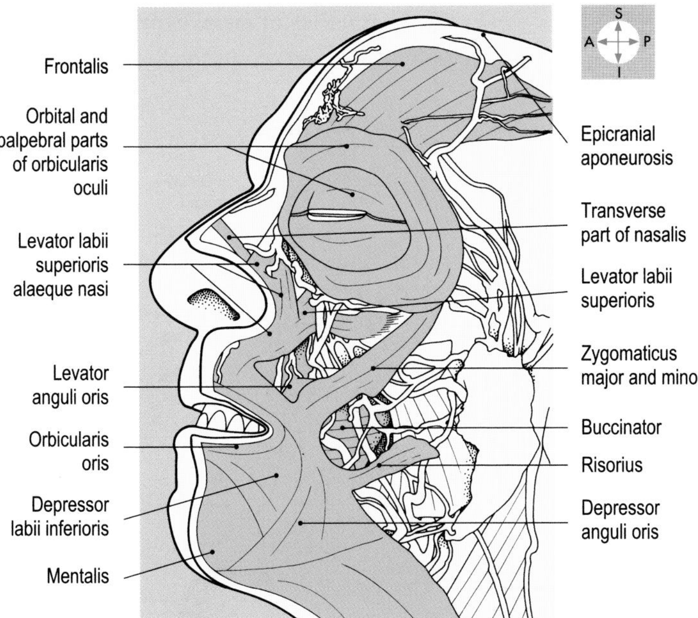

Fig. 7.18 Muscles of facial expression. The skin and subcutaneous fat have been removed.

Muscles of facial expression

In general, these muscles are arranged as sphincters or dilators around the orifices of the face (Fig. 7.18). Most are anchored to bone at one end and attached to skin at the other.

Palpebral fissure

The sphincter of the palpebral fissure (the gap between the eyelids) is orbicularis oculi, which is divided into inner palpebral and outer orbital parts. The palpebral part lies within the eyelids and is attached to the medial and lateral palpebral ligaments. The orbital portion is attached only to the medial palpebral ligament, and its fibres lie around the orbital margin. Both parts close the palpebral fissure, the palpebral part gently and the orbital part forcefully as when 'screwing up the eyes'. The palpebral part also helps sweep tears medially across the cornea from lacrimal gland to lacrimal canaliculi. The dilator components are provided by levator palpebrae superioris within the orbit (see p. 377), and by occipitofrontalis in the scalp. The latter muscle has two bellies, occipital and frontal, linked by an extensive intermediate tendon, the epicranial aponeurosis which forms a mobile layer over the vault of the skull. From its posterior extremity the occipital belly (occipitalis) descends to its attachment on the highest nuchal line of the occipital bone (Fig. 7.19); from its anterior end the frontal belly (frontalis) descends in the forehead and its fibres interdigitate with those of orbicularis oculi and attach to skin near the

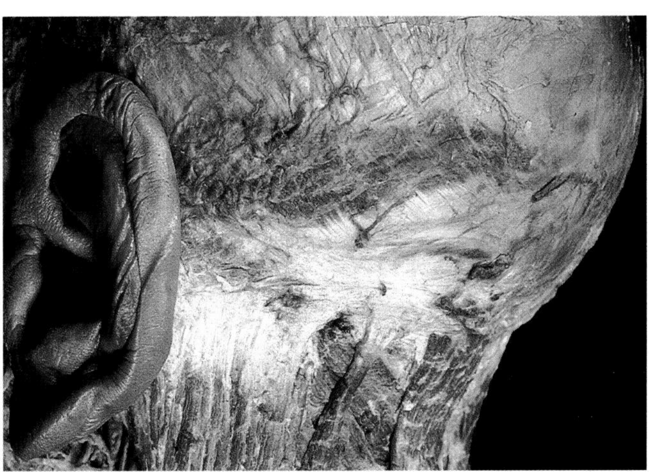

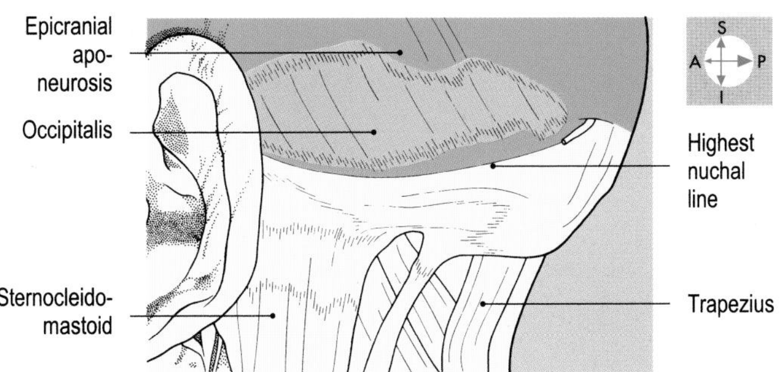

Fig. 7.19 Posterior view to show occipitalis and part of the epicranial aponeurosis.

eyebrow. Occipitalis fixes the epicranial aponeurosis allowing frontalis to raise the eyebrows.

Nostril

Around each nostril is nasalis with two feeble parts, alar and transverse, which dilate and compress the nostrils respectively.

Mouth

Orbicularis oris, the sphincter of the mouth, is embedded in the lips and attaches near the midline to the mandible and maxilla. In addition there are dilators around the mouth whose fibres continue into orbicularis oris. The most medial dilator of the upper lip is levator labii superioris alaeque nasi. This muscle attaches near the medial margin of the orbit and runs to the alar cartilage of the nose and to the upper lip. Levator labii superioris is attached to bone beneath the orbital margin, whereas levator anguli oris lies slightly deeper and its fibres incline towards the angle of the mouth. Two of the dilator muscles take attachment from the zygoma: zygomaticus major and minor. Attached to the mandible are three muscles, called, from lateral to medial, depressor anguli oris, depressor labii inferioris and mentalis.

The buccinator muscle (Figs 7.18 & 7.20) lies deep to the other dilator muscles in the wall of the cheek. Anteriorly it blends with the deep surface of orbicularis oris. Posteriorly it gains attachment to the outer surface of the mandible from the level of the first to the third molar teeth. Passing behind the third molar tooth, buccinator is attached to the pterygomandibular raphe and the pterygoid hamulus. The muscle attachment continues forwards along the outer surface of the maxilla as far as the first upper molar tooth. Buccinator controls the size of the vestibule of the mouth (that part of the buccal cavity lying between the cheek and the teeth).

The platysma (Fig. 7.21), the most extensive muscle of facial expression, descends in the subcutaneous tissue of the neck from the inferior border of the mandible and fades out on the anterior surface of the thorax. A few fibres may run horizontally from the angle of the mouth as risorius. Platysma is most easily seen in action during respiratory distress when the skin of the neck is pulled taut.

Ear

In the human the auricular muscles are almost vestigial.

Facial nerve

All the muscles of facial expression derive their motor nerve supply from the facial

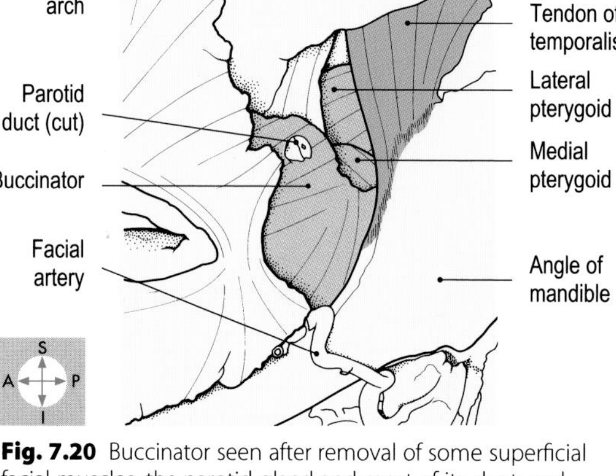

Fig. 7.20 Buccinator seen after removal of some superficial facial muscles, the parotid gland and most of its duct, and masseter.

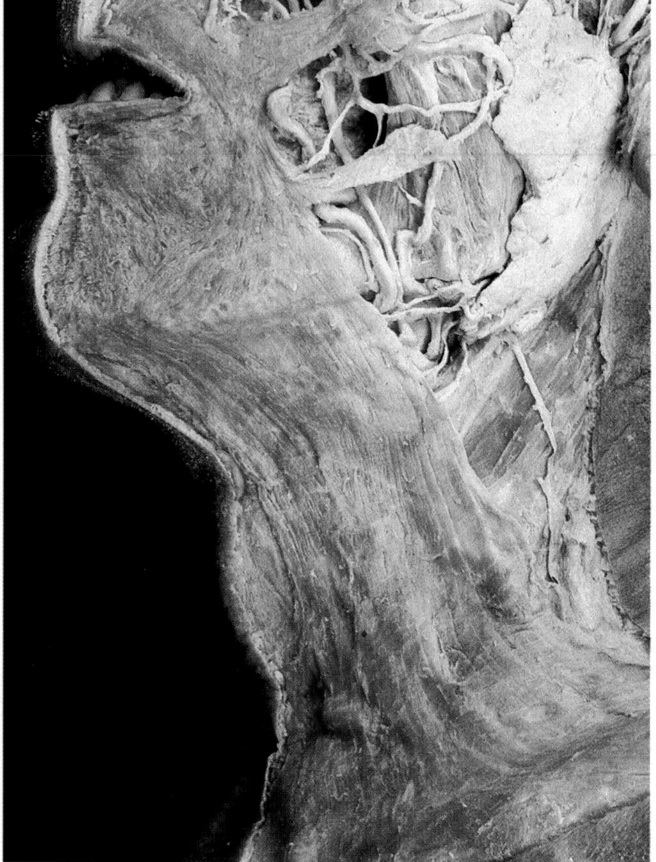

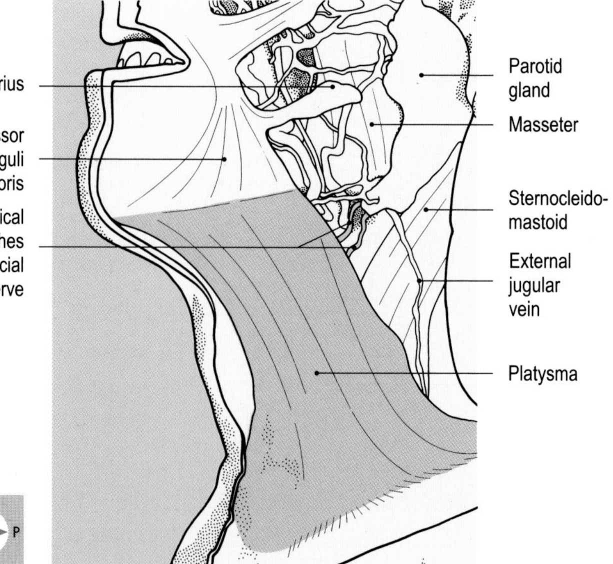

Fig. 7.21 Platysma, the largest muscle of facial expression, and its nerve supply.

(VII) nerve. Occipitalis and some of the auricular muscles are innervated by the posterior auricular branch of the nerve (see p. 338); the remaining muscles are supplied by the five sets of branches (Fig. 7.22) that emerge from the anterior border of the parotid gland (see p. 337). The temporal branch of the facial nerve ascends to supply the remaining auricular muscles and frontalis. The zygomatic branch is directed towards the eye and supplies muscles above and below the palpebral fissure. The third branch, the buccal, runs horizontally forwards to innervate buccinator and the muscles of the upper lip. The mandibular branch supplies the muscles of the lower lip, dipping below the mandible in its course. The cervical branch descends to supply platysma.

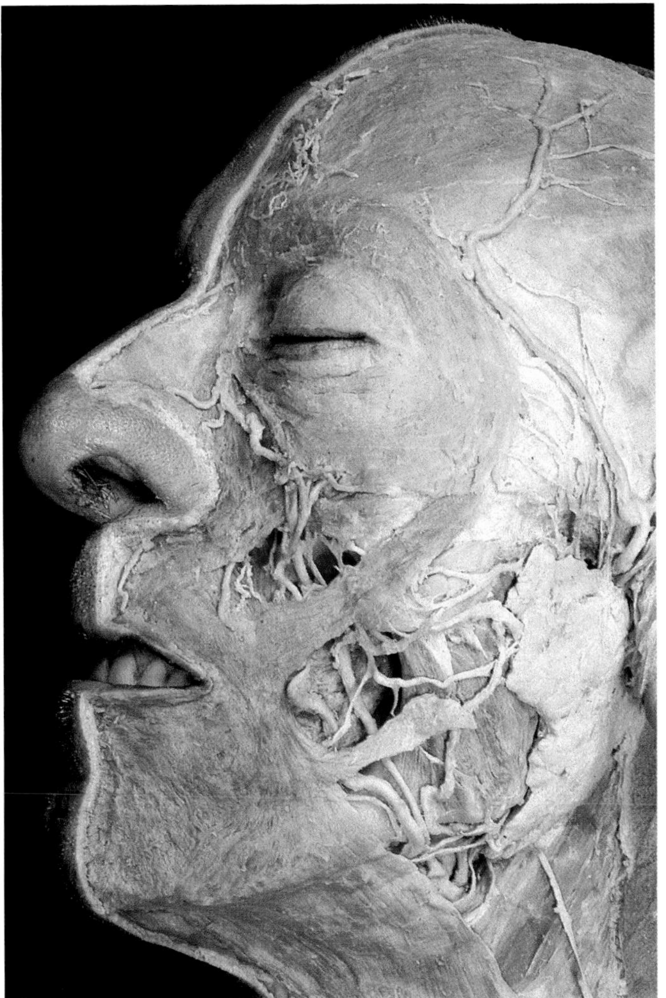

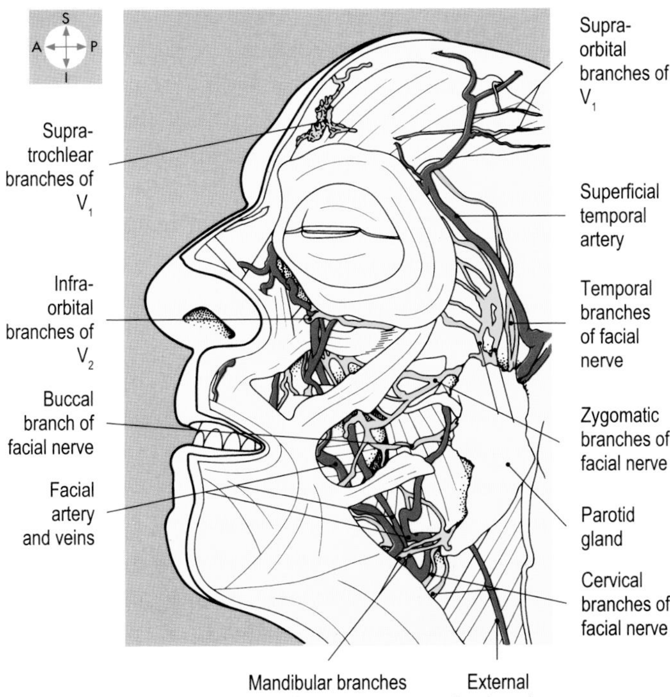

Fig. 7.22 Neurovascular structures of the face. In this specimen the facial vein is duplicated, a common variation.

Blood supply of face

Most of the superficial structures of the face obtain their blood supply from the facial artery (Fig. 7.22), a branch of the external carotid artery. The facial artery enters the face by hooking under the inferior border of the mandible where it is easily palpated. The vessel then pursues a tortuous course across the face towards the inner angle of the orbit. The area of the face in front of the ear is supplied by the transverse facial artery, an anterior branch of the superficial temporal artery. Emerging from the orbit to supply the forehead are the supraorbital and supratrochlear branches of the ophthalmic artery.

Blood from the face drains into the facial vein (Fig. 7.22), which accompanies the facial artery. The vein also receives the supratrochlear and supraorbital veins and thus communicates with ophthalmic veins in the orbit. Blood from the lateral part of the face drains into the superficial temporal vein.

Sensory supply

The sensory nerve supply of the face is conveyed in branches of the three divisions of the trigeminal (V) nerve (Fig. 7.23).

Scalp

The scalp (see Fig. 7.24) extends from the superior nuchal line posteriorly to the superior orbital margin anteriorly, and to the

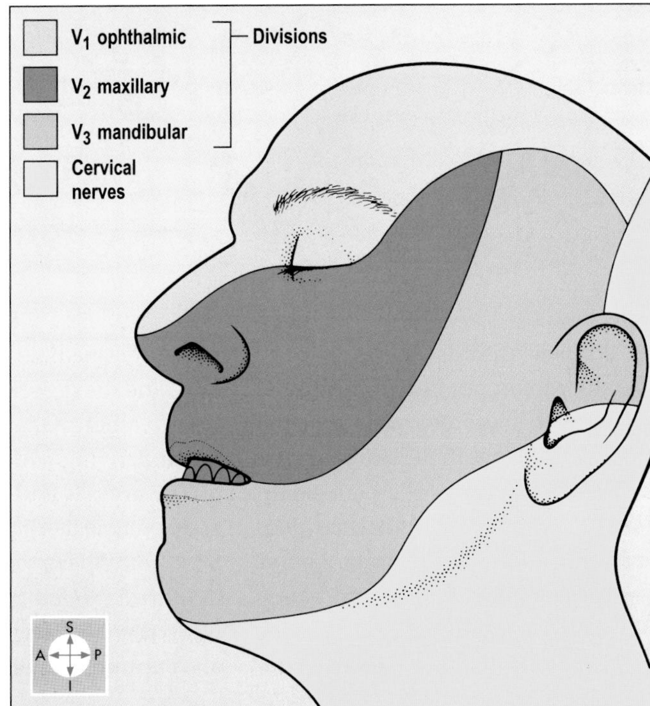

Fig. 7.23 Dermatomes of the face. Areas of the face are supplied with sensory fibres from the different divisions of the trigeminal nerve.

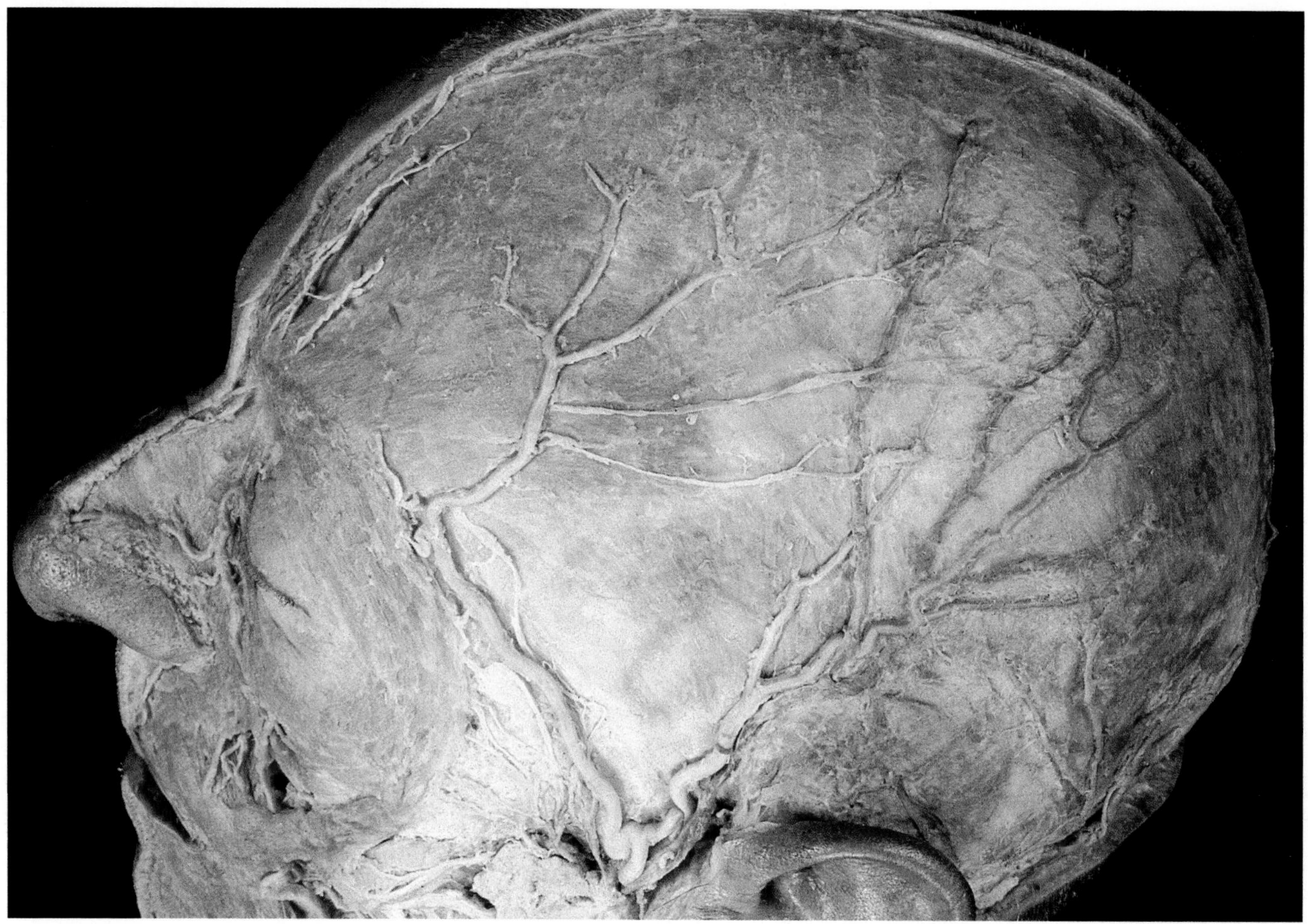

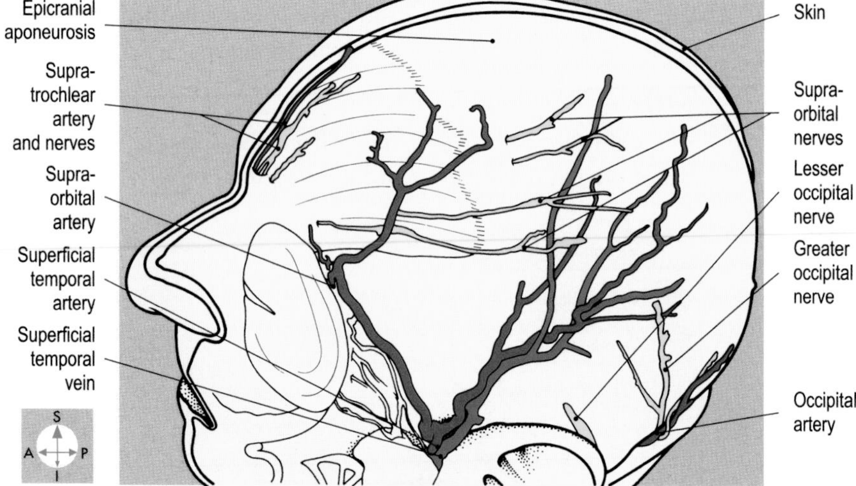

Fig. 7.24 Vessels and nerves of the scalp lying on the epicranial aponeurosis.

external acoustic meatus and zygomatic arch laterally. It comprises two functional layers applied to the outer surface of the vault of the skull. Close to the bones lies the pericranium, which forms the periosteum of the skull. This is loosely attached over each constituent bone but is firmly bound to the sutures so that subperiosteal bleeding is limited to the area of the bones involved. Superficial to the pericranium, but separated from it by a layer of loose connective tissue, lie the epicranial aponeurosis (intermediate tendon of occipitofrontalis) and the skin of the scalp, firmly bound to each other so that they move as one over the underlying pericranium and skull.

The arteries and nerves that supply the scalp enter at its circumference and because they accompany each other they will be described together, starting anteriorly. Near the midline are the supratrochlear and supraorbital nerves, arteries and veins. The nerves are derived from the ophthalmic division of the trigeminal (V) nerve. The vessels communicate with their ophthalmic counterparts within the orbit.

Lateral to the orbit the zygomaticotemporal nerve from the maxillary division of the trigeminal nerve, accompanied by its vessels, ascends a short distance into the scalp. Just in front of the ear the auriculotemporal nerve from the mandibular division of the fifth cranial nerve passes into the scalp. The superficial temporal artery and vein follow a similar course.

The area of the scalp behind the ear is supplied by the lesser occipital nerve (C2 anterior ramus) accompanied by the posterior auricular artery and vein. Posteriorly near the midline the scalp receives the greater occipital nerve (C2 posterior ramus) and the occipital artery and vein.

In addition, venous blood may drain via the diploic veins of the skull into the intracranial venous sinuses. Scalp wounds bleed profusely, making suturing difficult. To diminish bleeding circumferential pressure may be temporarily applied with an elastic bandage.

Parotid Gland

The parotid is the largest of the salivary glands and is pyramidal in shape (Fig. 7.25). Its base faces laterally between the anterior border of sternocleidomastoid and the ramus of the mandible, while its apex lies deeply against the styloid process. The gland extends upwards between the external acoustic meatus and the temporomandibular joint, movements of which may be painful when the parotid is inflamed.

The parotid gland is deeply indented in front by the mandible, masseter and medial pterygoid. Deep to the gland are the infratemporal fossa and the styloid apparatus, the latter separating it from the carotid sheath and the pharyngeal wall.

The investing fascia of the neck splits into two layers to enclose the gland (see p. 322). The superficial layer attaches above to the zygomatic arch whilst anteriorly it merges with the tissues of the cheek. The deep layer is attached to the tympanic part of the temporal bone and is thickened between the styloid process and the angle of the mandible to form the stylomandibular ligament. Swelling in the parotid is particularly painful because of the toughness of the surrounding fascia and its position between the mandible in front and the temporal bone behind.

The parotid duct (Fig. 7.26) passes forwards across the surface of masseter, turns medially and pierces buccinator to open obliquely into the vestibule of the mouth opposite the upper

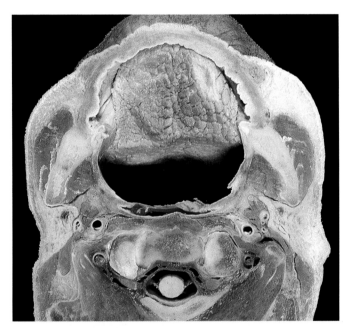

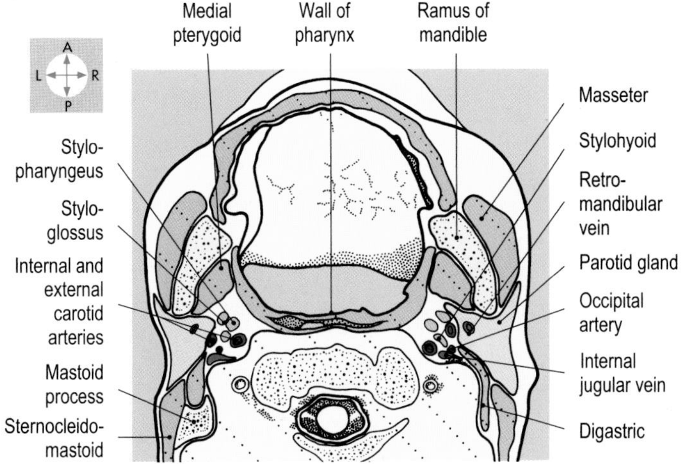

Fig. 7.25 Transverse section of the head through the parotid glands. Superior aspect. Compare Fig. 7.93.

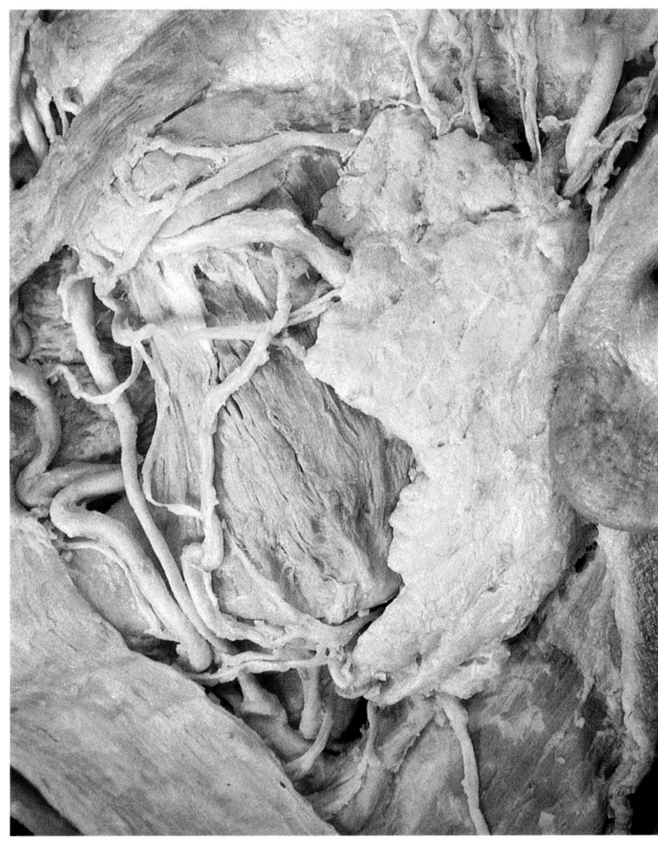

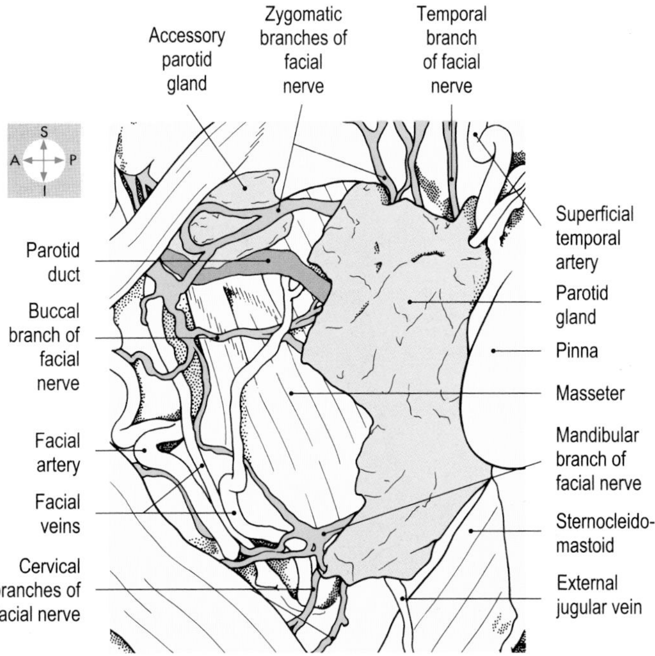

Fig. 7.26 Parotid gland and branches of the facial nerve, exposed by the removal of the superficial layer of parotid fascia.

second molar tooth. This oblique passage through the mucosa compresses the duct when intraoral pressure is raised. When masseter contracts, the duct may be palpated over the anterior edge of the muscle. An accessory part of the gland may lie alongside the duct.

Structures traversing parotid gland

Of these, the most superficial are branches of the facial (VII) nerve that run forwards to the face and pass superficial to the retromandibular vein and its tributaries. The deepest is the termination of the external carotid artery.

Facial (VII) nerve

The facial nerve emerges from the skull through the stylomastoid foramen and turns forwards to enter the posterior surface of the parotid gland. Before penetrating the gland it gives two branches. The posterior auricular branch passes behind the external acoustic meatus to supply occipitalis and the auricular muscles. The other supplies the posterior belly of digastric and stylohyoid. Within the gland the facial nerve forms a plexus from which five groups of branches (see Fig. 7.26) emerge at the periphery of the gland to supply the muscles of facial expression (see p. 333).

Retromandibular vein

Within the parotid gland the superficial temporal and maxillary veins unite to form the retromandibular vein (Fig. 7.27). Inferiorly this short vein terminates as anterior and posterior divisions which escape from the gland. The anterior division joins the facial vein, which drains into the internal jugular vein. The posterior division unites with the posterior auricular vein to form the external jugular vein (see p. 324).

Termination of external carotid artery

Entering the parotid from below, the external carotid artery ascends through the gland and at the level of the neck of the mandible divides into the maxillary and superficial temporal arteries (Fig. 7.28). The former runs anterosuperiorly to leave the

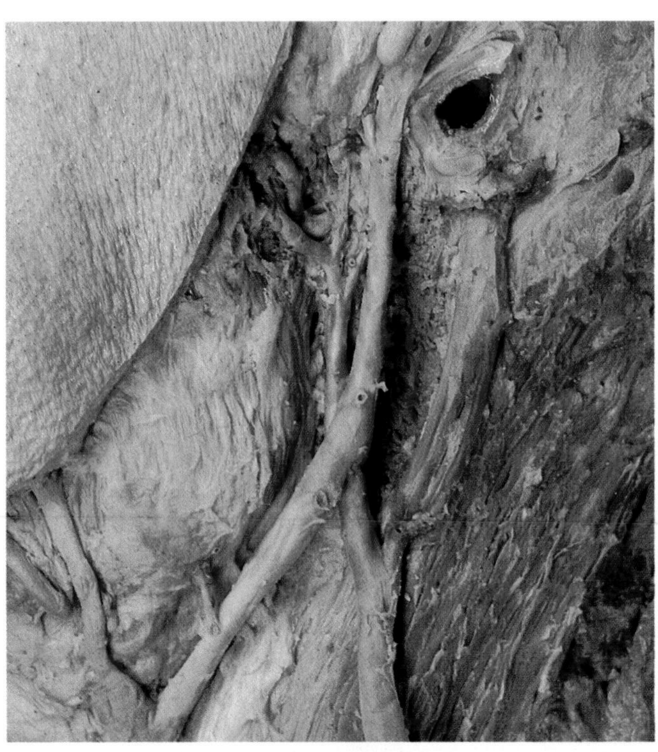

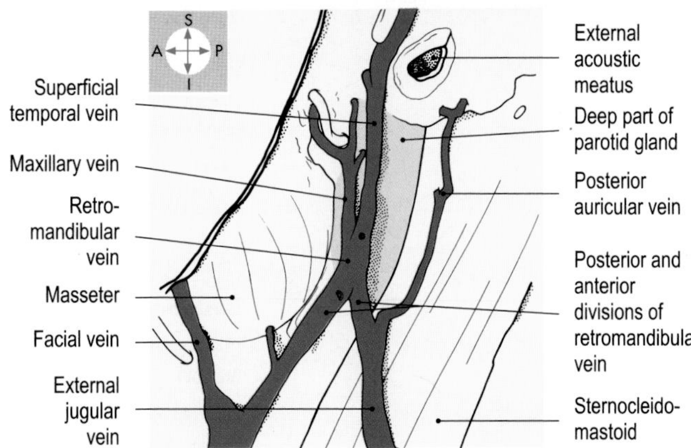

Fig. 7.27 Retromandibular vein and its communications, seen after removal of the superficial portion of the parotid gland.

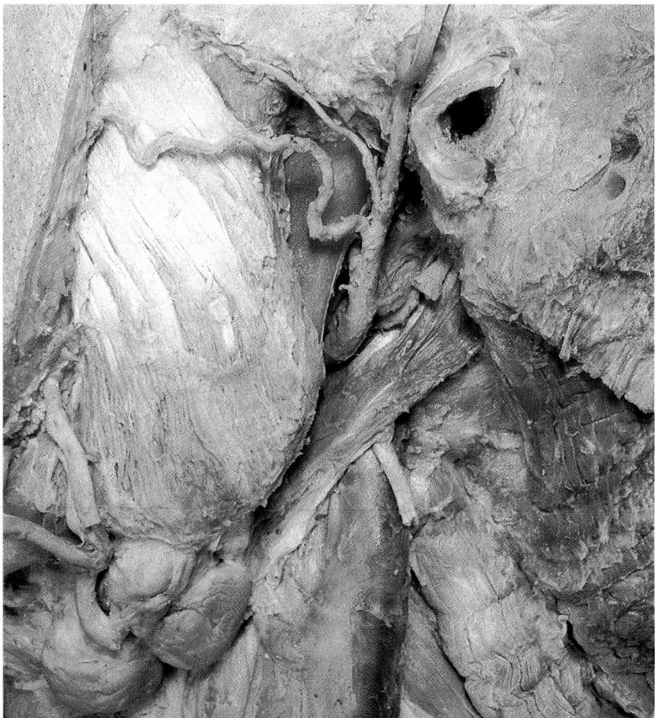

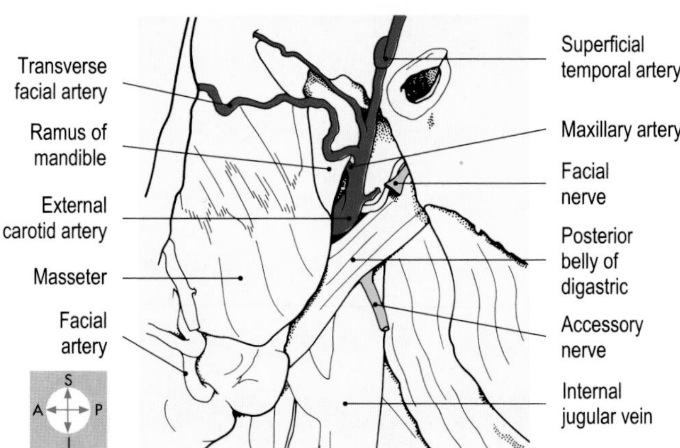

Fig. 7.28 External carotid artery and its terminal branches, revealed by complete excision of the parotid gland.

gland and enter the infratemporal fossa. The superficial temporal artery continues upwards between the external acoustic meatus and the temporomandibular joint to supply the temple. Its pulsation can be felt just above the joint.

Several lymph nodes lie just under the fascia covering the parotid gland or within the gland itself.

Neurovascular supply

The gland receives its vascular supply from the vessels traversing it. Parasympathetic secretomotor fibres follow a tortuous route to the gland. The preganglionic fibres arise from the inferior salivatory nucleus in the brainstem and pass in the tympanic branch of the glossopharyngeal (IX) nerve to the tympanic plexus in the middle ear, leaving the skull in the lesser petrosal nerve to synapse in the otic ganglion (see p. 343). Postganglionic parasympathetic fibres travel to the gland in the auriculotemporal branch of the mandibular (V_3) division. By contrast, postganglionic sympathetic nerves are conveyed in the plexus accompanying the external carotid artery.

Masseter, Temporalis and Infratemporal Fossa

Masseter

Masseter (Fig. 7.29) attaches along the length of the zygomatic arch and its fibres slope downwards and backwards to the lateral surface of the ramus of the mandible adjacent to the angle (Fig. 7.31). This muscle is a powerful elevator of the mandible and is easily palpated when the teeth are clenched. It is supplied by the masseteric branch of the mandibular (V_3) division of the trigeminal nerve.

Temporalis

Temporalis (Fig. 7.30) is a large fan-shaped muscle occupying the temporal fossa and taking attachment from the area of bone bounded by the inferior temporal line. The more superficial fibres arise from the temporal fascia that covers the muscle and is attached to the superior temporal line. All the fibres descend deep to the zygomatic arch to attach to the coronoid process and anteromedial aspect of the ramus of the mandible (Fig. 7.31). Temporalis elevates the mandible, as in closing the mouth, and its posterior fibres retract the mandible. The deep temporal branches of the mandibular (V_3) division of the trigeminal nerve supply the muscle from its deep surface.

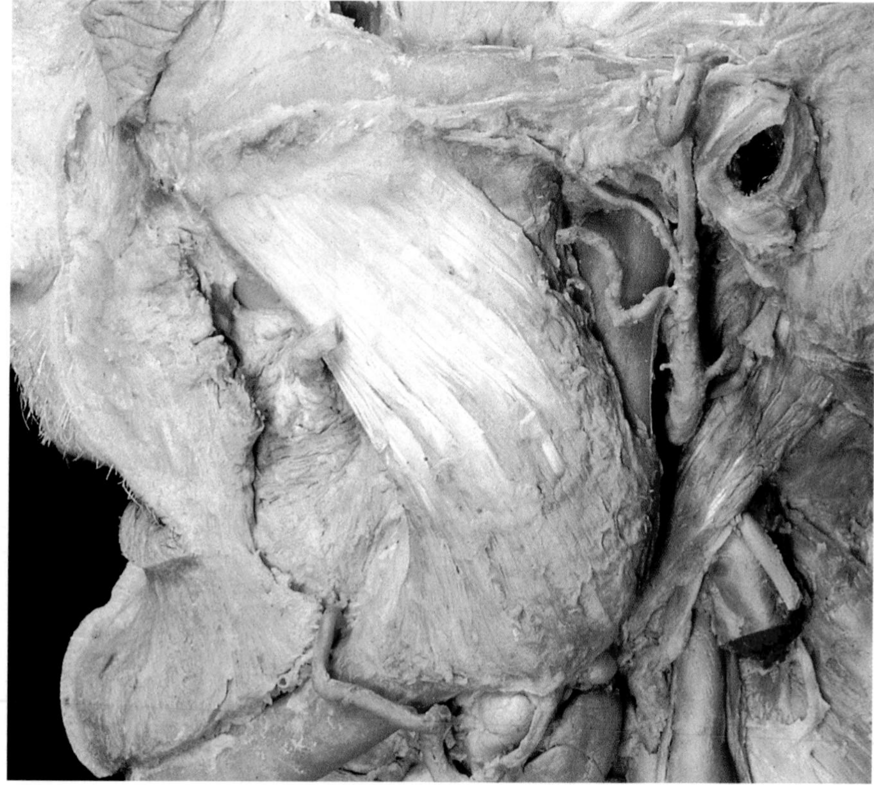

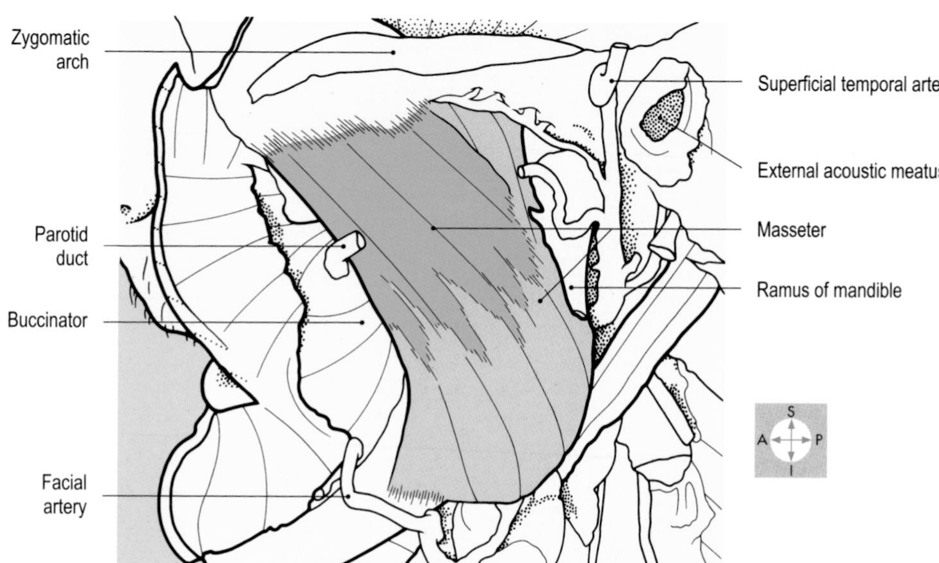

Fig. 7.29 Masseter, showing its attachment to the zygomatic arch and the angle of the mandible, after removal of the parotid gland.

Infratemporal fossa

This fossa lies deep to the ramus of the mandible and is limited on its medial aspect by the lateral wall of the pharynx and the medial pterygoid plate of the sphenoid bone. The fossa is bounded by the posterior surface of the maxilla in front and by the styloid process and its attached muscles behind. The roof is provided by the temporal and sphenoid bones in the base of the skull whilst inferiorly the fossa is continuous with the neck.

Within the fossa are the two pterygoid muscles, the mandibular (V_3) division of the trigeminal nerve and its branches, and the maxillary vessels and their branches. Adjacent to the fossa is the temporomandibular joint.

Pterygoid muscles

Each of the lateral and medial pterygoid muscles (see Figs 7.32–7.34) has two attachments to the skull. The upper head of the lateral pterygoid attaches to the inferior surface of the greater wing of the sphenoid. The lower head attaches to the lateral surface of the lateral pterygoid plate. Both heads converge on the neck of the mandible and the capsule of the temporomandibular joint. The lateral pterygoid pulls forward both the neck of the mandible and the articular disc, thus depressing the mandible and opening the mouth.

The lower head of the lateral pterygoid is clasped by the two heads of the medial pterygoid. The deep head of the latter is larger and attaches to the medial surface of the lateral pterygoid plate. The superficial head is attached to the tuberosity of the maxilla. The fibres of both heads incline obliquely down-wards and backwards to attach to the medial surface of the angle of the mandible. The muscle is a powerful elevator of the mandible.

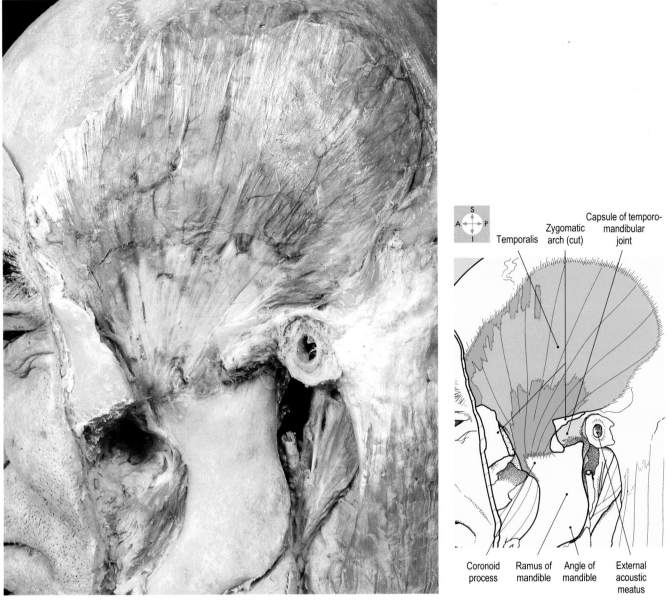

S
A P
I
Temporalis
Zygomatic arch (cut)
Capsule of temporo-mandibular joint
Coronoid process
Ramus of mandible
Angle of mandible
External acoustic meatus

Fig. 7.30 Temporalis, seen after removal of masseter, part of the zygomatic arch and the temporal fascia.

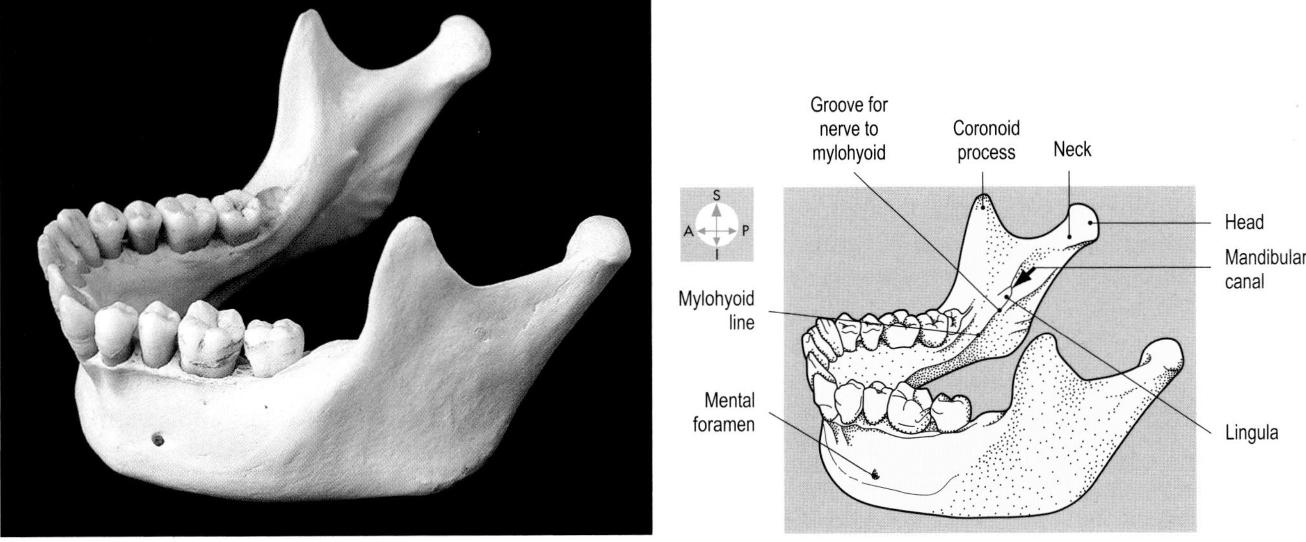

Fig. 7.31 Mandible. The right wisdom tooth is partially erupted.

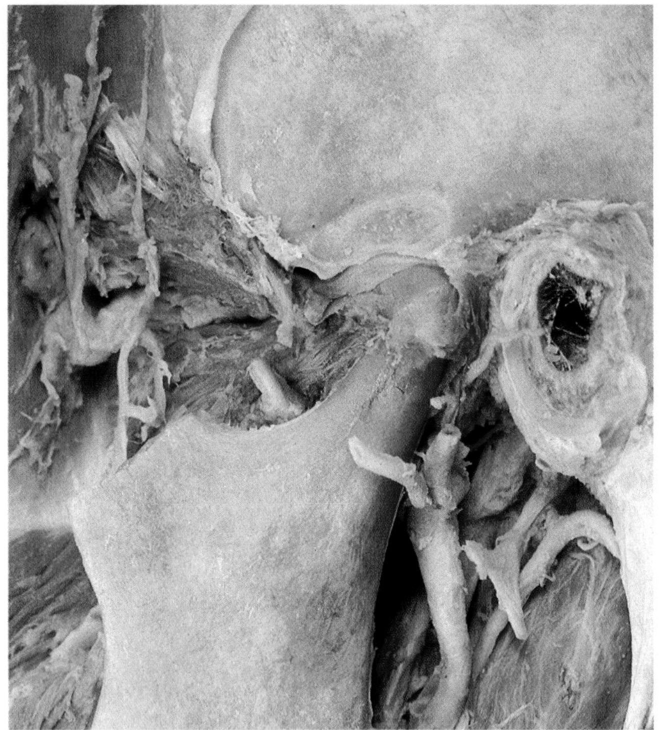

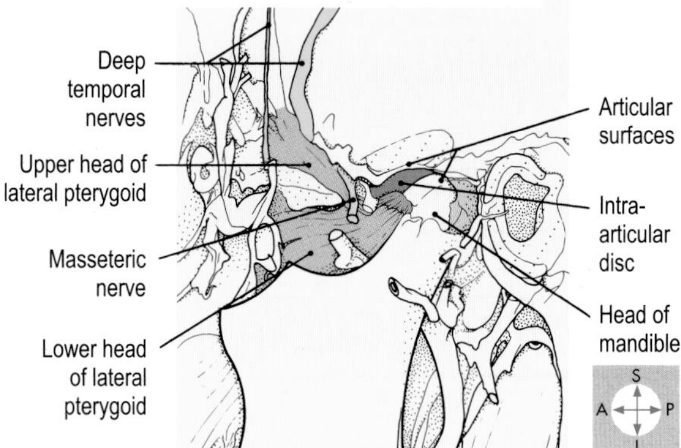

Fig. 7.32 Temporomandibular joint opened by excision of the lateral part of its capsule.

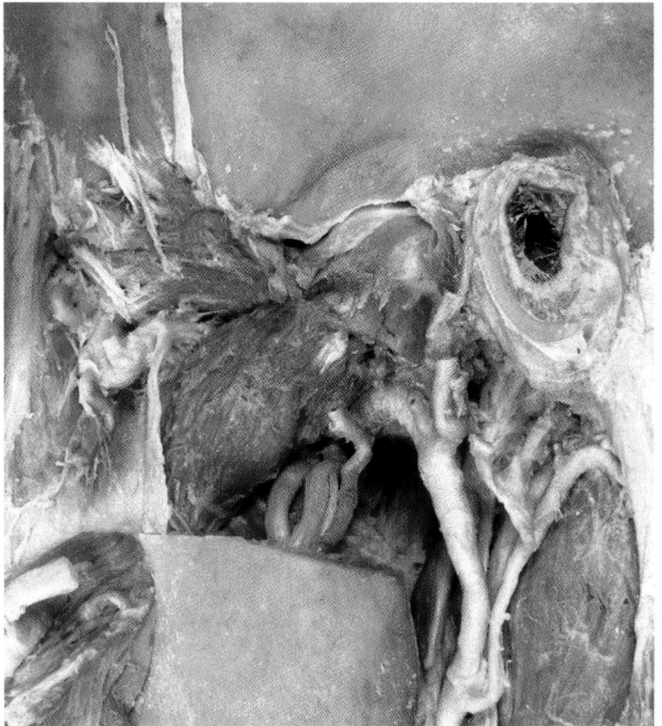

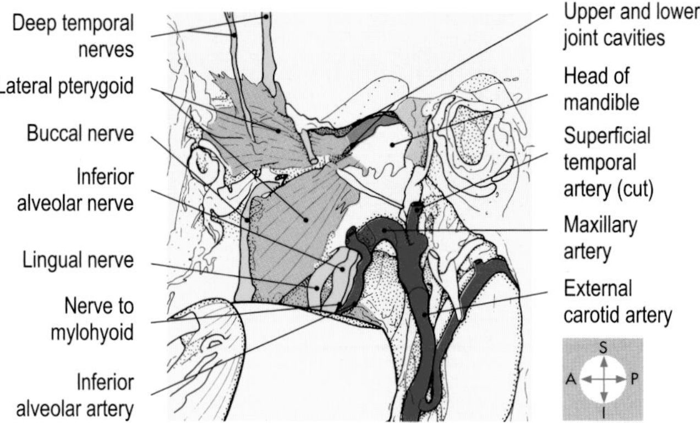

Fig. 7.33 Contents of the infratemporal fossa seen after excision of part of the mandible. In this specimen the maxillary artery passes deep to lateral pterygoid.

Temporomandibular joint

The temporomandibular joint (Fig. 7.32) is a synovial joint. The head of the mandible articulates with the articular fossa and eminence of the temporal bone. Fibrocartilage covers the articular surfaces and also forms an articular disc which divides the joint into two separate cavities. Within these cavities the non-cartilaginous surfaces are lined with synovial membrane.

The fibrous capsule surrounding the joint is attached to the margin of the articular cartilage and to the neck of the mandible. Anteriorly it receives the attachment of the lateral pterygoid while its deep surface is firmly adherent to the periphery of the articular disc.

Laterally the capsule (see Fig. 7.30) is thickened to form the lateral ligament, which inclines posteroinferiorly from the root of the zygomatic arch to the neck of the mandible. Two accessory ligaments lie medial to the joint, although not in contact with the capsule. The sphenomandibular ligament extends from the spine of the sphenoid to the lingula adjacent to the mandibular foramen. The stylomandibular ligament, a thickening of the parotid fascia, passes from the styloid process to the angle of the mandible.

The joint receives its nerve supply from the auriculotemporal and masseteric branches of the mandibular (V_3) division of the trigeminal nerve.

Movements at the joint include elevation, depression, protraction and retraction of the mandible. The head of the mandible does not merely rotate in the articular fossa but also moves forwards onto the articular eminence of the temporal bone, taking the articular disc with it. The alternate protraction and retraction of right and left sides produces the grinding movements used in chewing. The muscles responsible for these movements are known collectively as the muscles of mastication. The mouth is closed by contraction of masseter, temporalis and medial pterygoid. The lateral pterygoid protracts the mandible and, assisted by digastric and mylohyoid (see p. 346), also opens the mouth. Retraction is produced by the posterior fibres of temporalis. When the mandible is fully depressed the joint is relatively unstable and

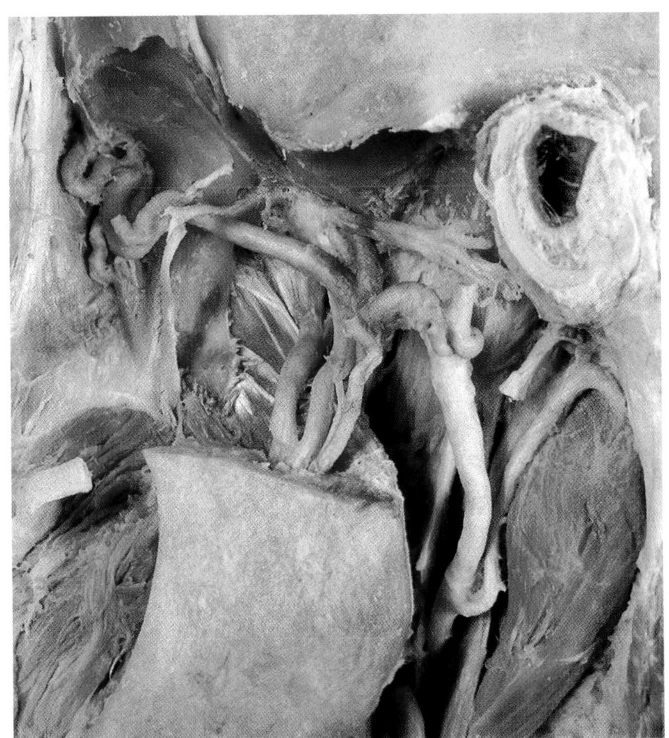

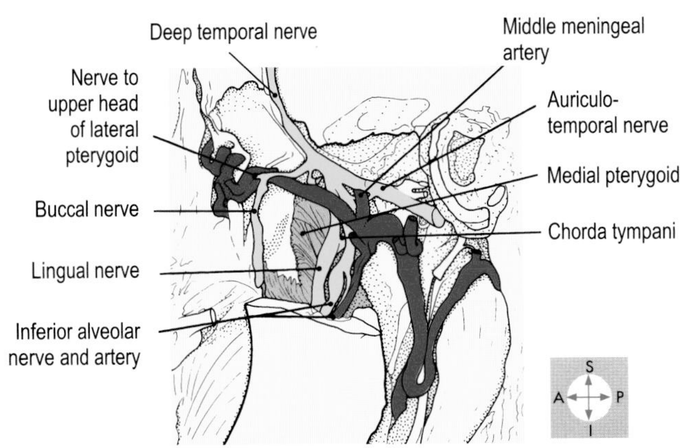

Fig. 7.34 Branches of the mandibular division of the trigeminal nerve and the maxillary artery, revealed by removal of the mandibular head and lateral pterygoid.

dislocation may occur, the head of the mandible moving in front of the articular eminence and resulting in an inability to close the mouth.

Mandibular (V_3) division of trigeminal nerve

The mandibular division of the trigeminal nerve (Figs 7.33 & 7.34) contains sensory and motor fibres and enters the infratemporal fossa through the foramen ovale in the sphenoid. Two small branches arise from the short main trunk of the nerve. The first branch ascends through the foramen spinosum to receive sensation from the meninges of the middle cranial fossa. The other branch is motor, supplying the medial pterygoid and giving a small branch that passes through the otic ganglion (lying just medial to the main trunk of the mandibular division) to supply tensor tympani and tensor veli palatini.

The main trunk descends between the lateral pterygoid and tensor palati muscles, dividing into anterior and posterior divisions. The anterior division is mainly motor and gives masseteric, deep temporal, lateral pterygoid and buccal branches. The masseteric nerve (Fig. 7.32) curves laterally above the lateral pterygoid to enter the deep surface of masseter. Two or three deep temporal nerves (Fig. 7.33) ascend deep to temporalis, which they supply, and further branches enter the deep surface of the lateral pterygoid. The buccal nerve (Figs 7.33 & 7.34) is a sensory branch that passes forwards between the two heads of the lateral pterygoid to supply the skin over the cheek and the mucosa lining the cheek, which it reaches by piercing, but not supplying, buccinator.

The posterior division of the main trunk is mainly sensory and has three branches, the auriculotemporal, lingual and inferior alveolar nerves. The auriculotemporal nerve (Fig. 7.34) arises by two roots, which clasp the origin of the middle meningeal artery. The nerve passes backwards before turning superiorly behind the temporomandibular joint to ascend in company with the superficial temporal vessels. It gives secretomotor branches to the parotid gland (see p. 337) and conveys sensation from the temporal region, the upper half of the pinna and most of the external acoustic meatus.

The lingual nerve (Figs 7.33 & 7.34) inclines downwards and forwards between the pterygoids, deviating medially to pass below the superior constrictor of the pharynx. In the floor of the mouth it runs forwards lateral to the hyoglossus muscle, at whose anterior border it again turns medially to pass inferior to the submandibular duct and enter the base of the tongue. It conveys general sensation from the anterior two-thirds of the tongue. Near the lower border of the lateral pterygoid the lingual nerve is joined by the chorda tympani (a branch of the facial nerve). Arising within the temporal bone, the chorda tympani emerges from the petrotympanic fissure. It carries taste fibres, which have travelled in the lingual nerve from the anterior two-thirds of the tongue and preganglionic parasympathetic fibres destined for the submandibular ganglion (see p. 350).

The inferior alveolar nerve (Figs 7.33 & 7.34) descends medial to the lateral pterygoid and gives rise to a motor branch that curves downwards to supply mylohyoid and the anterior belly of digastric. The inferior alveolar nerve then enters the mandibular foramen in the ramus of the mandible and runs forwards in the mandibular canal, supplying the lower teeth and alveolar ridge. Its mental branch emerges from the mental foramen to supply skin overlying the chin. Local anaesthetic injected near the inferior alveolar nerve as it enters the mandibular foramen will block sensation from the lower teeth and gums on that side of the mouth. Often there is loss of sensation in the same side of the tongue because of the proximity of the lingual nerve.

Maxillary artery

This artery (see Figs 7.33 & 7.34) arises in the parotid gland (see p. 337) as a terminal branch of the external carotid artery, passes anterosuperiorly across the infratemporal fossa, usually lateral to the lateral pterygoid, and traverses the pterygomaxillary fissure to enter the pterygopalatine fossa where terminal branches arise. These correspond to branches of the maxillary nerve (see p. 351).

In the infratemporal fossa the maxillary artery gives branches to supply masseter, temporalis and the pterygoid muscles. In addition, the middle meningeal artery arises deep to the lateral pterygoid, embraced by the two roots of the auriculotemporal nerve. It traverses the foramen spinosum and within the cranium supplies the meninges of the middle cranial fossa and the cranial vault.

The maxillary artery also gives rise to the inferior alveolar artery which accompanies the nerve into the mandibular canal. Further small branches supply the middle ear and the lining of the external acoustic meatus.

Pterygoid venous plexus

Veins within the pterygopalatine fossa form a plexus that extends through the pterygomaxillary fissure into the infratemporal fossa, where the plexus is related to the pterygoid muscles. This pterygoid plexus has important connections to the cavernous sinus in the skull and infraorbital and ophthalmic veins. The plexus drains by the maxillary vein into the retromandibular vein (see p. 338).

Digastric and Styloid Muscles

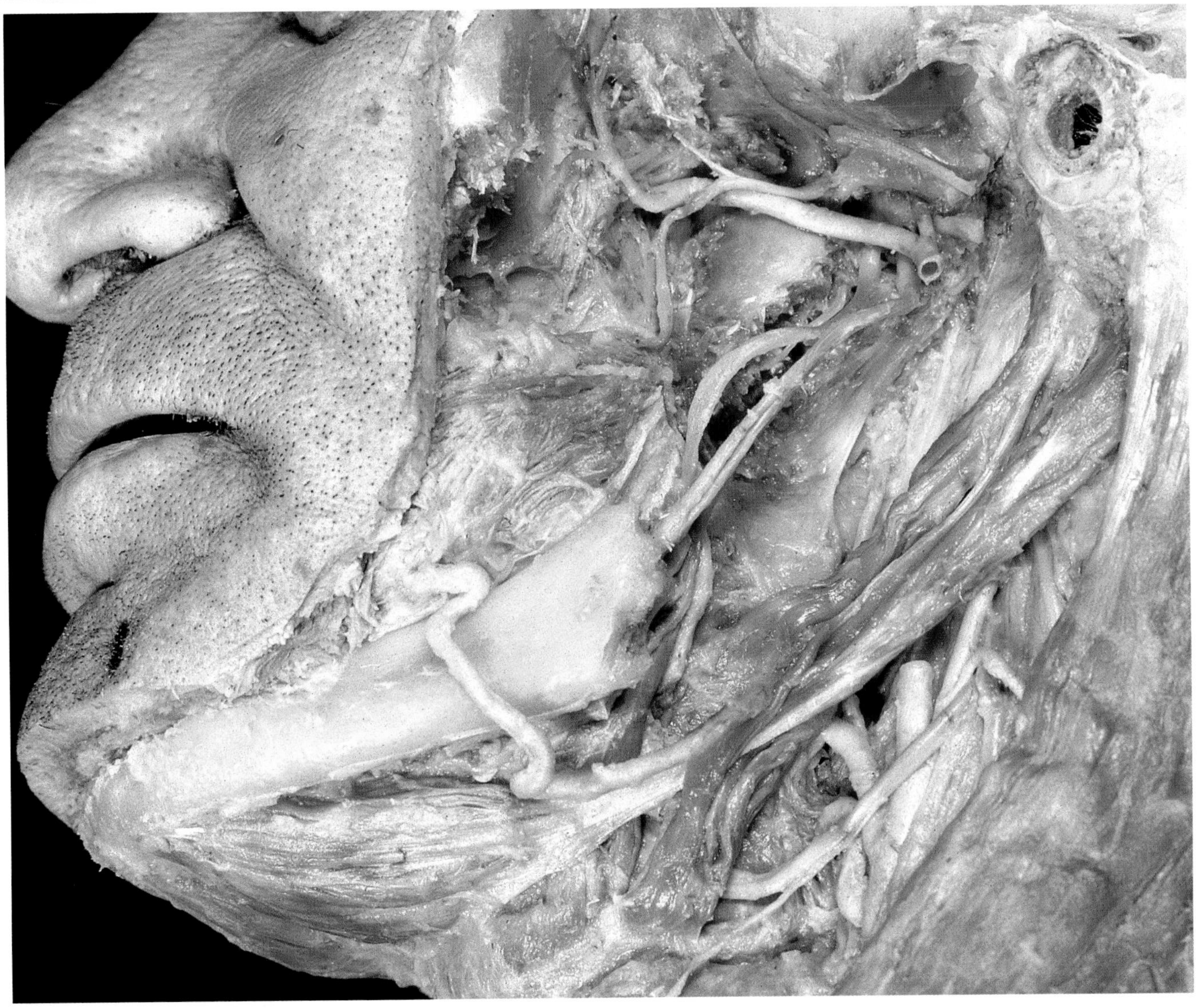

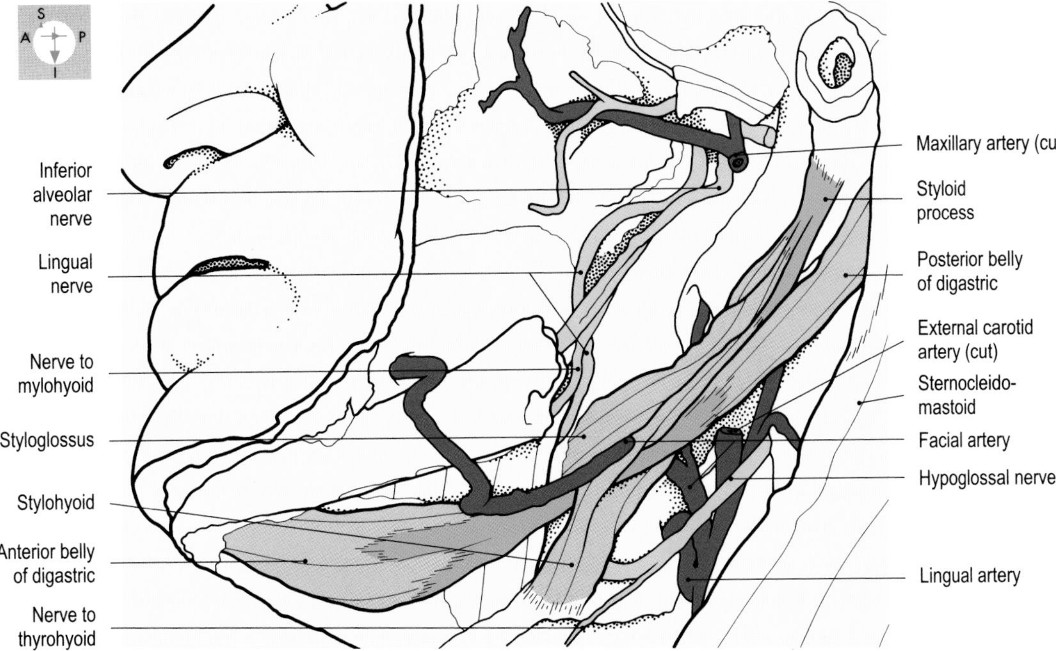

Fig. 7.35 Digastric and stylohyoid seen after removal of part of the mandible. The superficial part of the submandibular gland has also been excised.

Digastric

The digastric muscle (see Fig. 7.35) consists of anterior and posterior bellies united by an intermediate tendon. The posterior belly attaches to the medial surface of the mastoid process and inclines forwards and downwards, becoming continuous with the intermediate tendon close to the hyoid bone. This tendon pierces stylohyoid and is anchored by a fascial sling to the hyoid bone. The anterior belly continues forwards from the intermediate tendon to attach to the inferior border of the mandible near the midline. Digastric elevates the hyoid bone during swallowing and assists mylohyoid and the lateral pterygoid in depressing the mandible when opening the mouth. The posterior belly is innervated by the facial (VII) nerve (see p. 338). The anterior belly receives its motor supply from the mandibular (V_3) division of the trigeminal nerve via the mylohyoid branch of the inferior alveolar nerve (see p. 343).

Muscles of styloid process

Three muscles, stylohyoid, stylopharyngeus and styloglossus, attach to the styloid process but diverge to reach the hyoid bone, the pharynx and the tongue respectively.

Stylohyoid (see Fig. 7.35) inclines downwards and forwards from the posterior surface of the styloid process to attach to the body of the hyoid bone alongside the lesser horn. The muscle or its tendon is pierced by the intermediate tendon of digastric near the hyoid bone. Stylohyoid elevates the hyoid and is innervated by the facial (VII) nerve.

Stylopharyngeus (Fig. 7.36) is attached to the medial side of the root of the styloid process and passes inferomedially on the lateral surface of the superior pharyngeal constrictor. It enters the wall of the pharynx between the superior and middle constrictors and blends with the other longitudinal muscles of the pharynx. The muscle elevates the pharynx and larynx during swallowing and is the only muscle innervated by the glossopharyngeal (IX) nerve.

Styloglossus (Fig. 7.36) inclines anteromedially from the tip of the styloid process and upper end of the stylohyoid ligament and passes between the superior and middle constrictors of the pharynx to enter the tongue. It elevates and retracts the tongue and, in common with other muscles of the tongue, is supplied by the hypoglossal (XII) nerve.

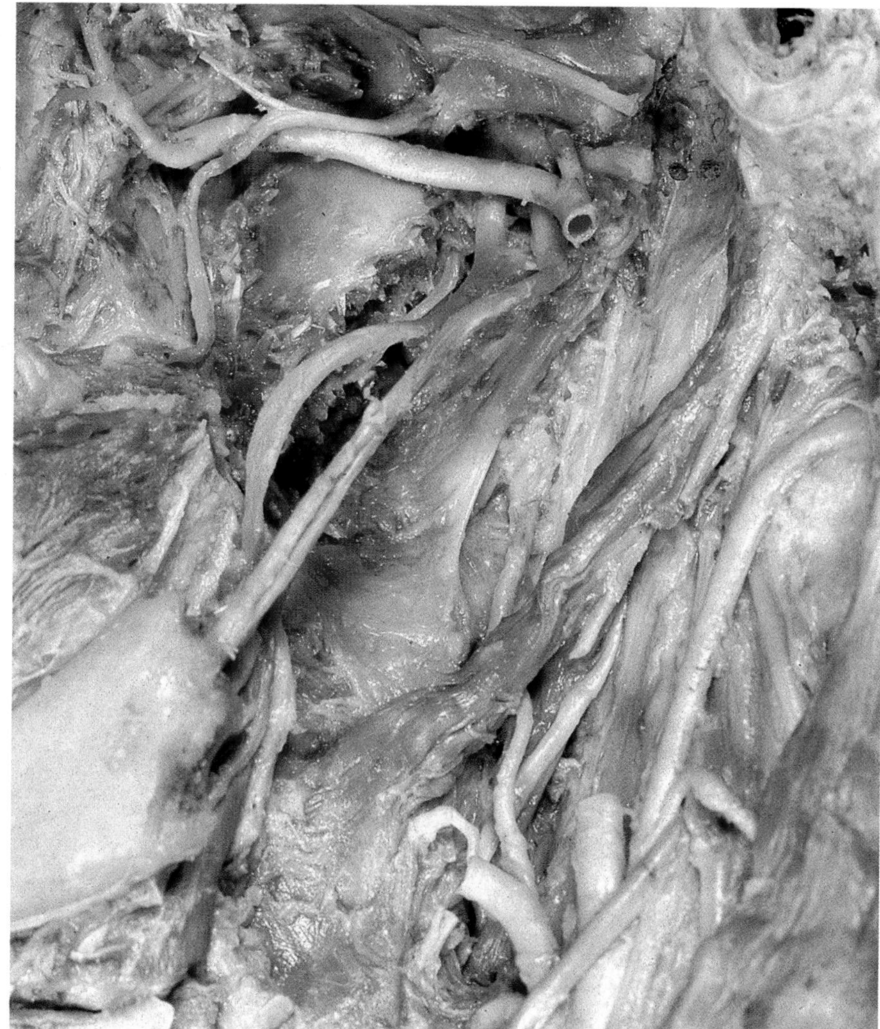

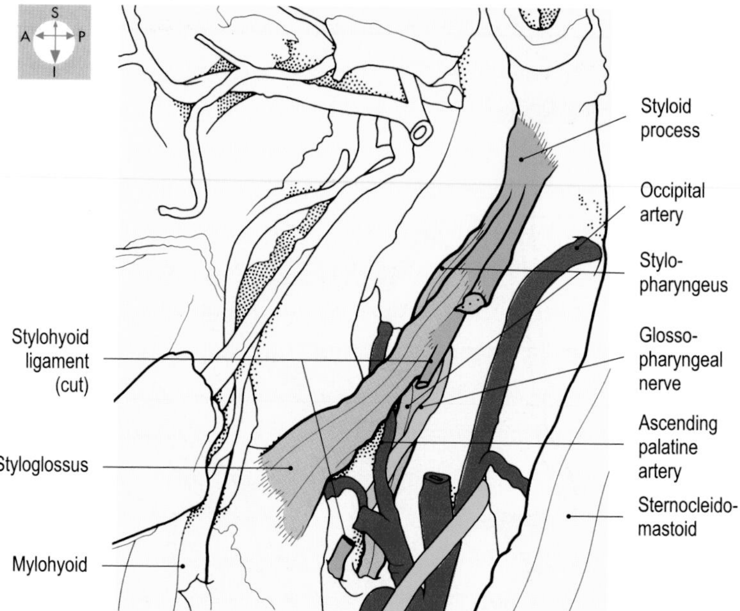

Fig. 7.36 Stylopharyngeus and styloglossus seen after excision of digastric, stylohyoid and the middle portion of the stylohyoid ligament.

Mylohyoid and Related Structures

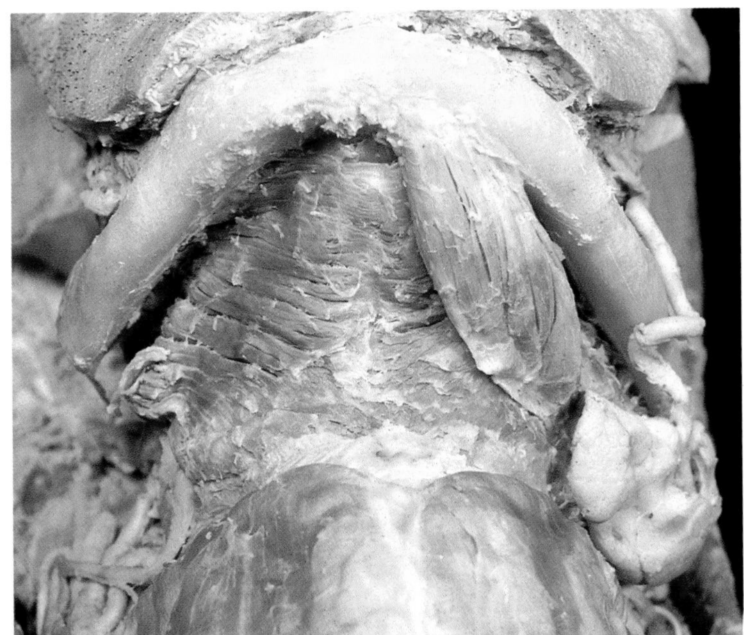

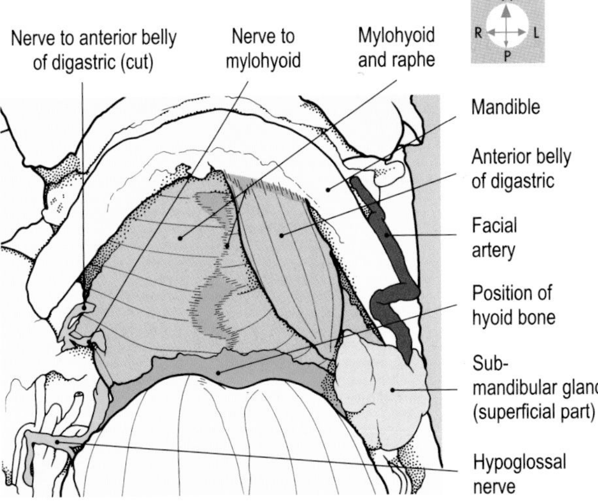

Fig. 7.37 Mylohyoid, revealed by removal of the right anterior belly of digastric and superficial part of the submandibular gland.

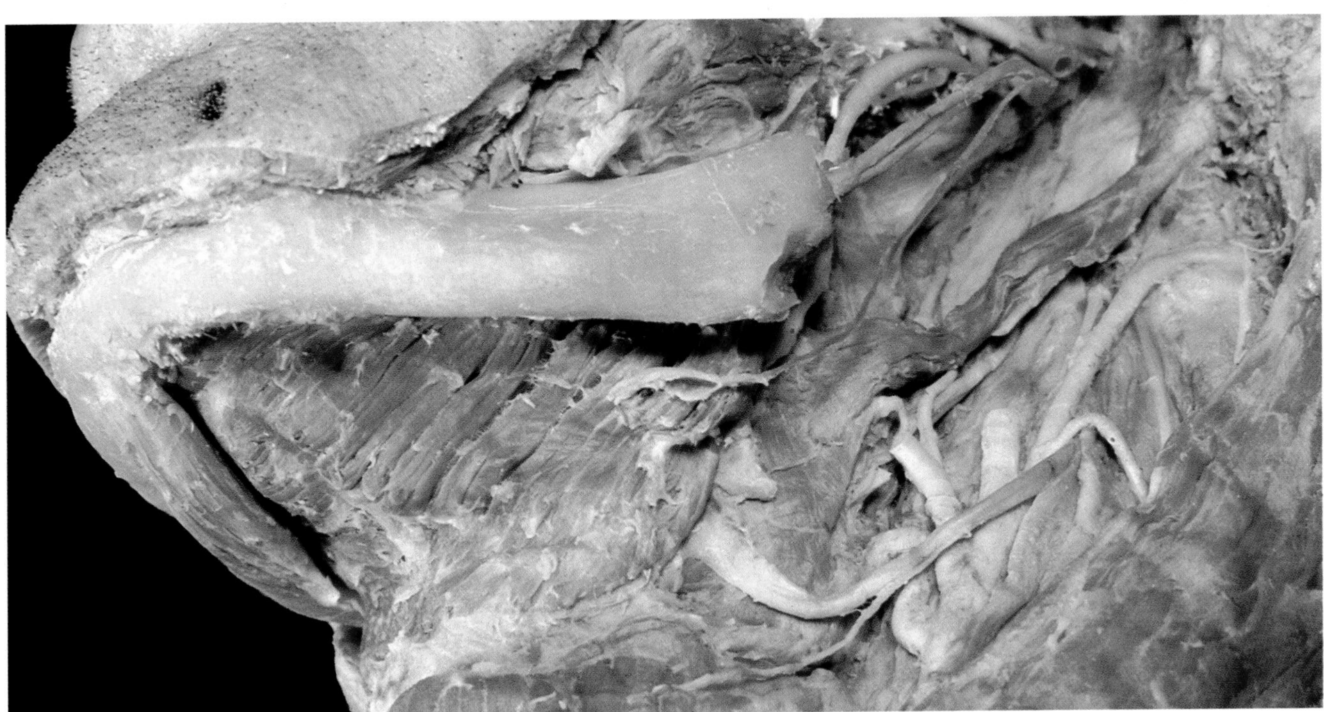

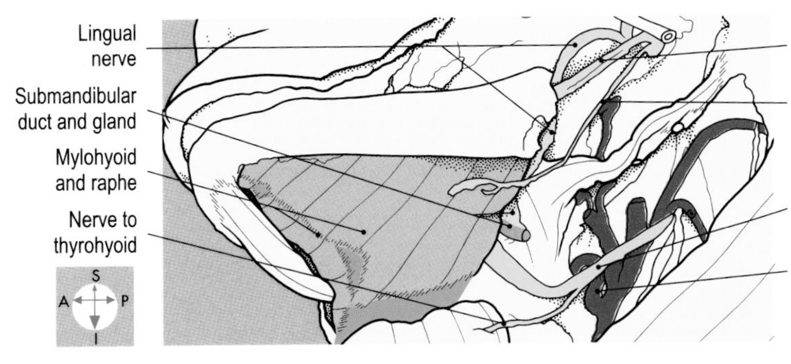

Fig. 7.38 The hypoglossal nerve, lingual nerve and submandibular duct passing above mylohyoid.

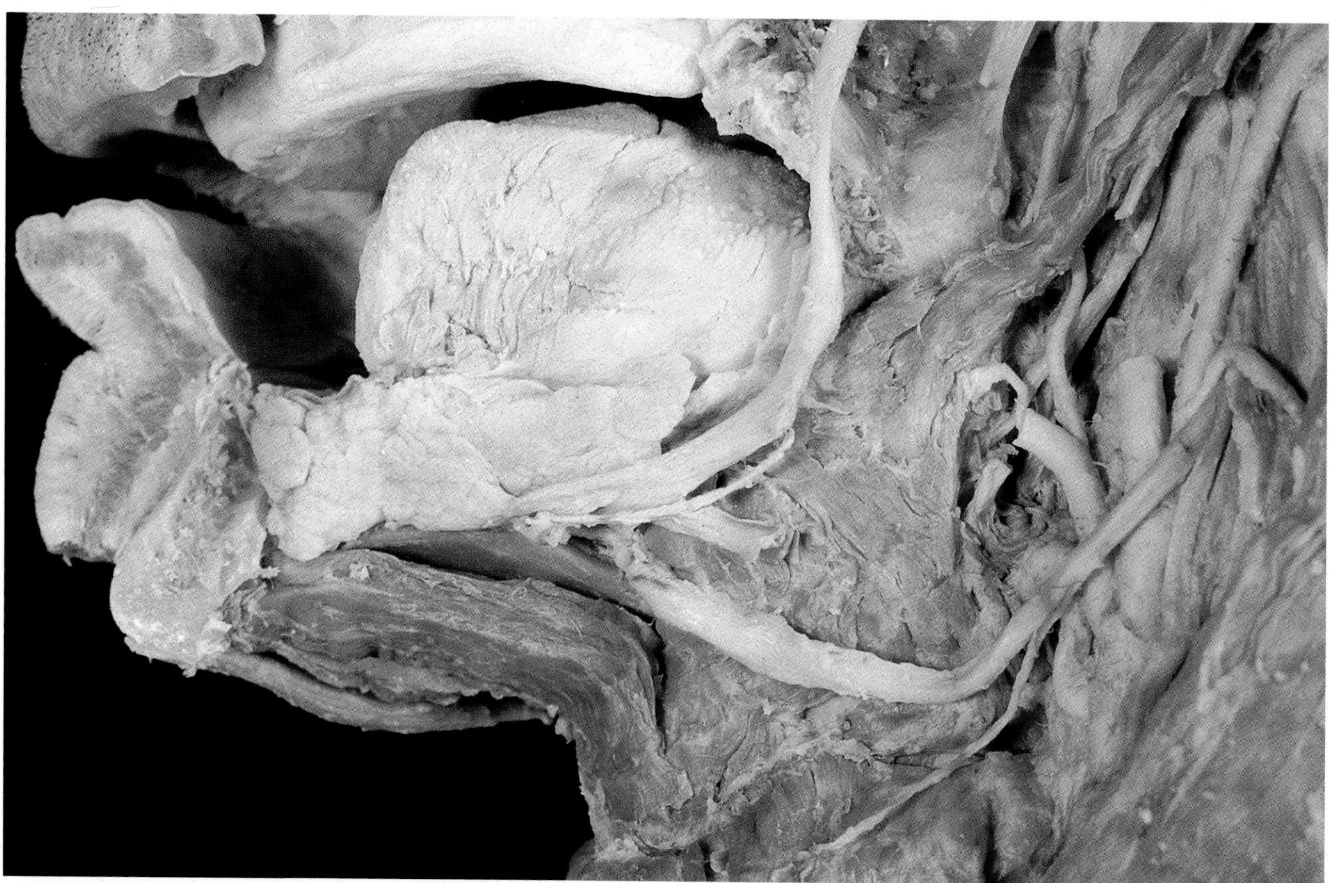

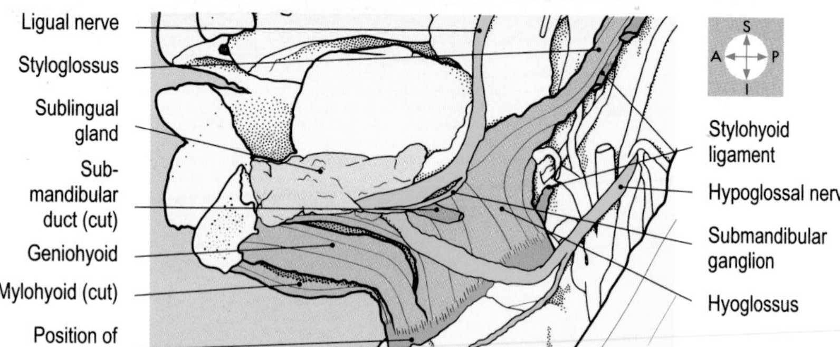

Fig. 7.39 Structures deep to mylohyoid, seen after partial removal of the mylohyoid and the mandible. The submandibular ganglion is elongated in this specimen.

Suspended from the body of the mandible is a thin sheet of muscle formed by the two mylohyoid muscles. The fibres of each muscle incline downwards and medially, meeting each other in the midline to form a shallow gutter. This gutter slopes downwards and backwards and ends at the free posterior borders of the two muscles on either side of the hyoid bone.

Each mylohyoid separates the superficial tissues in the upper part of the neck from the tongue and related structures within the mouth. Below the muscle lie the anterior belly of digastric (see p. 346), part of the platysma (see p. 334), the facial artery and vein, and the larger superficial part of the submandibular salivary gland (see Fig. 7.37). This gland curves around the posterior border of mylohyoid so that its deep part and the submandibular duct lie above the muscle. Also located on the superior aspect of mylohyoid are the sublingual glands, the tongue with its vessels and nerves and the geniohyoid muscles.

Mylohyoid

This muscle (see Figs 7.37 & 7.38) takes attachment from the mylohyoid line on the inner aspect of the body of the mandible. Most of its fibres reach a midline raphe, wherethey interdigitate with those from the opposite side. However, the posterior fibres descend to the body of the hyoid bone. The mylohyoid muscles raise the hyoid bone and the tongue during swallowing; they also help to depress the mandible when the hyoid bone is fixed from below. The muscle is innervated by the mylohyoid nerve, a branch of the inferior alveolar nerve from the mandibular division of the trigeminal nerve (V_3).

Geniohyoid

Above mylohyoid geniohyoid (Fig. 7.39) lies close to the midline, passing from the inferior mental spine (inferior genial tubercle) on the mandible to the body of the hyoid bone. Innervated by C1 spinal nerve fibres that are conveyed in the hypoglossal nerve, geniohyoid either elevates the hyoid or depresses the mandible.

Tongue

The tongue is a muscular organ and lies mostly within the oral cavity although its posterior part projects into the oropharynx.

Surface features

The tongue is covered by mucosa, which is reflected anteriorly and laterally onto the inferior surface. Under the tip of the tongue the mucous membrane forms a midline

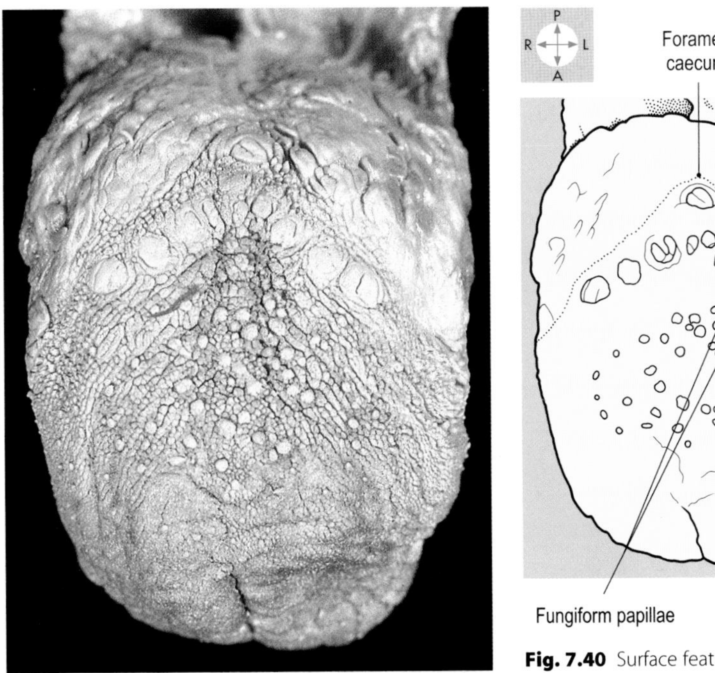

Fig. 7.40 Surface features of the tongue.

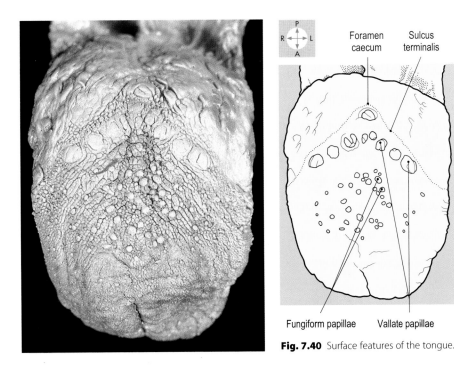

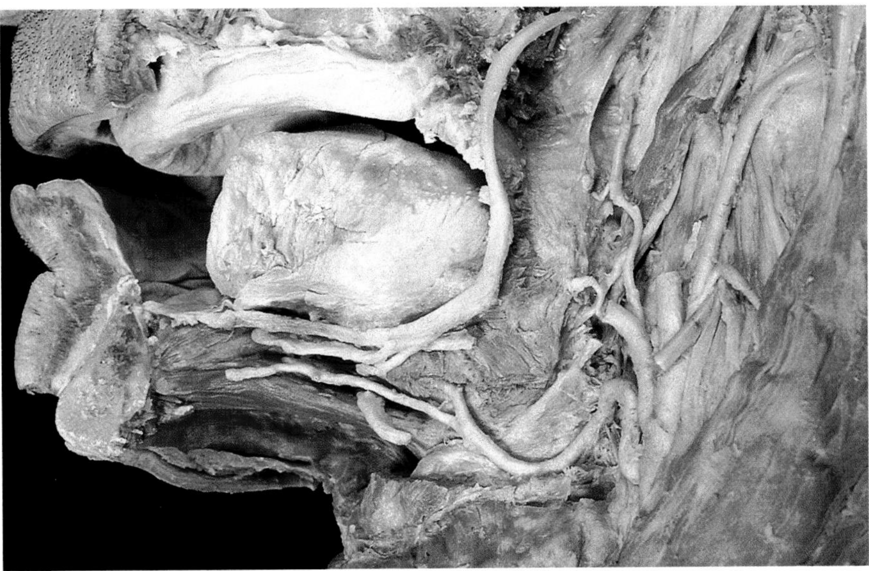

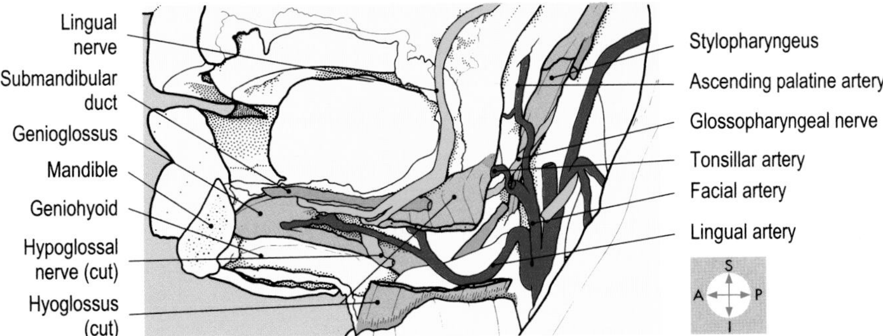

Fig. 7.41 Deeper structures in the base of the tongue, revealed after removal of the sublingual gland and part of hyoglossus.

fold, the frenulum. The upper surface of the tongue (Fig. 7.40) is divided into anterior two-thirds and posterior one-third by a V-shaped groove, the groove. A midline depression, the fora-men caecum, lies at the apex of the groove. A row of round elevations, the vallate papillae, lie just in front of the sulcus. From the mucosa of the tongue, somatic sensory and taste fibres pass centrally to reach the brain. From the anterior two-thirds of the tongue (and adjacent oral mucosa) these fibres travel in the lingual nerve (see p. 343). Somatic sensory fibres continue to the brain in the mandibular (V_3) division of the trigeminal nerve. However, taste fibres leave the lingual nerve and are conveyed via the chorda tympani nerve to the facial (VII) nerve (see p. 343). Both taste and somatic sensory nerve fibres from the posterior third of the tongue (including the vallate papillae) are conveyed in the glossopharyngeal (IX) nerve.

Muscles

The musculature of the tongue, divided into two functional halves by a fibrous septum, consists of both extrinsic and intrinsic muscles. In general, the extrinsic muscles alter the position of the tongue and the intrinsic muscles alter its shape.

The extrinsic muscles comprise styloglossus (see p. 346), hyoglossus and genioglossus. Hyoglossus (Fig. 7.39) is attached to the body and greater horn of the hyoid bone and its fibres pass upwards and forwards to reach the side of the tongue. Hyoglossus depresses the tongue, particularly at the sides. Genioglossus (Figs 7.41 & 7.42) forms much of the bulk of the tongue, its fibres radiating from the superior mental spine (superior genial tubercle). The superior fibres reach the tip whilst the inferior fibres pass into the posteroinferior part of the organ. Genioglossus draws the tongue forwards and downwards and its anterior fibres retract the tip.

Palatoglossus descends from the soft palate and enters the side of the tongue posteriorly. Although it helps to elevate the tongue it is usually considered to be a muscle of the palate (see p. 359).

The intrinsic muscles comprise interlacing longitudinal, transverse and vertical groups of fibres on either side of the midline fibrous septum. The shape of the tongue is changed by integrated contractions of the various groups.

The hypoglossal (XII) nerve (Fig. 7.39) supplies all the muscles of the tongue, both intrinsic and extrinsic. (The nerve supply to palatoglossus is described with the other muscles of the palate; see p. 359) Damage to the hypoglossal nerve causes the tongue to deviate to the injured side when protruded.

Blood supply

Arising from the front of the external carotid artery, the lingual artery (Fig. 7.41) loops upwards above the greater horn of the hyoid bone and continues forwards into the base of the tongue deep to hyoglossus. Having supplied structures in the tongue, the lingual artery terminates in the tip. Venous drainage follows a reciprocal course into the internal jugular vein.

Submandibular and sublingual glands

The superficial part of the submandibular salivary gland (see Fig. 7.37) lies inferior to mylohyoid and extends below the medial surface of the mandible. It is continuous around the posterior border of mylohyoid with the smaller deep part (see Fig. 7.38) of the gland that lies above the muscle. The lateral surface of the superficial part of the gland is indented by the facial artery as the vessel arches forwards to reach the inferior border of the mandible (see p. 335).

From the deep part of the gland the submandibular duct passes forwards and medially to open close to the midline at the base of the frenulum of the tongue. A number of small sublingual glands (see Fig. 7.39) lie beneath the mucosa adjacent to the submandibular duct. These glands are drained by ducts that open either into the submandibular duct or directly into the mouth. Calculi in the submandibular duct can often be palpated through the mucosa of the floor of the mouth. Both the sublingual and submandibular glands receive postganglionic parasympathetic secretomotor fibres from the submandibular ganglion (see Fig. 7.39). Preganglionic fibres reach the submandibular ganglion from the facial nerve by way of the chorda tympani and lingual nerves.

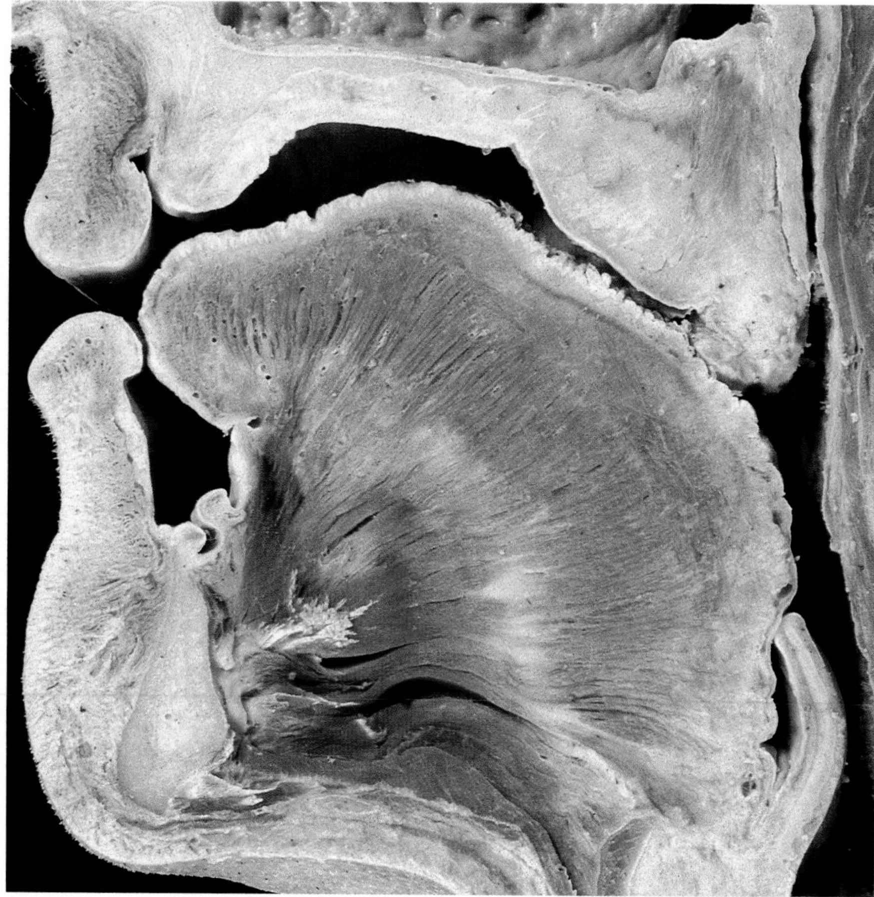

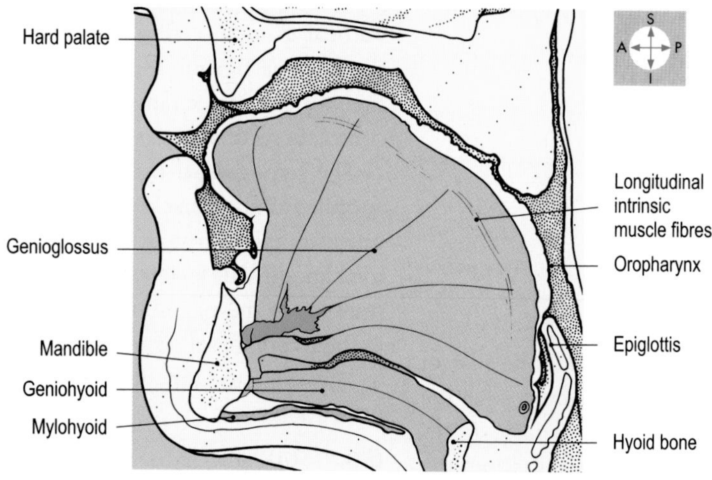

Fig. 7.42 Sagittal section through the tongue and surrounding structures.

Hypoglossal (XII) nerve

The twelfth cranial nerve (see Fig. 7.38) leaves the skull through the hypoglossal canal and descends between the internal jugular vein and internal carotid artery to turn forwards close to the origin of the occipital artery from the external carotid artery, where the superior root of the ansa cervicalis (see p. 327) arises. The hypoglossal nerve then continues forwards across the loop of the lingual artery and passes between mylohyoid and hyoglossus to enter the tongue whose muscles it supplies. The branches given to thyrohyoid and geniohyoid are composed of C1 fibres which are distributed via the hypoglossal nerve.

Glossopharyngeal (IX) nerve

The glossopharyngeal nerve (see Fig. 7.41) emerges from the skull through the jugular foramen. Initially contained within the carotid sheath, the nerve curves forwards around the stylopharyngeus muscle (which it also supplies) and passes between the superior and middle constrictors of the pharynx to enter the posterior part of the tongue. The glossopharyngeal nerve conveys both somatic and taste sensation from the posterior third of the tongue, oropharynx and lateral parts of the soft palate. The nerve has an autonomic sensory branch, the carotid sinus nerve, which ascends from the carotid sinus and carotid body. In addition, a tympanic branch passes to the tympanic plexus in the middle ear. The lesser petrosal nerve arises from this plexus.

Pterygopalatine Fossa

The pterygopalatine fossa lies between the pterygoid process of the sphenoid bone posteriorly, the palatine bone medially and the maxilla anteriorly (Fig. 7.43). It is slit-like and opens laterally through the pterygomaxillary fissure into the infratemporal fossa. It contains part of the maxillary (V_2) division of the trigeminal nerve, the pterygopalatine ganglion and its branches and the termination of the maxillary artery, together with accompanying veins and lymphatics. The pterygopalatine fossa communicates with the middle cranial fossa through the foramen rotundum, with the foramen lacerum through the pterygoid canal, with the orbit through the inferior orbital fissure, with the walls of the nasal cavity through the sphenopalatine foramen and with the palate via the greater and lesser palatine canals.

Maxillary (V_2) division of the trigeminal nerve

The maxillary division (Fig. 7.44) leaves the cranial cavity through the foramen rotundum, crosses the pterygopalatine fossa and continues forwards through the inferior orbital fissure into the orbit. It terminates as the infraorbital nerve, which traverses the infraorbital canal to reach the face. The maxillary division has several branches arising in the pterygopalatine fossa and the floor of the orbit. In the pterygopalatine fossa (see Fig. 7.45), two branches suspend the pterygopalatine ganglion from the parent nerve. Also arising in the fossa are the posterior superior alveolar nerves (Figs 7.44 & 7.45), which descend in the posterior wall of the maxillary air sinus to reach the upper molar teeth. In the floor of the orbit the middle and anterior superior alveolar nerves (Fig. 7.44) arise and descend in the lateral and anterior walls of the maxilla. Collectively the superior alveolar nerves

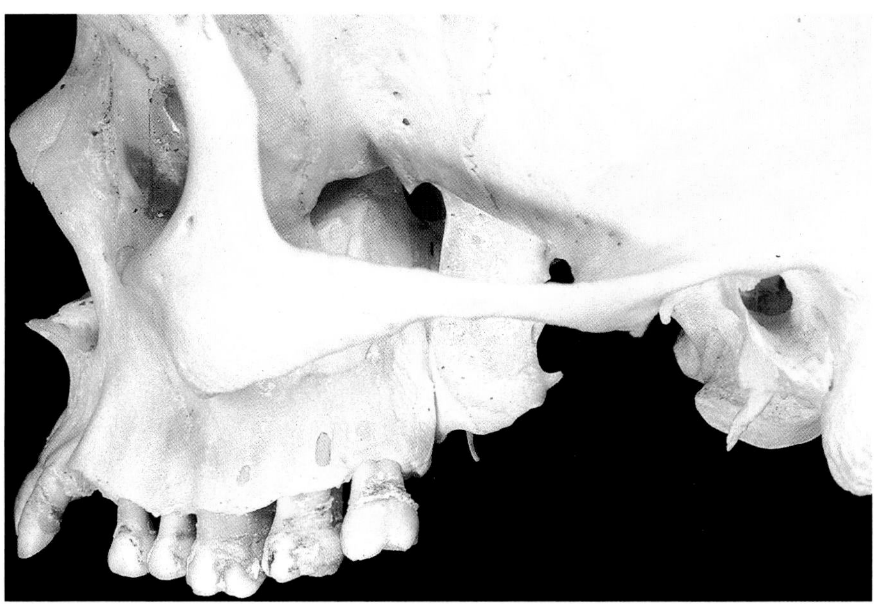

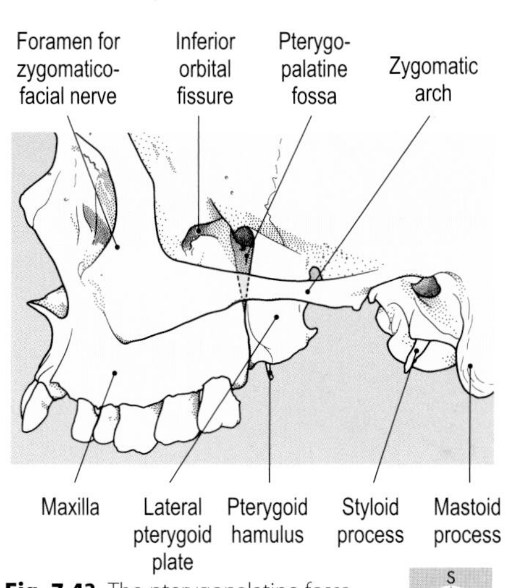

Fig. 7.43 The pterygopalatine fossa, bounded by the maxilla and lateral pterygoid plate.

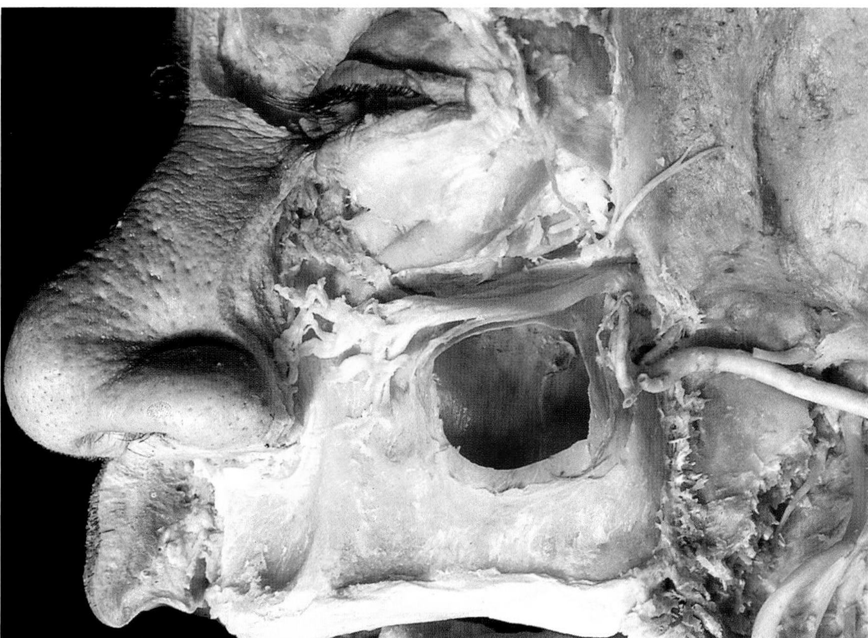

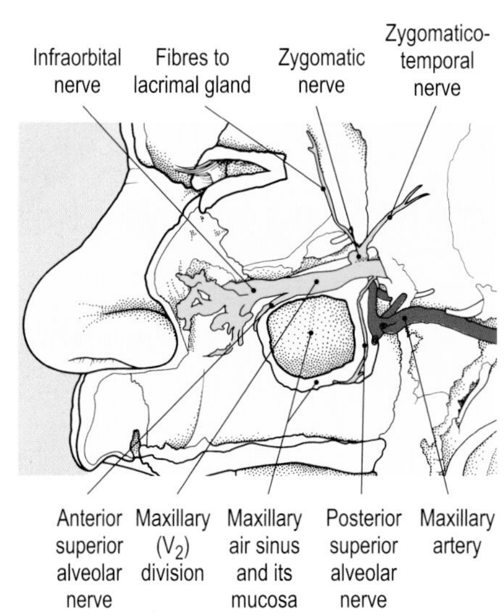

Fig. 7.44 The maxillary nerve and artery, seen after excision of part of the lateral walls of the orbit and maxillary air sinus.

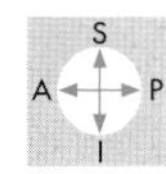

supply the maxilla and its air sinus, the alveolar ridge and all the upper teeth. The zygomatic nerve (see Fig. 7.44) also arises in the floor of the orbit and ascends on the lateral wall, dividing into zygomaticotemporal and zygomaticofacial nerves. These branches pierce the zygomatic bone to supply the overlying facial skin. A branch from the zygomaticotemporal nerve conveys postganglionic parasympathetic fibres from the pterygopalatine ganglion to the lacrimal gland. The infraorbital nerve (see Fig. 7.44) emerges onto the face through the infraorbital foramen and supplies the skin of the cheek, lower eyelid, upper lip and lateral surface of the external nose.

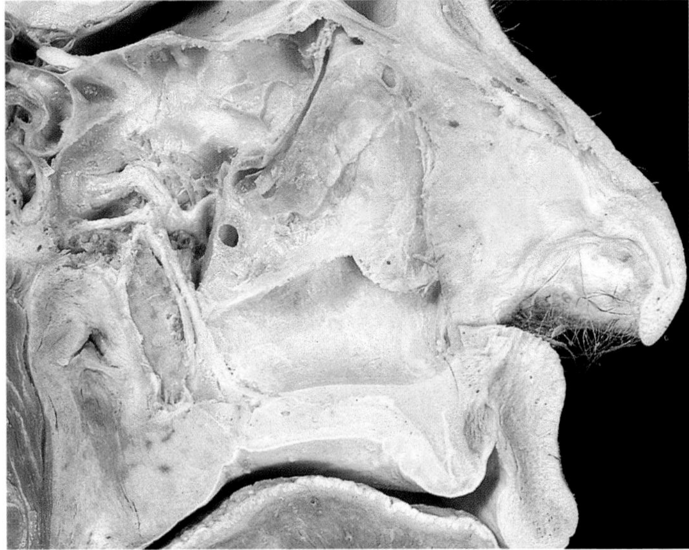

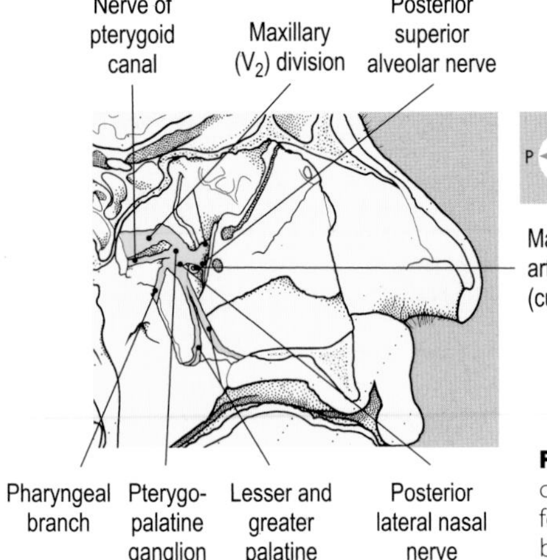

Fig. 7.45 Medial view of the contents of the pterygopalatine fossa, revealed by removal of bone from the lateral wall of the nose.

Pterygopalatine ganglion

The pterygopalatine ganglion (Fig. 7.45) is suspended from the maxillary division in the pterygopalatine fossa and transmits sensory, parasympathetic and sympathetic nerve fibres. Sensory fibres originating in the palate, nose and nasopharynx pass through the ganglion without synapsing to enter the maxillary division. Preganglionic parasympathetic fibres destined for the ganglion leave the brain in the facial (VII) nerve and travel via the greater petrosal nerve. These fibres emerge from the petrous temporal bone and pass along the floor of the middle cranial fossa to enter the foramen lacerum, where they accompany postganglionic vasomotor sympathetic fibres from the carotid plexus as the nerve of the pterygoid canal to reach the pterygopalatine ganglion. In the ganglion the parasympathetic fibres synapse, and postganglionic fibres are distributed through the appropriate branches of the ganglion to the mucous glands in the nose and palate. Secretomotor parasympathetic fibres destined for the lacrimal gland enter the maxillary division and travel in its zygomatic branch. The ganglion earns its nickname, the hay fever ganglion, by virtue of its parasympathetic component. Sympathetic fibres are also distributed in the branches of the ganglion.

There are five groups of branches from the pterygopalatine ganglion (Fig. 7.45): posterior lateral nasal, pharyngeal, nasopalatine, and greater and lesser palatine. Posterior lateral nasal nerves, entering via the sphenopalatine foramen, supply the lateral wall of the nasal cavity. The pharyngeal branch innervates the nasoph-arynx. The nasopalatine nerve (Fig. 7.46) crosses the anterior surface of the body of the sphenoid bone to enter the

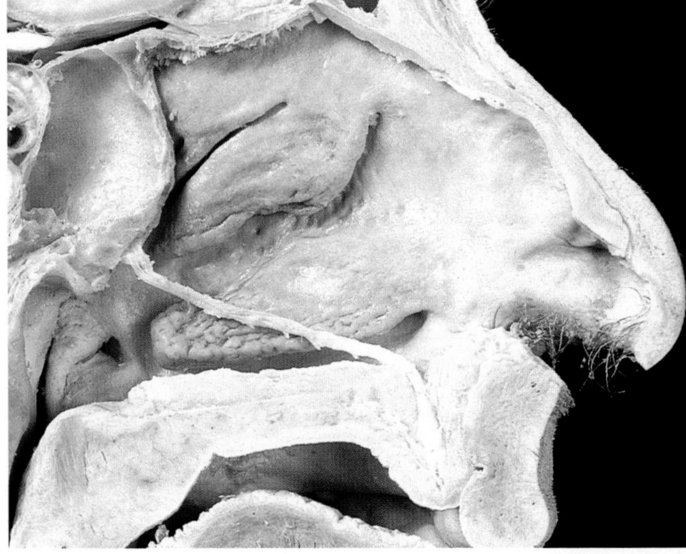

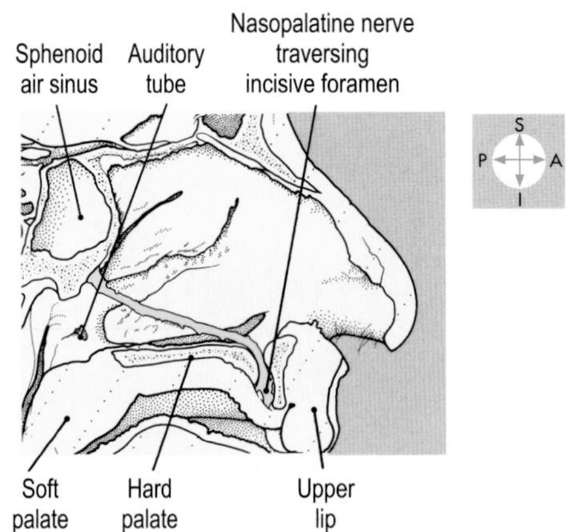

Fig. 7.46 Sagittal section showing the left nasopalatine nerve in situ after removal of the nasal septum.

nasal septum, then angles anteroinferiorly in a groove on the upper edge of the vomer, eventually passing through the incisive canal onto the lower surface of the anterior part of the hard palate. The nerve conveys sensation from the front of the palate and the inferior part of the nasal septum. The greater and lesser palatine nerves traverse the palatine canal to emerge from the appropriate palatine foramina on the lower surface of the hard palate. The greater palatine nerve supplies the hard palate whilst the lesser innervates the soft palate.

Vessels

The maxillary artery (Figs 7.44 & 7.45) enters the pterygopalatine fossa from the infratemporal fossa and divides into its terminal branches accompany the branches of the ganglion and which bear corresponding names. Venous blood drains into the pterygoid plexus, which continues into the infratemporal fossa and communicates with the cavernous sinus via the inferior and superior orbital fissures.

Nasal Cavities and Paranasal Air Sinuses

Nasal cavities

The paired nasal cavities lie centrally within the facial skeleton, medial to the orbits and the maxillary air sinuses (Fig. 7.47). They are separated from the oral cavity by the palate, from the anterior cranial fossa by the cribriform plates and from each other by the midline nasal septum. Anteriorly the cavities lead into the vestibules, which are surrounded by the cartilaginous external nose and open onto the face at the nostrils. Posteriorly the nasal cavities are limited by the free edge of the nasal septum at the choanae (posterior nasal apertures), which open into the nasopharynx. Each cavity is partially subdivided by three shelf-like projections from the lateral wall, the superior, middle and inferior conchae (Fig. 7.48). The parts of the nasal cavity beneath each of these are called correspondingly the superior, middle and inferior meatuses, whilst above the superior concha is the sphenoethmoidal recess. Into this recess and the meatuses drain the paranasal air sinuses and the nasolacrimal duct. Respiratory epithelium lines the cavity and paranasal air sinuses whilst the vestibule has a stratified squamous epithelium bearing nasal vibrissae (hairs).

Bony walls

The medial wall is the nasal septum (Fig. 7.49), common to both cavities and formed superiorly by the perpendicular plate of the ethmoid. This plate continues upwards as the crista galli, which projects into the anterior cranial fossa. The bony septum is completed posteroinferiorly by the vomer. Anteriorly the septum is composed of hyaline cartilage which extends into the external nose.

The roof of each cavity comprises, from in front backwards, the nasal and frontal bones, the cribriform plate of the ethmoid and, finally, the body of the sphenoid bone containing the sphenoidal air sinuses. Olfactory (I) nerves from the olfactory mucosa traverse the many small foramina in the cribriform plate to reach the olfactory bulbs in the anterior cranial fossa (see Fig. 7.50). These nerves are vulnerable to damage in head injuries with fracture of the cribriform plates, disrupting the sense of smell. Leakage of cerebrospinal fluid from the nose may also result from these fractures.

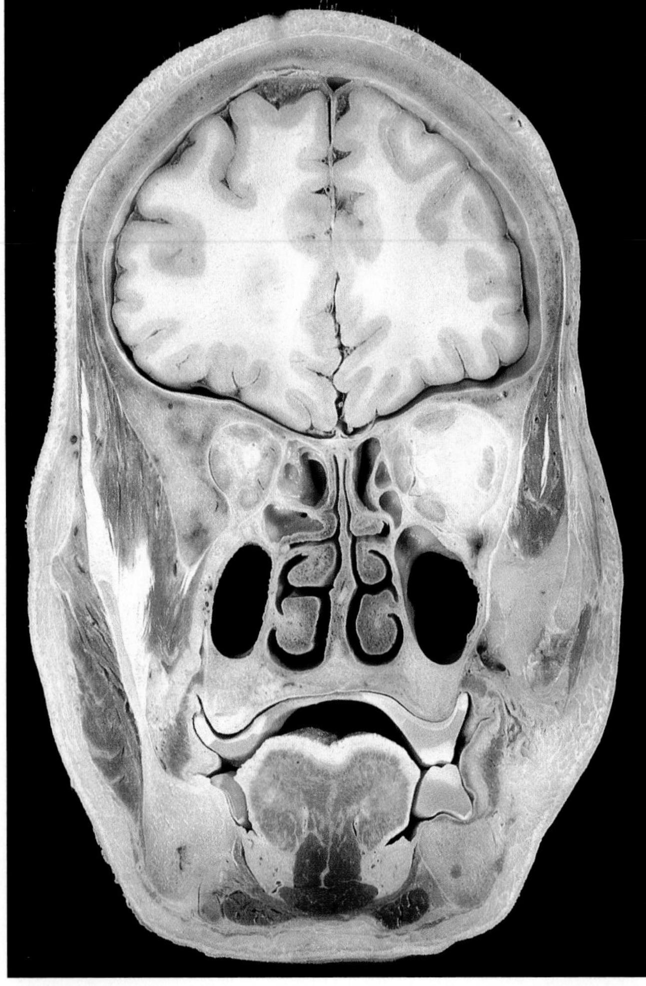

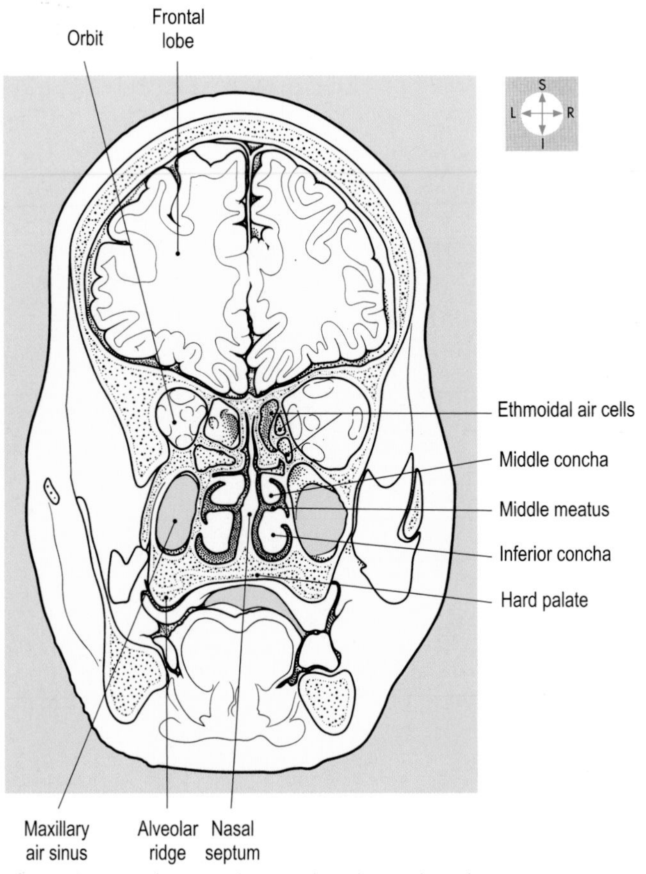

Fig. 7.47 Coronal section showing the orbits and nasal cavities. Posterior aspect. Compare Figs 7.83 & 7.91.

The floor of each nasal cavity is formed by the hard palate, consisting of the palatine process of the maxilla and the horizontal process of the palatine bone.

Numerous bones contribute to the lateral wall (Figs 7.48, 7.50 & 7.51), including the inferior concha and the maxilla, lacrimal, ethmoid, palatine and sphenoid bones. The maxilla forms the anteroinferior portion of the lateral wall and contains the maxillary air sinus. Between the maxilla and the ethmoid, part of the lacrimal bone covers the nasolacrimal canal, which opens into the inferior meatus. Each labyrinth (lateral mass) of the ethmoid is attached to the lateral part of the cribriform plate and contains numerous air cells. From the medial surface of the labyrinth project the small superior and the larger middle conchae. The ethmoidal air cells bulge into the middle meatus, forming the bulla, beneath which a curved groove, the hiatus semilunaris, separates the ethmoid from the maxilla. Forming the posterior limit of the hiatus semilunaris is the vertical plate of the palatine bone. The most posterior component of the lateral wall is the medial pterygoid plate of the sphenoid. Overlying the maxilla and palatine bones is a separate bone, the inferior concha.

Sensory nerve supply

The somatic sensory nerve supply to the walls of the nasal cavity is derived mainly from the maxillary (V_2) division of the trigeminal nerve. The lateral nasal nerves from the pterygopalatine ganglion (see p. 352) supply most of the lateral wall, while the nasopalatine nerve supplies the septum. Lesser and greater palatine nerves supply the posterior part of the lateral wall and the floor. In addition, fibres from the ophthalmic (V_1) division reach the nasal cavity via the anterior ethmoidal nerve. This nerve sup-

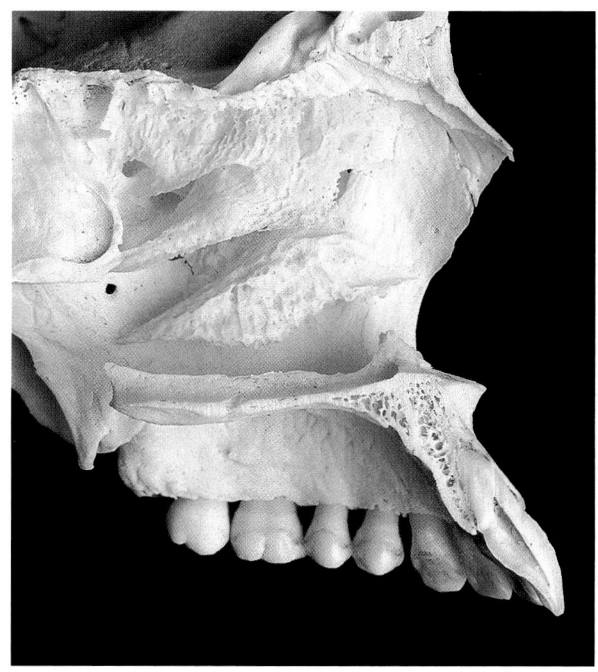

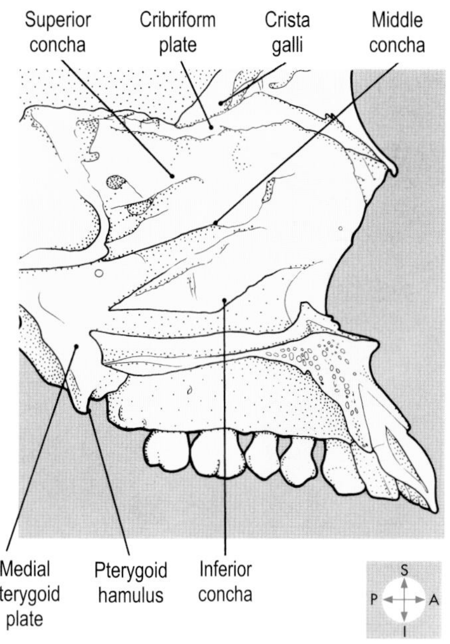

Fig. 7.48 Bony lateral wall of nasal cavity after sagittal section and removal of the septum.

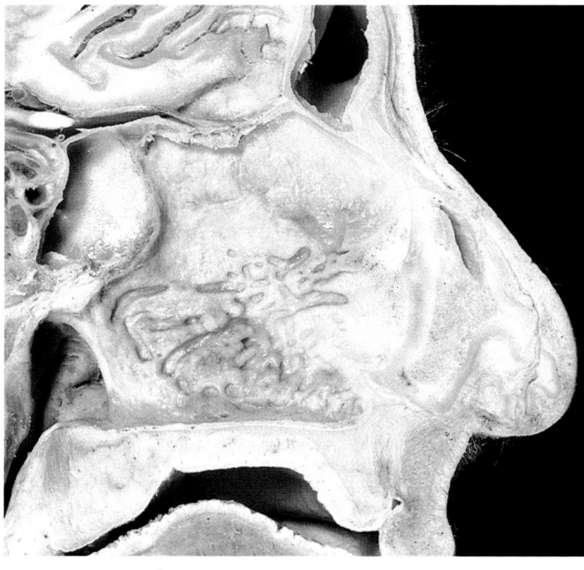

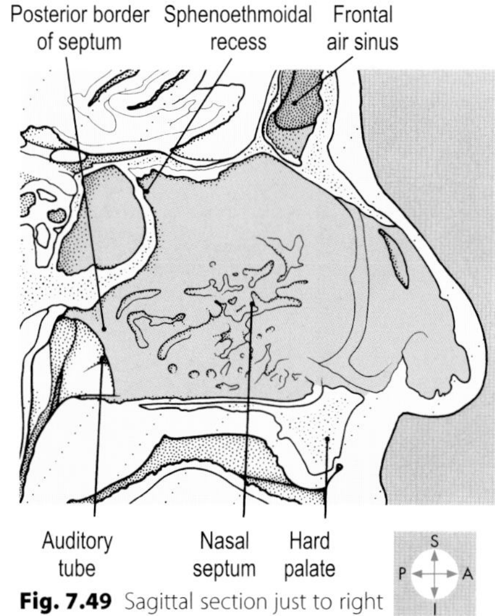

Fig. 7.49 Sagittal section just to right of midline with intact nasal septum.

plies the anterosuperior parts of the septum and the lateral wall and continues as the external nasal nerve to supply most of the external nose.

Blood supply

Most of the blood supply to the walls of the nasal cavity is provided by branches of the maxillary artery. These vessels arise in the pterygopalatine fossa and are named according to the branches of the pterygopalatine ganglion they accompany. The anteroinferior part of the nasal septum is highly vascular (Little's area) and commonly gives rise to nasal haemorrhage (epistaxis).

Venous blood passes to the pterygoid plexus, the facial vein and the ophthalmic veins.

Paranasal air sinuses

There are four paired groups of paranasal air sinuses (Figs 7.51, 7.52 & 7.53) contained within the frontal, maxillary, ethmoid and sphenoid bones. Each sinus communicates with the nasal cavity, is lined with mucous membrane and normally contains air. The frontal air sinuses are situated in the vertical and horizontal parts of the frontal bone, closely related to the frontal lobes of the brain. They are variable in size and open into the middle meatus at the infundibulum, the most anterior part of the hiatus semilunaris. The frontal air sinus is supplied by the supraorbital branch of the ophthalmic (V_1) division of the trigeminal nerve.

The maxillary air sinus (antrum) occupies the body of the maxilla, lying above the oral cavity and alveolar ridge and below

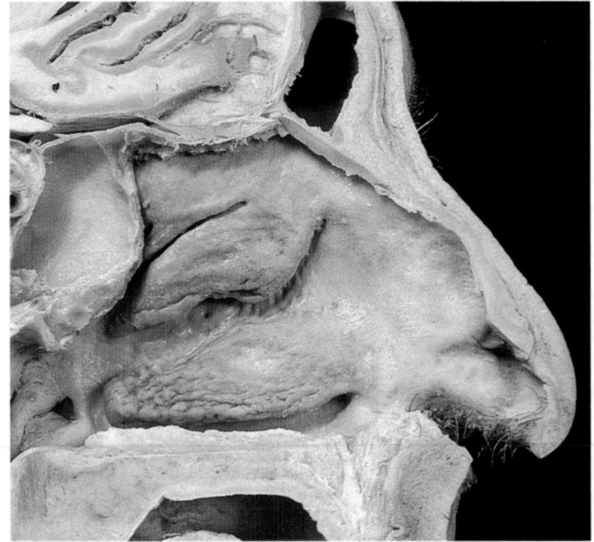

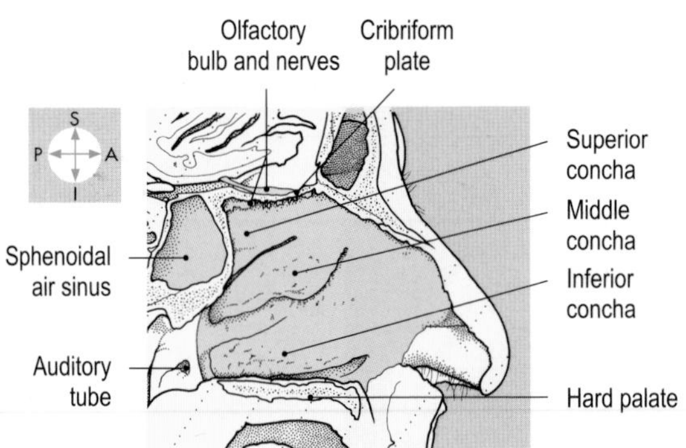

Fig. 7.50 Sagittal section with the nasal septum removed to show the lateral wall of the nasal cavity.

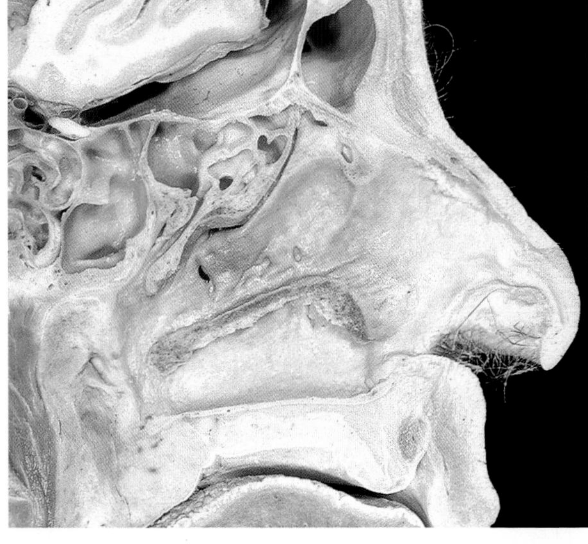

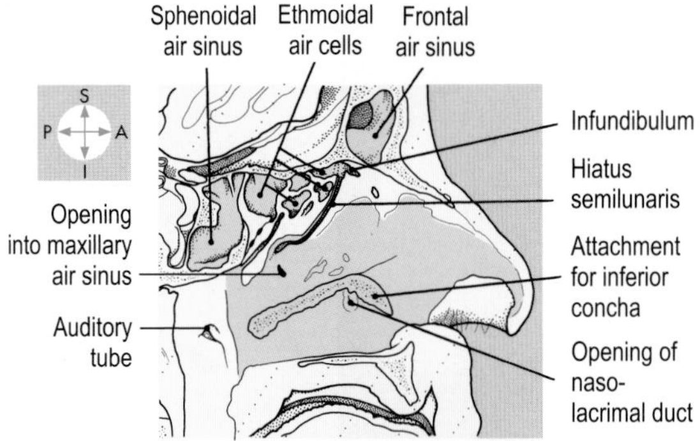

Fig. 7.51 Sagittal section after removal of the conchae, the ethmoid bulla and the upper part of the lateral nasal wall.

the orbit. Its opening at the posterior end of the hiatus semilunaris lies high on the medial wall of the antrum, permitting limited drainage for contents such as mucus or pus. Sensory innervation is from the superior alveolar nerves.

The ethmoidal air sinuses are subdivided into three groups of air cells, which communicate with the nose through many tiny foramina. The anterior cells open into the floor of the hiatus whilst the middle cells open onto the bulla, both groups being supplied by the anterior ethmoidal nerve. The posterior group, innervated by the posterior ethmoidal nerve, drains into the superior meatus under the superior concha.

The sphenoidal air sinuses lie just below the sella turcica in the body of the sphenoid, through the anterior wall of which they open into the sphenoethmoidal recess. The sensory supply is from the pharyngeal branch of the pterygopalatine ganglion.

Infection of the paranasal air sinuses (sinusitis) causes thickening of the mucosal lining which may block the openings into the nasal cavities.

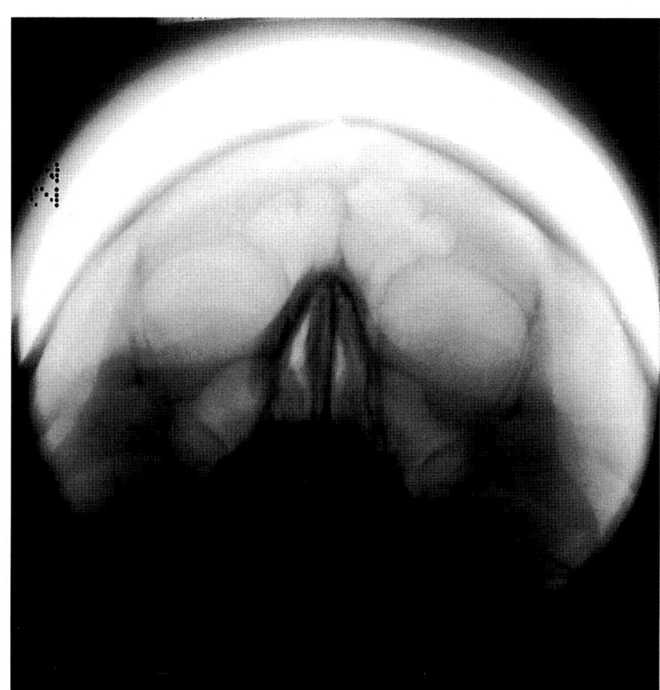

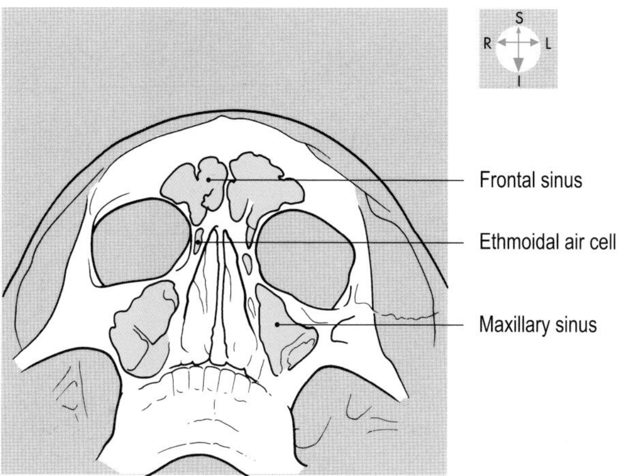

Fig. 7.52 Occipitomental radiograph showing paranasal air sinuses.

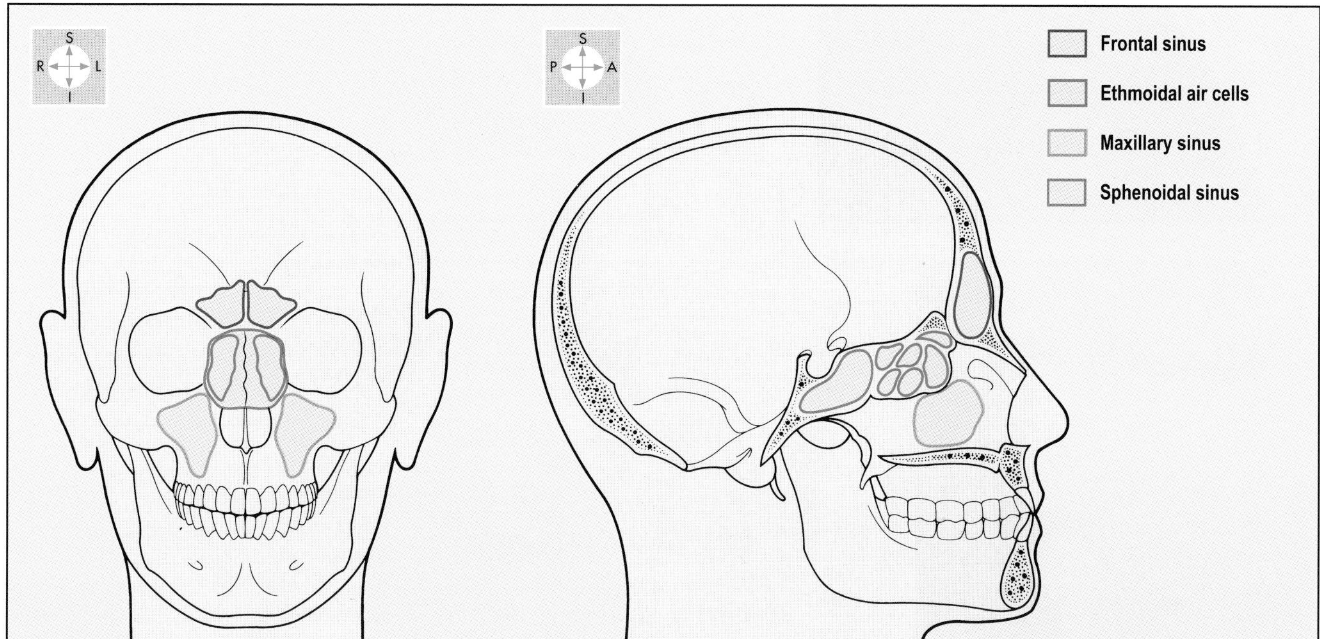

Fig. 7.53 Position of the paranasal air sinuses.

Palate

The palate consists of hard and soft parts covered by mucous membrane (Fig. 7.54). The hard palate separates the oral and nasal cavities whilst posteriorly the soft palate separates the nasopharynx from the oropharynx.

Hard palate

The bones that comprise the hard palate are the palatine processes of the maxillae anteriorly and the horizontal plates of the palatine bones posteriorly (see Fig. 7.81). The hard palate is bounded in front and laterally by the superior alveolar ridge. The soft palate is attached to the free posterior border of the hard palate. Sensory fibres reach the palate in branches of the maxillary (V_2) division of the trigeminal nerve. The nasopalatine nerve emerges from the incisive foramen and supplies the anterior part of the hard palate. The greater palatine nerve gains the hard palate via the greater palatine foramen and innervates its posterior portion.

Soft palate

The soft palate projects into the cavity of the pharynx from its attachment to the posterior edge of the hard palate. When elevated it separates the oropharynx from the nasopharynx. Five paired muscles attach to the soft palate and contribute to its structure. In the midline the uvula projects downwards from its posterior free border.

Muscles

Tensor veli palatini (Fig. 7.56) attaches to the scaphoid fossa and spine of the sphenoid and to the lateral surface of the cartilaginous portion of the auditory (Eustachian) tube. Its fibres descend

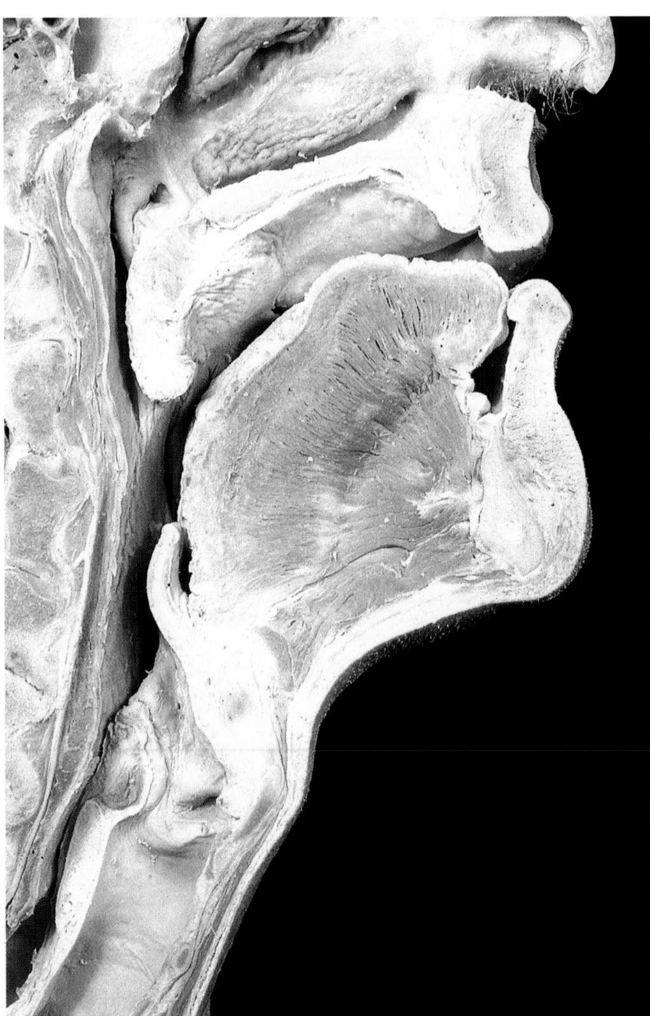

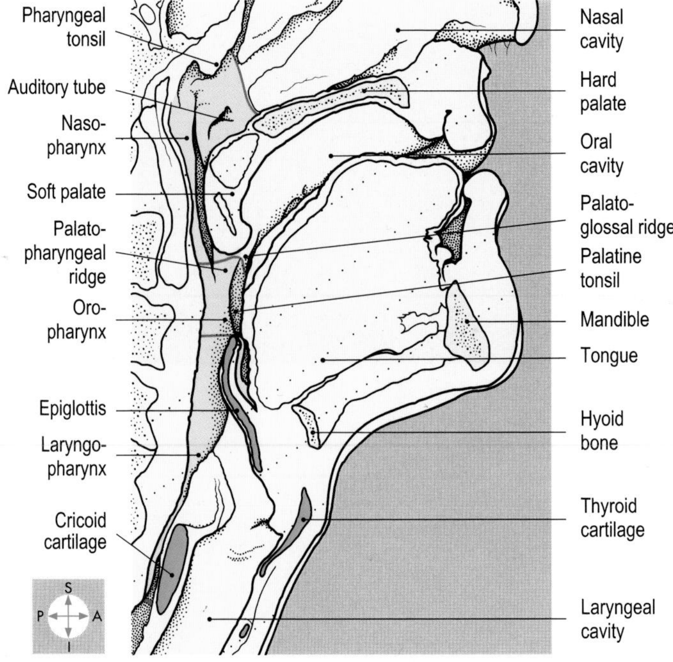

Fig. 7.54 Sagittal section through palate and pharynx showing communications with the nasal, oral and laryngeal cavities. Red line, boundaries of subdivisions of pharynx.

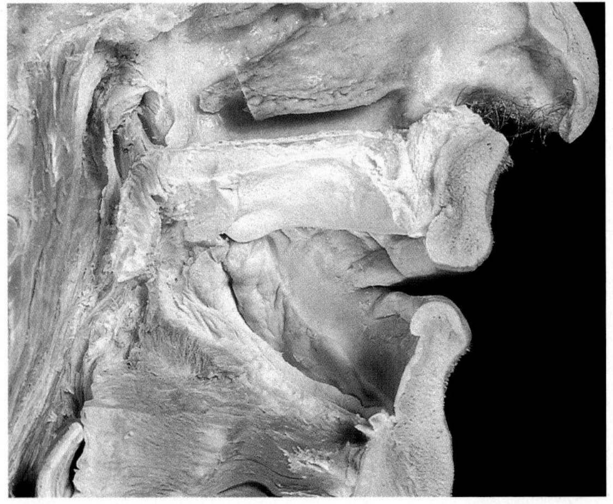

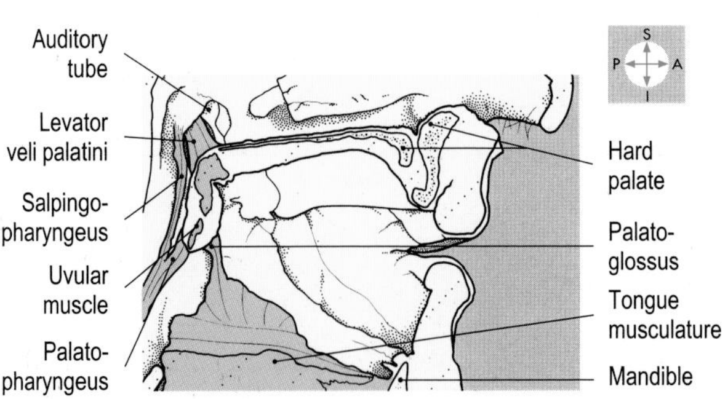

Fig. 7.55 Further dissection of Fig. 7.54 to show some of the muscles of the soft palate.

between the lateral and medial pterygoid plates on the lateral aspect of the pharyngeal wall and give way to a tendon just above the pterygoid hamulus. The tendon hooks under the hamulus and turns medially to enter the soft palate, where it forms the palatine aponeurosis by fanning out and attaching to the posterior border of the hard palate. The palatine aponeurosis forms the basic structure of the soft palate to which other muscles gain attachment. Tensor veli palatini is supplied by the mandibular (V_3) division of the trigeminal nerve and tenses the soft palate.

Levator veli palatini (Figs 7.55 & 7.56) attaches to the inferior surface of the petrous temporal bone just medial to the opening of the auditory tube and to the adjacent part of the tube. Its fibres descend medial to the medial pterygoid plate within the pharynx and attach to the upper surface of the palatine aponeurosis. The muscle is innervated by the pharyngeal plexus (see p. 361). Levator veli palatini elevates the soft palate during swallowing, preventing regurgitation of food into the nasal cavities.

Palatoglossus (Fig. 7.55) descends from the inferior surface of the palatine aponeurosis and inclines slightly forwards to enter the posterolateral part of the tongue. The position of palatoglossus is evident on the inner surface of the oral cavity as a mucosal elevation, the palatoglossal ridge (anterior pillar of the fauces; Fig. 7.54). The two palatoglossal ridges form the oropharyngeal isthmus, which marks the posterior boundary of the oral cavity. Innervated by fibres from the pharyngeal plexus, palatoglossus lowers the soft palate, raises the posterior part of the tongue and moves the palatoglossal ridge towards the midline, thus narrowing the isthmus.

Palatopharyngeus (Figs 7.55 & 7.56) attaches to the undersurface of the soft palate. Most of its fibres run posteroinferiorly as part of the longitudinal layer of muscle inside the pharynx and form the palatopharyngeal ridge (posterior pillar of the fauces). On contraction these fibres depress the soft palate. Other fibres pass horizontally backwards, raising the mucosa into a ridge against which the soft palate is elevated. Palatopharyngeus receives its motor supply from the pharyngeal plexus.

The uvular muscle (Figs 7.55 & 7.56), also supplied by the pharyngeal plexus, lies entirely within the soft palate and elevates the uvula. In cases of unilateral paralysis of the soft palate the uvula rises asymmetrically, being pulled away from the paralyzed side.

Sensory and secretomotor innervation to the soft palate is from the lesser palatine nerves of the maxillary (V_2) division of the trigeminal nerve, supplemented laterally on the undersurface of the palate by the glossopharyngeal (IX) nerve.

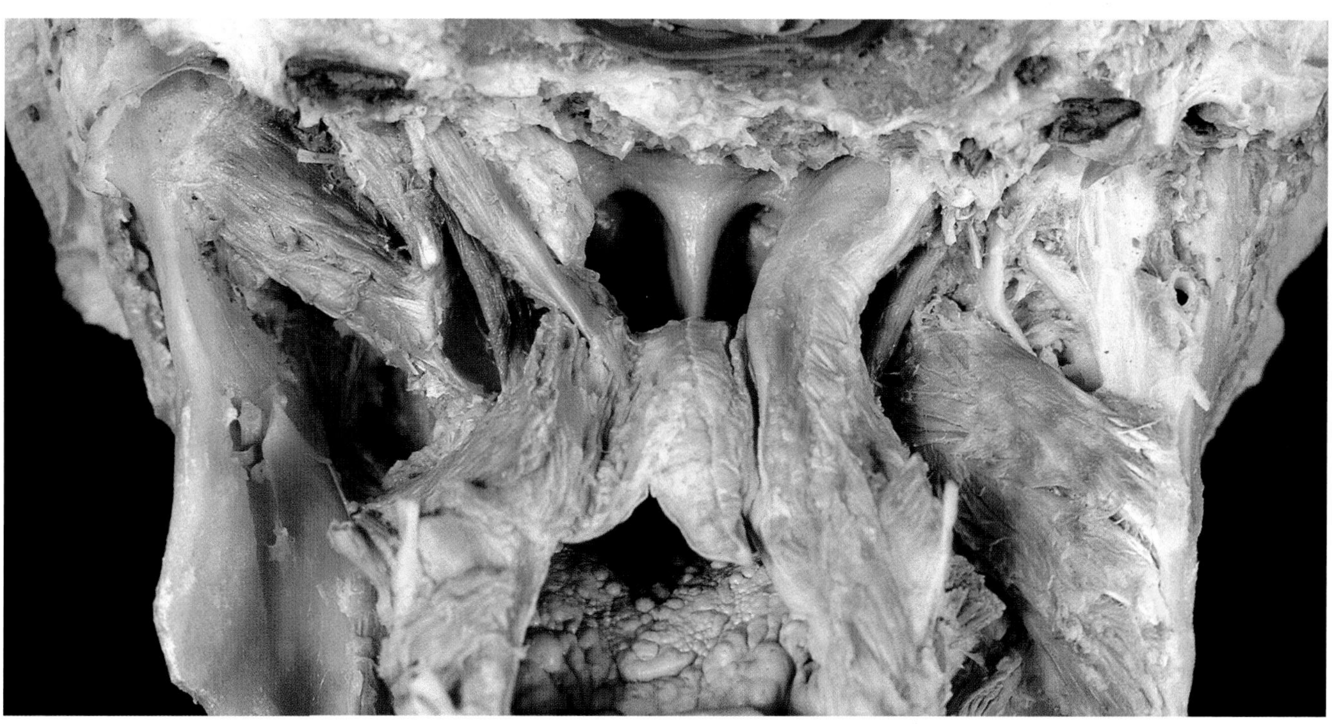

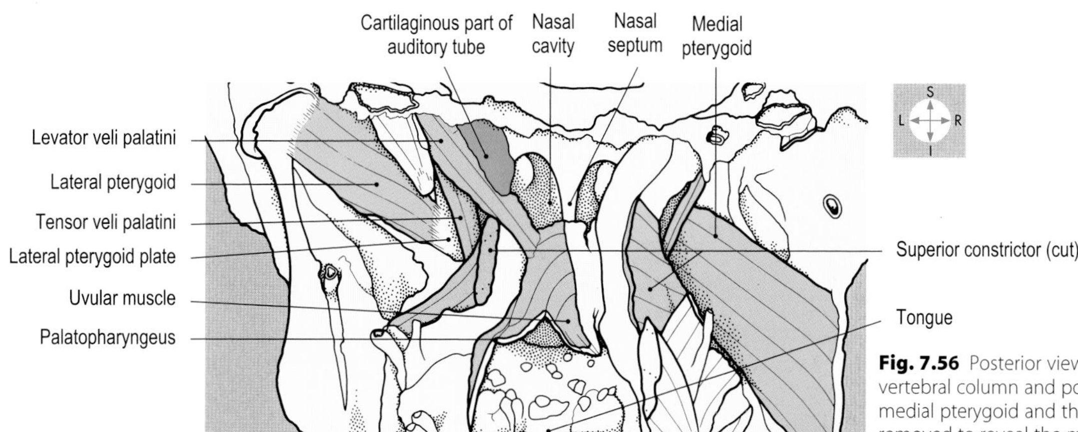

Fig. 7.56 Posterior view of soft palate after removal of cervical vertebral column and posterior wall of pharynx. On the left side, the medial pterygoid and the mucosa of the soft palate have been removed to reveal the muscles.

Pharynx

The pharynx is a muscular tube, which is continuous inferiorly with the oesophagus and into which the nasal, oral and laryngeal cavities open (Fig. 7.59). For descriptive purposes the pharynx is divided into nasopharynx, oropharynx and laryngopharynx (see Fig. 7.54). The nasopharynx is attached to the base of the skull and is bounded anteriorly by the choanae. Inferiorly it is continuous with the oropharynx at the level of the soft palate. The oropharynx begins anteriorly at the palatoglossal ridge and extends inferiorly to the level of the upper border of the epiglottis where it is in continuity with the laryngopharynx. The laryngopharynx lies behind the laryngeal inlet, the arytenoids and the cricoid lamina, and on either side of the inlet forms recesses, the piriform fossae (see Fig. 7.60). In normal deglutition these fossae are traversed by fluid and food which pass behind the cricoid cartilage in the terminal part of the laryngopharynx. Foreign bodies such as fish bones may lodge in these recesses during swallowing. At the inferior border of the cricoid cartilage, it is continuous with the oesophagus. The musculature of the pharynx consists of incomplete outer circular and inner longitudinal layers. The pharyngobasilar fascia lies internal to the muscle coat and is lined by mucous membrane.

Muscles

The circular layer of muscles comprises three overlapping constrictors, attaching posteriorly to the midline raphe (Figs 7.57 & 7.58), which is suspended from the pharyngeal tubercle of the occipital bone.

The superior constrictor attaches anteriorly to the lower part of the medial pterygoid plate, the pterygomandibular raphe (in company with buccinator; see p. 334) and the posterior end of the mylohyoid line on the mandible. Posteriorly its fibres attach to the pharyngeal tubercle and the pharyngeal raphe.

The middle constrictor attaches to the lower part of the stylohyoid ligament and to the angle between the greater and lesser horns of the hyoid bone. Posteriorly it attaches to the raphe, the upper fibres overlapping those of the superior constrictor.

The inferior constrictor has an anterior attachment to the oblique line on the thyroid cartilage, the lateral surface of the cricoid cartilage and the intervening fascia covering the cricothyroid muscle. Its superior fibres curve upwards to the pharyngeal raphe, overlapping those of the middle constrictor. The lower fibres, known as cricopharyngeus, pass horizontally around the lumen of the pharynx below the raphe.

The inner longitudinal layer consists of the stylopharyngeus, palatopharyngeus and salpingopharyngeus muscles. Stylopharyngeus (see p. 346) attaches to the styloid process and lies lateral to the superior constrictor. Its fibres descend between the superior and middle constrictors (Fig. 7.58) to blend with the other longitudinal muscles on the medial surface of the two lower constrictors. Palatopharyngeus inclines posteroinferiorly from the soft palate whilst salpingopharyngeus descends from the auditory tube, both muscles lying on the inner surface of the constrictors (see Fig. 7.55). The longitudinal muscles attach inferiorly to the posterior border of the lamina of the thyroid cartilage.

During swallowing, the pharyngeal constrictors contract sequentially from above downwards to propel the bolus of food into the oesophagus. Simultaneously the longitudinal muscles shorten the pharynx and elevate the larynx, thus closing its inlet against the base of the tongue. Due to the shape of the epiglottis, the bolus tends to traverse the piriform fossae. At the same time, the soft palate is raised to prevent food entering the nasopharynx and the cricopharyngeus relaxes to allow the bolus to enter the oesophagus.

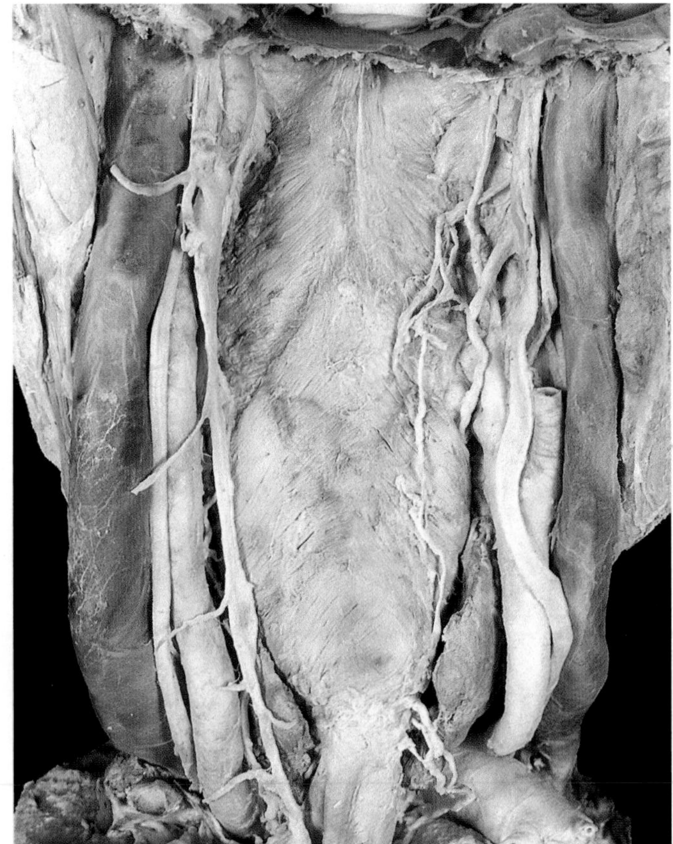

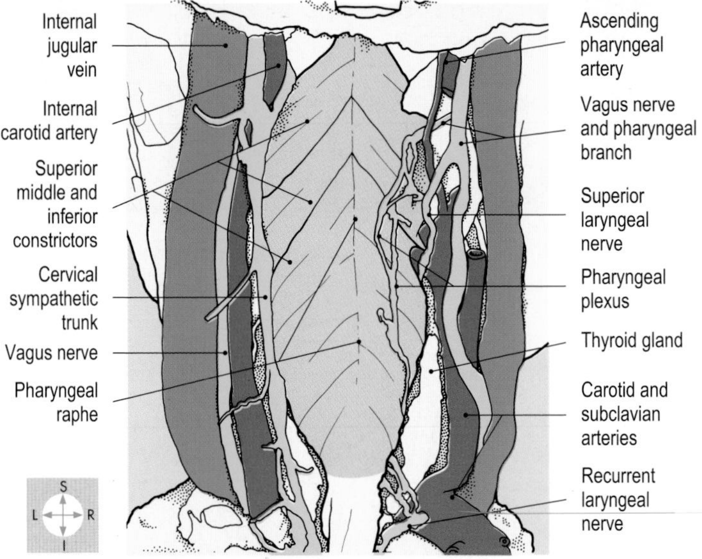

Fig. 7.57 Posterior view of pharyngeal musculature after removal of cervical vertebral column, posterior part of the skull, right sympathetic trunk and part of the right internal carotid artery.

Nerve supply

The pharyngeal plexus (Fig. 7.57) consists of nerve fibres lying on the outer surface of the pharynx and receives the pharyngeal branches of the glossopharyngeal (IX) and vagus (X) nerves. The motor component of the plexus is derived from the cranial part of the accessory (XI) nerve via the vagus nerve. It supplies the muscles of the pharynx except for stylopharyngeus (glossopharyngeal nerve, see p. 350).

Sensory fibres from the glossopharyngeal nerve traverse the plexus to supply the oropharynx whilst the vagal fibres of the plexus, assisted by those travelling in the laryngeal nerves (see p. 367), innervate the laryngopharynx. The sensory innervation of the nasopharynx is supplied by the maxillary (V_2) division of the trigeminal nerve via its pharyngeal branch from the pterygopalatine ganglion.

Pharyngobasilar fascia and auditory tube

The inner surface of the pharyngeal musculature is lined by the pharyngobasilar fascia. This fascial sheet completes the wall of the pharynx superiorly and forms a continuous attachment to the base of the skull. Inferiorly the fascia becomes gradually thinner, blending with the epimysium of the pharyngeal muscles.

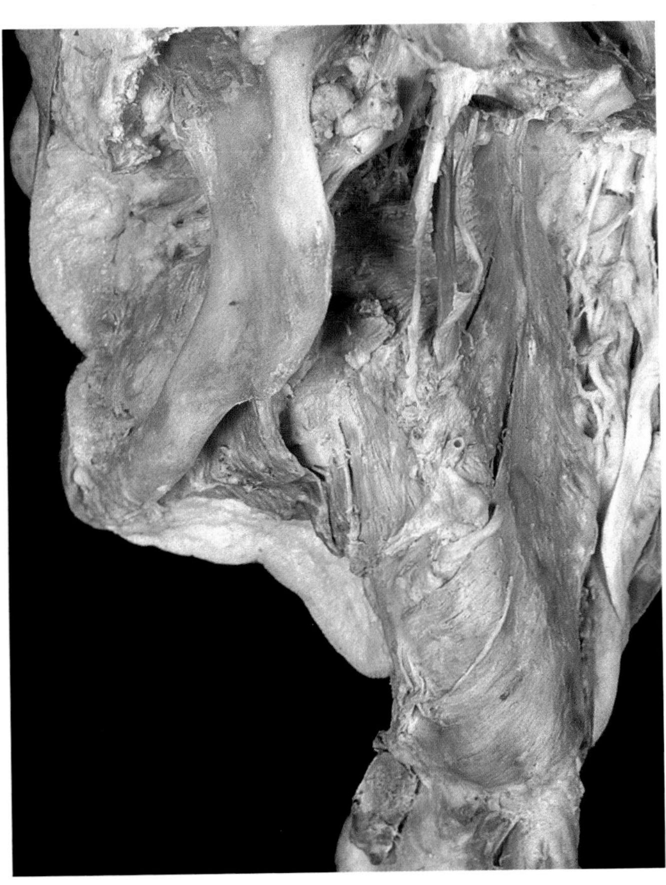

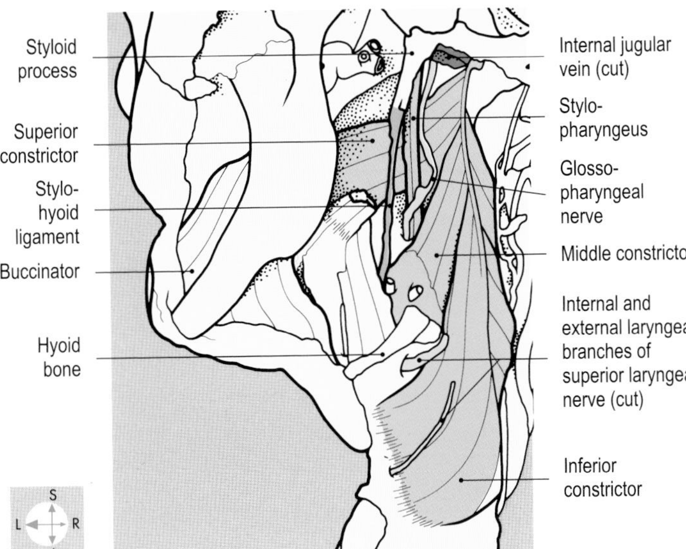

Fig. 7.58 Oblique posterior view of pharyngeal musculature.

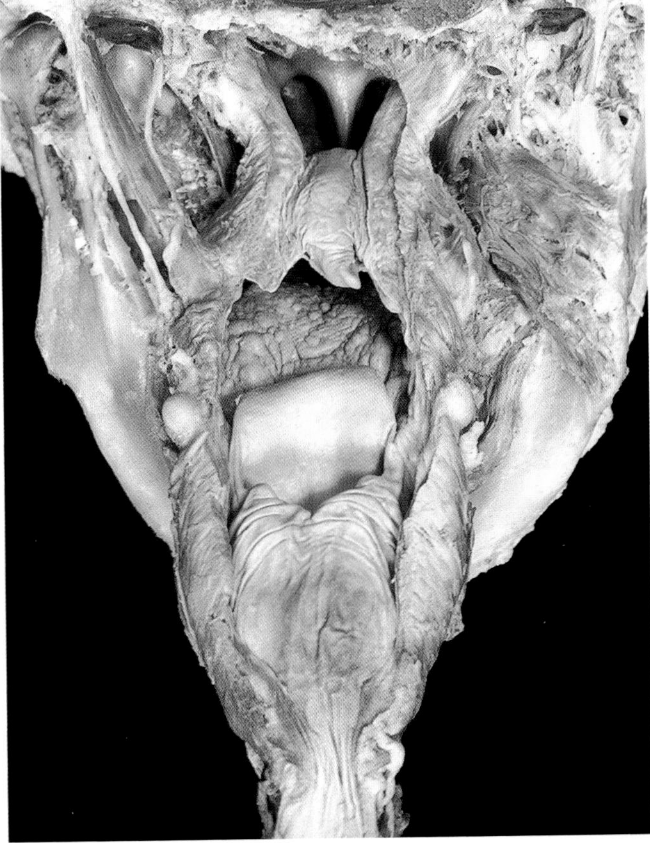

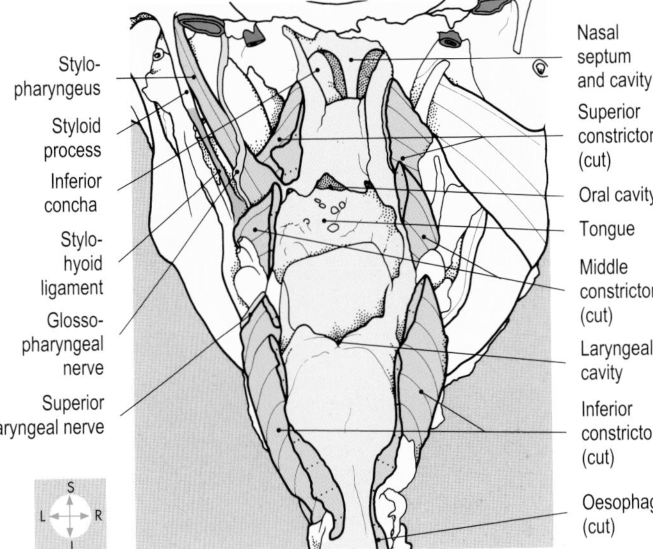

Fig. 7.59 Interior of the pharynx. This specimen retains medial pterygoid on the right and the styloid apparatus on the left.

The auditory (Eustachian) tube (see Figs 7.54–7.56) opens into the nasopharynx above the superior constrictor by piercing the pharyngobasilar fascia. Laterally the auditory tube leads into the cavity of the middle ear.

Lymphoid tissue

An incomplete ring of lymphoid tissue, the pharyngeal lymphoid ring (Waldeyer's ring) (see Fig. 7.54), lies in the wall of the pharynx between the mucosa and the muscles. This tissue is often subject to infection, particularly in children. On each side a palatine tonsil lies between the palatoglossal and palatopharyngeal ridges and has a rich blood supply, including its own tonsillar branch from the facial artery. The adenoids, or pharyngeal tonsils, are situated near the roof of the nasopharynx, close to the auditory tubes with their tubal tonsils. When enlarged, the adenoids may obstruct one or both tubes, giving rise to middle ear disease. The lingual tonsil lies under the mucosa of the posterior third of the tongue and comprises a diffuse collection of small lymphoid follicles.

Blood supply

The arterial supply to the pharynx is derived from branches of the facial, lingual and maxillary arteries (see p. 330). The ascending pharyngeal artery (see Fig. 7.57) is a direct branch of the external carotid artery and passes upwards medial to the styloid muscles on the lateral surface of the pharynx. Venous blood drains into the pterygoid plexus and the internal jugular vein.

Larynx

The larynx acts as a sphincter guarding the lower respiratory tract and is responsible for phonation. It lies in the neck and its inlet is continuous with the laryngopharynx (Figs 7.60 & 7.61). Inferiorly the larynx is continuous with the trachea. It consists of a framework of cartilages and bone, which supports the vocal and vestibular folds and the muscles that move them. Anteriorly lie the infrahyoid strap muscles.

Skeleton

The skeleton of the larynx comprises the thyroid, cricoid and arytenoid cartilages, the epiglottis and the hyoid bone.

The thyroid cartilage (see Figs 7.66 & 7.67) has two flat laminae joined anteriorly to form the midline laryngeal prominence ('Adam's apple'). The posterior margin of each lamina is free and bears a superior and an inferior horn. The tips of the inferior horns articulate by tiny synovial joints with the lateral surfaces of the cricoid cartilage.

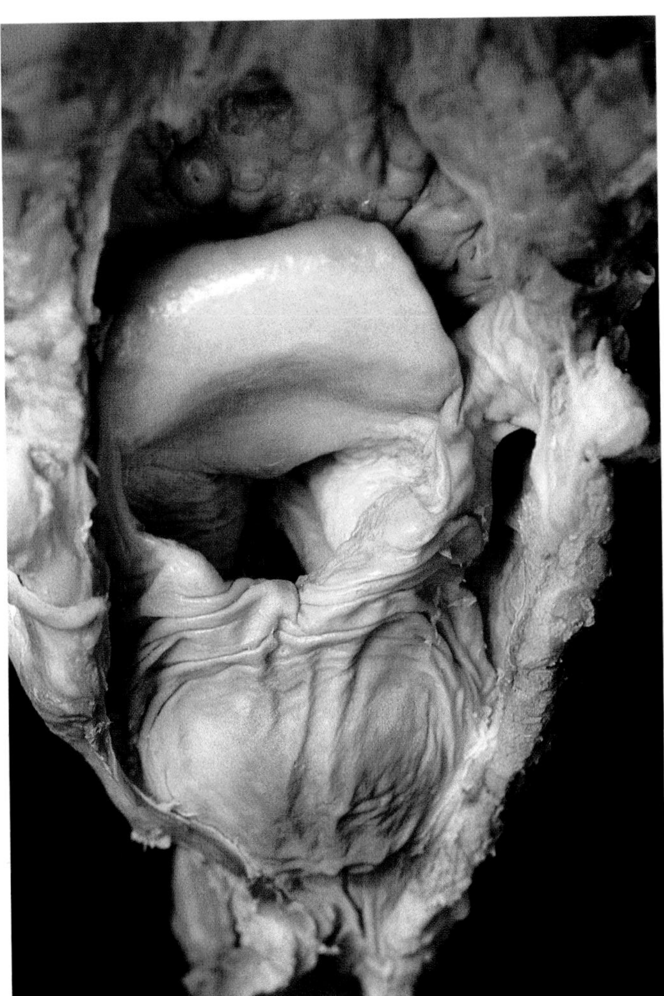

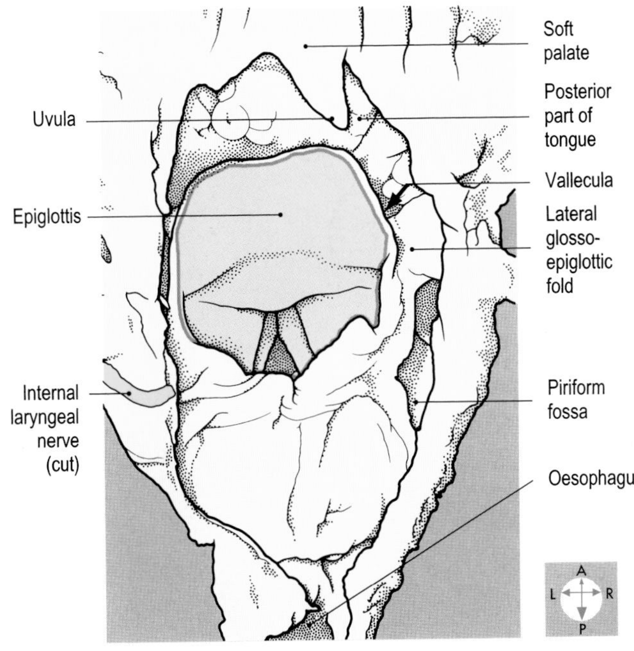

Fig. 7.60 Posterosuperior view of the larynx, seen through the opened laryngopharynx. The lumen of the larynx is visible through the laryngeal inlet (pink line).

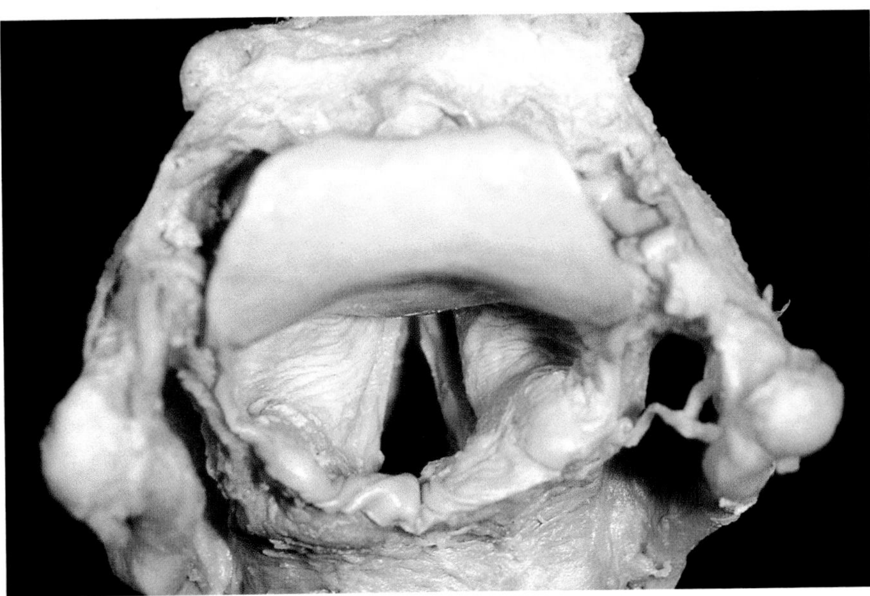

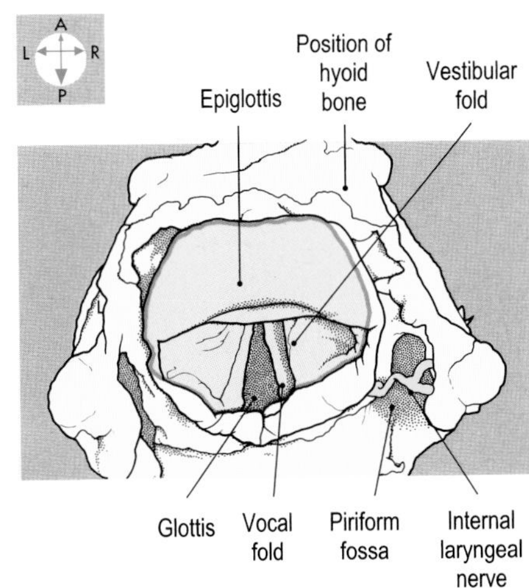

Fig. 7.61 Superior view into the larynx. The mucosa lining the laryngopharynx has been removed to reveal the internal laryngeal nerve (laryngeal inlet, pink line).

The cricoid cartilage (see Figs 7.66 & 7.70) lies below the thyroid cartilage and is shaped like a signet ring, with a narrow anterior arch and a wide posterior lamina. Its inferior border lies horizontally whilst the superior border slopes upwards posteriorly. Movement at the cricothyroid joints allows the arch of the cricoid to tip upwards whilst the lamina tips backwards.

In addition to its articulations with the thyroid cartilage, the upper border of the cricoid lamina bears articular surfaces, one on each side of the midline, for synovial joints with the two arytenoid cartilages. Each arytenoid (Figs 7.63, 7.66 & 7.70) is pyramidal in shape, with its base on the cricoid lamina and its apex superiorly. It has four surfaces (medial, posterior, anterolateral

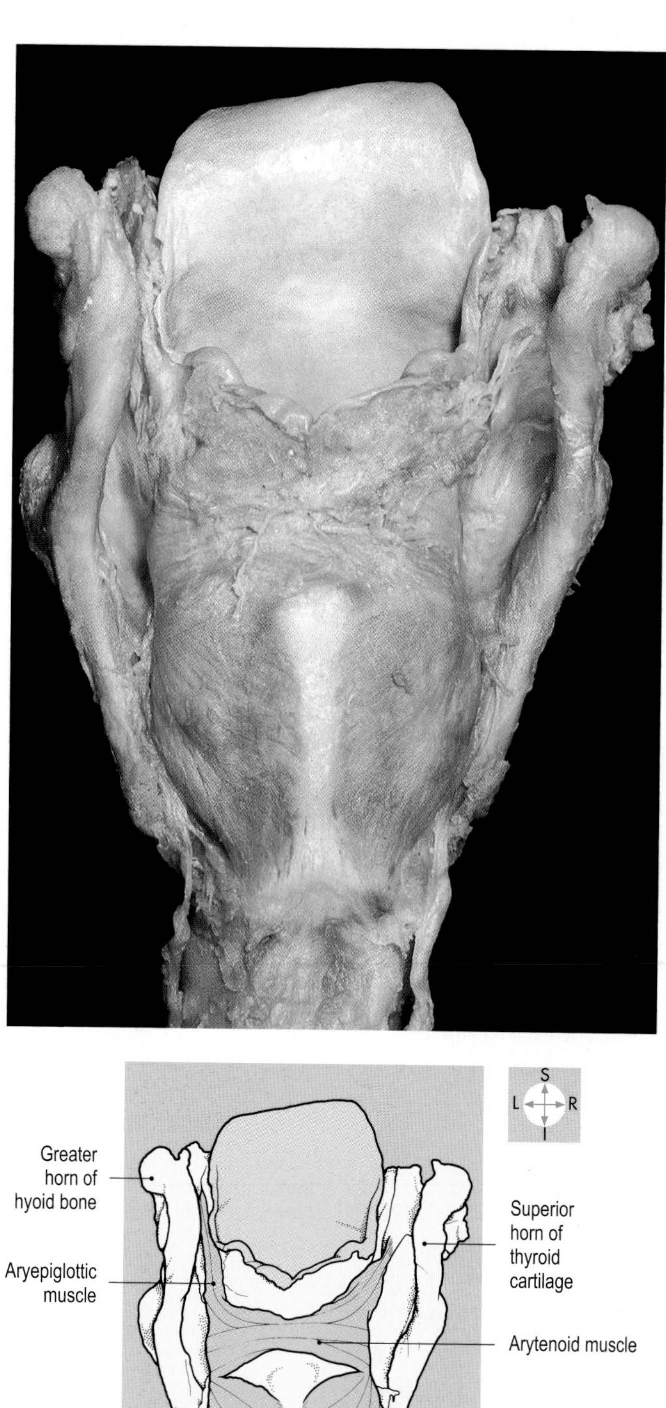

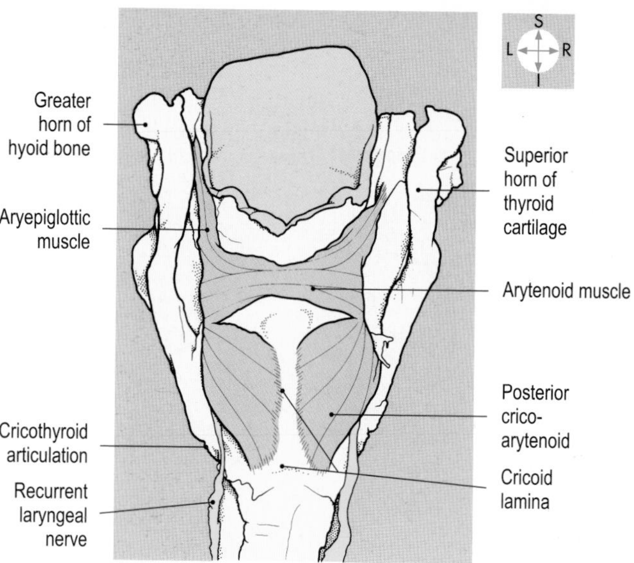

Fig. 7.62 Some of the intrinsic muscles of the larynx, seen after removal of the mucosa of the laryngopharynx.

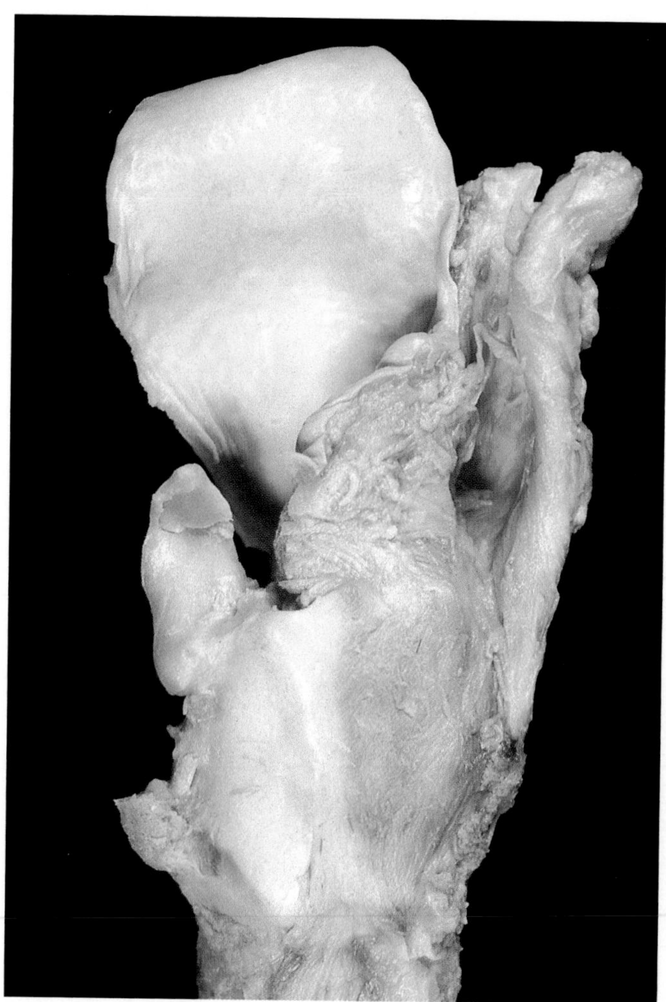

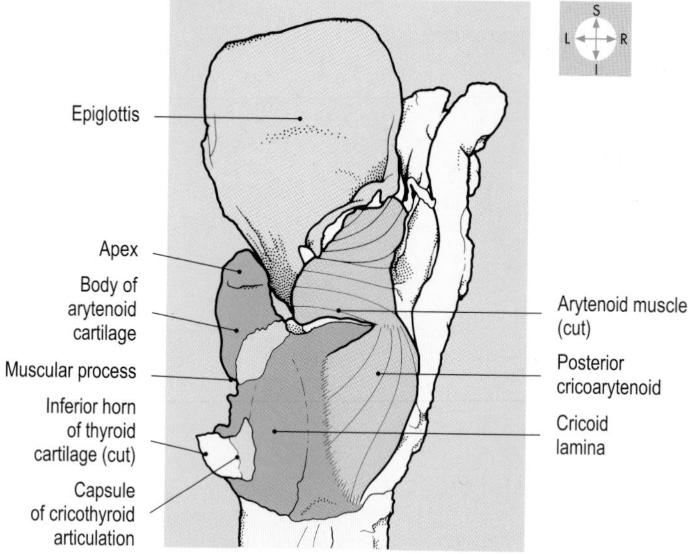

Fig. 7.63 Cricoid and arytenoid cartilages, exposed by removal of most of the soft tissues on the left of the larynx.

and inferior) and two processes. Anteriorly lies the vocal process, to which the vocal fold is attached, whilst its muscular process projects laterally. Each arytenoid is able to rotate around its own vertical axis. In addition, the arytenoids can slide laterally and downwards away from the midline on the slope of the articular surface on the cricoid.

The epiglottis (Figs 7.63 & 7.66) is attached in the midline to the inner surface of the thyroid cartilage, just below the laryngeal prominence. It extends upwards and backwards behind the tongue to which it is attached in the midline by the median glosso-epiglottic fold. From each side of the epiglottis a lateral glosso-epiglottic fold (see Fig. 7.60) extends to the side of the tongue. These folds bound a recess on each side of the midline, the vallecula (see Fig 7.60), which is a site where swallowed foreign bodies may lodge. The epiglottis overlies the laryngeal inlet when the larynx is raised against the tongue when swallowing.

The hyoid bone (see Figs 7.61 & 7.66) is the uppermost skeletal element of the larynx. It consists of a midline body bearing greater horns projecting posteriorly. On each side a lesser horn is located on the upper surface where the body and greater horn unite.

Membranes and ligaments

Several membranes are attached to the laryngeal framework and fill the gaps between the skeletal structures. The conus elasticus (cricovocal membrane) (see Fig. 7.65) is elastic and attaches inferiorly to the upper border of the cricoid cartilage. In the midline anteriorly, it reaches the inferior border of the thyroid cartilage, forming the inelastic cricothyroid ligament. Posteriorly it is attached to the vocal processes of the arytenoids. The membrane has a free upper border, which runs between the arytenoids and the thyroid cartilage and forms the basis of the vocal folds (true vocal cords).

The inelastic quadrangular (aryepiglottic) membrane (see Fig. 7.65) attaches posteriorly to the body and apex of the arytenoid and anteriorly to the lower part of the lateral edge of the epiglottis. It has a lower free border which forms the vestibular fold (false vocal cord) whilst the upper free edge forms the aryepiglottic fold (part of the laryngeal inlet).

The thyrohyoid membrane (see Fig. 7.67) fills the gap between the thyroid cartilage and the hyoid bone. Its posterior free edges are thickened to form the lateral thyrohyoid ligaments whilst the midline thickening is the median thyrohyoid ligament.

Mucous membrane (Fig. 7.64) lines the interior of the larynx. The epithelium is of the respiratory type, except over the vocal and aryepiglottic folds where it is stratified and squamous. A pouch of mucous membrane protrudes laterally between the vocal and vestibular folds, forming the saccule. It contains numerous mucous glands whose secretions moisten the vocal folds.

Intrinsic muscles

The intrinsic laryngeal muscles control the position and tension of the vocal and aryepiglottic folds, therefore modifying the shape of the airway through the larynx, acting both at the glottis (rima glottidis), the gap between the vocal folds, and at the inlet (see Fig. 7.61). During swallowing both openings narrow, but in coughing and phonation only the glottis narrows. The glottis

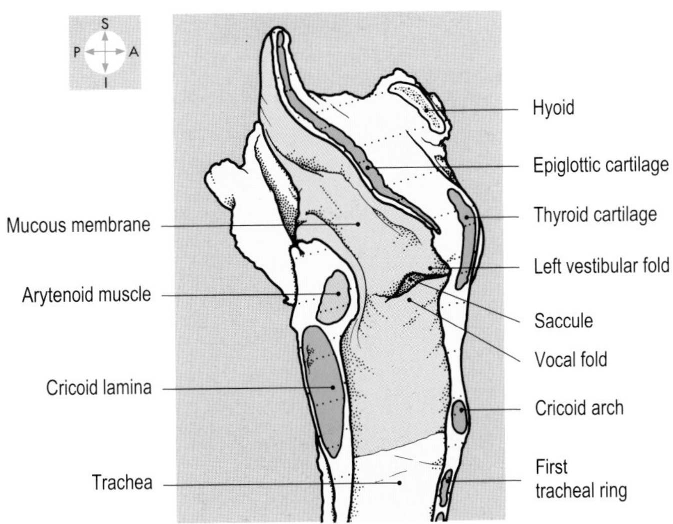

Fig. 7.64 Median sagittal section showing the lumen and mucous membrane of the larynx.

widens during inspiration, especially when deep. The muscles are symmetrical in their arrangement.

The cricothyroid muscle (see Fig. 7.67) attaches to the anterolateral surface of the cricoid cartilage and to the inferior edge of the thyroid cartilage and adjacent part of the inferior horn. It raises the arch of the cricoid cartilage, tipping the lamina backwards and thereby increasing the tension and length of the vocal folds. This has the effect of raising the pitch of the voice and narrowing the glottis.

The thyroarytenoid muscle (see Fig. 7.69) attaches to the posterior surface of the thyroid cartilage adjacent to the conus elasticus. Its fibres pass posteriorly to gain the vocal process and adjacent body of the arytenoid cartilage. The muscle opposes the action of cricothyroid, drawing the arytenoids forwards and relaxing the vocal folds. Part of the muscle (vocalis) lies in the free edge of the vocal fold. The vocalis gives rigidity to the edge of the fold and also modifies tension differentially along its length.

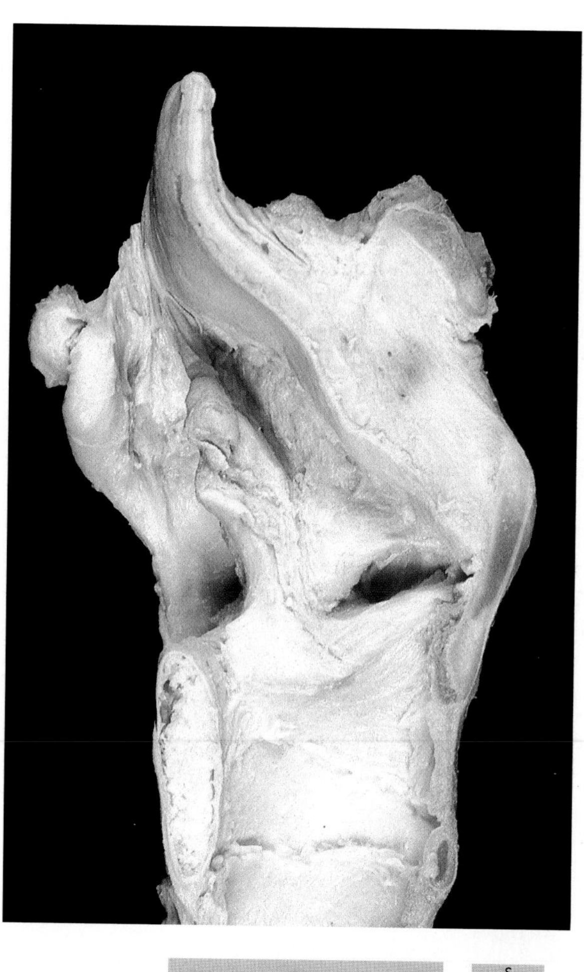

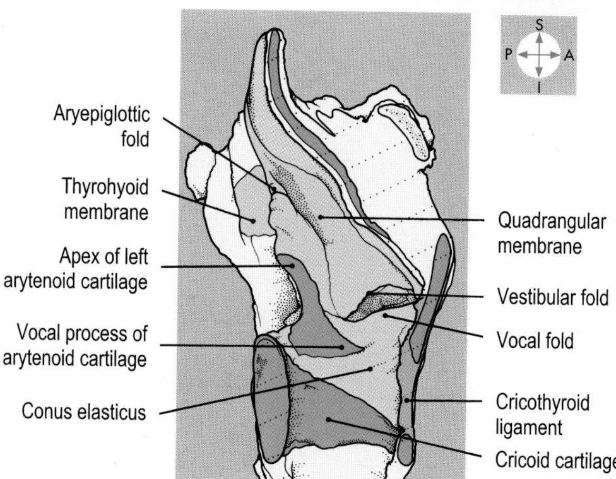

Fig. 7.65 Membranes and folds of the larynx, revealed by removal of most of the mucosa.

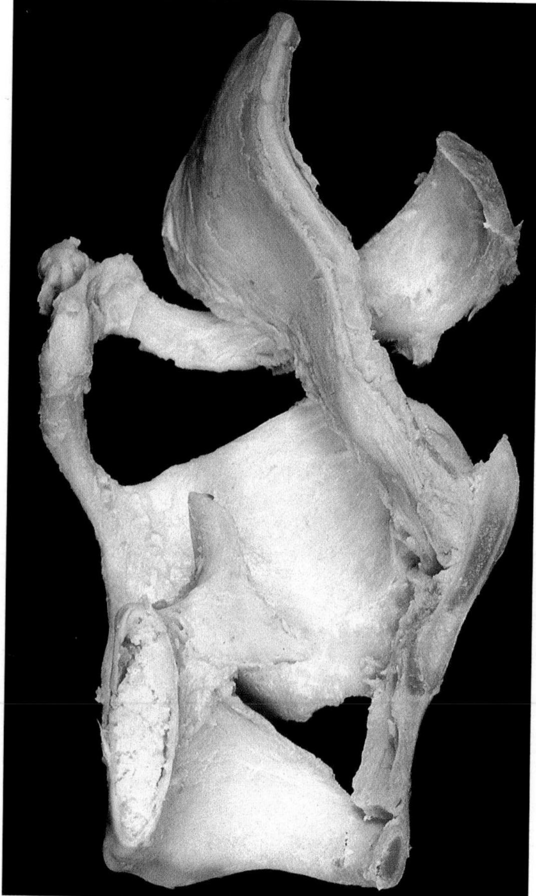

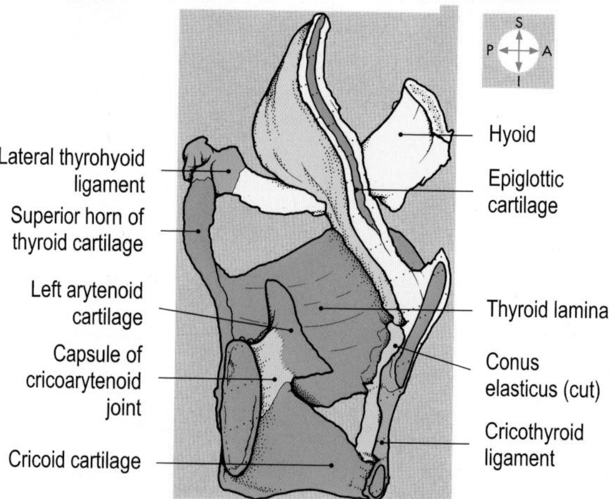

Fig. 7.66 Bisected skeleton of the larynx, revealed by removal of membranes.

Two muscles attach to the muscular process of each arytenoid. The lateral cricoarytenoid (Fig. 7.68) attaches to the lateral surface of the cricoid, its fibres passing posterosuperiorly to gain the muscular process of the arytenoid. The muscle rotates the arytenoid around its vertical axis, adducting the vocal folds and thereby closing the glottis. The posterior cricoarytenoid (see Figs 7.62 & 7.68) inclines anterosuperiorly from the lamina of the cricoid to the muscular process of the arytenoid. Its action opposes that of the lateral cricoarytenoid, rotating the arytenoid so that the folds are abducted and the glottis opened. Simultaneous contraction of the lateral and posterior cricoarytenoid muscles separates the arytenoids by sliding them down the cricoid lamina.

The arytenoid muscle (see Figs 7.62 & 7.64) spans the gap between the bodies of the arytenoid cartilages and has transverse and oblique parts. The muscle approximates the arytenoids, closing the glottis. The oblique arytenoids continue anterosuperiorly in the aryepiglottic fold as the aryepiglottic muscles (Fig. 7.68). These assist in closing the laryngeal inlet and are important during swallowing.

Nerve supply

The larynx is supplied by the right and left superior and recurrent laryngeal branches of the vagus (X) nerves. Each recurrent laryngeal nerve (Figs 7.67 & 7.68) ascends from the root of the neck (see

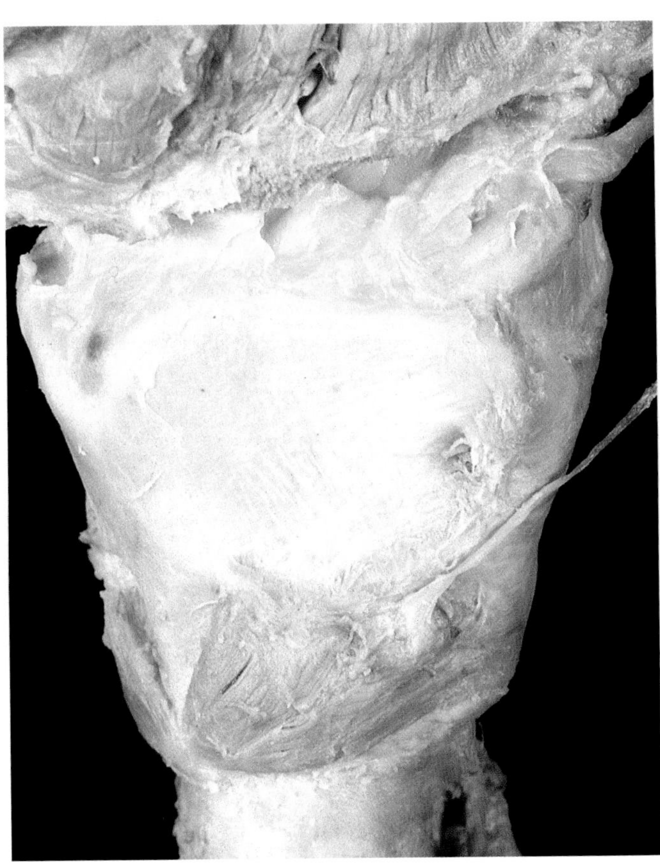

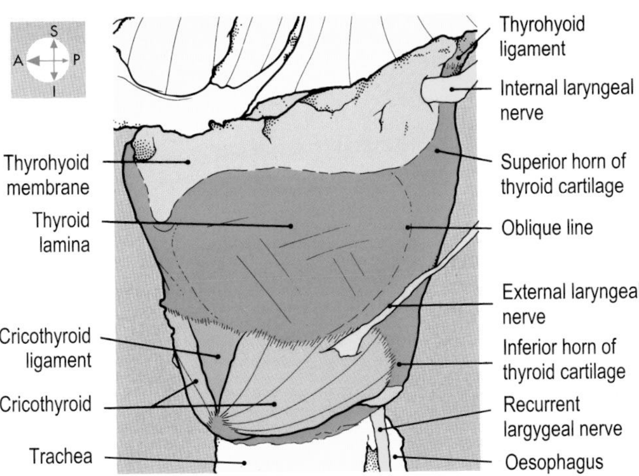

Fig. 7.67 Anterolateral view of the larynx.

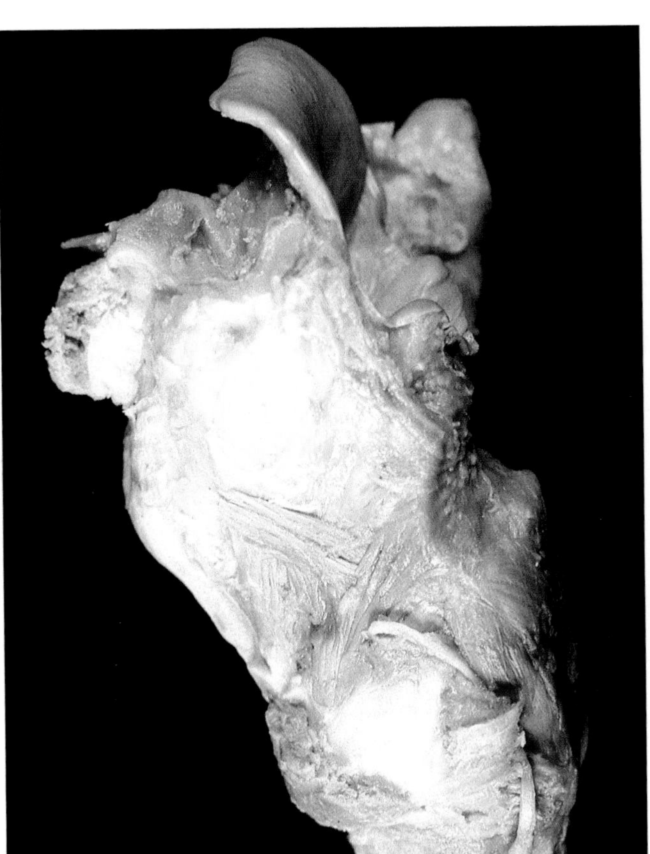

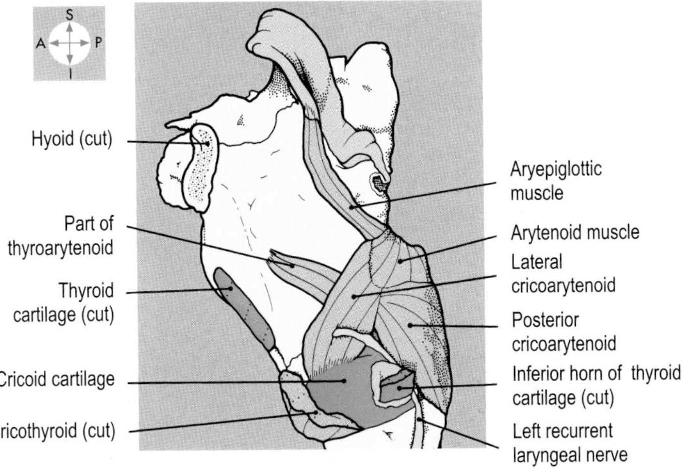

Fig. 7.68 Deeper intrinsic muscles seen after removal of half of the thyroid cartilage and the hyoid bone.

p. 329) in the groove between the trachea and oesophagus. Passing beneath the lower border of the inferior constrictor, the nerve enters the larynx behind the cricothyroid joint.

It supplies motor fibres to all of the intrinsic muscles (except cricothyroid) and carries sensory fibres from all of the structures within the larynx and laryngopharynx below the level of the vocal folds.

The superior laryngeal nerve (see Figs 7.57 & 7.67) arises from the vagus nerve just below the skull and descends to the thyrohyoid membrane where it divides, forming a motor external laryngeal branch and a sensory internal laryngeal branch. The external laryngeal nerve (see Fig. 7.67) descends on the outer surface of the larynx to supply the cricothyroid muscle. The internal laryngeal branch (see Figs 7.61 & 7.67) pierces the thyrohyoid membrane and provides sensory fibres to the larynx and laryngopharynx above the vocal folds.

Blood supply

The laryngeal branches of the superior and inferior thyroid arteries (see Figs 7.13 & 7.15) supply the larynx whilst venous blood drains via superior and middle thyroid vessels into the internal jugular veins.

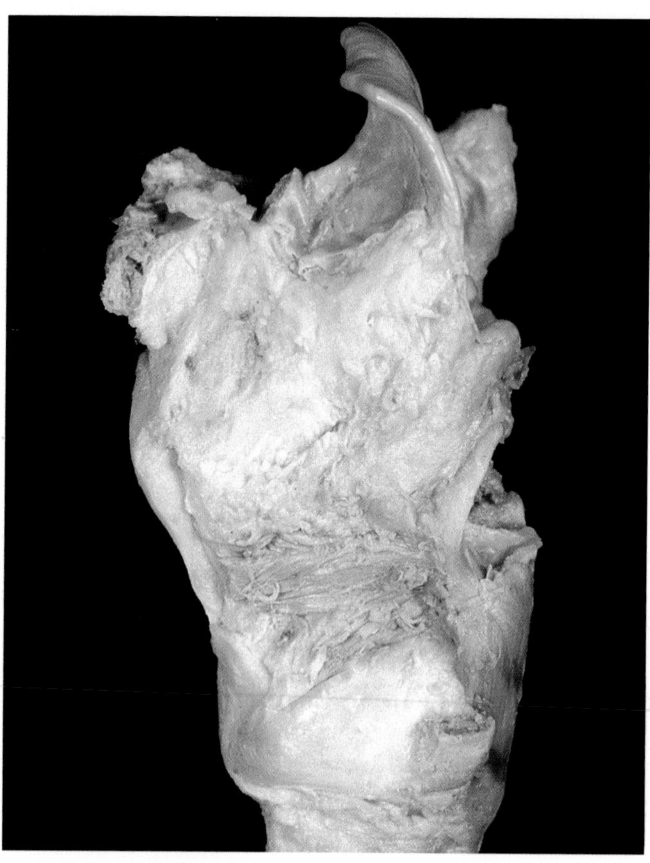

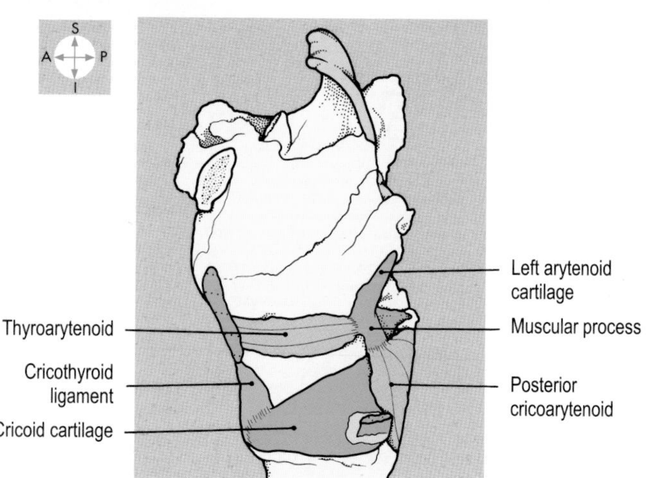

Fig. 7.69 Thryoarytenoid and the arytenoid cartilage after excision of the lateral cricoarytenoid, arytenoid and aryepiglottic muscles.

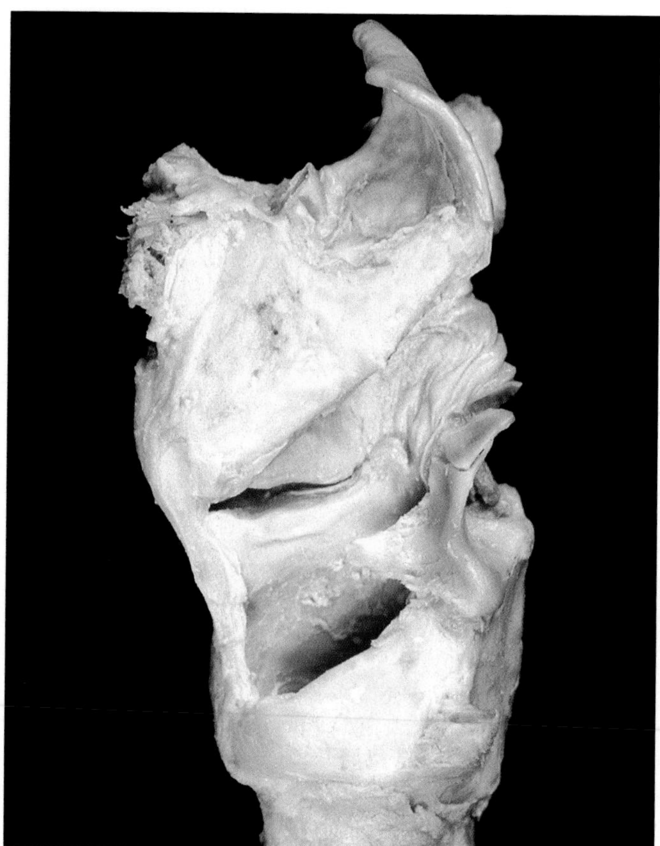

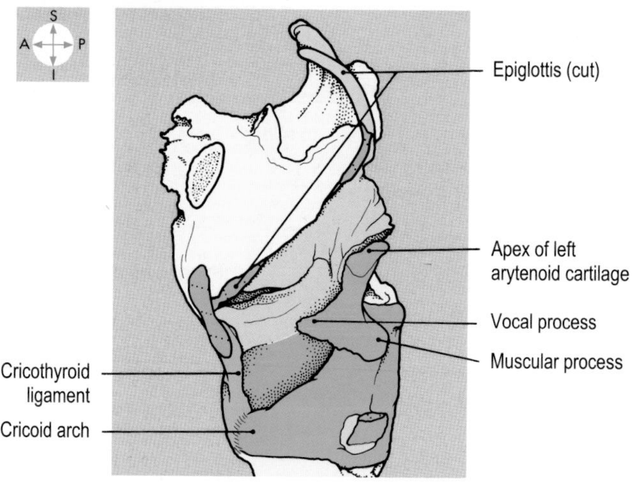

Fig. 7.70 Cartilages of the larynx, revealed by removal of muscles and membranes on the left side.

Cranium and Contents

The part of the skull that contains the brain and its immediate relations is called the neurocranium. Although the detailed anatomy of the central nervous system is outside the scope of this book, there are some important surface features of the brain (Figs 7.72 & 7.73) to which reference should be made when considering the bony features of the interior of the cranium.

Bony features

The vault of the skull consists of four flat bones. Anteriorly is the frontal bone, posteriorly the occipital bone and on each side is a parietal bone (Fig. 7.71). The frontal and parietal bones meet along the coronal suture, and the two parietal bones meet along the midline sagittal suture. Posteriorly the parietal bones meet the occipital bone at the lambdoid suture. The undersurface of the vault bears a long shallow midline groove for the superior sagittal

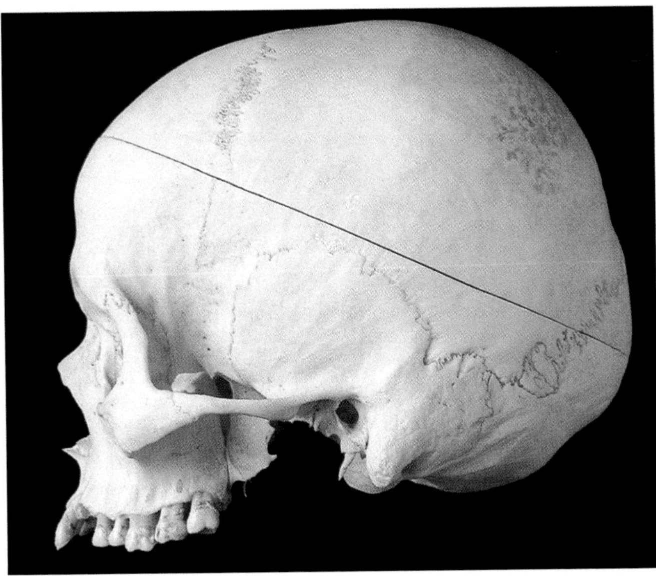

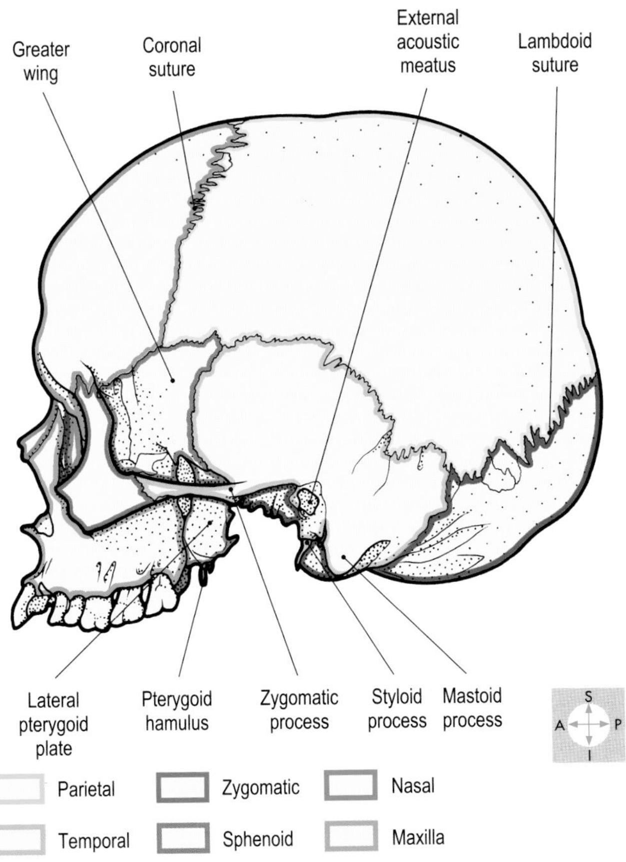

Fig. 7.71 Lateral view of the skull (without the mandible) showing the component bones.

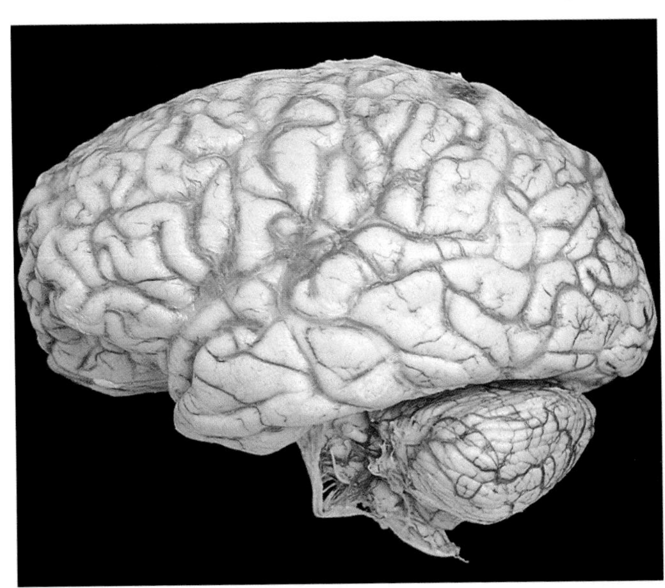

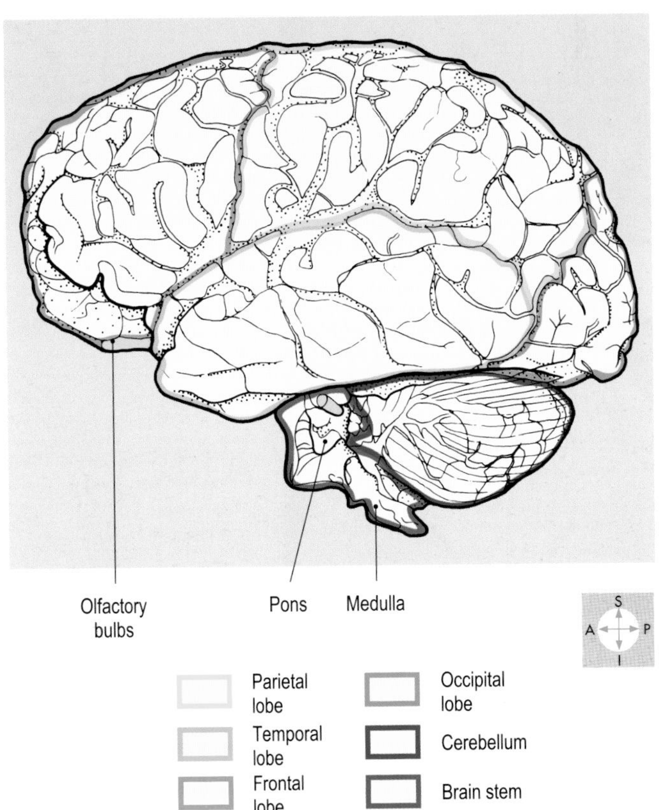

Fig. 7.72 Lateral view of the brain showing the cerebral hemisphere and the hindbrain.

venous sinus (see below), which terminates at a prominence, the internal occipital protuberance (Fig. 7.74). Below the level of each parietal bone, the greater wing of the sphenoid bone and the squamous part of the temporal bone complete the lateral wall of the vault.

The cranial base is characterized by the anterior, middle and posterior fossae, arranged in step-like sequence (Fig. 7.74), the anterior being superior. The anterior fossa, which accommodates the frontal lobes of the brain, is formed by the frontal bone laterally, the cribriform plates and crista galli of the ethmoid bone medially and is completed posteriorly by the lesser wings of the sphenoid bone. The numerous small foramina in the cribriform plates communicate with the nasal cavity (see p. 354).

The middle fossa, occupied by the temporal lobes of the brain, is formed by the greater wings and body of the sphenoid bone. Posteriorly the fossa is bounded by the petrous part of each temporal bone whilst anteriorly the fossa is completed by the lesser wings of the sphenoid. Each of the lesser wings is perforated by the optic canal, which continues forwards into the orbit. Between the lesser and greater wings is the superior orbital fissure, which also provides access to the orbit. The greater wing is traversed by the foramen rotundum (opening into the pterygopalatine fossa; see p. 351) and the foramina ovale and spinosum (both opening into the infratemporal fossa; see Fig. 7.81). Lying in the angle between the greater wing and body of the sphenoid and the apex of the petrous part of the temporal bone is the foramen lacerum, which forms part of the roof of the infratemporal fossa. In the midline the body of the sphenoid is hollowed, forming the sella turcica. This is limited by the paired anterior and posterior clinoid processes, and accommodates the pituitary gland.

The posterior cranial fossa contains the cerebellum, the pons and the medulla oblongata which is in continuity through the foramen magnum with the spinal cord. The floor of this fossa is formed mostly by the occipital bone, supplemented anteriorly by the body of the sphenoid and the posterior surface of the petrous part of each temporal bone. Anterior to the foramen magnum the occipital and sphenoid bones fuse to form a smooth incline, the clivus, on which the brainstem lies. The internal acoustic meatus opens onto the posterior surface of the petrous part of the temporal bone while in the suture between this bone and the occipital bone

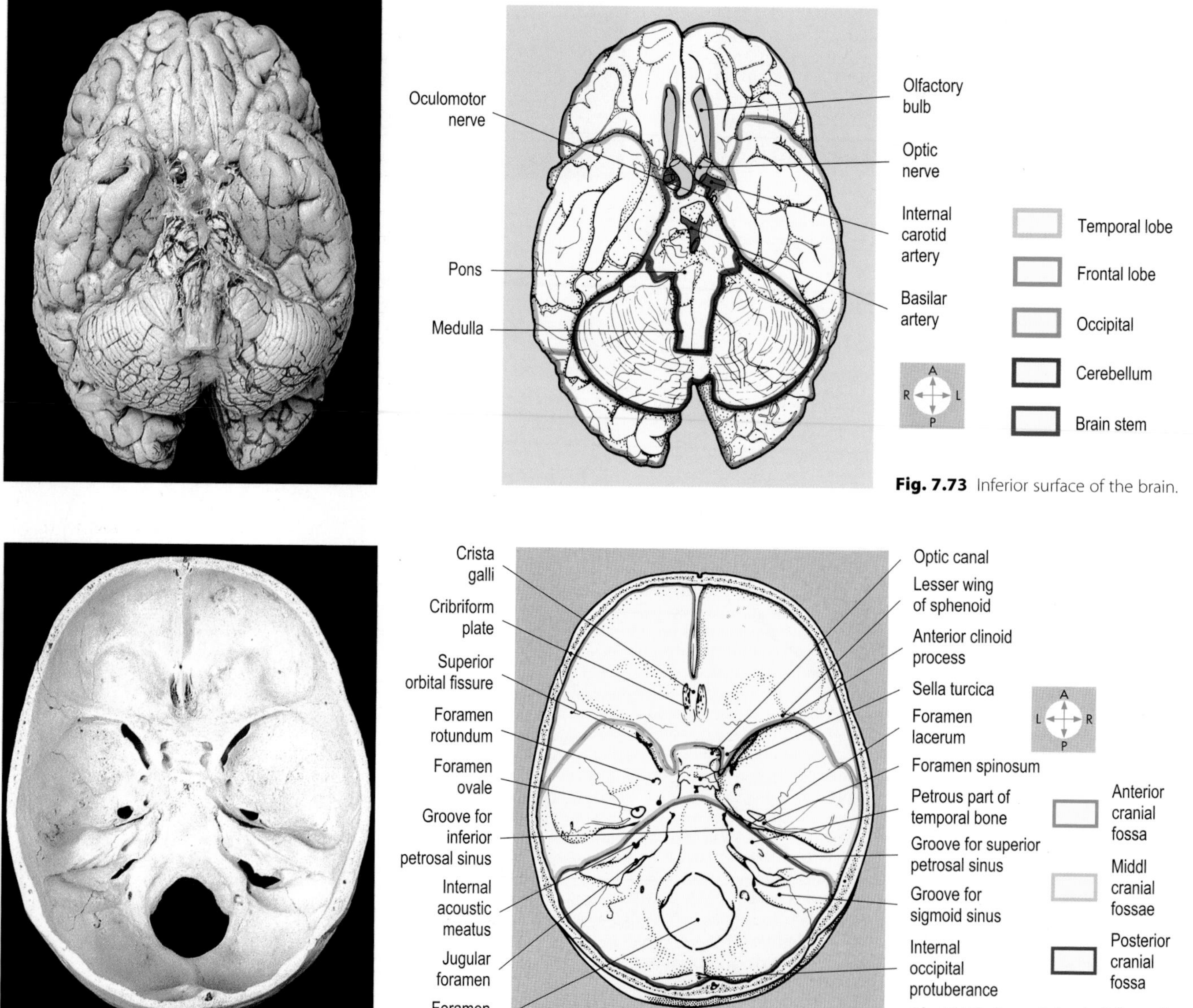

Fig. 7.73 Inferior surface of the brain.

Fig. 7.74 Base of the skull from above showing the cranial fossae.

is the jugular foramen. Running horizontally from the internal occipital protuberance is a groove for the transverse venous sinus. An S-shaped groove for the sigmoid sinus (Fig. 7.74) links the groove for the transverse sinus with the jugular foramen. The hypoglossal canal traverses the occipital bone anterolateral to the foramen magnum (see Fig. 7.81).

Meninges

Surrounding the brain are three membranes, the meninges, which comprise the dura mater, arachnoid mater and pia mater.

Dura mater

The dura mater consists of outer periosteal and inner meningeal layers. The periosteal dura attaches to and closely follows the bony contours of the cranial cavity and is continuous through the sutures and foramina with the periosteum (pericranium) on the outer surface of the skull. Although generally bound to the periosteal dura, the meningeal dura is raised in places as a double layer, forming the dural folds.

The largest of these folds is the midline falx cerebri (Figs 7.75 & 7.76), which projects downwards between the two cerebral hemispheres.

Anteriorly the falx cerebri is attached to the crista galli of the ethmoid bone. It arches over the corpus callosum and gains further attachment to the frontal, parietal and occipital bones. Posteriorly the falx ends by attaching to another dural fold, the tentorium cerebelli (Figs 7.75–7.77). The tentorium forms an incomplete roof over the posterior cranial fossa and separates the occipital lobes of the cerebrum from the cerebellum. Each side of the tentorium slopes upwards towards its midline attachment to the falx cerebri. Anteriorly there is a large aperture in the tentorium through which the brainstem passes. The thickened free edge of the tentorium surrounding this aperture continues forwards to reach the anterior clinoid process. The attached border of the tentorium runs laterally from the internal occipital protuberance along a horizontal groove on the inner surface of the occipital bone, then continues medially along the superior border of the petrous part of the temporal bone to reach the posterior clinoid process. Posteriorly the small falx cerebelli descends vertically from the tentorium and partially separates the two cerebellar hemispheres. The sella turcica in the middle fossa has a roof of dura called the diaphragma sellae, which is attached to the four clinoid processes and has a central aperture for the pituitary stalk.

Dural venous sinuses

Lying between the two layers of dura are endothelium-lined venous channels (see Fig. 7.76). These dural venous sinuses, which often groove the adjacent bones, collect blood from the brain and meninges. They also drain cerebrospinal fluid that has been secreted into the subarachnoid space by the choroid plexuses of the brain. A characteristic of these sinuses is the absence of valves.

The superior sagittal sinus lies in the attached margin of the falx cerebri (Figs 7.75 & 7.76). The sinus drains posteriorly and has along its length several dilatations called lacunae. These lacunae possess arachnoid granulations through which the reabsorption of cerebrospinal fluid takes place. The sinus also receives numerous cerebral veins. At the internal occipital protuberance the superior sagittal sinus turns laterally, usually to the right, and continues as the transverse sinus in the attached margin of the tentorium cerebelli (see Fig. 7.77). Just before reaching the petrous part of the temporal bone, the sinus turns inferiorly to continue as the sigmoid sinus (see Fig. 7.78). This follows an S-shaped course to reach the jugular foramen, through which it is continuous with the internal jugular vein.

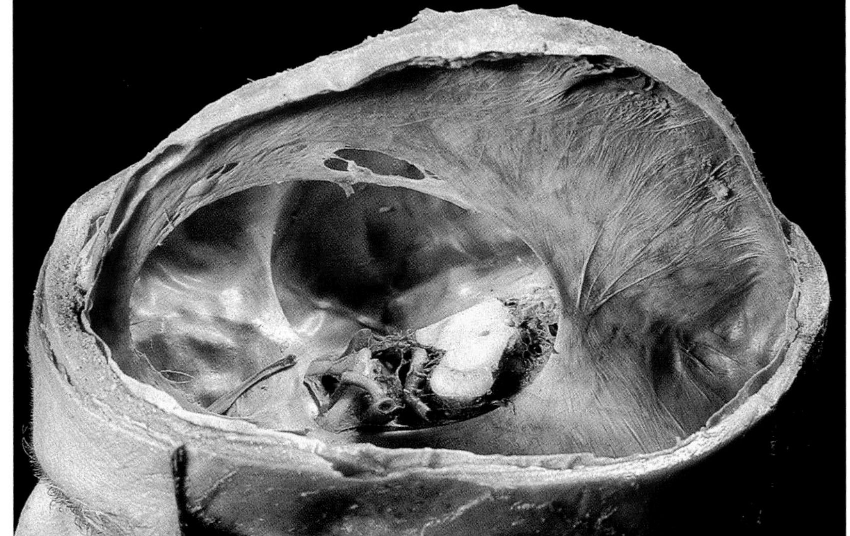

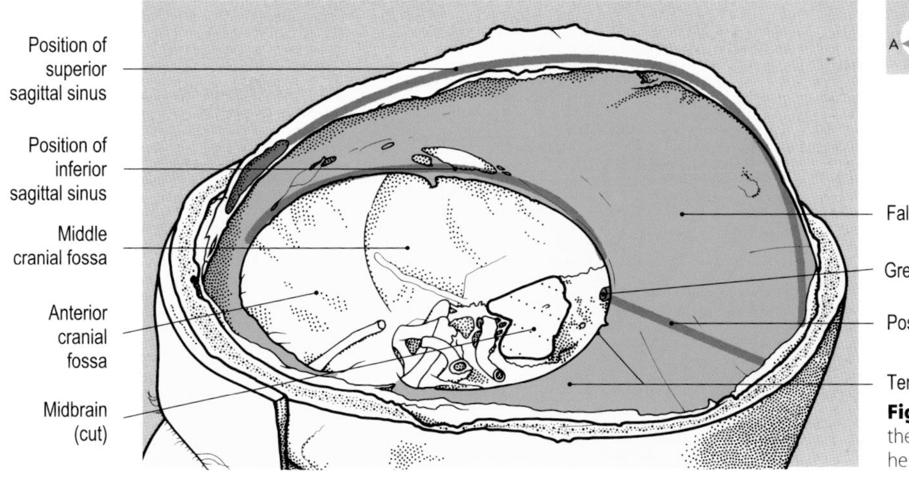

Fig. 7.75 Falx cerebri and tentorium cerebelli, revealed by removal of the vault of the cranium, associated dura and the cerebral hemispheres.

The smaller inferior sagittal sinus lies in the free border of the falx cerebri (see Fig. 7.75). The sinus runs posteriorly and at the tentorium cerebelli is joined by the great cerebral vein, which drains the deeper structures of the cerebral hemispheres. The union of these vessels forms the straight sinus (Figs 7.75–7.77), which continues posteriorly in the attachment of the falx cerebri to the tentorium as far as the internal occipital protuberance. Here the straight sinus usually turns to the left to form the transverse sinus, whose course mirrors that on the opposite side.

The cavernous venous sinuses (Figs 7.78 & 7.79) lie on either side of the pituitary gland and the body of the sphenoid bone. They contain numerous interconnected venous spaces, producing a spongy appearance. The two sinuses communicate with each

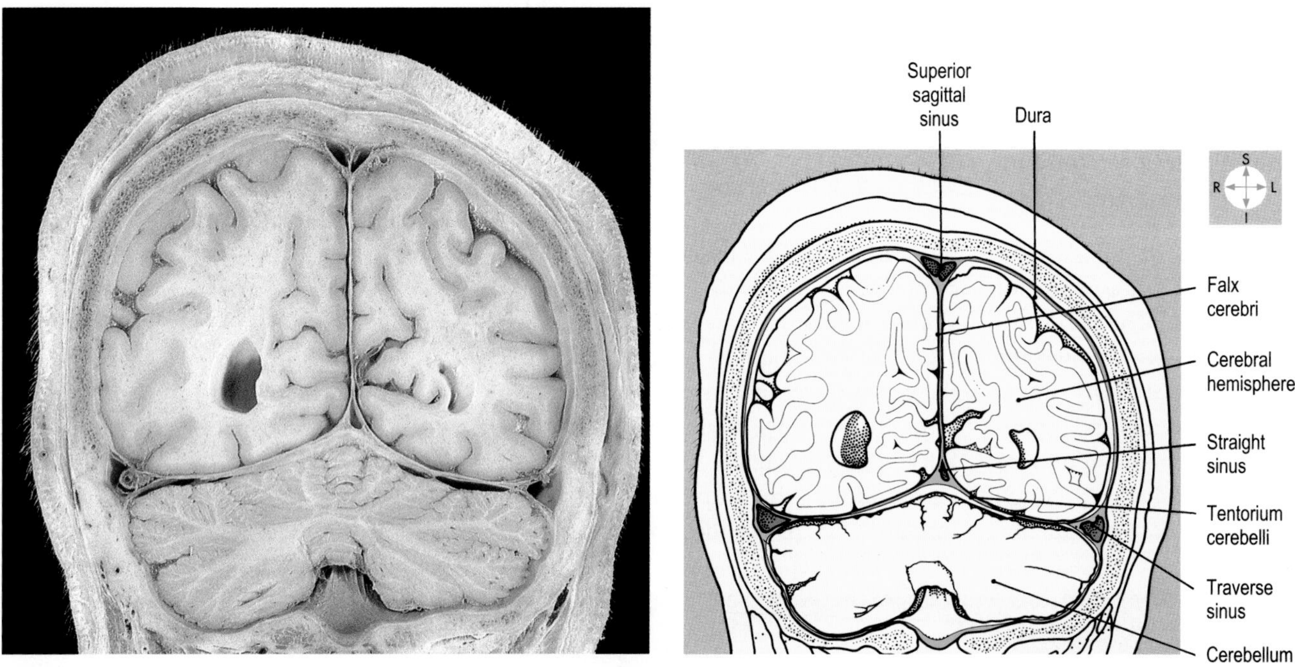

Fig. 7.76 Coronal section through the posterior cranial fossa, showing dura and its folds and venous sinuses. Anterior aspect.

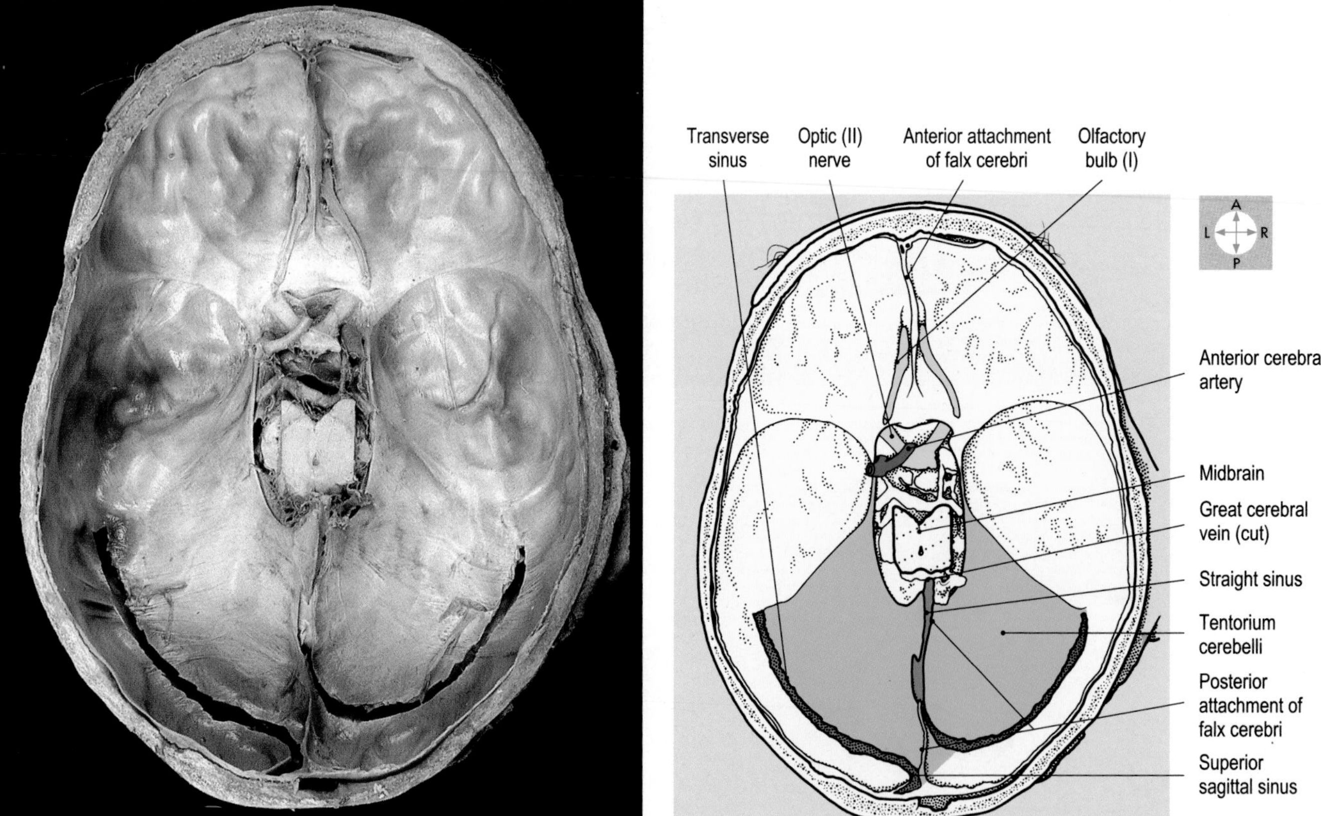

Fig. 7.77 Superior view of the tentorium cerebelli after removal of the falx cerebri and cerebral hemispheres. The venous sinuses have been opened. The straight sinus turns to the right and the superior sagittal sinus to the left in this specimen.

other and receive blood from the ophthalmic veins of the orbits via the superior orbital fissures. In addition, they receive vessels that pass through the superior and inferior orbital fissures from the ophthalmic veins and pterygoid venous plexuses. Posteriorly each cavernous sinus drains via the superior and inferior petrosal sinuses. The superior petrosal sinus runs along the superior border of the petrous part of the temporal bone to terminate in the junction of the transverse and sigmoid sinuses. The inferior petrosal sinus descends into the posterior cranial fossa and unites with the sigmoid sinus in the jugular foramen to form the internal jugular vein.

Arachnoid mater

The arachnoid mater, the middle of the meningeal layers, is loosely attached to the dura mater, generally following its folds. The arachnoid is separated from the deeper pia mater by the subarachnoid space, which contains cerebrospinal fluid and is traversed by the arteries of the brain and the cranial nerves.

Pia mater

The pia mater is the innermost of the meninges and clings to the surface of the brain, dipping into its numerous grooves or sulci.

Meningeal vessels

Of the many arteries entering the cranium to supply the meninges, one of particular importance is the middle meningeal artery, which arises from the maxillary artery (see p. 344) and enters through the foramen spinosum. This vessel runs laterally across the floor of the middle cranial fossa, grooving the bone, and divides on the squamous part of the temporal bone into frontal (anterior) and parietal (posterior) branches (Fig. 7.78). These branches arch superiorly on the inner surface of the lateral part of the skull and supply the meninges lining most of the vault. Meningeal veins follow the arteries and communicate with the dural venous sinuses and with veins lying outside the skull.

Bleeding from veins or arteries between the meningeal layers can raise intracranial pressure. An extradural (epidural) haematoma results from extravasation between the dura and the skull. A subdural haematoma is produced by bleeding between the dura and arachnoid layers, where normally no space exists. Blood leaking from the vessels that cross the subarachnoid space will give rise to a subarachnoid haemorrhage, the blood intermingling with cerebrospinal fluid.

Arterial supply to brain

The brain receives arterial blood from the vertebral and internal carotid arteries (see Fig. 7.79). The vertebral arteries (see p. 328) enter the posterior cranial fossa through the foramen magnum. Passing upwards and forwards they unite in the midline on the clivus to form the basilar artery. Branches to the brainstem and cerebellum arise from the vertebral and basilar arteries before the latter divides at the upper border of the pons to form the left and right posterior cerebral arteries. Before supplying the posterior part of the cerebral hemisphere, each of these vessels gives rise to

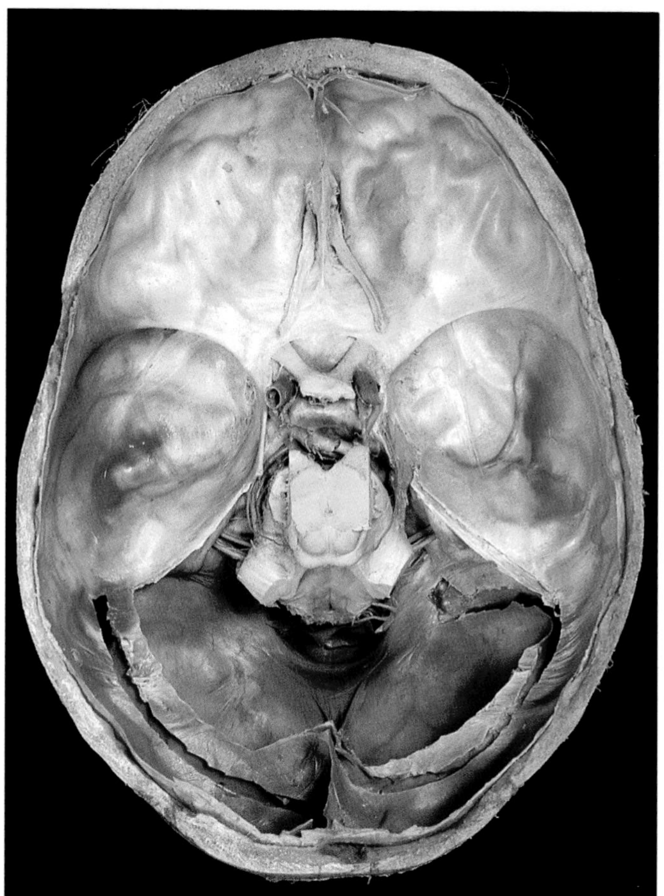

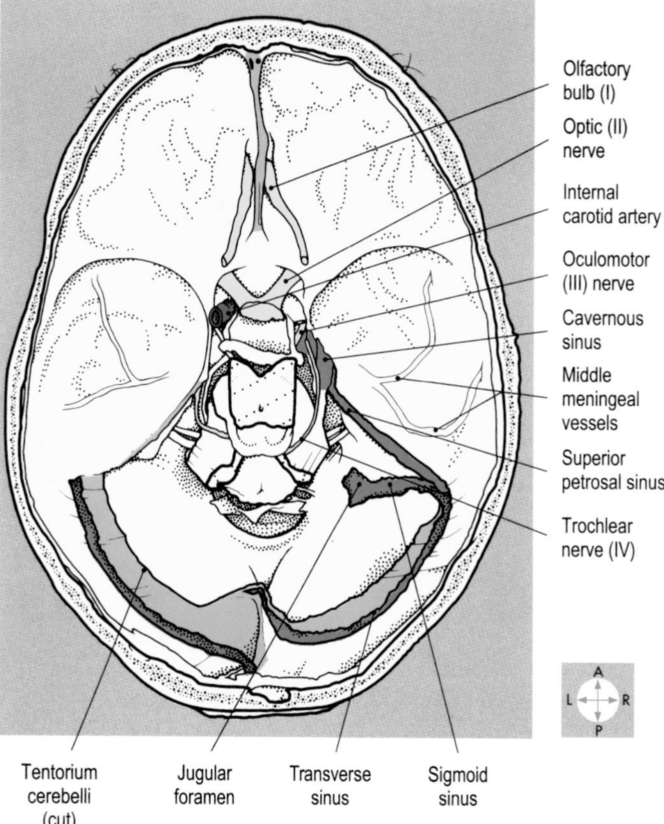

Fig. 7.78 Interior of posterior cranial fossa after removal of tentorium cerebelli and cerebellum. The venous sinuses have been further opened.

a posterior communicating artery, which passes forwards to form part of the cerebral arterial circle (circle of Willis) by anastomosing with the internal carotid artery.

The internal carotid artery traverses the carotid canal (Fig. 7.81) to enter the middle cranial fossa, emerging from the upper part of the foramen lacerum. The artery turns anteriorly to enter the cavernous sinus, then continues superiorly to leave the sinus through its roof. Here, near the anterior clinoid process, the ophthalmic artery arises and accompanies the optic nerve through the optic canal into the orbit. The internal carotid artery terminates as the anterior and middle cerebral arteries. The middle cerebral artery supplies the lateral portion of the cerebral hemisphere

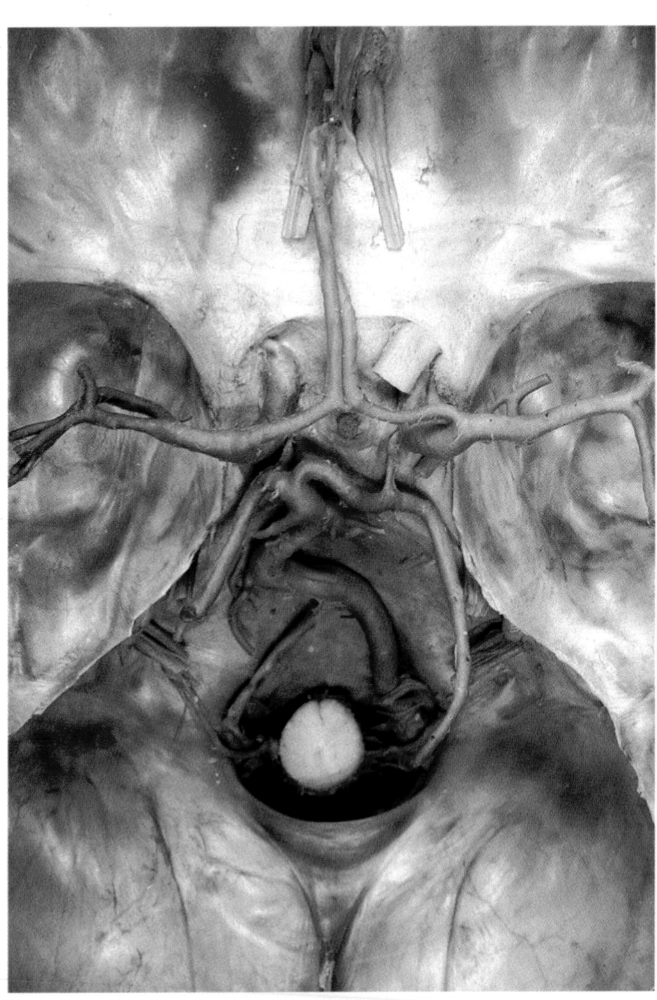

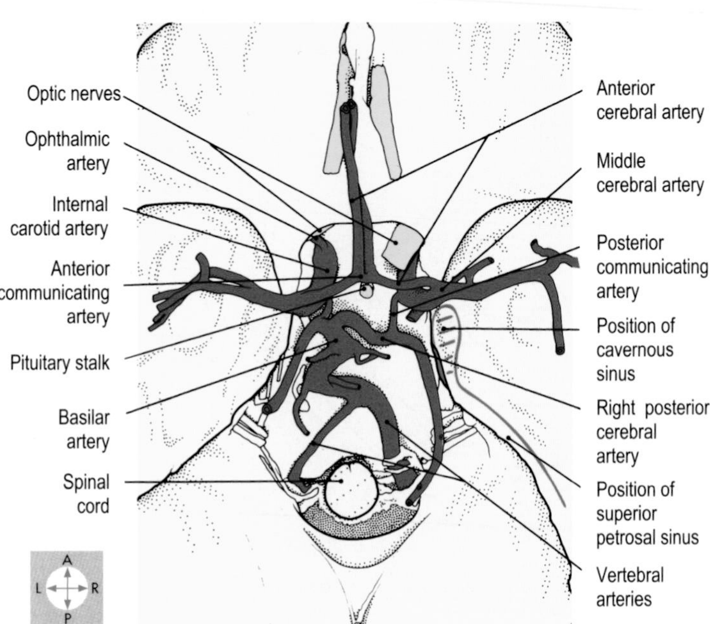

Fig. 7.79 Arterial circle, exposed by complete removal of the brain. The basilar and vertebral arteries are asymmetrical in this specimen.

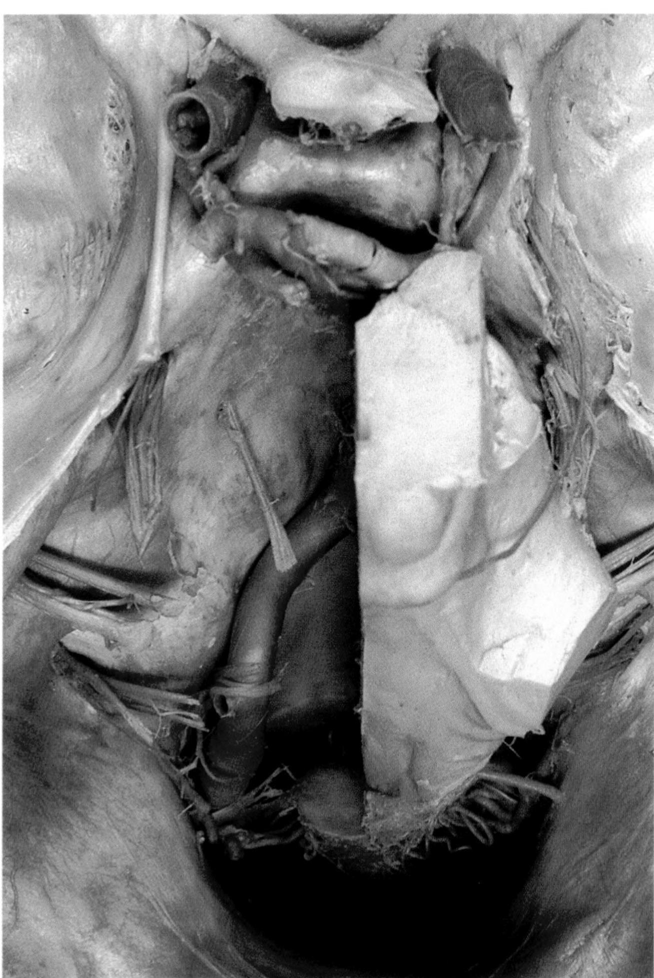

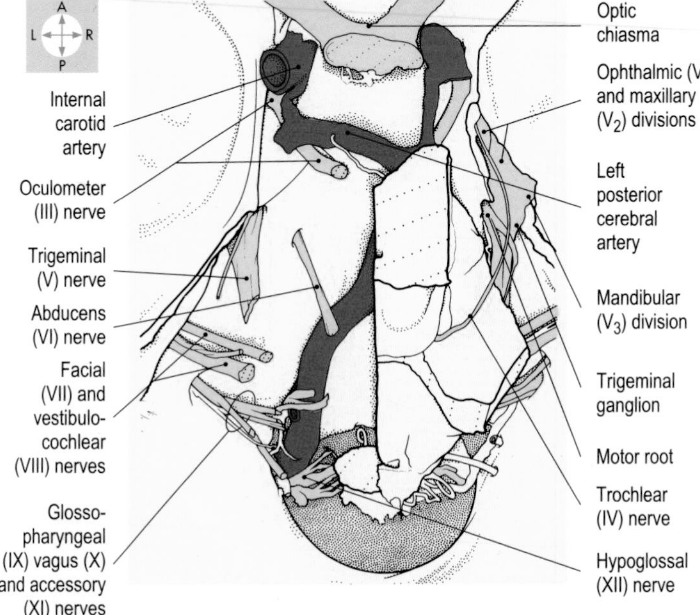

Fig. 7.80 Cranial nerves revealed by removal of most of the brain. The dura over the right trigeminal ganglion has been excised.

while the anterior cerebral artery ascends between the frontal lobes to supply the medial surface of the hemisphere.

The cerebral arterial circle is formed between the branches of the internal carotid and vertebral arteries (Fig. 7.79). The two anterior cerebral arteries are joined by the anterior communicating artery. On each side an anastomosis, via the posterior communicating artery, between the posterior cerebral branch of the basilar artery and the internal carotid artery completes the cerebral arterial circle.

Cranial nerves

The twelve pairs of cranial nerves enter or leave the skull through various foramina (Figs 7.78 & 7.80). The olfactory (I) nerves emerge from the nasal cavity as a number of short branches, which traverse the cribriform plates and terminate in the olfactory bulbs.

The optic (II) nerve leaves the orbit via the optic canal and joins the optic chiasma immediately anterior to the pituitary stalk. From the chiasma the optic tracts pass backwards to enter the brain.

Three cranial nerves enter the orbit through the superior orbital fissure. To reach the fissure the oculomotor (III) and trochlear (IV) nerves run forwards in the lateral wall of the cavernous sinus while the abducens (VI) nerve passes through the cavity of the sinus. Infection from the face can spread through veins to the cavernous sinus which may thrombose, causing damage to the abducens nerve and double vision.

The ganglion of the sensory part of the trigeminal (V) nerve lies covered in dura in a small depression on the apex of the petrous part of the temporal bone. The three divisions of the nerve converge on the anterior surface of the ganglion. From the orbit the ophthalmic (V_1) division traverses the superior orbital fissure and continues backwards, embedded in the lateral wall of the cavernous sinus, to reach the ganglion. The maxillary (V_2) division leaves the pterygopalatine fossa via the foramen rotundum and passes backwards along the lower edge of the sinus to the ganglion. The sensory part of the mandibular (V_3) division, accompanied by the motor root of the trigeminal nerve, ascends from the infratemporal fossa through the foramen ovale. The motor root passes beneath and not through the ganglion to traverse the foramen ovale.

The facial (VII) nerve enters, and the vestibulocochlear (VIII) nerve emerges from, the internal acoustic meatus in the petrous part of the temporal bone.

Three nerves leave via the jugular foramen to enter the carotid sheath, namely the glossopharyngeal (IX), vagus (X) and accessory (XI) nerves.

Finally, the hypoglossal (XII) nerve traverses the hypoglossal canal.

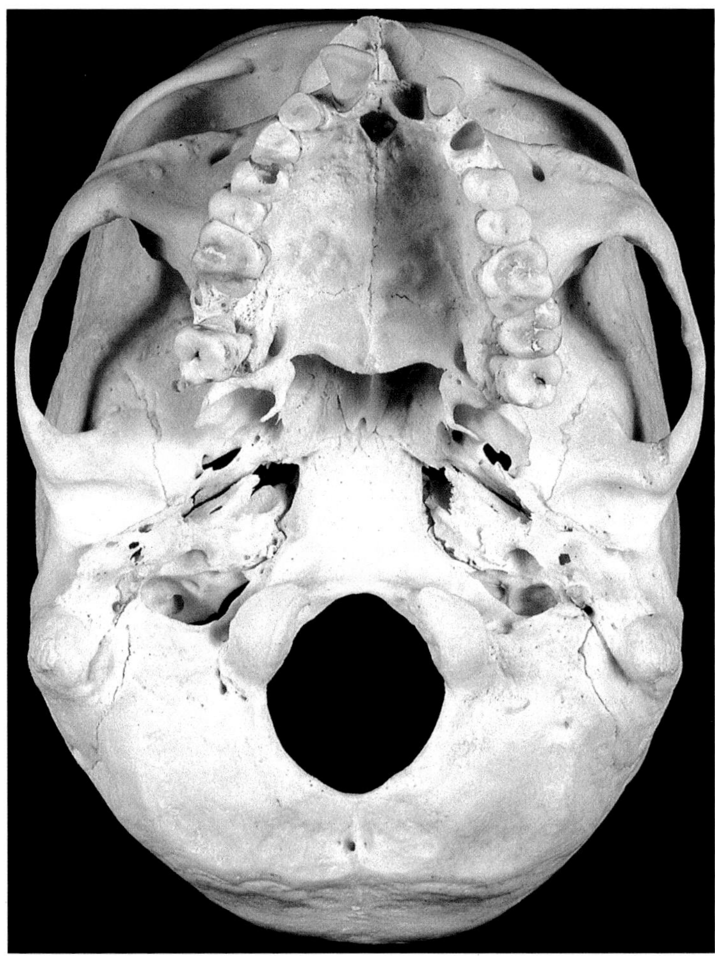

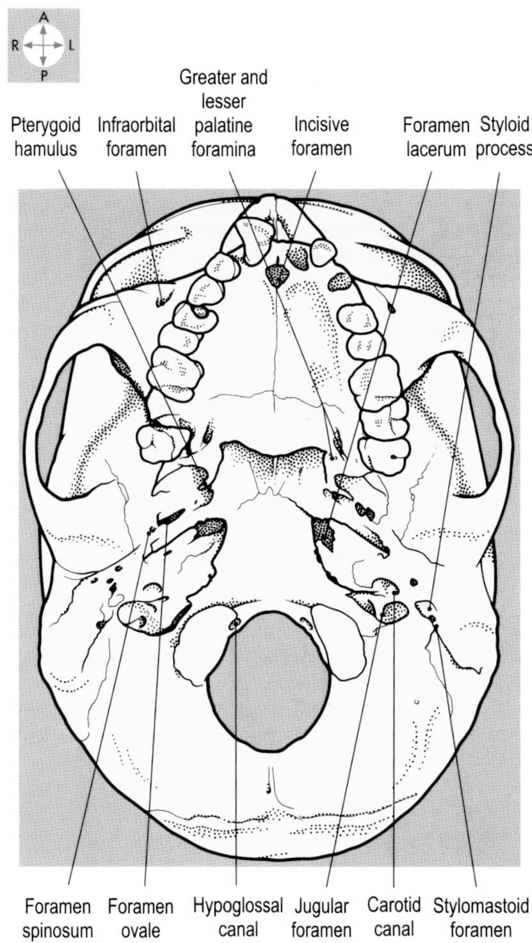

Fig. 7.81 Inferior view of the base of the skull showing the principal foramina.

Orbit

The orbit is a pyramidal cavity whose apex is directed posteriorly and base anteriorly (Fig. 7.82). Its bony walls separate it from the anterior cranial fossa above, the ethmoidal air cells and nasal cavity medially, the maxillary air sinus inferiorly and the lateral surface of the face and temporal fossa laterally (Fig. 7.83). Anteriorly the orbit presents a roughly rectangular aperture which is closed by the eyelids. Within the orbit are the eyeball, the extraocular muscles, cranial nerves II, III, IV, V (ophthalmic and maxillary divisions) and VI, and blood vessels, lymphatics and fat.

Bony walls

The roof of the orbit (Fig. 7.84) comprises the frontal bone, which anteriorly contains the frontal air sinuses. The lateral wall is formed anteriorly by the zygomatic bone and posteriorly by the greater wing of the sphenoid bone. The floor consists of the maxilla anteriorly and the greater wing of the sphenoid posteriorly. From

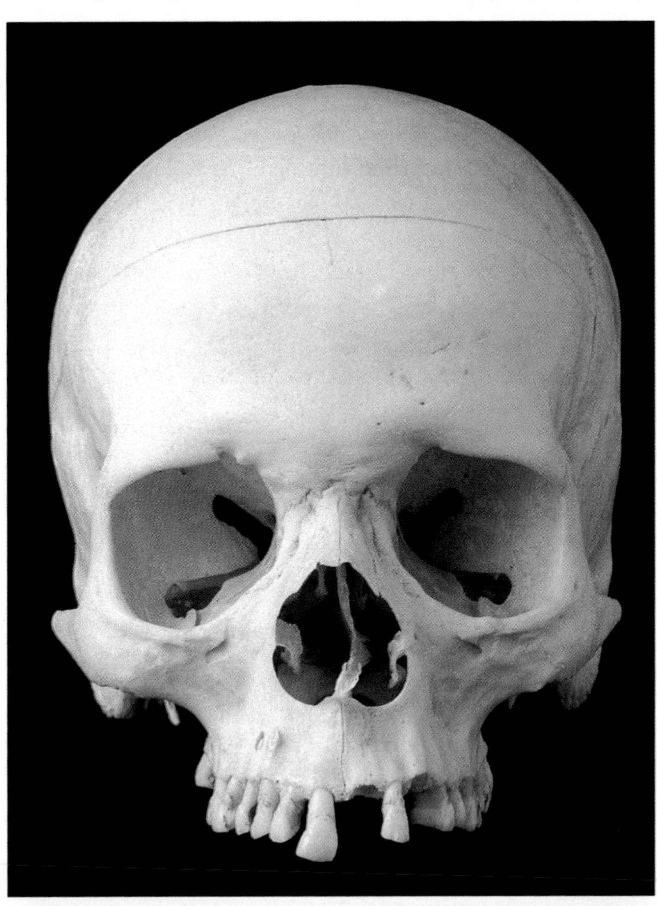

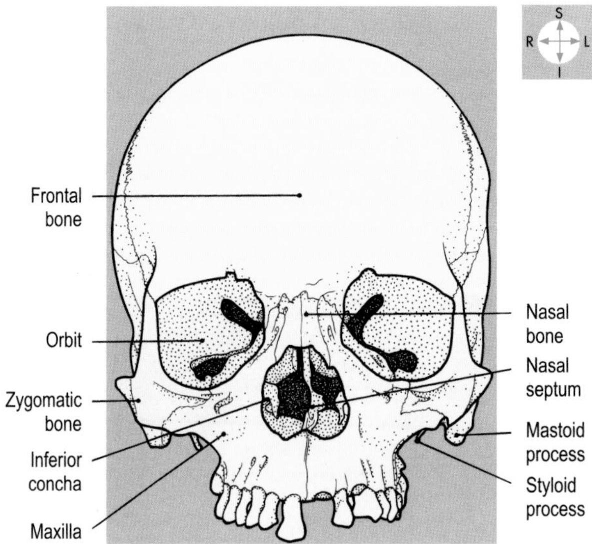

Fig. 7.82 Anterior view of the skull without the mandible.

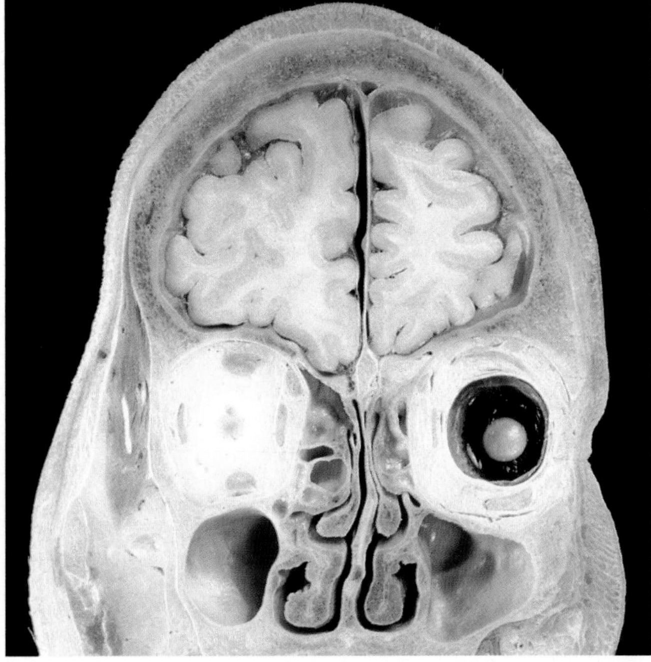

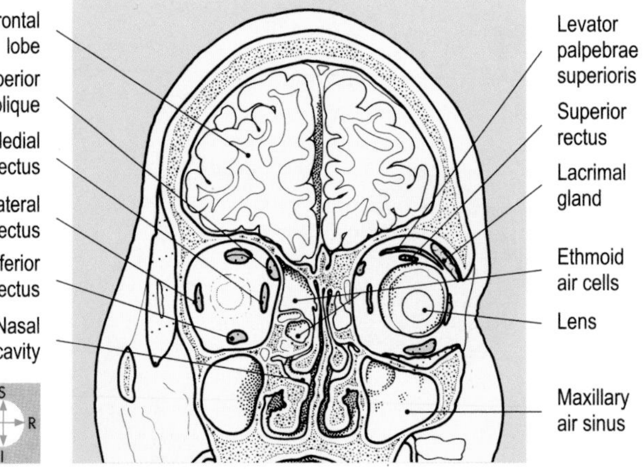

Fig. 7.83 Coronal section showing the extraocular muscles and the relations of the orbits. The section through the right orbit passes more anteriorly than on the left. Posterior aspect. Compare Figs 7.47 & 7.91.

anterior to posterior the medial wall comprises the maxilla, lacrimal, ethmoid and sphenoid bones. The medial walls of the two orbits lie parallel to the median plane while their lateral walls are directed forwards and laterally so that they lie at right angles to one another.

Several foramina and the superior and inferior orbital fissures (Fig. 7.84) allow various structures to enter and leave the orbit. On the medial wall, close to the orbital margin, is a depression called the lacrimal groove, bounded by the maxilla and the lacrimal bone. The nasolacrimal canal descends from this groove and opens into the inferior meatus of the nasal cavity. Anterior and posterior ethmoidal foramina perforate the medial wall and allow communication with the lateral wall of the nasal cavity. At the apex of the orbit are the optic canal and the superior and inferior orbital fissures, through which the orbit is in continuity with the middle cranial and pterygopalatine fossae.

Fascial layers

Movement of the eyeball is facilitated by its fascial sheath, the vagina bulbi (fascia bulbi) (see Fig. 7.89), which invests it but does not adhere to the sclera and is incomplete anteriorly. The vagina bulbi is attached to the eyeball around the margin of the cornea. Thickenings of the inferior part of the fascia (the suspensory ligament) extend laterally and medially to attach to the orbital walls (check ligaments). The fascia is pierced by the six muscles that move the eyeball. Anteriorly the orbit is closed by the orbital septum, which forms the fibrous layer of the eyelids.

Eyelids, conjunctiva and lacrimal apparatus

Within each eyelid the orbital septum is thickened to form a tarsal plate (see Figs 7.85 & 7.86) and is perforated between the eyelids by the palpebral fissure. Anterior to the septum lies orbicularis oculi and skin. Levator palpebrae superioris is attached to the upper edge of the superior tarsal plate while a few fibres of inferior rectus are attached to the lower edge of the inferior tarsal plate. Posteriorly each plate has tarsal (meibomian) glands and is covered by conjunctiva. The conjunctival epithelium is reflected onto the surface of the eyeball, where it blends with the margin of the cornea. Each eyelid carries a double row of eyelashes together with associated sebaceous glands (which when inflamed form a 'stye'). The lashes on each eyelid extend medially as far as a small elevation containing a central aperture, the lacrimal punctum, leading into the lacrimal canaliculus. The canaliculi carry tear fluid to the lacrimal sac in the lacrimal groove, and the sac in turn drains via the nasolacrimal duct, in the nasolacrimal canal, into the nasal cavity beneath the inferior concha (see Fig. 7.51).

The lacrimal gland (see Figs 7.85, 7.86 and 7.88) lies in the superolateral angle of the orbit behind the upper eyelid and is deeply indented by the lateral border of the tendon of levator palpebrae superioris. Small ducts open from the deep surface of the gland into the conjunctival sac. Fluid produced by the gland passes medially towards the lacrimal puncta across the surface of the cornea, assisted by blinking of the eyelid. Reflex blinking is initiated if the cornea is touched or becomes dry. Evaporation of the fluid is retarded by the oily secretion of the tarsal glands.

Extraocular muscles

Within the orbit most muscles comprise only striated fibres, but those that move the eyelids contain smooth fibres as well.

The extraocular muscles are the four recti, the two obliques and one muscle which attaches to the upper eyelids, levator palpebrae superioris (see Figs 7.85–7.87). This is the uppermost muscle in the orbit, and from its attachment to the lesser wing of the sphenoid it passes forwards to form a wide tendon, which enters the upper eyelid and blends with the superior tarsal plate.

The medial, lateral, superior and inferior recti (see Figs 7.86, 7.87, 7.89 & 7.90) attach posteriorly to the common tendinous ring that surrounds the optic canal and part of the superior orbital fissure. Passing forwards, these four muscles attach to the eyeball immediately behind the corneoscleral junction in positions corresponding to their names. Collectively they form a cone with

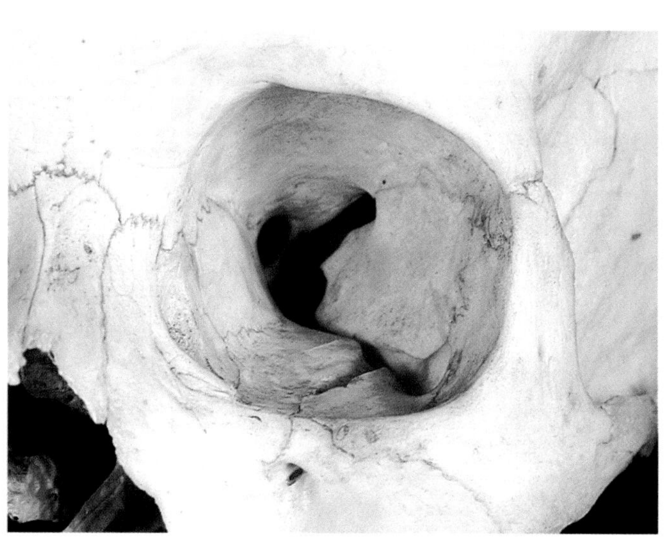

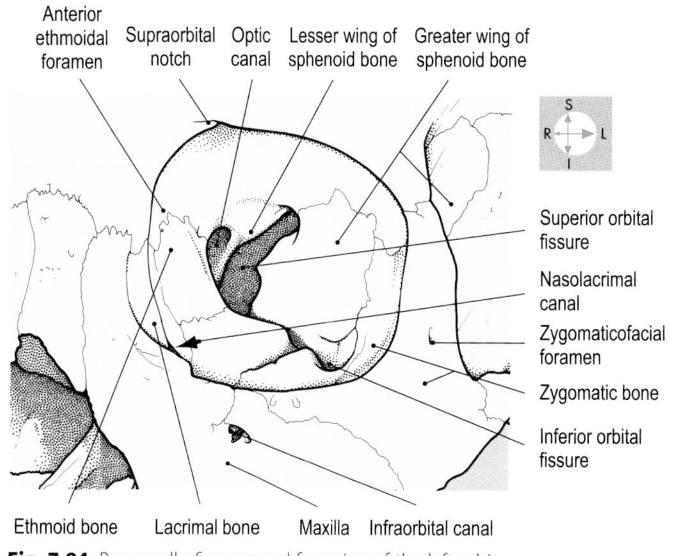

Fig. 7.84 Bony walls, fissures and foramina of the left orbit.

its apex at the optic canal and its base around the equator of the eyeball. Nerves and vessels entering the orbit run their course either within or outside this cone of muscle.

Superior oblique (Fig. 7.88) has a posterior attachment to the lesser wing of the sphenoid adjacent to the common tendinous ring. The muscle passes anteriorly along the junction between the medial wall and the roof of the orbit and forms a tendon which traverses a loop of fibrous tissue, the trochlea, which lies at the superomedial angle of the orbital margin and allows the tendon of superior oblique to turn backwards across the upper surface of the eyeball. The tendon lies beneath superior rectus and attaches to the superolateral part of the eyeball behind the equator.

Inferior oblique (Figs 7.85 & 7.86), lying entirely in the anterior part of the orbit, attaches to the floor of the orbit just lateral to the

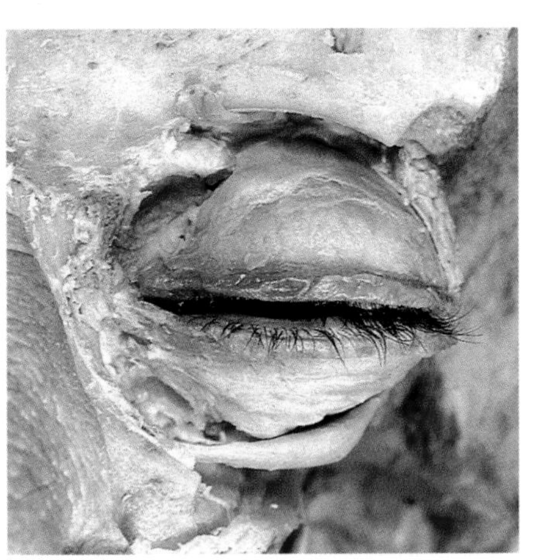

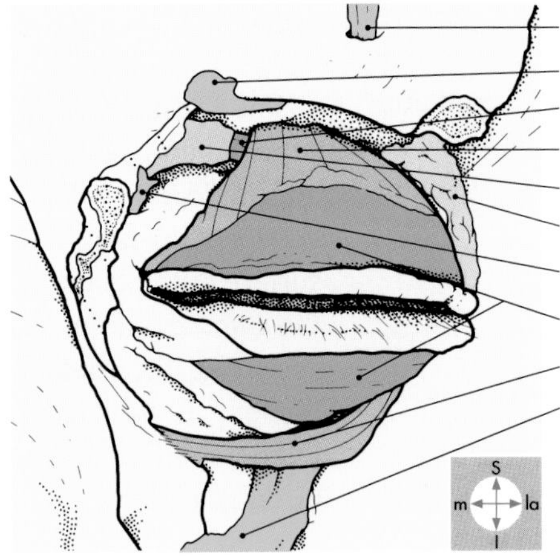

Fig. 7.85 Contents of the left orbit, revealed by removal of its lateral wall and floor and parts of the eyelids. The supraorbital nerve lies in a canal in the frontal bone.

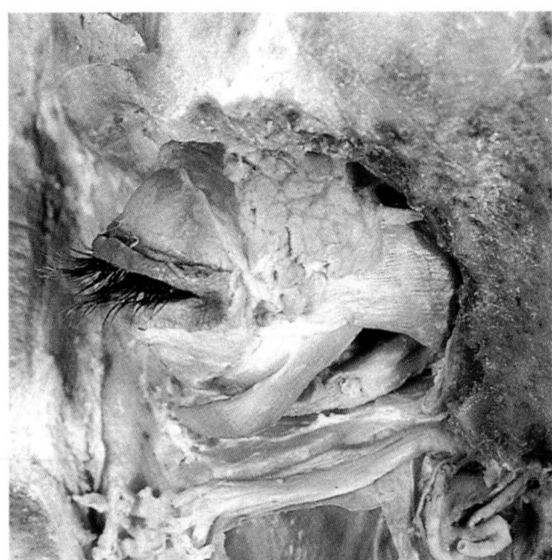

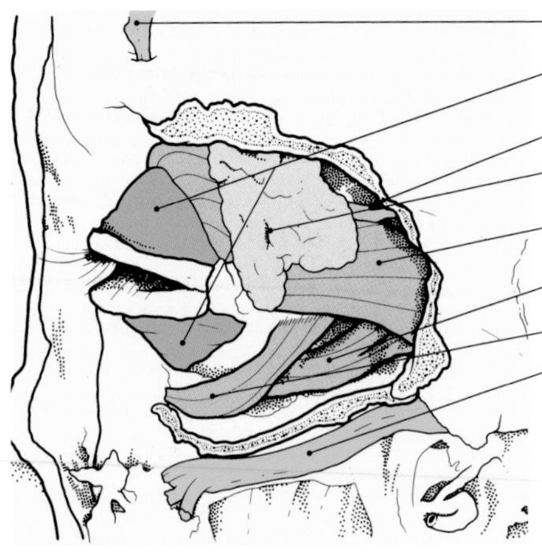

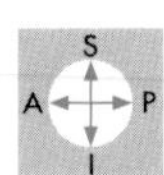

Fig. 7.86 Lateral view of specimen in Fig. 7.85.

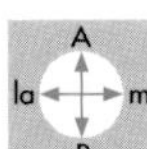

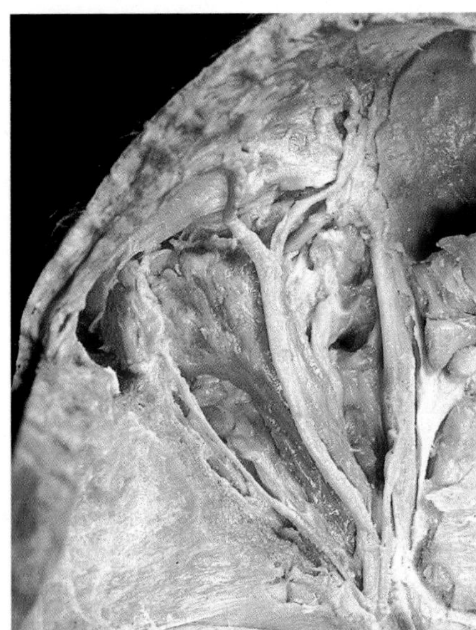

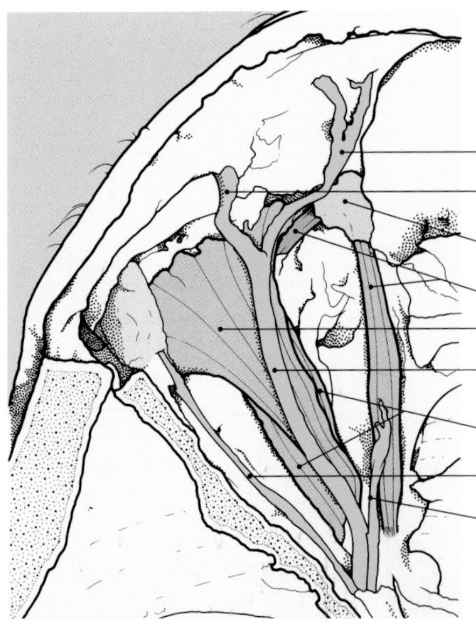

Fig. 7.87 Contents of the orbit seen from above after removal of the orbital plate of the frontal bone.

nasolacrimal canal. The muscle passes posterolaterally below the inferior rectus to attach to the inferolateral part of the eyeball behind the equator.

Three cranial nerves supply these muscles. The abducens (VI) nerve (see Figs 7.89 & 7.90) innervates lateral rectus while the trochlear (IV) nerve (Fig. 7.87) supplies superior oblique. All the remaining muscles receive motor branches from the oculomotor (III) nerve (Figs 7.88 & 7.90).

Movements of eyeball and eyelid

In defining the actions of individual extraocular muscles it is assumed that the eyeball is positioned so that the gaze is directed forwards into the distance. Within its fascial sheath the eyeball is rotated by the extraocular muscles, which displace the gaze upwards (elevation), downwards (depression), medially (adduction) and laterally (abduction). Rotation about an anteroposterior axis (torsion) may also occur. Collectively the extraocular muscles also contribute to the stability of the eyeball, the recti tending to pull the globe backwards and the obliques tending to pull it forwards.

The only actions of the medial and lateral recti are adduction and abduction respectively. Superior rectus elevates and adducts whilst inferior rectus depresses and adducts. Both oblique muscles produce abduction, the inferior oblique elevating the gaze and the superior oblique depressing it. Eye movements in general involve the coordinated contraction and relaxation of several individual muscles, and elevation and depression are accompanied by movement of the eyelids. Levator palpebrae superioris raises the upper eyelid (opposed by the orbicularis oculi) while inferior rectus depresses the lower eyelid.

Nerves

Several nerves reach the orbit from the middle cranial and pterygopalatine fossae. The optic (II) nerve (Fig. 7.88), which conveys visual sensation, traverses the optic canal with the ophthalmic artery. Enveloped by meninges and cerebrospinal fluid, the nerve passes forwards and laterally within the cone of rectus muscles and enters the eyeball just medial to its posterior pole. Increased intracranial pressure is transmitted through the cerebrospinal fluid to the eye, giving rise to the clinical sign called papilloedema. Other nerves gain the orbit through the orbital fissures.

The oculomotor (III) nerve (Figs 7.88 & 7.90) enters the cone of muscles via the superior orbital fissure. It has superior and inferior divisions, which are often formed before entering the orbit. The superior division supplies the superior rectus and levator palpebrae superioris while the inferior division gives branches to inferior rectus, inferior oblique, medial rectus and the ciliary ganglion. Sympathetic fibres to the smooth muscle in levator palpebrae superioris and inferior rectus enter the oculomotor (III) nerve in the cavernous sinus and travel with its branches to these muscles.

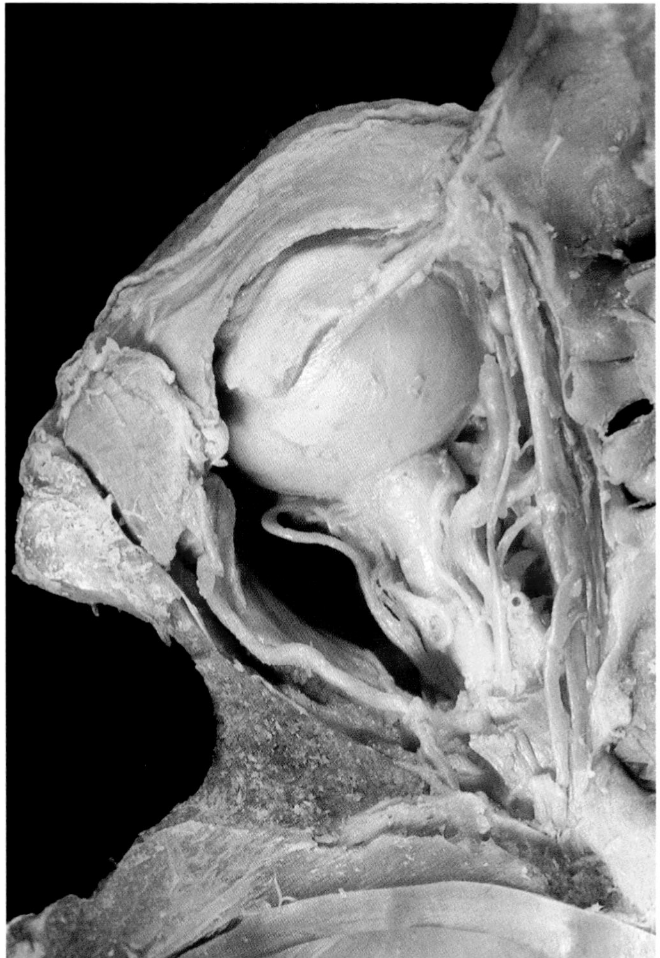

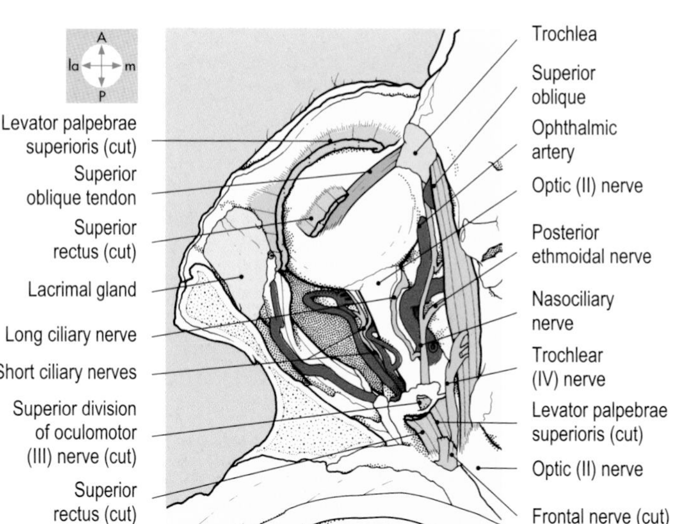

Fig. 7.88 Structures of the orbit seen following excision of superior rectus, levator palpebrae superioris and the superior division of the oculomotor nerve along with a quantity of orbital fat.

The trochlear (IV) nerve (see Fig. 7.88) enters the orbit via the superior orbital fissure, passing above the muscle cone to supply superior oblique.

The abducens (VI) nerve (Figs 7.89 & 7.90) gains the orbit via the superior orbital fissure and passes forwards on the inner surface of lateral rectus, which it supplies.

The ophthalmic (V_1) division of the trigeminal nerve divides into lacrimal, frontal and nasociliary nerves, each of which enters the orbit through the superior orbital fissure. The lacrimal nerve (see Fig. 7.87) passes forwards, outside the muscle cone, along the angle between the roof and lateral wall of the orbit. It is joined by parasympathetic secretomotor fibres from the zygomatic nerve (see p. 352), which are destined for the lacrimal gland. In addition, the lacrimal nerve conveys sensation from the lacrimal gland and the lateral part of the upper eyelid.

The frontal nerve (see Fig. 7.87) lies on the upper surface of levator palpebrae superioris and divides into supraorbital and supratrochlear nerves. The supraorbital nerve (see Figs 7.85 & 7.87) curves around the upper part of the orbital margin, occupying the supraorbital notch, and conveys sensation from the upper

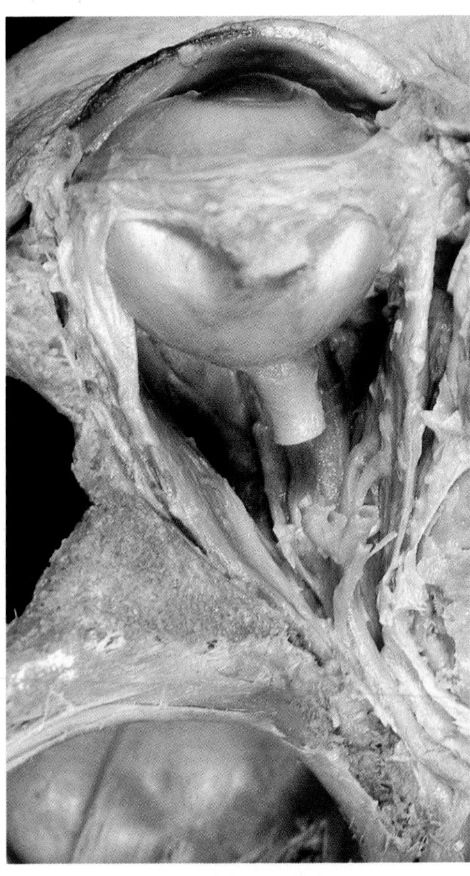

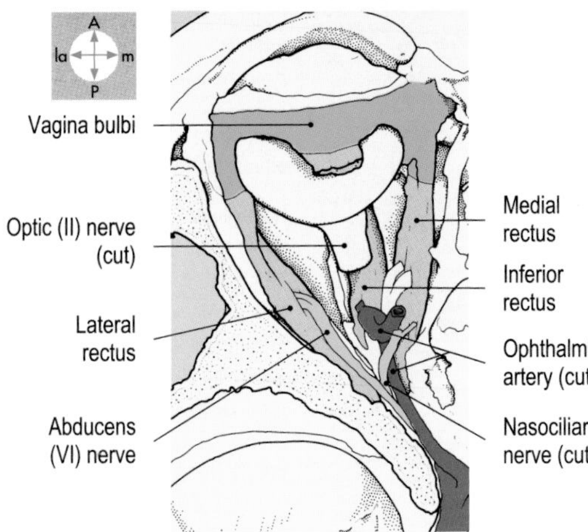

Fig. 7.89 Muscles of the orbit seen after removal of the upper eyelid, part of the optic nerve, and superior oblique.

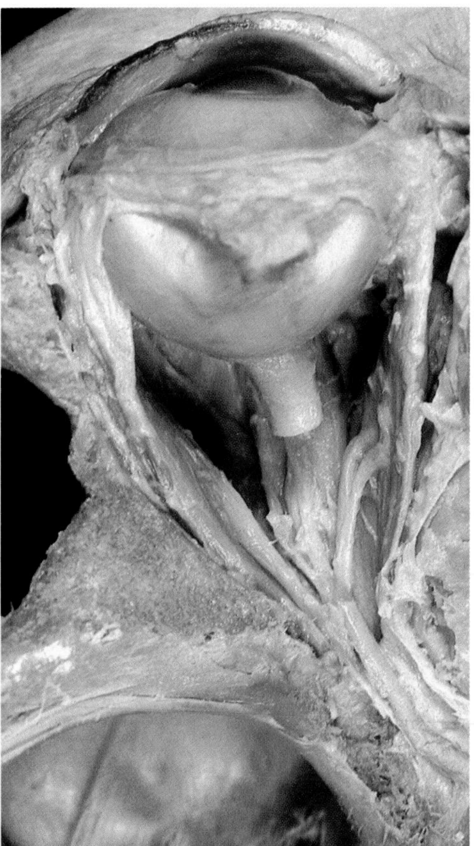

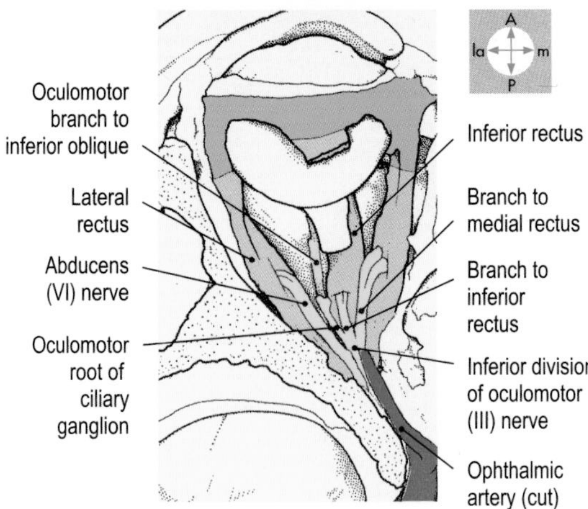

Fig. 7.90 Inferior division of the oculomotor nerve, revealed by excision of the distal part of the ophthalmic artery and the nasociliary nerve.

eyelid, forehead, scalp and frontal air sinus. The supratrochlear nerve (see Figs 7.85 & 7.87) lies more medially, leaving the orbit just above the trochlea to supply sensory fibres to the medial part of the upper eyelid, forehead and scalp.

The nasociliary nerve (see Fig. 7.88), lying within the muscle cone, crosses above the optic (II) nerve and continues forwards along the medial wall of the orbit to terminate below the trochlea. Its branches include one to the ciliary ganglion, two long ciliary nerves, posterior and anterior ethmoidal nerves and the infratrochlear nerve. The long ciliary nerves, which carry sympathetic vasoconstrictor fibres that join the nasociliary nerve in the cavernous sinus, pass forwards to supply vessels within the eyeball. The posterior and anterior ethmoidal nerves leave through their respective foramina, supplying ethmoidal air cells. The anterior ethmoidal nerve passes between the frontal and ethmoid bones and emerges on the upper surface of the cribriform plate. Leaving the anterior fossa, the nerve penetrates the plate to run on the inner surface of the nasal bone as the external nasal nerve and eventually reaches the tip of the nose. It conveys sensation from a strip of nasal skin close to the midline and from the nasal septum. The infratrochlear nerve supplies the medial part of the upper eyelid (see Fig. 7.85).

Autonomic nerves

The ciliary ganglion lies just behind the eyeball, lateral to the optic (II) nerve. It receives sensory fibres from the nasociliary nerve, sympathetic fibres from the internal carotid plexus in the cavernous sinus and parasympathetic fibres from the oculomotor (III) nerve. Only the last synapse in the ganglion. From the anterior part of the ganglion, short ciliary nerves (see Fig. 7.88) pass forwards into the eyeball, conveying general sensory fibres from the eyeball (including the cornea), parasympathetic fibres to the ciliary muscle and sphincter pupillae and sympathetic fibres to dilator pupillae.

Vasoconstrictor sympathetic fibres reach the eyeball in the long ciliary branches of the nasociliary nerve. Other intraorbital sympathetic fibres travel in the oculomotor (III) nerve to the smooth muscle component of levator palpebrae superioris and inferior rectus. Parasympathetic fibres reach the lacrimal gland via the lacrimal nerve, which communicates with the zygomatic branch of the maxillary (V_2) division of the trigeminal nerve. The cell bodies of these fibres lie in the pterygopalatine ganglion (see p. 352).

Vessels

The ophthalmic artery (Figs 7.88 & 7.89), a branch of the internal carotid artery in the middle cranial fossa, enters the orbit through the optic canal inferior to the optic (II) nerve. The artery then accompanies the nasociliary nerve, passing above the optic nerve and continuing forwards along the medial wall of the orbit. Its first branch, the central retinal artery, enters the optic nerve and passes into the eyeball to supply the retina. Occlusion of this artery results in blindness. Other branches of the ophthalmic artery accompany those of the ophthalmic (V_1) division of the trigeminal nerve. In addition, there are posterior and anterior ciliary branches to the eyeball, and branches to the extraocular muscles.

Venous blood from the eyeball and adjacent structures drains into inferior and superior ophthalmic veins. The superior ophthalmic vein terminates posteriorly in the cavernous venous sinus while the inferior vein passes through the inferior orbital fissure into the pterygoid venous plexus in the pterygopalatine fossa. Both superior and inferior ophthalmic veins communicate with veins on the face.

Exam Skills

Each of the incomplete statements below is followed by five suggested answers or completions. Decide which are true and which are false. The answers are supplied on page 415.

1. The internal carotid artery:

a) arises from the brachiocephalic artery on the right.
b) traverses the foramina transversaria of cervical vertebrae 1–6.
c) has a branch entering the orbit.
d) forms the basilar artery.
e) gives rise to the anterior cerebral artery.

2. In the larynx:

a) sensation from the vestibular fold travels in the superior laryngeal nerve.
b) contraction of cricothyroid lowers pitch.
c) the cricoid cartilage forms a complete ring.
d) interarytenoid muscle adducts the vocal folds.
e) the vocal fold is covered with respiratory epithelium.

3. The internal jugular vein:

a) is a continuation of the sigmoid sinus.
b) drains into the brachiocephalic vein.
c) receives blood from the lingual vein.
d) communicates with the retromandibular vein.
e) has the ansa cervicalis on its anterolateral surface.

4. The head of the mandible:

a) is moved medially by lateral and medial pterygoid acting together.
b) is separated from the temporal bone by an intra-articular disc.
c) is moved posteriorly by the lateral pterygoid muscle.
d) is moved posteriorly by temporalis.
e) most often dislocates backwards.

5. The intracranial dura mater:

a) is easily separated into endosteal and meningeal layers.
b) forms the tentorium cerebelli.
c) contains the sigmoid sinus in the free edge of the falx cerebri.
d) is separated from the arachnoid mater by cerebrospinal fluid.
e) forms the diaphragma sellae.

6. The thyroid gland:

a) has an isthmus at the level of the second and third tracheal rings.
b) receives blood from a branch of the subclavian artery.
c) is enclosed in prevertebral fascia.
d) is closely related to both recurrent laryngeal nerves.
e) rises on swallowing.

7. The hypoglossal nerve:

a) leaves the skull through the jugular foramen.
b) conveys touch sensation from the anterior two-thirds of the tongue.
c) innervates the genioglossus muscle.
d) carries C1 fibres for the ansa cervicalis.
e) when damaged results in the protruded tongue deviating to the damaged side.

8. Transection of the facial nerve in the internal acoustic meatus gives rise to:

a) paralysis of buccinator.
b) loss of taste in the anterior two-thirds of the tongue.
c) paralysis of masseter.
d) loss of secretion by the parotid gland.
e) paralysis of stapedius.

9. The maxillary air sinus:

a) extends below the level of the hard palate.
b) has a sensory supply from the ophthalmic division of the trigeminal nerve.
c) is indented by the root of the canine tooth.
d) has a roof formed by the floor of the orbit.
e) opens into the inferior meatus.

10. The maxillary division of the trigeminal nerve:

a) is related to the cavernous venous sinus.
b) conveys sensation from the lower eyelid.
c) passes through the foramen rotundum.
d) conveys sensation from part of the nasal septum.
e) conveys sensation from the hard palate.

11. The vagus nerve:

a) passes through the jugular foramen.
b) is contained in the carotid sheath.
c) conveys touch sensation from the laryngopharynx.
d) is motor to the stylopharyngeus muscle.
e) carries fibres destined for the submandibular gland.

12. In the neck:

a) the phrenic nerve crosses posterior to the subclavian artery.
b) the left vagus nerve gives rise to the recurrent laryngeal nerve.
c) the scalenus anterior muscle lies posterior to the subclavian vein.
d) the thoracic duct drains into the junction of the subclavian and internal jugular veins on the left.
e) the sternohyoid muscle is supplied by the ansa cervicalis.

13. The glossopharyngeal nerve:

a) is motor to the pharyngeal constrictor muscles.
b) traverses the parotid gland.
c) conveys touch sensation from the posterior third of the tongue.
d) is motor to stylopharyngeus.
e) carries sensory fibres from the larynx.

14. Concerning the nasal cavity and its walls:

a) the nasolacrimal duct opens in the middle meatus.
b) the inferior concha is part of the ethmoid bone.
c) the septum is supplied by the mandibular division of the trigeminal nerve.
d) the vomer forms the anterior part of the septum.
e) the sphenoidal air sinus opens into the middle meatus.

15. Concerning the cranial cavity:

a) the superior sagittal sinus drains into the transverse sinus.
b) bleeding from the middle meningeal artery gives rise to extradural/epidural haematoma.
c) the trigeminal ganglion is closely related to the apex of the petrous temporal bone.
d) the internal carotid artery gives rise to the posterior cerebral artery.
e) the temporal lobe lies in the anterior cranial fossa.

16. Concerning the orbit:

a) lateral rectus is supplied by the fourth cranial nerve.
b) superior oblique produces adduction of the eye.
c) the oculomotor nerve carries parasympathetic fibres to sphincter pupillae.
d) secretomotor fibres for the lacrimal gland travel in the nasociliary nerve.
e) the ophthalmic artery enters through the superior orbital fissure.

Clinical Skills

The answers are supplied on page 418.

Case Study 1

A 50-year-old woman presented to her doctor with a pain-free swelling in the right side of her face. Examination indicated that this was a benign parotid tumour, and the woman had a partial parotidectomy at a later date. On recovering from the anaesthetic, the patient was observed to dribble from the right side of her mouth and to have difficulty with closing her right eye. Over a period of a few weeks both these signs disappeared, but the patient now noticed that when she ate she experienced sweating from the skin overlying the area from which the tumour was removed.

Questions:

1. How would you test for normal function in the parotid gland?
2. Why did the patient experience problems with her mouth and eye after surgery?
3. Why did the initial postsurgery symptoms recover?
4. Explain why the patient experienced sweating with eating.

Case Study 2

The morning after a particularly good party, a 20-year-old student awoke and yawned widely. He heard a click and found that he could not close his mouth. He also experienced sharp, severe pain on both sides of his face just in front of the ear. The student was now unable to speak clearly or eat.

Questions:

1. What had happened?
2. What anatomical features are responsible for the condition?
3. On anatomical grounds, what is the treatment?

Case Study 3

A 35-year-old female visited her doctor with weight loss, anxiety and tremor. The doctor observed that she had exophthalmos (protruding eyes) and correctly made the diagnosis of thyrotoxicosis (overactive thyroid gland). In order to examine the gland he stood behind the sitting patient and felt her neck just below the laryngeal prominence.

Questions:

1. What would the doctor ask the patient to do in order to make his examination of the gland complete?
   The prescribed treatment in this patient was partial thyroidectomy. Following surgery the patient was noticed to have a husky voice.
2. What is the likely cause of the change in voice?
3. How may the surgeon have avoided the problem?
4. What other nearby structures are particularly liable to damage in this operation?

Case Study 4

A general practitioner referred a 14-year-old boy to hospital for urgent admission. The boy had suffered acne for some months and in the previous few days had experienced an exacerbation of the condition. He admitted to squeezing pustules on his left cheek and 36 hours later noticed double vision on looking to the left. In the previous few hours he had pain in the middle third of his face on the left and then complained of double vision on looking in most directions.

Questions:

1. What was the diagnosis?
2. Why did the boy experience double vision on looking to the left?
3. What is the anatomical explanation for the progression of events?
4. If allowed to progress untreated, what would be the likely next problem?

Observation Skills

Identify the structures indicated. The answers are supplied at the foot of the page.

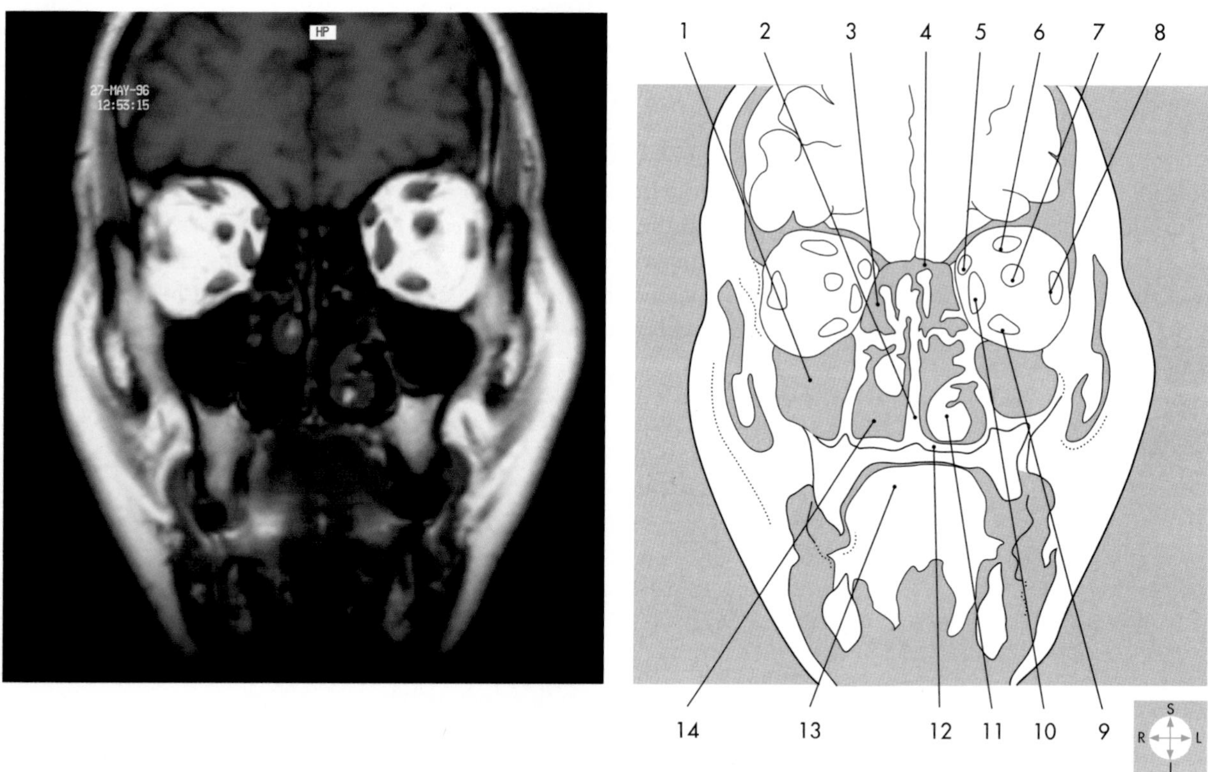

Fig. 7.91 Coronal MR image showing the orbits and nasal cavities. Compare Figs 7.47 & 7.97.

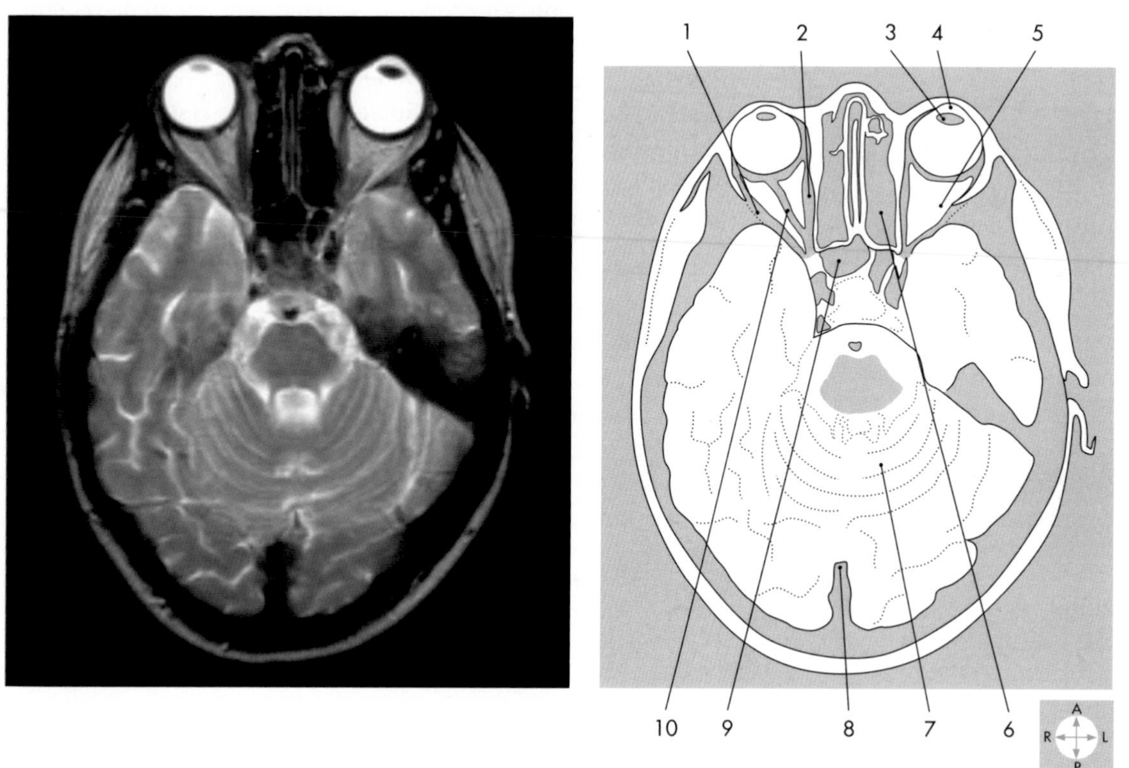

Fig. 7.92 Transverse MR image showing the orbits. Compare Fig. 7.99.

Answers

Fig. 7.91 1 = maxillary sinus; 2 = nasal septum; 3 = ethmoid air cells; 4 = cribriform plate; 5 = superior oblique; 6 = superior rectus; 7 = optic nerve; 8 = lateral rectus; 9 = inferior rectus; 10 = medial rectus; 11 = inferior concha; 12 = hard palate; 13 = tongue; 14 = nasal cavity.

Fig. 7.92 1 = lateral rectus; 2 = medial rectus; 3 = lens; 4 = anterior chamber; 5 = retrobulbar fat; 6 = ethmoid air cells; 7 = cerebellum; 8 = posterior cerebellar notch containing falx cerebelli; 9 = sphenoid sinus; 10 = optic nerve.

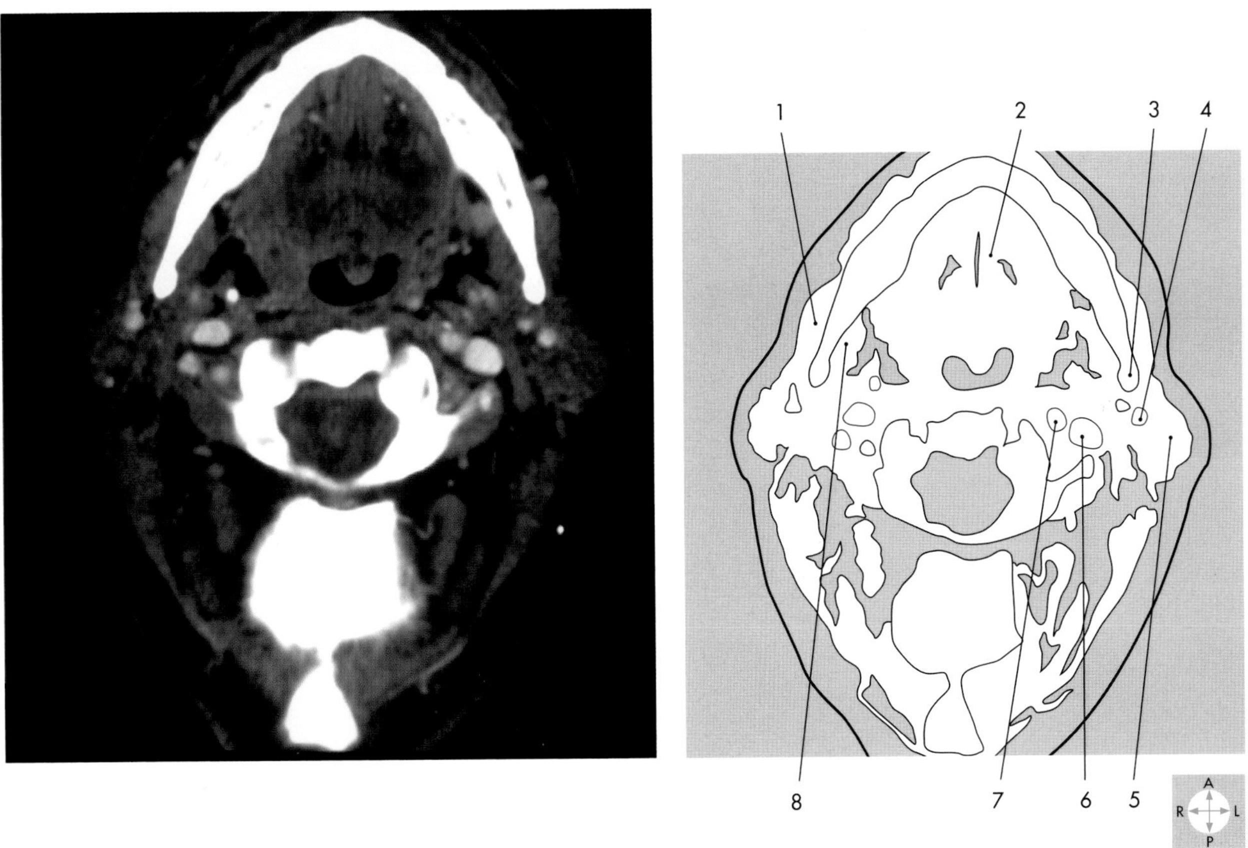

Fig. 7.93 Transverse CT image at the level of the second cervical vertebra. Compare Figs 7.25 & 7.101.

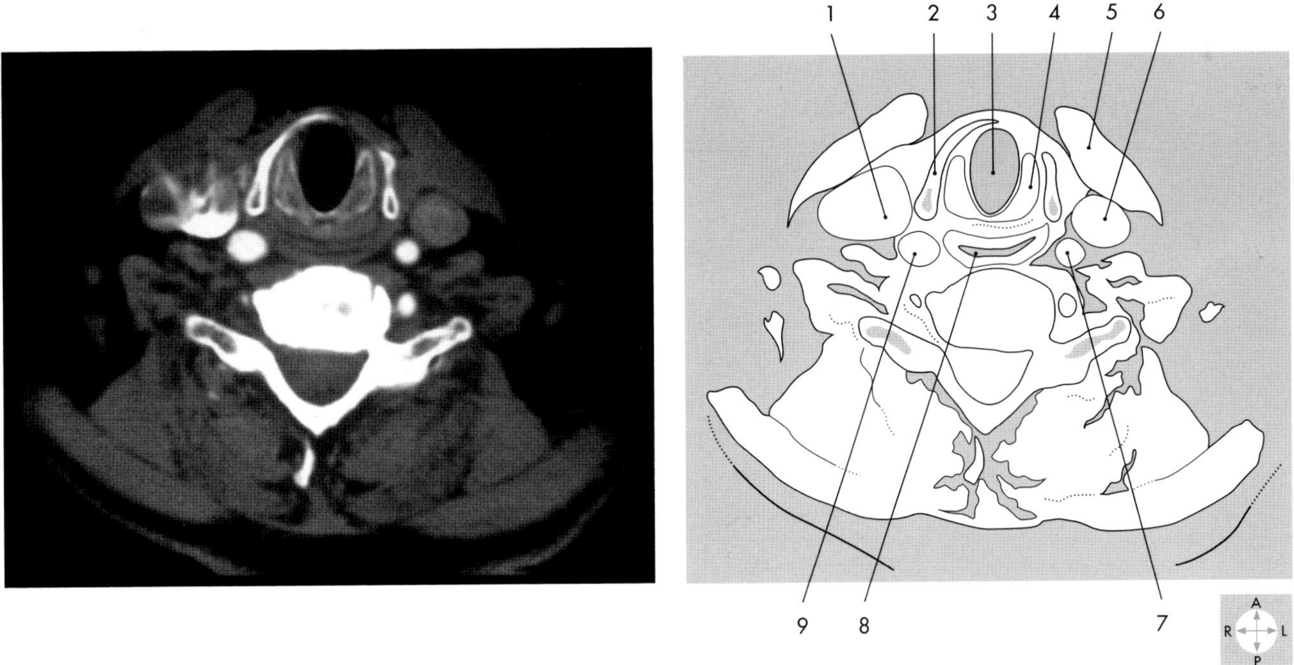

Fig. 7.94 Transverse CT image at the level of the fifth cervical vertebra. Compare Fig. 7.5.

Answers

Fig. 7.93 1 = masseter; 2 = genioglossus; 3 = ramus of mandible; 4 = external carotid artery; 5 = parotid gland; 6 = internal jugular vein; 7 = internal carotid artery; 8 = medial pterygoid.

Fig. 7.94 1 = right internal jugular vein; 2 = lamina of thyroid cartilage; 3 = cavity of larynx; 4 = cricoid cartilage; 5 = sternocleidomastoid; 6 = left internal jugular vein; 7 = left common carotid artery; 8 = laryngopharynx; 9 = right common carotid artery.

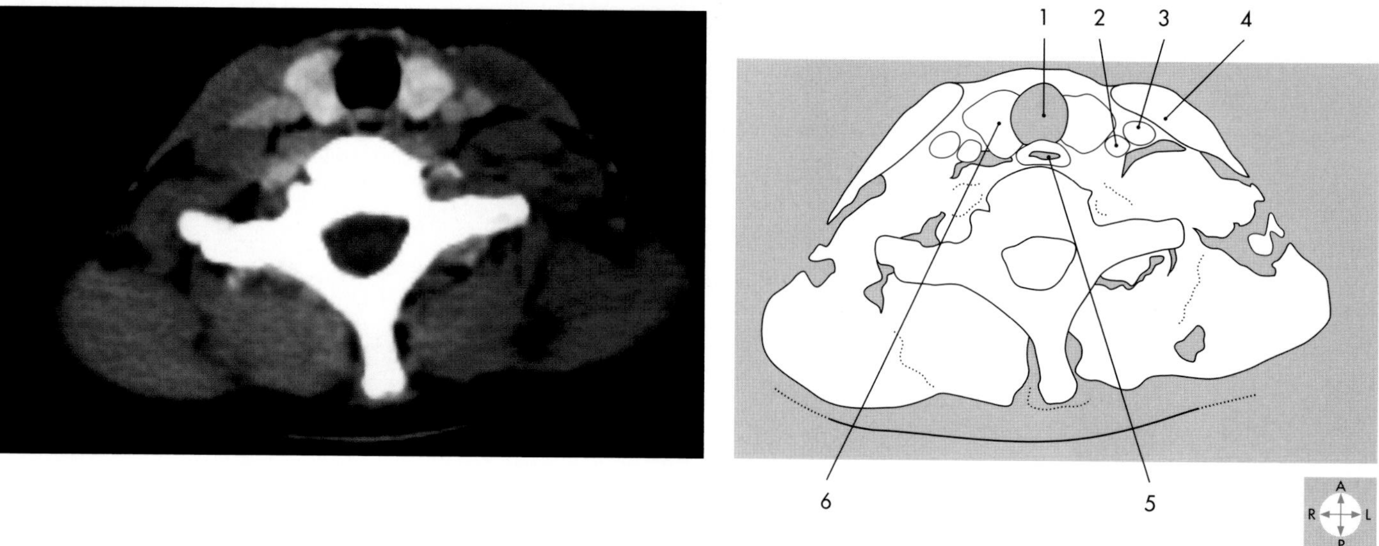

Fig. 7.95 Transverse CT image at the level of the sixth cervical vertebra. Compare Fig. 7.102.

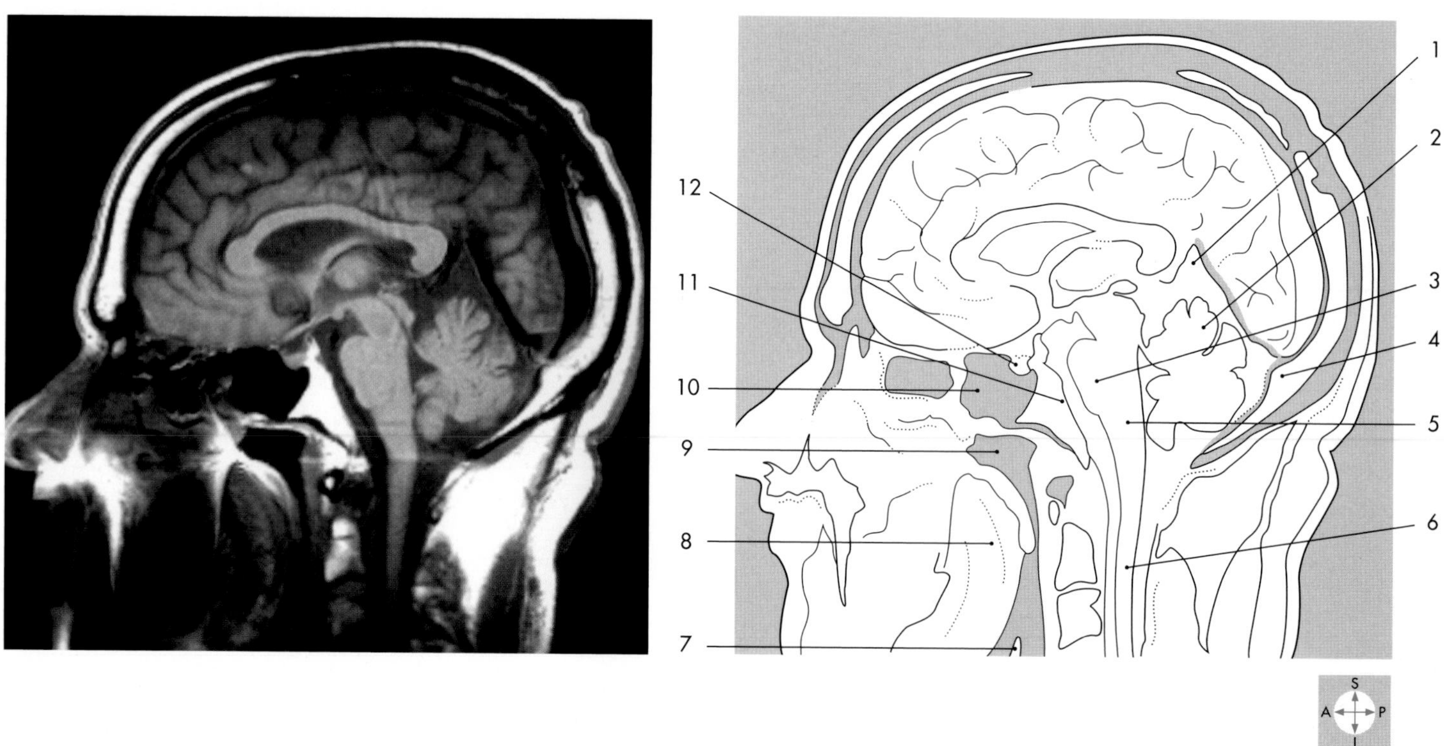

Fig. 7.96 Sagittal MR image of the head near the midline.

Answers

Fig. 7.95 1 = trachea; 2 = common carotid artery; 3 = internal jugular vein; 4 = sternocleidomastoid; 5 = oesophagus; 6 = lateral lobe of thyroid gland.

Fig. 7.96 1 = tentorium cerebelli; 2 = cerebellum; 3 = pons; 4 = internal occipital protuberance; 5 = medulla oblongata; 6 = cervical spinal cord; 7 = epiglottis; 8 = tongue musculature; 9 = nasopharynx; 10 = sphenoid sinus; 11 = clivus; 12 = pituitary gland.

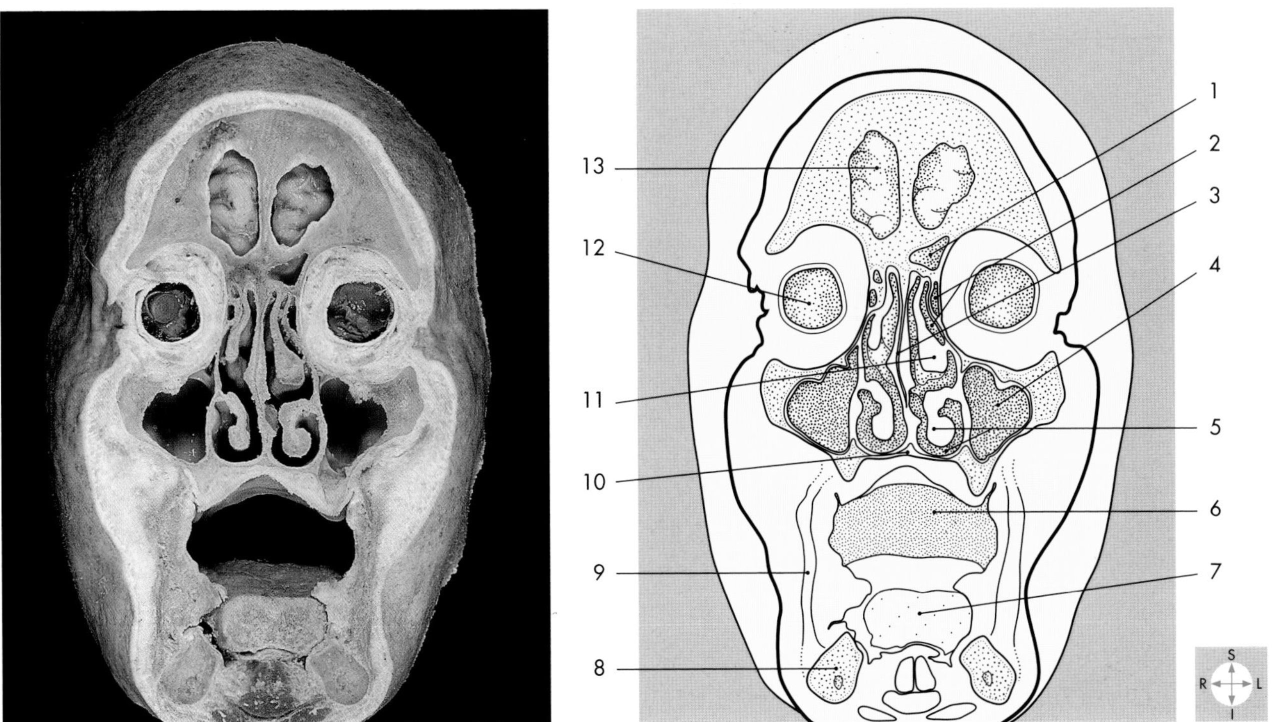

Fig. 7.97 Coronal section showing the orbits and nasal cavities. Anterior aspect. Compare Fig. 7.91.

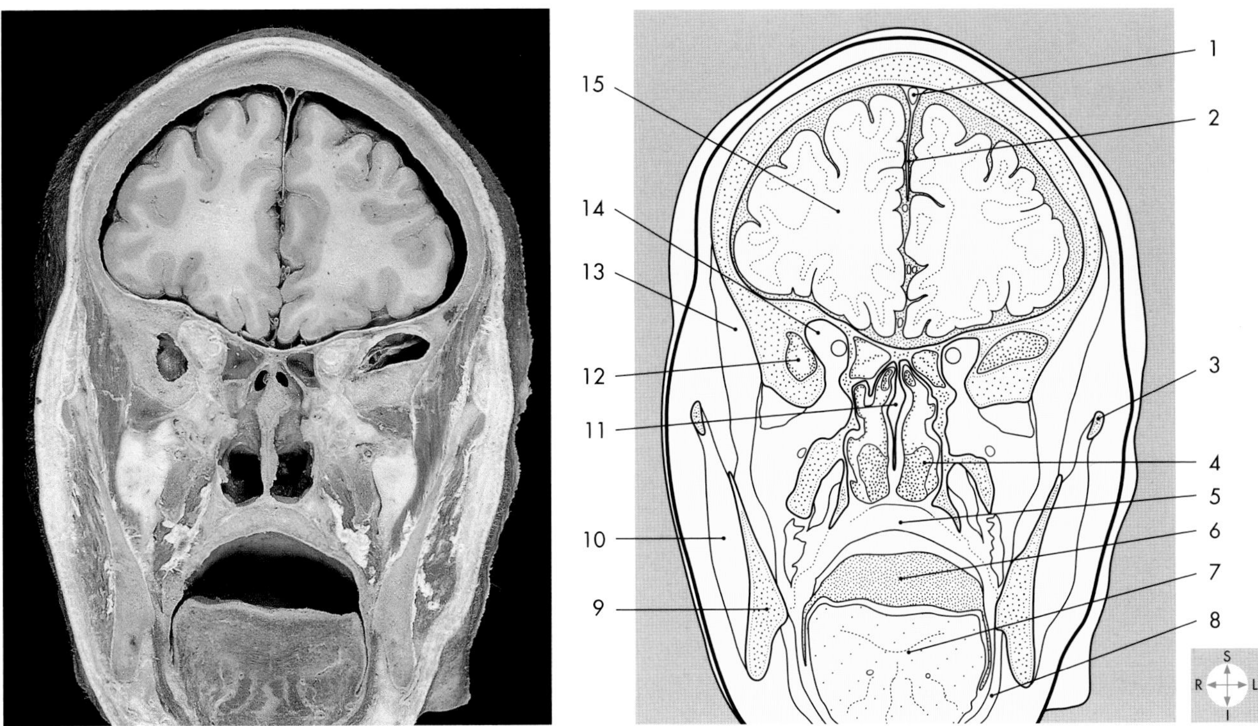

Fig. 7.98 Coronal section at the choanae showing the soft palate. Anterior aspect.

Answers

Fig. 7.97 1 = frontal sinus; 2 = ethmoid air cells; 3 = nasal septum; 4 = maxillary sinus; 5 = inferior concha and meatus; 6 = oral cavity (distended); 7 = tongue; 8 = mandible; 9 = buccinator; 10 = hard palate; 11 = middle concha; 12 = eyeball; 13 = frontal lobe.

Fig. 7.98 1 = superior sagittal sinus; 2 = falx cerebri; 3 = zygomatic arch; 4 = nasopharynx; 5 = soft palate; 6 = oral cavity (distended); 7 = tongue; 8 = mylohyoid; 9 = mandible; 10 = masseter; 11 = nasal septum; 12 = temporal lobe; 13 = temporalis; 14 = apex of orbit; 15 = cerebral hemisphere.

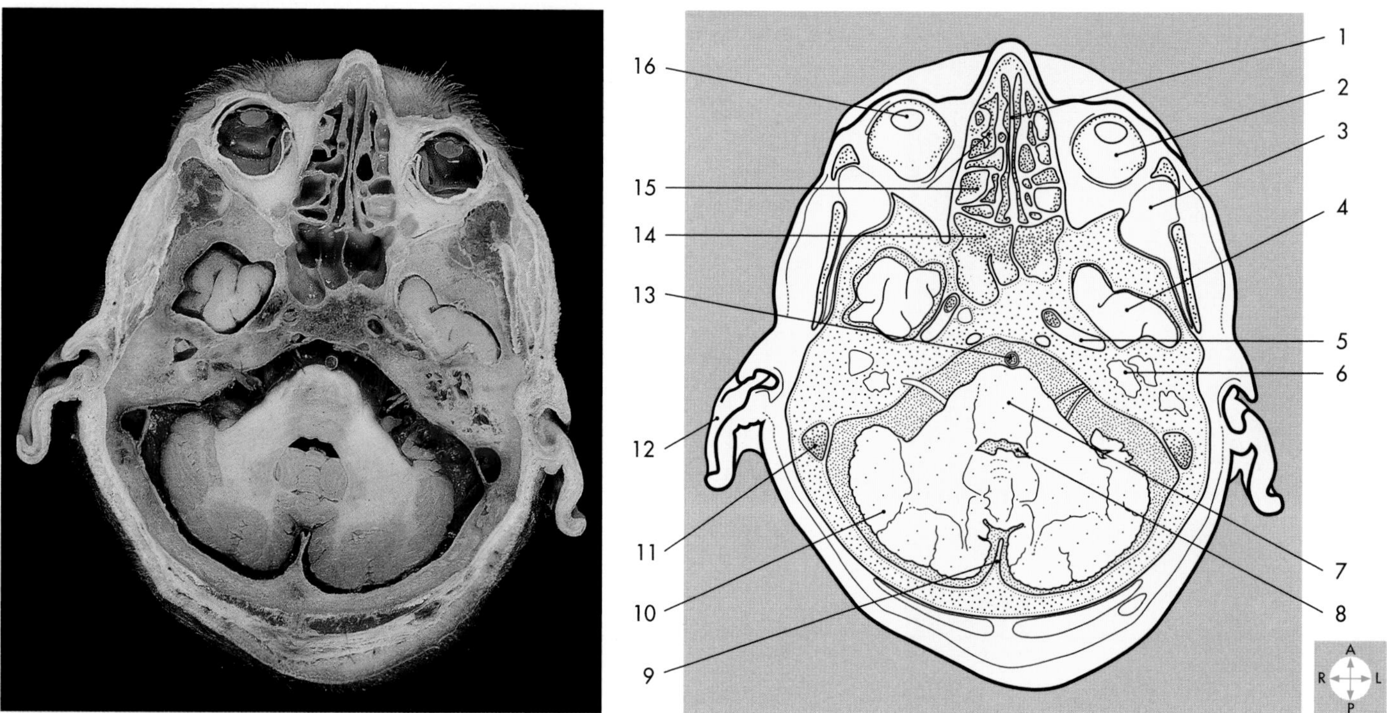

Fig. 7.99 Transverse section showing the orbits and posterior cranial fossa. Inferior aspect. Compare Fig. 7.92.

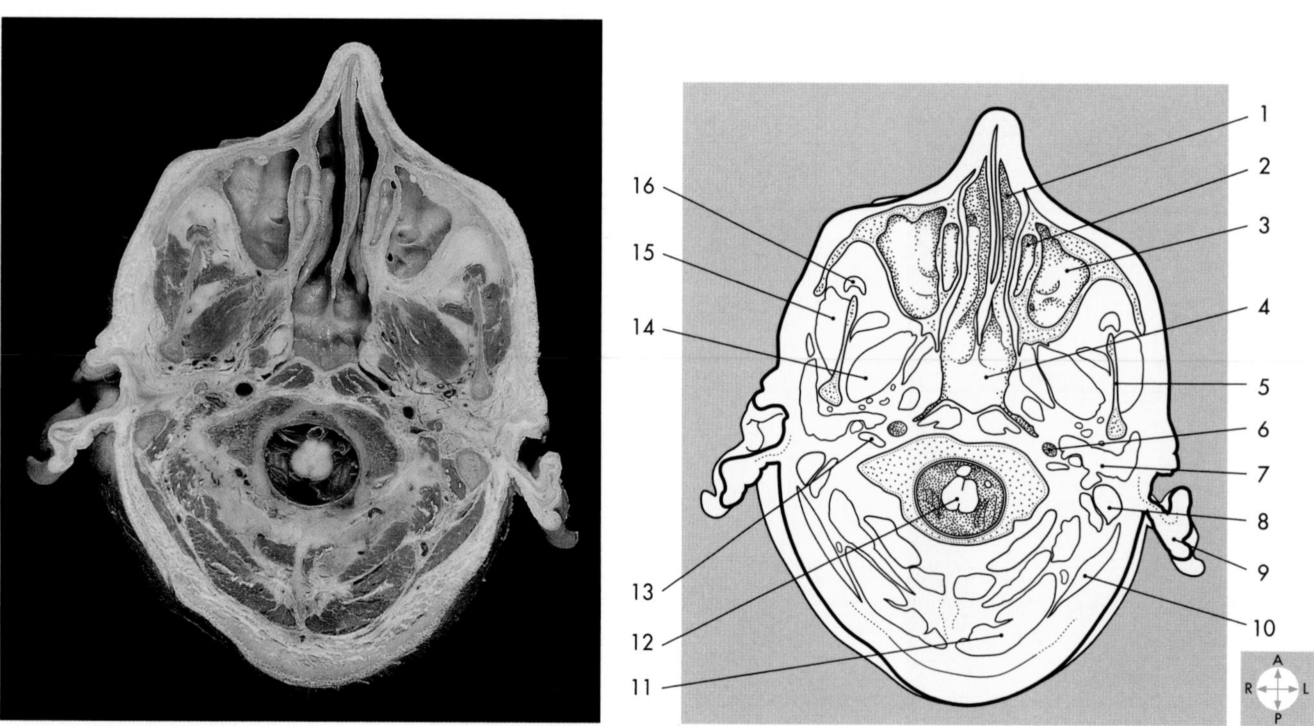

Fig. 7.100 Transverse section showing the maxillary sinuses and nasal cavities. Inferior aspect.

Answers

Fig. 7.99 1 = nasal septum; 2 = eyeball; 3 = temporalis; 4 = temporal lobe; 5 = carotid canal; 6 = inner ear; 7 = pons; 8 = fourth ventricle; 9 = falx cerebelli; 10 = cerebellum; 11 = sigmoid sinus; 12 = pinna; 13 = basilar artery; 14 = sphenoid sinus; 15 = ethmoid air cells; 16 = lens.

Fig. 7.100 1 = nasal cavity; 2 = ethmoid air cells; 3 = maxillary sinus; 4 = nasopharynx; 5 = mandible; 6 = internal carotid artery; 7 = parotid gland; 8 = mastoid process; 9 = pinna; 10 = sternocleidomastoid; 11 = trapezius; 12 = cervical spinal cord; 13 = internal jugular vein; 14 = lateral pterygoid; 15 = masseter; 16 = temporalis.

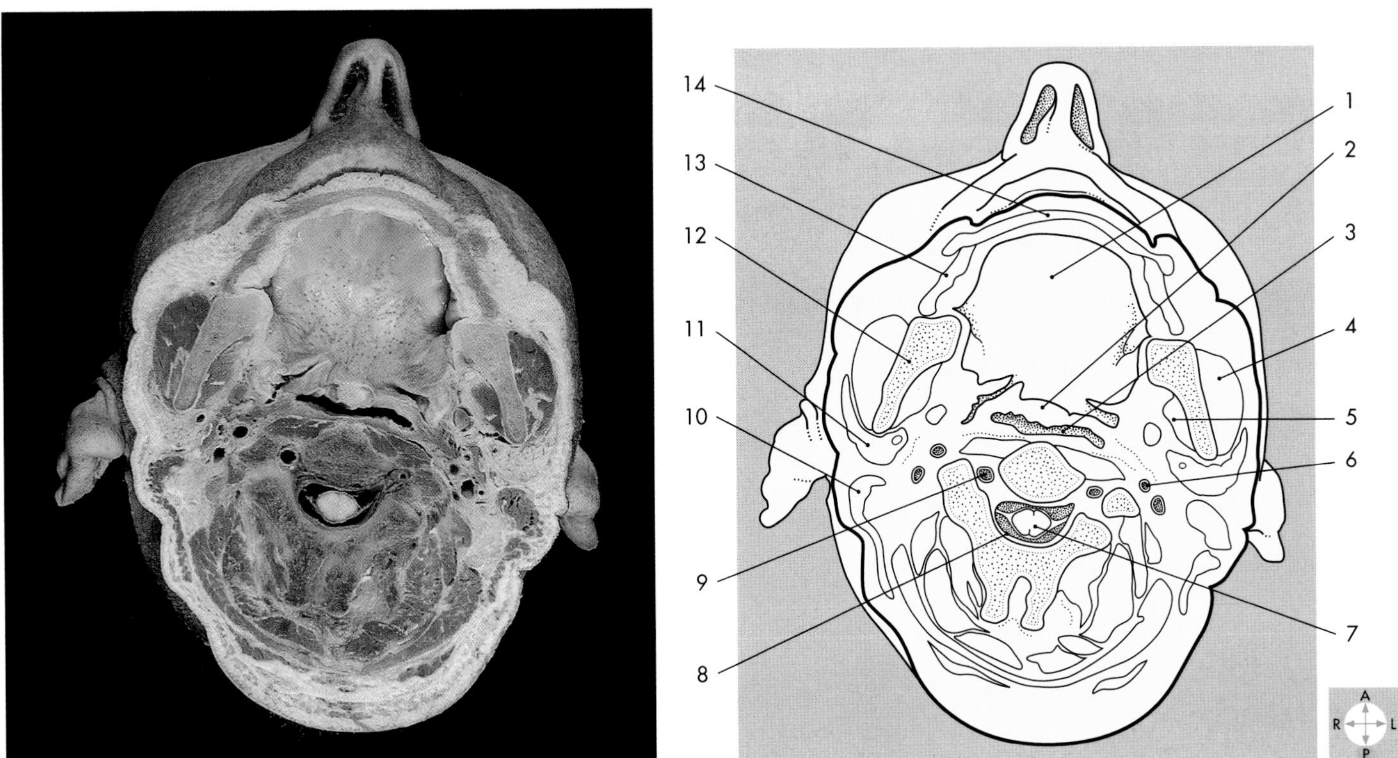

Fig. 7.101 Transverse section at the level of the second cervical vertebra. Inferior aspect. Compare Fig. 7.93.

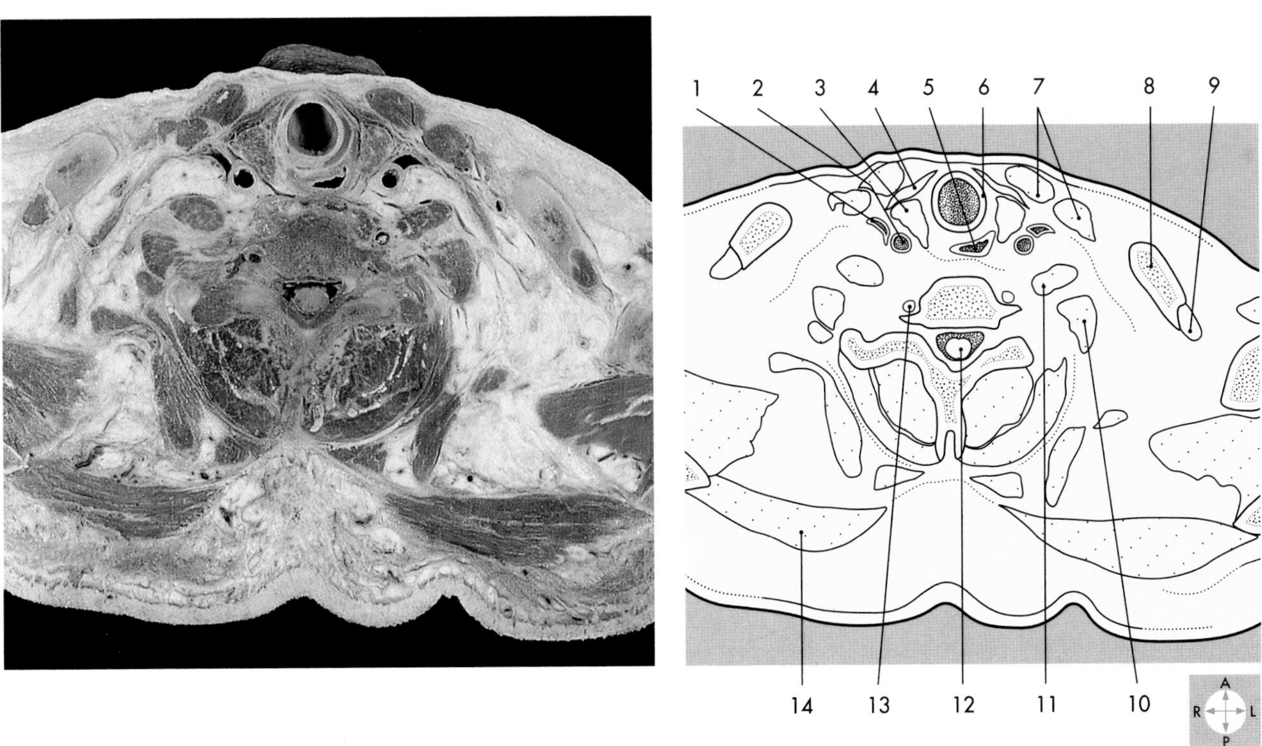

Fig. 7.102 Transverse section at the level of the sixth cervical vertebra. Inferior aspect. Compare Fig. 7.95.

Answers

Fig. 7.101 1 = hard palate; 2 = soft palate; 3 = oropharynx; 4 = masseter; 5 = medial pterygoid; 6 = internal carotid artery; 7 = cervical spinal cord; 8 = dura mater; 9 = vertebral artery; 10 = sternocleidomastoid; 11 = parotid gland; 12 = mandible; 13 = buccinator; 14 = orbicularis oris in lower lip.

Fig. 7.102 1 = internal jugular vein; 2 = common carotid artery; 3 = thyroid gland; 4 = strap muscle; 5 = laryngopharynx; 6 = cricoid cartilage; 7 = sternocleidomastoid; 8 = clavicle; 9 = subclavius; 10 = scalenus medius; 11 = scalenus anterior; 12 = spinal cord; 13 = vertebral artery; 14 = trapezius.

Back

CHAPTER 8

Introduction

The back consists of the vertebrae, the intervertebral joints and ligaments, and the muscles that clothe their posterior and lateral aspects (Fig. 8.1). The vertebral column encloses the spinal cord and its meninges.

The vertebral column comprises vertebrae which are classified regionally as cervical (7), thoracic (12), lumbar (5), sacral (5 vertebrae fused to form the sacrum) and coccygeal (3–5) (Fig. 8.5). Typically, a vertebra consists of a body, two pedicles, two laminae, two transverse processes and a single spinous process (Fig. 8.6). The body and vertebral arch, formed by the pedicles and laminae, surround the vertebral canal which encloses the meninges and spinal cord (see Fig. 8.8). Pairs of superior and inferior articular processes form synovial joints with corresponding processes on adjacent vertebrae. The vertebral bodies are united by fibrocartilaginous discs (Fig. 8.5) and anterior and posterior longitudinal ligaments (see p. 402). Each vertebra usually possesses features characteristic of its region.

The vertebral column is curved anteroposteriorly. In the adult, the thoracic and sacral/coccygeal vertebrae form curves that are concave anteriorly (primary or kyphotic curves), whereas in the cervical and lumbar regions the curves are concave posteriorly (secondary or lordotic curves) (Fig. 8.5).

The movements between adjacent vertebrae are relatively limited although summation enables the vertebral column as a whole to achieve a wide range of motion (Figs 8.2–8.4). Both flexion and extension occur throughout the length of the vertebral column, particularly in the cervical region. Lateral flexion is greatest in the cervical and lumbar regions and rotation occurs mainly in the upper thoracic region.

The muscles of the back (see Fig. 8.7) may be classified into superficial, intermediate and deep groups. The superficial muscles

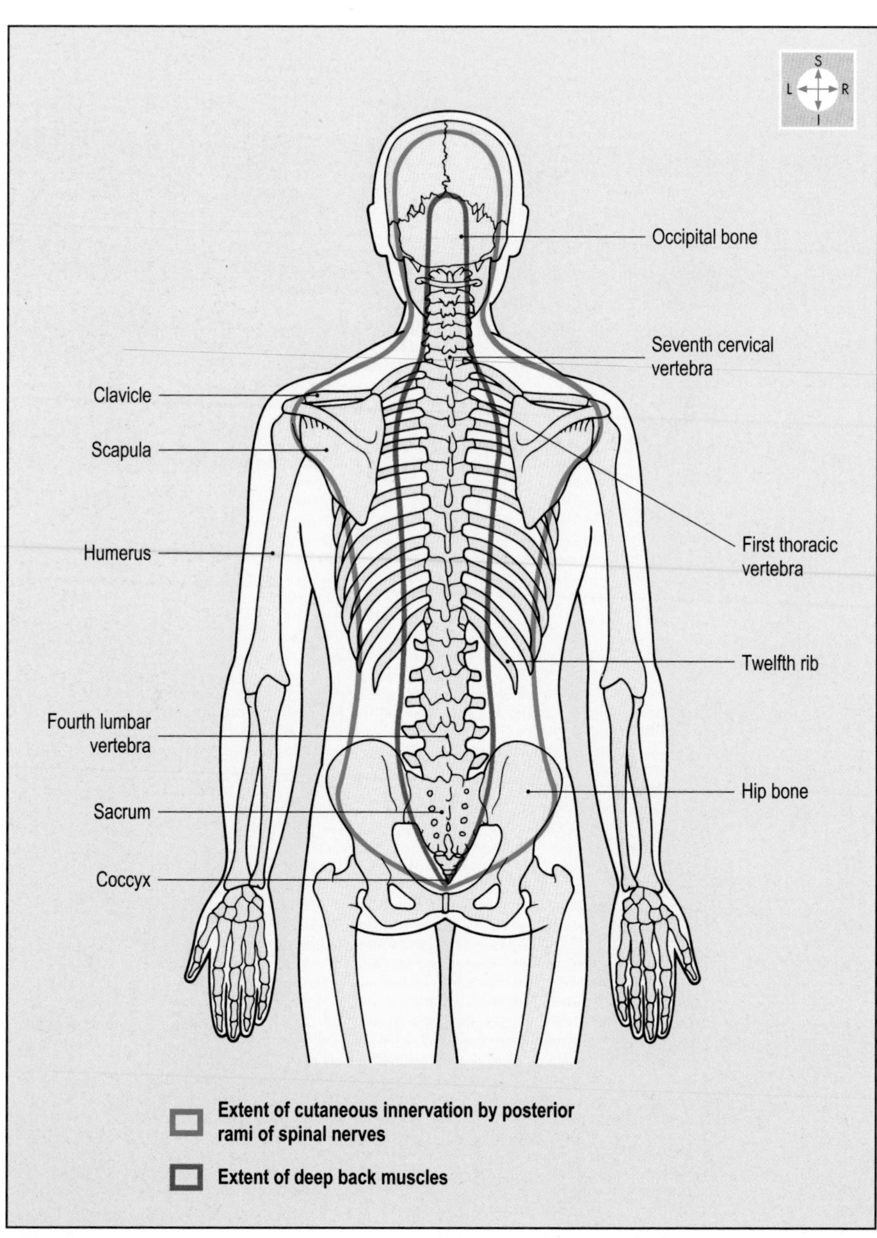

Fig. 8.1 Posterior aspect of the back.

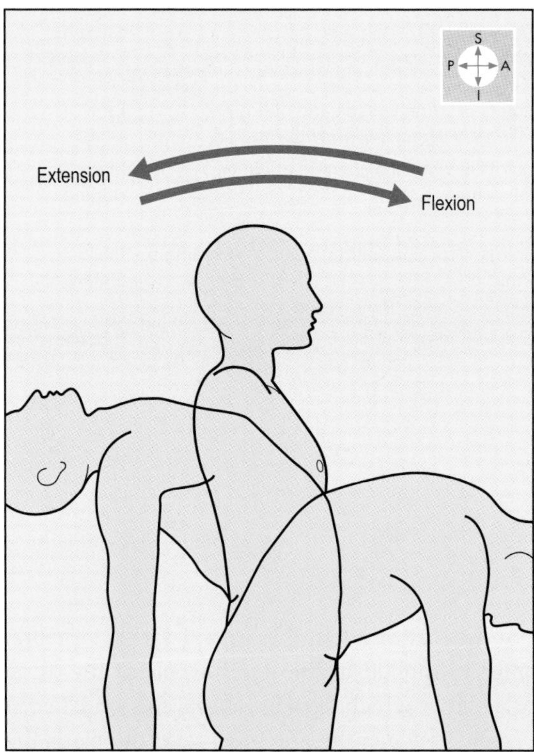

Fig. 8.2 Flexion and extension of the vertebral column from the anatomical position.

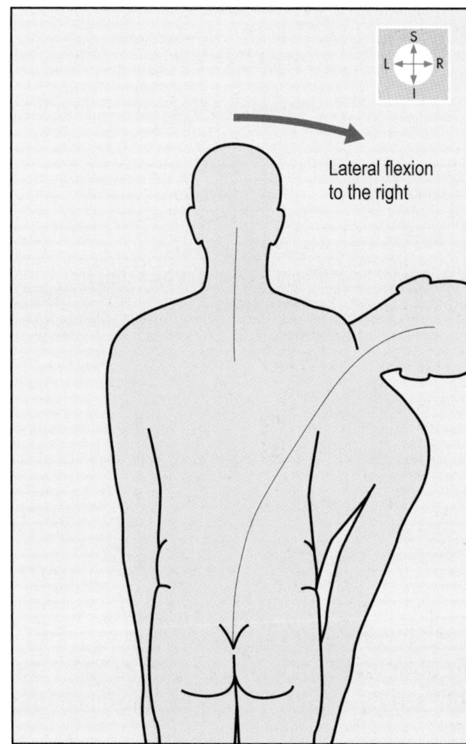

Fig. 8.3 Lateral flexion of the vertebral column to the right from the anatomical position.

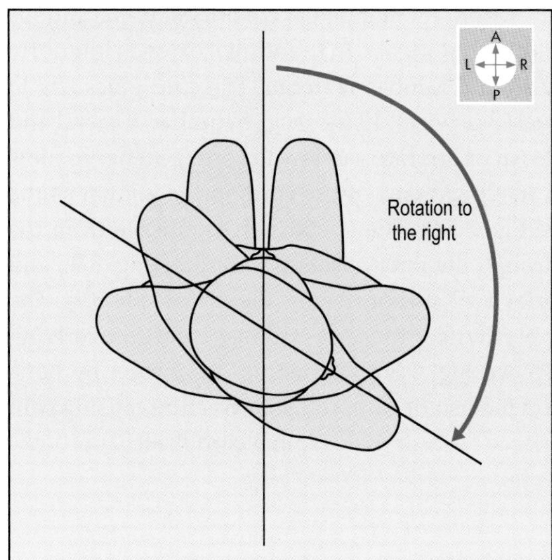

Fig. 8.4 View from above of a seated person showing rotation of the vertebral column to the right. The head rotates with respect to the shoulders, and the shoulders rotate with respect to the pelvis.

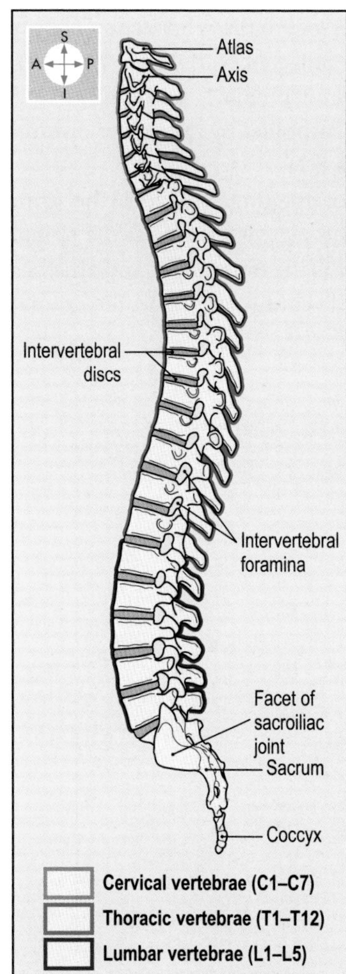

Fig. 8.5 Lateral view of the vertebral column.

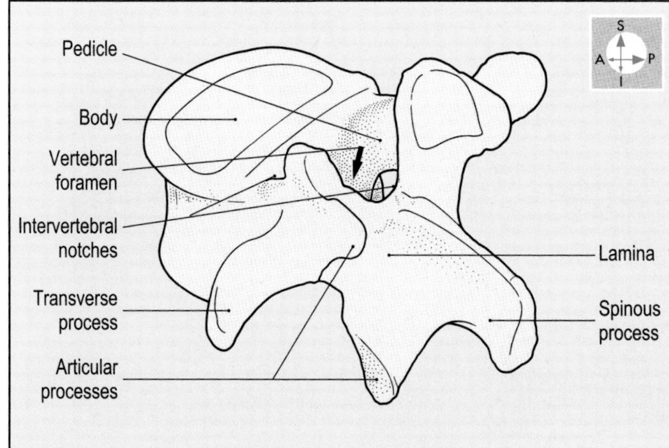

Fig. 8.6 Oblique view of a lumbar vertebra to show its processes, vertebral foramen and intervertebral notches.

	Vertebral Bodies	Transverse Processes	Vertebral Foramina	Articular Processes	Spinous Processes
Cervical Vertebrae	small	**foramina transversaria present**	triangular	joints in coronal plane and oblique, allowing lateral flexion with rotation	**bifid** short
Thoracic Vertebrae	heart-shaped **costal facets present**	**costal facets present** no foramina transversaria incline posterolaterally	circular	joints in vertical plane and oblique, allowing rotation	long sloping
Lumbar Vertebrae	massive kidney shaped	**no costal facets** incline laterally and slightly posteriorly	triangular	joints vertical in sagittal plane, preventing rotation	thick rectangular
Sacral Segments	**fused**	**fused**	canal		tubercles

Table 8.1 Features of typical vertebrae in the regions of the vertebral column

(trapezius, latissimus dorsi, levator scapulae, rhomboid major and minor) act mainly on the shoulder girdle (see pp 100 & 102). The intermediate group (the two serratus posterior muscles) are respiratory.

The deep muscles (see p. 404), including splenius, erector spinae and transversospinalis, interconnect the base of the skull, the sacrum and the intervening vertebrae. Erector spinae is subdivided into named components, including iliocostalis, longissimus and spinalis, which usually span several vertebrae. Deep to erector spinae is the transversospinalis, whose components usually run obliquely, attaching adjacent vertebrae (Fig. 8.7). Transversospinalis comprises semispinalis, multifidus and rotatores. The deep muscles are all supplied by the posterior rami of the spinal nerves (Fig. 8.8; Table 8.1).

Within the vertebral canal three meningeal layers, the dura mater, the arachnoid mater and the pia mater, invest the spinal cord (see Fig. 8.33). The dura mater is the outer layer and attaches to the foramen magnum where it is continuous with the cranial dura. Inferiorly the dura attaches to the second sacral vertebra. The arachnoid mater is applied to the inner aspect of the dura. The pia is a vascular layer which closely invests the spinal cord and spinal nerve roots. Between the arachnoid and the pia is the subarachnoid space containing cerebrospinal fluid.

The spinal cord, within its meningeal coverings, is continuous above with the medulla oblongata. In the adult it extends inferiorly to the level of the second lumbar vertebra. The cord gives rise to paired spinal nerves: 8 cervical, 12 thoracic, 5 lumbar, 5 sacral and 3 coccygeal. The leash of lumbar, sacral and coccygeal nerve roots descends beyond the lower end of the cord and is known as the cauda equina (see Fig. 8.34). The spinal nerves emerge from the vertebral canal through the intervertebral foramina (Fig. 8.9), and divide into posterior and anterior rami (Fig. 8.8; Table 8.2). The posterior rami supply the deep muscles of the back and the overlying skin (Fig. 8.1, also see Fig. 1.36). Vertebrae, weakened by bone disease or growth of metastatic tumours, may fracture causing pain and injury to the nerve roots or to the spinal cord itself.

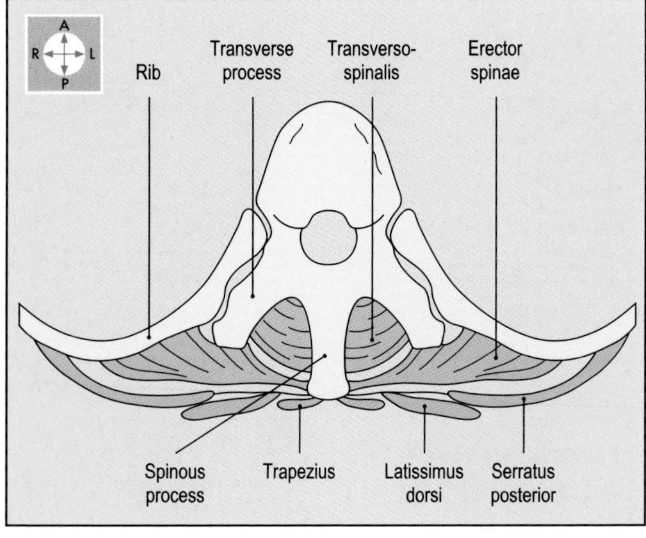

Fig. 8.7 A thoracic vertebra with the main groups of back muscles. Inferior aspect.

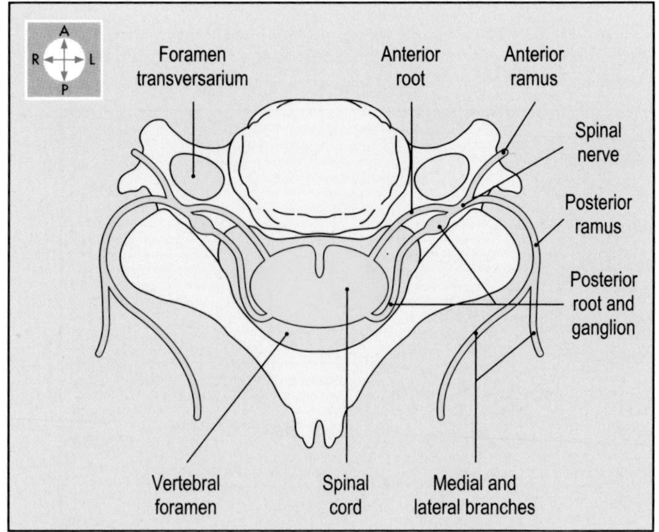

Fig. 8.8 A cervical vertebra with the spinal cord and a pair of spinal nerves. Inferior aspect.

The vertebral arch develops from right and left parts which normally fuse across the midline posteriorly. Failure of fusion, most commonly in the lumbar region, results in spina bifida. Often the condition affects only the bones (spina bifida occulta) but more severe forms may leave the spinal meninges exposed or involve maldevelopment of the spinal cord, associated with weakness or paralysis of muscles in the lower limbs.

Spinal Nerves	Principle Areas of Distribution
Cervical 1–4	via the cervical plexus (page 324) to the neck, and via the phrenic nerves (page 59) to the diaphragm.
Cervical 5–8 and thoracic 1	via the brachial plexus (page 80) to the upper limbs.
Thoracic 1–11	via the intercostal nerves (page 35) to the thoracic and abdominal walls.
Thoracic 12	via the subcostal nerves (page 201) to the lower abdominal wall.
Lumbar 1	via ilioinguinal and iliohypogastric nerves (page 145) to the lower abdominal wall.
Lumbar 1–4	via the lumbar plexus (page 203) to the lower limbs.
Lumbar 4 and 5	via the lumbo-sacral trunk (page 203) to the sacral plexus.
Sacral 1–4	via the sacral plexus (page 237) to the pelvis and lower limbs.
Sacral 5 and coccygeal 1	via the coccygeal plexus (page 237) to skin over the coccyx.

Table 8.2 Summaries of the main areas of distribution of the anterior rami of spinal nerves

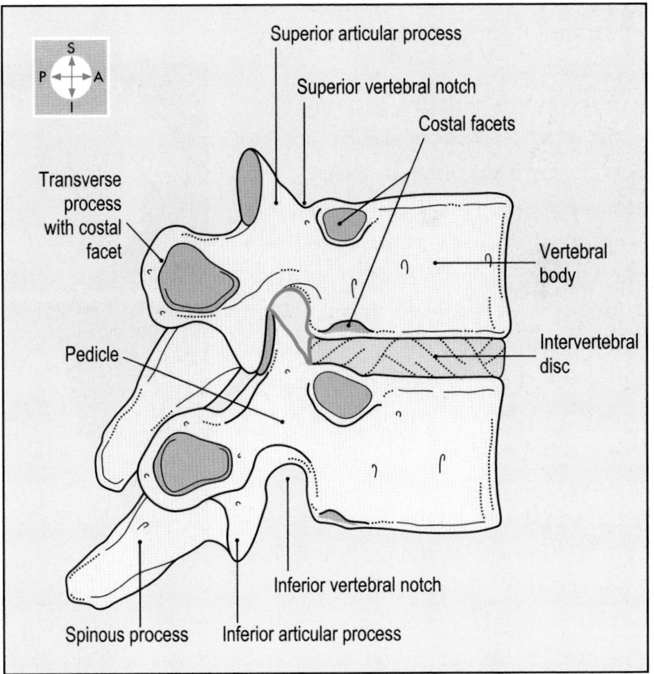

Fig. 8.9 Intervertebral foramen (pink) between two typical thoracic vertebrae. The facet joints between the superior and inferior articular processes of adjacent vertebrae lie posterior to the segmental nerve in the foramen.

Vertebrae and Joints

Cervical vertebrae

The seven cervical vertebrae are relatively small and enclose a wide vertebral canal with adequate space for the cervical part of the spinal cord. Each transverse process is perforated by a foramen transversarium transmitting the vertebral vessels. The spinous processes all give attachment to a strong midline elastic ligament, the ligamentum nuchae.

Four of the cervical vertebrae (numbers 3–6) have a typical appearance whereas the first, second and seventh are modified. The typical vertebrae (Fig. 8.10) possess short bifid spines and their transverse processes have anterior and posterior tubercles. Often the upper and lower surfaces of the vertebral bodies are not flat but curve upwards at their lateral edges. The facets on the superior articular processes face obliquely backwards and upwards and therefore rotation and lateral flexion always occur together.

The first cervical vertebra, the atlas (Fig. 8.11), has anterior and posterior arches, relatively large transverse processes and two lateral masses. The atlas has no body and its spinous process is represented by a tubercle. On the superior surface of each lateral mass is a concave facet which articulates with the convex occipital condyle of the skull. The atlanto-occipital joints permit flexion and extension (nodding movements).

The second cervical vertebra, the axis (Fig. 8.12), possesses some of the features of a typical cervical vertebra but it has a unique vertical projection, the dens (odontoid process). This projects superiorly from the upper surface of its body and represents the body of the atlas. The dens articulates by a synovial joint with a facet on the posterior surface of the anterior arch of the atlas, where it is retained by the alar, apical and transverse ligaments (see Figs 8.14 & 8.15). The planes of the lateral atlantoaxial joints and the pivot joint of the dens (Fig. 8.13) allow rotation of the head as in looking from side to side.

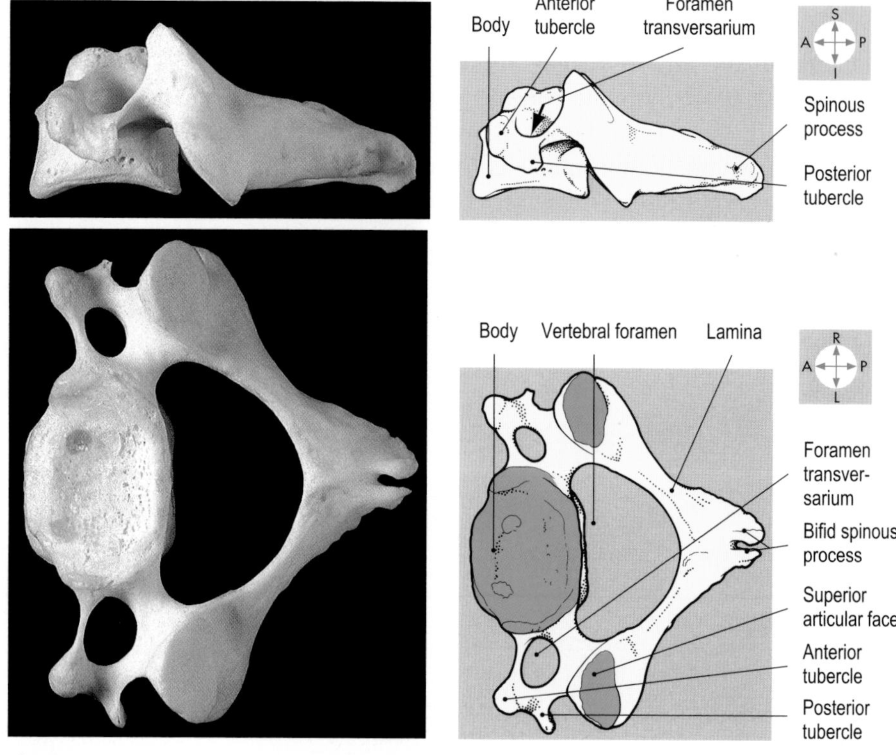

Fig. 8.10 Lateral and superior views of a typical (fourth) cervical vertebra.

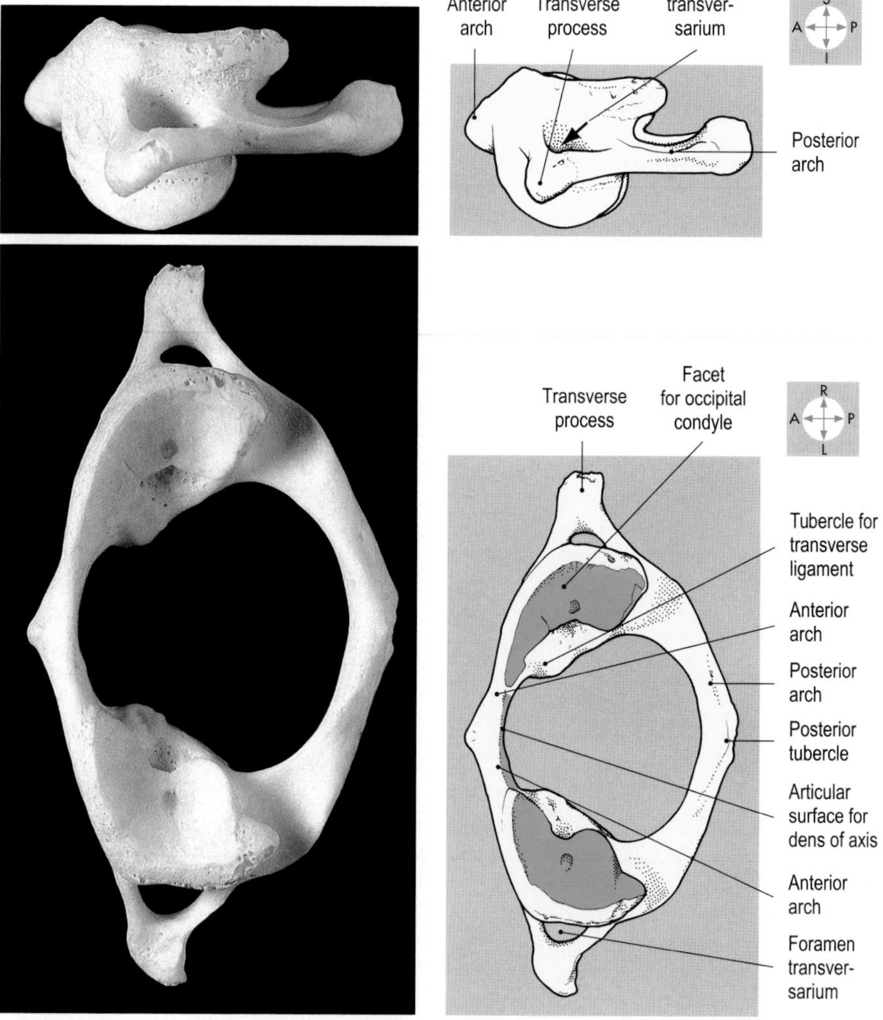

Fig. 8.11 Lateral and superior views of the first cervical vertebra, the atlas.

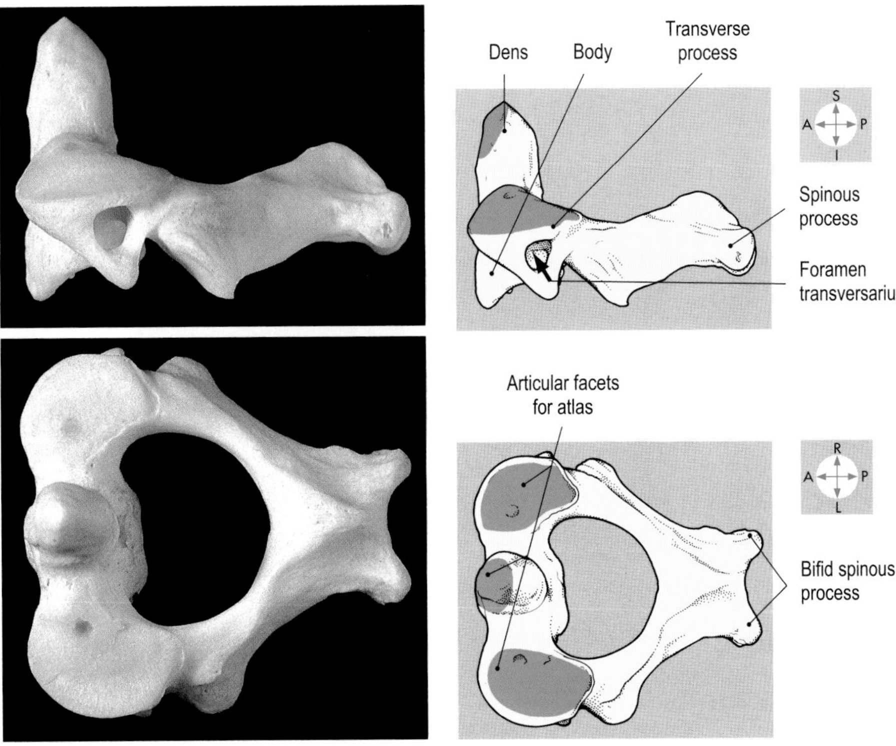

Fig. 8.12 Lateral and superior views of the second cervical vertebra, the axis.

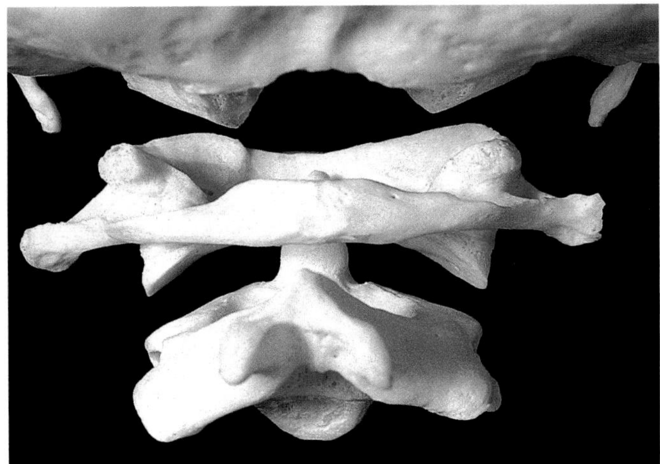

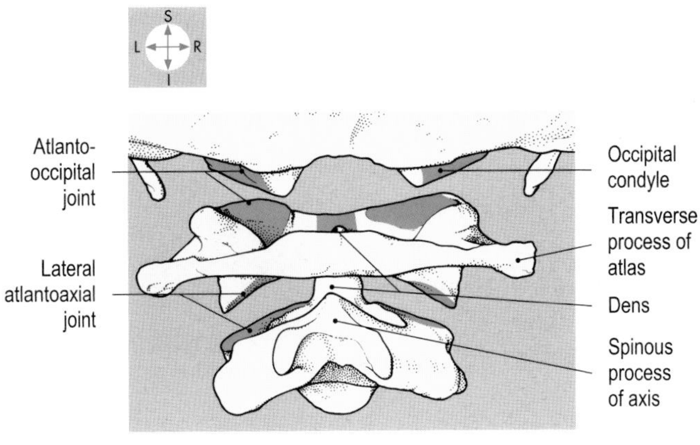

Fig. 8.13 Base of the skull, atlas and axis, seen in an expanded posterior view.

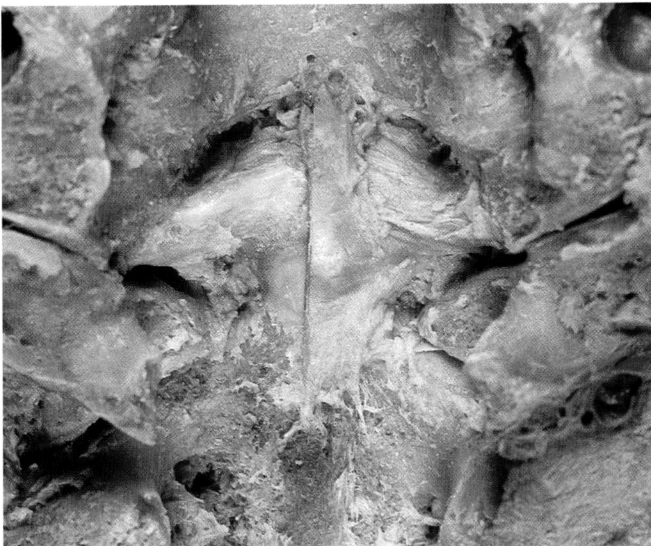

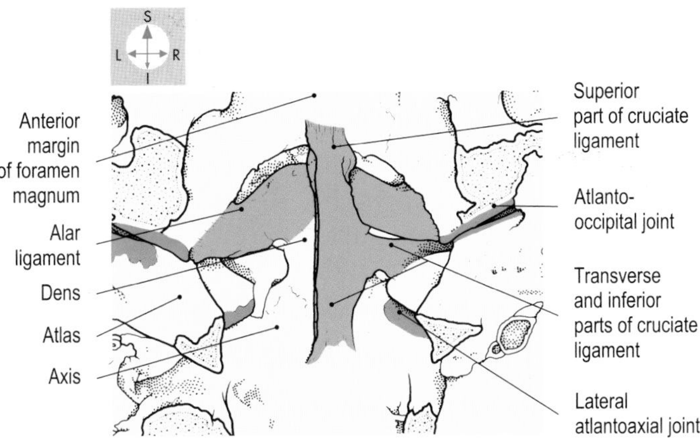

Fig. 8.14 Ligaments of the atlantoaxial joint. The posterior longitudinal ligament, spinal cord and meninges, vertebral arches and the posterior part of the skull have been removed. On the left side part of the cruciate ligament has been excised. The view is oblique.

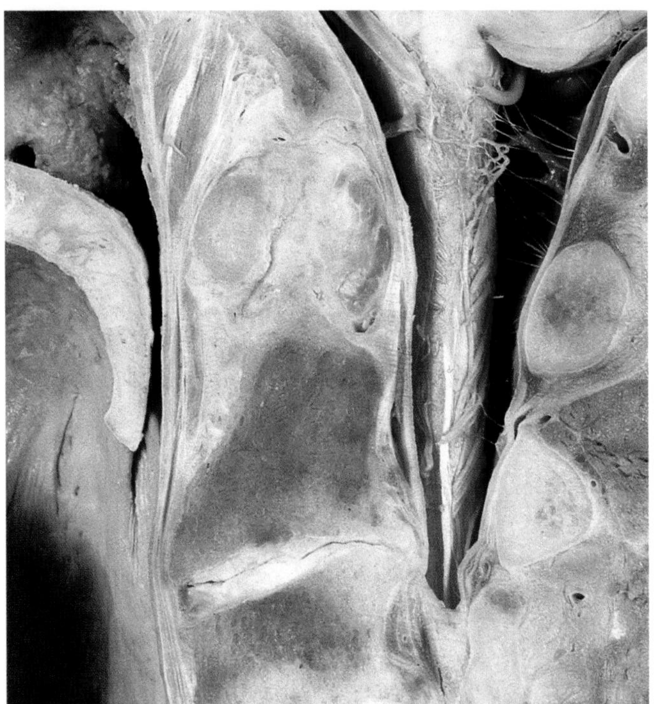

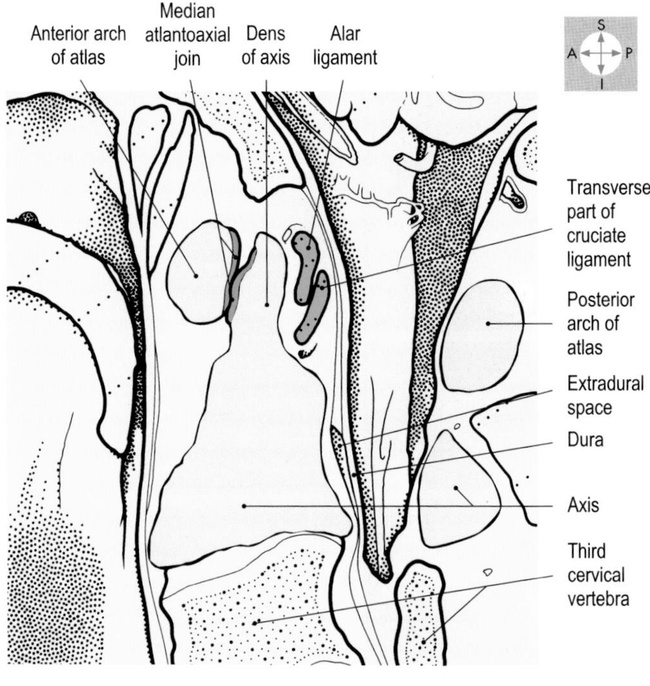

Fig. 8.15 Near sagittal section through the median atlantoaxial joint.

The seventh cervical vertebra (Fig. 8.16) possesses a long, non-bifid spine, which provides the inferior attachment for the ligamentum nuchae. The spinous process is easily palpable and hence the vertebra is called the vertebra prominens. The foramina transversaria of this vertebra are traversed by the vertebral veins but not by the arteries.

The joints of the whole cervical column allow movements of flexion, extension, rotation and lateral flexion. These movements are brought about by the prevertebral and postvertebral muscles (Fig. 8.17), assisted by sternocleidomastoid and trapezius. The prevertebral muscles comprise the scalene group (see p. 329) and the longus colli group. The latter passes from the base of the skull down the anterior surface of the vertebral column into the thorax. The prevertebral muscles are much smaller than the postvertebral group which has an antigravity action in keeping the head upright.

Arthritis involving joints of the cervical spine is often associated with the formation of bony outgrowths (osteophytes) which may compress the nerve roots that contribute to the brachial plexus (see p. 80). Injuries to the cervical column, particularly involving fracture or dislocation of vertebrae, may result in spinal cord injury leading to quadriplegia or death. The atlantoaxial joint is particularly liable to disruption in hyperextension injuries.

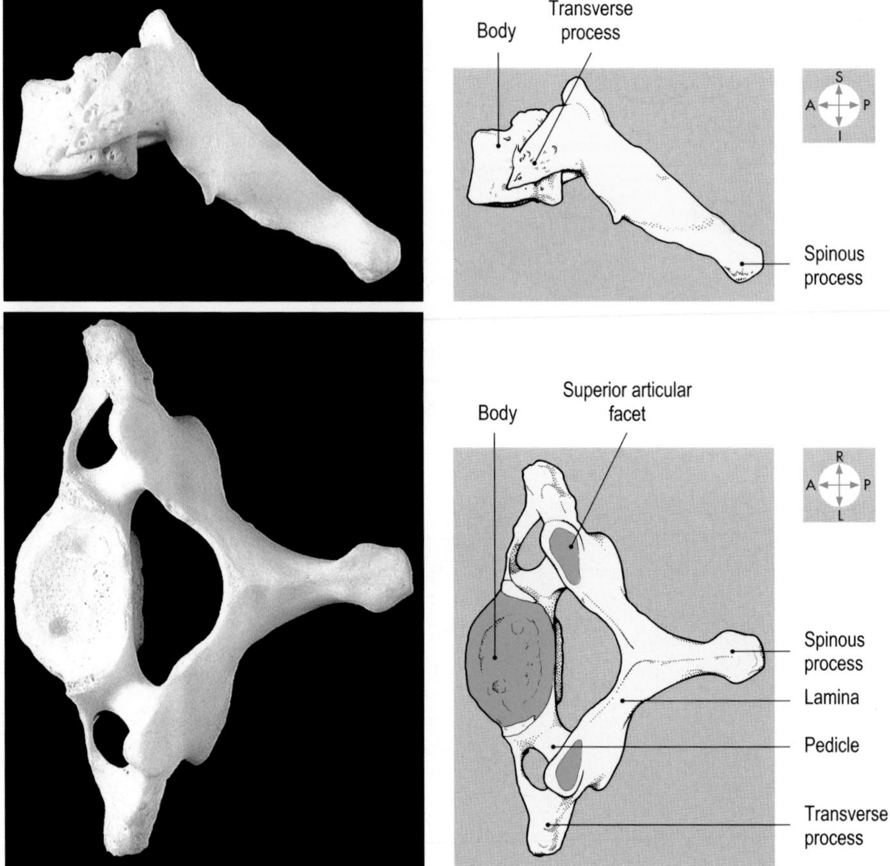

Fig. 8.16 Lateral and superior views of the seventh cervical vertebra, the vertebra prominens.

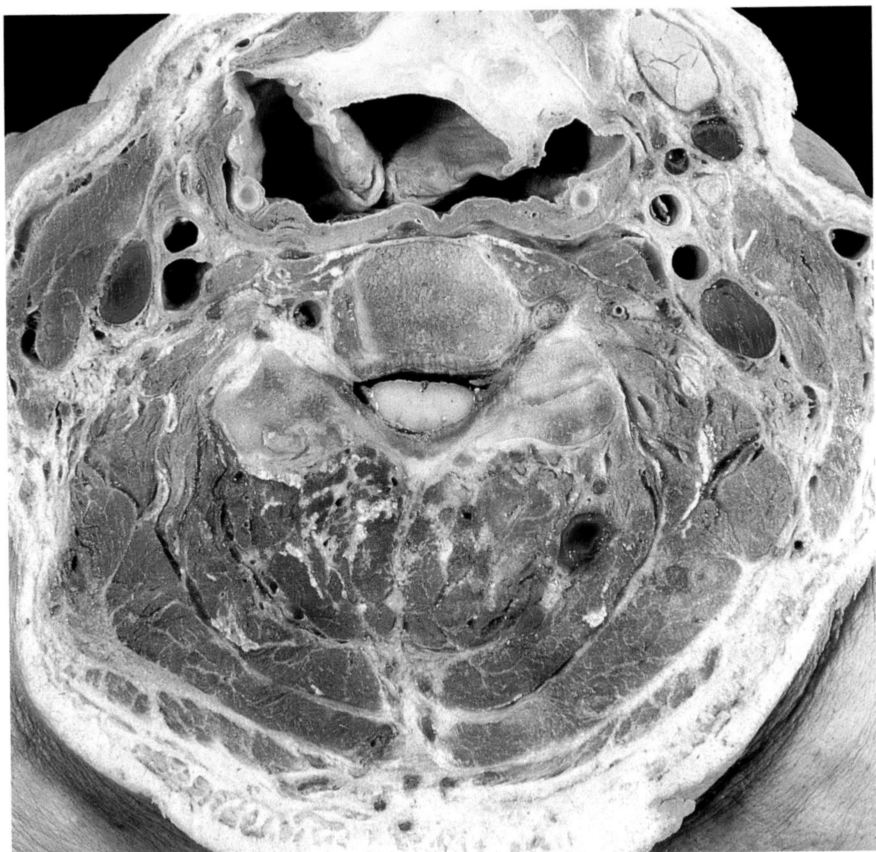

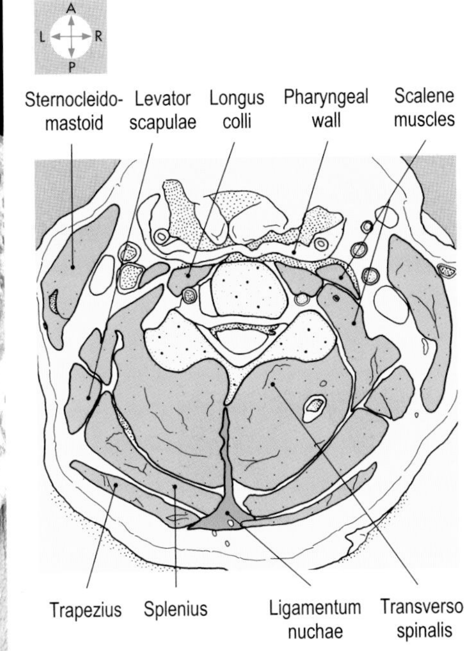

Fig. 8.17 Transverse section at the level of the fourth cervical vertebra, showing the muscles of the neck. Superior aspect. Compare Fig. 7.94.

Thoracic vertebrae

The bodies of the twelve thoracic vertebrae increase in size from above downwards. The bodies bear characteristic costal facets (Fig. 8.18), which form synovial joints with the heads of the ribs. Typically a vertebral body possesses one pair of facets (superior and inferior costal facets) on each side adjacent to the attachment of the pedicle. The upper facet receives the rib whose number corresponds to the vertebra, whilst the lower facet articulates with the rib below. However the tenth, eleventh and twelfth vertebrae possess facets on each side, which are for articulation with their own ribs. The vertebral canal is smaller than in any other region.

The transverse processes project laterally and backwards and typically each bears near its tip a facet for the tubercle of the corresponding rib. The spinous processes are long and slope steeply downwards. The plane of the joints between the facets on the articular processes is almost vertical and permits rotation. However, all movements in the thoracic region are restricted by the rib cage.

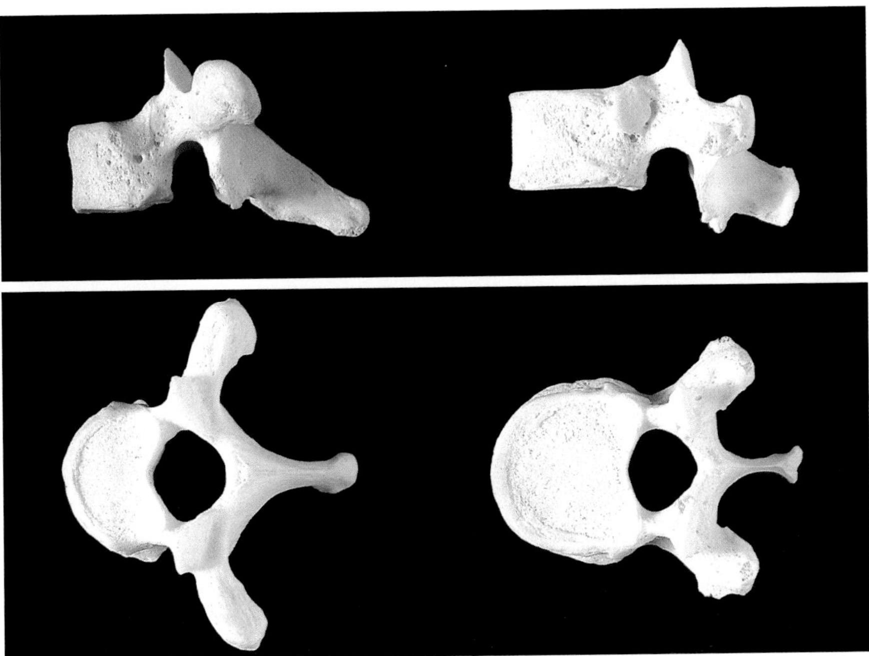

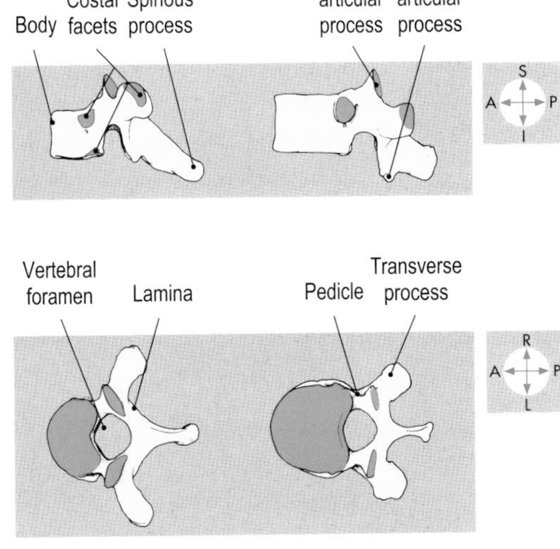

Fig. 8.18 Lateral and superior views of the second and tenth thoracic vertebrae.

Lumbar vertebrae

The upper four lumbar vertebrae are very similar. The vertebral foramina are moderate in size (Fig. 8.19) but the bodies are comparatively large, with concave sides. The transverse processes taper and are directed laterally and slightly backwards. The spinous processes are deep and rectangular. Facets on the superior articular processes face medially and 'grasp' the laterally directed inferior facets of the vertebra above, permitting wide ranges of flexion, extension and lateral flexion but severely restricting rotation.

The fifth lumbar vertebra has shorter transverse processes and a less angular spinous process. Its inferior articular facets are widely separated and face anteriorly. They articulate with the sacrum (Fig. 8.20) and prevent forward displacement of the vertebra. One or both transverse processes may be fused with the upper part of the sacrum (sacralization of the fifth lumbar vertebra), which can cause difficulty in the interpretation of radiographs.

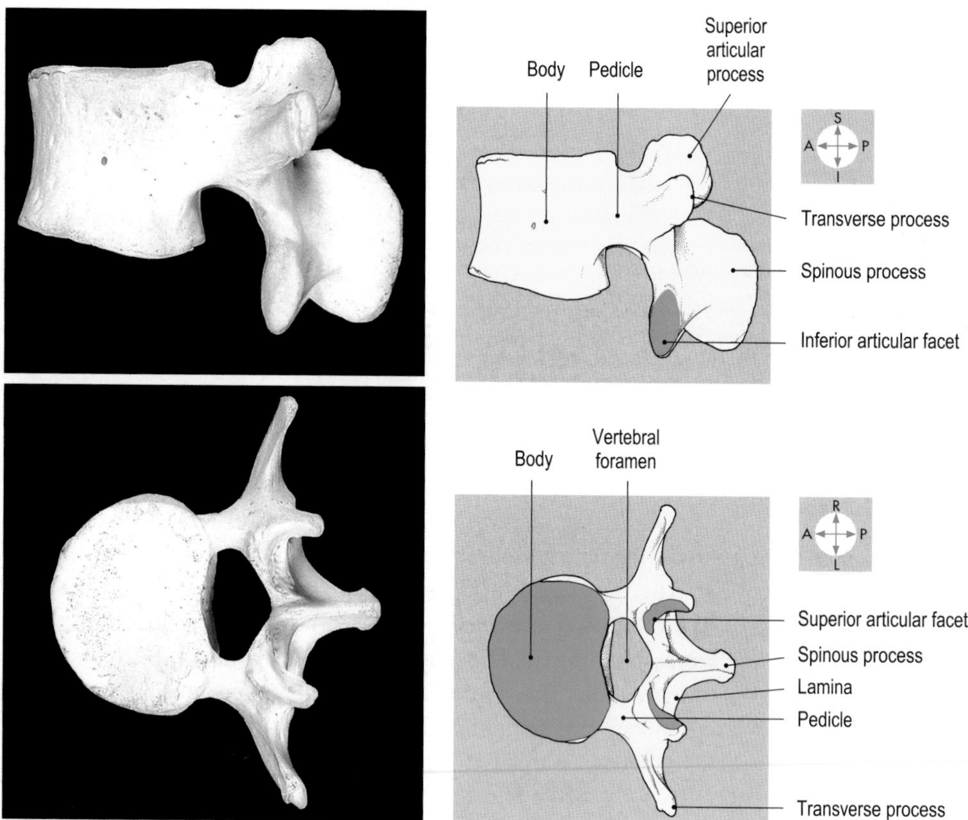

Fig. 8.19 Lateral and superior views of a typical (third) lumbar vertebra.

Sacral and coccygeal vertebrae

The sacrum is a triangular bone formed by the fusion of five vertebrae (Figs 8.20 & 8.21). The upper surface of the sacrum resembles that of a lumbar vertebra and carries the lumbosacral disc. Below the apex of the sacrum lies the coccyx (Fig. 8.22), which may be a small single bone or up to four rudimentary vertebrae. The coccyx and the sacrum usually articulate via a small intervertebral disc, although they may be fused. The sacrum slopes backwards and downwards and is concave anteriorly. The bone in the female has relatively small joint surfaces and larger alae whilst in the male the larger sacral promontory often creates a 'heart-shaped' pelvic inlet (see p. 214). The fused pedicles and laminae enclose the sacral canal, triangular in cross-section, which opens posteroinferiorly at the V-shaped sacral hiatus. The canal contains the lower part of the cauda equina, comprising the roots of the sacral and coccygeal nerves. The anterior rami of the upper four sacral nerves pass into the pelvis via the anterior sacral foramina and contribute to the sacral plexus. The posterior rami traverse the posterior sacral foramina (Fig. 8.21). Lateral to the foramina are the lateral masses, each of which

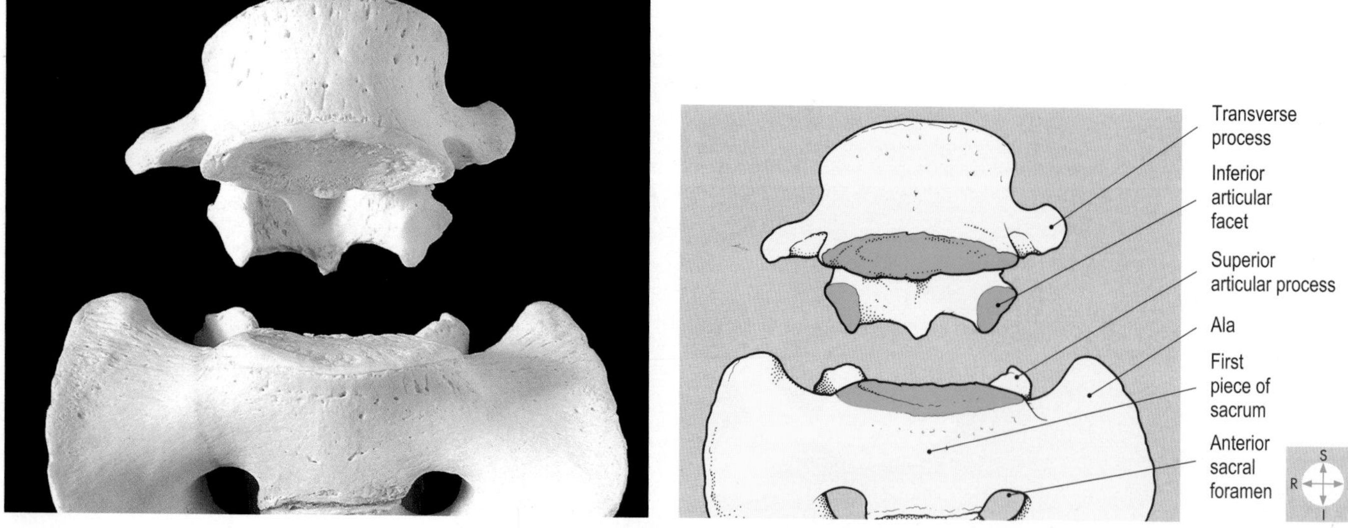

Fig. 8.20 Fifth lumbar vertebra and the upper part of the sacrum, seen in an expanded anterior view.

bears an auricular surface for articulation with the ilium (Fig. 8.22).

The sacroiliac joint is synovial but allows very little movement because of the irregularity of the articulating surfaces and the thick posterior interosseous ligament. Each joint is further supported by the anterior and posterior sacroiliac ligaments and the iliolumbar, sacrospinous and sacrotuberous ligaments. Body weight, acting downwards through the lumbosacral disc, tends to rotate the lower part of the sacrum backwards, a movement prevented by the sacrospinous and sacrotuberous ligaments (see Fig. 8.24).

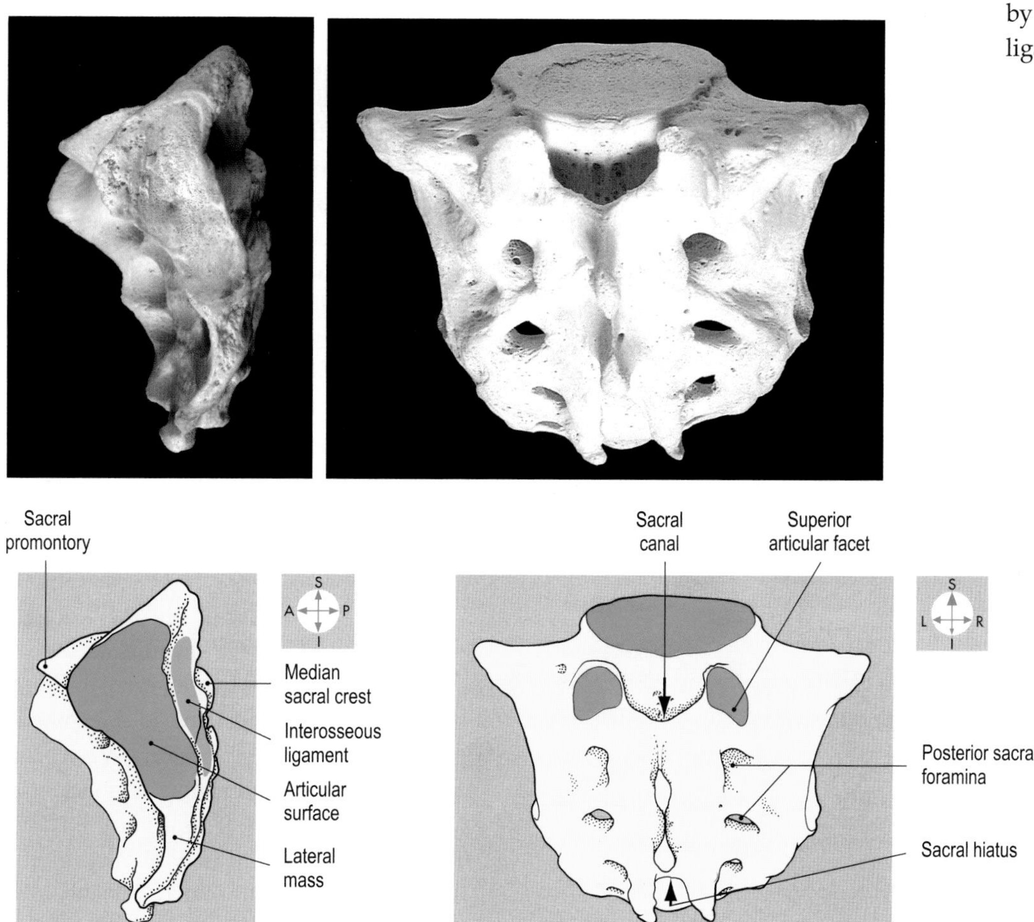

Fig. 8.21 Lateral and posterosuperior views of the sacrum.

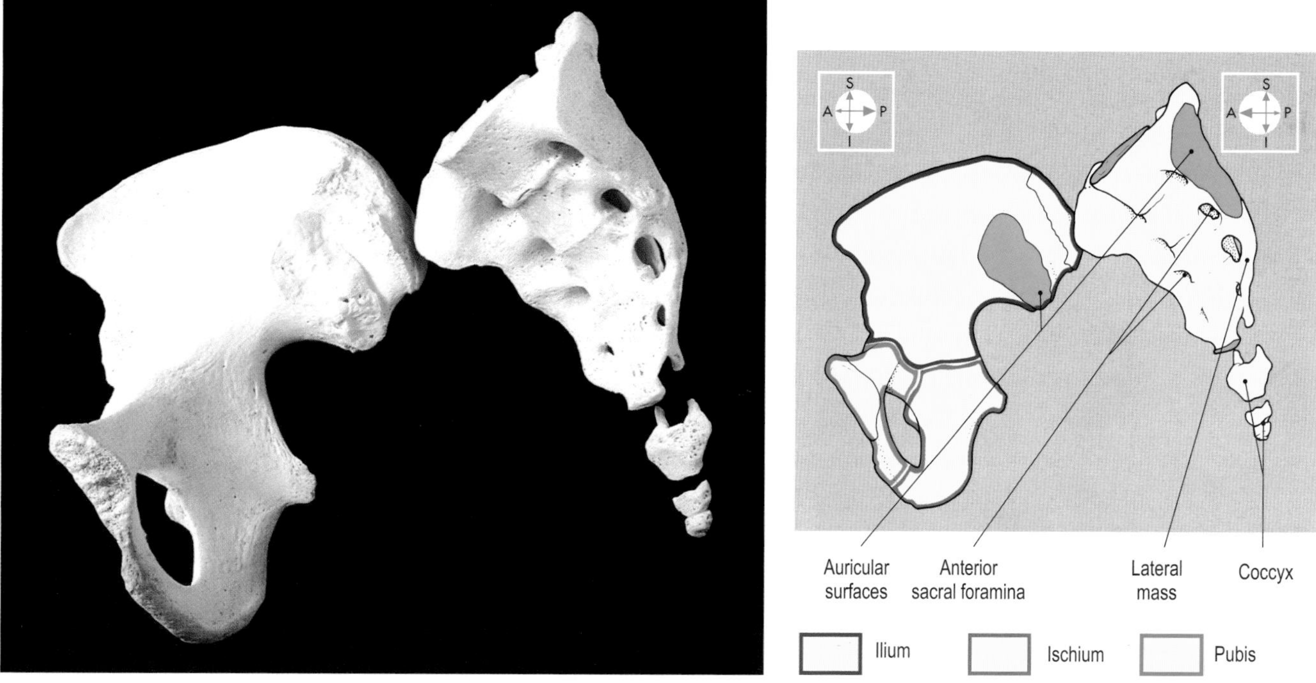

Fig. 8.22 Oblique view of the sacrum, coccyx and right hip bone.

Intervertebral discs

Intervertebral discs connect adjacent vertebral bodies (Fig. 8.23) and act as fibrocartilaginous joints along the whole length of the vertebral column. Like the vertebral bodies, the discs gradually increase in size from above downwards, the largest being the lumbosacral disc between the fifth lumbar vertebra and the sacrum (Fig. 8.24). The discs contribute about one-fifth of the length of the vertebral column. Each disc consists of a laminated anulus fibrosus surrounding a gelatinous nucleus pulposus (Fig. 8.27). The nucleus pulposus lies closer to the posterior surface of the disc and thus is more liable to posterior herniation when the disc is damaged. This herniation, often called 'a slipped disc', may occur near the midline and compress the spinal cord, causing loss of bladder control. Posterolateral herniation may compress nerves near the intervertebral foramen (see p. 394) and cause muscle weakness and referred pain in the lower limb (sciatica). Herniation of lumbar discs affects nerve roots passing through the intervertebral foramen below the level of the disc (for example, L4–L5 disc herniation affects nerve L5).

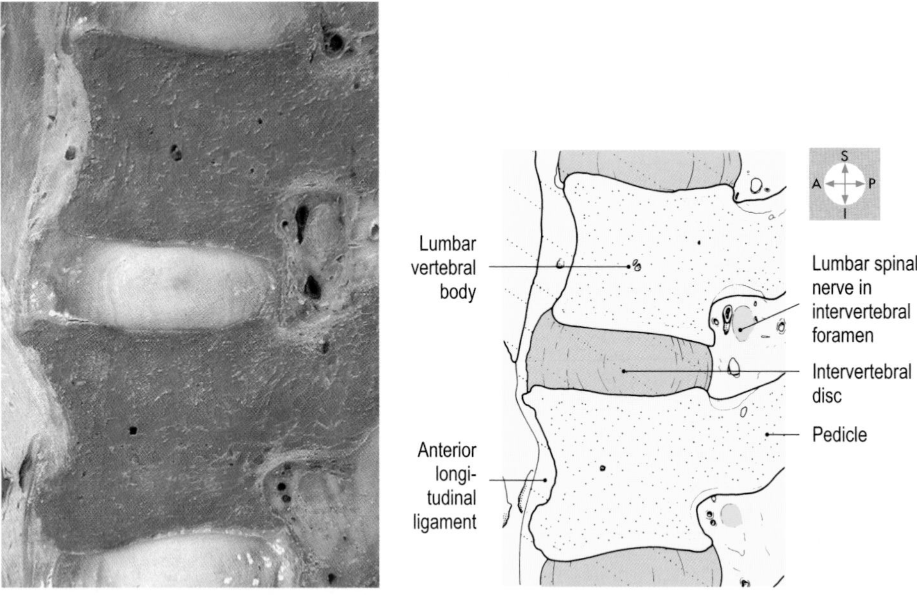

Fig. 8.23 Sagittal section of the lumbar vertebral column.

Intervertebral ligaments

The intervertebral discs are reinforced by posterior and anterior longitudinal ligaments (Figs 8.25 & 8.26). These ligaments attach to vertebral bodies and intervertebral discs and anchor inferiorly to the sacrum and superiorly to the cervical vertebrae or skull. Other ligaments interconnect the laminae, spinous processes and transverse processes of adjacent vertebrae. Ligamenta flava interconnect the laminae within the vertebral canal. The high content of elastic tissue gives these ligaments their yellow appearance and they assist return of the vertebral column to the erect position following flexion. Supraspinous and interspinous ligaments connect adjacent spinous processes of thoracic and lumbar vertebrae. It is through these ligaments that a needle is inserted to withdraw cerebrospinal fluid during lumbar puncture.

The supraspinous and interspinous ligaments are replaced in the cervical region by the ligamentum nuchae, which attaches to the skull at the external occipital protuberance and crest and to the spinous processes of all the cervical vertebrae. Intertransverse ligaments connect the transverse processes of adjacent vertebrae. The lumbosacral joint is reinforced by the iliolumbar ligament which attaches the transverse process of the fifth lumbar vertebra to the iliac crest (Fig. 8.27).

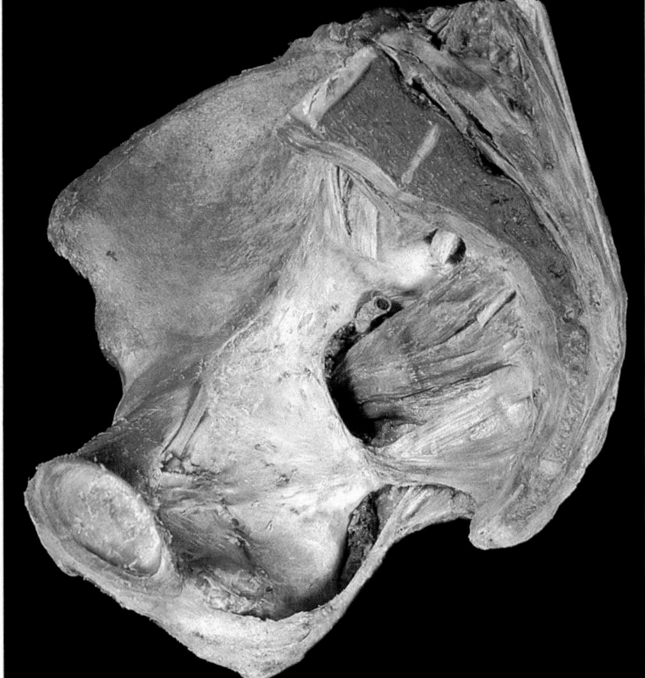

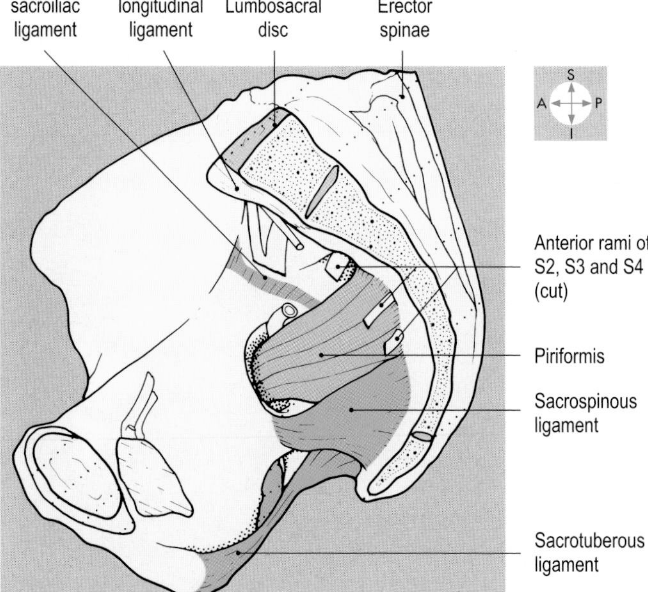

Fig. 8.24 Right hemipelvis, showing the sacrum and coccyx in sagittal section.

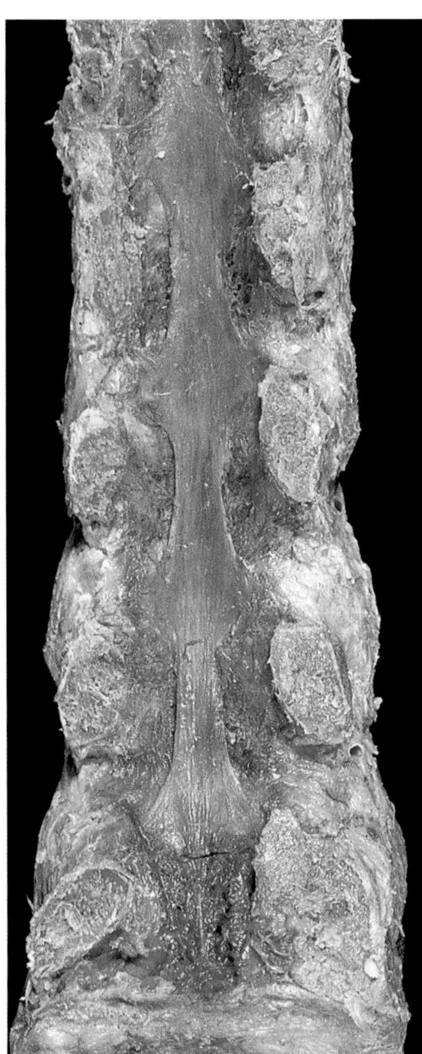

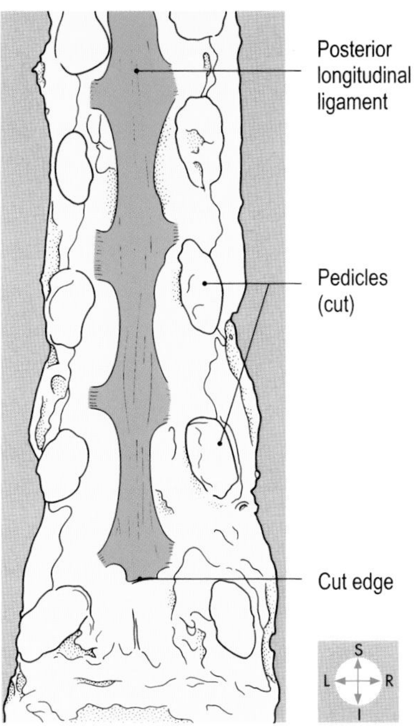

Fig. 8.25 Posterior longitudinal ligament, exposed by removal of the vertebral arches, meninges and spinal cord.

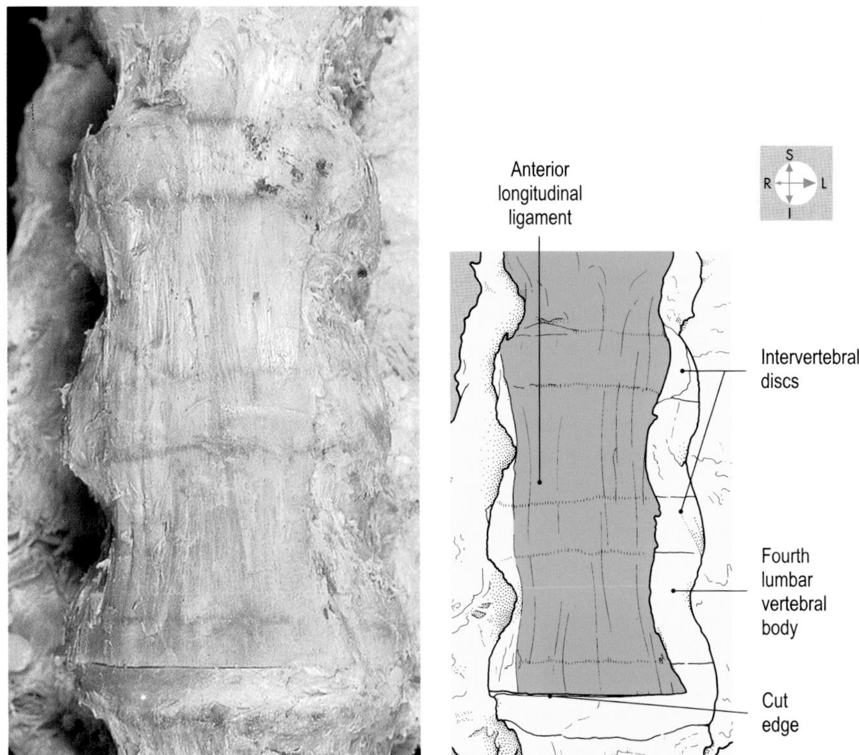

Fig. 8.26 Oblique view of anterior longitudinal ligament of the lumbar spine.

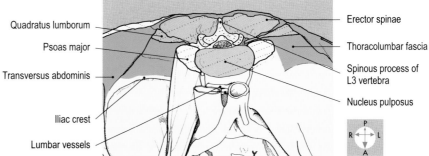

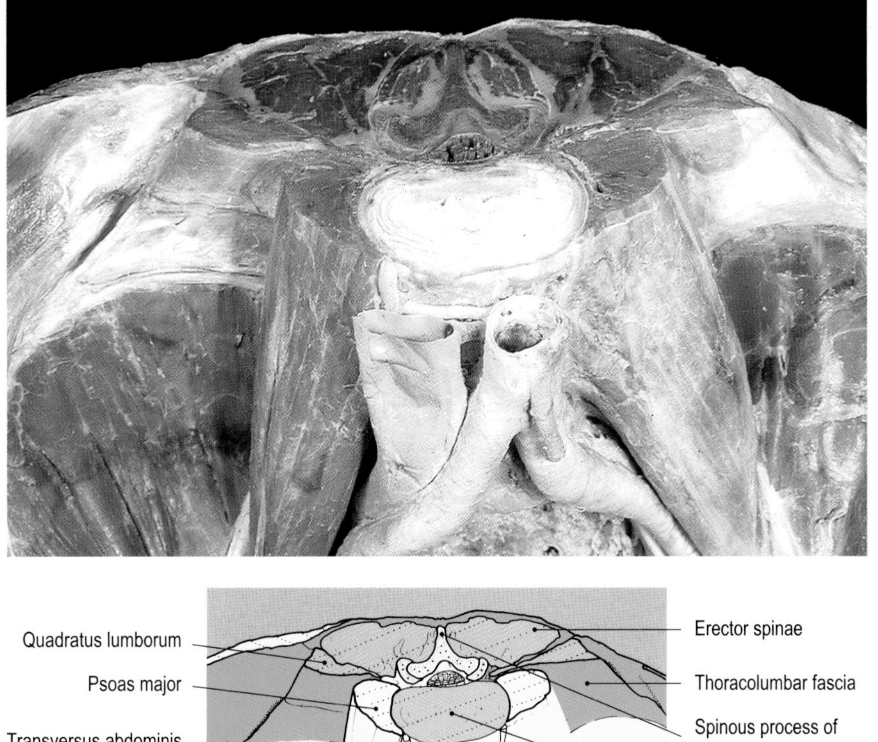

Fig. 8.27 Oblique view of a transverse section of the lumbar spine and muscles at the level of the disc between the third and fourth lumbar vertebrae.

Muscles

The muscles of the erector spinae group are covered in the lumbar region by the thoracolumbar fascia, in the lumbar and thoracic regions by the serratus posterior muscles and in the neck by the splenius muscles.

In the lumbar region the thoracolumbar fascia is trilaminar and encloses erector spinae posteriorly and quadratus lumborum anteriorly (see Fig. 8.27). At the lateral margins of both muscles the laminae of the fascia fuse and give attachment to the transversus abdominis (see Fig. 8.27).

Serratus posterior superior and inferior (Figs 8.28 & 8.29) are weak respiratory muscles which connect lower cervical and upper thoracic spines with upper ribs, and lower thoracic and upper lumbar spines with lower ribs respectively. They are supplied by branches of anterior rami of thoracic spinal nerves (intercostal nerves).

Splenius muscles

Splenius (Fig. 8.30) attaches medially to the lower part of the ligamentum nuchae and to the upper thoracic spinous processes. The superior part, splenius capitis, attaches laterally to the mastoid process and superior nuchal line. The inferior part, splenius cervicis, attaches laterally to the transverse processes of the upper cervical vertebrae.

Erector spinae

On each side erector spinae (see Fig. 8.32) occupies the groove between the spinous and transverse processes of vertebrae. The muscle attaches inferiorly to the posterior surface of the sacrum and the posterior part of the iliac crest. In the lumbar region it forms a prominent vertical muscle mass (see Fig. 8.36) and attaches to the spinous and transverse processes of the lumbar vertebrae. In the upper lumbar region the

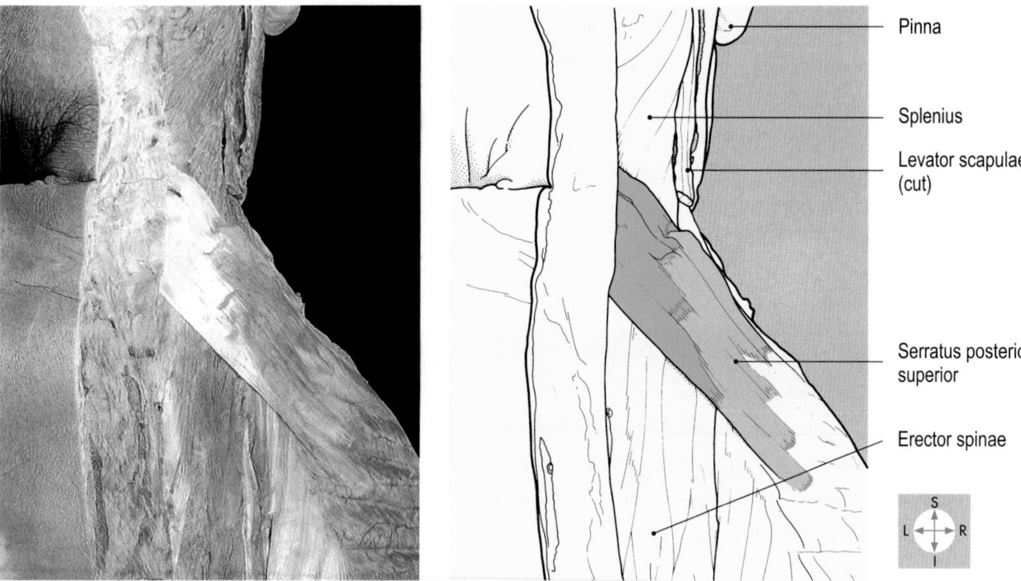

Fig. 8.28 Serratus posterior superior. The upper limb girdle and its muscles have been removed.

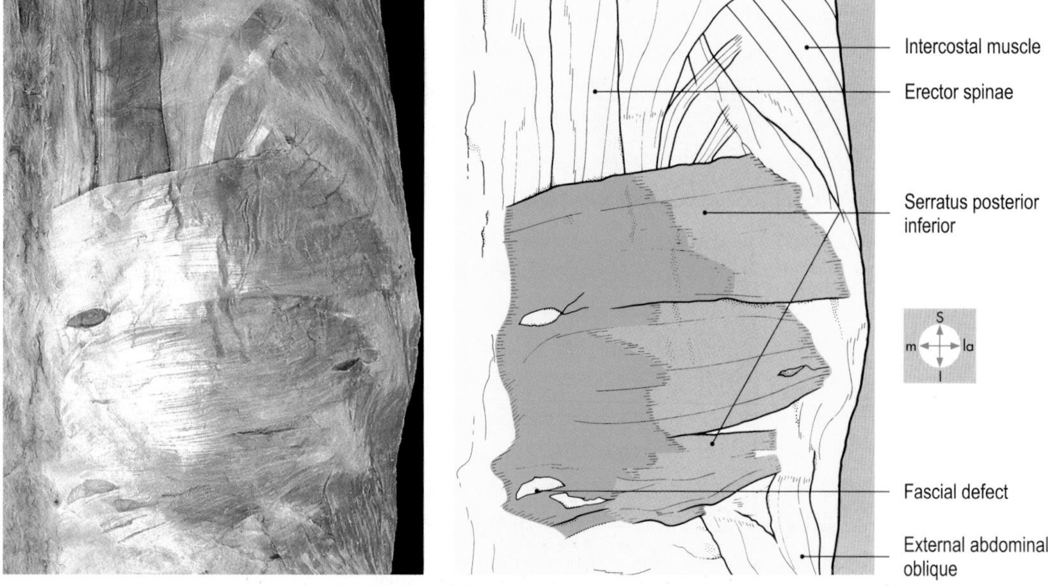

Fig. 8.29 Serratus posterior inferior revealed by removal of latissimus dorsi.

muscle divides into three columns. The lateral column forms iliocostalis, which attaches to the angles of the ribs and transverse processes of the lower cervical vertebrae. The intermediate column forms the longissimus, which attaches to the ribs and the transverse processes of the thoracic and cervical vertebrae. The medial part of the erector spinae forms the spinalis, which attaches to the spinous processes of the upper lumbar, thoracic and lower cervical vertebrae.

Erector spinae is innervated by branches from the posterior rami of spinal nerves.

Transversospinalis

The muscles of this group lie obliquely (Fig. 8.31), covered by erector spinae (see Fig. 8.7). They interconnect transverse processes and spinous processes of vertebrae at higher levels. Semispinalis forms the longest and most superficial member of this group and interconnects lower thoracic transverse processes and upper thoracic and cervical spinous processes. Multifidus lies deep to semispinalis. Its fibres attach the transverse process of each vertebra to the spinous processes of one to three vertebrae above. The deepest fibres of transversospinalis form the rotatores, which connect the lamina of one vertebra to the transverse process of the vertebra below. The rotatores are best developed in the thoracic region.

The transversospinalis muscles are supplied by the posterior rami of the spinal nerves.

Actions

Simultaneous contraction of the deep muscles of both sides extends the vertebral column and regulates or prevents flexion. Unilateral contraction produces lateral flexion and rotation, assisted by the abdominal oblique muscles. The deep muscles have a very important role in achieving and maintaining the fully upright posture.

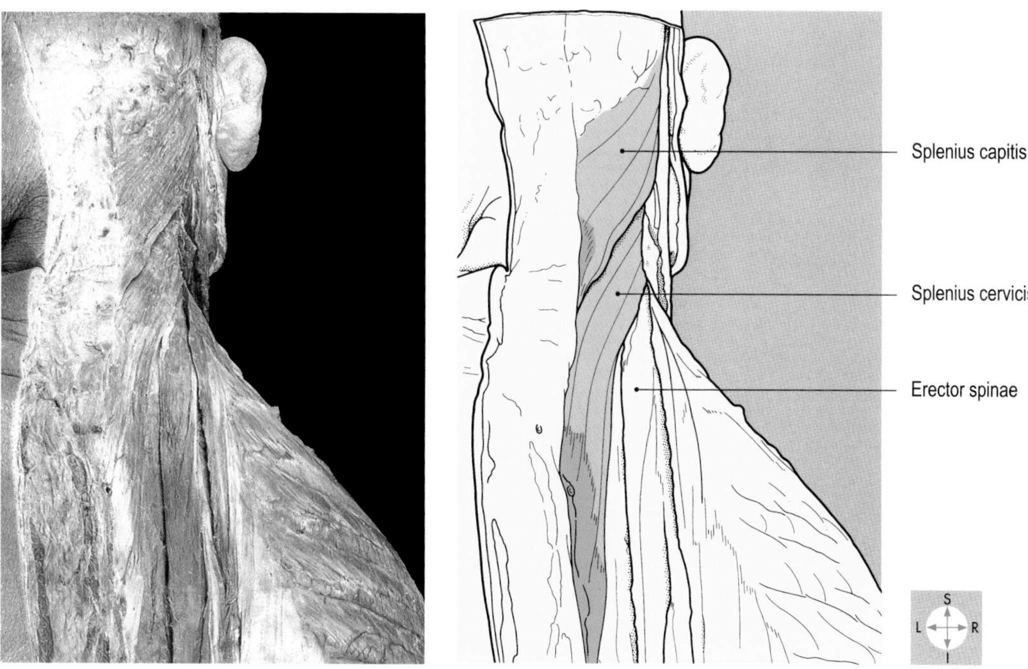

Fig. 8.30 Splenius cervicis and capitis after excision of serratus posterior superior.

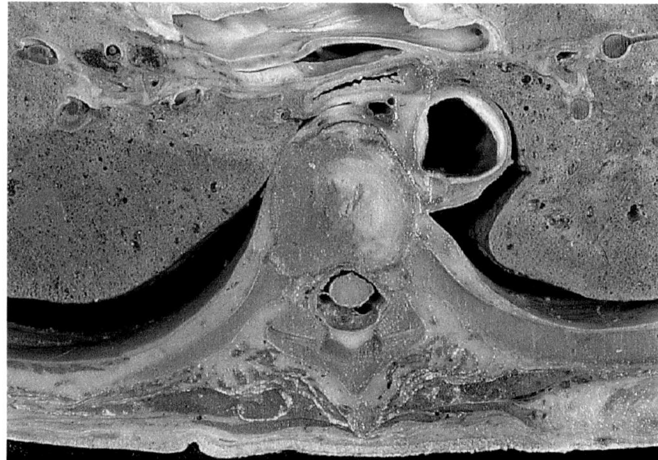

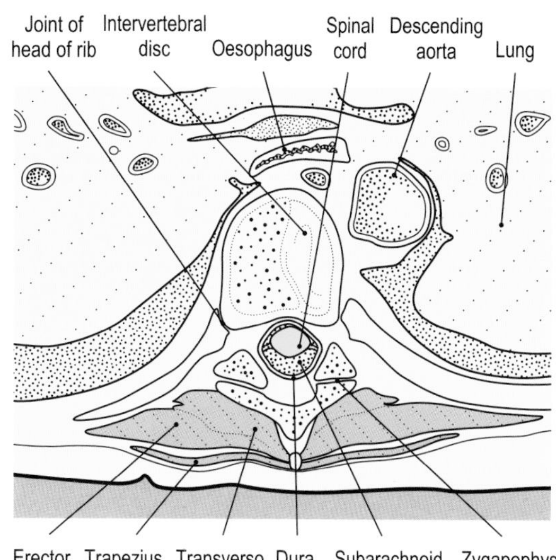

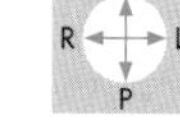

Fig. 8.31 Transverse section at the level of the sixth thoracic vertebra to show the back muscles and the vertebral foramen. Inferior aspect.

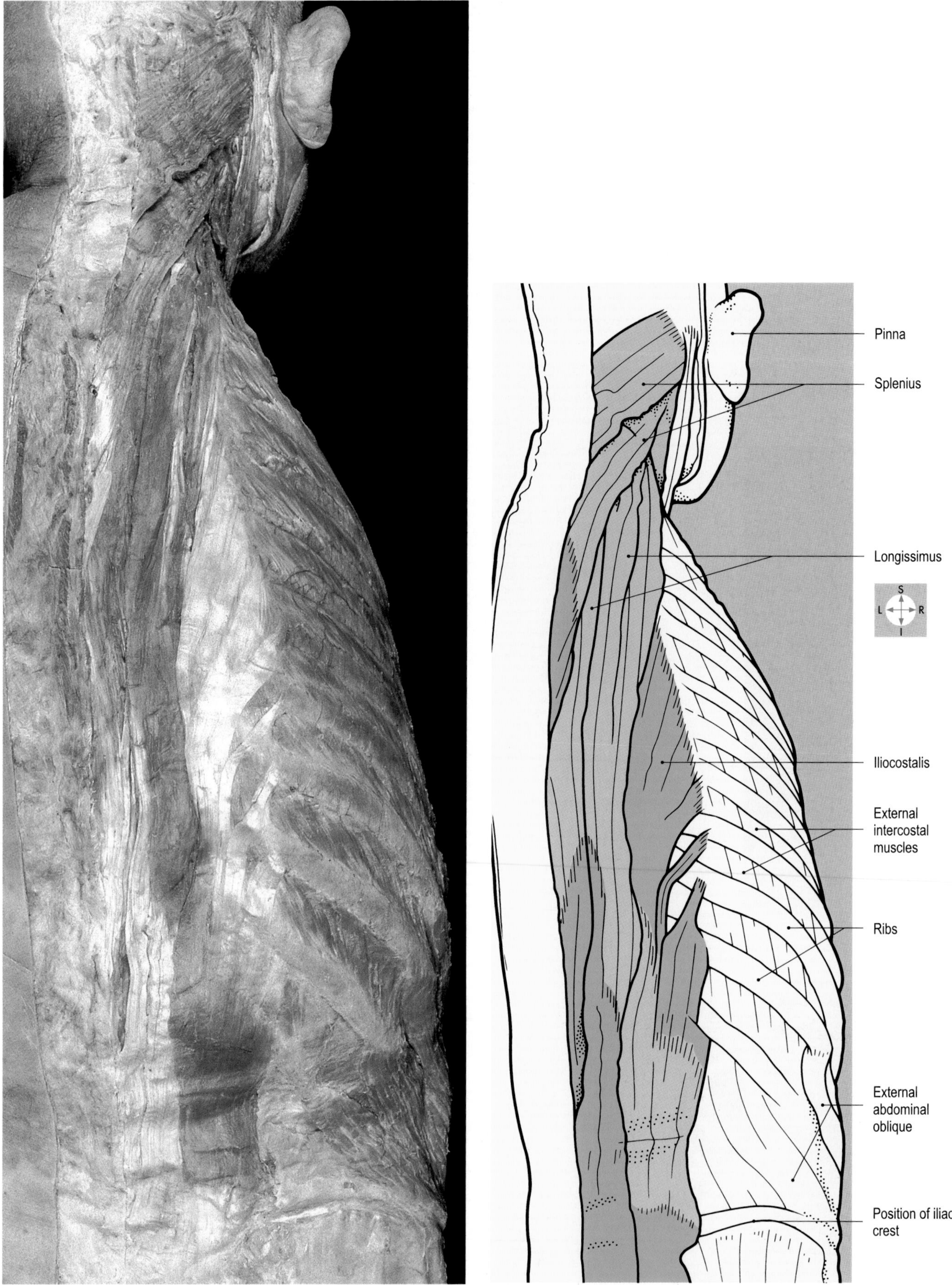

Fig. 8.32 Splenius and erector spinae exposed by removal of overlying muscles and fasciae.

Meninges

The spinal cord is surrounded by three membranes (dura mater, arachnoid mater and pia mater; Fig. 8.33), which are continuous through the foramen magnum with the cranial meninges.

Dura mater

The dura mater surrounding the spinal cord forms a sheath that corresponds to the inner (meningeal) layer of the cranial dura (see p. 371). The spinal dura is separated from the periosteum of the vertebral canal by the extradural (epidural) space (see Figs 8.15 & 8.31), which contains fat, vessels and loose connective tissue. Anaesthetic agents are instilled into this space to produce epidural anaesthesia. Spinal dura is attached to the margins of the foramen magnum and via fibrous slips to the posterior longitudinal ligament within the vertebral canal. Inferiorly the dura covers the filum terminale (Fig. 8.34). At the level of the second sacral vertebra the dura attaches to the filum terminale and these continue onto the back of the coccyx to fuse with the periosteum.

Each spinal nerve root is surrounded by a sleeve of dura mater which extends through the intervertebral foramen before fusing with the epineurium of the spinal nerve.

Arachnoid mater

The arachnoid mater is a delicate membrane that surrounds the spinal cord and the nerves within the vertebral canal. Above it is continuous with the cranial arachnoid through the foramen magnum and below it ends at the level of the second sacral

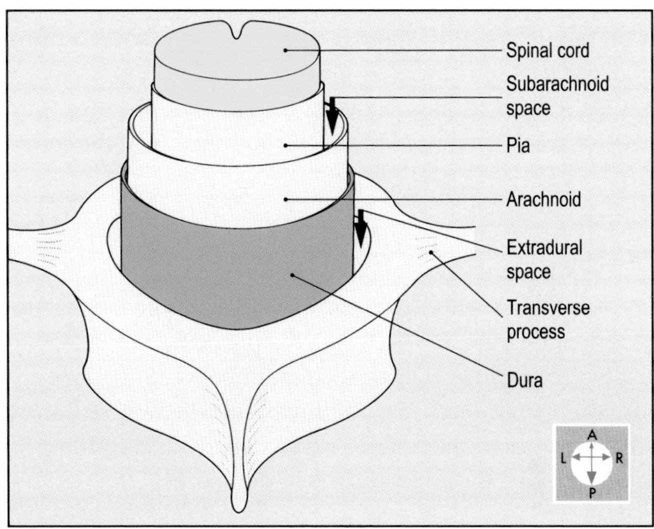

Fig. 8.33 Spinal meninges.

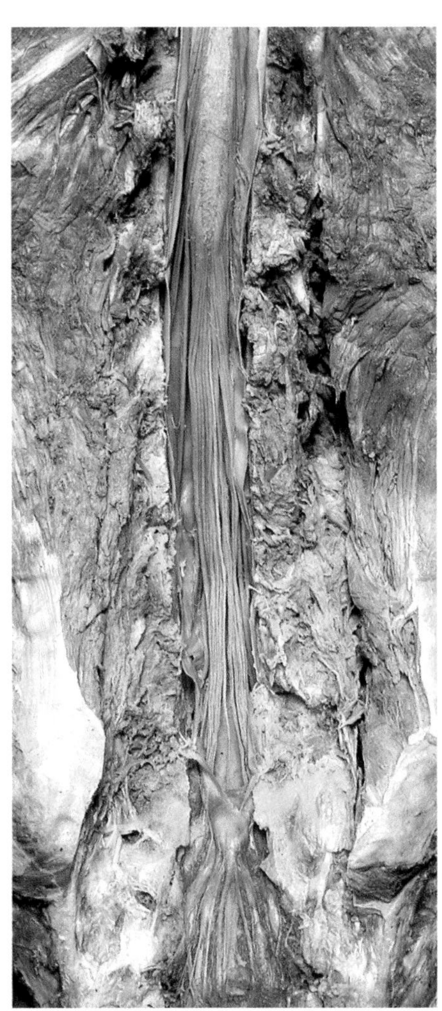

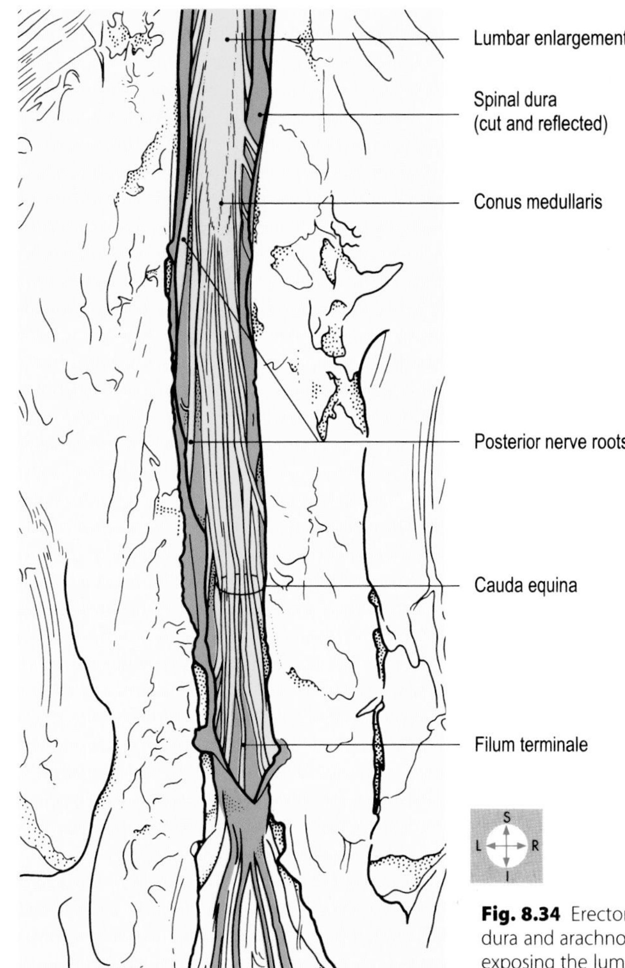

Fig. 8.34 Erector spinae and neural arches removed; spinal dura and arachnoid opened posteriorly and reflected laterally, exposing the lumbar enlargement, conus medullaris and cauda equina.

vertebra. The arachnoid is connected to the pia mater by numerous delicate strands that cross the subarachnoid space between the two meninges. This space is filled with cerebrospinal fluid and also contains blood vessels, which supply the spinal cord. The cerebrospinal fluid is produced in the ventricular system of the brain and circulates in the subarachnoid space around the spinal cord and brain (see p. 373). Cerebrospinal fluid is usually sampled by inserting a needle between the arches of the third and fourth or fourth and fifth lumbar vertebrae. In this procedure, which is called a spinal tap or lumbar puncture, the needle is carefully orientated to pass between the spinous processes and enter the subarachnoid space below the termination of the spinal cord.

Pia mater

The pia mater is a highly vascular layer that closely invests the spinal cord and nerves. On each side the pia mater is attached to the dura by the ligamentum denticulatum between the anterior and posterior spinal roots. The pia surrounds the termination of the spinal cord (conus medullaris) and continues as the filum terminale as far as the posterior surface of the coccyx.

Spinal Cord	Level in Vertebral Canal	Meninges
C1 segment	Foramen magnum of skull	
Cervical enlargement	C4–T2 bodies	
C8 segment	C7 body	
L3 segment	T12 body	
Lumbo-sacral enlargement	T12, L1 bodies	
Lowest extent of spinal cord in adults	L2 body	
Lowest extent of spinal cord in infants	L3 body	
	L3-S2 bodies	Subarachnoid space below spinal cord containing cauda equina
	L3/L4 and L4/L5 spaces	Obtain sample of CSF by lumbar puncture
	S3 segment	Lowest extent of subarachnoid space

Table 8.3 Levels of spinal cord segments and meninges

Spinal Cord

Surface features

At the level of the upper border of the atlas the spinal cord is directly continuous with the medulla oblongata. Inferiorly the cord usually extends as far as the first lumbar intervertebral disc, where it terminates as the conus medullaris. In transverse section the spinal cord is oval, with its smaller diameter anteroposteriorly. The cord is especially wide at the cervical and lumbar enlargements due to increased numbers of nerve cell bodies within the spinal cord which innervate the upper and lower limbs.

On the anterior aspect of the cord lies the anterior median fissure, whereas posteriorly there is a relatively shallow posterior median sulcus. On each side a posterolateral sulcus marks the site of attachment of the posterior nerve roots.

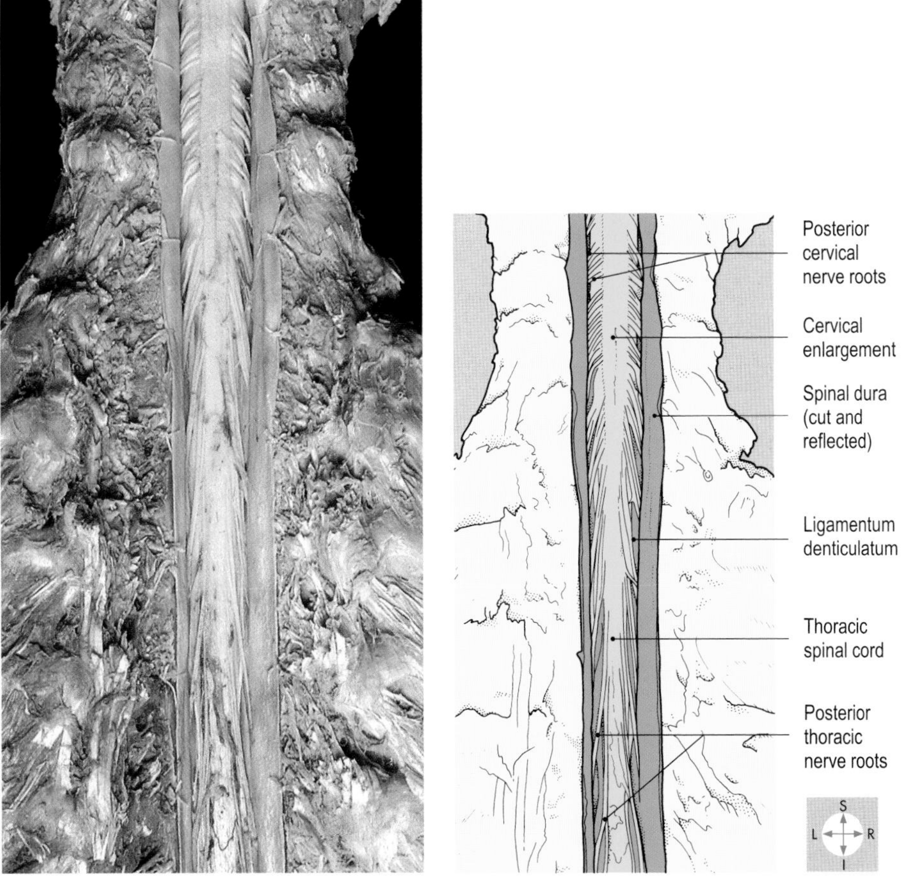

Fig. 8.35 Cervical spinal cord and dorsal nerve roots. Erector spinae and neural arches removed; the spinal dura has been reflected laterally.

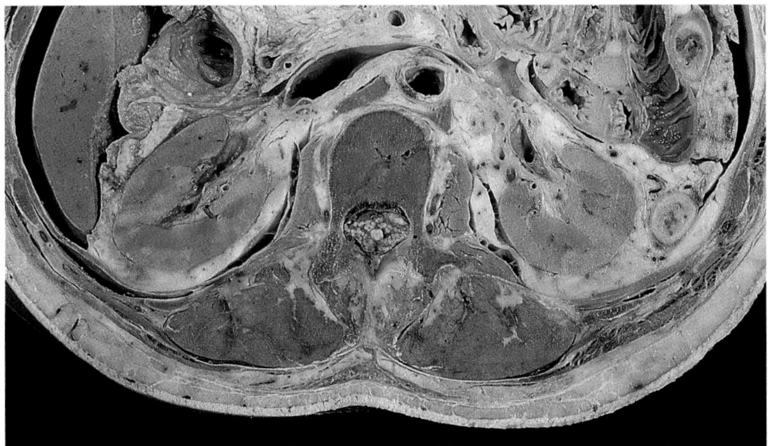

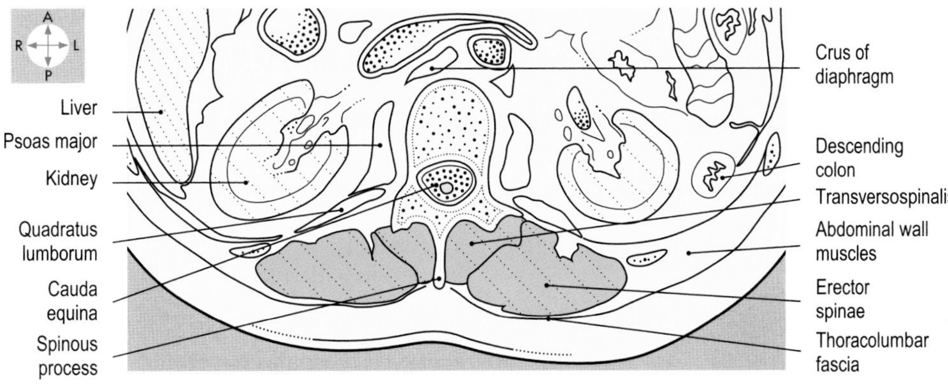

Fig. 8.36 Transverse section at the level of the first lumbar vertebra to show the back muscles and the contents of the vertebral foramen. Inferior aspect.

Spinal nerve roots

The spinal nerves are attached to the spinal cord by anterior and posterior nerve roots (Fig. 8.35). The region of the spinal cord to which one pair of anterior and posterior nerve roots attaches is called a spinal segment (Table 8.3).

Each anterior spinal root emerges from the cord as a series of small rootlets while similar branches from each posterior spinal root sink into the posterolateral sulcus. The anterior and posterior roots cross the subarachnoid space and unite in the appropriate intervertebral foramen to form a spinal nerve. Each posterior root is characterized by a ganglion just proximal to the union of anterior and posterior roots.

Because the spinal cord is shorter than the vertebral column the lower spinal nerve roots descend within the vertebral canal before leaving through their intervertebral foramina (Table 8.3). These lumbar, sacral and coccygeal nerve roots are clustered around the conus medullaris and filum terminale to form the cauda equina (see Fig. 8.34 and Fig. 8.36).

Blood supply

The spinal cord receives its arterial supply from anterior and posterior spinal arteries that arise from vertebral arteries and are reinforced by branches of the deep cervical, intercostal and lumbar arteries. These vessels form a longitudinal anastomosis that runs the length of the spinal cord. One main branch from an upper lumbar or lower thoracic artery often provides an important supply to the spinal cord. Damage to this vessel, the artery of Adamkiewicz, may threaten the viability of part of the spinal cord. The venous return from the spinal cord drains into a series of longitudinal anastomosing channels, which empty into veins corresponding to the arteries.

Exam Skills

Each of the incomplete statements below is followed by five suggested answers or completions. Decide which are true and which are false. The answers are supplied on page 415.

1. During walking and/or running the following normally occur:

a) lateral flexion at the lumbar intervertebral joints.
b) movement at the hip joints.
c) contraction of the gluteal muscles.
d) movement at the sacroiliac joints.
e) rotation of the thoracic vertebral column.

2. Concerning the joints between the atlas and the axis:

a) they are all synovial.
b) they allow rotation of the head.
c) they are supported by the alar ligaments.
d) dislocation is usually fatal.
e) they are closely related to the first cervical nerves.

3. The sacroiliac joint:

a) is a fibrous joint.
b) allows rotation in which the lower part of the sacrum moves anteriorly.
c) is stabilized by the sacrotuberous ligament.
d) is a posterior relation of the common iliac artery.
e) is stabilized by the iliolumbar ligament.

4. The lumbar region of the vertebral column:

a) is the least mobile region of the spinal column.
b) has vertebrae which possess mamillary processes.
c) is flexed by the rectus abdominis.
d) has a secondary curvature.
e) has spinous processes which overlap the body of the adjacent vertebra below.

5. The spinal cord:

a) gives rise to eight pairs of cervical spinal nerves.
b) is continuous above with the medulla oblongata.
c) is intimately related to the pia mater.
d) extends throughout the length of the vertebral canal.
e) is separated from CSF by the arachnoid mater.

6. The intervertebral disc between vertebrae L3 and L4:

a) is the smallest intervertebral disc.
b) is related anteriorly to the abdominal aorta.
c) provides attachment for psoas major.
d) is related posteriorly to the cauda equina.
e) is closely related to the second lumbar nerves.

7. The atlas vertebra:

a) has no spinous process.
b) possesses no foramina transversaria.
c) has a vertebral body.
d) permits nodding movements at its joints with the cranium.
e) has large transverse processes.

8. Intervertebral discs:

a) occur between the bodies of adjacent vertebrae.
b) are intimately related to the anterior and posterior longitudinal ligaments.
c) are secondary cartilaginous joints.
d) form part of the borders of the intervertebral foramina.
e) contribute to the curvatures of the vertebral column.

9. The sacrum:

a) usually consists of fused components of five vertebrae.
b) is concave anteriorly.
c) is attached by ligaments to the ilium and ischium.
d) forms synovial joints with the articular processes of the fifth lumbar vertebra.
e) possesses on each side an ala which is crossed by the anterior ramus of the fifth lumbar nerve.

10. The thoracic vertebral column:

a) has a primary curvature which is concave anteriorly.
b) includes 12 vertebrae.
c) articulates with the heads of ribs.
d) throughout its length is related anteriorly to the oesophagus.
e) permits lateral flexion which is restricted by the ribs.

11. The thoracolumbar fascia:

a) provides attachment for transversus abdominis.
b) encloses psoas major muscle.
c) has no attachment to bone.
d) provides attachment for external abdominal oblique muscle.
e) provides attachment for latissimus dorsi.

12. The spinal dura mater:

a) is attached to the vertebral periosteum.
b) lies deep to the spinal arteries.
c) lies superficial to the vertebral venous plexus.
d) terminates at the level of vertebra L2.
e) attaches to the margins of the foramen magnum.

13. A typical cervical vertebra possesses:

a) two pairs of synovial joints.
b) a bifid spinous process.
c) a relatively wide vertebral foramen.
d) a relatively small body.
e) foramina transversaria.

14. The vertebral canal:

a) transmits the vertebral artery.
b) contains ligamenta flava.
c) contains a venous plexus.
d) is narrowed by rotation of the head.
e) lies anterolateral to the cervical vertebral discs.

15. The following relate to lumbar puncture at vertebral level L4/L5:

a) the spinal cord terminates at a higher vertebral level.
b) at this level the ligaments are thinner and easier to penetrate.
c) there is no overlap of the spinous processes.
d) the spinal nerves that exit from the vertebral column below this level are of little importance.
e) the subarachnoid space extends inferiorly to below vertebral level L5.

16. The joints between vertebrae C4 and C5 allow:

a) rotation.
b) flexion with rotation.
c) pure extension.
d) lateral flexion.
e) lateral flexion with rotation.

Clinical Skills

The answers are supplied on page 418.

Case Study 1

A 45-year-old man began to experience headaches which spread over the back of his head. He had no previous medical problems other than a whiplash injury following a car accident several years previously. His physician paid particular attention to the man's neck and found nothing remarkable on examination other than some restriction of neck movement. Cervical spine radiographs were reported to show early degenerative changes with occasional small osteophytes.

A physiotherapist friend visited the man and was disappointed to find him sitting slumped in a low easy chair but straining forwards and upwards to watch television. The friend tactfully suggested that it might be more comfortable if the television were placed at a lower level and how comfortable cushions were when placed in the hollow of the back. When the physiotherapist called again, she was pleased to discover that the television had been repositioned, the cushions were in use and the man had not experienced any more headaches. He later became re-employed as a gardener.

Questions:

1. At which joints do the movements in the cervical spine occur?
2. Which curvatures are present in the normal vertebral column and what are the effects of sitting as described?
3. What was the cause of the pain felt over the back of the head?

Case Study 2

A 40-year-old man had suffered from intermittent low backache which started soon after he had helped a neighbour move furniture two years previously. He had some tingling along the outside of his left leg which usually lasted for only a few days. He found that lying flat on the carpeted floor of his living room relieved his backache.

A few days later when bending he felt a sudden severe pain in his back, and tingling along the outside and back of his left leg below the knee. His physician found the man's spine was held in a curve convex to the right and noted that any movement of his lumbar spine produced pain and was restricted by muscle spasm. His lower limbs showed no sensory deficit or muscle weakness and his reflexes were normal apart from an absent left ankle jerk. Straight leg raising aggravated the backache and subsequently, radiography of his lumbar spine showed probable disc space narrowing at L5/S1. Magnetic resonance imaging confirmed a small posterolateral disc protrusion at that level.

Questions:

1. Which dermatome is associated with the posterolateral surface of the leg below the knee?
2. Which segmental level is tested by the ankle jerk?
3. Which spinal nerve traverses the intervertebral foramen immediately below L5 vertebra.
4. What are the boundaries of an intervertebral foramen?
5. Why should disc protrusion at L4/L5 involve S1 nerve?

Case Study 3

A 50-year-old man had been unwell for about three months and was losing weight. He suddenly developed severe abdominal pain and was admitted to hospital with suspected peritonitis.

The surgeon took a detailed history and discovered that, although abdominal pain was the main feature, the patient had had backache for several weeks and this was now worse. The abdomen revealed no distension or localized signs and normal bowel sounds were heard. Results of blood tests showed that the white cell count was normal but that haemoglobin was low. Chest and abdominal radiographs were accompanied by additional films because the radiologist had noticed spinal disease. Several vertebrae showed areas of increased bone formation (sclerosis), others showed areas of bone destruction (lysis), and T10 and T11 showed collapse of their bodies. Subsequent tests revealed high plasma levels of acid and alkaline phosphatases and the man was referred to a urologist who obtained fragments of prostatic tissue-containing tumour.

Questions:

1. What was the cause of the 'abdominal' pain?
2. What is the route of spread of disease from pelvic organs such as the prostate to the vertebral bodies?
3. Why was the patient anaemic?

Case Study 4

A previously healthy 30-year-old mother collapsed after taking her children to school. In Accident & Emergency she appeared confused and complained bitterly of a severe generalized headache and that the room lights were too bright. Abnormal findings on physical examination were limited to blood pressure 180/110 and apparent restriction of cervical spine movements.

After admission to hospital a neurologist confirmed photophobia, neck stiffness and raised blood pressure. He performed a lumbar puncture and found blood in the cerebrospinal fluid (CSF).

Questions:

1. Where is CSF located?
2. How are samples of CSF usually obtained?
3. What is a safe vertebral level to attempt lumbar puncture and what layers are traversed?
4. Why was the patient's neck stiff even though she had no history of cervical spine disease?

Observation Skills

Identify the structures indicated. The answers are supplied at the foot of the page.

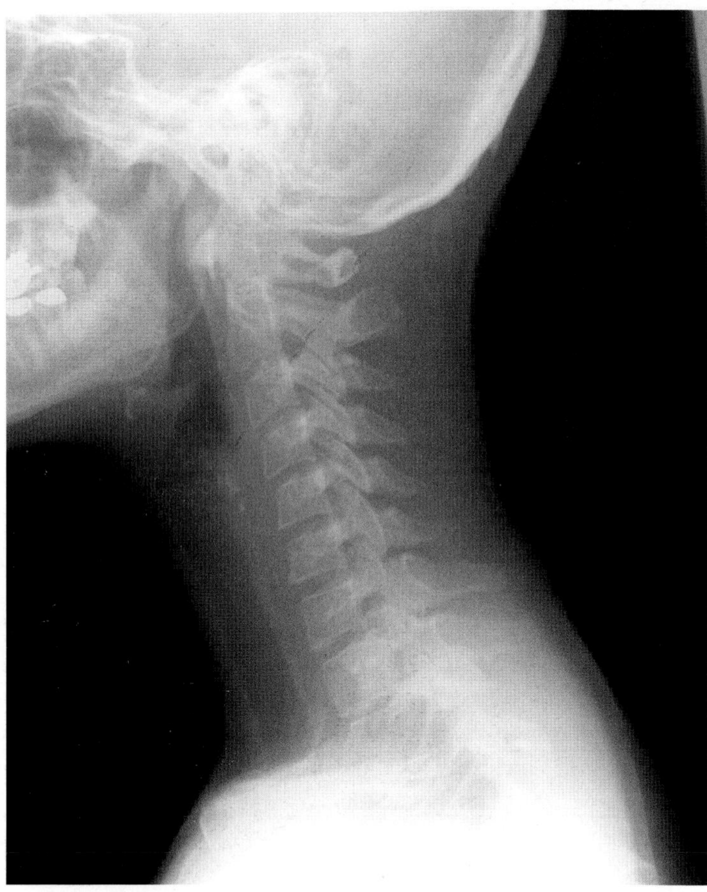

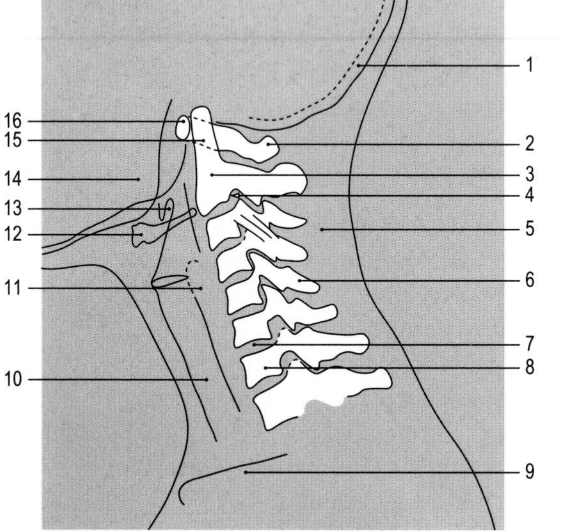

Fig. 8.37 Lateral radiograph of cervical spine.

Answers

Fig. 8.37 1 = occipital bone; 2 = posterior arch of atlas; 3 = body of axis; 4 = intervertebral foramen; 5 = soft tissue shadow of postvertebral muscles; 6 = spinous process of fifth cervical vertebra; 7 = intervertebral disc; 8 = body of seventh cervical vertebra; 9 = clavicle; 10 = tracheal air shadow; 11 = calcification in laryngeal cartilage; 12 = hyoid bone; 13 = epiglottis; 14 = mandible; 15 = odontoid process; 16 = anterior arch of atlas.

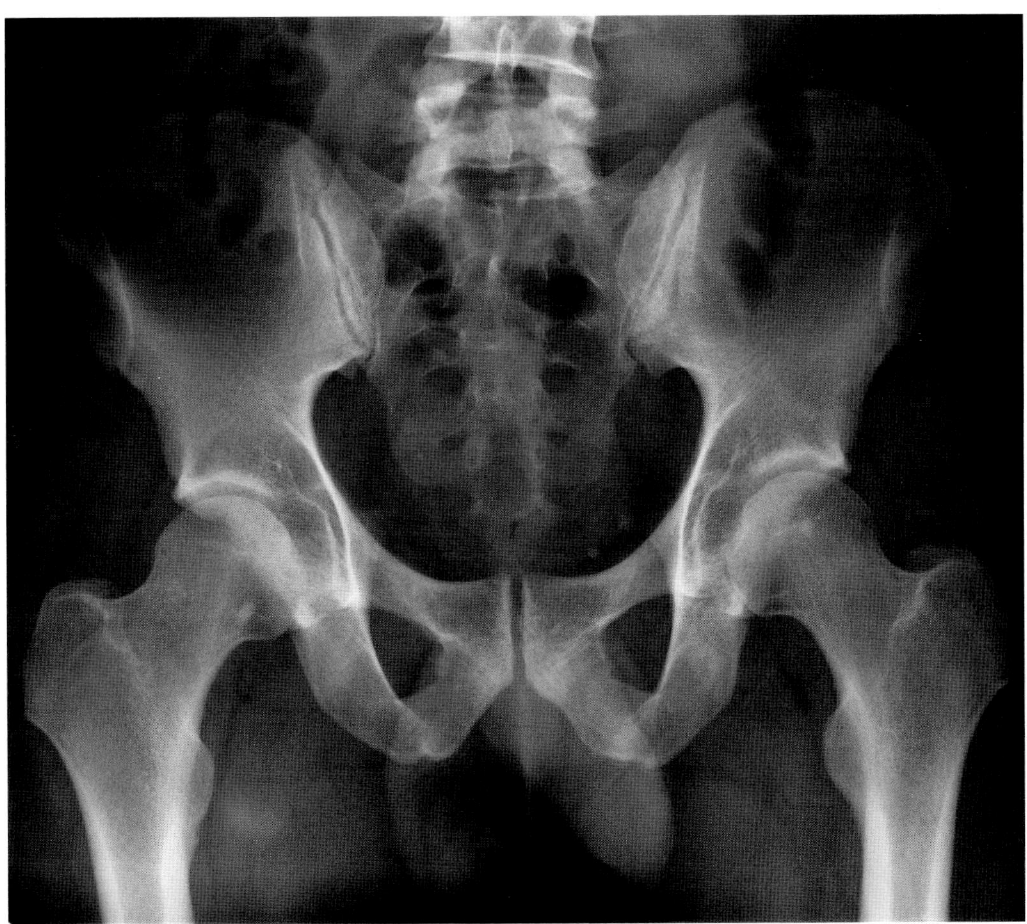

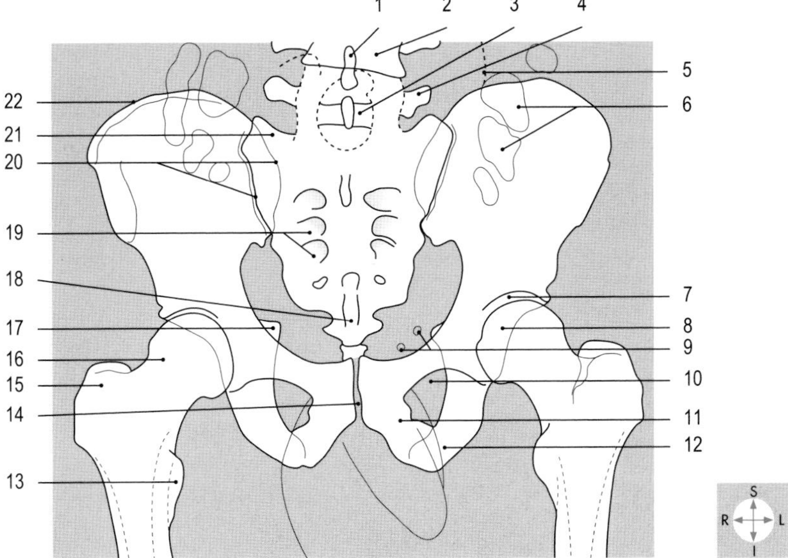

Fig. 8.38 Anteroposterior radiograph of male pelvis and lumbar spine.

Answers

Fig. 8.38 1 = spinous process; 2 = body of fourth lumbar vertebra; 3 = lamina; 4 = transverse process; 5 = edge of soft tissue shadow of psoas major; 6 = gas in colon; 7 = coxal joint; 8 = head of femur; 9 = phleboliths; 10 = obturator foramen; 11 = inferior ramus of pubis; 12 = ischial tuberosity; 13 = lesser trochanter; 14 = pubic symphysis; 15 = greater trochanter; 16 = neck of femur; 17 = ischial spine; 18 = coccyx; 19 = sacral foramina; 20 = sacroiliac joint; 21 = lateral mass of sacrum; 22 = iliac crest

Exam and Clinical Skills Answers

Thorax

1 a) T; b) T; c) T; d) F; e) F
2 a) F; b) T; c) T: d) T; e) T
3 a) T; b) F; c) T; d) T; e) F
4 a) T; b) T; c) T; d) T; e) T
5 a) T; b) F; c) T; d) F; e) T
6 a) F; b) T; c) T; d) F; e) T
7 a) T; b) F; c) T; d) T; e) F
8 a) T; b) F; c) T; d) F; e) T
9 a) T; b) T; c) T; d) T; e) T
10 a) T; b) T; c) F; d) T; e) F
11 a) F; b) T; c) F; d) T; e) T
12 a) F; b) T; c) T; d) T; e) T
13 a) T; b) T; c) F; d) F; e) F
14 a) F; b) T; c) T; d) F; e) T
15 a) F; b) T; c) T; d) F; e) T
16 a) F; b) F; c) T; d) T; e) F

Upper Limb

1 a) T; b) F; c) T; d) T; e) T
2 a) F; b) T; c) T; d) F; e) T
3 a) T; b) T; c) F; d) T; e) T
4 a) T; b) T; c) T; d) T; e) T
5 a) T; b) T; c) T; d) T; e) F
6 a) F; b) F; c) T; d) T; e) T
7 a) T; b) T; c) F; d) F; e) T
8 a) F; b) T; c) F; d) T; e) F
9 a) T; b) F; c) T; d) T; e) F
10 a) T; b) T; c) F; d) F; e) T
11 a) T; b) F; c) F; d) F; e) F
12 a) F; b) T; c) T; d) T; e) T
13 a) F; b) T; c) T; d) F; e) F
14 a) F; b) F; c) T; d) T; e) F
15 a) F; b) T; c) T; d) T; e) T
16 a) T; b) T; c) T; d) T; e) F

Abdomen

1 a) T; b) T; c) T; d) F; e) F
2 a) F; b) T; c) T; d) T; e) F
3 a) F; b) T; c) T; d) T; e) F
4 a) T; b) T; c) T; d) F; e) F
5 a) T; b) F; c) T; d) F; e) T
6 a) F; b) T; c) T; d) T; e) F
7 a) T; b) T; c) F; d) F; e) T
8 a) F; b) F; c) F; d) T; e) T
9 a) T; b) T; c) F; d) T; e) T
10 a) T; b) T; c) T; d) F; e) T
11 a) T; b) T; c) T; d) F; e) T
12 a) T; b) F; c) T; d) T; e) F
13 a) T; b) T; c) T; d) T; e) T
14 a) T; b) T: c) F; d) T; e) F
15 a) F; b) T; c) T; d) T; e) F
16 a) T; b) T; c) F; d) T; e) F

Pelvis and Perineum

1 a) F; b) T; c) F; d) T; e) T
2 a) F; b) T; c) T; d) F; e) T
3 a) T; b) F; c) T; d) T; e) F
4 a) T; b) F; c) T; d) F; e) T
5 a) T; b) T; c) F; d) T; e) T
6 a) T; b) T; c) F; d) T; e) F
7 a) T; b) F; c) T; d) T; e) F
8 a) T; b) F; c) T; d) T; e) F
9 a) F; b) T; c) T; d) T; e) T
10 a) F; b) T; c) T; d) T; e) F
11 a) T; b) T; c) T; d) F; e) F
12 a) T; b) T; c) F; d) T; e) T
13 a) T; b) T: c) T; d) F; e) T
14 a) T; b) T; c) T; d) F; e) T
15 a) F; b) T; c) T; d) T; e) F
16 a) T; b) T; c) F; d) T; e) F

Lower Limb

1 a) T; b) T; c) F; d) T; e) T
2 a) T; b) T; c) T; d) F; e) T
3 a) T; b) F; c) F; d) T; e) T
4 a) T; b) T; c) T; d) T; e) F
5 a) T; b) T; c) T; d) F; e) T
6 a) T; b) T; c) F; d) T; e) T
7 a) T; b) T; c) T; d) T; e) T
8 a) T; b) T; c) T; d) T; e) F
9 a) F; b) T; c) T; d) T; e) T
10 a) T; b) T; c) T; d) F; e) T
11 a) T; b) T; c) T; d) T; e) F
12 a) T; b) F; c) F; d) T; e) T
13 a) T; b) T; c) T; d) T; e) F
14 a) T; b) T; c) T; d) F; e) T
15 a) T; b) F; c) T; d) T; e) T
16 a) F; b) T; c) T; d) T; e) T

Head and Neck

1 a) F; b) F; c) T; d) F; e) T
2 a) T; b) F; c) T; d) T; e) F
3 a) T; b) T; c) T; d) T; e) T
4 a) T; b) T; c) F; d) T; e) F
5 a) F; b) T; c) F; d) F; e) T
6 a) T; b) T; c) F; d) T; e) T
7 a) F; b) F; c) T; d) T; e) T
8 a) T; b) T; c) F; d) F; e) T
9 a) T; b) F; c) T; d) T; e) F
10 a) T; b) T; c) T; d) T; e) T
11 a) T; b) T; c) T; d) F; e) F
12 a) F; b) F; c) T; d) T; e) T
13 a) F; b) F; c) T; d) T; e) F
14 a) F; b) F; c) F; d) F; e) F
15 a) T; b) T; c) T; d) F; e) F
16 a) F; b) F; c) T; d) F; e) F

Back

1 a) T; b) T; c) T; d) F; e) T
2 a) T; b) T; c) T; d) T; e) F
3 a) F; b) F; c) T; d) T; e) T
4 a) F; b) T; c) T; d) T; e) F
5 a) T; b) T; c) T; d) F; e) F
6 a) F; b) T; c) T; d) T; e) F
7 a) T; b) F; c) F; d) T; e) T
8 a) T; b) T; c) T; d) T; e) T
9 a) T; b) T; c) T; d) T; e) T
10 a) T; b) T; c) T; d) F; e) T
11 a) T; b) F; c) F; d) F; e) T
12 a) F; b) F; c) F; d) F; e) T
13 a) T; b) T; c) T; d) T; e) T
14 a) F; b) T; c) T; d) F; e) F
15 a) T; b) F; c) T; d) F; e) T
16 a) T; b) T; c) T; d) T; e) T

Thorax

Case Study 1

1. The physical examination should be directed at the (i) axilla, (ii) opposite breast, (iii) supra-and infraclavicular regions, and (iv) the parasternal region. Malignancies of the breast commonly spread via lymphatics to these areas.
2. Pectoralis major.
3. During surgery the nerve supply to the serratus anterior (long thoracic nerve) must have been damaged.
4. Surgery removes most of the lymphatic drainage of the limb through the axilla.

Case Study 2

1. The left recurrent laryngeal nerve has been damaged by the lesion, thereby affecting the innervation of laryngeal muscles.
2. Left phrenic nerve, aortic arch, left bronchus, left pulmonary artery and vein.
3. Phrenic nerve.
4. The left upper lobe would collapse as air is absorbed from the bronchial tree within the lobe.

Case Study 3

1. Pain referred via autonomic nerves to the eighth cervical and first thoracic spinal cord segments.
2. Reduction in coronary blood flow causes damage to heart muscle and conduction tissue.
3. The right coronary artery usually supplies both SA and AV nodes.
4. Between the right and left coronary arteries in the coronary sulcus and between the anterior and posterior interventricular arteries at the apex of the heart.

Case Study 4

1. Coarctation of the aorta at a site beyond the origin of the left subclavian artery.
2. Intercostal arteries. Blood was flowing from the anterior into the posterior intercostal arteries and then into the descending thoracic aorta.
3. Both anterior and posterior intercostal arteries in the first two intercostal spaces are branches from vessels which arise proximal to the coarctation (internal thoracic artery and costocervical trunk respectively).
4. Yes. Turbulence caused by the narrowed segment of the aorta particularly during ventricular contraction.

Upper Limb

Case Study 1

1. Mitral valve, left ventricle, aortic valve, ascending aorta, aortic arch, brachiocephalic, right subclavian and axillary arteries.
2. Sudden reduction of arterial lumen at major branches such as profunda brachii.
3. Lack of sensation and movement are obvious: amputation of her hand would probably have been necessary.
4. Anastomoses and collaterals involving branches of the scapular arteries.

Case Study 2

1. Loss of muscle bulk (wasting) in lower motor neurone problems: median nerve in carpal tunnel.
2. Cut thumb without pain: impaired sensation of anterior thumb, index, middle fingers.
3. Incisions parallel to Langer's lines following skin creases produce less obvious scars.
4. Recurrent branch of median nerve, in hand and ulnar nerve.

Case Study 3

1. Shallow glenoid fossa, lax joint capsule.
2. Axillary nerve at surgical neck: cutaneous sensation over insertion of deltoid.
3. To prevent external rotation, which produces instability.
4. Pain promotes disuse atrophy (wasting) resulting in muscle weakness making further injury more likely.
5. Strength of rotator cuff muscles acting as 'adjustable ligaments'.

Case Study 4

1. Superficial extensor muscles of the forearm at common extensor origin and supracondylar ridge.
2. Extension with lateral deviation (abduction) at the wrist joint.
3. Extensors carpi radialis longus and brevis.
4. Any powerful grip requires extension at the wrist produced by three carpal extensor muscles.

Abdomen

Case Study 1

1. Indirect inguinal hernia.
2. There must be a persistent processus vaginalis along the inguinal canal into the scrotum: a tubular communication between the general peritoneal cavity and the tunica vaginalis anterior to the testis.
3. The hernia had been present only at times of high intra-abdominal pressure (e.g. during coughing or crying). The intestine can slide to and fro along the processus vaginalis.
4. Most likely a loop of small intestine.
5. The gut loop became trapped in the hernial sac and its lumen became obstructed.
6. He will replace the gut in the abdomen and close off the processus at the deep inguinal ring.

Case Study 2

1. In addition to the general signs of shock there was the tender abdomen and the pain in the left shoulder, the latter very likely a referred pain from irritation (by blood) of the inferior surface of the diaphragm.
2. The organ is readily ruptured because of its delicate consistency. It may be trapped against the left lower ribs that lie posterior to it. It has a rich blood supply and may therefore bleed profusely.
3. Greater sac.

Case Study 3

1. Hepatitis due to alcohol poisoning.
2. In addition to the history, the liver is enlarged and tender.
3. The liver lies immediately inferior to the diaphragm and it therefore descends when the diaphragm contracts.
4. Obstruction to portal blood flow through the liver leads to a rise in pressure in the portal vein and its tributaries. Portacaval anastomoses dilate, providing alternative routes for blood to reach the heart. One site of anastomosis is in the wall of the oesophagus where submucosal veins (oesophageal varices) become dilated.
5. In the wall of the rectum and anal canal; within the falciform ligament and in the abdominal wall radiating from the umbilicus (caput medusae); between the posterior abdominal wall and any retroperitoneal digestive organ, such as the duodenum.

Case Study 4

1. The right ureter: he has ureteric colic: the pain of a kidney stone passing down the ureter.
2. The patient has signs indicating a problem with the genitourinary system. Rectal examination enables the prostate gland, part of that system, to be palpated. In addition, it might help to suggest or eliminate other causes of such pain: an inflamed appendix within the pelvis would produce tenderness to the right of the rectum.
3. A vertical line near the tips of the lumbar vertebral transverse processes, across the sacroiliac joint and then sweeping past the ischial spine to curve medially towards the bladder.
4. The films will show the bladder, and provided the kidney is excreting, the kidney itself, the calices, renal pelvis and ureter on each side.

Pelvis and Perineum

Case Study 1

1. The pudendal nerve supplies most of the perineum. It gives branches to the skin around the anus (inferior rectal branches) and to most of the vulva (posterior labial branches).
2. The ischial spines, around which the pudendal nerves runs to enter the perineum from the gluteal regions.

Case Study 2

1. The pregnancy was in the right uterine tube and the bleeding was irritating the adjacent peritoneum.
2. Tenderness in the right vaginal fornix. The dilated and bleeding uterine tube lay close to the vagina.
3. He suspected bleeding into the peritoneal cavity. If the patient is being nursed lying flat, blood might track from the pelvis to the subphrenic area to give the classic referred pain due to the phrenic nerve's innervation of the inferior surface of the diaphragm.

Case Study 3

1. The maintenance of a higher pressure in the urethra than in the bladder.
2. The external urethral sphincter (sphincter urethrae) and the levator ani (pelvic floor). These muscles compress the urethra and support its upper part within the pelvic cavity where it is subjected to the same increases in pressure, for example during laughing, as the bladder. The planned exercises are intended to strengthen these muscles.
3. The pelvic floor is stretched during childbirth. Thus the gap between the pubococcygeus muscles gets wider and the bladder sinks to a lower level. The prostate contributes to urinary continence in men, unless it is diseased or damaged.
4. Parasympathetic nerves arising from the spinal cord segments S2, S3 and S4.

Case Study 4

1. The cancer may already have spread via the lymphatic vessels accompanying the mesenteric vessels and abdominal aorta, then the thoracic duct, to the root of the neck.
2. He may have been testing for enlargement of the liver, a likely site for blood-borne secondary cancer because of the portal venous system.
3. The sacrum, vagina, prostate and bladder.

Lower Limb

Case Study 1

1. Applying firm downward pressure over the quadriceps just above the patella forces fluid from the suprapatellar pouch behind the patella towards the general synovial cavity. The extra fluid accumulates behind the patella which 'floats' forwards away from the femur. On displacing the patella backwards it can be felt to tap against the patella surface of the femur.
2. The medial meniscus.
3. The tibial collateral ligament.
4. Extracapsular: ligamentum patellae, tibial and fibular collateral, oblique popliteal ligament. Intracapsular: anterior and posterior cruciate, oblique popliteal. Collaterals provide medial and lateral stability, and limit over-extension. Cruciates provide anteroposterior stability and resist over-extension, as does the oblique popliteal ligament. The meniscofemoral ligament holds the lateral meniscus onto the lateral femoral condyle as the femur rotates.

Case Study 2

1. Great saphenous vein.
2. The swelling is a ballooning out of the wall of the great saphenous vein just where it goes deeply to drain into the femoral vein. The thrill on coughing results from transmission of a pressure wave down the venous system as the result of raised intra-abdominal pressure.
3. The 'muscle pump' mechanism operates in the foot, calf and thigh. Muscle contractions squeeze and empty the deep veins, the blood being propelled upwards towards the heart, valves ensuring unidirectional flow.

Case Study 3

1. Femoral artery which is located superficially just below the mid-point of the inguinal ligament.
2. Femoral in the groin, popliteal behind the knee, posterior tibial behind medial malleolus, dorsalis pedis on dorsum of foot.
3. Superior medial, superior lateral, inferior medial and inferior lateral genicular from popliteal; recurrent genicular from anterior and posterior tibials; descending genicular from femoral.

Case Study 4

1. Sciatic nerve. Tibial nerve.
2. Involvement of anterior horn cell, anterior nerve root, spinal nerve or its anterior ramus. These comprise the 'lower motor neurone', characterized by muscle wasting and flaccid paralysis.

Head and Neck

Case Study 1

1. Give the patient something acidic to suck, and then observe the opening of the parotid duct (in the cheek, opposite the second upper molar tooth) for the production of secretions.
2. The facial nerve, motor nerve to muscles of facial expression, lies within the parotid gland and is often disturbed during surgery.
3. The nerve was not interrupted, more likely just stretched, so recovery of function occurred.
4. Some parasympathetic nerve fibres to the parotid gland were interrupted during surgery, and during the healing process they were able to innervate sweat glands in the skin. Thus when they would be expected to stimulate salivation, they gave rise to 'gustatory sweating'.

Case Study 2

1. The student had dislocated his temporomandibular joints on both sides.
2. The head of the mandible has moved further forward than usual, and is now in front of the articular prominence of the joint. Contraction of muscles normally associated with closure of the mouth only raises the head more firmly in front of the prominence.
3. Relaxing the closing muscles, and putting downward pressure on the mandible to allow the head to slip back into the fossa of the joint.

Case Study 3

1. He would ask the patient to swallow. Swallowing raises the larynx, and as the thyroid gland is enclosed in the pretracheal fascia which is itself attached to the larynx, the thyroid gland also rises on swallowing.
2. The recurrent laryngeal nerve lies posterior to the thyroid gland and is likely to be damaged during surgery.
3. Good surgical practice is to positively identify a vulnerable structure, so that subsequent manipulation of tissues avoids damage to it.
4. The parathyroid glands also lie embedded in the posterior surface of the lateral lobes of the thyroid gland.

Case Study 4

1. Cavernous venous sinus thrombosis on the left side.
2. The abducent nerve (VI) runs through the body of the cavernous sinus, and supplies the lateral rectus muscle of the orbit which abducts the eye.
3. Infection from the pustules on the surface of the face has been carried by the veins of the face through the ophthalmic veins, or deep facial veins to the cavernous sinus where thrombosis has occurred. Infection enters the veins when pustules are squeezed.
4. The thrombosis has already involved oculomotor, trochlear and maxillary nerves, and will probably begin to affect the arterial supply to the orbit. Ultimately, meningitis and death are the probable outcomes without treatment.

Back

Case Study 1

1. Atlantoaxial, rotation; atlanto-occipital, nodding; other intervertebral joints, flexion, extension, lateral flexion with rotation.
2. Cervical convex anteriorly, thoracic concave anteriorly, lumbar convex anteriorly: loss of normal lumbar and cervical curves, but increased extension of upper cervical joints.
3. Irritation of roots of upper cervical nerves.

Case Study 2

1. Fifth lumbar.
2. First sacral.
3. Fifth lumbar.
4. Upper and lower vertebral notches (pedicles), intervertebral disc, facet joint.
5. First sacral nerve roots lie close to L5 disc as they pass inferolaterally.

Case Study 3

1. Pain referred from lower thoracic spine involving nerves T10, T11, T12.
2. Valveless veins linking pelvic venous plexuses, internal and external vertebral plexus, basivertebral veins.
3. Normal haemopoetic marrow in vertebrae replaced by metastatic tumour.

Case Study 4

1. In the subarachnoid space bathing spinal cord and brain, and in the ventricular system of brain.
2. By lumbar puncture with the vertebral column flexed to open the interval between vertebral arches.
3. Inferior to the conus medullaris between vertebrae L3/L4 or L4/L5. Skin, fascia, supra- and interspinous ligaments or ligamenta flava, extradural space, dura, arachnoid.
4. Neck movements stimulate reflex contraction of muscles because meningeal irritation by the subarachnoid bleeding increases sensitivity of dural receptors.

Alternative terms

Eponyms

Achilles tendon	Tendo calcaneus
Adam's apple	Laryngeal prominence
Alcock's canal	Pudendal canal
Astley Cooper's ligaments (breast)	Suspensory ligaments of breast
Aschoff-Tawara node	Atrioventricular node
Bartholin's gland	Greater vestibular gland
Bell's nerve	Long thoracic nerve
Bigelow's ligament	Iliofemoral ligament
Buck's fascia	Deep fascia of penis
Camper's fascia	Fatty layer of subcutaneous tissue of abdominal wall
Cloquet's node	Deep inguinal node in femoral canal
Colles' fascia	Membranous layer of subcutaneous tissue of perineum
Cooper's fascia	Cremasteric fascia
Cooper's ligaments (breast)	Suspensory ligaments of breast
Cowper's glands	Bulbourethral glands
Denonvillier's fascia	Rectovesical septum
Douglas, Line of	Arcuate line of rectus sheath
Douglas, Pouch of	Rectouterine pouch
Drummond, Marginal artery of	Marginal artery of colon
Dupuytren's fascia	Palmar aponeurosis
Eustachian tube	Auditory tube
Fallopian tube	Uterine tube
Galen, Vein of	Great cerebral vein
Gasserian ganglion	Trigeminal ganglion
Gimbernat's ligament	Lacunar ligament
Harvey's ligament	Ligamentum arteriosum
Highmore, Antrum of	Maxillary air sinus
His, Bundle of	Atrioventricular bundle
Houston's valve	Horizontal/transverse rectal fold
Hunter's canal	Adductor canal, Subsartorial canal
Jacobson's nerve	Tympanic branch of glossopharyngeal nerve
Keith-Flack, Node of	Sinuatrial node
Koch's node	Sinuatrial node
Langerhans, islets of	Pancreatic islets
Langer's lines	Cleavage lines of skin
Lisfranc, Tubercle of	Scalene tubercle
Lister's tubercle	Dorsal tubercle of radius
Lockwood, Ligament of	Suspensory ligament part of vagina bulbi (of eyeball)
Louis, Angle of	Sternal angle
Marshall's vein	Oblique vein of left atrium
Meckel's cave	Trigeminal cave
Meckel's diverticulum	Ileal diverticulum
Meibomian glands	Tarsal glands
Morison, Pouch of	Hepatorenal recess
Müller's muscle	Smooth muscle component of levator palpabrae superioris
Nuck, canal of	Processus vaginalis
Oddi, Sphincter of	Hepatopancreatic ampullary sphincter
Pachionian bodies	Arachnoid granulations
Peyer's patches	Aggregated lymphoid nodules in ileum
Poupart's ligament	Inguinal ligament
Purkinje fibres	Cardiac conducting tissue
Retzius, Cave of	Retropubic space
Rosenmüller, Fossa of	Pharyngeal recess
Santorini's duct	Accessory pancreatic duct
Scarpa's fascia	Membranous layer of subcutaneous tissue of abdominal wall
Scarpa's triangle	Femoral triangle
Sibson's fascia	Suprapleural membrane
Spence, Tail of	Axillary tail of breast
Stensen's (Stenoni) duct	Parotid duct
Tenon's capsule	Vagina bulbi, Fascia bulbi (of eyeball)
Thebesian veins	Small cardiac veins
Vater, Ampulla of	Hepatopancreatic ampulla
Vidian nerve	Nerve of pterygoid canal
Waldeyer's ring	Pharyngeal lymphoid ring
Wharton's duct	Submandibular duct
Willis, Circle of	Cerebral arterial circle
Winslow, Foramen of	Omental or epiploic foramen
Wirsung, Duct of	Main pancreatic duct
Wrisberg, Ligament of	Meniscofemoral ligament

Older terms still used in clinical practice

Anterior primary ramus	Anterior ramus (of spinal nerve)
Auditory nerve	Vestibulocochlear nerve
Circumflex nerve	Axillary nerve
Common femoral artery	Femoral artery
Common peroneal nerve	Common fibular nerve
Costophrenic recess	Costodiaphragmatic recess
Dental nerves	Alveolar nerves
Descendens cervicalis	Inferior root of ansa cervicalis
Descendens hypoglossi	Superior root of ansa cervicalis
Dorsal nerve	Thoracic nerve
Dorsal vertebra	Thoracic vertebra
Innominate artery/vein	Brachiocephalic artery/vein
Innominate bone	Hip bone
Internal mammary artery	Internal thoracic artery
Ischiorectal fossa	Ischioanal fossa
Left anterior descending artery (LAD)	Anterior interventricular artery
Lesser sac	Omental bursa
Lienogastric ligament	Gastrosplenic ligament
Lienorenal ligament	Splenorenal ligament
Ligamentum teres	Round ligament

Lumbocostal arch	Arcuate ligament
Pelvic colon	Sigmoid colon
Peroneal artery	Fibular artery
Pharyngotympanic tube	Auditory tube
Posterior facial vein	Retromandibular vein
Posterior primary ramus	Posterior ramus (of spinal nerve)
Spiral groove	Radial groove (of humerus)
Sternocostalis	Transversus thoracis
Sternomastoid	Sternocleidomastoid
Subsartorial canal	Adductor canal
Superficial fascia	Subcutaneous tissue
Superficial femoral artery	Femoral artery
Supinator longus	Brachioradialis
Suprasternal notch	Jugular notch
Utero-vesical pouch	Vesico-uterine pouch

Index

Note: The index does not list eponyms. Readers should refer to the list of alternative terms to find the currently used term.